179—

CLINICAL NEUROTOXICOLOGY

Syndromes, Substances, Environments

CLINICAL NEUROTOXICOLOGY

Syndromes, Substances, Environments

MICHAEL R. DOBBS, MD
Assistant Professor of Neurology and Preventive Medicine
University of Kentucky College of Medicine
Neurology Residency Program Director
University of Kentucky Chandler Medical Center
Lexington, Kentucky

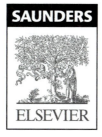

SAUNDERS

ELSEVIER

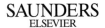

1600 John F. Kennedy Blvd.
Ste 1800
Philadelphia, PA 19103-2899

CLINICAL NEUROTOXICOLOGY:
SYNDROMES, SUBSTANCES, ENVIRONMENTS   ISBN: 978-0-323-05260-3

Notice

Knowledge and best practice in this field are constantly changing. As new research and experience broaden our knowledge, changes in practice, treatment, and drug therapy may become necessary or appropriate. Readers are advised to check the most current information provided (i) on procedures featured or (ii) by the manufacturer of each product to be administered, to verify the recommended dose or formula, the method and duration of administration, and contraindications. It is the responsibility of the practitioner, relying on their own experience and knowledge of the patient, to make diagnoses, to determine dosages and the best treatment for each individual patient, and to take all appropriate safety precautions. To the fullest extent of the law, neither the Publisher nor the Authors assume any liability for any injury and/or damage to persons or property arising out of or related to any use of the material contained in this book.

The Publisher

Library of Congress Cataloging-in-Publication Data

Clinical neurotoxicology : syndromes, substances, environments /
[edited by] Michael R. Dobbs. — 1st ed.
    p. ; cm.
  Includes bibliographical references and index.
  ISBN 978-0-323-05260-3
  1. Neurotoxicology. I. Dobbs, Michael R.
  [DNLM: 1. Neurotoxicity Syndromes. 2. Nervous System—drug effects.
3. Neurotoxins. WL 140 C6413 2009]
  RC347.5.C65 2009
  616.8'0471—dc22
                              2008043221

Acquisitions Editor: Adrianne Brigido
Developmental Editor: Joan Ryan
Project Manager: Mary Stermel
Design Direction: Gene Harris
Marketing Manager: Courtney Ingram

Printed in the United States of America

Last digit is the print number: 9 8 7 6 5 4 3 2 1

To Elizabeth and Catherine

Joseph R. Berger, MD
Professor and Chairman, Department of Neurology, University of Kentucky Medical Center, Lexington, Kentucky, USA

Delia Bethell, BM, BCh, MRCPCH
Clinical Trials Investigator, Armed Forces Research Institute of Medical Sciences, Bangkok, Thailand

Peter G. Blain, BMedSci, MB, BS, PhD, FBiol, FFOM, FRCP(Edin), FRCP(Lond)
Professor of Environmental Medicine, Medical Toxicology Centre, Faculty of Medical Sciences, Newcastle University, Newcastle upon Tyne, United Kingdom; Consultant Physician (Internal Medicine), Royal Victoria Infirmary, Newcastle Hospitals NHS Foundation Trust, Newcastle upon Tyne, United Kingdom

John C.M. Brust, MD
Department of Neurology, Harlem Hospital Center, New York, New York, USA

D. Brandon Burtis, DO
Chief Resident, Department of Neurology, University of Kentucky College of Medicine, Lexington, Kentucky, USA

Mary Capelli-Schellpfeffer, MD, MPA
Assistant Professor, Department of Medicine, Stritch School of Medicine, Loyola University Chicago, Chicago, Illinois, USA; Medical Director, Occupational Health Services, Loyola University Health System, Chicago, Illinois, USA

Sarah A. Carr, MS
Department of Neurology, Sanders-Brown Center on Aging, University of Kentucky Medical Center, Lexington, Kentucky, USA

Jane W. Chan, MD
Associate Professor, Department of Neurology, University of Kentucky College of Medicine, Lexington, Kentucky, USA

Pratap Chand, MD, DM, FRCP
Professor of Neurology, Department of Neurology and Psychiatry, St. Louis University School of Medicine, St. Louis, Missouri, USA

Sundeep Dhillon, MA, BM, BCh, MRCGP, DCH, *Dip*IMC, RCS*Ed*, FRGS
Centre for Altitude Space and Extreme Environment Medicine, Institute of Human Health and Performance, University College London, London, United Kingdom

Michael R. Dobbs, MD
Assistant Professor of Neurology and Preventive Medicine, University of Kentucky College of Medicine, Neurology Residency Program Director, University of Kentucky Chandler Medical Center, Lexington, Kentucky, USA

Peter D. Donofrio, MD
Professor of Neurology, Vanderbilt University Medical Center, Nashville, Tennessee, USA

Thierry Philippe Jacques Duprez, MD
Associate Professor, Department of Neuroradiology, Associate to the Head of the Department of Radiology, Cliniques St-Luc, Université Catholique de Louvain, Louvain-la-Neuve, Brussels, Belgium

Tracy J. Eicher, MD
United States Air Force Medical Corps, Wright-Patterson Medical Center, WPAFB, Ohio, USA

Alberto J. Espay, MD, MSc
Assistant Professor of Neurology, Department of Neurology, University of Cincinnati, Cincinnati, Ohio, USA

Jeremy Farrar, MBBS, DPhil, FRCP, FMedSci, OBE
Honorable Professor of International Health, London School of Hygiene and Tropical Medicine, Professor of Tropical Medicine, Oxford University, Director of the Clinical Research Unit, Hospital for Tropical Diseases, Ho Chi Minh City, Vietnam

Dominic B. Fee, MD
Assistant Professor, Department of Neurology, University of Kentucky Chandler Medical Center, Lexington, Kentucky, USA; Staff Physician, Department of Neurology, VA Hospital, Lexington, Kentucky, USA

Larry W. Figgs, PhD, MPH, CHCE
Associate Professor, College of Public Health, University of Kentucky, Lexington, Kentucky, USA

Jordan A. Firestone, MD, PhD, MPH
Assistant Professor of Medicine and Environmental and Occupational Health, University of Washington School of Medicine and Public Health Services, Seattle, Washington, USA; Clinic Director of Occupational and Environmental Medicine, University of Washington Med-Harborview Medical Center, University of Washington, Seattle, Washington, USA

Arthur D. Forman, MD
Associate Professor, Department of Neuro-Oncology, University of Texas M.D. Anderson Cancer Center, Houston, Texas, USA

Brent Furbee, MD
Associate Clinical Professor, Department of Emergency Medicine, Indiana University School of Medicine, Indianapolis, Indiana, USA; Medical Director, Indiana Poison Center, Clarian Health Partners, Indianapolis, Indiana, USA

Ray F. Garman, MD, MPH
Associate Professor of Preventive Medicine, University of Kentucky, Lexington, Kentucky, USA; College of Public Health, Kentucky Clinic South, Lexington, Kentucky, USA

Des Gorman, BSc, MBChB, MD (Auckland), PhD (Sydney)
Head of the School of Medicine, University of Auckland, Auckland, New Zealand

Sidney M. Gospe, Jr., MD, PhD
Herman and Faye Sarkowsky Endowed Chair, Head, Division of Pediatric Neurology, Professor, Departments of Neurology and Pediatrics, University of Washington, Seattle Children's Hospital, Seattle, Washington, USA

David G. Greer, MD
Assistant Clinical Professor, University of Alabama Birmingham, Huntsville, Alabama, USA;
Neurologist, Huntsville Hospital, Huntsville, Alabama, USA

Patrick M. Grogan, MD
Program Director, Neurology Residency, Department of Neurology/SG05N, Wilford Hall Medical Center, Lackland Air Force Base, Texas, USA; Assistant Professor of Neurology, Department of Neurology, University of Texas Health Science Center, San Antonio, San Antonio, Texas, USA

Philippe Hantson, MD, PhD
Professor of Toxicology, Université Catholique de Louvain, Professor, Department of Intensive Care, Cliniques St-Luc, Brussels, Belgium

Tran Tinh Hien, MD, PhD, FRCP
Professor of Tropical Medicine, University of Medicine and Pharmacy, Oxford University, Vice Director, Hospital for Tropical Diseases, Ho Chi Minh City, Vietnam

Michael Hoffmann, MBB*Ch*, MD, FCP (SA) Neurol, FAHA, FAAN
Professor of Neurology, Department of Neurology, University of South Florida School of Medicine, Tampa, Florida, USA

Christopher P. Holstege, MD
Associate Professor, Department of Emergency Medicine and Pediatrics, University of Virginia School of Medicine, Charlottesville, Virginia, USA; Medical Director, Blue Ridge Poison Center, University of Virginia Health System, Charlottesville, Virginia, USA; Chief, Division of Medical Toxicology, University of Virginia School of Medicine, Charlottesville, Virginia, USA

Amber N. Hood, MS
Senior Research Assistant, Department of Forensic Science, Oklahoma State University Center for Health Sciences, Tulsa, Oklahoma, USA

Maria K. Houtchens, MD
Department of Neurology, Brigham and Women's Hospital, Boston, Massachusetts, USA

J. Stephen Huff, MD
Associate Professor of Emergency Medicine and Neurology, Department of Emergency Medicine, University of Virginia School of Medicine, Charlottesville, Virginia, USA

Col. (S) Michael S. Jaffee, MD, NSAF
Assistant Professor of Neurology, Lieutenant Colonel, USAF Medical Corps, Lackland Air Force Base, Texas, USA

David A. Jett, PhD, MS
Program Director for Counterterrorism Research, National Institutes of Health, National Institute of Neurological Disorders and Stroke, Bethesda, Maryland, USA

Gregory A. Jicha, MD, PhD
Assistant Professor, Department of Neurology, Sanders-Brown Center on Aging, University of Kentucky College of Medicine, Lexington, Kentucky, USA

Bryan S. Judge, MD
Assistant Professor, Grand Rapids Medicine Education and Research Center, Michigan State University Program in Emergency Medicine, Associate Medical Director, Helen DeVos Children's Hospital Regional Poison Center, Grand Rapids, Michigan, USA

Jonathan S. Katz, MD
California Pacific Medical Center, San Francisco, California, USA

Kara A. Kennedy, DO
Resident, Department of Neurology, University of Kentucky School of Medicine, Lexington, Kentucky, USA

Hani A. Kushlaf, MBBCh
Chief Neurology Resident, Department of Neurology, University of Kentucky, Lexington, Kentucky, USA

David Lawrence, DO
Department of Emergency Medicine, Division of Medical Toxicology, University of Virginia School of Medicine, Charlottesville, Virginia, USA

Victor A. Levin, MD
Professor, Department of Neuro-Oncology, Bernard W. Biedenham Chair in Cancer Research, University of Texas M.D. Anderson Cancer Center, Houston, Texas, USA

Elizabeth Lienemann, MS
Research Technician, MEDTOX Scientific, Inc., St. Paul, Minnesota, USA

Steven B. Lippmann, MD
Professor, Department of Psychiatry, University of Louisville School of Medicine, Louisville, Kentucky, USA

Nancy McLinskey, MD
Clinical Instructor, Department of Neurology, University of Virginia School of Medicine, Charlottesville, Virginia, USA

Christina A. Meyers, PhD, ABPP
Professor of Neuropsychology, Department of Neuro-Oncology, The University of Texas M.D. Anderson Cancer Center, Houston, Texas, USA

Puneet Narang, MD
Psychiatry Resident, Hennepin County Medical Center, Minneapolis, Minnesota, USA

Jonathan Newmark, MD, COL, MC, USA
Adjunct Professor of Neurology, F. Edward Hébert School of Medicine, Uniformed Services University of Health Sciences, Bethesda, Maryland, USA; Deputy Joint Program Executive Officer, Medical Systems, Joint Program Executive Office for Chemical/Biological Defense, U. S. Department of Defense, Consultant to the U. S. Army Surgeon General for Chemical Causality Care, Falls Church, Virginia, USA

John P. Ney, MD
Clinical Instructor, Department of Neurology, University of Washington, Seattle, Washington, USA; Chief, Clinical Neurophysiology, Department of Medicine, Neurology Service, Madigan Army Medical Center, Tacoma, Washington, USA

Lawrence K. Oliver, PhD
Assistant Professor of Laboratory Medicine, Mayo College of Medicine, Mayo Clinic, Co-Director, Cardiovascular Laboratory, Co-Director, Metals Laboratory, Director, Assay Development Lab, Division of Central Clinical Lab Services, Department of Laboratory Medicine and Pathology, Mayo Clinic, Rochester, Minnesota, USA

Peter J. Osterbauer, MD
Chief, Neurology Services, USAF Medical Corps, Elmendorf Air Force Base, Arkansas, USA

Sumit Parikh, MD
Neurogenetics and Metabolism, Cleveland Clinic, Cleveland, Ohio, USA

L. Cameron Pimperl, MD
Medical Director, Oncologics Inc. Cancer Center, Laurel, Mississippi, USA; Consulting Staff, South Central Regional Medical Center, Laurel, Mississippi, USA; Consulting Staff, Jeff Anderson Cancer Center, Meridian, Mississippi, USA

Terri L. Postma, MD
Chief Resident, Department of Neurology, University of Kentucky College of Medicine, Lexington, Kentucky, USA

T. Scott Prince, MD, MSPH
Associate Professor, Department of Preventive Medicine and Environmental Health, University of Kentucky, Lexington, Kentucky, USA

Leon Prockop, MD
Professor and Chair Emeritus, Department of Neurology, University of South Florida School of Medicine, Tampa, Florida, USA

Jason R. Richardson, MS, PhD
Assistant Professor of Environmental and Occupational Medicine, Robert Wood Johnson Medical School, Resident Member, Environmental and Occupational Health Sciences Institute, University of Medicine and Dentistry-New Jersey, Piscataway, New Jersey, USA

Daniel E. Rusyniak, MD
Associate Professor of Emergency Medicine, Associate Professor of Pharmacology and Toxicology, Adjunct Associate Clinical Professor of Neurology, Indiana University School of Medicine, Indianapolis, Indiana, USA

Melody Ryan, PharmD, MPH
Associate Professor, Department of Pharmacy Practice and Science, College of Pharmacy and Department of Neurology, University of Kentucky College of Medicine, Clinical Pharmacy Specialist, Veterans Affairs Medical Center, Lexington, Kentucky, USA

Redda Tekle Haimamot, MD, FRCP(C), PhD
Faculty of Medicine, Addis Abba University, Addis Abba, Ethiopia

Brett J. Theeler, MD
Chief Resident, Department of Medicine, Neurology Service, Madigan Army Medical Center, Tacoma, Washington, USA

Asit K. Tripathy, MD
Neurogenetics and Metabolism, Cleveland Clinic, Cleveland, Ohio, USA

Anand G. Vaishnav, MD
Assistant Professor, Department of Neurology, University of Kentucky School of Medicine, Lexington, Kentucky, USA

David R. Wallace, PhD
Professor of Pharmacology and Forensic Sciences, Oklahoma State University Center for Health Science, Tulsa, Oklahoma, USA; Assistant Dean for Research and Director, Center for Integrative Neuroscience, Tulsa, Oklahoma, USA

Michael R. Watters, MD, FAAN
Director of Resident Education, Division of Neurology, Professor of Neurology, Queens' Medical Center University Tower, Hohn A. Burns School of Medicine, University of Hawaii at Manoa, Honolulu, Hawaii, USA

Brandon Wills, DO, MS
Clinical Assistant Professor, Division of Emergency Medicine, University of Washington, Seattle, Washington, USA; Attending Physician, Department of Emergency Medicine, Madigan Army Medical Center, Tacoma, Washington, USA; Associate Medical Director, Washington Poison Center, Seattle, Washington, USA

Recently, when interviewing candidates for neurology residency, I was asked by one applicant what subspecialty was not represented in our large, multidivisional department. After some thought, my answer was neurotoxicology. The applicant was surprised that I considered this a deficit, as she had never been exposed to the area in her otherwise excellent medical school experience, but every clinical neurologist knows how ubiquitous the effect of toxins or a question of their contribution to a patient's difficulties is in everyday practice.

Neurology, like internal medicine before it, has increasingly differentiated into various subspecialties. The core of neurology consists of fields such as epilepsy, stroke, dementia, neuromuscular diseases, and movement disorders. These are illnesses that are cared for and studied virtually entirely by neurologists. However, in the real-world general hospital and ambulatory practice, the vast majority of neurology occurs at the interfaces with other disciplines. These include otoneurology, vestibular neurology, cancer neurology, neuroophthalmology, pain neurology, sleep neurology, critical care neurology, neuropsychiatry, uroneurology, neurological complications of general medical disease, and neurological infectious diseases. Most modern academic neurology departments now have some people, often entire divisions, devoted to these areas. Strikingly missing is the increasingly important area of neurotoxicology.

The field of neurotoxicology, of course, has existed for some time and there is a rich literature on the effects on the nervous system of various toxins and environmental factors, including warfare. However, this literature has not penetrated the curriculum of the standard neurology residency, and most otherwise competent neurologists would admit to a severe deficit in their knowledge in this area beyond the most rudimentary understanding. For example, the effects of ethyl alcohol on the nervous system have been extensively studied and this area is reasonably well understood by most neurologists. Several encyclopedic textbooks exist, some of which are on my own bookshelf, and I refer to them periodically when I think that a toxin may be responsible for a patient's problem. Beyond these small islands, understanding of this important aspect of neurology is sorely lacking in the academic centers and in the practices of neurology worldwide. In particular, neurologists have no working knowledge of the concepts and approaches to neurotoxicology, and usually cannot recognize a toxic syndrome when they see one.

Michael Dobbs has skillfully addressed this important lacune in the neurology curriculum with his book,

Clinical Neurotoxicology: Syndromes, Substances, Environments. This multi-authored, but carefully edited, text provides a clinical approach to the field of neurotoxicology, using a systems-oriented symptomatic approach. For example, a neurologist faced with a cryptic case of optic neuropathy can go to the chapter on that subject and learn whether his or her patient fits any of the known patterns for this particular syndrome. There are also very useful chapters on testing patients for toxic disorders and on the common clinical syndromes of the various neurotoxic substances, such as metals, drugs, organic, bacterial, and animal neurotoxins. Finally, various environmental conditions, including warfare, are covered in specific chapters.

This kind of symptom-oriented approach has worked well before for complex and difficult areas such as metabolic diseases of the nervous system, and it has worked very well here. Rather than trying to grasp all of the basic science of neurotoxicity and build one's clinical knowledge up from that base, a clinician can approach a specific patient in a logical and practical manner. This is the only pragmatic manner in which a physician can hope to begin to approach an area as broad and complex as neurotoxicology. Dr. Dobbs has been inclusive in choosing his chapter authors. Rather than limiting himself to the relatively small number of neurologists with real expertise in this area, he has invited emergency physicians, pharmacists, and other experts to provide what is truly an authoritative approach to specific problems—to avoid the usual review of the literature in which there is no evidence of personal clinical experience. For example, reading John Brust's approach to the neurotoxicity of illicit drugs and the alcohols gives the reader the advantage of his vast experience in these areas, which includes the nuances of real world patient care. No one physician could hope to accumulate a substantial personal experience in any one, let alone all, of the disorders covered in Dobbs's book.

Dobbs's *Clinical Neurotoxicology* will become a must-have reference for all clinical neurologists, emergency physicians, and internists. Anyone who sees patients will find it an invaluable source of practical and authoritative information, which will guide the physician in evaluating patients with potential toxic disorders.

Martin A. Samuels, MD, FAAN, MACP
Chairman
Department of Neurology
Brigham and Women's Hospital
Professor of Neurology
Harvard Medical School

Neurotoxicology as a medical specialty has not yet reached its pinnacle. Indeed, there are very few specialists who, if asked, would say that their primary interest is neurotoxicology. Perhaps this is because neurotoxicology encompasses several medical fields—neurology, emergency medicine, pharmacology, and public health. Perhaps it is because neurotoxicology is not taught as part of most residency programs. Maybe it is because there aren't enough patients available to a physician to make it a focus of a clinical practice.

There are many scientists and practitioners who lay claim to this mantle, but who exactly are neurotoxicologists? Neurotoxicologists are the basic scientists who, in the laboratory, study the toxic effects of substances in cells, tissues, and animal models. Neurotoxicologists are the neurologists who seek out clinical neurotoxicology cases. These neurologists may not have formal neurotoxicology training, but they have developed an interest in the field and acquired significant expertise that is augmented by their skills in neurodiagnostic thinking. Neurotoxicologists are the emergency medicine practitioners who have either undergone formal training in medical toxicology or developed an independent interest in toxicology, of whom a small minority would call themselves "neurotoxicologists." Neurotoxicologists are the practitioners of the public health medical specialties of preventive medicine, occupational medicine, and similar veins that focus on neurotoxicology.

This textbook, *Clinical Neurotoxicology*, is an attempt to address the underrepresented discipline of clinical neurotoxicology in a logical, comprehensible, and comprehensive manner. It would not be possible to include all aspects of this immensely broad field of study in a single text. This work focuses on clinical aspects of neurotoxicology germane to medical practitioners. It is largely not concerned with basic science, except where currently clinically relevant. The work is divided into six sections. The first section, Neurotoxic Overview, is an overview of clinical neurotoxicology, with chapters encompassing basic science relevant to clinical practitioners, the approach to neurotoxic patients, and overviews of the development, industrial, and occupational medicine aspects of the field. The second section, Neurotoxic Syndromes, contains detailed descriptions of toxic syndromes such as toxic movement disorders, seizures, coma, or neuropathy. This is where a reader using this as a reference text might start. Suppose a clinician was seeing a patient whom they suspect to have tremor secondary to some toxic exposure. This clinician would turn to the "Toxic Movement Disorders" chapter, and may discover several possible substances that could be implicated based on the patient's clinical picture. For additional details of testing or treatment of specific neurotoxic substances, they would then seek more information in the third and fourth sections of this book (Neurotoxic Testing and Neurotoxic Substances, respectively). The fifth and sixth sections of the book (Neurotoxic Environments and Conditions, and Neurotoxic Weapons and Warfare, respectively) address potentially neurotoxic environments and conditions, as well as neurotoxic weapons and warfare.

Clinical Neurotoxicology is contributed to by experts from around the world, including neurologists, critical care specialists, emergency physicians, pharmacists, public health physicians, psychiatrists, and radiation oncologists. Our diverse group of authors includes a world-class mountain climber who is also a first-rate physician and another physician who is a world authority on barotrauma. There are also eminent basic scientists among the writers. I am very proud that many contributing authors are physicians- and scientists-in-training, including several of my own residents.

Michael R. Dobbs, MD
2009

ACKNOWLEDGMENTS • • • •

First I would like to acknowledge the work of the contributors, many of whom were working in previously "uncharted waters" as they wrote their chapters. Their efforts made compiling and editing this book fairly easy.

I owe a debt of gratitude as well to the acquisitions editors at Elsevier, Susan Pioli and Adrianne Brigido. Their vision and faith in the idea of a comprehensive clinical neurotoxicology textbook got this project off the ground and kept it running.

This book would not have been physically possible without the tireless work and extraordinary skills of Joan Ryan, developmental editor at Elsevier Saunders, and her team. I could not possibly acknowledge her enough. Thank you, Joan. Also, Mary Stermel at Elsevier worked very hard on the production end of the book.

Joe Berger, my department chair, teacher, and mentor wrote material for this book. More importantly, however, he supported my efforts in this project wholeheartedly. He is a trusted advisor to me in my academic life.

Acknowledgments would hardly be complete without recognizing those who truly worked behind the scenes on this book. I mean of course the families and friends who supported our time away from them as we worked. My wife, Betsy, frequently proofread my work and gave me advice, and she showed me a great deal of patience. Our 4-year-old daughter, Cate, often played with me when I was able to take breaks from the computer. Sometimes, little Cate even sat in my lap as I wrote or edited. Those will be fond memories.

CONTENTS · · · · ·

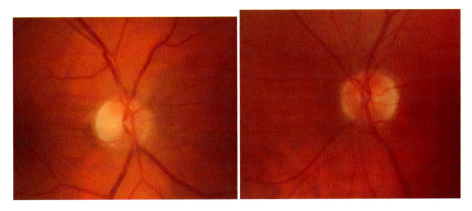

Figure 9-1. The optic nerves have mild temporal pallor (right optic disc, *left;* left optic disc, *right*).

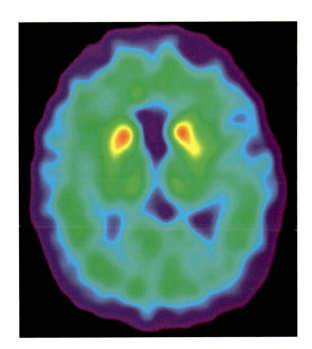

Figure 19-3. ^{18}F-dopa positron emission tomography scan performed 3.5 months after methanol poisoning in a patient who developed early extrapyramidal signs. Reduced uptake of the tracer occurs symmetrically in both putamina *(orange)*. (Adapted from Airas L, Paavilainen T, Marttila RJ, et al. Methanol intoxication-induced nigrostriatal dysfunction detected using 6-[^{18}F]fluoro-L-dopa PET. *Neurotoxicology.* 2008;29:671–674.)

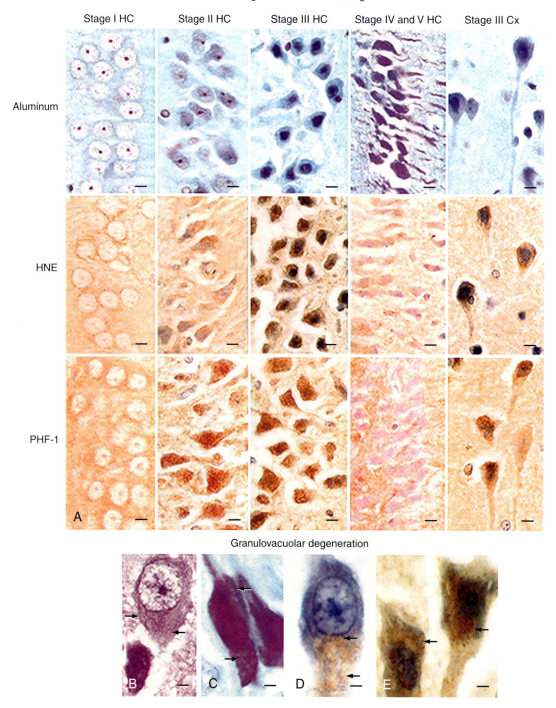

Figure 25-2. *(A)* Stages of aluminum loading, oxidative damage, and the hyperphosphorylated protein τ in hippocampal (HC) neurons (columns 1–4) and layer V cortical (Cx) neurons (column 5). Row 1: neurons stained for aluminum at increasing stages of aluminum loading. In column 4, hippocampal neurons with Stage IV aluminum loading are recognizable by their magenta nuclei and blue cytoplasm (upper part of micrograph), whereas those at Stage V aluminum loading have a magenta nucleus and magenta cytoplasm (lower part of micrograph). Row 2: Immunostaining with 4-hydroxy-2-nonenal (HNE), a marker for oxidative damage. Row 3: Immunostaining with plant homeodomain finger protein 1 (PHF-1), a marker for the hyperphosphorylated protein τ. The micrographs in rows 2 and 3 illustrate equivalent cells in sections adjacent to those shown in row 1. Scale bars = 10 μm. *(B–E)* granulovacuolar degeneration (GVD) in hippocampal neurons from cognitively damaged rats. Arrows designate some vacuoles that contain visible GVD granules within the plane of focus: *(B)* Stained with hematoxylin and eosin; *(C)* Stained for aluminum; *(D)* Immunostained for HNE-associated oxidative damage; *(E)* Immunostained with PHF-1 for the hyperphosphorylated protein τ. Scale bars = 2 μm. (Walton JR. An aluminum-based rat model for Alzheimer's disease exhibits oxidative damage, inhibition of PP2A activity, hyperphosphorylated τ, and granulovacuolar degeneration. *J Inorg Biochem.* 2007;101[9]:1275–1284.)

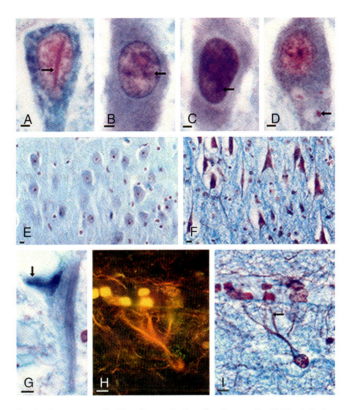

Figure 25-4. Features of human brain tissue revealed by the stain for aluminum. *(A–C)* Nuclei of neurons in transition between Stages III and IV have aluminum staining in the form of straight *(A,* arrow) or radiating *(B,* arrow) fibrils or as an amorphous substance *(C,* arrow). Scale bar = 2.5 μm. *(D)* Granules (e.g., arrow) stain for aluminum in vacuoles of a Stage II neuron with early-stage granulovacuolar degeneration. Scale bar = 2.5 μm. *(E)* and *(F)* Extremes of aluminum staining in CA1 hippocampal neurons from aged human brain tissue. *(E)* Stage I neurons from a nondemented control brain exhibit minimal staining (nucleoli only) for aluminum. *(F)* Stage V neurons from an AD brain exhibit maximal staining for aluminum (nucleus and cytoplasm). Scale bar = 20 μm. *(G)* The nucleus (arrow) appears to be extruding from this neurofibrillary tangle–bearing neuron. Scale bar = 2.5 μm. Fluorescent image *(H)* and bright field image *(I)* of an astrocyte with processes containing aluminum that abuts a capillary containing erythrocytes that stain for aluminum. The arrow indicates an astrocyte process. Scale bar = 5 μm. (Walton JR. An aluminum-based rat model for Alzheimer's disease exhibits oxidative damage, inhibition of PP2A activity, hyperphosphorylated τ, and granulovacuolar degeneration. *Neurotoxicology.* 2006;27[3]:385–394.)

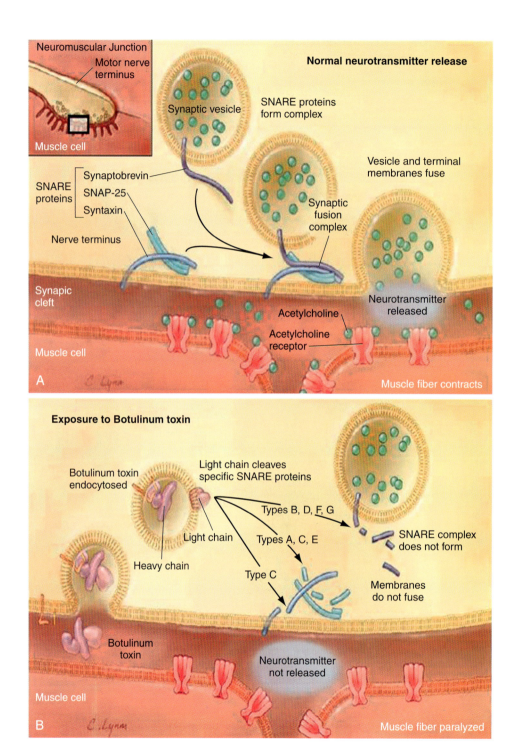

Figure 37-1. Mechanism of action of botulinum neurotoxin. (Horowitz BZ. Botulinum toxin. *Crit Care Clin.* 2005;21:825–839.)

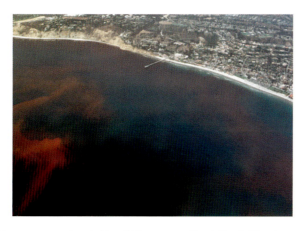

Figure 40-1. A red tide off the coast of La Jolla, California. (Courtesy of Wikipedia.)

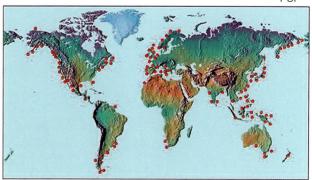

• PSP

Figure 40-2. Worldwide prevalence of paralytic shellfish poisoning in 2006. (Courtesy of U.S. National Office for Harmful Algal Blooms/Woods Hole Oceanographic Institution.)

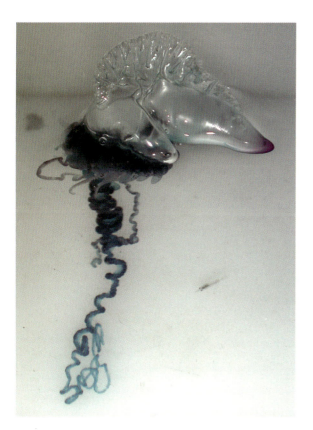

Figure 42-2. Portuguese man-of-war, *Physalia physalis*. (Courtesy of Wikipedia.)

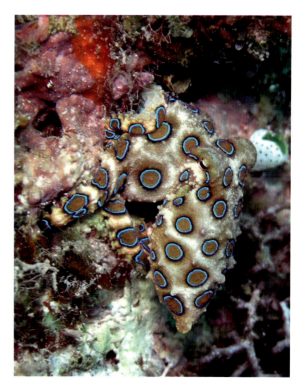

Figure 42-3. Greater blue-ringed octopus, *Hapalochlaena lunulata*. (Courtesy of Wikipedia.)

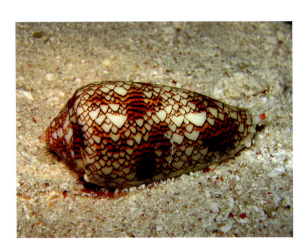

Figure 42-5. Sea snake, *Laticauda colubrina*. (Courtesy of Wikipedia.)

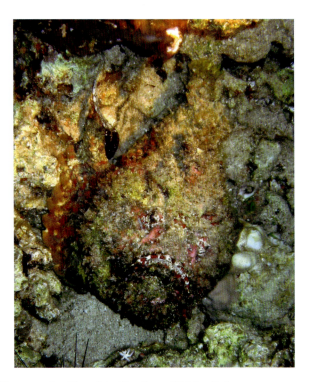

Figure 42-6. Stonefish. (Courtesy of Wikipedia.)

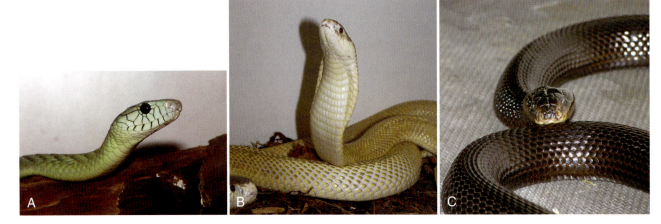

Figure 43-6. Examples of highly neurotoxic species of snake: the Western green mamba *(Dendroaspis viridis; A)*; the monocled cobra *(Naja kaouthia,* Suphan phase) shown rearing and beginning to hood *(B)*; and the black desert cobra *(Walterinnesia aegyptia; C)*. (Courtesy of KRZ, T. Postma.)

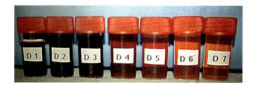

Figure 46-4. Discoloration of urine induced by a 10-g dose of hydroxocobalamin in a patient with normal renal function (patient 13). Urine samples from 7 days (D1–D7) are shown. (Borron SW, Baud FJ, Mégarbane B, Bismuth C. Hydroxocobalamin for severe acute cyanide poisoning by ingestion or inhalation. *Am J Emerg Med.* 2007;25(5):551–558.)

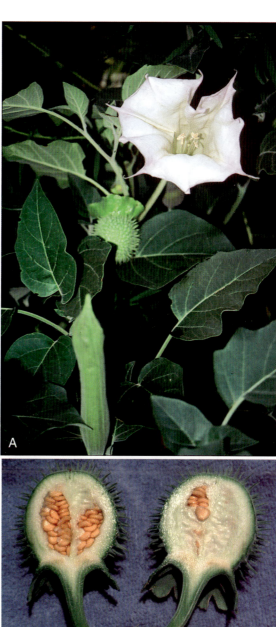

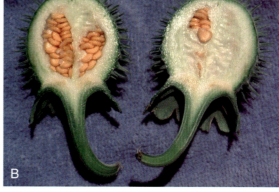

Figure 47-3. Anticholinergics. *(A) Datura meteloides.* *(B) Datura metalloids* seed pod.

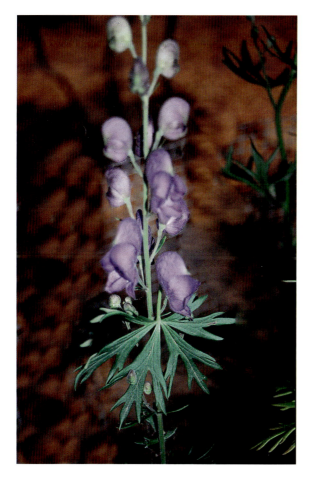

Figure 47-1. Aconitine. *Aconitum napellus.*

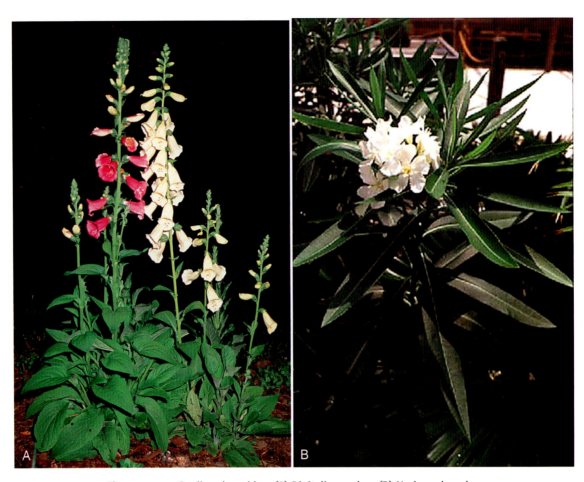

Figure 47-4. Cardiac glycosides. *(A) Digitalis species. (B) Nerium oleander.*

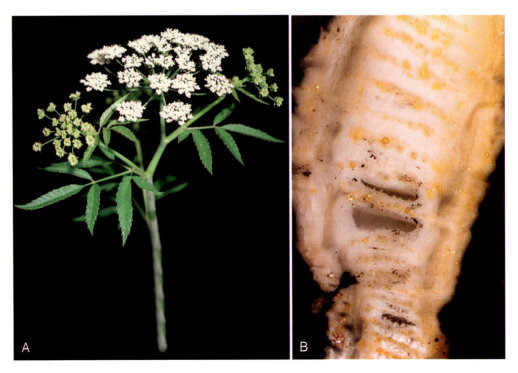

Figure 47-5. Cicutoxin. *(A) Cicuta douglasii. (B)* Water hemlock root.

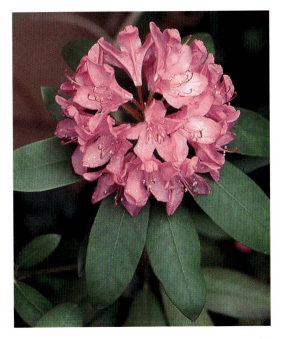

Figure 47-6. Grayanotoxins. *Rhododendron* species.

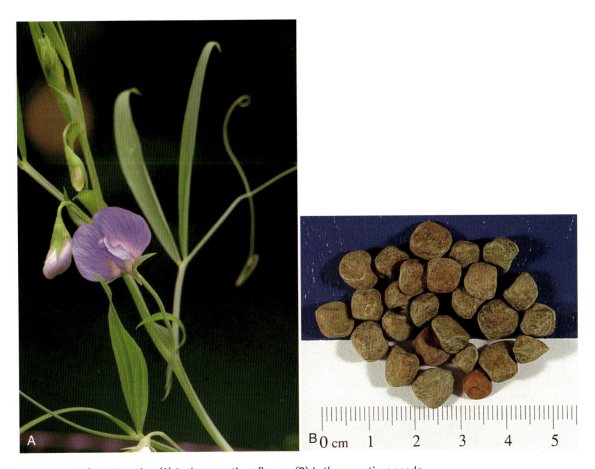

Figure 47-7. *Lathyrus* species *(A) Lathyrus sativus* flower. *(B) Lathyrus sativus* seeds.

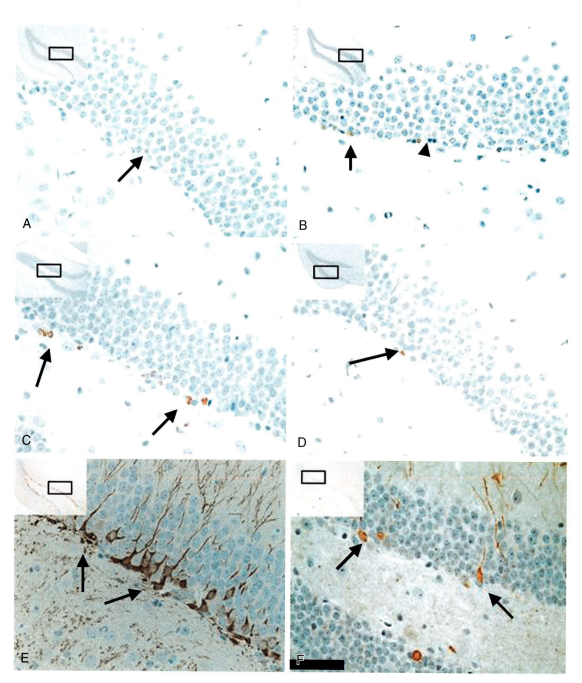

Figure 48-1. Photomicrographs depicting specific cellular responses in mouse dentate gyrus before irradiation *(A, C,* and *E)* and either 12 hours *(B)* or 48 hours *(D* and *E)* after 10 Gy. Panels include apoptosis *(A* and *B)*, proliferating cells (Ki-67; *C* and *D)*, and immature neurons (Dcx; *E* and *F)*. The SGZ is a narrow band of cells between the hilus *(H)* and granule cell layer. Apoptotic nuclei are characterized by TUNEL *(arrows, A* and *B)* or dense chromatin or nuclear fragmentation *(arrowhead, B)*. Although an occasional apoptotic nucleus was seen in tissues from unirradiated mice *(A)*, a significant increase in apoptosis was seen in the SGZ 12 hours after irradiation *(B)*. Proliferating Ki-67-positive cells *(arrows, C)* are spread out within the SGZ in tissues from unirradiated animals; only an occasional Ki-67-positive cell was found after 10 Gy *(D)*. Dcx-positive cells are highly concentrated in the SGZ and lower regions of the granule cell layer of unirradiated mice *(arrows, E)*. After 10 Gy, there are substantially fewer Dcx-positive cells *(F;* scale bar = 50 μm). All micrographs are ×40. The inset in each panel is a low-power image (×10) of the dentate gyrus; black boxes are the areas photographed at ×40. TUNEL, terminal deoxynucleotidyl transferase–mediated 2′-deoxyuridine 5′-triphosphate nick end labeling. (Mizumatsu S, Monje ML, Morhardt DR, et al. Extreme sensitivity of adult neurogenesis to low doses of x-irradiation. *Can Res.* 2003;63:4021–4027.)

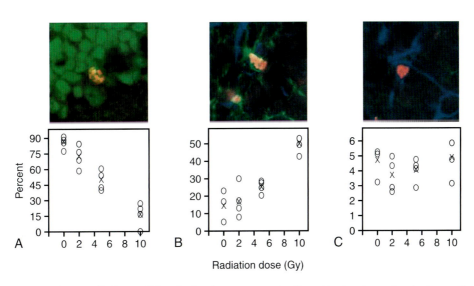

Figure 48-2. Two months after irradiation, cell fate in the dentate gyrus is altered by low to moderate doses of x-rays. Confocal images *(top)* were used to quantify the percentage of BrdUrd-positive cells that coexpressed mature cell markers. Proliferating cells were labeled with BrdUrd (red or orange stain in confocal images), and 3 weeks later, the relative proportion of cells adopting a recognized cell fate was determined as a function of radiation dose *(bottom)*. Neurons (green cells in *A, top*), oligodendrocytes (green cells in *B, top*), and astrocytes (blue cells in *C, top*) were labeled with antibodies against NeuN, NG2, and GFAP, respectively. Each confocal image shows a double-labeled cell. The production of new neurons *(A, bottom)* was reduced dose dependently ($p < 0.001$), whereas there was no apparent change in the production of GFAP with dose *(C, bottom)*. In contrast, the percentage of BrdUrd-positive cells adopting an oligodendrocyte fate *(B, bottom)* appeared to increase, particularly after 10 Gy. In the graphs, each circle represents the value from an individual animal; each X represents the mean value for a given dose group. BrdUrd, bromodeoxyuridine. (Mizumatsu S, Monje ML, Morhardt DR, et al. Extreme sensitivity of adult neurogenesis to low doses of x-irradiation. *Can Res.* 2003;63:4021–4027.)

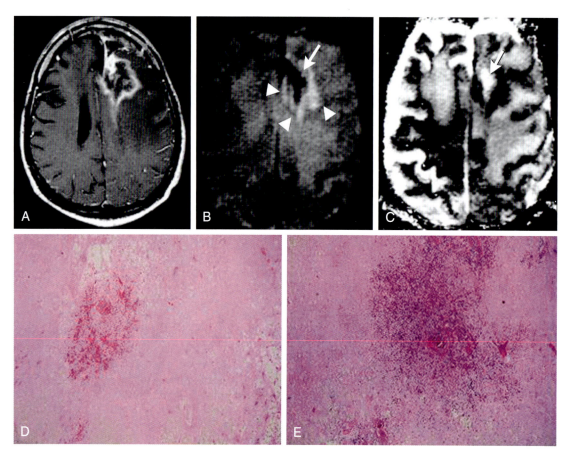

Figure 48-3. Images obtained in a 54-year-old man with biopsy-proven radiation necrosis after receiving radiation and chemotherapy for anaplastic oligodendroglioma. *(A)* Gadolinium-enhanced T$_1$-weighted image shows an irregular ring-enhancing lesion with mass effect. *(B)* Diffusion-weighted image obtained at the same level as panel A shows a mixed signal intensity pattern *(arrowheads)*, with marked hypointensity *(arrow)*, which is typical for radiation necrosis. Radiation necrosis may have various signal intensity patterns on diffusion-weighted images, reflecting the development of necrosis. Marked diffusion-weighted imaging hypointensity is probably attributable to liquefactions in late-stage necrosis. *(C)* ADC map, which corresponds to panel B, shows a mixed SI pattern, with a markedly high ADC value *(arrow)*. *(D and E)* Histopathological specimens (hematoxylin and eosin, ×20, D, and ×40, E) show total parenchymal necrosis with hemorrhage. No evidence of viable tumor cells was found. (Asao C, Korogi Y, Kitajima M, et al. Diffusion-weighted imaging of radiation-induced brain injury for differentiation from tumor recurrence. *Am J Neuroradiol.* 2005;26:1455–1460.)

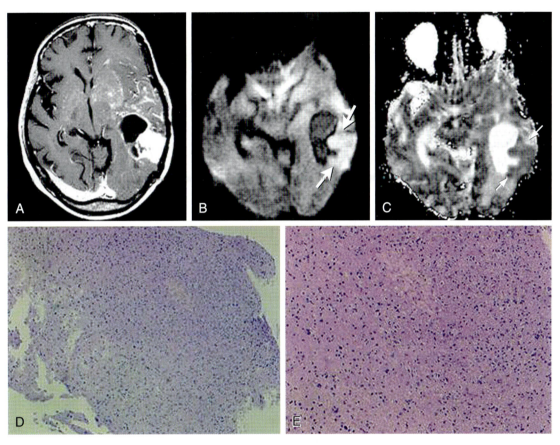

Figure 48-5. Images obtained in a 53-year-old woman with biopsy-proven tumor after receiving radiation and chemotherapy for anaplastic astrocytoma. *(A)* Gadolinium-enhanced T_1-weighted image shows a ring-enhancing lesion with a solid enhancing component in the left temporal lobe. Multiple patchy enhancements with mass effect are also seen in the left basal ganglia and insula, suggestive of tumor infiltration. *(B)* Diffusion-weighted image obtained at the same level as that of panel A shows the solid enhancing component of predominant hyperintensity *(arrows),* which usually represents densely packed tumor cells. *(C)* ADC map, which shows the relatively low apparent diffusion coefficient value of the lesion *(arrows). (D and E)* Histopathological specimens (hematoxylin and eosin, $\times 20$, *D,* and $\times 80$, *E*) show tumor tissues with increased cellular density corresponding to anaplastic astrocytoma. No evidence of necrotic tissue was found. (Asao C, Korogi Y, Kitajima M, et al. Diffusion-weighted imaging of radiation-induced brain injury for differentiation from tumor recurrence. *Am J Neuroradiol.* 2005;26:1455–1460.)

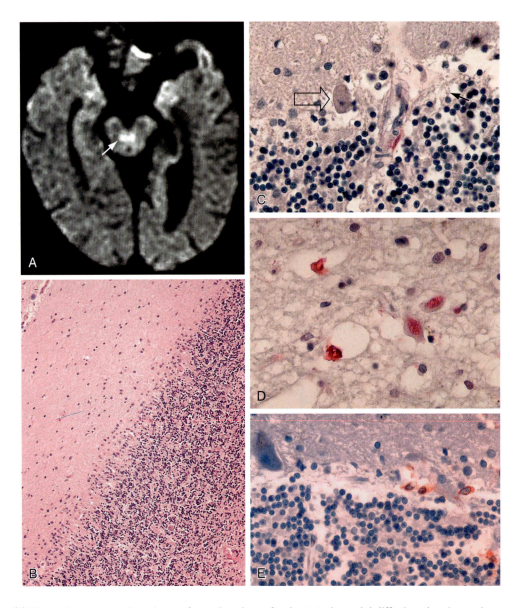

Figure 49-1. *(A)* Magnetic resonance imaging performed 12 days after heatstroke; axial diffusion showing an increased signal *(arrow)* in the central tegmentum of the midbrain at the anterior aspect of the periaqueductal gray matter, corresponding to Wernekinck's commissure. *(B)* Cerebellar cortex showing complete loss of Purkinje cells with proliferation of Bergmann glia. Note that the granule cells and molecular layers are relatively spared (hematoxylin and eosin, ×100). *(C)* In situ end labeling in the cerebellar cortex showing that one remaining Purkinje cell with pyknotic nucleus and homogenized cytoplasm is not stained *(large empty arrow),* whereas an endothelial cell serving as internal controls is stained *(thin arrow;* Apoptag kit, ×400). *(D)* In situ end labeling in the centromedian nucleus of the thalamus showing positivity of the nuclei of remaining neurons; cellular remnants within vacuoles are also positively stained (Apoptag kit, ×400). *(E)* Immunostaining for heat shock protein 70 in the cerebellar cortex showing positively stained astrocytes of Bergmann glia around a necrotic Purkinje cells (avidin–biotin complex, peroxidase–antiperoxidase technique, ×400). (Bazille C, Megarbane B, Bensimhon D, et al. Brain damage after heatstroke. *J Neuropathol Exp Neurol.* 005;64[11]:970–975.)

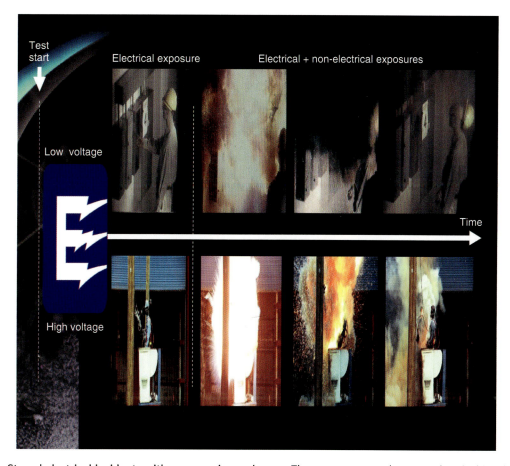

Figure 50-1. Staged electrical incidents with mannequin employees. The top sequence shows an electrical incident staged as a maintenance employee at a low-voltage (480 V) installation.[3] Peak monitored temperature exceeded 225°C within 10 msec at the mannequin's hand and at 120 msec at the neck. Peak pressure estimate was at 2160 lb/ft² and a 141.5-dB sound. Cooling of the hand to 70°C required more than 2500 msec. The bottom sequence was staged as a high-voltage (>1000 V) illustration of a line worker in a bucket at an overhead cable, with video images courtesy of ConEd frame captured for visual comparison.

NEUROTOXIC OVERVIEW

CONTENTS

Introduction to Clinical Neurotoxicology

Michael R. Dobbs

INTRODUCTION

Toxins are causes of neurological diseases from antiquity to contemporary times. Pliny described "palsy" from exposure to lead dust in the 1st century AD, one of the earliest known medical neurotoxic descriptions.[1] Although carbon monoxide has long been known to cause acute central nervous system (CNS) damage, it is only recently that we are finding delayed CNS injury in people poisoned by this molecule.[2]

Toxins and environmental conditions are important and underrecognized causes of neurological disease. In addition to chemical toxins, extremes of cold, heat, and altitude all can have adverse effects on our bodies and nervous systems. As medical developments occur and scientific knowledge advances, new toxic and environmental causes of diseases are discovered.

EPIDEMIOLOGY

Conservative estimates in the 1980s acknowledged that about 8 million people worked full-time with substances known to be neurotoxic.[3,4] At that time, about 750 chemicals were suspected to be neurotoxic to humans based on available scientific evidence.[5] We do not know how many there are today, but an unadventurous estimate might suggest more than 1000.

The level of evidence for whether something is truly toxic to the human nervous system varies from substance to substance. Some evidence is purely experimental, whereas in others there is a strong clinical association.

Spencer and Schaumburg, in the second edition of their encyclopedic neurotoxicology text, used evidence-based criteria in deciding which toxins to include.[6] They assigned each toxin a "neurotoxicity rating." A rating of "A" indicated a strong association between the substance and the condition; "B" denoted a suspected but unproven association; and "C" meant probably not causal. They separated evidence into clinical and experimental. Based on their criteria, the editors chose to include 465 items in their alphabetized list of substances with neurotoxic potential.[6]

CLINICAL NEUROTOXICOLOGY

Although the CNS is somewhat protected by the blood–brain barrier, and the peripheral nervous system by the blood–nerve barrier, the nervous system remains susceptible to toxic injury (Table 1). Generally, nonpolar,

Table 1:	**Factors Rendering the Nervous System Susceptible to Toxic Injuries**
1.	Neurons and their processes have a high surface area, increasing their exposure risk.
2.	High lipid content of neuronal structures results in accumulation and retention of lipophilic substances.
3.	Neurons have high metabolic demands and are strongly affected by energy or nutrient depletion.
4.	High blood flow in the central nervous system increases effective exposure to circulating toxins.
5.	Chemical toxins can interfere with normal neurotransmission by mimicking structures of endogenous molecules.
6.	Following toxic injury, recovery of normal, complex interneuronal and intraneuronal connections is typically imperfect.
7.	Neurons typically are postmitotic and do not divide.

Modified from Firestone JA, Longstreth WT. Central Nervous System Diseases, In: Rosenstock L, et al., eds. *Textbook of Clinical Occupational and Environmental Medicine.* 2nd ed. London: Elsevier Saunders; 2004.

highly lipid–soluble substances may gain access to the nervous system most easily.

The effects of neurotoxic agents on the CNS present wide-ranging disturbances. This can include mental status disturbances (mood disorders, psychosis, encephalopathy, coma), myelopathy, focal cerebral lesions, seizures, and movement disorders. Neurotoxic effects on the peripheral nervous system, however, typically present with neuropathy, myopathy, or neuromuscular junction syndromes.

Some disorders of neurotoxicology are not easily definable as being caused by a single, specific toxin, such as toxic axonopathies and encephalopathies seen with exposure to mixed organic solvents. Most neurotoxins manifest through effects on a single, specific part of the nervous system cortex, cord, extrapyramidal neurons, peripheral nerves, etc., and the syndromes can be somewhat defined by these presentations. However, sometimes toxins affect the nervous system in more than one sphere.

Practitioners

It makes sense that clinical neurotoxicologists would be neurologists, and arguably, every fully trained neurologist should have sufficient expertise to diagnose and manage common neurotoxic disorders. However, formal clinical neurotoxicology training is lacking in most neurology residency programs, and no neurology fellowships are available to study clinical neurotoxicology. Therefore, most neurologists are uncomfortable with neurotoxicology. Consequentially, a serious knowledge gap exists in this field.

It is exciting that this void is being filled to some extent by emergency medicine physicians who complete additional training in medical toxicology fellowships. It

is hardly surprising that this has happened. Emergency physicians must be able to immediately recognize and treat toxic emergencies, and the medical toxicology fellowship was conceived somewhat out of that necessity. Medical toxicology fellowships are also available to other general medical physicians. Of course, in the comprehensive study of general toxicology, it follows that physicians must gain some expertise in clinical neurotoxicology. Therefore, emergency medicine toxicologists and other medical toxicologists are sometimes incredibly proficient practitioners in recognizing and treating syndromes of clinical neurotoxicology.

However, what most emergency medicine doctors and other nonneurologists lack is a core of training that centers on precise localization and differential diagnosis of a nervous system problem. Many clinical neurotoxicology syndromes can be quite challenging to diagnose, and some are still being defined neurologically. Therefore, a role is available today for competent clinical neurologists in evaluating, diagnosing, and treating patients with neurotoxic disorders. It follows that there should also be room in neurology training programs for some time dedicated to studying clinical neurotoxicology.

Common Toxic Syndromes or "Toxidromes" of the Nervous System

While the term *toxidrome* is commonly reserved to refer to signs and symptoms seen with a particular class of poisons (e.g., the cholinergic syndrome), clinicians might also find it useful to group neurotoxic syndromes based on the system preferentially affected. We might call these *neurotoxidromes.* All of these systemic neurological syndromes can be caused be various nontoxic states, which

Table 2: Major Categories of Neurotoxic Substances

Category	Examples
Metals	Lead, arsenic, thallium
Pharmaceuticals	Tacrolimus, phenytoin
Biologicals (noniatrogenic)	Tetanus toxin, tetrodotoxin
Organic industrials	Toluene, styrene, n-hexane
Miscellaneous	Radiation, nerve agents

is one of the things that makes clinical neurotoxicology so challenging to practice.

Encephalopathy Syndromes

Acute toxic encephalopathies exhibit confusion, attention deficits, seizures, and coma. Much of this is from CNS capillary damage, hypoxia, and cerebral edema.[7] Sometimes, depending on the toxin and dose, with appropriate care, neurological symptoms may resolve. Permanent deficits can result, however, even with a single exposure.

Chronic, low-level exposures may cause insidious symptoms that are long unrecognized. Such symptoms incorporate mood disturbances, fatigue, and cognitive disorders. Permanent residual deficits may remain, especially with severe symptoms or prolonged exposure, although improvement may occur following removal of the toxin. Significant progress to recovery may take months to years to transpire.

Spinal Cord Syndromes

Myelopathy is seen with exposure to a few toxins and fairly characterizes the associated syndromes. Lathyrism, due to ingestion of the toxic grass pea, is an epidemic neurotoxic syndrome seen during famine in parts of the world where this legume grows. It characteristically presents as an irreversible thoracic myelopathy with upper motor neuron signs. Nitrous oxide is another spinal cord toxin. Exposure to nitrous oxide typically affects the posterior columns of the spinal cord in a manner that can be indistinguishable from vitamin B_{12} deficiency.

Movement Disorder Syndromes

Some toxic agents are selective in toxicity to lenticular or striatal neurons. These toxins produce signs and symptoms related to these structures, such as parkinsonism, dystonia, chorea, and ballismus. Some classic toxins in

this category include manganese, carbon monoxide, and phenothiazine drugs. Intoxications causing movement disorder abnormalities may also show symptoms related to injury to other parts of the nervous system.

Neuromuscular Syndromes

The neuromuscular syndromes can be divided into neuropathy, myopathy, and toxic neuromuscular junction disorders. However, within those broad categories is a need for further characterization. The ancillary tests of electromyography, nerve conduction studies, and nerve or muscle biopsy (in select cases) can be quite useful. Refer to the appropriate chapters for more details on toxic neuromuscular diseases.

Chronic Neuropathy

Sometimes, it is difficult to sort out whether a chronic, peripheral polyneuropathy is from a toxic agent or from some other cause. This is particularly compounded in patients who have underlying illnesses that are prone to neuropathy (such as diabetes mellitus or acquired immune deficiency syndrome) and are on multiple medications that can cause neuropathy as well. Chronic toxic neuropathies can present as axonopathies, myelinopathies, or mixed pictures depending on the individual toxic agent.

Acute Neuropathies

Acute toxic neuropathies can be focal or diffuse. Lead intoxication in adults presents as a mononeuropathy, typically of a radial nerve. Buckthorn (coyotillo) berry intoxication demonstrates the classic acute peripheral polyneuropathy and is clinically indistinguishable from the acute inflammatory demyelinating polyneuropathy (AIDP) of Guillain-Barré syndrome. Diphtheria toxin and tick paralysis toxin are two other toxins that can mimic AIDP.

Neuromuscular Junction Disorders

Botulinum toxin and organophosphates are among the toxic agents that act at the neuromuscular junction. Cranial nerve palsies superimposed on diffuse muscular weakness are commonly seen. Respiratory muscle weakness can be so severe as to cause respiratory failure.

Myopathies

The toxic myopathies are often secondary to prescription drugs. Familiar drugs implicated include 3-hydroxy-3-methylglutaryl–coenzyme–A reductase inhibitors (statins) and antipsychotic agents. Resolution is common after discontinuation of the offending agent.

ENVIRONMENTAL NEUROLOGY

Aside from neurological disorders caused by toxins, many environments are known to either directly cause or predispose an individual for neurological problems. Some environments also place humans at risk for unique or unusual neurological troubles. Potentially neurotoxic environments include mountains (altitude sickness), marine environments (envenomations, barotrauma), locations of extreme temperature (heat stroke, dehydration, frostbite), and flight (airplanes, spacecraft).

CONTROVERSIES

As a young field of study, clinical neurotoxicology is naturally rife with controversies. The available potential for ongoing discovery is part of what makes clinical neurotoxicology so stimulating to study and to practice. Some ongoing major controversies include whether there are toxic roots for neurodegenerative diseases such as Parkinson's disease, Alzheimer's disease, and amyotrophic lateral sclerosis.

CONCLUSION

At present, neurotoxins are important but underrecognized causes of neurological illness. There is a need for more training in clinical neurotoxicology during neurology residency. Current practitioners include select neurologists and medical toxicologists.

Human society continues to advance technologically. As it progresses, we will most likely place ourselves into unfamiliar situations and environments and expose ourselves to novel substances. Some of these environments and substances may be harmful. It is reasonable to expect that we will continue to experience diseases caused by toxins and environments throughout our future as a species. It is reasonable to expect that many of these will be toxic to the human nervous system.

REFERENCES

1. Hunter D. *The Diseases of Occupations.* 6th ed. London: Hodder and Stoughton; 1978:251.
2. Kwon OY, Chung SP, Ha YR, Yoo IS, Kim SW. Delayed postanoxic encephalopathy after carbon monoxide poisoning. *Emerg Med J.* 2004;21(2):250–251.
3. Anger WK. Workplace exposures. In: Annau Z, ed. *Neurobehavioral Toxicology.* Baltimore: John's Hopkins; 1986.
4. National Institute for Occupational Safety and Health. National Occupational Hazard Survey, 1972–74. DHEW Publication No. (NIOSH) 78-114. Cincinnati, Ohio: NIOSH; 1977.
5. Anger WK. Neurobehavioral testing of chemicals: impact on recommended standards. *Neurobehav Toxicol Teratol.* 1984;6: 147–153.
6. Spencer PS, Schaumburg HH. *Experimental and Clinical Neurotoxicology.* New York: Oxford University Press; 2000.
7. Feldman RG. *Approach to Diagnosis: Occupational and Environmental Neurotoxicology.* Philadelphia: Lippincott-Raven; 1999.

CHAPTER 2

Cellular and Molecular Neurotoxicology: Basic Principles

David R. Wallace

HISTORICAL PERSPECTIVE OF NEUROTOXICOLOGY

It has been long known that a variety of compounds and insults can be toxic to the central nervous system (CNS). Only in the last 20 to 25 years has the study of neurotoxicology intensified and focused attention on specific agents and diseases. A good indicator of the growth of neurotoxicology is the examination of the number of societies and journals devoted wholly or partly to the subject (Table 1).

In addition to the societies and journals, more than 150 books have been published since the late 1970s that deal with some aspect of neurotoxicology. As we have become more aware of our surrounding environment, it has become clear that numerous agents, pharmaceuticals, chemicals, metals, and natural products can have toxic effect on the CNS. An estimated 80,000 to 100,000 chemicals are in use worldwide, most of which have received little toxicity testing for the CNS. There are thousands of potential pharmaceuticals and natural product supplements, which may have good toxicity testing, but neurotoxicity testing is weak or lacking. The sheer weight of the hundreds of thousands of compounds that can be found in the environment (heavy metals, pesticides, ionizing radiation, etc.) and in the workplace (industrial pollution, combustion by-products, etc.) also suggests that the broad area of neurotoxicology will only continue to grow. Another source of CNS-acting toxins is via bacteria and viruses. Proteins from the human immunodeficiency virus (HIV) have been shown to have neurotoxic properties.[1,2] Our laboratory, as well as others, has shown that HIV-related neurotoxicity affects the dopaminergic system, which could underlie symptoms of psychosis and Parkinson's-like symptoms in late-stage acquired immune deficiency syndrome (AIDS).[1] One of the newest areas of neurotoxicological interest involves the use of biological weapons or weapons of mass destruction. Better understanding of the agents used for these devices would also provide insight into the actions of other neurotoxic agents. Another complicating issue in the field of neurotoxicology is that some agents at "normal" concentrations are harmless and do not elicit any overt neurologic symptoms. In healthy adults, most exogenous agents are metabolized to inactive compounds, eliminated, or both. In some instances, however, agents may accumulate over time or dose to levels that are toxic, which could be due to chronic exposure or to inadequate metabolism or elimination. In addition, brief exposure may initiate changes that are not clearly observed early in exposure but may appear much later. Our work has shown that concentrations of heavy metals such as mercury or lead, which are below concentrations normally considered toxic, can alter the function of the dopaminergic

Table 1: Societies and Journals with Neurotoxicology Emphasis in 2008

Societies	Journals
Behavioral Toxicology Society	*Neurotoxicity Research*
International Neurotoxicology Association	*Neurotoxicology*
Neurobehavioral Teratology Society	*Neurotoxicology and Teratology*
Neurotoxicity Society	
Neurotoxicology Specialty Section of the Society of Toxicology	
Scientific Committee on Neurotoxicology and Psychophysiology of the International Commission on Occupational Health	

system.[3] Under these conditions, an individual may be entirely asymptomatic but could be predisposed to degeneration of dopaminergic neurons later or could exhibit increased sensitivity to other toxins. This effect could interfere with the appropriate diagnosis of exposure versus neurodegenerative disease that exhibits similar neurological symptoms. As a population, we continue to lengthen our life span, which increases our exposure to toxins that may exert neurologic effects. With an ever-expanding population and increasing industrialization of additional countries, the number and amount of pollutants that are toxins will continue to increase. In this situation, we enter a complex and possibly vicious cycle that could potentially become self-limiting. To break this cycle, we need to research further the mechanism of action, diagnosis, and potential treatment following exposure to these agents. Therefore, the need to examine and understand neurotoxic agents is vital. As our understanding of these agents grows, our ability to develop and provide potential pharmacotherapies increases.

NEUROTOXIC ENDPOINTS, BIOMARKERS, AND MODEL SYSTEMS

To determine whether a compound is neurotoxic, an endpoint to assess neurotoxicity must be determined and accepted. In 1998 the U.S. Environmental Protection Agency (EPA) published Guidelines for Neurotoxicity Risk Assessment, which outlined some common endpoints for the neurotoxic effects of an exogenous compound (Table 2). Regarding human studies, it has been difficult to accurately determine neurotoxicity except upon postmortem examination. Recent advances in functional magnetic resonance imaging (fMRI) and positron emission tomography (PET) imaging have improved clinical ability to determine neurological damage, but the need for relatively noninvasive and accurate biomarkers remains. Correlates between brain imaging and other secondary analyses have been attempted with manganese exposure.[4,5] Their findings have suggested that individuals with a strong MRI signal, in conjunction with elevated manganese content in red blood cells, could be a predictor of future neurological damage associated with manganese exposure.[4] Another issue that has plagued neurotoxicology research has been the use of appropriate and comparable animal or nonanimal model systems.[6] Due to the complexity of the human CNS, it is difficult to find appropriate model systems in which modifications can be directly correlated to effects in the human CNS. Rodents are relatively inexpensive, widely used, and well characterized, but our understanding of the rodent CNS has led us to the conclusion that this may not be the best model system for all comparative studies. Some factors and issues that need to be considered when selecting an animal model are applicability to the human CNS, commonality to the human CNS, similar pathways, and neural systems compared to the human CNS. In some instances, however, rodents are used to the exclusion of other systems, even when it is understood that their use is not the best model for the system in question.[7] Alternative testing methods have been a topic of discussion for the last 2 decades. Slowly, the old dogma is evolving and there is an understanding that other species may provide as much, if not more, information compared to mammalian and vertebrate species. This effort of finding alternative testing models is supported by the federal agencies responsible for regulatory and funding matters.[8,9] Research into other species (*Drosophila, Caenorhabditis elegans,* and zebra fish) has more fully elucidated the neural systems of such species, and it has become evident to the neurotoxicology community that these species can provide powerful model systems to study specific interactions of toxic agents within the CNS. These systems are significantly simpler than human, primate, or rodent CNS yet have enough complexity to examine toxic effects and neural interactions on a more focused level. The human genome project has revealed that many human genes are similar, if not exact, to our ancient ancestors.

Table 2: Measurable Endpoints for the Determination of Neurotoxic Effects

Category	Measurable Outcome
Structural or neuropathological	• Gross changes in morphology, including brain weight • Histological changes in neurons or glia (neuronopathy, axonopathy, myelinopathy)
Neurochemical	• Alterations in synthesis, release, uptake, degradation of neurotransmitters • Alterations in second-messenger-associated signal transduction • Alterations in membrane-bound enzymes regulating neuronal activity • Inhibition and aging of neuropathy enzyme • Increases in glial fibrillary acidic protein in adults
Neurophysiological	• Changes in velocity, amplitude, or refractory period of nerve conduction • Changes in latency or amplitude of sensory-evoked potential • Changes in electroencephalographic pattern
Behavioral and neurological	• Increases or decreases in motor activity • Changes in touch, sight, sound, taste, or smell sensations • Changes in motor coordination, weakness, paralysis, abnormal movement or posture, tremor, or ongoing performance • Absence or decreased occurrence, magnitude, or latency of sensorimotor reflex • Altered magnitude of neurologic measurement, including grip strength and hindlimb splay • Seizures • Changes in rate or temporal patterning of schedule-controlled behavior • Changes in learning, memory, and attention
Developmental	• Chemically induced changes in the time of appearance of behaviors during development • Chemically induced changes in the growth or organization of structural or neurochemical elements

Therefore, many species previously thought of as being too "primitive" are now known to express the genes of interest in neurotoxicity testing. Ballatori and Villalobos[6] provide an excellent review of alternative species used in neurotoxicity testing.

Another concern with extrapolating in vitro work to in vivo work is the conditions in which the in vitro work is performed. Caution must be exercised when interpreting in vitro concentrations to in vivo effects, the use of immortalized cell lines to primary neuronal culture,[10] and the employment of newly developed techniques without fully understanding the connection between in vitro and in vivo studies. In most cases, parallel in vitro and in vivo studies are most advantageous.[11] The intent of this chapter is to provide a view on neurotoxicology as this field relates on a cellular and molecular. Examination of these topics clearly demonstrates that molecular and cellular (as well as genetic) aspects of neurotoxicology are not mutually exclusive but are intimately interrelated. The molecular and cellular changes that occur following exposure to exogenous agents that may provide protection and the molecular and cellular environments that

may facilitate neurotoxicity are discussed. The genetic effects of toxic agents are also briefly discussed from the perspectives of genetic alterations following exposure and genetic alterations or defects present before exposure that may predispose an individual to a toxic insult following exposure.

CELLULAR NEUROTOXICOLOGY

The field of cellular neurotoxicology can involve a single cellular process or multiple cascading processes. With the complexity of the human brain, many toxin actions involve multiple processes and act upon many neurotransmitter systems. Processes that are affected can be involved with the following:

1. Energy homeostasis—production or utilization of adenosine triphosphate
2. Electrolyte homeostasis—alterations in key cations; Na^+, K^+, Ca^{++}, and anions; Cl^-

3. Intracellular signaling—alterations in G-protein coupling, phosphoinositol turnover, intracellular protein scaffolding

4. Neurotransmitters—alterations in neurotransmitter release, uptake, storage

Since toxins can interfere with cellular function on multiple levels, the development of biomarkers for neurotoxins has been slow. By definition, a *biomarker* is obtained by the analysis of bodily tissue and/or fluids for chemicals, metabolites of chemicals, enzymes, and other biochemical substances as a result of biological-chemical interactions. The measured response may be functional and physiological, biochemical at the cellular level, or a molecular interaction. Biomarkers may be used to assess the exposure (absorbed amount or internal dose) and effects of chemicals and susceptibility of individuals, and they may be applied whether exposure has been from dietary, environmental, or occupational sources. In general, there is a complex interrelationship among the factors involved with exposure, the host, and the measurable outcome (Table 3). Biomarkers may be used to elucidate cause–effect and dose–effect relationships in health risk assessment, in clinical diagnosis, and for monitoring purposes.

Ideally, the desired biomarker is one that could easily be measured in a living subject and would accurately represent the toxin exposure. While a single marker probably does not exist, a combination of markers, examined together, might provide a more accurate assessment of toxin exposure. Further complicating the interpretation of toxicant–CNS effects are the various classifications of biomarkers. There are biomarkers of exposure, effect, and susceptibility.[12] Finding the appropriate biomarker for a particular toxin is a daunting task. Recent work has examined subchronic exposure to acrylamide and methylmercury, followed by blood and urine sampling. Using surface-enhanced laser desorption/ionization time-of-flight mass spectrometry (SELDI-TOF MS), specific proteins were found in both serum and urine with mass-to-charge (*m/z*) ratios that correctly classified each of the treatment and control groups.[13] A novel method involves the use of metabolomics, which is an in vitro method that uses the metabolic or biochemical "fingerprint" of the cell to determine whether a toxin has altered the metabolic actions of the cell before visible damage or symptomology.[14] As an extension to earlier studies, which examined glial fibrillary acidic protein as a marker of trimethyltin (TMT) toxicity, the production of autoantibodies has been examined as a potentially new and less invasive way to determining TMT exposure.[15] Collectively, these three methods are advancing what was previously understood and accepted for neurochemical biomarkers.

The CNS undergoes many phases of development before adulthood. During each phase, particular biomarkers would be important for one phase but not another.[16] Developmental neurotoxicology is one of the more difficult disciplines to assess for toxin exposure. Initially, there is fetal development, when the CNS is most susceptible to toxins that cross the placental barrier. Postnatal development is also a vulnerable period,

Table 3:	Factors That Can Affect Interactions Among the Exposure Compound, the Host, and the Measurable Outcome[64]			
Source →	**Chemical** →	**Exposure Route** →	**Host** →	**Response**
DISTRIBUTION	PROPERTIES	ROUTE		
• Air • Water • Soil • Food		• Air • Oral • Derma • Parental	• Age • Race • Gender • Health status	• Immediate • Delayed
		EXPOSURE		
		• Dose • Concentration • Amount • Rate • Single or multiple chemicals • Absorption		

although much less so than fetal development. Lastly, prepubescent and adolescent development periods are also temporal time points that warrant monitoring and investigation. These variations have been demonstrated with the toxic effects of amphetamine on the developing brain.[16] Barone et al.[17] reviewed the biomarkers and methods used for assessing exposure to pesticides during these periods of development. A difficulty that requires attention is the use of an appropriate model system and interpretation of databases at the appropriate stages of development.[17] The use of oligodendrocytes, or oligodendroglia, has attracted attention due to the influence of some environmental toxins such as lead that affect the myelination of neurons.[18] Alterations in myelination change conduction speeds of myelinated neurons and thus affect neuronal function. Oligodendrocytes possess a variety of ligand- and voltage-gated ion channels and neurotransmitter receptors. The best characterized of the neurotransmitters that assist in shaping the developing oligodendrocytes population is glutamate.[19,20] The primary receptor classes expressed in oligodendrocytes are the ionotropic glutamate receptors (α-amino-3-hydroxy-5-methyl-4-isoxazolepropionic acid and kainate). In addition to glutamate receptors, γ-aminobutyric acid, serotonin, glycine, dopamine, nicotinic, β-adrenergic, substance P, somatostatin, and opioid receptors are also expressed. Calcium, sodium, and potassium channels have also been identified in oligodendrocytes (see Deng and Poretz[18] and references cited within). In addition, the use of oligodendrocytes may provide a useful model system for the study of toxicant–CNS action. Biomarkers of exposure include such combinations (biomarker–toxin) as follows[12,21]:

- Mercapturates—styrene
- Hemoglobin—carbon disulfide
- Porphyrins—metals
- Acetylcholinesterase—organophosphates
- Monoamine oxidase B—styrene and manganese
- Dopamine-β-hydroxylase—manganese and styrene
- Calcium—mercury

The advantage to these biomarker–toxin combinations is they can be detected and measured shortly following exposure and before overt neuroanatomic damage or lesions. The measurement of acetylcholinesterase activity can be accomplished through blood sampling, although a less invasive method has been tested.[22] Intervention at this point, shortly following exposure, may prevent or attenuate further damage to the individual.[23]

Susceptibility markers include d-aminolevulinic acid dehydratase for lead and aldehyde dehydrogenase for alcohol.[12,21] Although these biomarkers can be used for examining toxin exposure in the CNS, they are difficult to measure directly. Therefore, there is a need for establishing biomarkers that can be easily measured in the periphery and that are similar to the targets of toxic substances in the CNS.[24] Parameters that can be measured in the periphery include receptors (muscarinic, β-adrenergic, benzodiazepine, α1- and α2-adrenergic), enzymes (acetylcholinesterase, monoamine oxidase B), signal transduction systems (calcium, adenylyl cyclase, phosphoinositide metabolism), and uptake systems (serotonin), which can be found in human blood cells.[21,24] The most common blood cell types that have been studied to date are lymphocytes, platelets, and erythrocytes. Conventional markers of dopaminergic function have been the assessment of dopaminergic enzymes such as dopamine-β-hydroxylase activity, monoamine oxidase activity, and the dopamine transporter function. Although dopamine-β-hydroxylase and monoamine oxidase activity have been shown to be reliable markers of manganese exposure, the measurement of plasma prolactin levels has been reported to be just as accurate when assessing early exposure to manganese.[25] The use of peripheral biomarkers has numerous advantages in addition to the obvious, eliminating the need to biopsy brain tissue from a living individual. These advantages included time-course analysis, elimination of ethical concerns, less invasive procedures, and ease of performance compared to CNS biopsies. If the appropriate biomarker is discovered for a particular toxin exposure, it may be possible to detect the toxin exposure before clear clinical symptoms becoming present. Yet several significant obstacles must be overcome for a peripheral biomarker to reflect an accurate representation of CNS effects[26-28]:

- CNS and peripheral markers must exhibit the same pharmacologic and biochemical characteristics under control situations and following toxin exposure.
- Time-course response profiles must be performed to determine whether the peripheral tissue responds in the same fashion as the CNS tissue.
- The complexity of the CNS allows for adaptation that may not be present in the periphery. Other neuronal systems or neurotransmitters may adapt or compensate for toxin-related CNS changes following exposure.
- Inherent in many human studies is inter- and intragroup variability that may in some instances be large.

These factors must be considered when attempting to accurately determine whether a potential biomarker has been changed. In most instances, hypothesis-driven research is preferred, yet mechanistic research still has a place in the field neurotoxicology. Work on the actions of organophosphate pesticides and their mechanisms of action are probably the best described.[29-31] The value of mechanistic studies in neurotoxicology is to facilitate the development of biomarkers for future use in detecting toxin exposure.[31] When one considers the thousands of toxins and the additional thousands of potential toxins that an individual may be exposed to in a lifetime, it is startling that only a handful of reliable biomarkers exist. Increased use of mechanistic studies, in a fashion similar to what has been accomplished with organophosphate exposure, would further advance our understanding of toxin effects and could lead to earlier detection of exposure.[27,31] Use of existing data to formulate nonhuman studies characterizing the actions of a toxin would also be extremely valuable. Using existing information on exposure of domoic acid, a glutamate agonist, in a population in which toxicity to this endogenous toxin was reported was used in a quantitative fashion and was able to yield an accurate dose–response model for domoic acid toxicity that is biologically based.[32,33] Using this method would allow the use of nonhuman experimental units and provide information comparable to a comprehensive human study.[32]

A cellular extension of the protein–protein interactions involves the release of neurotransmitters. It is possible to measure neurotransmitter release in vitro using synaptosomal, brain slice, and culture methodologies. In these methods, the brain would have to be removed from the subject before experimentation, which would prove to be a drawback in nonterminal studies. With the use of a carbon microelectrode and amperometry, real-time release of neurotransmitters can be measured.[34] The use of amperometry focuses on presynaptic effects of toxins and alterations of neurotransmitter release. Numerous protein–protein interactions (docking, exocytosis) must occur for proper release of neurotransmitters after stimulation (see Burgoyne and Morgan[35] for review). Proteins involved in the stimulation–exocytosis process can be soluble N-ethylmaleimide sensitive fusion protein attachment protein receptors (SNARE). SNARE proteins can be further classified as being associated with vesicles (synaptobrevins) or plasma membrane (syntaxin and synaptosomal-associated protein-25). Disruption of the activity of any of these proteins could result in robust changes in transmitter release. Many classes of drugs, and abused psychostimulants such as amphetamine and methamphetamine, have been shown to increase dopamine release and elicit toxicity partly through a presynaptic mechanism. The organic solvent toluene has also been reported to increase the presynaptic release of dopamine in a calcium-dependent manner.[34] Polychlorinated biphenyls and heavy metals (lead, mercury, manganese) have also been reported to increase presynaptic neurotransmitter release through calcium-dependent and calcium-independent mechanisms.[34] The ability of toxins to possess both direct and indirect effects complicates the interpretation of biomarker changes. For example, with the use of amperometry, only catecholamine and indolamine release can be measured[34]; however, actions of the toxin at another site may in turn alter the release of the catecholamine or indolamine being measured through an indirect mechanism. In sum, outstanding biomarkers in cellular neurotoxicology have yet to be identified, especially in light of the thousands of potential toxins known to exist. Recently, the advancement in the "omics," such as proteomics, genomics, and metabolomics, has provided us with tools to study protein–protein interactions. By examining the effect of a potential toxin on protein–protein interactions on an intracellular level, we can begin to describe the cellular changes that occur following toxin exposure that are devoid of obvious clinical symptoms. It is clear that additional work is needed, but research methodologies are available to expand the current mechanistic literature and develop valuable and reliable biomarkers for particular toxins.

MOLECULAR NEUROTOXICOLOGY

Past work in the field of neurotoxicology has emphasized the outcomes following exposure to a toxic agent. This emphasis was partly because of the limitations of the technology available at the time. Most work was categorized into three groups: molecular mechanistic, correlative, and "black box."[36] The superficial nature of this work led to questions and concerns from the more established fields of neuroscience. This trend has slowly evolved and changed with the acceptance of the interdisciplinary nature of the neurotoxicology field. Areas of neurophysiology, neurochemistry, neuroscience, and molecular biology have demonstrated areas of overlap that have assisted in furthering our understanding of neurotoxicology. Further advances in neurotoxicology will come from additional molecular research and increased understanding of CNS injury from endogenous and exogenous agents.[37] Recently, there has been a substantial expansion and diversification in technology that has facilitated the study of neurotoxicology on molecular and cellular levels. Previous work in "molecular biology" has emphasized the studies of messenger RNA and gene expression. One area of study that has gained significant attention in the past few years has been the field of proteomics. Lubec et al.[38] provides a review of the potential and the limitations of proteomics, or the protein outcome from the genome. Genetic expression leads to the synthesis and degradation of proteins that are integrally involved in normal neuronal function. Agents that interfere with this protein processing could lead to neuronal damage, death, or predisposition to further insults. Oxidative or covalent modification of proteins could lead to alterations in tertiary structure and loss of protein function. The advantage to proteomics over "classical" protein chemistry is that proteomics examines multiple steps in the cycle of protein synthesis, function, and degradation whereas protein chemistry focuses on the sequence of amino acids that form the protein. Therefore, proteomics focuses on a more comprehensive view of cellular proteins and provides considerable more information about the effects of toxins on the CNS.[39] Effects of possible toxic agents can be detected at the posttranslational level following exposure.[40,41] The most applicable use for proteomics in assessing the effects of a possible toxin is mapping posttranslational modifications of proteins.[39] Posttranslational processing involves many processes, including protein phosphorylation, glycosylation, tertiary structure, function, and turnover. Modifications of proteins influence protein trafficking, which could have significant impact on the movement and insertion of proteins such as neurotransmitter receptors and transporters. In addition to alteration in posttranslational processing, many potential toxic agents are electrophilic and covalently bind to groups on proteins, such as thiol groups, thus altering their structure, function, and subsequent degradation and elimination.[42,43] Oxidation of proteins is believed to be involved in many toxic insults and degenerative diseases of the CNS.[44,45] The measurement of oxidized proteins, or carbonyls, is an accepted method for the determination of oxidized proteins in brain tissue.[46] In addition to posttranslational modifications, protein-expression profiling and protein-network mapping can be employed. The method of protein-expression profiling has been used to assess protein changes in head trauma, and hypoxia and during the aging process.[47–49] A limitation for the use of protein-expression profiling is the amount of protein being measured. Large quantities of the protein would need to be obtained, and in many cases, extraction from blood would not yield enough protein to profile. Therefore, a more invasive procedure would need to be performed. An improvement on this method used liquid chromatography–mass spectrometry (LC-MS) detection of isotope-labeled proteins.[50] Protein-network mapping is an enormously powerful tool for identifying changes in multiprotein complexes induced by exposure to a possible toxin. There are two approaches to measuring protein-network mapping. First, the "two-hybrid" system uses a reporter gene to detect the interaction of protein pairs within the yeast cell nucleus. The two-hybrid system can be used to screen potential toxic agents that disrupt specific protein–protein interactions. This method is not without limitations regarding data interpretation. Second, "pull-down" studies use immunoprecipation of a protein that, in turn, precipitates associated or interactive proteins. Collectively, each method (posttranslational

modification, protein-expression profiling, and protein-network mapping) builds on each of the previous methods. Taken together, these methods provide a more complete and powerful image of protein modifications following potential toxin exposure.

The role of genetics and neurotoxic susceptibility is only briefly discussed here as it relates to alterations in protein production. A sizable body of work is accessible regarding causal peripheral effects of toxins, genetic polymorphisms, and cancer.[51–53] These publications have emphasized the occurrence of cancers of the breast, lung, and bladder, among other organs. The cytochrome P450 enzymes (CYPs) are found throughout the body and exhibit numerous polymorphisms. Polymorphisms have been identified in human CYP1A1, CYP1B1, CYP2C9, CYP2C18, CYP2D6, and CYP3A4. Polymorphic changes in CYP3A4 or in glutathione S-transferase may increase or decrease an individual's susceptibility to organophosphate pesticides[54] and may predispose an individual to increased risk for heart disease.[55] Past dogma has been that any toxin must be mutagenic, genotoxic, or both for symptoms to appear, yet more recent work has suggested that a toxin may be epigenetic and still elicit damaging effects.[56] Similar to protein–protein interactions, a toxin interruption of extra-, inter-, or intracellular communication would disrupt the homeostatic regulation of the cells and may be an underlying cause for toxin-induced disease.[56] Oxidative stress is also a form of epigenetic event because many compounds are known to increase the generation of reactive oxygen species but are not overtly genotoxic.[56–59] Toxins that are not genotoxic but that cause an epigenetic event could be as important in the field of neurotoxicology as agents that are genotoxic or cytotoxic. The use of microarray technology has demonstrated immense usefulness in toxicity studies.[60] Recent work has examined the effects of toxic compounds on DNA expression in the CNS. A group of genes that may contribute to methamphetamine-induced toxicity in the ventral striatum of the mouse has been identified.[61,62] In addition, the use of microarray technology has demonstrated alterations in gene expression in animals exposed to the dopaminergic toxin N-methyl-4-phenyl-1,2,3,6-tetrahydropyridine and experiencing chronic alcoholism.[60] It is clear that the microarray technology is an extremely powerful tool but more work needs to be done to refine the method.

SUMMARY AND CLINICAL CONSIDERATIONS

The field of neurotoxicology is not only rapidly growing but also rapidly evolving. As the number of drugs and environmental, bacterial, and viral agents with potential neurotoxic properties has grown, the need for additional testing has increased. Only recently has the technology advanced to a level that neurotoxicological studies can be performed without operating in a black box. Upon comparative analysis of where the field was nearly 15 years ago versus where it is today, it becomes obvious that more work is needed.[63] Examination of the effects of agents suspected of being toxic can occur on the molecular (protein–protein), cellular (biomarkers, neuronal function), or both levels. Proteomics is rapidly growing and developing as a tool that can be used in neurotoxicology, yet it can be constrained with limitations just as any of the neurotoxicology subdisciplines can be.[38] Proteomics is more comprehensive than some of the other subdisciplines because it focuses on a more comprehensive view of cellular proteins and their interactions, and as such it will provide significantly greater amounts of information regarding the effects of toxins on the CNS.[39] Proteomics can be classified into three focuses:

1. Posttranslational modification
2. Protein-expression profiling
3. Protein-network mapping

Collectively, these methods present a more complete and powerful image of protein modifications following potential toxin exposure. Cellular neurotoxicology involves alterations in cellular energy homeostasis, ion homeostasis, intracellular signaling function, and neurotransmitter release, uptake, and storage. From a clinical perspective, the development of a reliable biomarker, or series of biomarkers, has been remained elusive. The need is to develop appropriate biomarkers that are reliable, reproducible, and easy to obtain. The three broad classes of biomarkers are biomarkers of exposure, effect, and susceptibility.[12] The advantage to biomarker–toxin combinations is they can be detected and measured shortly following exposure and before overt neuroanatomic damage or lesions. Intervention at this point, shortly following exposure, may prevent or at least attenuate further damage to the individual.[23] The use of peripheral biomarkers to assess toxin damage in the CNS has numerous advantages:

1. Time-course analysis may be performed.
2. Ethical concerns with the use of human subjects can partially be avoided.
3. Procedures to acquire samples are less invasive.
4. Peripheral studies are easier to perform.

It has is becoming increasingly apparent that interactions between toxins and DNA are not as straightforward as eliciting mutations. Numerous agents cause epigenetic responses (cellular alterations that are not mutagenic or cytotoxic). This finding suggests that many agents that may originally have been thought of as nontoxic should be reexamined for potential "indirect" toxicity. With the advancement of the human genome project and the development of a human genome map, the effects of potential toxins on single or multiple genes can be identified. As technology and methodology advances continue and cooperation with other disciplines such as neuroscience, biochemistry, neurophysiology, and molecular biology is improved, the mechanisms of toxin action will be further elucidated. With this increased understanding, improved clinical interventions to prevent neuronal damage following exposure to a toxin can be developed before the development of symptoms.

REFERENCES

1. Wallace DR, Dodson S, Nath A, et al. Estrogen attenuates gp120- and TAT_{1-72}-induced oxidative stress and prevents loss of dopamine transporter function. *Synapse*. 2006;59:51–60.
2. Wallace DR, Dodson SL, Nath A, et al. δ-Opioid agonists attenuate TAT_{1-72}-induced oxidative stress in SK-N-SH cells. *Neurotoxicology*. 2006;27:101–107.
3. Hood AN, Wallace DR. Co-exposure of heavy metals and psychostimulants alter dopamine transporter (DAT) density without changes in DAT function. *Neurotoxicology*. 2009; revised submission.
4. Jiang Y, Zheng W, Long L, et al. Brain magnetic resonance imaging and manganese concentrations in red blood cells of smelting workers: search for biomarkers of manganese exposure. *Neurotoxicology*. 2007;28:126–135.
5. Erikson KM, Dorman DC, Lash LH, et al. Duration of airborne-manganese exposure in rhesus monkeys is associated with brain regional changes in biomarkers of neurotoxicity. *Neurotoxicology*. 2008;29:377–385.
6. Ballatori N, Villalobos AR. Defining the molecular and cellular basis of toxicity using comparative models. *Toxicol Appl Pharmacol*. 2002;183:207–220.
7. Olson H, Betton G, Robinson D, et al. Concordance of the toxicity of pharmaceutics in humans and animals. *Reg Toxicol Pharmacol*. 2000;32:56–67.
8. Goss LB, Sabourin TD. Utilization of alternative species for toxicity testing: an overview. *J Appl Toxicol*. 1985;5:193–219.
9. Bonaventura C. NIEHS Workshop: unique marine/freshwater models for environmental health research. *Environ Health Perspect*. 1999;107:89–92.
10. Stacey G, Viviani B. Cell culture models for neurotoxicology. *Cell Biol Toxicol*. 2001;17:319–334.
11. Tiffany-Castiglioni E, Ehrich M, Dees L, et al. Bridging the gap between in vitro and in vivo models for neurotoxicology. *Toxicol Sci*. 1999;51:178–183.
12. Costa LG, Manzo L. Biochemical markers of neurotoxicity: research strategies and epidemiological applications. *Toxicol Lett*. 1995;77(1–3):137–144.
13. Fang M, Boobis AR, Edwards RJ. Searching for novel biomarkers of centrally and peripherally acting neurotoxicants, using surface-enhanced laser desorption/ionization time-of-flight mass spectrometry (SELDI-TOF MS) *Food Chem Toxicol*. 2007;45:2126–2137.
14. Van Vliet E, Morath S, Eskes C, et al. A novel in vitro metabolomics approach for neurotoxicity testing, proof of principle for methyl chloride and caffeine. *Neurotoxicology*. 2008;29:1–12.
15. El-Fawal HAN, O'Callaghan JP. Autoantibodies to neurotypic and gliotypic proteins as biomarkers of neurotoxicity: assessment of trimethyltin (TMT) *Neurotoxicology*. 2008;29:109–115.

16. Slikker W, Bowyer JF. Biomarkers of adult and developmental neurotoxicity. *Toxicol Appl Pharmacol.* 2005;206:255–260.

17. Barone S Jr, Das KP, Lassiter TL, et al. Vulnerable processes of nervous system development: a review of markers and methods. *Neurotoxicology.* 2000;21(1–2):15–36.

18. Deng W, Poretz RD. Oligodendroglia in development and neurotoxicity. *Neurotoxicology.* 2003;24:161–178.

19. Gallo V, Ghiani CA. Glutamate receptors in glia: new cells, new inputs and new functions. *Trends Pharmacol Sci.* 2000;21:252–258.

20. Matute C, Alberdi E, Domercq M, et al. The link between excitotoxic oligodendroglial death and demyelinating diseases. *Trends Neurosci.* 2001;24:224–230.

21. Manzo L, Castoldi AF, Coccini T, et al. Assessing effects of neurotoxic pollutants by biochemical markers. *Environ Res Sect A.* 2001;85:31–36.

22. Henn BC, McMaster S, Padilla S. Measuring cholinesterase activity in human saliva. *J Toxicol Environ Health A.* 2006;69:1805–1818.

23. Manzo L, Castoldi AF, Coccini T, et al. Mechanisms of neurotoxicity: applications to human biomonitoring. *Toxicol Lett.* 1995;77:63–72.

24. Manzo L, Artigas F, Martinez M, et al. Biochemical markers of neurotoxicity: basic issues and a review of mechanistic studies. *Hum Exp Toxicol.* 1996;15 (Suppl 1):20–35.

25. Smargiassi A, Mutti A. Peripheral biomarkers and exposure to manganese. *Neurotoxicology.* 1999;20(2–3):401–406.

26. Castoldi AF, Coccini T, Rossi AD, et al. Biomarkers in environmental medicine: alterations of cell signaling as early indicators of neurotoxicity. *Funct Neurol.* 1994;9:101–109.

27. Costa LG. Biomarker research in neurotoxicology: the role of mechanistic studies to bridge the gap between the laboratory and epidemiological investigations. *Environ Health Perspect.* 1996;104 (Suppl 1):55–67.

28. Duman RS, Heninger GR, Nestler EJ. Molecular psychiatry: adaptations of receptor coupled signal transduction pathways underlying stress- and drug-induced neural plasticity. *J Nerv Ment Dis.* 1994;182:692–700.

29. Lotti M. The pathogenesis of organophosphate polyneuropathy. *Crit Rev Toxicol.* 1992;21:465–488.

30. Costa LG. Basic toxicology of pesticides. *Occup Med State Art Rev.* 1997;12:251–268.

31. Costa LG. Biochemical and molecular neurotoxicology: relevance to biomarker development, neurotoxicity testing and risk assessment. *Toxicol Lett.* 1998;102–103:417–421.

32. Slikker W Jr, Scallet AC, Gaylor DW. Biologically based dose–response model for neurotoxicity risk assessment. *Toxicol Lett.* 1998;102–103:429–433.

33. Scallet AC, Schmued LC, Johannessen JN. Neurohistochemical biomarkers of the marine neurotoxicant, domoic acid. *Neurotoxicol Teratol.* 2005;27:745–752.

34. Westerink RHS. Exocytose: using amperometry to study presynaptic mechanisms of neurotoxicity. *Neurotoxicology.* 2004;25:461–470.

35. Burgoyne RD, Morgan A. Secretory granule exocytosis. *Physiol Rev.* 2003;83:581–632.

36. Lotti M. Neurotoxicology: the Cinderella of neuroscience. *Neurotoxicology.* 1996;17(2):313–321.

37. Verity MA. Introduction: a coming of age for molecular neurotoxicology. *Brain Pathol.* 2002;12:472–474.

38. Lubec G, Krapfenbauer K, Fountoulakis M. Proteomics in brain research: potentials and limitations. *Prog Neurobiol.* 2003;69:193–211.

39. LoPachin RM, Jones RC, Patterson TA, et al. Application of proteomics to the study of molecular mechanisms in neurotoxicology. *Neurotoxicology.* 2003;24:761–775.

40. Ficarro SB, McCleveland ML, Stukenburg PT, et al. Phosphoproteome analysis by mass spectrometry and its application to *Saccharomyces cerevisiae. Nat Biotechnol.* 2002;20:301–305.

41. Goshe MB, Conrads TP, Panisko EA, et al. Phosphoprotein isotope-coded affinity tag approach for isolating and quantitating phosphopeptides in proteome-wide analysis. *Anal Chem.* 2001;73:2578–2586.

42. Harding JJ. Non-enzymatic covalent post-translational modification of proteins in vivo. In: Anfinsen CB, Edsall JT, Richards FM, eds. *Advances in Protein Chemistry.* New York, NY: Academic Press; 1985:247–334.

43. Hinson JA, Roberts DW. Role of covalent and non-covalent interactions in cell toxicity: effects on proteins. *Ann Rev Pharmacol Toxicol.* 1992;32:471–510.

44. Butterfield DA, Stadtman ER. Protein oxidation processes in aging brain. *Adv Cell Aging Gerontol.* 1997;2:161–191.

45. Butterfield DA, Drake J, Pocernich C, et al. Evidence of oxidative damage in Alzheimer's disease brain: central role for amyloid β-peptide. *Trends Mol Med.* 2001;7:548–554.

46. Castegna A, Aksenov M, Aksenov M, et al. Proteomic identification of oxidatively modified proteins in Alzheimer's disease brain: I. Creatine kinase BB, glutamine synthase and ubiquitin carboxy-terminal hydrolase L-1. *Free Rad Biol Med.* 2002;33:81–91.

47. Jenkins LW, Peters GW, Dixon CE, et al. Conventional and function proteomics using large format two dimensional gel electrophoresis 24 h after controlled cortical impact on postnatal day 17 rats. *J Neurotrauma.* 2002;19:715–740.

48. Gozal E, Gozal D, Pierce WM, et al. Proteomic analysis of the CA1 and CA3 regions of rat hippocampus and differential susceptibility to intermittent hypoxia. *J Neurochem.* 2002;83:331–345.

49. Fountoulakis M, Hardmaier R, Schuller E. Differences in protein level between neonatal and adult brain. *Electrophoresis.* 2000;21:673–678.

50. Gygi SP, Rist B, Gerber SA, et al. Quantitative analysis of complex protein mixtures using isotope-coded affinity tags. *J Neurochem.* 1999;17:994–999.

51. Vineis P, Bartsch H, Caporaso N, et al. Genetic based N-acetyltransferase metabolic polymorphism and low-level environmental exposure to carcinogens. *Nature.* 1994;369:154–156.

52. Millikan RC, Pittman GS, Newman B, et al. Cigarette smoking, N-acetyltransferases 1 and 2, and breast cancer risk. *Cancer Epidemiol Biomarkers Prev.* 1998;7(5):371–378.

53. Portier CJ, Bell DA. Genetic susceptibility: significance in risk assessment. *Toxicol Lett.* 1998;102–103:185–189.

54. Eaton DL. Biotransformation enzyme polymorphism and pesticide susceptibility. *Neurotoxicology.* 2000;21(1–2):101–111.

55. Furlong CE, Li WF, Richter RJ, et al. Genetic and temporal determinants of pesticide sensitivity: role of paraoxonase (PON1). *Neurotoxicology.* 2000;21(1–2):91–100.

56. Trosko JE, Chang CC, Upham B, et al. Epigenetic toxicology as toxicant-induced changes in intracellular signaling leading to altered gap junctional intercellular communication. *Toxicol Lett.* 1998;102–103:71–78.

57. Trosko JE. Challenge to the simple paradigm that "carcinogens" are "mutagens" and to the in vitro and in vivo assays used to test the paradigm. *Mutat Res.* 1997;373:245–249.

58. Martinez JD, Pennington ME, Craven MT, et al. Free radicals generated by ionizing radiation signals nuclear translocation of p53. *Cell Growth Diff.* 1997;8:941–949.

59. Maniatis T. Catalysis by a multiprotein IjB kinase complex. *Science.* 1997;278:818–819.

60. Vrana KE, Freeman WM, Aschner M. Use of microarray technologies in toxicology research. *Neurotoxicology.* 2003;24:321–332.

61. Barrett T, Xie T, Piao Y, et al. A murine dopamine neuron-specific cDNA library and microarray: increased COX1 expression during methamphetamine neurotoxicity. *Neurobiol Dis.* 2001;8:822–833.

62. Xie T, Tong L, Barrett T, et al. Changes in gene expression linked to methamphetamine-induced dopaminergic neurotoxicity. *J Neurosci.* 2002;22:274–283.

63. Silbergeld EK. Neurochemical approaches to developing biochemical markers of neurotoxicity: review of current status and evaluation of future prospects. *Environ Res.* 1993;63:274–286.

64. World Health Organization. IPCS Environmental Health Criteria 155. Biomarkers and Risk Assessment: Concepts and Principles. Geneva, Switzerland: WHO; 1993:57p.

CHAPTER 3

Approach to the Outpatient with Suspected Neurotoxic Exposure

Michael R. Dobbs

INTRODUCTION

Patients often claim that their symptoms may have been caused by an exposure, either recent or remote. Some more common claims include exposures to chemicals or metals at industrial jobs or during military service. Other allegations include accidental or intentional poisonings. Oftentimes, the patient is incorrect about the source of their problem. Many alleged cases of neurotoxic exposure turn out to be other illnesses, such as diabetic peripheral polyneuropathy, Parkinson's disease, or Alzheimer's disease. Conversion disorder and malingering may also sometimes explain the problem. Accurate diagnosis of a patient with a neurotoxic syndrome is usually difficult. However, it is important to not miss cases of true neurotoxicity. Many of these syndromes can be successfully treated, and even fully reversed, if caught early in the course.

LIMITS IN NEUROTOXICOLOGY

There are limits in diagnostic testing. For many potentially toxic exposures, the thresholds for developing symptoms are unknown and may vary among individuals. Many

tests, such as electromyography and electroencephalography, lack specificity for toxins. Some laboratory studies are not routinely available, such as whole-blood manganese, and patients must therefore be sent to highly specialized centers.

Several ongoing controversies in clinical neurotoxicology remain to be settled. Several well-characterized diseases have been demonstrated to have a remote and/or chronic toxic contributor in their pathogenesis. These include Alzheimer's dementia, Parkinson's disease, motor neuron disease, cryptogenic peripheral polyneuropathy, primary brain cancer, and some cases of epilepsy. Some of these exposures have been determined to cause a disorder in epidemiological studies, where specific dose and duration of offending agent are poorly understood (e.g., occupational manganese toxicity and parkinsonism).

In addition, many people believe several nosological entities are related to neurotoxins. For example, Gulf War syndrome has the symptom constellation of generalized fatigue, muscle and joint pain, headaches, loss of memory, and poor sleep. Veterans of the Gulf War were exposed to various potentially hazardous substances and conditions. These include pyridostigmine bromide pretreatment to mitigate nerve agent exposure, possible chemical weapons exposures, insecticides and repellants, depleted uranium, petroleum-based fuels, and various vaccines. While a systematic review of the problem did show that deployment to the Persian Gulf region was probably causal of the poorly defined Gulf War syndrome, the data were inadequate and conflicting in pinpointing a toxic cause.[1]

LEGAL ISSUES

In many cases of neurotoxic exposures, the victims feel unjustly harmed and there are questions of culpability. Patients who perceive that they have been injured by toxic exposures may believe they have a right to collect damages. Litigation may ensue. These legal points could obscure the picture.

Practitioners may be asked to testify or provide a deposition about toxic exposure on a patient's behalf or, alternatively, to document a claimant's lack of objective neurological dysfunction by the party being challenged. In the United States, unless subpoenaed, the choice of whether to participate is up to the practitioner. Keep in mind that unless a practitioner is well versed in clinical neurotoxicology, including the latest medical literature, an accurate picture may be elusive. The case may be wrongly skewed in one direction by such "expert" testimony. Also, as there are so many controversies in clinical neurotoxicology, expert witnesses risk being discredited with the potential for damage to their reputations. I advise caution.

ISSUES OF IMPAIRMENT AND DISABILITY

Impairment and disability are not interchangeable terms. A person may be impaired functionally but not disabled from doing his or her job. Disability is job dependent, and what may be disabling to one person may not be to another. As a clinical neurologist, if I lost my right index finger to an accident, although I would be impaired I could still probably swing a reflex hammer well enough to do my job. A surgeon, however, might well be disabled from performing surgery if he were to lose an index finger. Our impairments (the loss of a finger) would be equal, but our disabilities would be different.

Neurotoxins may cause impairments or disabilities to differing degrees depending on the toxin, exposure route, dose, treatment, and individual susceptibility. Most toxic exposures are dynamic processes. Impaired or disabled neurotoxic patients today may be back to normal at some time. Then again, they may not.

There is also often apprehension on returning to a place of exposure for fear that exposure may occur again. If exposure occurred at the workplace, this phobia could truly be disabling. In these cases, it is important not only to treat the patient's fears through appropriate medication and counseling but also to assure the patient that the risks of future exposures are reduced to the fullest possible extent by the patient's place of work.

OTHER PROFESSIONALS

There are medical and mental health professionals who claim to have special expertise in diagnosing and treating neurotoxic exposures. Many of them do. However, be cautious in referring your patients.

An incorrect diagnosis could lead to hardship and suffering in various ways. Patients incorrectly labeled with neurotoxic syndromes may try to seek legal compensation only to be disappointed when their weak case is thrown out of court. If an incorrect diagnosis proceeds to definitive treatment, many therapies for neurotoxic syndromes are not benign themselves, such as some chelating agents. Since clinical neurotoxicology is a burgeoning field of study with potentially high financial stakes in the legal arena, there is also a real risk of hucksterism.

INTENTIONAL POISONINGS

Cases of intentional neurotoxic poisonings throughout history are legion. Case reports are also scattered throughout the medical literature. Here are a few examples of neurotoxins used as poisons.

Thallium poisoning should be considered in any patient with a rapidly progressing peripheral neuropathy with or without alopecia.[2] Arsenic has been a popular poison in history, both in fictional media and in the real world. Ethylene glycol, found in automobile antifreeze, has been used to poison humans and animals. Cyanide-laced acetaminophen capsules were used to murder random consumers in the Chicago area in the 1980s, and cyanide has been used to intentionally poison many others in recent history.

CONSUMER ISSUES

In the United Kingdom in 2007, quantities of counterfeit toothpaste, labeled as a popular brand, were found to contain diethylene glycol in amounts that were reported as potentially toxic to individuals with impaired liver or kidney function. These items were being sold in market stalls and discount shops.[3]

Children may be especially vulnerable to exposures from consumer sources. As an isolated case, in Oregon in 2003, a 4-year-old boy surreptitiously ingested a small toy necklace he had acquired from a vending machine (Figure 3-1). After developing cryptic signs and symptoms, including a possible seizure, and visits to more than one physician, a blood lead level was found to be 123 µg/dL (the Centers for Disease Control and Prevention level of concern is more than 10 µg/dL). The necklace's contents were 38.8% lead (388,000 mg/kg), 3.6% antimony, and 0.5% tin. A national recall of the necklaces ensued. The child underwent successful chelation without further neurological problems.[4]

Chinese imports have been a hot-button topic in toxicology lately. The *Journal of the American Medical Association,* in June 2007, reported multiple episodes of potentially neurotoxic imported products from China. This included "monkfish" soup containing high levels of tetrodotoxin and oral care products containing diethylene glycol. Two people reportedly became ill from the tetrodotoxin-containing soup (probably puffer fish rather than monkfish), and the diethylene glycol–tainted products have been blamed for dozens of deaths in Panama.[5] Some children's toys from China continue to show unacceptably high levels of lead containing paint as of this writing. It is unknown how many children are at risk.

These are just a few examples. Many other neurotoxins have come into contact with unsuspecting consumers, including intentional cyanide poisoning and occasional unintentional outbreaks of botulism. It is more likely than not that additional neurotoxic compounds will be found in consumer goods.

Neurotoxins can come from unexpected, commonly trusted sources. If not caught early, irreversible damage or death may occur. Clinicians therefore must maintain not only a high index of suspicion but also a sound knowledge base for neurotoxic syndromes—both common and uncommon.

DIFFERENTIAL DIAGNOSIS

Differentiating neurotoxic disorders from those of other causes is probably the most challenging aspect of clinical neurotoxicology. As toxins can affect all spheres of the nervous system, there is a toxic mimic for nearly every neurological syndrome. Clinicians may find mnemonic devices (Table 1) helpful but ultimately clinical neurotoxicology requires a substantial knowledge base to approach the suspected intoxicated patient and achieve a diagnosis successfully. As in other disciplines, chance favors the prepared mind.

It is not enough to ascertain that a patient was in the area of a neurotoxic substance to diagnose a neurotoxic syndrome. Without knowledge of epidemiology for particular disorders, dose effect, and individual susceptibility factors, it is not reasonable to state that a neurotoxic cause for symptoms and signs is more than likely. The overriding principle for the diagnosis of a possible neurotoxic syndrome is establishing causation.

Sir Austin Bradford Hill's principles for distinguishing association from causation in epidemiological studies can also be applied to the neurotoxic patient as a guideline (Table 2).[6] However, testing is not available for various neurotoxic compounds, and laboratory criteria for normal levels are inconsistent. Temporality varies from toxin to toxin, with some not showing symptoms until years after exposure begins. Individuals vary in

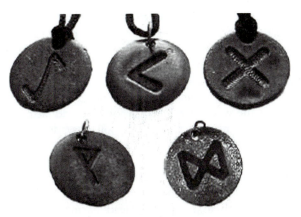

Figure 3-1. Medallions from recalled toy necklaces that were sold in vending machines in Oregon and linked to lead poisoning. (Oregon Department of Health Services.)

Table 1: "Vitamin D & E" Mnemonic Aid for Differential Diagnosis	
V	Vascular
I	Infectious
T	Toxic or traumatic
A	Autoimmune or amyloid
M	Metabolic
I	Inflammatory
N	Neoplastic
D	Degenerative
& E	Epileptic

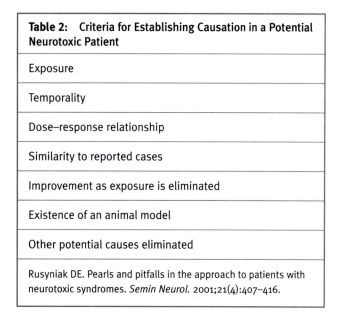

Table 2: Criteria for Establishing Causation in a Potential Neurotoxic Patient

Exposure
Temporality
Dose–response relationship
Similarity to reported cases
Improvement as exposure is eliminated
Existence of an animal model
Other potential causes eliminated
Rusyniak DE. Pearls and pitfalls in the approach to patients with neurotoxic syndromes. *Semin Neurol.* 2001;21(4):407–416.

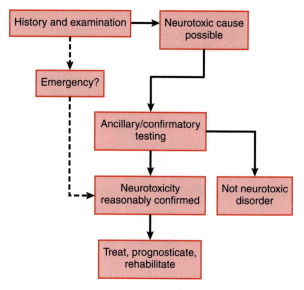

Figure 3-2. Algorithm for approach to neurotoxic disease. In an emergency situation, it is sometimes prudent to proceed to treatment without waiting for confirmatory testing if the potential benefit-to-risk ratio is high.

their susceptibility to neurotoxins, depending on genetics, protective equipment, and states of health. Clinical symptoms improve with elimination of exposure, but this is not true for all neurotoxins (methylmercury as an example). Many neurotoxic exposure syndromes are emerging entities without corresponding animal models, and case reports for clinical comparison may be sparse, contradictory, or nonexistent.

It is not uniformly possible to eliminate other causes. Cases of neurotoxicity may be complicated by other disease states that contribute to the overall clinical picture, such as mental disorders and underlying peripheral polyneuropathies from metabolic or systemic diseases.

Reading this may make you feel as if reliably diagnosing neurotoxic syndromes is a bleak prospect at best. It is not futile, however. With established, well-characterized neurotoxic syndromes, it may be fairly straightforward to determine causation. Although all criteria for causation might not be met with emerging or partially understood neurotoxic syndromes, it may well be possible to determine at least whether a toxic cause for a patient's problem is more (or less) than likely.

TAKING THE HISTORY

Perhaps nowhere in medicine is it more important, or sometimes more challenging, to obtain an accurate and complete patient history than in clinical neurotoxicology (Figure 3-2). Sometimes, however, it is simple. The patient will have a known exposure and either will have not developed symptoms or will have classical clinical symptoms of intoxication (see Case Study 1). At the other end of the spectrum are patients who cannot provide a history, such as the comatose patient, and those who have no idea that they have been exposed to something toxic (see Case Study 2). Most patients fall somewhere between these extremes.

Marshall et al. developed the CH2OPD2 mnemonic (community, home, hobbies, occupation, personal habits, diet, and drugs) as a tool to identify a patient's history of exposures to potentially toxic environmental contaminants.[7] You may find this useful when screening for potential neurotoxic exposures in your patients (Table 3).

Social History

All too often, practitioners gloss over social history, an important window into the patient's life. However, clinicians simply cannot afford to minimize the social history in cases of possible neurotoxic exposures, for many times therein lies the answer.

Work history is vital, because many toxic exposures occur in the workplace.[8] At-risk jobs include farmers or farmworkers (pesticides), painters (solvents), deep miners (raw ore such as manganese), and warehouse workers (carbon monoxide).

However, sometimes equally important is the patient's home environment. Houses built in prior eras may contain paint with toxic levels of lead or may have been framed with arsenic-treated wood. If a patient drinks water from a well, there is the potential for minerals to seep

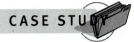

CASE STUDY

A 3-year-old swallowed a lead musket ball at day care (Figure 3-3). A radiograph revealed the ball retained in the stomach. The lead ball was removed by endoscopy without complication. A venous blood lead level approximately 48 hours postingestion was elevated (89 mg/dL). The child was treated with a course of succimer, and a repeat lead level 1 week after chelation was 5 mg/dL. The child never developed symptoms. (Courtesy of Christopher Holstege, MD.)

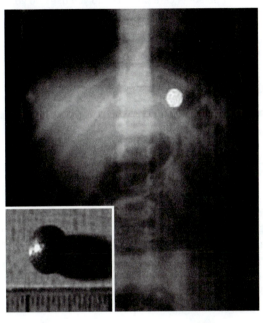

Figure 3-3. Radiograph of a 3-year-old child who swallowed a lead musket ball at day care. (Courtesy of Christopher Holstege, MD.)

CASE STUDY

A 67-year-old Pakistani man was visiting relatives in the United States. He spoke no English. He was found ataxic and confused after being left alone at home for a few hours. He was brought in for acute stroke. The on-call neurologist saw him. His examination showed truncal ataxia. The examiner thought he appeared to be intoxicated. However, he denied drinking (or other exposures). He was not dyspneic, but he was repeatedly puffing out breaths between his lips, which his family also found strange. Laboratory studies were normal except for high partial pressure of CO_2. A toxicological screen, including serum alcohols, was normal. Magnetic resonance imaging (MRI) of the brain was normal. He was admitted for close observation. Shortly thereafter, his son returned urgently to the bedside. He had changed the antifreeze in his car the day prior and placed the used coolant into empty soft drink bottles for storage. One bottle appeared to be missing some fluid. His father confirmed that he had drunk a "sweet drink" from a bottle in the garage while home alone that afternoon. He was treated with antidote urgently, and he made a full recovery, although he did experience transient kidney failure requiring dialysis.

in from groundwater. High inorganic arsenic levels have been found in wells around the world. Many people use reverse osmosis filters to reduce arsenic concentrations from private water sources. However, such filters do not guarantee safe drinking water, and despite regulatory standards, some people continue to be exposed to very high arsenic concentrations.[9]

Outside interests and hobbies are sometimes other sources for exposure. The recreational welder may be exposed to manganese, the antique firearms aficionado may encounter toxic amounts of lead while making bullets, and builders of models can be exposed to toluene or other solvents. There have also been many casual gardeners who have unintentionally become intoxicated from neurotoxic pesticides. Other people in the homes of these hobbyists may also be at risk of toxicity from these substances (see Case Study 1).

Travel history can be important, as many toxins are derived from restricted environments. Travelers may also venture into dangerous territories or try local cuisine or traditions to which they are unaccustomed. Travelers' naïve physiology may not be tolerant of exposure to toxins that locals have come to coexist with.

Special Information to Collect

Be sure to ask about the source of the putative exposure, the amount of toxic substance, the length of exposure time, the environmental conditions, and the route of contact. Be aware that the patient may have been exposed to other toxic compounds that complicate the issue at hand. Patients exposed to organic toxins in industry, for example, are rarely exposed to just a single potentially toxic chemical substance. In complicated cases, it may be necessary to obtain records of compounds used at the patient's place of exposure.

Table 3: The CH2OPD2 Mnemonic for Taking a Neurotoxic Exposure History

Code	Category	Example Questions
C	Community	Do you live near a hazardous waste site or industrial facilities?
H	Home	Is your home more than 30 years old? Have you done renovations? Do you use well water? Do you use pesticides?
H	Hobbies	What are your hobbies? Do you work with lead or solvents?
O	Occupation	What do you do? What is your workplace air quality? Do you work with any known toxic substances?
P	Personal habits	Do you or family members smoke? What sort of personal care products do you use? Do you drink alcohol? How much?
D	Diet	How often do you eat tuna or sportfish? Do you use any supplements? Do you eat any unusual foods or game?
D	Drugs	Are you taking any over-the-counter drugs or home remedies? Do you use any illicit drugs or substances?

Modified from Marshall L, Weir E, Abelsohn A, Sanborn MD. Identifying and managing adverse environmental health effects: I. Taking an exposure history. *CMAJ.* 2002;166(8):1049–1055.

CLINICAL EXAMINATION

General

A complete physical examination in a possible neurotoxic condition is especially important. Many signs of toxic exposure are seen in the skin, membranes, hair, and nails. For example, inorganic arsenic exposure may lead to the development of Mees' lines. Mees' lines are transverse white bands across the beds of the nails from arsenic deposits. Arsenic may additionally cause hyperpigmentation, hyperkeratosis, and exfoliative dermatitis. Elemental mercury can cause acrodynia, and thallium exposure leads to alopecia. Acute exposure to cyanide or carbon monoxide may result in reddening of the mucous membranes and skin from unused oxygen-rich arterial blood saturating the venous system.

The teeth and gums can provide important clues. Bluish discoloration of the gums may be seen in chronic lead exposure. Cadmium is reported to cause yellowing of teeth, as well as anosmia.

Neurotoxins may also cause cardiovascular complications. Heart dysfunction is seen with intoxication by arsenic, ergot, aconitine (monkshood), and others. High-dose acute arsenic exposure patients may have signs of acute cardiopulmonary collapse, such as associated hypotension, pulmonary edema, and heart failure. Ergot exposure may show diminished peripheral pulses from vasoconstriction.

Shortness of breath is a common sign of exposure to various substances and is not itself a helpful item for narrowing a differential diagnosis. However, it is prudent to keep in mind that the toxic patient who is having trouble breathing may quickly decompensate and needs urgent medical care.

Neurological

The standard, complete neurological examination should be performed in all suspected neurotoxic patients (Table 4). The table lists components of the neurological examination, as well as some representative toxins associated with abnormal examination findings. It should be clear that although vital in organizing the overall picture, most isolated examination findings are not diagnostic of specific intoxications.

Focal versus Diffuse Deficits

People who use sympathomimetic drugs such as cocaine or amphetamines often show focal deficits from brain ischemia, and victims of cadmium exposure may experience focal neurological deficits from brain hemorrhage. Diffuse neurological deficits are seen with many neurotoxins. A few include organic solvents, lead, arsenic, and botulinum toxin. Some toxins may show focal neurological deficits superimposed on a

Table 4: The Neurological Examination and Representative Toxins by System

System and Testing	Representative Toxins
MENTAL STATUS	Radiation, chemotherapies, toluene, methanol, ethanol, lead, mercury
LANGUAGE	
CRANIAL NERVES	
I (Olfactory)	
II (Optic)	
Pupils afferent Color vision Acuity Visual fields Funduscopy	Mercury, toluene, methanol, styrene, vigabatrin
III (Oculomotor)	
Pupils efferent	Botulinum toxin, organophosphates, opiates
III (Oculomotor), IV (Trochlear), and VI (Abducens)	
Eye movements	Botulinum toxin, tetrodotoxin, tick toxin, some arachnid and reptile venoms
V (Trigeminal)	
Sensory face and scalp (V1–V3)	Trichloroethylene
MOTOR MUSCLES OF MASTICATION	
VII (Facial)	
Motor facial expression Salivation and lacrimation Taste anterior 1/3 of tongue Corneal reflex efferent	Thallium, arsenic, botulinum toxin, buckthorn berry, barotrauma (environmental)
VIII (Vestibulocochlear)	
Vestibular testing Hearing	Lead, carbon monoxide, aspirin, quinine, macrolides
IX (Glossopharyngeal) and X (Vagus)	
Gag, palatal elevation	Tetanus and botulinum toxins; vomiting induced by many agents via cranial nerve X
XI (Accessory)	
Trapezius and sternocleidomastoid power	
XII (Hypoglossal)	
Motor-intrinsic tongue muscles	Tetanus and botulinum toxins

Continued

Table 4: The Neurological Examination and Representative Toxins by System—cont'd

System and Testing	Representative Toxins
MOTOR	
Drift Bulk and tone Muscular power Fisher's test	Lead (focal), thallium, organophosphates, buckthorn berry, lathyrus, botulinum toxin, tetrodotoxin, tick toxin, some arachnid and reptile venoms, tetanus toxin
REFLEXES	
Deep tendon reflexes Abdominal reflexes Plantar responses Hoffmann's responses Other sacral reflexes	Lathyrus, barbiturates, physostigmine, buckthorn berry, tetanus toxin
COORDINATION	
Finger-to-nose and heel-to-shin testing Rapid alternating movements	Ethylene glycol, ethanol, phenytoin, methylmercury
SENSORY	
Pinprick Light touch Vibration Proprioception Graphesthesia	Ethanol, arsenic, nitrous oxide
GAIT AND STATION	
Standing at rest Stand in tandem Walking normally Walking on heels, toes, and heel to toe	Manganese, ethanol, ethylene glycol, phenytoin
FRONTAL RELEASE SIGNS	
Glabellar Rooting Snout Palmomental Grasp	Carbon monoxide
TREMOR AND OTHER ABNORMAL MOVEMENTS	Carbon monoxide, manganese, mercury, caffeine, cocaine
AUTONOMIC	
Orthostatic testing Perspiration level Salivation/lacrimation	Organophosphates, muscarine (mushrooms), tetanus toxin
MALINGERING AND CONVERSION TESTING	Pseudotoxicity

generalized encephalopathy. Manganese and carbon monoxide, as examples, may exhibit focal parkinsonism from basal ganglia damage while showing general cerebral or psychiatric symptoms.

Mental Status

Myriad toxins cause mental status abnormalities. These can range from severe encephalopathy to simply mild complaints of memory loss or slowed thinking. In the office setting, chronic encephalopathic states on the milder side of the spectrum are probably more likely to be encountered.

Virtually all classes of neurotoxins can have encephalopathic effects. A few representative classic syndromes are acute neuromanganism, chronic lead encephalopathy in children or adults, encephalopathy seen in survivors of carbon monoxide exposure, Korsakoff's syndrome in long-term alcoholics, and dementia in those whose brains have been exposed to significant amounts of radiation.

There are also those patients who have complaints of cognitive dysfunction but in whom routine mental status testing in the office does not show abnormalities. In these cases, if an exposure is plausible, it may be reasonable to go ahead and order specialized cognitive testing.

Language

Language deficits are not typically found in isolation in neurotoxic syndromes. If aphasia is present, it may suggest localization to a particular region of the brain. Dysarthria may be seen in cases of toxicity affecting the brainstem or cranial nerves.

Cranial Nerves

Cranial Nerve I

Hundreds of substances have been implicated in causing or contributing to disorders of smell (and taste). Importantly, loss of sense of smell (anosmia) for whatever reason may increase risk of toxic exposure, since many toxins have characteristic or noxious odors.

Cranial Nerve II

The visual system can be affected by various toxins and potentially at all levels.

Gobba and others have described loss of color vision as an early indicator of neurotoxic damage from several substances, including mercury, toluene, and styrene (Table 5).[10] Typically, there seems to be blue–yellow discrimination loss or, less often, combined blue–yellow and red–green loss. This is in contrast to other neurological diseases such as multiple sclerosis, where

Table 5: Some Toxins Causing Color Vision Loss
SIGNIFICANT INDUSTRIAL SOLVENTS
Styrene
Perchlorethylene
Toluene
Carbon disulfide
n-Hexane
Solvent mixtures
SIGNIFICANT INDUSTRIAL METALS AND OTHER CHEMICALS
Mercury
Organophosphates
2-*t*-Butylazo-2-hydroxy-5-methylxane
Modified from Gobba F, Cavalleri A. Color vision impairment in workers exposed to neurotoxic chemicals. *Neurotoxicology.* 2003;24(4–5):693–702. Review.

red desaturation is most common. The eyes may be unequally involved, and the course is variable.[10–15] The localization of toxic color vision loss in otherwise apparently healthy eyes remains elusive, and damage anywhere from the retina to color vision areas of the visual cortex has been postulated. Color vision loss may be a fairly common effect of exposure to organic neurotoxins. It is advisable to examine for loss of color vision in all toxic exposure cases.

Other substances are implicated in toxic disorders of vision. The effective antiepileptic medication, vigabatrin, was shown by Frisén and Malmgren to cause irreversible diffuse atrophy of the retinal nerve fiber layer in a retrospective study of 25 patients.[16] Vigabatrin has its greatest effect on the peripheral retina leading to constricted visual fields. Vigabatrin can also cause blue–yellow colorblindness.

Many substances can cause toxic optic neuropathy. Refer to Chapter 9 for details.

Botulism tends to preferentially affect muscles of the cranial nerves, and a hallmark is pupillary dilation (unresponsive to light) secondary to paralysis of the ciliary muscle. Atropine and other anticholinergic agents can also cause pupillary dilation. Pupillary miosis is characteristic of the cholinergic state of organophosphate intoxication and is commonly seen in opiate overdose.

Cranial Nerves III, IV, and VI

Botulism commonly causes ophthalmoplegia, but so do many other biological toxins. A few include tetrodotoxin, tick paralysis neurotoxin, and certain arachnid and reptile venoms.

Cranial Nerve V

The classic clinical syndrome of exposure to trichloroethylene is bilateral trigeminal sensory neuropathy.

Cranial Nerve VII

Inner ear barotrauma can sometimes affect a facial nerve, causing unilateral facial nerve weakness. Bilateral facial nerve paralysis may be seen in intoxications with thallium, arsenic, botulinum toxin, and buckthorn berry ingestion. Bifacial paralysis is not a specific sign of any toxin but instead reflects systemic dysfunction.

Cranial Nerve VIII

Toxins affecting the eighth cranial nerve are numerous. These include quinine, chloroform, chemotherapeutic agents, macrolide antibiotics, aspirin, lead, barbiturates, and carbon monoxide.

Cranial Nerves IX and X

Palatal elevation and the gag reflex are controlled by cranial nerves IX and X. Botulinum toxin can impair gag. The "spatula test" showing hyperactive gag can be useful in clinically confirming tetanus.

The vagus nerve (cranial nerve X) and nucleus or tractus solitarius are important mediators of nausea and emesis in response to toxic substances in the gut. Chemoreceptors and mechanoreceptors in the stomach and small intestine probably respond to toxins and irritants and communicate via vagal afferents with the nucleus solitarius, meeting with fibers from the area postrema, inducing retching. Clinically relevant toxins such as radiation and cancer chemotherapeutic agents have been found to provoke vomiting through stimulation of serotonin (5-HT$_3$) receptors in the digestive tract.[17,18] There is also evidence of a role in emesis for substance P and its receptor (neurokinin, or NK-1) in the brainstem.[19] The neural emetic mechanism serves a protective function in cases of toxic ingestion.

Cranial Nerve XI

Weakness of the sternocleidomastoid and trapezius muscles is typically nonspecific. It can be seen with toxins that affect the motor neurons or neuromuscular junction.

Cranial Nerve XII

Botulinum toxin can cause weakness of the intrinsic tongue muscles innervated by the hypoglossal nerve. This would typically be bilateral. Tetanus toxin can cause tongue spasms that interfere with swallowing.

Nystagmus

Toxic nystagmus is usually coarse, rhythmic, horizontal, and worsened with lateral gaze. Many toxic compounds can cause nystagmus. These include barbiturates, lead, quinine, and alcohol. Phenytoin intoxication may manifest with nystagmus as the earliest sign. Barbiturates, paradoxically, can also inhibit or alter nystagmus. Wernicke's syndrome related to alcoholism or malnutrition may present with nystagmus alone (or in combination with ophthalmoplegia, mental status changes, and ataxia).

Occupational nystagmus is an uncommon occupational hazard of people who work in low light (such as deep miners) or at close vision occupations (jewelers, artists, etc.). This nystagmus is typically pendular but may be rotary. It usually develops after many years of eyestrain. There may be associated blepharospasm, as well as tremor, vertigo, and photophobia.

Motor System

Acute muscular weakness with twitching and fasciculations is characteristic of cholinergic overload, as is seen in organophosphate intoxication.

Focal motor neuropathy is commonly seen in adult lead overexposure. This palsy is classically of the radial nerve and causes wrist drop, although other motor nerves can be affected.

Fine, rapid tremors are seen in many toxic states, including alcohol, lead, mercury, and various drug compounds (caffeine, bromides, barbiturates, cocaine, amphetamine, ephedrine). A coarser resting tremor (2 to 6 Hz), similar to that seen in Parkinson's disease, may be present in states following carbon monoxide or manganese exposure.

Myoclonus is not common in toxic states. It has often been reported after ingestion of Sugihiratake mushrooms. However, most of these cases had preexisting nephropathy.[20] Sugihiratake mushroom–intoxicated patients may also demonstrate other neurological conditions such as encephalopathy and status epilepticus. Other substances reported to cause myoclonus include lithium, pseudoephedrine, tricyclic antidepressants, bismuth subsalicylate, carbamazepine, aniline oils, methyl bromide, strychnine, chloralose, and lead. It is worth noting that myoclonus in many cases of toxicity results from metabolic derangement rather than the toxin itself and that myoclonus is rarely the sole neurological symptom or sign present in intoxication.

Reflexes

A detailed reflex examination is important to help exclude peripheral neuropathic processes. Typically, the deep tendon reflexes are diminished in a glove-and-stocking pattern in toxic peripheral polyneuropathies. A patient may be completely areflexic in cases of toxicity from buckthorn (coyotillo) berry ingestion, which can mimic Guillain-Barré syndrome, as well as in severe intoxication with arsenic.

The Babinski (plantar) response has been reported in normal individuals intoxicated with scopolamine or barbiturates. Physostigmine and similar compounds may abolish the Babinski response.

Sensory

Sensory systems should be assessed in a comprehensive manner. Many toxins cause sensory neuropathy (see Chapter 14). Nitrous oxide affects the posterior columns of the spinal cord preferentially, leading to deficits in position and vibratory sensation. Patients with nitrous oxide poisoning could demonstrate a spinal sensory level in severe cases.

Coordination

Coordination abnormalities are largely nonspecific and are seen with intoxication from various substances. The alcohols are especially common toxins causing coordination deficits. Phenytoin also characteristically affects coordination.

Gait and Station

Besides intoxication with ethanol, manganese intoxication is perhaps the most classic example of a substance producing a toxic gait abnormality. The "cock-walk gait" of neuromanganism manifests as a gait with plantar flexion and flexion of the elbows. Manganese also produces features of parkinsonism.

Tests for Malingering or Conversion

Clinical tests such as Hoover sign, sensory testing for "splitting the midline," and others are useful if embellishment is suspected. Although these findings may be seen in malingering or conversion pseudotoxic states, positive tests for embellishment do not necessarily mean that the patient is not intoxicated.

Specialized Cognitive Testing

When assessing for subtle cognitive abnormalities in a patient, there is no substitute for dedicated psychometric testing administered and interpreted by a skilled neuropsychologist. Care should be taken to ensure that the choice of tests is such that they can be repeated over time to assess for clinical worsening or improvement. These tests may help quantify the degree of deficit so that adaptive strategies can be made. This is especially important in cases where patients depend on their mind for their livelihood (see Case Study 3).

CONFIRMATORY TESTS

Many testing resources are available to the neurotoxicologist, the utility of which may vary from situation to situation. Blood level tests are available, accurate, and standardized for many toxins, such as certain of the heavy metals, alcohols, and drugs of abuse. Urine testing is also available. It becomes, for many, a challenging question of when to use blood testing versus urine testing. Hair or fingernail testing is useful to document exposure for some toxins, such as arsenic. In addition, useful ancillary tests may help guide diagnosis and treatment in several neurotoxic exposures. Consider the example of lead.

If lead poisoning is suspected, a whole-blood lead level confirms the diagnosis. A blood level greater than

CASE STUDY

A 20-year-old woman who was an excellent premedical student had completed chemotherapy for lymphoma and her disease was in remission. A few weeks after chemotherapy was completed, her grades had started to decline. She was noticing trouble concentrating in classes, and the quality of her note taking had suffered. A screen for depression was normal, as was a rudimentary mental status testing in the office. The remainder of her neurological examination was unremarkable. MRI of the brain was normal. Neuropsychometric testing revealed relative inefficiency on tasks of processing speed, auditory attention, divided attention, sentence repetition, sustained attention, naming, and verbal fluency superimposed on superior intellectual abilities. No global intellectual decline was evident. She was counseled that her problem was likely to be a temporary encephalopathy from chemotherapy. Special arrangements were made to allow her extra time to complete tests in her classes, and she adopted a mildly lighter course schedule. She continued to have significant concentration problems, and she was started on methylphenidate. Her grades improved back to baseline. A few months later, she was able to discontinue methylphenidate and did fine academically with a full course load.

10 μg/dL is cause for concern, but like many neurotoxins, actual levels for toxicity are not known and may vary. It is noteworthy that in adults 20 μg/dL is the threshold for neurotoxicity, and encephalopathy is usually not seen until levels of 100 μg/dL are reached. Testing a hemogram may show a microcytic hypochromic anemia. Chemistry profiles may reveal uric acid derangements or other abnormalities. Uric acid is usually low in lead-poisoned children, while it is high in lead-poisoned adults. Historically, it is believed that much of the ancient Roman aristocracy suffered from gout due to lead exposure. Lead may also cause liver or kidney damage. Radiographs of the abdomen may show lead foreign bodies. Radiographs of long bones may show characteristic findings of lead poisoning. A computerized tomography scan or MRI scan of the brain may be useful to look for cerebral edema in cases of acute intoxication with encephalopathy. During treatment of lead poisoning with chelation therapy, urine levels to monitor excretion followed by repeat blood levels to assess for recurrence are useful.

Laboratory Testing

It can be exceptionally difficult to decide on methods of confirmatory testing in neurotoxic cases. Unfortunately, a simple whole-blood or serum level is not always reflective of the amount of toxin in someone's body. Some toxins, particularly certain metals in the chronic state, can accumulate in body structures such as bone or nervous tissue, leading to a falsely low serum or urine level. Many organic toxins have no reliable confirmatory tests. For details on choosing laboratory tests, see Chapter 17.

Blood and Serum

Blood testing is probably useful in intoxications due to thallium, ethanol, methanol, ethylene glycol, certain anticonvulsants, and other medications. Whole-blood-level testing is useful for cyanide, manganese, mercury, and lead. Arsenic may be underestimated in blood or serum testing and should be used only for acute exposure. Elevated carboxyhemoglobin indicates exposure to carbon monoxide, with a level greater than 10% likely being toxic.

Surrogate blood tests are available for organophosphate insecticide intoxication—red blood cell cholinesterase and serum pseudocholinesterase—but these tests are not commonly available quickly in an emergency setting. Testing for red blood cell cholinesterase or serum pseudocholinesterase is therefore not useful for acute organophosphate poisonings but is worthwhile to document and follow in cases of chronic exposure.

Because blood and serum testing for many toxins is not well standardized, it is prudent to become familiar with the ranges and limits for abnormal values in your patient population. Your local clinical laboratory supervisor and poison control center may be able to help.

Urine

In general, a 24-hour urine collection is preferred over a random sample. Some toxins are released in a diurnal pattern, and collection over 24 hours maximizes the likelihood of a positive study. Urine testing is the preferred test for arsenic intoxication. Urine drug screens may be useful for establishing recent ingestion of illicit substances. See specific chapters for details.

Hair

Several laboratories offer hair analysis for traces of minerals and other toxins. It is used by health-care providers and promoted by laboratories as a clinical tool to identify toxic exposures. The validity of these tests is questionable, and reproducibility of similar values among laboratories has been questioned by multiple scientific studies.[21,22] If a clinician uses hair analysis as a clinical assessment tool, extreme caution is advised.

Neurophysiological

Only in rare instances will a neurophysiology study such as electroencephalography or electromyography definitively diagnose a neurointoxication. Such studies' sensitivity far outweighs their specificity. For example, many intoxications show diffuse, generalized slowing suggestive of encephalopathy on the electroencephalogram. This does not suggest a particular toxic exposure; it merely provides objective evidence of encephalopathy in the intoxicated patient. It is also vital to remember that the absence of any abnormality on appropriately ordered neurophysiological tests argues against an organic, toxic cause for the patient's symptoms. The utility of neurophysiological testing in the practice of clinical neurotoxicology is largely that of an ancillary role, albeit an important one.

Imaging

Normal computerized tomography or MRI scanning of the central nervous system does not rule out a toxic central nervous system disorder. On the other hand, certain neurotoxic syndromes are recognized largely because of characteristic findings on neuroimaging. As an illustration, manganese can deposit in the basal ganglia, showing as hyperintense regions on T_1-weighted imaging.

CONCLUSION

After reasonable diagnostic procedures are completed, the clinician must establish a probability that the patient's disorder is due to exposure to a neurotoxin. Then the clinician should treat as indicated. Often, it is difficult to establish neurotoxicity with certainty because of a lack of biomarkers for most toxins. However, when reasonably established, it is obligatory to inform the appropriate authorities of the nature and source of exposure so that others can be protected. As clinical neurotoxicologists, we should continue to follow the patient throughout the course of the illness. If additional signs or symptoms develop over time that point to another cause, then we should be ready to backtrack and consider other possible etiologies for the patient's problem.

REFERENCES

1. Gronseth GS. Gulf war syndrome: a toxic exposure? A systematic review. *Neurol Clin.* 2005;23(2):523–540.
2. Rusyniak DE, Furbee RB, Kirk MA. Thallium and arsenic poisoning in a small midwestern town. *Ann Emerg Med.* 2002;39(3):307–311.
3. Fake toothpaste found. *Br Dent J.* 2007;203(2):68.
4. Centers for Disease Control and Preventions. Lead poisoning from ingestion of a toy necklace: Oregon, 2003. *MMWR.* 2004;53(23):509–511.
5. Hampton T. Deadly fish, tainted toothpaste spur scrutiny of products from China. *JAMA.* 2007;297(23):2577.
6. Rusyniak DE. Pearls and pitfalls in the approach to patients with neurotoxic syndromes. *Semin Neurol.* 2001;21(4):407–416.
7. Marshall L, Weir E, Abelsohn A, Sanborn MD. Identifying and managing adverse environmental health effects: I. Taking an exposure history. *CMAJ.* 2002;166(8):1049–1055.
8. National Institute for Occupational Safety and Health. National Occupational Hazard Survey, 1972–74. DHEW Publication No. (NIOSH) 78-114. Cincinnati, Ohio: NIOSH; 1977.
9. George CM, Smith AH, Kalman DA, Steinmaus CM. Reverse osmosis filter use and high arsenic levels in private well water. *Arch Environ Occup Health.* 2006;61(4):171–175.
10. Gobba F, Cavalleri A. Color vision impairment in workers exposed to neurotoxic chemicals. *Neurotoxicology.* 2003;24(4–5):693–702. Review.
11. Urban P, Gobba F, Nerudová J, Lukás E, Cábelková Z, Cikrt M. Color discrimination impairment in workers exposed to mercury vapor. *Neurotoxicology.* 2003;24(4–5):711–716.
12. Gobba F, Cavalleri A. Evolution of color vision loss induced by occupational exposure to chemicals. *Neurotoxicology.* 2000;21(5):777–781.
13. Cavalleri A, Gobba F, Nicali E, Fiocchi V. Dose-related color vision impairment in toluene-exposed workers. *Arch Environ Health.* 2000;55(6):399–404.
14. Gobba F, Righi E, Fantuzzi G, Predieri G, Cavazzuti L, Aggazzotti G. Two-year evolution of perchloroethylene-induced color-vision loss. *Arch Environ Health.* 1998;53(3):196–198.
15. Campagna D, Gobba F, Mergler D, et al. Color vision loss among styrene-exposed workers neurotoxicological threshold assessment. *Neurotoxicology.* 1996;17(2):367–373.
16. Frisén L, Malmgren K (2003). Characterization of vigabatrin-associated optic atrophy. *Acta Ophthalmol Scand.* 81(5):466–473.
17. Lang IM. Noxious stimulation of emesis. *Dig Dis Sci.* 1999;44"(8 Suppl):58S–63S.
18. Carpenter DO. Neural mechanisms of emesis. *Can J Physiol Pharmacol.* 1990;68(2):230–236.
19. Saito R, Takano Y, Kamiya HO. Roles of substance P and NK(1) receptor in the brainstem in the development of emesis. *J Pharmacol Sci.* 2003;91(2):87–94.
20. Nishizawa M. Acute encephalopathy after ingestion of "Sugihi-ratake" mushroom. *Rinsho Shinkeigaku.* 2005;45(11):818–820.
21. Seidel S, Kreutzer R, Smith D, McNeel S, Gilliss D. Assessment of commercial laboratories performing hair mineral analysis. *JAMA.* 2001;285(1):67–72.
22. Shamberger RJ. Validity of hair mineral testing. *Biol Trace Elem Res.* 2002;87(1–3):1–28.

CHAPTER 4

Toxin-Induced Neurologic Emergencies

David Lawrence, Nancy McLinskey, J. Stephen Huff, and Christopher P. Holstege

INTRODUCTION

Exposure to toxins may cause several common neurological emergencies, including toxin-induced seizures, acute change in mental status, and muscle weakness (see also specific chapters for these problems in the Neurotoxic Syndromes section of this book). When a patient presents with a known or suspected poisoning, knowledge of the potential complications associated with that toxin or toxins will enable the health-care team to clearly manage those poisoned patients. This chapter reviews commonly encountered neurologic emergencies associated with poisonings and reviews the appropriate initial management of the poisoned patient.

GENERAL MANAGEMENT

When evaluating a patient who has presented with a potential toxicological emergency it is important not to limit the differential diagnosis. A comatose patient who smells of alcohol may be harboring an intracranial hemorrhage, while an agitated patient who appears anticholinergic may actually be encephalopathic from an infectious etiology. Patients must be thoroughly assessed and appropriately stabilized. It is vital not to miss easily treatable conditions. For example, hypoglycemia may appear to mimic many toxin-induced neurologic abnormalities, including delirium, coma, seizure, or even focal neurological deficits.[1,2] Patients with altered mental status should receive rapid determination and, if necessary, correction of serum glucose levels. There is often no specific antidote or treatment for a poisoned patient, and careful supportive care may be the most important intervention.

In any medical emergency, the first priority is to assure that the airway is patent and that the patient is ventilating adequately. If necessary, endotracheal tube intubation should be performed. Physicians are often lulled into a false sense of security when a patient's oxygen saturations are adequate on high-flow oxygen. However, if the patient has either inadequate ventilation or impairment of protective airway reflexes, then the patient may be at risk for subsequent CO_2 narcosis with worsening acidosis or aspiration. If clinical judgment suggests that a patient will not be able to protect the airway, endotracheal intubation should be considered.

The patient's cardiovascular status should be assessed. A large-bore peripheral intravenous line should be considered in all poisoned patients. A second line placed in either the peripheral or the central venous system may be required if the patient is symptomatic. The initial treatment of hypotension consists of intravenous fluids. Close monitoring of the patient's pulmonary status should be performed to assure that pulmonary edema does not develop as fluids are infused. Patients are recommended to be placed on continuous cardiac monitoring. An initial electrocardiogram (ECG) may serve several purposes. For one, it can help identify the class of toxin involved and identify the risk for future complications. For example, a prolonged QT interval suggests the presence of a toxin that blocks myocardial potassium efflux channels (i.e., phenothiazines, venlafaxine), and the QT prolongation may result in the patient suddenly progressing to torsades de pointes. The ECG can also guide early treatment, such as the need to initiate sodium bicarbonate therapy in a patient with a prolonged QRS interval to prevent arrhythmias, improve hypotension, or both.[3]

A combative intoxicated patient must be sedated in a safe and efficient manner to expedite the evaluation and protect the patient and staff members. Benzodiazepines are the preferred initial agent for sedation because of relative safety and lack of significant interactions with other medications.

A key vital sign sometimes overlooked in the management of the poisoned patient is the temperature. A core temperature (either rectal or Foley catheter) should be obtained and aggressive cooling measures should be initiated for markedly hyperthermic patients.[4] A safe and efficient method of cooling is evaporative cooling using water misting and large fans. Active cooling should be continued until the patient's core temperature is 39°C. Cooling below this point is discouraged as it may lead to overshoot hypothermia.[5,6]

Health-care providers have a low threshold to consider carbon monoxide (CO) exposure in the patient presenting with altered mental status. CO is a relatively common, potentially deadly, and easily missed poisoning. Patients can be exposed in multiple ways. Incomplete combustion of carbonaceous fuel produces CO, and machines using these fuels in poorly ventilated spaces can cause dangerous concentrations to accumulate.[7] Individuals may also intentionally expose themselves to CO as a method of suicide. CO poisoning may present with multiple vague and nonspecific findings. Initial symptoms include headache, dizziness, nausea, and confusion. As exposure increases, progression to altered mental status, syncope, seizures, coma, and cardiac disturbances may occur.[7] Seizure activity may be the initial presentation of CO poisoning in children; therefore, this should be considered in the differential diagnosis of a pediatric patient with a first-time seizure.[8] Standard oxygen saturation monitors will not detect the presence of CO. The diagnosis is confirmed by testing either venous or arterial blood for carboxyhemoglobin. A normal baseline level in a nonsmoker is 1% to 3%. There are several pitfalls to be considered when interpreting a carboxyhemoglobin level. The level is useful to confirm CO exposure but correlates poorly with clinical effects. Smokers and those recently exposed to automobile exhaust may have elevated levels as high as 10%.[7] Perhaps the most important reason to diagnose CO poisoning is to avoid further exposure. Patients returning to a home, place of business, or vehicle with elevated CO levels may suffer devastating consequences.

A number of common but readily preventable complications are encountered in the poisoned patient. For example, aspiration pneumonia can occur in the overdose patients,[9,10] and can significantly increase morbidity and mortality. Aspiration can result when an obtunded patient cannot adequately protect the airway. Endotracheal intubation does not completely protect a patient from aspiration but may aid in preventing this complication. Poisoned patients are also at risk for rhabdomyolysis[11] because of profound sedation or direct myotoxic effects. Levels of creatinine phosphokinase, myoglobin, or both should be performed in obtunded or markedly agitated patients. It should be noted that a delayed rise in creatinine phosphokinase may occur after hydration. Early identification and treatment with aggressive hydration are the keys to minimizing renal damage due to rhabdomyolysis.

Gastrointestinal decontamination must also be considered in patients presenting with acute toxic ingestions. The most important consideration before gastrointestinal decontamination is to assure a well-protected airway, either by the patient's intact defenses or by endotracheal intubation. Several methods are available to attempt gastrointestinal decontamination. Inducing emesis with syrup of ipecac is no longer recommended.[12] Gastric lavage is rarely indicated due to significant associated risks and the lack of evidence that it improves outcomes[13]; it should only be considered in carefully selected cases. Activated charcoal is an effective agent for reducing the absorption of many poisons and is a reasonable therapy for patients in whom serious toxicity can be anticipated.[14] It is most effective within an hour and has decreasing efficacy over time with most regular-release products. Administration of activated charcoal to a patient who has or is at risk for developing diminished protective airway reflexes may predispose the patient to aspiration. Although endotracheal intubation does not eliminate the risk of aspirating charcoal, it has been shown to be effective in minimizing the risk of significant aspiration pneumonia.[10,15] Whole-bowel irrigation is performed by administering large volumes (100–200 ml/hr in adults) of polyethylene glycol–electrolyte solution either by mouth or by nasogastric tube. This can be considered in patients with large overdoses of poisons, particularly sustained release products, products not bound by activated charcoal (lithium and iron), and body packers (persons who transports illicit drugs by internal concealment) or stuffers (persons who hastily ingest illicit drugs to avoid detection).[16]

Once the poisoned patient has been adequately stabilized, it is then appropriate to begin the process of toxin identification and treatment. Oftentimes, history from the patient, a family member, or a bystander is the most important step in this process. However, the history often is incomplete or unreliable and a thorough physical exam and focused laboratory analysis provides an opportunity to discover the toxin involved.

TOXICOLOGY-DIRECTED PHYSICAL EXAM

In the known or suspected poisoned patient, note all vital signs, including blood pressure, heart rate, respiratory rate and effort, and temperature. The skin must be examined for diaphoresis, dryness, piloerection, and any sign of skin breakdown. As previously mentioned, a cardiovascular and respiratory exam should be performed. The presence or absence of bowel sounds should be determined. A neurological exam should make special note of the presence or absence of clonus, hyperreflexia, or rigidity. The level of consciousness and or responsiveness should be determined. Examine the eyes, noting pupil size, pupil reactivity, and the presence or absence of nystagmus. Several aspects of the physical exam are especially important when evaluating a poisoned patient and may reveal a particular toxidrome.

The neurologic examination may be quite helpful but may be misleading. In general, physical examination signs are symmetric in toxidromes; asymmetry of physical findings (pupillary asymmetry, hemiparesis) suggests structural etiologies of altered mental status. However, if the patient is profoundly unresponsive, absence of physical examination signs does not allow a determination of structural versus metabolic or toxicologic coma. For example, an unresponsive patient, flaccid, with no spontaneous muscle movement and nonreactive pupils may have barbiturate or other overdose or have a structural cause of coma. In addition, truly pinpoint pupils (the size the point of a pin makes when touched to paper) suggest severe pontine damage, but the pupils in the narcotic toxidrome are small but not pinpoint. Abnormal posturing may occur at times with toxic syndromes, and drug-induced dystonias and dyskinesia may simulate seizures. Extraocular eye movements may be lost in some toxic overdoses, such as tricyclic antidepressants (TCAs) and carbamezepine; thus, a comatose patient with these overdoses may not have oculocephalic or oculovestibular reflexes.

TOXIDROMES

Toxidromes are toxic syndromes or the constellation of signs and symptoms associated with a class of poisons. Rapid recognition of a toxidrome, if present, can help determine whether a specific poison or class of toxin is involved. Table 1 lists selected toxidromes and their characteristics. It is important to note that patients may not present with all components of a toxidrome and that mixed ingestions may cloud the classic characteristics.

Specific aspects of a toxidrome may have great significance when evaluating a patient. For example, noting the presence of dry axilla in a markedly agitated patient may be the only way of differentiating an anticholinergic patient from a sympathomimetic patient. Similarly, miosis may be the only sign distinguishing opioid toxicity from a benzodiazepine overdose.

Not all drugs fit completely in these drug classes. For example, meperidine and tramadol, despite their classification as opioids, do not cause miosis. Also, medications in the phenothiazine class can cause significant anticholinergic toxicity, but because of concurrent $\alpha 1$-antagonism, miosis occurs.

Although in most cases a toxidrome will not indicate a specific poison, recognition is important for several reasons. Identification of the class of toxin can aid in directing therapeutic actions, as well as narrowing the differential diagnosis. This can be especially useful when a patient has access to multiple potential poisons.

DIAGNOSTIC TESTING

The use of diagnostic testing should be carefully considered when managing the acutely poisoned. Certain tests can offer valuable information. However, many commonly ordered tests do not aid in the acute management of poisoned patients.

Urine drug screens should not be ordered on a routine basis due to the possibility of misleading information.[17–19] The potential for false positives and false negatives[20] often confuse the picture. Most assays rely on the antibody identification of drug metabolites, which can remain positive days after use and thus may not be related to the patient's current clinical picture. The positive identification of drug metabolites is likewise influenced by chronicity of ingestion, fat solubility, and co-ingestions. In one such example, Perrone et al.[21] showed a cocaine retention time of 72 hours following its use. Conversely, many drugs of abuse are not detected on most urine drug screens, including γ-hydroxybutyric acid (GHB), fentanyl, and ketamine. For these reasons, routine drug screening of those with altered mental status, abnormal

Table 1: Selected Toxidromes

Toxidrome	Signs and Symptoms	Examples of Potential Agents
Opioid	Sedation, miosis, decreased bowel sounds, decreased respirations	Heroin, methadone, morphine, oxycodone, fentanyl, clonidine
Anticholinergic	Mydriasis, dry skin, dry mucous membranes, tachycardia, decreased bowel sounds, altered mental status, hallucinations, urinary retention	Antihistamines, cyclic antidepressants, jimsonweed, cyclobenzaprine, scopolamine, atropine
Sedative–hypnotic	Sedation, decreased respirations, normal pupils, normal vital signs	Benzodiazepines, barbiturates, ethanol
Sympathomimetic	Agitation, mydriasis, tachycardia, hypertension, hyperthermia, diaphoresis, normal bowel sounds	Ampheta mines, cocaine, phencyclidine, ephedrine, methylphenidate
Cholinergic	Miosis, increased secretions, bronchorrhea, bronchospasm, vomiting, diarrhea, bradycardia	Organophosphates, carbamates

vital signs, or suspected ingestion is not warranted and rarely guides patient treatment or disposition.

Certain tests are vital to the evaluation of a poisoned patient. An ECG should be obtained upon presentation. Potential toxins can be placed into broad classes based on their cardiac effects. Two such classes, agents that block the cardiac fast sodium channels and agents that block cardiac potassium efflux channels, can lead to characteristic changes in cardiac indices consisting of QRS prolongation and QT prolongation respectively. The recognition of specific ECG changes can direct treatment and be potentially lifesaving. Administering sodium bicarbonate to a patient with QRS widening after poisoning with a sodium channel blocker will both provide a sodium load, helping overcome the blockade of sodium channels, and alkalinize the serum, providing inhibition of drug binding to the sodium channel. This will shorten the QRS interval, correct hypotension, and prevent arrhythmias.[3] Sodium bicarbonate has been effective in treating cardiotoxicity due to many agents that cause sodium channel blockade. These include TCAs, propoxyphene, diphenhydramine, and cocaine.[22–24]

Patients with QT prolongation are at greater risk for developing torsades de pointes. Arrhythmias are most commonly associated with a QTc of more than 500 ms. However, the likelihood of arrhythmia will vary for individuals.[25] Administration of magnesium sulfate is reasonable in patients with QT prolongation to prevent the occurrence of torsades de pointes. It is also important to maintain potassium in the high normal range in patients with evidence of QT prolongation.[26] Patients with sustained or unstable torsades will require cardioversion. If torsades is recurrent and refractory to treatment, overdrive pacing either electrically or with isoproteranol can be effective.

ECG findings in association with other clinical manifestations may help narrow the differential diagnosis. For example, the findings of QRS prolongation, an anticholinergic syndrome, and an associated seizure narrow the differential diagnosis to agents such as cyclic antidepressants and diphenhydramine. ECG changes have also been shown to predict the degree of toxicity and subsequent risk for other noncardiac adverse outcomes. For example, there is evidence that following TCA poisoning a QRS interval duration of more than 100 ms predicts a 30% greater risk of seizures.[27] Also, having a terminal R wave in lead aVR amplitude of more than 3 mm is predictive for seizures or arrhythmias.[28]

A basic chemistry profile should be obtained in a poisoned patient. Evidence of metabolic acidosis can be an important clue for several poisonings. For example, an obtunded patient with metabolic acidosis should raise the possibility of methanol or ethylene glycol poisoning. Also, profound acidosis in a seizing patient can be a clue in diagnosing isoniazid poisoning. A variation of the classic mnemonic MUDPILES, MULESKI can be used to generate a differential for the patient with metabolic acidosis (Table 2).

All patients with a suspected intentional overdose should have a serum acetaminophen level tested. This is an easily obtained potential toxin found in many combination products. Initial clinical symptoms may be vague (e.g., nausea, vomiting, abdominal pain) or even absent in the first 24 hours.[29] A small but significant

Table 2: Potential Toxic Causes of Increased Anion Gap Metabolic Acidosis

M	Methanol
U	Uremia
L	Lactic acidosis (i.e., sepsis, seizures, cyanide, carbon monoxide, metformin)
E	Ethylene glycol
S	Salicylates, NSAIDs, sympathomimetics, solvents (i.e., toluene)
K	Ketoacidosis (alcoholic, diabetic, starvation)
I	Iron, ibuprofen, isoniazid
NSAID, nonsteroidal antiinflammatory drug.	

number of poisoned patients will have a detectable acetaminophen level that is not suspected based on history.[30] The antidote, N-acetylcysteine, is extremely effective in preventing hepatic injury if given within 8 hours.[31] Therefore, early detection and treatment is important.

There is controversy regarding the routine testing for salicylates in patients who intentionally overdose. Some studies conclude that obtaining levels is unnecessary[30–33] due to low yield unless there is a history of salicylate ingestion or a clinical suspicion. While universal screening may be unnecessary, a low threshold for testing for this easily obtained and potentially serious poison should be maintained. The diagnosis of salicylate poisoning based solely on clinical exam is, however, not without pitfalls. Numerous cases have been reported pertaining to a delayed or mistaken diagnosis in the face of significant salicylate toxicity. These cases present with nonspecific symptoms including neurologic complaints such as confusion and delirium, as well as fever and abdominal pain. Possible misdiagnoses include encephalitis, surgical abdomen, myocardial infarction, sepsis, and alcoholic ketoacidosis.[34–36] One study revealed that a delayed diagnosis (up to 72 hours) of chronic salicylate poisoning is associated with higher morbidity and mortality rates compared to those diagnosed on admission.[37]

Clinical effects of toxins do not usually correlate well with specific levels and results are often not available in time to make real-time decisions. However, for a select group of medicines, levels should be obtained if the history or physical indicates they may be contributing to the patient's condition. The drugs for which serum levels are often clinically useful are lithium, digoxin, phenytoin,

carbamazepine, valproic acid, phenobarbital, and in select cases, ethanol.

Lithium intoxication can present with many nonspecific symptoms, including nausea, vomiting, ataxia, confusion, tremor, myoclonus, and possibly coma or seizures. It is reasonable to check a lithium level in patients presenting with a questionable history and any of these complaints if there is a history of either current or past lithium use or a family member taking lithium. Lithium levels do not accurately reflect the degree of toxicity in chronic exposure, and it is possible to have significant symptoms with near-normal serum levels.

Patients who have overdosed on valproic acid or have developed toxic levels during chronic treatment can present with symptoms ranging from confusion, malaise, and ataxia to coma with respiratory depression. In these patients, it is also important to order an ammonia level. Valproic acid both in chronic use and overdose can cause marked hyperammonemia. This can cause symptoms of confusion and weakness even with therapeutic valproic acid levels. Marked hyperammonemia can lead to cerebral edema.[38] The hyperammonemia is believed to be partly due to a depletion in carnitine. Treatment with L-carnitine has been recommended for patients who present with coma after a valproic acid overdose, have rising ammonia levels, or have a valproic acid level of more than 450 mg/L.[39] Although this practice appears to be safe and potentially beneficial, it has not been validated with randomized controlled trials.[38]

SEIZURES

Many toxins have the ability to cause seizures. Some agents cause seizures directly by altering the balance between inhibitory and excitatory neurotransmission. Many other agents promote seizure activity indirectly by causing profound systemic derangements, such as hypoglycemia, hemodynamic collapse, or hypoxia. Table 3 provides a list of agents that may cause seizures directly.

In general, toxin-induced seizures are treated in a similar fashion to those not associated with toxin ingestion. Clinicians should assure the patient maintains a patent airway, and blood glucose should be measured. Most toxin-induced seizures are self-limiting and do not require loading with antiepileptic medications. However, in the event of status epilepticus or prolonged seizures, parenteral benzodiazepines have been recognized as first-line agents. If seizures are refractory to standard doses of benzodiazepines, second-line agents such as barbiturates or propofol may be employed. Additional benzodiazepines such as midazolam are another option. Most evidence is based on case reports. Propofol has been used successfully to treat toxin-induced seizures.[43,44] This agent has several attractive

Table 3: Agents Causing Seizures[40–42]

Category	Specific Agents	Mechanism
Analgesics	Propoxyphene Tramadol Meperidine	Unknown
Antimicrobials	Isoniazid Penicillin	GABA depletion GABA antagonism
Drugs of abuse	Amphetamines Cocaine Phencyclidine	Adrenergic agonism
Psychiatric medications	Cyclic antidepressants Venlafaxine Bupropion	GABA antagonism and histamine antagonism Unknown
Pesticides	Organophosphate Organochlorine (lindane) Type 2 pyrethroids DEET	Cholinergic excess GABA antagonism Unknown Unknown
Botanicals	*Gyrometra esculenta* mushroom Cicutoxin (water hemlock) Nicotine (tobacco) Aconitine (monk's hood) *Gingko biloba*	GABA depletion GABA antagonism Nicotine agonism Sodium channel opener GABA depletion
Over the counter	Antihistamines Caffeine	Histamine antagonism Adenosine antagonism
Withdrawal	Antiepileptic medications Ethanol Benzodiazepines Baclofen	Multiple GABA receptor down-regulation and NMDA receptor upregulation GABA$_A$ receptor down-regulation GABA$_B$ receptor down-regulation
Others	Camphor Carbamazepine Theophylline Lidocaine Benzoate Baclofen Tiagabine	Unknown Adenosine antagonism Adenosine antagonism Sodium channel blockade Unknown GABA$_B$ agonism Unknown

DEET, N,N-diethyl-meta-toluamide; GABA, γ-aminobutyric acid; NMDA, *N*-methyl-d-aspartate.

features, which include its ability to act as both a γ-aminobutyric acid (GABA) agonist and an *N*-methyl-d-aspartate (NMDA) antagonist,[45] providing two potential mechanisms in seizure prevention. Propofol is also short acting, allowing for easy titration. In cases of toxin-induced seizures, phenytoin is generally not recommended. Phenytoin is considered to be ineffective for treating toxin-induced seizures[40–42] and may add to the underlying toxicity of some agents. Animal studies have demonstrated a detrimental effect when phenytoin is used to treat theophylline-induced seizures[46] and when given to prevent arrhythmias in TCA poisoning.[47] Phenytoin has also been shown to be ineffective in animal models of cocaine and nerve agent–induced seizures.[48,49] If a poisoned patient requires intubation, it is important to avoid the use of long-acting paralytic agents because these agents may mask developing seizures. Delayed treatment of seizures may inhibit seizure abortment and thereby propagate further neuronal damage.[50] Unfortunately, use of paralytic agents remains common practice. In one study, 10% of intubated poisoned patients had received a long-acting paralytic agent.[51] Several toxin-induced seizures have unique treatments that should be employed in addition to standard treatment. These are shown in Table 4.

Several seizure-provoking agents require special mention due to their unique management.

Organophosphates

Organophosphate poisoning may cause significant morbidity and mortality due to seizure activity. Organophosphates (i.e., nerve agents) induce seizures that progress through three stages. The first 5 minutes of exposure precipitates seizures due to cholinergic overstimulation. During this period, agents with central anticholinergic properties can abort or prevent these seizures. Beyond 5 minutes of exposure, other changes are noted, such as decreased brain norepinephrine levels, increased gluta-minergic response, and NMDA receptor activation. In this mixed cholinergic and noncholinergic stage, anticholinergic treatment alone will not terminate seizures. Seizure activity continuing 40 minutes after exposure is mediated by noncholinergic mechanisms and results in structural neuronal injury that is difficult to stop with pharmaceutical agents.[58–60]

When dealing with patients poisoned by organophosphates, it is important to remember the effect of nicotinic overstimulation on the neuromuscular junction. Patients may exhibit muscle fasciculations, weakness, and frank paralysis. In this setting, seizures may not be evident. Therefore, patients presenting with unresponsiveness and flaccid paralysis after organophosphate exposure should be assumed to be experiencing seizure activity until proved otherwise.[61] Aggressive management at stopping seizures (atropine and benzodiazepines), electroencephalogram monitoring, and pralidoxime should be initiated immediately in these cases.

Methylxanthines

Seizures are a known manifestation of poisoning with methylxanthines (i.e., theophylline, caffeine). The primary mechanism for seizure activity in this drug class is adenosine antagonism.[62,63] However, other mechanisms, including pyridoxine depletion, may be involved.[54] In addition to seizures, poisoning with methylxanthines can cause nausea, vomiting, tremor, mental status changes, tachycardia, and hypotension.[62,64] Increased cerebral blood flow may serve as a compensatory mechanism for high metabolic demand during seizure activity. Adenosine aids this process by serving as a cerebral vasodilator.[62] However, in the event of adenosine blockade, which occurs with methylxanthine toxicity, cerebral blood flow may be restricted, thus causing additional cerebral damage. Benzodiazepines are a reasonable treatment in methylxanthine-induced seizure activity; however, phenobarbital appears to be more effective in treating theophylline-induced seizures,[56] which may be due to theophylline acting as an antagonist to benzodiazepines. There is some evidence that pyridoxine may also be helpful and that it is reasonable to administer this to patients with methylxanthine-related seizures that fail to stop with benzodiazepine or phenobarbital.[65]

Antidepressants

Many antidepressant medications have been reported to cause seizures. However, most of these, including the serotonin-specific reuptake inhibitors, rarely cause seizures. Several agents are well known to promote seizure activity, such as cyclic antidepressants, venlafaxine, and bupropion. TCAs deserve special discussion due to their complex pharmacologic and toxicological mechanisms. Seizures secondary to TCAs are directly caused by GABA antagonism, as well as antihistamine effects. TCAs have other toxic effects, which include antimuscarinic effects leading to profound anticholinergic symptoms. In addition, TCAs may cause multiple cardiovascular effects,

Table 4: Seizure-Causing Agents Requiring Specific Treatments	
Agent	**Treatments**
Gingko biloba	Pyridoxine[52,53]
Gyrometra esculenta (false morel) mushroom	Pyridoxine[54]
Isoniazid	Pyridoxine[54]
Organophosphates Nerve agents	Atropine has added benefit when used with benzodiazepines[55]
Theophylline	Barbiturates are more effective than benzodiazepines[56] Hemodialysis may be required to speed drug elimination[57]; pyridoxine may be considered

such as cardiac sodium channel blockade leading to QRS interval prolongation, decreased inotropy, and arrhythmias. Potassium efflux blockade may cause QT interval prolongation predisposing to torsades de pointes, and antagonism at peripheral α1 receptors may cause vasodilation with tachycardia, hypotension, or both. Finally, depletion of biogenic amines may exacerbate hypotension.[66,67] Seizures caused by TCAs may contribute to cardiotoxicity.[68] Prolonged seizure activity may produce serum acidosis and thus the loss of the cardioprotective effect of serum alkalinization.[3] Prophylactic or additional bicarbonate administration to a patient with prolonged seizures is therefore recommended. Alkalinization will not help terminate or prevent seizures but will help prevent cardiovascular decompensation.

Bupropion has a high risk of causing seizures both in overdose and in therapeutic doses.[69] The mechanism of action is unclear; however, up to 8% of patients presenting with a bupropion overdose will develop a seizure,[70] and in recent a study 23% of toxin-induced seizures were due to bupropion.[71]

Venlafaxine is more toxic than other serotonergic antidepressants.[72] It can cause seizures, as well as QRS and QT interval prolongation in overdose.[73,74] One study determined venlafaxine was responsible for 6% of drug-related seizures reported to a poison center.[71]

Antiepileptic Medications

Several antiepileptic medications are implicated in causing seizures when taken in overdose. Phenytoin is reported to cause seizures when taken in overdose. However, this is usually only with extreme overdoses with serum levels of more than 50 mg/L[75] and in those patients with preexisting seizure disorders. Carbamazapine may cause seizures in overdose, which is due to adenosine receptor antagonism. Tiagabine has been reported to cause seizures and myoclonus in overdose.[76–78] Tiagabine exerts its therapeutic effect by blocking GABA reuptake, resulting in increased GABA activity in the brain.[78] Overdoses can result in lethargy, confusion, or coma. However, patients may also present with manifestations of GABA depletion such as agitation and seizures.[79] Possible mechanisms include depletion of presynaptic GABA or stimulation of presynaptic GABA_B receptors inhibiting GABA release.[77]

Baclofen

Baclofen is another agent that can cause seizures both in overdose[80,81] and withdrawal.[82] Seizures are possibly caused by excessive presynaptic GABA_B stimulation inhibiting GABA release.[83] Severe withdrawal often results from a malfunction of an intrathecal pump. Benzodiazepine can help relieve symptoms, but intrathecal baclofen should be reinstituted as soon as possible.[82]

Isoniazid

Isoniazid, gyrometra mushrooms (false morels), and hydrazine (found in rocket fuel) can cause treatment refractory seizures by inhibiting pyridoxine phosphokinase, which leads to a depletion of GABA. These seizures will also result in profound lactic acidosis due to isoniazid poisoning inhibiting conversion of lactate to pyruvate.[84] The treatment initially involves administration of benzodiazepines, fluid resuscitation, and correction of acidosis. However, due to GABA depletion, benzodiazepines are ineffective.[85] Patients will require administration of pyridoxine restore GABA synthesis. Pyridoxine administration will also correct confusion and coma caused by isoniazid poisoning.[86,87] The recommended dose for pyridoxine is 1 g of pyridoxine for every gram of isoniazid ingested. An empiric dose of 5 g or 70 mg/kg (up to 5 g) in children is recommended if the exact amount of the ingestion is not known. Give slowly over 5 to 10 minutes. This dose can be repeated at 20-minute intervals if seizures do not resolve or mental status remains altered.[54,84] Avoid giving large doses of pyridoxine for a prolonged period of time because this can result in severe peripheral neuropathy.[54]

Strychnine

Strychnine poisoning should be suspected in patients presenting with first-time seizure-like activity with intact consciousness. Strychnine is a competitive antagonist of the inhibitory neurotransmitter glycine,[88] resulting in disinhibition of motor neurons in the spinal cord. This can lead to increased motor neuron impulses reaching the muscles, producing muscle activity. Apprehension, hyperreflexia, and muscle spasms can begin 15 to 30 minutes after ingestion or inhalation. This may progress to painful, generalized convulsions lasting 30 seconds to 2 minutes that are often precipitated by even mild stimuli.[86,88] Consciousness is usually preserved, consistent with the site of action of the toxin. Rhabdomyolysis, hyperthermia, and lactic acidosis may develop as muscle spasms progressively intensify. Death is due to spasm of the respiratory muscles, resulting in respiratory failure. Prompt aggressive treatment with benzodiazepines, barbiturates, hydration, and possibly endotracheal intubation with neuromuscular blockade can decrease morbidity and mortality.[86,88,89]

ACUTE ALTERATION OF MENTAL STATUS

Alteration of mental status is a broad term and a common finding in patients presenting to the health-care setting. Presentations may range from frank coma to a profound agitated delirium and should be specifically defined. *Agitated delirium* is a condition marked by disorientation, behavioral disturbance, and hyperexcitability. *Confusion* is a condition in which the patient demonstrates clouded or slow mentation. *Stupor* is defined as a semiconscious state in which the patient requires active or noxious stimulation to illicit a response. *Coma* is marked by unresponsiveness despite active stimulation.

Table 5 provides a list of clinical presentations and the agents classically associated with them. Caution must be used in interpreting this table. Only the presentations classically caused by the agents are included. It is important to note that many agents can produce a wide range of mental status changes depending on individual reactions and the severity of poisoning or time of presentation. Often patients are on multiple medications, and

drug interactions may be the source of the confusion. There are several important examples. Patients poisoned with anticholinergic agents will classily present with agitated delirium. However, patients poisoned with cyclic antidepressants or antihistamines may also present with sedation or coma depending on the degree of poisoning. Phenytoin usually presents with ataxia or confusion. However, extremely high levels can cause coma.

Profound agitated delirium requires adequate sedation to prevent harm to both the patient and the staff members. In addition, sedation of these patients will allow further evaluation and treatment, as well as prevention of complications such as rhabdomyolysis and hyperthermia. Benzodiazepines are the first-line agents of

Table 5: Agents that can Cause Acute Alterations of Mental Status	
Presentation	**Common Agents**
Agitated delirium	Amphetamines, cocaine, phenycyclidine, anticholinergic agents, serotonin syndrome, caffeine, nicotine, pemoline, ethanol withdrawal
Confusion, stupor, or coma	Benzodiazepines, alcohols, barbiturates, opioids, valproic acid, clonidine, γ-hydroxybyric acid, phenytoin, carbamazepine, lithium
Hallucinations	Lysergic acid diethylamide, anticholinergic agents, nutmeg, psilocybin, fluoroquinolones
DIFFERENTIAL FOR SEDATION OR COMA	
Associated Findings	Agents
Horizontal nystagmus	Benzodiazepines, ethanol, ethylene glycol, phenytoin, carbamazepine
Miosis with normal heart rate	Opiates, valproic acid
Miosis and bradycardia	Clonidine, imidazoline receptor agonist (tetrahydrozaline, oxymetazaline)
Miosis and tachycardia	Phenothiazines (i.e., thorazine), olanzapine, quetiapine
DIFFERENTIAL FOR AGITATED DELIRIUM	
Associated Findings	Agents
Mydriasis, diaphoresis, normal or active bowel sounds	Amphetamines, cocaine, caffeine, ethanol withdrawal, benzodiazepine withdrawal
Mydriasis, dry axilla and mucous membranes, decreased bowel sounds	Antihistamines, anticholinergics (i.e., TCAs, jimsonweed, cyclobenzaprine)
Mydriasis, piloerection, yawning	Opiate withdrawal
Rotary nystagmus	Phencyclidine
TCA, tricyclic antidepressant.	

emergency sedation; however, haloperidol can be used in low doses (less than 10 mg to prevent the development of extrapyramidal symptoms) as an adjunct. Haloperidol may be useful in cases of poisonings resulting in dopaminergic hyperstimulation (i.e., pemoline toxicity) or where hallucinations are a significant feature. In general, patients presenting with decreased level of consciousness should be treated primarily with supportive care. In cases in which a patient exhibits adequate airway protection and sufficient respiratory effort, it is unnecessary and often undesirable to awaken the patient. Also in patients with mixed overdoses or poisoning with long-acting agents, it is often desirable to endotracheally intubate the patient and provide ventilatory support rather than attempt to reverse the sedation.

Antidotes

Several antidotes can be used to reverse alteration of mental status due to overdoses or toxic ingestion of specific substances. However, these antidotes should not be used indiscriminately. They include physostigmine, flumazenil, and naloxone and are discussed below.

Physostigmine

Profound altered mental status due to anticholinergic poisoning may be reversed by physostigmine. Physostigmine is a cholinesterase inhibitor that finds its primary application in the treatment of severe isolated anticholinergic poisoning.[90] When indicated, physostigmine is administered preferably in small incremental doses of 1 to 2 mg. The pediatric dose ranges from 0.05 mg/kg to 0.5 mg[90] given by slow intravenous infusion. If administered in select cases, it is recommend that the physostigmine dose be combined with 10 ml of normal saline and administering slowly over 10 minutes due to the risk of cholinergic crisis with rapid injection or the administration of large doses. Physostigmine has limited uses today in overdose management. Importantly, a clear anticholinergic toxidrome must be demonstrated. Administering physostigmine to a patient without anticholinergic toxicity could have severe consequences. These include, seizures, arrhythmias, asystole, and bronchorrhea.[91] Therefore, it should not be given routinely to altered patients. Also, it is important to perform an ECG before administration of physostigmine. Prolongation of the PR interval (>200 ms), QRS interval (>100 ms), or the QTc interval are considered contraindications for physostigmine use.[90,92]

Physostigmine has also been proposed as an agent to reverse coma caused by GHB.[93,94] However, recent reviews and animal work have suggested that this is ineffective and potentially harmful; therefore, this practice should be discouraged.[91,95]

Flumazenil

Benzodiazepines are involved in many intentional overdoses. While these overdoses are rarely fatal when a benzodiazepine is the sole ingestant, they often complicate overdoses with other central nervous system depressants (e.g., ethanol, opioids, other sedatives) due to their synergistic activity. Flumazenil finds its greatest utility in the reversal of benzodiazepine-induced sedation following iatrogenic administration. The initial flumazenil dose is 0.2 mg and should be administered intravenously over 30 seconds. If no response occurs after an additional 30 seconds, a second dose is recommended. Additional incremental doses of 0.5 mg may be administered at 1-minute intervals until the desired response is noted or until a total of 3 mg has been administered. It is important to note that resedation may occur[96] and patients should be observed carefully after requiring reversal. Flumazenil should not be administered as a nonspecific coma-reversal drug and should be used with extreme caution after intentional benzodiazepine overdose since it has the potential to precipitate withdrawal in benzodiazepine-dependent individuals, induce seizures in those at risk, or both.[97–99]

Naloxone

Opioid poisoning from the abuse of morphine derivatives or synthetic narcotic agents may be reversed with the opioid antagonist naloxone.[100] Naloxone is commonly used in comatose patients as a therapeutic and diagnostic agent. The standard dosage regimen is to administer from 0.4 to 2.0 mg slowly, preferably intravenously. Intramuscular administration is an alternative parenteral route, but if the patient is hypotensive, naloxone may not be absorbed rapidly from the intramuscular injection site. The intravenous dose should be readministered at 5-minute intervals until the desired endpoint is achieved: restoration of respiratory function, ability to protect the airway, and improved level of consciousness.[101] If the intravenous route of administration is not viable, alternative routes include intramuscular injection, intraosseous infusion, and pulmonary via the endotracheal tube, intranasally, or via nebulization.[101] Patients may fail to respond to naloxone administration for a variety of reasons: an insufficient dose of naloxone, the absence of an opioid exposure, a mixed overdose with other central nervous and respiratory system depressants, or medical or traumatic reasons.

Naloxone can precipitate profound withdrawal symptoms in opioid-dependent patients. Symptoms include agitation, vomiting, diarrhea, piloerection, diaphoresis, and yawning.[101] Health-care providers should use care when administering this agent. Only give the amount necessary to restore adequate respiration and airway protection.

Naloxone's clinical efficacy can last for as little as 45 minutes.[100] Therefore, patients are at risk for recurrence of narcotic effect. This is particularly true for patients exposed to methadone or sustained-release opioid products. Patients should be observed for resedation for at least 4 hours after reversal with naloxone. If a patient does resedate, it is reasonable to administer naloxone as an infusion. An infusion of two-thirds the effective initial bolus per hour is usually effective.[101] These patients should be observed closely in a monitored setting: they may develop withdrawal symptoms or worsening sedation as drug is either metabolized or absorbed.

WEAKNESS

Generalized weakness is a common presenting complaint. It is often a subjective complaint caused by illnesses or poisons with systemic effects. In this section, we will address poisons that cause true decreases in muscle strength (Table 6). This includes focal and generalized weakness.

Botulism

Botulism is a progressive paralytic illness caused by botulinum toxin produced by the bacteria *Clostridium botulinum*.[102] Botulinum toxin is an extremely potent neurotoxin. There are seven distinct subtypes of clostridia neurotoxins (A, B, C1, D, E, F, and G), of which only A, B, E, and rarely F cause illness in humans.[103] These cause

several syndromes, namely, foodborne botulism, infant botulism, wound botulism, and adult intestinal botulism. Foodborne botulism is caused by ingestion of preformed botulinum toxin, while the other syndromes are caused by germination of *C. botulinum* spores and elaboration of the toxin, which is then absorbed. Once botulinum toxin is systemically absorbed, it attacks cholinergic presynaptic nerve endings. The toxin cannot cross the blood–brain barrier and therefore only affects the peripheral nervous system.[104] The toxin is taken up into the nerve by endocytosis and prevents the fusion of the acetylcholine-containing synaptic vesicle with the nerve terminus. Ultimately, the nerve cannot release acetylcholine and neurotransmission is interrupted,[104,105] resulting in paralysis. Paralysis caused by botulinum toxin will persist until the cleaved proteins are regenerated. Therefore, if a patient's condition progresses to the point of requiring mechanical ventilation, ventilator dependency for several months may result.[106] For this reason, it is important to recognize botulism and initiate treatment with antitoxin as early as possible. Antitoxin treatment will not reverse any paralysis that has already occurred but will arrest further paralysis, limit disability, and hopefully prevent the need for mechanical ventilation.[104]

A classic pentad for diagnosing botulism consists of nausea and vomiting, dysphagia, diplopia, dry mouth, and dilated and fixed pupils.[107] In a study of 705 patients with botulism, 68% of patients had at least three symptoms on admission while only 2% had all five symptoms.[102] Therefore, patients often will not present with all classic clinical effects. It is important to note that patients presenting with some or all symptoms consistent with botulism should be closely observed for progression. Death due to botulism toxin is most often secondary to paralysis of respiratory muscles and therefore may be prevented with adequate supportive care.

Tick Paralysis

Tick paralysis is caused by neurotoxins secreted by feeding female ticks. Ataxia may be the initial sign, but ascending weakness will develop if untreated. Full paralysis may ascend to affect muscles of respiration and those innervated by the cranial nerves. Patients may complain of sensory symptoms as well. On exam patients may demonstrate weakness, often more pronounced in the lower extremities, and diminished or absent deep tendon reflexes. Objective sensory abnormalities are rarely found.

Similarities in presentation may lead to the misdiagnosis of Guillain-Barré syndrome. However, cerebrospinal fluid protein levels will not be elevated in cases of tick paralysis.

The diagnosis is ascertained by finding the tick attached to the patient. This may entail a thorough search

Table 6: Toxin Induced Weakness	
Bulbar weakness, with associated mydriasis and dry mouth	Botulism
Ataxia, ascending weakness	Tick paralysis
Paresthesias progressing to ascending weakness	Tetrodotoxin, saxitoxin
Following apparent recovery from organophosphate poisoning, the development of weakness of neck flexors and proximal limb muscles	Organophosphate-induced intermediate syndrome

involving the hair, axilla, perineum, and ear canal. Treatment requires tick removal, which will likely produce symptom resolution within 24 hours.[108]

Tetrodotoxin

Tetrodotoxin is a water-soluble toxin that binds to receptor site 1 of voltage-dependent Na channels. Inhibition of sodium flux through Na ion channels renders excitable tissues such as nerves and muscle nonfunctional.[109]

The severity and speed of clinical effects due to tetrodotoxin ingestion varies depending be reported, usually beginning within an hour after ingestion.[110] Paresthesias initially affect the tongue, lips, and mouth and progress to involvement of the extremities. Gastrointestinal symptoms may be seen and include nausea, vomiting, and less often, diarrhea. Muscle weakness, headache, ataxia, dizziness, urinary retention, floating sensations, and feelings of doom may occur.[99,111] An ascending flaccid paralysis can also develop. Other reported effects include diaphoresis, pleuritic chest pain, fixed dilated pupils, dysphagia, aphonia, seizures, bradycardia, hypotension, and heart block. Death can occur within hours secondary to respiratory muscle paralysis or dysrhythmias. Clinical effects in the mildest of cases resolve within hours, whereas the more severe cases may not resolve for days. Treatment is supportive; there is no specific antitoxin. Patients who have progressed to having generalized paresthesias, extremity weakness, pupillary dilation, or reflex changes should be admitted to the hospital for observation until peak effects have passed.[99] Those with respiratory failure should be intubated and placed on mechanical ventilation. Vasopressor support may be necessary for hypotension refractory to intravenous fluids. Atropine has been used for symptomatic bradycardia.[110]

Intermediate Syndrome

Intermediate syndrome is the development of profound muscle weakness 24 to 96 hours after exposure to organophosphates. It occurs after resolution of the initial cholinergic syndrome.[112] Patients will present with weakness of neck flexion and proximal muscle weakness. Respiratory muscle weakness may also occur, leading to respiratory insufficiency. Although there is no specific antidote available, early recognition of the syndrome and initiation of supportive care can prevent death due to respiratory failure. Appropriate supportive care provides recovery in 5 to 18 days.[89]

Hyperthermic Syndromes

Altered mentation and fever may be the initial presentation of a toxin-induced hyperthermic syndrome. However, the differential diagnosis for hyperthermic syndromes is broad and includes infectious etiologies, endocrine disarray, and environmental heatstroke. Early recognition of a hyperthermic syndrome may aid in facilitating accurate treatment. Many medications or poisons have the potential to produce such a syndrome and are listed in Table 7. Cornerstone therapy for hyperthermic syndromes is aggressive hydration, sedation with benzodiazepines, and active cooling. Specific treatments have been proposed for several hyperthermic syndromes. However, most of these treatments have not been definitively proved to be safe and efficacious in humans. The most important step in management is recognizing which hyperthermic syndrome may be present and discontinuing any possible culprit medications. Prompt initiation of aggressive supportive care may help prevent rhabdomyolysis, coagulopathy, multisystem organ failure, and other potential consequences of hyperthermia.[4,115]

Malignant Hyperthermia

Malignant hyperthermia is a relatively rare complication caused by administration of volatile anesthetic agents, succinylcholine, or both, leading to an abnormal release of calcium from the cytoplasmic reticulum.[116] It is heralded by a rise in end tidal CO_2 and progresses to manifest with hypercarbia, tachypnea, tachycardia, hyperthermia, muscle rigidity, hyperthermia, metabolic acidosis, skin mottling, and rhabdomyolysis.[116,117] If not treated promptly, sustained hypermetabolism can cause rhabdomyolysis due to cellular hypoxia. This can lead to profound hyperkalemia, resulting in arrhythmias or myoglobinuric renal failure.

Other complications of malignant hyperthermia include compartment syndrome due to muscle edema, mesenteric ischemia, congestive heart failure, and disseminated intravascular coagulation.

Treatment involves immediate discontinuation of the offending agent, hyperventilation with 100% oxygen, administration of dantrolene, active cooling, and correction of hyperkalemia.[116,117] Due to the etiologic agents involved, it is extremely unlikely this condition will present outside of the operating room.

Serotonin Syndrome

Serotonin syndrome is caused by an overdose of a serotonergic drug or an interaction between two or more drugs with serotonergic actions. This syndrome often presents with the triad of altered mental status, autonomic instability, and neuromuscular changes.[118] A distinguishing characteristic of this syndrome is the presence of clonus, which is more prominent in the lower extremities. However, it can present subtly with agitation, akathisia, or tachycardia.[119,120] Many agents have the potential to induce serotonin syndrome; therefore, a low threshold of suspicion is warranted for this entity. Discontinuation of any serotonergic medication at an early stage may prevent the progression.

Table 7: Hyperthermic Syndromes[4,113,114]

Syndrome	Clinical Features	Examples
Malignant hyperthermia	Increased CO_2 production, rigidity, hyperthermia, metabolic acidosis, rhabdomyolysis	Volatile anesthetic gases, succinylcholine
Serotonin syndrome	Altered mental status, tachycardia, hypertension, diaphoresis, hyperreflexia, clonus, hyperthermia	Combination or overdose of serotonergic agents (i.e., SSRIs), TCAs, dextromethorphan, MAO inhibitors, meperidine
Neuroleptic malignant syndrome	Altered mental status, hyperthermia, rigidity	Neuroleptics including phenothiazines (promethazine, thioridazine, chlorpromazine and fluphenazine), butyrophenones (haloperidol), clozapine, quetiapine, risperidone, olanzapine, aripiprazole, cessation of anti-Parkinson's medications
Anticholinergic syndrome	Mydriasis, dry skin, dry mucous membranes, decreased bowel sounds, sedation, altered mental status, hallucinations, urinary retention	Antihistamines, TCAs, jimsonweed, cyclobenzaprine, atropine
Sympathomimetic syndrome	Agitation, tachycardia, mydriasis, diaphoresis, hypertension	Amphetamines, cocaine, phencyclidine
Uncoupling	Metabolic acidosis, hyperthermia, tachypnea	Salicylates, dinitrophenol

MAO, monoamine oxidase; SSRI, serotonin-specific reuptake inhibitor; TCA, tricyclic antidepressant.

The first diagnostic criteria for serotonin syndrome were introduced by Sternbach in 1991.[121] Diagnosis requires the addition or increase in a known serotonergic agent, which leads to the development of at least 3 of the following 10 symptoms: mental status changes (confusion, hypomania), agitation, myoclonus, hyperreflexia, diaphoresis, shivering, tremor, diarrhea, incoordination, or fever. The diagnosis also requires ruling out other etiologies and establishing that there was no recent use of neuroleptic agents. New diagnostic criteria were developed in 2003.[120,122] The Hunter Serotonin Toxicity Criteria was designed as a flowchart and thought to be more specific and simpler to use. In summary, a patient with a known exposure to a serotonergic agent can be considered to have serotonin toxicity if that patient has one of the following criteria: (1) spontaneous clonus; (2) inducible or ocular clonus in combination with agitation, diaphoresis, hypertonia with pyrexia, or hyperreflexia; and (3) tremor and hyperreflexia. Without any of the preceding findings or combinations of findings, clinically significant serotonin toxicity cannot be diagnosed.

Treatment involves cessation of any serotonergic agents and supportive care. Several specific pharmacological interventions have been suggested. Unfortunately, data on their use comes primarily from case reports rather than controlled trials. It is therefore difficult to distinguish effectiveness of the antidote from natural resolution of the syndrome.[120] Cyproheptadine is an antihistamine, which also acts as a 5HT-2 antagonist, and is the most widely used medication for serotonin syndrome. It is administered orally and therefore difficult to administer to patients with severe toxicity and may cause additional sedation.[120]

Neuroleptic Malignant Syndrome

Neuroleptic malignant syndrome (NMS) is a potentially life-threatening complication caused by dopamine antagonists. It is characterized by hyperthermia, muscular rigidity, autonomic instability, and altered mental status.[123] Research criteria have been published by the American Psychiatric Association.[98] The criteria include the following:

1. Development of severe muscle rigidity and hyperthermia associated with the use of neuroleptic medications
2. Presence of at least two of the following: diaphoresis, dysphagia, incontinence, change in level of

consciousness, mutism, tachycardia, increased or labile blood pressure, leukocytosis, or laboratory evidence of muscle injury

3. Symptoms not caused by another ingestion or a neurological or medical condition

4. Symptoms not better accounted for by a mental disorder

Despite specific criteria, the diagnosis can often be challenging. A distinguishing feature is lead pipe rigidity in which passive movement is resisted in all directions.

The most vital step in treating NMS is early recognition of the syndrome and immediate withdrawal of the responsible agent, along with supportive care. Dehydration is commonly found in these patients and must be corrected with intrevenous fluids.[124] Several proposed pharmacological treatments for this condition can be considered but are not consistently effective.[123] Bromocriptine and amantadine are dopamine agonists, which have been reported in case reports to reduce recovery time and mortality.[123] Both bromocriptine and amantadine are considered serotonergic medications and therefore should be avoided if there is any possibility that the differential diagnosis includes serotonin syndrome.[125–127] Dantrolene may be beneficial as it will attenuate the tonic muscle contractions seen in NMS.[128] However, it can cause muscle weakness and respiratory insufficiency.[128] Electroconvulsive therapy may be effective for treatment resistant cases or if lethal catatonia is possible diagnosis.[123,124] An NMS-like syndrome can be seen in Parkinson's disease patients who abruptly discontinue levodopa therapy. The prompt reinstitution of levodopa will treat the condition.[129,130]

Anticholinergic-Induced Hyperthermia

Anticholinergic toxicity can induce hyperthermia due to muscarinic antagonism, which impairs perspiration in patients with marked agitation and hyperactivity.[90] The principle diagnostic feature that distinguishes anticholinergic syndrome is dry skin, best determined by noting dry axilla.

Sympathomimetic-Induced Hyperthermia

Sympathomimetic poisoning can induce hyperthermia through excessive neuromuscular activity, resulting in increased thermogenesis.[115] Ethanol and benzodiazepine withdrawal can present in a similar fashion. Aggressive treatment with benzodiazepines is the first-line treatment. However, in cases not responsive to benzodiazepines, treatment with haloperidol or droperidol may be effective. This is especially true in methamphetamine toxicity, for which haloperidol[131] and droperidol[132] have been found safe and effective. If these medications are used, the patient should be monitored for prolongation of the QT interval and development of torsades de pointes.

Uncoupling of Oxidative Phosphorylation

Some agents (i.e., salicylates and dinitrophenol) can cause hyperthermia by uncoupling oxidative phosphorylation. Clinical clues to salicylate poisoning are tinnitus, tachypnea, respiratory alkalosis, and metabolic acidosis.[133] Treatment includes prompt initiation of serum and urinary alkalinization with sodium bicarbonate and arranging urgent dialysis for patients with profound toxicity.

Dinitrophenol is occasionally used as a diet aid. Poisoning with this agent will present with hyperthermia, tachypnea, and tachycardia and can progress to agitation, delirium, coma, muscular rigidity, and death.[134,135]

CONCLUSION

Neurological emergencies caused by poisoning are often encountered. Toxic exposure or overdose should be considered in any patient presenting with seizures of unknown etiology, unexplained mental status changes, acute progressive weakness, and hyperthermic syndromes. Early recognition that a patient's symptoms are caused by a poison or a toxic syndrome can prompt an efficient diagnostic workup and ultimately facilitate timely treatment.

REFERENCES

1. Malouf R, Brust J. Hypoglycemia: causes, neurological manifestations, and outcome. *Ann Neurol*. 1985;17(5):421–430.
2. Luber SD. Acute hypoglycemia masquerading as head trauma: a report of four cases. *Am J Emerg Med*. 1996;14(6):543–547.
3. Kolecki PF, Curry SC. Poisoning by sodium channel blocking agents. *Crit Care Clin*. 1997;13(4):829–848.
4. Rusyniak DE, Sprague JE. Toxin-induced hyperthermic syndromes. *Med Clin North Am*. 2005;89(6):1277–1296.
5. Jardine DS. Heat illness and heat stroke. *Pediatr Rev*. 2007;28(7):249–258.
6. Lugo-Amador NM, Rothenhaus T, Moyer P. Heat-related illness. *Emerg Med Clin North Am*. 2004;22(2):315–327.
7. Kao LW, Nanagas KA. Carbon monoxide poisoning. *Med Clin*. 2005;89(6):1161–1194.
8. Herman LY. Carbon monoxide poisoning presenting as an isolated seizure. *J Emerg Med*. 1998;16(3):429–432.
9. Isbister GK, Downes F, Sibbritt D, et al. Aspiration pneumonitis in an overdose population: frequency, predictors, and outcomes. *Crit Care Med*. 2004;32(1):88–93.
10. Liisanantti J, Kaukoranta P, Martikainen M, Ala-Kokko T. Aspiration pneumonia following severe self-poisoning. *Resuscitation*. 2003;56(1):49–53.
11. Talaie H, Pajouhmand A, Abdollahi M, et al. Rhabdomyolysis among acute human poisoning cases. *Hum Exp Toxicol*. 2007;26(7):557–561.
12. O'Malley GF, Seifert S, Heard K, et al. Olanzapine overdose mimicking opioid intoxication. *Ann Emerg Med*. 1999;34(2):279–281.

13. Eddleston M, Mohamed F, Davies JO, et al. Respiratory failure in acute organophosphorus pesticide self-poisoning. *QJM*. 2006;99(8):513–522.

14. Toxicology, A.A.o.C., E.A.o.P. Centres, and C. Toxicologists. Position paper: single-dose activated charcoal. *Clin Toxicol*. 2005;43(2):61–87.

15. Moll J, Kerns W 2nd, Tomaszewski C, Rose R. Incidence of aspiration pneumonia in intubated patients receiving activated charcoal. *J Emerg Med*. 1999;17(2):279–283.

16. Toxicology, A.A.o.C. and E.A.o.P.C.a.C. Toxicologists. Position paper: whole bowel irrigation. *Clin Toxicol*. 2004;42(6):843–854.

17. Belson MG, Simon HK. Utility of comprehensive toxicologic screens in children. *Am J Emerg Med*. 1999;17(3):221–224.

18. Brett AS. Implications of discordance between clinical impression and toxicology analysis in drug overdose. *Arch Intern Med*. 1988;148(2):437–441.

19. Mahoney JD, Gross PL, Stern TA, et al. Quantitative serum toxic screening in the management of suspected drug overdose. *Am J Emerg Med*. 1990;8(1):16–22.

20. George S, Braithwaite RA. A preliminary evaluation of five rapid detection kits for on site drugs of abuse screening. *Addiction*. 1995;90(2):227–232.

21. Perrone J, et al. Drug screening versus history in detection of substance use in ED psychiatric patients. *Am J Emerg Med*. 2001;19(1):49–51.

22. Marraffa JM, De Roos F, Jayaraman S, Hollander JE. Diethylene glycol: widely used solvent presents serious poisoning potential. *J Emerg Med*. 2008; 35(4): 401–406.

23. Kerns W, Garvey L, Owens J. Cocaine-induced wide complex dysrhythmia. *J Emerg Med*. 1997;15(3):321–329.

24. Clark RF, Vance MV. Massive diphenhydramine poisoning resulting in a wide-complex tachycardia: successful treatment with sodium bicarbonate. *Ann Emerg Med*. 1992;21(3):318–321.

25. Yap YG, Camm AJ. Drug-induced QT prolongation and torsades de pointes. *Heart*. 2003;89(11):1363–1372.

26. Gupta A, Lawrence AT, Krishnan K, et al. Current concepts in the mechanisms and management of drug-induced QT prolongation and torsades de pointes. *Am Heart J*. 2007;153(6):891–899.

27. Boehnert MT, Lovejoy FH. Value of the QRS duration versus the serum drug level in predicting seizures and ventricular arrhythmias after an acute overdose of tricyclic antidepressants. *N Engl J Med*. 1985;313(8):474–479.

28. Liebelt EL, Francis PD, Woolf AD. ECG lead aVR versus QRS interval in predicting seizures and arrhythmias in acute tricyclic antidepressant toxicity. *Ann Emerg Med*. 1995;26(2):195–201.

29. Rowden AK, Norvell J, Eldridge DL, Kirk MA. Updates on acetaminophen toxicity. *Med Clin North Am*. 2005;89(6):1145–1159.

30. Sporer KA, Khayam-Bashi H. Acetaminophen and salicylate serum levels in patients with suicidal ingestion or altered mental status. *Am J Emerg Med*. 1996;14(5):443–446.

31. Smilkstein MJ, Knapp GL, Kulig KW, Rumack BH. Efficacy of oral N-acetylcysteine in the treatment of acetaminophen overdose: analysis of the national multicenter study (1976 to 1985). *N Engl J Med*. 1988;319(24):1557–1562.

32. Chan T, Chan AY, Ho CS, Critchley JA. The clinical value of screening for salicylates in acute poisoning. *Vet Hum Toxicol*. 1995;37:37–38.

33. Wood DM, Dargan PI, Jones AL. Measuring plasma salicylate concentrations in all patients with drug overdose or altered consciousness: is it necessary? *Emerg Med J*. 2005;22(6):401–403.

34. Paul BN. Salicylate poisoning in the elderly: diagnostic pitfalls. *J Am Geriatr Soc*. 1972;20(8):387–390.

35. Leatherman JW, Schmitz PG. Fever, hyperdynamic shock, and multiple-system organ failure: a pseudo-sepsis syndrome associated with chronic salicylate intoxication. *Chest*. 1991;100(5):1391–1396.

36. Chui PT. Anesthesia in a patient with undiagnosed salicylate poisoning presenting as intraabdominal sepsis. *J Clin Anesth*. 1999;11(3):251–253.

37. Anderson RJ, Potts DE, Gabow PA, et al. Unrecognized adult salicylate intoxication. *Ann Intern Med*. 1976;85(6):745–748.

38. Lheureux P, Penaloza A, Zahir S, Gris M. Science review: carnitine in the treatment of valproic acid–induced toxicity—what is the evidence? *Crit Care*. 2005;9(5):431–440.

39. Russell S. Carnitine as an antidote for acute valproate toxicity in children. *Curr Opin Pediatr*. 2007;19(2):206–210.

40. Shannon M, McElroy EA, Liebelt EL. Toxic seizures in children: case scenarios and treatment strategies. *Pediatr Emerg Care*. 2003;19(3):201–210.

41. Wills B, Erickson, T. Drug- and toxin-associated seizures. *Med Clin North Am*. 2005;89(6):1297–1321.

42. Wallace K. Antibiotic-induced convulsions. *Crit Care Clin*. 1997;13(4):741–762.

43. Wang YC, Liu BM, Supernaw RB, et al. Management of star fruit–induced neurotoxicity and seizures in a patient with chronic renal failure. *Pharmacotherapy*. 2006;26(1):143–146.

44. Merigian KS, Browning RG, Leeper KV. Successful treatment of amoxapine-induced refractory status epilepticus with propofol (diprivan). *Acad Emerg Med*. 1995;2(2):128–133.

45. Marik P. Propofol: therapeutic indications and side-effects. *Curr Pharm Des*. 2004;10:3639–3649.

46. Blake KV, Massey KL, Hendeles L, et al. Relative efficacy of phenytoin and phenobarbital for the prevention of theophylline-induced seizures in mice. *Ann Emerg Med*. 1988;17(10):1024–1028.

47. Callaham M, Schumaker H, Pentel P. Phenytoin prophylaxis of cardiotoxicity in experimental amitriptyline poisoning. *J Pharmacol Exp Ther*. 1988;245(1):216–220.

48. McDonough J, Benjamin A, McMonagle JD, et al. Effects of fosphenytoin on nerve agent–induced status epilepticus. *Drug Chem Toxicol*. 2004;27(1):27–39.

49. Derlet RW, Albertson TE. Anticonvulsant modification of cocaine-induced toxicity in the rat. *Neuropharmacology*. 1990;29(3):255–259.

50. Fountain NB. Status epilepticus: risk factors and complications. *Epilepsia*. 2000;41(s2):S23-S30.

51. Lawrence D, Dobmeier S, Kirk M. Long-acting neuromuscular blocking agents are commonly administered during the treatment of overdose patients. *Clin Toxicol*. 2007;45(6):614.

52. Kajiyama Y, Fujii K, Takeuchi H, Manabe Y. Ginkgo seed poisoning. *Pediatrics*. 2002;109(2):325–327.

53. Kastner U, Hallmen C, Wiese M, et al. The human pyridoxal kinase, a plausible target for ginkgotoxin from *Ginkgo biloba*. *FEBS J*. 2007;274(4):1036–1045.

54. Lheureux P, Penaloza A, Gris M. Pyridoxine in clinical toxicology: a review. *Eur J Emerg Med*. 2005;12(2):78–85.

55. Shih T-M, Rowland TC, McDonough JH. Anticonvulsants for nerve agent–induced seizures: the influence of the therapeutic dose of atropine. *J Pharmacol Exp Ther*. 2007;320(1):154–161.

56. Yoshikawa H. First-line therapy for theophylline-associated seizures. *Acta Neurol Scand*. 2007;115(s186):57–61.

57. de Pont A-CJM. Extracorporeal treatment of intoxications. *Curr Opin Crit Care*. 2007;13(6):668–673.

58. McDonough JH, Shih T-M. Neuropharmacological mechanisms of nerve agent–induced seizure and neuropathology. *Neurosci Biobehav Rev*. 1997;21(5):559–579.

59. Myhrer T, Enger S, Aas P. Pharmacological therapies against soman-induced seizures in rats 30 min following onset and anticonvulsant impact. *Eur J Pharmacol*. 2006;548(1–3):83–89.

60. Sanada M, Zheng F, Huth T, Alzheimer C. Cholinergic modulation of periaqueductal grey neurons: does it contribute to epileptogenesis after organophosphorus nerve agent intoxication? *Toxicology.* 2007;233(1–3):199–208.

61. Holstege CP, Miller MB, Wermuth M, et al. Crotalid snake envenomation. *Crit Care Clin.* 1997;13(4):889–921.

62. Holstege CP, Hunter Y, Baer AB, et al. Massive caffeine overdose requiring vasopressin infusion and hemodialysis. *Clin Toxicol.* 2003;41(7):1003–1007.

63. Shannon M, Maher T. Anticonvulsant effects of intracerebroventricular adenocard in theophylline-induced seizures. *Ann Emerg Med.* 1995;26(1):65–68.

64. Shannon M. Life-threatening events after theophylline overdose: a 10-year prospective analysis. *Arch Intern Med.* 1999;159(9):989–994.

65. Bonner AB, Peterson SL, Weir MR. Seizures induced by theophylline and isoniazid in mice [see comment] *Vet Hum Toxicol.* 1999;41(3):175–177.

66. Tan C, Pillai S, Manning PG. Electrocardiographical case: a man found unconscious. *Singapore Med J.* 2006;47(8):730–734; quiz 735.

67. Scharman EJ, Erdman AR, Cobaugh DJ, et al. Methylphenidate poisoning: an evidence-based consensus guideline for out-of-hospital management. *Clin Toxicol.* 2007;45(7):737–752.

68. Taboulet P, Michard F, Muszynski J, et al. Cardiovascular repercussions of seizures during cyclic antidepressant poisoning. *Clin Toxicol.* 1995;33(3):205–211.

69. Pesola GR, Avasarala J. Bupropion seizure proportion among new-onset generalized seizures and drug-related seizures presenting to an emergency department. *J Emerg Med.* 2002;22(3):235–239.

70. Belson MG, Kelley TR. Bupropion exposures: clinical manifestations and medical outcome. *J Emerg Med.* 2002;23(3):223–230.

71. Thundiyil J, Kearney T, Olson K. Evolving epidemiology of drug-induced seizures reported to a poison control center system. *J Med Toxicol.* 2007;3(1):15–19.

72. Whyte IM, Dawson AH, Buckley NA. Relative toxicity of venlafaxine and selective serotonin reuptake inhibitors in overdose compared to tricyclic antidepressants. *QJM.* 2003;96(5):369–374.

73. Blythe D, Hackett LP. Cardiovascular and neurological toxicity of venlafaxine. *Hum Exp Toxicol.* 1999;18(5):309–313.

74. Mazur JE, Doty JD, Krygiel AS. Fatality related to a 30-g venlafaxine overdose. *Pharmacotherapy.* 2003;23(12):1668–1672.

75. Craig S. Phenytoin poisoning. *Neurocrit Care.* 2005;3(2):161–170.

76. Jette N, Cappell J, VanPassel L, Akman CI. Tiagabine-induced nonconvulsive status epilepticus in an adolescent without epilepsy. *Neurology.* 2006;67(8):1514–1515.

77. Fulton JA, Hoffman RS, Nelson LS. Tiagabine overdose: a case of status epilepticus in a non-epileptic patient. *Clin Toxicol.* 2005;43(7):869–871.

78. Forbes RA, Kalra H, Hackett LP, Daly FF. Deliberate self-poisoning with tiagabine: an unusual toxidrome. *Emerg Med Australas.* 2007;19(6):556–558.

79. Spiller HA, Winter ML, Ryan M, et al. Retrospective evaluation of tiagabine overdose. *Clin Toxicol.* 2005;43(7):855–859.

80. Perry HE, Wright RO, Shannon MW, Woolf AD. Baclofen overdose: drug experimentation in a group of adolescents. *Pediatrics.* 1998;101(6):1045–1048.

81. Leung NY, Whyte IM, Isbister GK. Baclofen overdose: defining the spectrum of toxicity. *Emerg Med Australas.* 2006;18(1):77–82.

82. Kao LW, Amin Y, Kirk MA, Turner MS. Intrathecal baclofen withdrawal mimicking sepsis. *J Emerg Med.* 2003;24(4):423–427.

83. Hansel DE, Hansel CR, Shindle MK, et al. Oral baclofen in cerebral palsy: possible seizure potentiation? *Pediatr Neurol.* 2003;29(3):203–206.

84. Topcu I, Yentur EA, Kefi A, et al. Seizures, metabolic acidosis and coma resulting from acute isoniazid intoxication. *Anaesth Intensive Care.* 2005;33(4):518–520.

85. Morrow LE, Wear RE, Schuller D, Malesker M. Acute isoniazid toxicity and the need for adequate pyridoxine supplies. *Pharmacotherapy.* 2006;26(10):1529–1532.

86. Smith BA. Strychnine poisoning. *J Emerg Med.* 1990;8(3):321–325.

87. Salkind AR, Hewitt CC. Coma from long-term overingestion of isoniazid. *Arch Intern Med.* 1997;157(21):2518–2520.

88. Wood D, Webster E, Martinez D, et al. Case report: survival after deliberate strychnine self-poisoning, with toxicokinetic data. *Crit Care.* 2002;6(5):456–459.

89. Libenson MH, Yang JM. Case 12-2001: a 16-year-old boy with an altered mental status and muscle rigidity. *N Engl J Med.* 2001;344(16):1232–1239.

90. Frascogna N. Physostigmine: is there a role for this antidote in pediatric poisonings? *Curr Opin Pediatr.* 2007;19(2):201–205.

91. Bania TC, Chu J. Physostigmine does not effect arousal but produces toxicity in an animal model of severe γ-hydroxybutyrate intoxication. *Acad Emerg Med.* 2005;12(3):185–189.

92. Burns MJ, Linden CH, Graudins A, et al. A comparison of physostigmine and benzodiazepines for the treatment of anticholinergic poisoning. *Ann Emerg Med.* 2000;35(4):374–381.

93. Caldicott DGE, Kuhn M. γ-Hydroxybutyrate overdose and physostigmine: teaching new tricks to an old drug? *Ann Emerg Med.* 2001;37(1):99–102.

94. Yates W, Viera A. Physostigmine in the treatment of γ-hydroxybutyric acid overdose. *Mayo Clin Proc.* 2000;75(4):401–402.

95. Zvosec DL, Smith SW, Litonjua R, Westfal RE. Physostigmine for γ-hydroxybutyrate coma: inefficacy, adverse events, and review. *Clin Toxicol.* 2007;45(3):261–265.

96. Seger DL. Flumazenil: treatment or toxin. *J Toxicol Clin Toxicol.* 2004;42(2):209–216.

97. Haverkos GP, DiSalvo RP, Imhoff TE. Fatal seizures after flumazenil administration in a patient with mixed overdose. *Ann Pharmacother.* 1994;28(12):1347–1349.

98. Charles PD, Davis TL. Neuroleptic malignant syndrome. In: Robertson D, Low PA, Polinsky RJ eds. *Primer on the Autonomic Nervous System.* 2nd ed. San Diego, CA: Academic Press; 2004:302–305.

99. How C-K, Chern CH, Huang YC, et al. Tetrodotoxin poisoning. *Am J Emerg Med.* 2003;21(1):51–54.

100. Chamberlain JM, Klein BL. A comprehensive review of naloxone for the emergency physician. *Am J Emerg Med.* 1994;12(6):650–660.

101. Clarke SFJ, Dargan PI, Jones AL. Naloxone in opioid poisoning: walking the tightrope. *Emerg Med J.* 2005;22(9):612–616.

102. Varma JK, Katsitadze G, Moiscrafishvili M, et al. Signs and symptoms predictive of death in patients with foodborne botulism: Republic of Georgia, 1980–2002 [see comment] *Clin Infect Dis.* 2004;39(3):357–362.

103. Sobel J. Botulism. *Clin Infect Dis.* 2005;41(8):1167–1173.

104. Horowitz BZ. Botulinum toxin. *Crit Care Clin.* 2005;21(4):825–839.

105. Cherington M. Botulism: update and review. *Semin Neurol.* 2004;24(2):155–163.

106. Arnon SS, Schechter R, Inglesby TV, et al. Botulinum toxin as a biological weapon: medical and public health management. *JAMA.* 2001;285(8):1059–1070.

107. Wainwright RB, Heyward WL, Middaugh JP, et al. Food-borne botulism in Alaska, 1947–1985: epidemiology and clinical findings. *J Infect Dis.* 1988;157(6):1158–1162.

108. Li Z, Turner RP. Pediatric tick paralysis: discussion of two cases and literature review. *Pediatr Neurol.* 2004;31(4):304–307.

109. Kiernan MC, Isbister GK, Lin CS, et al. Acute tetrodotoxin-induced neurotoxicity after ingestion of puffer fish. *Ann Neurol.* 2005;57(3):339–348.

110. Hwang D, Noguchi T. Tetrodotoxin poisoning. In: Taylor SL, ed. *Advances in Food and Nutrition Research.* San Diego: Academic Press; 2007:141–236.

111. Isbister GK, Kiernan MC. Neurotoxic marine poisoning. *Lancet Neurol.* 2005;4(4):219–228.

112. Aygun D, Erenler AK, Karatas AD, Baydin A. Intermediate syndrome following acute organophosphate poisoning: correlation with initial serum levels of muscle enzymes. *Basic Clin Pharmacol Toxicol.* 2007;100(3):201–204.

113. Halloran LL, Bernard DW. Management of drug-induced hyperthermia. *Curr Opin Pediatr.* 2004;16(2):211–215.

114. Hadad E, Weinbroum A, Ben-Abraham R. Drug-induced hyperthermia and muscle rigidity: a practical approach. *Eur J Emerg Med.* 2003;10(2):149–154.

115. Prosser JM, Naim M, Helfaer MA. A 14-year-old girl with agitation and hyperthermia. *Pediatr Emerg Care.* 2006;22(9): 676–679.

116. Litman RS, Rosenberg H. Malignant hyperthermia: update on susceptibility testing. *JAMA.* 2005;293(23):2918–2924.

117. Rosenberg H, Davis M, James D, et al. Malignant hyperthermia. *Orphanet J Rare Dis.* 2007;2(1):21.

118. Isbister GK, Buckley NA. The pathophysiology of serotonin toxicity in animals and humans: implications for diagnosis and treatment. *Clin Neuropharmacol.* 2005;28(5):205–214.

119. Boyer EW, Shannon M. The serotonin syndrome. *N Engl J Med.* 2005;352(11):1112–1120.

120. Isbister J, Buckley NA, Whyte IM. Serotonin toxicity: a practical approach to diagnosis and treatment. *Med J Aust.* 2007;187(6):361–365.

121. Sternbach H. The serotonin syndrome. *Am J Psychiatry.* 1991;148(6):705–713.

122. Dunkley EJC, Isbister GK, Sibbritt D, et al. The hunter serotonin toxicity criteria: simple and accurate diagnostic decision rules for serotonin toxicity. *QJM.* 2003;96(9):635–642.

123. Strawn JR, Keck PE Jr, Caroff SN. Neuroleptic malignant syndrome. *Am J Psychiatry.* 2007;164(6):870–876.

124. Nisijima K, Shioda K, Iwamura T. Neuroleptic malignant syndrome and serotonin syndrome. *Prog Brain Res.* 2007;162:81–104.

125. Cheng P-L, Hung SW, Lin LW, et al. Amantadine-induced serotonin syndrome in a patient with renal failure. *Am J Emerg Med.* 2008;26(1):112.e5–112.e6.

126. Kaufman KR, Levitt MJ, Schiltz JF, Sunderram J. Neuroleptic malignant syndrome and serotonin syndrome in the critical care setting: case analysis. *Ann Clin Psychiatry.* 2006;18(3): 201–204.

127. Gillman PK. The serotonin syndrome and its treatment. *J Psychopharmacol.* 1999;13(1):100–109.

128. Krause T, Gerbershagen MU, Fiege M, et al. Dantrolene: a review of its pharmacology, therapeutic use and new developments. *Anaesthesia.* 2004;59(4):364–373.

129. Gordon P, Frucht S. Neuroleptic malignant syndrome in advanced Parkinson's disease. *Mov Disord.* 2001;16(5):960–962.

130. Serrano-Duenas M. Neuroleptic malignant syndrome-like, or—dopaminergic malignant syndrome—due to levodopa therapy withdrawal: clinical features in 11 patients. *Parkinsonism Relat Disord.* 2003;9(3):175–178.

131. Ruha A, Yarema M. Pharmacologic treatment of acute pediatric methamphetamine toxicity. *Pediatr Emerg Care.* 2006;22(12):782–785.

132. Richards JR, Derlet RW, Duncan DR. Methamphetamine toxicity: treatment with a benzodiazepine versus a butyrophenone. *Eur J Emerg Med.* 1997;4(3):130–135.

133. O'Malley GF. Emergency department management of the salicylate-poisoned patient. *Emerg Med Clin North Am.* 2007;25(2):333–346.

134. McFee R, Caraccio TR, McGuigan MA, et al. Dying to be thin: a dinitrophenol-related fatality. *Vet Hum Toxicol.* 2004;46(5):251–254.

135. Miranda E, McIntyre IM, Parker DR, et al. Two deaths attributed to the use of 2,4 dinitrophenol. *J Anal Toxicol.* 2006;30:219–222.

CHAPTER 5

Occupational and Environmental Neurotoxicology

T. Scott Prince

INTRODUCTION

Thousands of chemicals are in regular use in occupational settings. Most of these have undergone only limited toxicological testing, and only a few have been studied specifically for their neurological effects. Clinicians and the public may generally picture heavy-industry sites, with dirty work areas and poor safety conditions, when they think of hazardous workplace exposures. However, many modern jobs, from agriculture to engineering to medical care, involve risk from chemicals with potential neurotoxic effects. On a recent list of approximately 85 commonly used types of chemicals, half listed significant neurological effects possible following exposure.[1] In addition to chemical exposure, workers are regularly exposed to physical and infectious agents that can result in neurological disease.

In a speech about risk communication given to a group of physicians, Dr. Vincent Covello from Columbia University told of a law firm recruiting members for a class-action lawsuit regarding exposure to water containing organic solvents. In the neighborhoods near the contamination, they distributed a recruitment questionnaire that asked respondents whether they, or any of their family members, had ever had a symptom such as headache, fatigue, drowsiness, loss of concentration, difficulty remembering, or unusual sensations. While many in the audience appreciated the humor of the attorneys' casting such a broad net for clients, those who evaluate patients with these symptoms may also value the story for its reflection of the difficulty faced in making specific diagnoses or determining etiology. Certainly, occupational exposures may cause well-recognized neurological syndromes that have fairly specific signs and symptoms. However, even in these cases the diagnosis is often more readily apparent if the exposure is known and the physician is aware of it.

Raising the awareness of occupational and environmental causes of disease is a challenge in the graduate and continuing education of health-care providers. A lack of emphasis during formal training, limited time for a thorough occupational and environmental history during patient visits, complexity of diagnosis, and limited research all contribute in reducing recognition of the possible links between exposure and symptoms in clinical practice.[2] Although occupational exposures can contribute to an array of common medical diagnoses, studies indicate that relatively few physicians include even basic occupational factors as part of their medical history.[3,4]

CLINICAL AND PUBLIC HEALTH APPROACH

Simply asking patients what their job is and what the significant hazards are at work[5] can provide valuable insight into exposure risk. Even more effective would

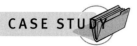

CASE STUDY

Our clinic was involved in the case of a gentleman who was hospitalized three times over the course of 6 months with severe headache, colic, numbness of the feet, and new-onset hypertension. He was diagnosed with recurrent gastrointestinal bleeding, even though no blood was ever detected in his gastrointestinal tract with multiple studies. His other symptoms were attributed primarily to his anemia and elevated blood pressure. Following his second hospitalization, he volunteered to his physicians that he had recently begun working scraping old paint off a farmhouse and even asked if the paint could contain something harmful. It was not until much later, after a veterinarian diagnosed two dogs on the farm with lead poisoning, that he was tested and found to have a blood lead level of more than 100 µg/dL. By the time this test was performed, the patient had stopped working with the paint approximately 2 months prior and was asymptomatic, with only mildly elevated blood pressure. No treatment, other than recommended continued avoidance, was given, and his blood lead level and blood pressure gradually returned to normal over the next few months.

developed countries continue to be at risk from envenomation, wild plants, trauma from animals and machinery, and exposure to agrochemicals.[14,15] High-risk exposures on the farm, particularly pesticide use, are often sporadic throughout the year, and this may contribute to less familiarity with appropriate safety precautions and personal protective equipment (PPE) use. Although agricultural production is becoming concentrated onto larger and more mechanized farms, there remain numerous part-time farmers, many of whom farm where they live. This puts the farm family, whose members often assist with the work, at risk of exposure. Even if appropriate precautions are employed during use, agrochemicals and other farm hazards remain dangerous if located near the home or if the home environment becomes contaminated.[16]

Table 1 briefly lists examples of work settings and occupations with an increased level of neurotoxin exposure. It is meant to provide an overview but is certainly not complete, nor is it as detailed as other chapters in this text. For instance, the production (mining or manufacture) of the chemical neurotoxins on the list is not included as a separate occupation, even though overexposure is clearly a concern for those workers.

If occupational exposures are suspected as a factor in a patient's condition, or if there has been an exposure and the patient is concerned about future effects, sources of information can aid in identifying the specifics of workplace exposure and its toxicity.[7,8] At many workplaces, particularly those that employ few workers or work with frequently changing chemical requirements, it is difficult for the physician or patient to discover all chemical exposures. Labels may list ingredients, although it may only be the "active" ingredients in terms of primary use while the other ingredients may still have health effects. The label may also list a contact number or Internet site for the manufacturer. If a worker is exposed while working for a company, the employer should be able to provide material safety data sheets (MSDSs) for the chemicals used. The quality of the information on the MSDSs varies, however, and may serve only as a starting point for further investigation. In addition, these do not include the intermediate products (or byproducts) of a process. Sampling of the work environment may be indicated, and an industrial hygienist can be consulted (as described later), although this typically requires the cooperation of the employer.

Uncontrolled exposures, such as those from unplanned mixtures or spills, combustion byproducts, or emergency response, may be impossible to completely specify. Knowledge of the chemistry involved of such an event, along with any available reports from similar events, can help develop a list of potential exposures. In rare instances, recreating the circumstances of the event—in a highly controlled setting and usually on a

be using one of the several available standardized questionnaires covering occupational and environmental exposure.[6–8] These may used either during the first visit for all patients or as an aid in evaluating those patients for whom toxic exposure might be a concern. Such questionnaires may also be valuable in specific settings involving ongoing exposure for which medical surveillance is indicated.

Examples exist of neurological cases involving unusual toxic exposures or sensitivities occurring across various occupational settings. However, certain occupations have been long known to carry a substantially increased risk of neurological disease. Traditional industrial manufacturing may involve exposure to numerous solvents, fumes, dusts, physical hazards, and metals. Some of these, like the combination of solvents and loud noise, have been shown to be additive or synergistic in their damage to their target organs.[9–11] Unfortunately, research into the toxicity of mixtures or combined exposures has been extremely limited.[12,13]

Another broad occupational category with significant risk from neurotoxic exposures is agriculture. Although now representing a much smaller percentage of working adults than before the industrial revolution, farmers in

Table 1: Examples of Occupational Exposures with Potential for Neurotoxic Effects

Industry or General Job Category	Specific Task or Setting	Hazardous Exposure
Agriculture	Pesticide use[17,18] Manure pits	Anticholenergics Arsenic Strychnine Hydrogen sulfide
Aviation[19]	Altitude Space flight	Hypoxia, decompression sickness Microgravity
Battery manufacture or recycling	Handling battery plates	Lead
Diving[19]	Pressure change Contaminated tanks	Decompression sickness, nitrogen narcosis, oxygen toxicity Carbon monoxide
Dry cleaning[20]	General environment	Perchloroethylene, other solvents
Electronics manufacture	Semiconductors Switches Solder	Arsenic Mercury Lead
Electroplating	Various	Arsenic, mercury, solvents
Fiberglass or rigid polyester manufacture	Resin application	Styrene[21]
Health care	Amalgams,[22] instruments Sterilizers	Mercury Ethylene oxide
Metalworking	Various	Solvents, manganese[23]
Painting or paint removal	Various	Solvents,[24] lead, arsenic
Petrochemical	Various	Solvents, fuels
Textile	Rayon production	Carbon disulfide[25]
Waste-water plant	Treatment pools	Hydrogen sulfide
Welding	Welding rods	Manganese[23]

smaller scale—may allow sampling to help determine the chemicals involved.

If a list of chemicals is known, and there is not an obvious candidate toxin for the clinical presentation, it can take effort to narrow down the potential suspects. In dealing with more organized employers, who keep lists of all their chemicals electronically, the problem may be too much nonspecific information. Patients who have obtained lists of chemicals from their place of employment may bring in multiple pages containing all chemicals used in the business. One recent patient at our clinic brought in a list supplied by the employer containing 7960 products, with more than 15,000 different chemical constituents. Faced with such a list, the patient, family member, coworkers, supervisor, or health and safety official at the company may need to be enlisted in narrowing down the number of suspect chemicals to those that represent significant exposures for the particular patient.

Evaluating exposures from work in the more distant past presents its own set of challenges. Patients may not remember their exposures, which may be complicated because their exposures may have affected their ability to remember (or, rarely, even made them delusional). Records are typically not as detailed; route, frequency, duration, and extent of exposure usually have to be estimated based on incomplete information. Again, the employer, family members, or coworkers; union records; or general knowledge of the processes used in that job or industry in the past may be required to characterize the possible degree of exposure. In the case of industrial exposure, there may be a public record of prior inspections of the company, usually by either the National Institute of Occupational Safety and Health (NIOSH) or the Occupational Safety and Health Administration (OSHA). (Note: The state in which the industry is located may have a state "OSHA" program rather than use the federal program.) This record can provide at least a snapshot of information about past hazards.

INDUSTRIAL HYGIENE

If available, usually the most valuable resource to assist in identifying relevant industrial exposures, as well as providing estimates of dose and duration, is an industrial hygienist familiar with the facility or specific process. Industrial hygienists can quantify the degree to which specific exposures are present and are likely to be significant for each of the processes or areas in a facility. They may be the best source for details of past chemicals that were used and types of risks that existed in prior processes. They can also detail the frequency and routes of present and past exposure. The route of exposure is often important for determining the toxic effects expected, assessing the ability of environmental sampling methods to accurately estimate the dose, and directing preventive measures to reduce future exposures.

While often not available, industrial hygiene sampling results from the worksite can be extremely valuable is characterizing exposure and risk. When considering a workplace sampling, several issues must be kept in mind, both in analyzing past results and, when possible, in obtaining additional samples. While most sampling is done to measure airborne concentrations, many neurotoxins, particularly solvents and other lipophilic compounds, readily penetrate the skin. Thus, skin absorption may contribute a larger part of the total dose than does inhalation. For the chemicals for which the American Conference of Industrial Hygienists has recommended threshold limit values, there is a special "skin" designation.[26] Ingestion of the toxin may also be a concern, especially if eating and drinking are allowed in the work area, there is cross-contamination of workers' dining or break areas, or potentially contaminated clothing is worn away from the work area.

Environmental results must also be considered by the *who, what, when,* and *where* used in obtaining the sample. Samples should be from the workers performing the same tasks (with the same methods and equipment) as the patient. Analysis should include which chemicals were sampled during which process and whether other possible contributing exposures were not sampled. Ideally, samples should be taken during both typical and peak exposure conditions, with the industrial hygienist calculating appropriate time-weighting of the exposure. Based on the hours worked, adjustments may also be needed to the recommended levels used for comparison to the sampling results, as these are often based on a 40-hour workweek and need to be adjusted downward for longer exposure times. This is particularly important when the combination of the chemicals' biological half-life and a significantly increased workday or workweek could prevent the worker from clearing a metabolized toxin before the next set of exposures. Finally, respiratory samples taken from the worker's breathing zone are more useful than the less specific "monitor on a pole" work area results.

When possible to obtain, biological sampling bypasses many of these problems. Generally performed on blood, exhaled air, or urine, these tests measure the presence of a chemical, its metabolite, or an associated biochemical alteration. While such tests can estimate the dose received by the individual more accurately than environmental samples, tests are not available for all substances and the timing and handling of samples is important. In addition, one must be aware of *other* substances and metabolic pathways that could contribute to the resultant level of the measured chemical because it may be a marker for several different exposures. Even when a toxin or its marker metabolite is detected, good reference data for what is typical, which distinguishes a normal or nonhazardous result from a toxic result, is often lacking, especially for newer or less studied compounds. For instance, a measurement may indicated the presence of a toxin at a level greater than the background environmental level expected, but it may be unknown as to whether the level measured is definitively linked to neurotoxic outcomes. Use of specific biological tests for diagnosis and their issues of interpretation are discussed further in the relevant chapters.

Beyond assisting with the diagnosis, the industrial hygienist can aid in reducing or eliminating any harmful exposure discovered. Typically, the approach is to control a hazardous exposure, which involves reducing or eliminating the exposure broadly for the area or task at risk and thus potentially prevents disease in many other workers.[27] The first and most definitive option is to eliminate the exposure by changing the process, often by substituting a less toxic alternative. While this procedure often makes discovering exposures from the distant past difficult, it is generally effective in reducing future risk for workers. Altering the process through engineering controls such as enclosures, enhanced ventilation, or reduced liquid or dust buildup can be effective and does not rely on worker compliance. When the concentration of the toxin in the work environment cannot be effectively lowered, workers should use PPE. The choice of PPE must be evaluated carefully by the industrial hygienist to match the type, route, and frequency of exposure, and workers must be trained and supported in the proper sizing, use, and maintenance of the PPE. In addition, administrative controls, such as limiting the time an employee can be in an area, may be employed, but this is more difficult to monitor and enforce and should not replace the more effective methods described previously. However, in the rare case of an individual patient with a particularly high sensitivity or susceptibility to an exposure level that is otherwise felt to clearly be safe and acceptable for the other workers, the appropriate administrative response might be to move the affected worker to an area with no exposure.

ADDITIONAL RESOURCES

When trying to garner additional information regarding an exposure and its effects, government, professional, and academic institutions, often working in partnership, provide several avenues for efficiently and quickly accessing information. The NIOSH and the Agency for Toxic Substances and Disease Registry sections of the Centers for Disease Control's Web site (www.cdc.gov) have extensive information on occupational hazards and links to several toxicology databases. The National Library of Medicine has the familiar PubMed (www.pubmed.gov) searches of the medical literature and offers Toxnet (toxnet.nlm.nih.gov), which searches multiple databases and has links to other toxicology resources. One particularly useful strategy on these National Library of Medicine sites is to perform searches from both directions of your clinical case: searching by symptoms, clinical findings, or diagnosis for etiologic factors and by exposures, looking for reported cases with similar clinic presentation. Other valuable online sources include the Extension Toxicology Network (extoxnet.orst.edu/ghindex.html; extensive information on pesticides), the U.S. Environmental Protection Agency (www.epa.gov), and OSHA (www.OSHA.gov). While poison control centers typically focus on acute exposures and their effects, they may also be helpful with questions regarding specific chronic exposures.

DEVELOPING COUNTRIES

The task of discovering and evaluating toxicity from occupational exposures becomes even more challenging in less developed areas of the world. Before industrialization, a significant majority of the working population of an area was involved in obtaining food through subsistence farming, fishing, and hunting. These activities, while quite hazardous from a trauma or injury perspective, only rarely resulted in exposure to significant amounts of neurotoxins (particularly if biotoxins, such as venoms, are excluded). As more industry developed in an area, there was the corresponding increased risk of exposure to industrial chemicals.[28] Even those workers who remained in farming become more focused on cash crops, with increased use of manufactured fertilizers and pesticides.

Risk of industrial exposure in less developed countries is usually greater because of several factors.[28,29] There may be fewer legal restrictions on workplace hazards, as well as fewer resources to enforce the regulations that do exist, including allowing children to work in areas in which they may be particularly sensitive to the exposures. There may be no required worker education for known hazards; even labels for ingredients may be missing, incomplete, or in a language unfamiliar to the worker. Engineering controls are less advanced, and PPE is generally less available. Hours may be long, allowing less recovery time from the exposures. The metabolism and excretion of toxins may be adversely affected by factors external to the work, such as malnutrition or other environmental exposures.

In addition, occupational health services and medical surveillance in less developed areas is uncommon, allowing conditions to progress further before detected. Limited medical treatment resources, for treatment of both acute emergency exposures and chronic conditions, worsen outcomes and lead to greater morbidity and mortality. Financial and social pressure to work may be great,[30] with few social support systems to assist those who should not or cannot continue to work. An unfortunate corporate response to increasing cost of production, including improved occupational and environmental health and safety regulations, may be to move production to countries (or areas within a country) with less regulation. While this may lower corporate costs for labor and legal compliance, it results in more worker exposure, greater environmental contamination, and higher human and societal costs.

CONCLUSION

While occupationally related neurological disease may present in an obvious fashion, symptoms, clinical findings, and their association to the relevant exposure are often subtle. Tracing the condition back to the workplace can require knowledge, willingness to maintain a reasonable index of suspicion, additional time and effort in taking the history, investigation of other information resources, and assistance of other health and safety professionals. In addition to correctly identifying the cause of the disease and perhaps providing the opportunity for more specific clinical treatment, this effort is worthwhile because reducing or eliminating the exposure is a critical, and sometimes the only option available, to preventing disease progression. Identification can also have a beneficial multiplier effect, protecting many other workers with similar exposures and preventing future disease through industrial hygiene measures. The preventive emphasis on avoidance of known neurotoxic exposure is especially important in developing areas of the world where resources for worker protection, surveillance, diagnosis, and treatment are limited.

REFERENCES

1. Frumkin H, McCunney R, Barbanel C. Health effects of common substances. In: McCunney R, ed. *A Practical Approach to Occupational and Environmental Medicine* (ed 2). Boston, Mass: Little, Brown; 1994:709–733.
2. Harber P, Merz B. Time and knowledge barriers to recognizing occupational disease. *J Occup Environ Med.* 2001;43:285–288.
3. Demers RY, Wall SJ. Occupational history-taking in a family practice occupational setting. *J Med Educ.* 1983;58:151–153.
4. Politi BJ, Arena VC, Schwerha J, Sussman N. Occupational medical history taking: how are today's physicians doing? A cross-sectional investigation of the frequency of occupational history-taking by physicians in a major U.S. teaching center. *J Occup Environ Med.* 2004;46:550–555.
5. Goldstein, B. The second question of the occupational history: what is the riskiest part of your job? *J Occup Environ Med.* 2007;49:1060–1062.
6. Rosenstock L, Logerfo J, Heyer NJ, Carter WB. Development and validation of a self-administered occupational health history questionnaire. *J Occup Med.* 1984;26:50–54.
7. Frank AL. Taking an exposure history. In: Balk S, ed. *Case Studies in Environmental Medicine.* Atlanta: Agency for Toxic Substances and Disease Registry; 1992:1–55.
8. Feldman R. *Occupational and Environmental Neurotoxicology.* Philadelphia: Lippincott-Raven; 1999:466–474.
9. Barregård L, Axelsson A. Is there an ototraumatic interaction between noise and solvents? *Scand Audiol.* 1984;3:151–155.
10. Prasher D, Al-Hajjaj H, Aylott S, Aksentijevic A. Effects of exposure to a mixture of solvents and noise on hearing and balance in aircraft maintenance workers. *Noise Health.* 2005;7:31–39.
11. Hodgkinson L, Prasher D. Effects of industrial solvents on hearing and balance: a review. *Noise Health.* 2006;8:114–133.
12. Hansen H, De Rose CT, Pohl H, et al. Public health challenges posed by chemical mixtures. *Environ Health Perspect.* 1998;106:1271–1280.
13. Cory-Slechta, DA. Studying toxicants as single chemicals: does this strategy adequately identify neurotoxic risk? *Neurotoxicology.* 2005;26:491–510.
14. Frank AL, Mcknight R, Kirkhorn S, Gunderson P. Issues of agricultural safety and health. *Annu Rev Public Health.* 2004;25:225–245.
15. Prince, S. Overview of hazards for those working in agriculture. In: Lessenger J, ed. *Agriculture Medicine.* Porterville, CA: Springer; 2006:29–34.
16. Curwin BD, Hein MJ, Sanderson WT, et al. Urinary pesticide concentrations among children, mothers and fathers living in farm and non-farm households in Iowa. *Ann Occup Hyg.* 2007;51:53–65.
17. Ahasan MR, Partanen T. Occupational health and safety in the least developed countries: a simple case of neglect. *J Epidemiol.* 2001;11:74–80.
18. Katz NB, Katz O, Mandel S. Neurotoxicity of chemicals commonly used in agriculture. In: Lessenger J, ed. *Agriculture Medicine.* Porterville, CA: Springer; 2006:300–323.
19. Jaffee MS. The neurology of aviation, underwater, and space environments. *Neurol Clin.* 2005;23:541–552.
20. Echeverria D, White RF, Sampaio C. A behavioural evaluation of PCE exposure in patients and dry cleaners: a possible relationship between clinical and preclinical effects. *J Occup Environ Med.* 1995;37:667–680.
21. Viaene MK, Pauwels W, Veulemans H, et al. Neurobehavioural changes and persistence of complaints in workers exposed to styrene in a polyester boat building plant: influence of exposure characteristics and microsomal epoxide hydrolase phenotype. *Occup Environ Med.* 2001;58:103–112.
22. Joshi A, Douglass CW, Kim HD, et al. The relationship between amalgam restorations and mercury levels in male dentists and nondental health professionals. *J Public Health Dent.* 2003;63:52–60.
23. Levy BS, Nassetta WJ. Neurologic effects of manganese in humans: a review. *Int J Occup Environ Health.* 2003;9:153–163.
24. Trieberg G, Barocka A, Erbguth F, et al. Neurotoxicity of solvent mixtures in spray painters: II. Neurologic psychiatric, psychological, and neuroradiological findings. *Int Arch Occup Environ Health.* 199;64:361–372.
25. Agency for Toxic Substances and Disease Registry. *Toxicological Profile for Carbon Disulfide.* Atlanta: ATSDR; 1992:36–145.
26. American Conference of Governmental Industrial Hygienists. 2007 TLVs and BEIs. Cincinnati, Conn: ACGIH; 2007:10–73.
27. Futlon L (revision by Hammond SK). Gases, vapors, and solvents. In: Polg, B, ed. *Fundamentals of Industrial Hygiene.* 5th ed. National Safety Council; 2002:164–167.
28. London L, Kisting S. Ethical concerns in international health and safety. *Occup Med.* 2000;17:587–600.
29. Frumkin H, Levy BS, Levenstein C. Occupational and environmental health in eastern Europe: challenges and opportunities. *Am J Ind Med.* 1991;20:265–270.
30. Levy BS. Global occupational health issues: working in partnership to prevent illness and injury. *AAOHN J.* 1996;44:244–247.

Developmental Neurotoxicity

Asit K. Tripathy and Sumit Parikh

INTRODUCTION

There is growing concern over worsening environmental chemical exposures. Industrial and agricultural activities continue to produce increasing amounts of potentially toxic waste, with the U.S. Environmental Protection Agency (EPA) reporting 4.44 billion pounds of waste released into the environment in 2003.[1] Multiple chemicals are routinely used in food, clothing, personal care, and household goods. Hazardous waste sites are appearing ever closer to communities, with the Agency for Toxic Substances and Disease Registry (ATSDR) estimating 3 million to 4 million children living within 1 mile of at least one such site.[2]

At the same time, the incidence of congenital malformations; neurological, developmental behavioral disorders such as attention-deficit/hyperactivity disorder (ADHD) and autism; and systemic disorders such as asthma and cancer are increasing.[3] It is by no means a stretch of the imagination to connect these increasing pediatric morbidities to ever-increasing neurotoxic exposures. In fact, environmental conditions are likely one of the key determinants of a child's developmental and neurological health.[4]

The child's brain is more vulnerable to the harmful effects of these exposures than is the brain of an adult. Pediatric brain growth is occurring at its fastest during fetal development and childhood. This time represents a critical period for brain formation and maturation. Chemical exposures at this time directly interfere with the developing cerebral architecture by altering gene expression and protein production. It is this effect that leads to the focused vulnerability in the pediatric population. This risk of injury extends to include the preconception and prenatal periods.

Add to these facts the consideration that the pediatric patient has developing organs, altered metabolic capabilities, a smaller physical size, and risky behaviors, and it is easy to understand why the fetus and child are prime targets for toxin-mediated neural injury. These particular characteristics of the fetus and child lead to a neurological vulnerability that does not exist in the adult patient. And without ways yet to reverse the injury or block the effects of the exposure, the consequences include long-standing and chronically disabling neurological problems.

CHILDREN ARE UNIQUE

Age-independent Vulnerabilities

Even before considering the child's developing brain and its critical vulnerability, several aspects of the developing child's milieu lead to a unique susceptibility to toxin-mediated morbidity.

The Parent and Caregiver

A child, even before conception and birth, is at the parent's mercy—both in regards to being shielded from toxins in the environment and in regards to receiving the proper evaluation and care after an exposure. Common exposures such as secondhand tobacco smoke, excessive sunlight, pesticides at home, and take-home occupational exposures all occur without the child's direct involvement.[5] What the pregnant mother ingests is out of the child's hands. The dependence of the child on the adult to provide a safe environment for brain growth both in utero and through development cannot be understated.

Supermetabolism

Infants and children breathe more air, drink more water, and eat more food per kilogram of body weight than adults. An infant breathes twice as fast as an adult. A child in the first year drinks seven times more water per kilogram

---

Table 1:   Physiological Differences Between Children and Adults

	Infants	Children	Teens	Adults
Surface area–to–body mass ratio (m²/kg)[a]	Newborn = 0.067	Young child = 0.047	Older child = 0.033	Adult = 0.025
RESPIRATORY VENTILATION RATES				
Respiratory volume (mL/kg/breath)[b] Alveolar surface area (m²)[c] Respiration rate (breaths/min)[d] Respiratory minute ventilation rate[e]	10 3 40 133	— — — —	— — — —	2 10 75 2
DRINKING WATER (TAP)				
Mean intake (mL/kg/day)[f]	<1 year 43.5	1–10 years 35.5	11–19 years 18.2	20–64 years 19.9
FRUIT CONSUMPTION (G/KG/DAY)[G]				
Citrus fruit Other fruit (including apples) Apples	<1 year 1.9 12.9 5.0	3–5 years 2.6 5.8 3.0	12–19 years 1.1 1.1 0.4	40–69 years 0.9 1.3 0.4
SOIL INGESTION (MG/DAY)[H] **PICA (IN CHILD)**				
Outdoor[h] Indoor[h]	— — — —	5000 2.5 years 50 60	— — — —	— — 20[i] 0.4
Difference in gastrointestinal absorption of lead	0–2 years 42–53%	2–6 years 30–40% 6–7 years 18–24%	— —	— 7–15%

[a]Square meters per kilogram.
[b]Milliliters per kilogram per breath.
[c]Per square meter.
[d]Breaths per minute.
[e]Milliliters per kilogram of body weight per square meter of lung surface area per minute.
[f]Milliliters per kilogram per day.
[g]Grams per kilogram per day.
[h]Milligrams per day.
[i]Gardening for adults.
Adapted from the Agency for Toxic Substances and Disease Registry. (www.atsdr.cdc.gov)

than an adult. Compared to an adult, a child, in the first several years of life, consumes up to four times more food per kilogram. These characteristics all allow a higher level of environmental exposure, whether through inhalation or ingestion.[6] Additional details are provided in Table 1.

The infant is also vulnerable to dermal toxins—and with a highly permeable skin and developing dermal layer, toxins such as lindane and hexachlorophene easily enter the bloodstream and enter the brain.[6]

As children grow older, their evolving body composition and biochemistry continue to affect the absorption, distribution, storage, metabolism, and excretion of chemicals differently than they do for their adult counterparts.[7] Organ system function, such as hepatic detoxification, improves over time but often at different rates. The child's detoxification immaturity may even be a mixed blessing. While caffeine often persists in the infant for longer than in the adult, the infant's inability to metabolize substances such as acetaminophen can offer resistance to fatal hepatic injury. Thus, the toxicity of a certain compound may vary significantly due to the altered pharmacokinetics in the child.[8]

Risky Behaviors

Infants and children maintain a fairly homogenous diet that often allows for focused exposure—especially if a toxin is unique to the most frequently ingested food.[9] Children spend more time on the ground and in the outdoors than do adults. Their lack of mobility leads to repeat exposures, often in an area with a concentrated exposure to a toxin. With an evolving sense of judgment, certain ingestions and environmental exposures only occur during adolescence.

Long Life

Since children have longer to live than adults, an exposure to a certain chemical or toxin has a longer time to express injury. Certain toxins leech into bones and adipocytes, which cause symptoms over time.[10] Children may present with symptoms much later in life than when the exposure occurred. A commonly cited example of this phenomenon is the radiation exposure in Russia from the Chernobyl plant meltdown in 1996. These children had a higher rate of adult-onset thyroid cancer.[11] A more common exposure such as tobacco smoke can accumulate over time as well, increasing the child's risk of morbidity from asthma and cancer later in life.[12]

Age-dependent Vulnerabilities

In addition to the risks described in the preceding section, each stage of brain development and transition through the various milestones of childhood brings with it unique dangers that evolve as the child develops. A summary of the risks associated with each milestone is provided in Table 2.

Preconception Period

Oogonia only fully develop during fetal life; thus, they remain vulnerable to environmental injury until ovulation. Spermatogonia are also at risk of toxin-mediated deleterious effects. Paternal exposures can also cause transmission of certain toxins in seminal fluid. These exposures can lead to varying amounts of male and female infertility, increased spontaneous abortion rates, and genetic damage that may produce a chromosomal abnormality.[13]

Fetal and Newborn Periods

The fetus is unique in that it is undergoing the most critical brain development and is at the mercy of its host—the mother-to-be. This relationship leads to certain vulnerabilities that can only occur during this period. All nutrients needed for development and growth come from the placenta. While the placenta offers some protection against unwanted exposures, it is not an effective barrier against many toxins. This was quickly discovered after the consequences of in utero thalidomide exposure in the 1950s and 1960s.[14]

The placenta easily permits low-molecular-weight substances such as carbon monoxide and fat-soluble substances such as hydrocarbons and ethanol. Its ability to provide a detoxifying role is limited.[15] Placental characteristics such as blood flow, permeability, and metabolism all affect the transfer of chemicals to the fetus. These characteristics do not remain static during the pregnancy but change as the gestation progresses.[15] Many compounds identified as neurotoxins in adults can pass through the placenta rapidly and reach the fetal circulation upon exposure of the mother—including exposures in the workplace.[16] In addition, lipophilic substances, including specific pesticides and halogenated compounds such as polychlorinated biphenyls (PCBs), accumulate in the maternal adipose tissue, resulting in sustained exposure to the developing infant that exceeds the mother's own exposure by a 100-fold on the basis of body weight.[17]

Certain fetal exposures also occur independently of the placenta—including heat, noise, and ionizing radiation.[18] Apart from the immature and developing brain and placenta, the blood–brain barrier is developing. While an effective guardian against certain toxins in adults, it is not completely formed until 12 months after birth and thus offers ineffective protection to the developing newborn and infant.[19]

Infant and Toddler Periods

Infants and toddlers eat more and grow faster than children do during any other point in life. To allow optimal nutrient absorption, the intestines have a larger vascular supply. Infants and toddlers breathe faster and have a larger intake of food and water per kilogram of body weight compared to adults.[6] These "normal"

Table 2: Hazardous Exposure Susceptibility and Anticipatory Guidance by Age

Developmental Stage	Developmental Characteristics	Vulnerabilities	Anticipatory Guidance
Preconception	—	Male and female parental reproductive systems Occupational, environmental, and vocational exposures Pharmaceuticals Substance abuse	Dietary advisories (mercury and PCBs)
Fetal	Rapid	Dividing cells sensitive to transplacental carcinogens Developing reproductive system that can lead to transgenerational effects Critical periods of organ development Brain development: Immature blood–brain barrier Placenta as semipermeable membrane	Dietary advisories (mercury and PCBs) Occupational, environmental, and vocational exposures Take-home occupational exposures Pharmaceuticals and herbal and alternative remedies Substance abuse Topical insect repellants Baseline household environmental survey Maternal exposures during preparation of nursery and other remodeling (lead and volatile organic compounds)
Newborn (birth–2 months)	Nonambulatory Restricted environment High calorie and water intake High air intake Highly permeable skin Alkaline gastric secretions (low gastric acidity)	Brain development • Immature blood–brain barrier • Synapse formation Lungs • Alveolar development • Lung fluid cleared by pulmonary lymphatic system High respiratory rate Gastrointestinal tract: Highly permeable, increased pH Immature detoxification capacity of liver, kidney, and digestive system Skin • Permeable with large surface-to-volume ratio • Contaminants used or deposited on floor, specially household products, pesticides, and take-home occupational agents	Consider day care and home indoor and outdoor environments Ingestion • Breast milk • Infant formula (tap- or well-water contaminants) Respiratory • Indoor air contaminants, especially those layering near the floor (e.g., mercury, pesticides, allergens, radon, asbestos, take-home occupational agents) • Outdoor air pollutants, especially ozone and particulates

Table 2: Hazardous Exposure Susceptibility and Anticipatory Guidance by Age—cont'd

Developmental Stage	Developmental Characteristics	Vulnerabilities	Anticipatory Guidance
Infant or toddler (2 months–2 years)	Crawling and early walking Oral exploration Limited diet High intake of fruits and vegetables	Brain development • Immature blood–brain barrier • Synapse formation Lungs: Alveolar development High respiratory rate Skin: Permeable with large surface-to-volume ratio Small intestine that avidly absorbs lead if diet is deficient in iron or calcium Immature detoxification Capacity of liver, kidney, and digestive system	Consider day care and home indoor and outdoor environments Ingestion • Pesticides on fruit and vegetables • Tap-water contaminants • Contaminants on floor and within easy reach, especially medicines, household products, pesticides, lead, and take-home occupational agents • Pica Respiratory • Indoor air contaminants, especially those layering near the floor (e.g., mercury, pesticides, allergens, radon, asbestos, take-home occupational agents) • Outdoor air pollutants, especially ozone and particulates Skin • Contaminants on floor and within reach, especially household products, pesticides, and take-home occupational agents • Topical insect repellents
Young child (2–6 years)	Expanded environment, still includes significant time on floor Increased independence High intake of fruits and vegetables	Brain developing Lungs: Alveolar development and increasing volume Small intestine that avidly absorbs lead if is diet deficient in iron or calcium Immature detoxification capacity of liver, kidney, and gastrointestinal system	Consider home, day care, and preschool, and playmates' indoor and outdoor environments Ingestion • Pesticides on fruit and vegetables • Tap-water contaminants • Contaminants on floor and within easy reach, especially medicines, household products, pesticides, lead, and take-home occupational agents • Pica Respiratory • Indoor air contaminants, especially those layering near the floor (e.g., mercury, pesticides, allergens, radon, asbestos, take-home occupational agents) • Outdoor air pollutants, especially ozone and particulates Skin • Contaminants on floor and within reach, especially household products, pesticides, and take-home occupational agents • Topical insect repellents

Continued

Chapter 6 • Developmental Neurotoxicity

Table 2:	Hazardous Exposure Susceptibility and Anticipatory Guidance by Age—cont'd		
Developmental Stage	Developmental Characteristics	Vulnerabilities	Anticipatory Guidance
School-age child (6–12 years)	Increased number of environments and less supervised play: school, playground, friends' houses	Brain developing Lungs: Increased volume	Consider home, school, friends', and afterschool programs' indoor and outdoor environments Ingestion • Tap water • Food Respiratory • Indoor and outdoor air quality • Hazards associated with hobbies and school crafts • Take-home occupational hazards Skin • Hazards associated with hobbies and school crafts • Take-home occupational hazards • Topical insect repellants
Adolescent (12–18 years)	Puberty Accelerated growth Experimentation with controlled substances Independence and exposure to multiple environments Possible employment, such as work in family business or training in hazardous trades	Brain and lungs continue to develop Muscles and bones grow rapidly Gonadal maturation Breast development Ova and sperm maturation	Consider home, school, friends, occupational, and trade school environments Ingestion • Tap water • Food • Occupational hazards ingested because of poor hygiene • Substance abuse Respiratory • Indoor and outdoor quality • Occupational and trade school hazards • Take-home occupational exposures • Hazards associated with hobbies and school crafts • Substance abuse Skin • Occupational and trade school hazards • Take-home occupational exposures • Hazards associated with hobbies and school crafts • Topical insect repellents

PCB, polychlorinated biphenyl.
Adapted from Bearer CF. Environmental health hazards: how children are different from adults. *Future Child*. 1995;5(2):11–26.

physiological functions work against the child in relation to neurotoxin exposure.

A child's higher respiratory rate leads to increased exposures to inhaled pollutants. Early respiratory exposures to air contaminants such as insect antigens have shown a higher incidence of asthma compared to exposures later in life.[3] With more time spent on the ground or close to the floor, certain inhalants, such as mercury, may be taken in at higher concentrations.[20]

The infant's and child's menu of food choices is limited in variety, sometimes by choice and sometimes by necessity. The infant's primary means of sustenance is either breast milk or formula. Breast milk may be contaminated by both historic and current maternal exposures—including occupational ones.[16] DDT, hexachlorobenzene, PCBs, and metals like lead and mercury can be found in human milk.[21] Lactation can mobilize sequestered fat-soluble toxins such as dioxins, PCBs, and bone lead. Breast milk concentrations of certain chemicals, such as methylmercury, are 3- to 10-fold higher than corresponding maternal blood levels.[22,23]

The bulk of infant formula comes in powdered form and is prepared by adding a fixed quantity of water. An infant's daily intake of water may be up to 180 mL/kg/day, which is the equivalent of an adult drinking 35 cans of soda per day (considering a typical soda can is 12 fluid ounces).[18] Heavy metal contaminants in water supplies, typically from lead in old pipe joints and fixtures, are ingested. When private well water is used, the amount of contaminants from surrounding water sources is often not known since wells are typically unregulated.[24]

The older infant and child has a larger per kilogram body weight ingestion of fruits, grains, and vegetables compared to adults.[6] Any exposure to residual pesticides in these items is thus higher as well. For these reasons, the U.S. Food Quality Protection Act of 1996 set separate pesticide limits to account for levels ingested by infants and children.[25]

Infants and children have a larger surface area of skin per kilogram of body weight than do adults, allowing for a higher surface area for potential dermal exposures. Their skin is not as protected due to a still-developing keratin layer.[6] An infant's and young child's skin thus absorbs faster and larger amounts of applied chemicals. Examples of such exposures include the use of hexachlorophene in the 1950s in skin cleansers for newborns (to prevent staphylococcal infection), which then led to vacuolizations forming in the nervous system.[26,27] Today, betadine scrubs are known to cause hypothyroidism in infants.[28]

Other behaviors unique to the infant and child include mouthing of objects and frequent hand–mouth contact. Thus, exposures to oral nonfood items are common and may include outright pica. Outdoors, this exposure may be soil.[1] The indoor and outdoor environment may also be contaminated with lead paint, chips, or dust particles; pesticides; take-home contaminants; and home-cleaning products.[29]

Childhood Period

Since exploratory behaviors only expand as the child develops, the susceptibility to environmental exposures only increases. Again, with more time spent outdoors, air pollutants and exposure to soil and dust contaminants remains high. While their respiratory drive and food intake has decreased some, it is still higher than adult amounts. With time spent at schools, playgrounds, and afterschool centers, unique exposures exist that do not occur for the rest of the family.[22]

Adolescent Period

The statement that adolescents are known risk-takers is an understatement. Their nature of exploring takes an exponential leap over that of young children. These behaviors include exposures to new environments beyond the home and school (abandoned buildings, warehouses, factories) and experimentation with drugs and alcohol. Some of these exposures may include items not typically considered drugs of abuse, such as inhalants from glue, gasoline, and aerosol cans.[24] Some of these are items used for advanced hobbies, such as model-building. With increasing use of alternative and performance-enhancing supplements, these substances can also lead to neurological symptoms. For example, creatine ingestion has been known to cause headaches, migraines, and renal injury.

With the teen years come afterschool jobs and the added need to consider exposures in a work environment. Adolescents, for various reasons, have more occupational injuries than adults.[30]

CHILDREN'S BRAINS ARE UNIQUE

To add insult to injury, aside from the pediatric vulnerabilities discussed earlier, the fetus, infant, and child has a brain that is immature. The adult brain has many mechanisms in place to protect itself from exposures that do not yet exist in the child. With mature cellular-tight junctions, active cerebrospinal fluid production and resorption, normal neurotransmitter function, and a functional blood–brain barrier, the adult brain maintains a resistance to toxins not possible in the fetus and child. In fact, the blood–brain barrier does not even mature until a child is a year old, and neurotransmitter function normalizes over the first several years.[31]

The fetus and child have a brain undergoing what is perhaps the most critical period of growth and development. The fetus undergoes a finely tuned and carefully choreographed set of genetic events allowing the sequential expression of unique proteins involved in brain development. These genes allow the almost simultaneous but well-synchronized and essential processes of neural tube formation, prosencephalon development, neuronal migration, and cortical organization.[32] The bulk of this development occurs in the first trimester, especially during the initial 6 weeks of gestation. Disruption of this sequence has devastating consequences. Later gestational development involves further neuronal maturation and cell growth, which is also critical to the neurologically functional child.

In the postnatal years, brain development involves neuronal pruning, arborization, and maturation of myelination.[33] The number of synaptic connections between neurons reaches a peak around 2 years. Similarly, great postnatal activity occurs in the development of receptors and transmitter systems, as well as in the production of myelin. Progressive myelination of axons results in considerable increases in cortical white matter through adolescence and into adulthood, along with improved signal transmission speeds and the ability to develop higher levels of cortical functioning.[33]

Toxic agents that injure the developing brain typically interfere with one or more of these tasks. It is often assumed that the impact of toxins on the developing brain is an all-or-none phenomenon. However, neurotoxins typically produce a range of problems—from mild to severe, impairing either one or many of the previously described developmental milestones.[31,34,35]

The severity of the injury often depends on the timing of the exposure. Typically, the earlier in development the exposure occurs, the larger the neurological deficit. The first month of gestation, being a time of critical brain organo- and histogenesis, is that key period—with exposures then leading to gross malformations of cortex development.[36] Exposures in the second half of gestation, even by the same toxin, impair growth and differentiation, often leading to altered functions of the mature structure.[36] However, the overall brain structures form intact. If the exposure occurs at a key portion of early brain formation, the effect often outweighs what is expected for the typical dose response.[37]

For example, both lead and alcohol cause more injury to the early developing brain, typically during the first 6 weeks of gestation, than the amount of injury sustained after an identical exposure in the second or third trimesters.[38] Early exposure to alcohol affects overall brain size and may lead to varying amounts of structural brain defects, along with the systemic fetal alcohol syndrome. Exposures to alcohol during later developmental periods alter central nervous system function in a manner that causes severe neuronal and behavioral changes but spares overall brain and fetal growth.[39] While these children are often learning impaired, there are minimal morphological findings indicating this exposure occurred.[40]

Heavy metals such as lead, mercury, and manganese directly disrupt biochemical processes, interrupt neural cell migration, and prevent synaptogenesis but do not cause gross structural malformation.[1,41] Such disruptions impair learning, coordination, and fine neurological tasks. Late exposure to radiation is known to mostly affect cell differentiation, while alcohol impairs cell migration.[37]

SYMPTOMS OF BRAIN DYSFUNCTION

Symptoms exhibited by a child, as in adults, can be wide and varied. Certain toxins can lead to acute or subacute onset of almost any neurological symptoms.

These include encephalopathy and delirium, movement disorders, focal neuropathies, and seizures.[42]

Long-term exposures, however, lead to behavioral problems and cognitive difficulties. As discussed earlier, in utero exposures lead to varying amounts of malformations, growth disruption, and more subtle cellular changes in neurological function. These alterations lead to behavior, learning, and attention problems.[43] The consequences of these chronic problems are school failure, diminished economic productivity, and risk of antisocial and criminal behavior.[19]

Of the 4 million children born in the United States each year, 3% to 8% have neurological developmental problems.[44] In addition, among all live births, 3% have one or more congenital malformations at birth. Up to 10% of these findings appear to be related to in utero exposures to exogenous factors like drugs, infections, ionizing radiations, and environmental factors.[45] With increasing numbers of autism spectrum disorders, attention deficit disorder, and learning disabilities, estimated to be up to 17% of the U.S. pediatric population by the Centers for Disease Control and Prevention (CDC), there is a concern that the etiology in some of these individuals is due to the increasing chemical exposures.[14]

Various toxins, after chronic exposure, can lead to alterations in neurocognitive functioning, including impaired attention, memory, and emotional lability. These effects may also coexist with other focal neurological abnormalities, including neuropathies with arsenic, tremors with mercury, and incoordination with organophosphates.[4] The same toxin may contribute to either acute or chronic symptoms based on the dose to which the child is exposed. For example, lead's effect on the developing brain of infant and toddler is well known, and toxicity in childhood often leads to short attention span, deficit in intellectual function, and increased risk of antisocial behavior.[41] Acute lead poisoning, on the other hand, leads to listlessness, drowsiness, and irritability, followed by seizures and increased intracranial pressure.[46]

Lists of the most common toxic exposures in the United States are shown in Tables 3 and 4. Acute and chronic symptoms of a variety of these neurotoxins are explored in detail in other sections of this book.

EVALUATION AND TESTING

Most patients, including the pediatric ones, present with various signs and symptoms that may include a toxin exposure in the differential diagnosis. When presented with an intoxicated or encephalopathic-appearing individual, toxin exposures are often at the forefront of the differential. However, when presented with a child with

Table 3: The 10 Categories of Pediatric Exposures Most Commonly Reported to Pediatric Environmental Health Specialty Units (PEHSUs) in the United States[*]

PEHSU Category	Total U.S. Exposures Reported
Lead	219
Fungus or mold	112
Gases or fumes	55
Mercury	48
Indoor air contaminants	48
Pesticides	35
Arsenic	28
Water toxins	23
Perchlorate	7
Soil toxins	7
Total	**582**

[*]These 10 categories account for 582 (94%) of the 616 children involved in calls to PEHSUs between April 1, 2004, and March 31, 2005. Data from Wilborne-Davis P Agency for Toxic Substances and Disease Registry quarterly reports for PEHSU Program (through cooperative agreement U50/ATU 300014 with the Association of Occupational and Environmental Clinics). Submitted October 2005.

Table 4: The 20 Most Dangerous Nonpharmaceutical Environmental Substances[*]

Substance	Overall Outcome
Ethanol (beverage)	532
Carbon monoxide	181
Bleach: Hypochlorite (liquid and dry)	153
Mushroom: Hallucinogenic	115
Lamp oil	107
Gasoline	81
Plant: Anticholinergic	67
Wall, floor, tile, or all-purpose cleaner: Alkali	66
Freon or other propellant	61
Unknown mushroom	59
Chlorine gas	53
Other acid	49
Cyanoacrylate	49
Alkali (excluding cleaners, bleach, etc.)	48
Pyrethroid	47
Other hydrocarbon	46
Miscellaneous cleaning agents: Alkali	45
Penlight, flashlight, or dry cell battery	45
Industrial cleaner: Alkali	41
Ammonia (excluding cleaners)	40

[*]Based on numbers of death and major and moderate outcomes of children's exposures to them. These 20 substances account for 44.8% of the 4205 significant outcomes reported for 2004. Data from Watson WA, Litovitz TL, Rodgers GC Jr, et al. 2004 annual report of the American Association of Poison Control Centers Toxic Exposure Surveillance System. *Am J Emerg Med.* 2005;23(5):589–666.

a learning disability or developmental delays, it may not be the first consideration.

The evaluation of the pediatric patient with a potential chronic neurotoxicity begins with an environmental history.[24] The regular use of a standardized environmental database form may be beneficial.[2] A physician may not have the luxury of a patient who has a clinical presentation that is "classical" for a certain condition such as fetal hydantoin or fetal alcohol syndrome. A history of prematurity, behavioral problems, intellectual deficits, malformations, hearing or vision loss, or additional focal neurological complaints should trigger the need to obtain additional environmental information.[4] The key areas of questioning include a detailed account of all chemicals the child is exposed to, duration of exposure, severity of exposure, and any protective measures taken.[14] Screening for underlying metabolic, nutritional, or degenerative diseases is also necessary.[44]

For the sick child for whom toxin exposure may not have previously been considered, an exposure history should be obtained if an illness is not responding to therapy.[47]

These questions should include an assessment of whether the symptoms subside or worsen in a particular location, on specific days, or with certain activities.[14] Clinicians should remain aware of other individuals with similar symptoms presenting to the area. Further focused testing should be obtained using patient blood, urine, or other body fluid specimens. If a specific toxin is identified, further information must be gathered on its characteristics,

along with the patient's burden of exposure to it, including dose intensity, frequency, and duration.[48]

If the history points to a possible environmental toxin exposure, consultation with a pediatric environmental specialist should be considered. The local poison control center or toxicologists are key resources. The health department should be notified. Environmental samples might be collected. If further management by a more experienced group is needed, the United States has formed Pediatric Environmental Health Specialty Units (PEHSUs). An updated list of these units is provided by the Association of Occupational and Environmental Clinics (AOEC) at www.aoec.org. The association's most recent map of contacts as of this publication is provided in Figure 6-1.

TREATMENT

Treating neurotoxic injuries should be easy: remove the toxins. But this is easier said than done. In the case of acute symptoms, hospitalizing the patient is the first

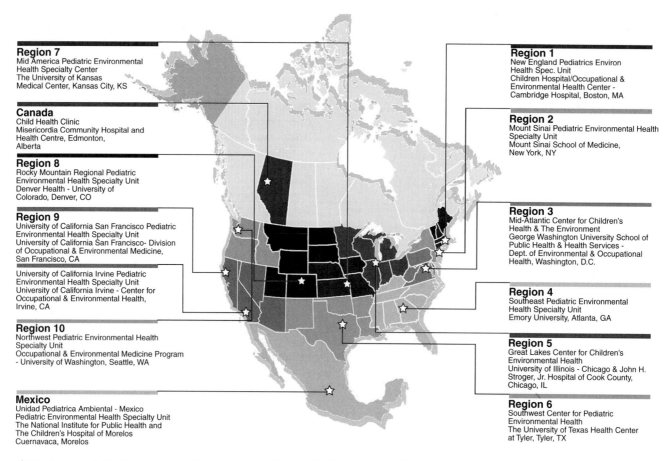

Region 7
Mid America Pediatric Environmental
Health Specialty Center
The University of Kansas
Medical Center, Kansas City, KS

Canada
Child Health Clinic
Misericordia Community Hospital and
Health Centre, Edmonton,
Alberta

Region 8
Rocky Mountain Regional Pediatric
Environmental Health Specialty Unit
Denver Health - University of
Colorado, Denver, CO

Region 9
University of California San Francisco Pediatric
Environmental Health Specialty Unit
University of California San Francisco- Division
of Occupational & Environmental Medicine,
San Francisco, CA

University of California Irvine Pediatric
Environmental Health Specialty Unit
University of California Irvine - Center for
Occupational & Environmental Health,
Irvine, CA

Region 10
Northwest Pediatric Environmental Health
Specialty Unit
Occupational & Environmental Medicine Program
- University of Washington, Seattle, WA

Mexico
Unidad Pediatrica Ambiental - Mexico
Pediatric Environmental Health Specialty Unit
The National Institute for Public Health and
The Children's Hospital of Morelos
Cuernavaca, Morelos

Region 1
New England Pediatrics Environ
Health Spec. Unit
Children Hospital/Occupational &
Environmental Health Center -
Cambridge Hospital, Boston, MA

Region 2
Mount Sinai Pediatric Environmental Health
Specialty Unit
Mount Sinai School of Medicine,
New York, NY

Region 3
Mid-Atlantic Center for Children's
Health & The Environment
George Washington University School of
Public Health & Health Services -
Dept. of Environmental & Occupational
Health, Washington, D.C.

Region 4
Southeast Pediatric Environmental
Health Specialty Unit
Emory University, Atlanta, GA

Region 5
Great Lakes Center for Children's
Environmental Health
University of Illinois - Chicago & John H.
Stroger, Jr. Hospital of Cook County,
Chicago, IL

Region 6
Southwest Center for Pediatric
Environmental Health
The University of Texas Health Center
at Tyler, Tyler, TX

Figure 6-1. Pediatric Environmental Health Specialty Units available in the United States as of 2007. Map provided by the Association of Occupational and Environmental Clinics. An updated version might be available at www.aoec.org.

step. Next, all affected clothing should be removed and the child should be decontaminated, typically by a shower. Medical interventions should be used as deemed appropriate, tailored to the type of toxin identified or suspected. These interventions include gastric lavage, activated charcoal, and emetics.[48] Standard supportive care, including respiratory and cardiovascular support, is often necessary. Both the local poison control center and the ATSDR online resources offer immediate and expert guidance on the medical management of individual toxins. A call can also be placed to a regional PEHSU (see Figure 6-1). When known, substance specific therapy can help prevent further complications, reverse current symptoms, and reduce mortality. In addition, clinicians should ascertain whether or not other individuals in the vicinity of the patient have been exposed and need treatment.[48]

Before returning home, the local health department must screen the child's environment and begin complete removal of the toxin. If it is not feasible to completely remove the toxin, reducing exposure is the next goal.

Lead paint can be stripped and unleaded paint applied.[49] Asbestos can be sheathed in plastic covering, preventing entry into the living space. Polluted water or air can be treated.[22] Simple behaviors such as increasing hand-washing before meals and wiping down contaminated areas are effective. Smokers can be asked to leave the indoors when smoking and bathe or change their clothing before interacting with the child.[50] Household chemicals can be locked away out of a child's reach.

It is critical that a trained professional, public health agency, or both be enlisted so that further exposure to the toxin to the parent, child, or health-care worker does not occur in the attempt at removal.

Since an environmental exposure is often location dependent, removing the child, toxin, or both from the locale may help prevent continued exposure and injury, but any injury to the growing brain that has already occurred may not be reversed.[51] In addition, some exposures, such as radiation, can have a continued effect over many years, with symptoms often showing decades after the insult.[40]

PUBLIC HEALTH

Prevention is the best cure. In regard to avoidable exposures, providing parents with information during their visits, in the form of anticipatory guidance, can reduce preventable injuries from occurring.[52] Much of this guidance can occur during the well-child visit, and age-appropriate guidelines are provided by the American Academy of Pediatrics (AAP). While such visits do have time constraints, simple questions such as where the child lives, whether there is tobacco smoke exposure, and the source of the water supply are quick and easy ways to screen for potential environmental exposures.[14] As per the AAP, the most common areas leading to pediatric environmental toxin exposure include the home, tobacco smoke, and take-home contaminants from the work environment. The infant and toddler years add the risk of injury from common household pesticides and chemicals and lead poisoning. The young child has the addition of school and art and craft exposures. The teen years bring occupational and hobby exposures.[14] Relatively simple items for a busy physician to quickly screen for and provide guidance on in a brief office visit include ensuring a safe food and water supply, limiting exposures to lead and other toxins in the home, and preventing the transfer of chemicals from the workplace into the home.[53]

The AAP and the CDC also recommend reviewing potential environmental hazards before the arrival of a baby, and they provide a standardized checklist to allow for quick office screening.[14] By ascertaining behavior risks that can be curbed or changed, such as alcohol, tobacco, and illicit substance intake, permanent injury to a growing fetus and newborn might be prevented. Although seemingly naïve, a simple reminder and review of the harmful effects of alcohol and drug use during pregnancy is often effective. Simple modifications such as avoiding fish contaminated with mercury during the pregnancy and nursing period are useful.[54]

On international and national levels, both the World Health Organization (WHO) and the U.S. EPA have developed exposure evaluation and treatment guidelines.[1] The U.S. National Institute of Health Statistics and CDC maintain databases for issues related to developmental neurotoxicities.[55] Laws such as the U.S. Food Quality Protection Act have required stricter food standards to ensure that pesticide exposure is limited to values tolerated by infants.[25] With these efforts over the past 2 decades, the proportion of U.S. children who have blood lead concentrations of 10 mcg/dL or higher declined by more than 80% after the elimination of leaded gasoline and lead solder from canned foods and a ban on leaded paint used in housing and other consumer products.[56] The incidence of neural tube defects has declined with dietary folic acid fortification in grains and flour. Child-resistant safety caps on medications, lowered hot-water furnace temperatures, and restricting public exposure to tobacco smoke have added to the success in reducing pediatric neurotoxin exposures.[57]

CONCLUSION

With the continued use of myriad chemicals in common household products, food, and clothing, both children and adults are continually exposed to potential neurotoxins. With the pediatric brain in its formative stages of development, neurotoxin exposures have grave consequences. The normal variations of pediatric physiology and the child's developmental idiosyncrasies lead to a higher amount of and novel toxin exposures when compared with adults. These ingredients all culminate in creating a recipe in which the fetus and child are at a high risk of neurotoxin-mediated neurological injury, injuries that typically lead to long-lasting neurological symptoms and lifelong problems.

An awareness of these vulnerabilities allows clinicians to help families in preventing these exposures from occurring. If an exposure to a toxin has occurred, they can then target the appropriate treatments and use the correct resources in helping the child and family return to normalcy.

Excellent and continually updated resources on pediatric environmental health are available through the CDC environmental health Web site, in association with the ATSDR and the AAP (www.aap.org).

REFERENCES

1. U.S. Environmental Protection Agency. *America's Children and the Environment: Measures of Contaminants, Body Burdens, and Illnesses.* Washington, DC: U.S. EPA; 2003.
2. Agency for Toxic Substances and Disease Registry. Annual Reports 2003. www.atsdr.cdc.gov: ATSDR; 2003.
3. Veal K, Lowry JA, Belmont JM. The epidemiology of pediatric environmental exposures. *Pediatr Clin North Am.* 2007;54:15–31.
4. Landrigan PJ, Garg A. Chronic effects of toxic environmental exposures on children's health. *J Toxicol Clin Toxicol.* 2002;40:449–456.
5. Lemasters GK, Perreault SD, Hales BF, et al. Workshop to identify critical windows of exposure for children's health: reproductive health in children and adolescents work group summary. *Environ Health Perspect.* 2000;108 (Suppl 3):505–509.
6. Snodgrass WR. Physiological and biochemical differences between children and adults as determinants of toxic response to environmental pollutants. In: Guzelian PS, Henry CJ, Olin SS, eds. *Similarities and Differences between Children and Adults: Implications for Risk Assessment.* Washington, DC: ILSI Press; 1992:35–42.

7. Behrman RE, Kliegman RM, Arvin AM, eds. *Nelson Textbook of Pediatrics.* 15th ed. Philadelphia: WB Saunders; 1996.

8. Nebert DW, Gonzalez FJ. P450 genes: structure, evolution, and regulation. *Annu Rev Biochem.* 1987;56:945–993.

9. National Research Council. Pesticides in the diets of infants and children. *Neurol Clin.* 2000;18(3):541–562.

10. Silbergeld EK. Lead in bone: implication for toxicology during pregnancy and lactation. *Environ Health Perspect.* 1991;91: 63–70.

11. DeVita R, Olivieri A, Spinelli A, et al. Health status and internal radiocontamination assessment in children exposed to the fallout of the Chernobyl accident. *Arch Environ Health.* 2000;55(3):181–186.

12. DeBaun MR, Gurney JG. Environmental exposure and cancer in children: a conceptual framework for the pediatrician. *Pediatr Clin North Am.* 2001;48(5):1215–1222.

13. Paul M, ed. *Occupational and Environmental Reproductive Hazards: A Guide for Clinicians.* Baltimore: Williams & Wilkins; 1993.

14. American Academy of Pediatrics Committee on Environmental Health. *Pediatric Environmental Health.* 2nd ed. Elk Grove Village, Illinois: American Academy of Pediatrics; 2003.

15. Slikker W, Miller RK. Placental metabolism and transfer: role in developmental toxicity. In: Kimmel CA, Buelke-Sam J, eds. *Developmental Toxicology.* 2nd ed. New York: Raven Press; 1994:245–283.

16. Wolff MS. Occupationally derived chemicals in breast milk. *Am J Ind Med.* 1983;4:259-281.

17. Andersen HR, Nielsen JB, Grandjean P. Toxicologic evidence of developmental neurotoxicity of environmental chemicals. *Toxicology.* 2000;144(1–3):121–127.

18. Paulson JA. Pediatric advocacy. *Pediatr Clin North Am.* 2001;48(5):1307–1318.

19. Grandjean P, Landrigan PJ. Developmental neurotoxicity of industrial chemicals. *Lancet.* 2006;368(9553):2167–2178.

20. Aronow R, Cubbage C, Weiner R, Johnson B, Hesse J, Bedford J. Mercury exposure from interior latex paint: Michigan. *MMWR.* 1990;39(8):125–126.

21. Fisher J, Mahle D, Bankston L, Greene R, Gearhart J. Lactational transfer of volatile chemicals in breast milk. *Am Ind Hyg Assoc J.* 1997;58(6):425–431.

22. Etzel RA. Indoor air pollutants in homes and schools. *Pediatr Clin North Am.* 2001;48(5): 1153-1165.

23. Schreiber JS. Parents worried about breast milk contaminants: what is best for baby? *Pediatr Clin North Am.* 2001;48(5): 1113–1128.

24. Balk SJ, Walton-Brown S, Pope A. Environmental history-taking. In: *Training Manual on Pediatric Environmental Health: Putting It Into Practice.* Washington, DC: Children's Environmental Health Network; 1999:82–95.

25. *Food Quality Protection Act of 1996.* Public Law 104-170. Aug 3, 1996.

26. Graubarth J, Bloom CJ, Coleman FC, Solomon HN. Dye poisoning in the nursery: a review of seventeen cases. *JAMA.* 1945;128:1155–1157.

27. Howarth BE. Epidemic of aniline methaemoglobinaemia in newborn babies. *Lancet.* 1951;1(17):934–935.

28. Chai S, Bearer CF. A developmental approach to pediatric environmental health. In: *Training Manual on Pediatric Environmental Health: Putting It Into Practice.* Washington, DC: Children's Environmental Health Network; 1999:57–75.

29. Centers for Disease Control and Prevention. Screening Young Children for Lead Poisoning: Guidance for State and Local Public Health Officials. Atlanta: U.S. Department of Health and Human Services; 1997.

30. Goldman LR, Koduru S. Chemicals in the environment and developmental toxicity to children: a public health and policy perspective. *Environ Health Perspect.* 2000;108 (Suppl 3):443–448.

31. Levitt, P. Structural and functional maturation of the developing primate brain. *Pediatrics.* 2003;143:S35–S45.

32. Volpe JJ. *Neurology of the Newborn.* 4th ed. Philadelphia: Saunders; 2001.

33. Weiss B. Vulnerability of children and the developing brain to neurotoxic hazards. *Environ Health Perspect.* 2000;108 (Suppl 3):375–381.

34. Lanphear BP, Wright RO, Dietrich KN. Environmental neurotoxins. *Pediatr Rev.* 2005;26(6)191–197.

35. National Research Council. Scientific Frontiers in Developmental Toxicology and Risk Assessment. Washington, DC: National Academy Press; 2000.

36. Rodier PM. Environmental causes of central nervous system maldevelopment. *Pediatrics.* 2004;113 (Suppl 4):1076.

37. Rice D, Barone S Jr. Critical periods of vulnerability for the developing nervous system: evidence from humans and animal models. *Environ Health Perspect.* 2000;108 (Suppl 3):511–533.

38. Rodier PM. Developing brain as a target of toxicity. *Environ Health Perspect.* 1995;103 (Suppl 6):73–76.

39. Rodier PM, Reynolds SS, Roberts WN. Behavioral consequences of interference with CNS development in the early fetal period. *Teratology.* 1979;19(3):327–336.

40. Anderson LM, Diwan BA, Fear NT, Roman E. Critical windows of exposure for children's health: cancer in human epidemiological studies and neoplasms in experimental animal models. *Environ Health Perspect.* 2000;108 (Suppl 3):573–594.

41. Cory-Slechta, DA. Interactions of lead exposure and stress: implications for cognitive dysfunction. In: Davidson PW, Myers GJ, and Weiss B, eds. *Neurotoxicity and Developmental Disabilities.* San Diego, Calif: Elsevier Academic Press; 2006.

42. Walsh LE, Garg BP. Poisoning and drug-induced neurologic diseases. In: Swaiman KF, Ashwal A, Ferriero DM, eds. *Pediatric Neurology: Principles and Practice.* vol 11. 4th ed. Philadelphia: Mosby; 2006:2173–2206.

43. Trask CL, Kosofsky BE. Developmental considerations of neurotoxic exposures. *Neurol Clin.* 2000;18(3):541-562.

44. Boyle CA, Decouflé P, Yeargin-Allsopp M. Prevalence and health impact of developmental disabilities in U.S. children. *Pediatrics.* 1994;93(3):399–403.

45. Shepard TH, Wilson JG. Embryotoxicity of drugs in man. In: Wilson JG, Fraser FC, eds. *Handbook of Teratology.* New York: Plenum Press; 1997:309–355.

46. Shannon MW, Graef JW. Lead intoxication in infancy. *Pediatrics.* 1992;89:87–90.

47. Balk SJ. The environmental history: asking the right questions. *Contemp Pediatr.* 1996;3:19–36.

48. Borak J, Callan M, & Abbott W. *Hazardous Materials Exposure: Emergency Response and Patient Care.* Englewood Cliffs, NJ: Brady–Prentice Hall; 1991.

49. Baker EL, Folland DS, Taylor TA, et al. Lead poisoning in children of lead workers: home contamination with industrial dust. *N Engl J Med.* 1977;296(5):260–261.

50. Cook DG, Strachan DP. Health effects of passive smoking: summary of effects of parental smoking on the respiratory health of children and implications for research. *Thorax.* 1999;54: 357–366.

51. Selevan S, Kimmel CA, Mendola P. Identifying critical windows of exposure for children's health. *Environ Health Perspect.* 2000;108 (Suppl 3):451–455.

52. Stickler GB, Simmons PS. Pediatricians' preferences for anticipatory guidance topics compared with parental anxieties. *Clin Pediatr (Phila).* 1995;34(7):384–387.

53. Mayer JL, Balk SJ. A pediatrician's guide to environmental toxins. *Contemp Pediatr.* 1988. Pt 1:5(7):22–40 and Pt 2:5(8): 63–76.

54. U.S. Environmental Protection Agency and the Agency for Toxic Substances and Disease Registry. Should I Eat the Fish I Catch? Washington, DC: U.S. EPA; 2001.

55. National Institute for Occupational Safety and Health. Report to Congress on Worker's Home Contamination Study Conducted under the Workers' Family Protection Act (29 USC 671A). Cincinnati, Ohio: U.S. Department of Health and Human Services; 1995. Publication 95-123.

56. Lanphear BP, Dietrich KN, Berger O. Prevention of lead toxicity in U.S. children. *Ambul Pediatr.* 2003;3(1):27–36.

57. Weiss B, Landrigan PJ. The developing brain and the environment: an introduction. *Environ Health Perspect.* 2000;108 (Suppl 3):373–374.

SECTION 2

NEUROTOXIC SYNDROMES: SYMPTOMATIC, SYSTEMS-ORIENTED APPROACH IN CLINICAL NEUROTOXICOLOGY

CONTENTS

CHAPTER 7

Toxic Encephalopathies I: Cortical and Mixed Encephalopathies

Tracy J. Eicher

INTRODUCTION

Optimal cognitive processing depends on a complex interplay among neurotransmitters, electrolytes, and numerous other molecules in the brain's milieu. This delicate balance can be disrupted by many substances encountered in the environment, whether ingested, inhaled, or absorbed through the skin. An encephalopathy can result from either direct assault on the neurons themselves or damage to the white matter tracts devoted to communication between neurons. Neurotoxic agents known to strike primarily white matter are addressed separately in the chapter on toxic leukoencephalopathies. This chapter focuses on toxins causing cortical, mixed cortical, and white matter encephalopathies.

SIGNS AND SYMPTOMS

Victims of a toxin-induced encephalopathy may exhibit various symptoms, most of which are nonspecific and can lead the clinician to an incorrect diagnostic conclusion. The acuity and severity of the presenting symptoms furthermore depend not only on the toxin itself but also on the dose and duration of exposure. In addition, the baseline cerebral function of the exposed individual affects the clinical presentation. It is therefore imperative for the investigator to remain vigilant to the possibility of toxic exposure while taking a thorough history. A basic awareness of the more common features of neurotoxic encephalopathy can aid in identification and timely treatment of the exposure.

Cortical and Mixed-type Encephalopathies

A purely cortical encephalopathy most commonly results from acute exposure to toxins that cause anoxic injury to the neurons. Diffuse injury to cortical and cerebellar gray matter is the rule in such situations. Moreover, the structures of the basal ganglia are exquisitely sensitive to this type of insult. Perhaps the most pure example of this situation occurs with carbon monoxide (CO) exposure. The CO molecule competes with oxygen for binding by hemoglobin in the blood, causing a lack of oxygenation to the brain. Bilateral necrosis of the globus pallidus is widely recognized as the hallmark of CO poisoning, although it is seen in other hypoxic injuries as well (Figure 7-1).

Purely cortical injury from toxin exposures is uncommon. More common is a combination of cortical and

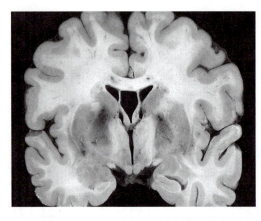

Figure 7-1. Bilateral necrosis of the globus pallidus is widely recognized as the hallmark of carbon monoxide poisoning, although it is seen in other hypoxic injuries. (Reprinted with permission from Gray F, De Girolami U, Poirier J. Escourolle and Poirier Manual of Basic Neuropathology, 4th edition. Philadelphia: Butterworth-Heinemann, an Imprint of Elsevier, 2004.)

white matter injury. Even in the case of CO exposure, pathological studies show extensive zones of demyelination in subcortical white matter.[1]

The symptoms following most forms of toxic injury are generally a reflection of injury to both gray and white matter and include memory disturbance, decreased or slowed cognition, mood disturbance, fatigue, and headache. Damage to gray matter in the basal ganglia may produce symptoms of parkinsonism, and cerebellar insults may manifest as ataxia and disequilibrium. Symptoms referable to specific areas of cortical gray matter, including aphasia, apraxia, and neglect, are rarely prominent among the presenting complaints but may accompany the other clinical signs.

It should also be recognized that the symptoms of toxic encephalopathy exist as a continuum from mild to severe and are influenced not only by the identity and amount of the toxin involved but also by the time course of the exposure. Prognosis for recovery similarly depends on these same factors. For example, low levels of exposure to toxin A that occurs chronically for weeks or months may result in significant and permanent neurocognitive impairment (see Figure 7-1), while a much-higher-level, one-time exposure to the same toxin has a much better outcome. Conversely, a one-time exposure to a moderate to high dose of toxin B may have devastating results, while low-level chronic exposure is comparatively well tolerated.

DIAGNOSTIC APPROACH

The initial differential diagnosis of an encephalopathic patient is broad, but the consideration of toxic exposure should be considered early. The first critical step

in narrowing the list of possible causes is the clinical history. In acute exposures, details regarding the victim and the setting often provide the best leads. For instance, a teenager known to be fully functioning hours earlier who was found in a severely encephalopathic state in his garage quickly raises the suspicion of exposure to solvents (via "huffing"), whereas a toddler found in a similar setting is likely to have ingested ethylene glycol, pesticides, or other toxins found at the scene. The cause of a chronic encephalopathy can be far more difficult to identify. Potential exposures in the workplace and home environment should be asked about. Water-supply source, hobbies, and use of herbal supplements should not be overlooked.

Once the list of possibilities has been narrowed, confirmatory investigation may be possible. Laboratory tests may reveal the specific toxin or its metabolites in the blood or urine, while other toxins leave more subtle and often less specific clues such as blood dyscrasias, bone marrow suppression, or alterations in liver function. Certain physical examination findings can also provide clues or supportive evidence of the offending agent. For example, Mees' lines on the fingernails suggests arsenic or thallium poisoning; bradykinesia occurs with acute exposure to CO but may also occur with exposure to carbon disulfide or manganese; and altered color vision has been reported in toxicity from carbon disulfide, *n*-hexane, perchlorethylene, and styrene. Neuroimaging studies may help narrow the differential as some neurotoxins have a high affinity for specific areas of the brain. Other toxins are less specific, but neuroimaging studies may nonetheless prove useful in that they can show the extent of white matter damage or cerebral atrophy. Electrophysiological studies may be helpful in narrowing the list of offenders or in differentiating among possible toxins. Many substances damage both central and peripheral nerves, whereas others affect only the central nervous system (CNS).

It should be stressed that, if available, treatment should not be delayed while confirmatory testing is done. Especially in an acute setting, when a specific toxin is strongly suspected, steps to remove or reverse the effects of the toxin should be initiated as soon as possible.

Neuropsychiatric testing is commonly used in analysis of the toxin-exposed patient. The overlapping neuropsychiatric and neurocognitive sequelae of toxic encephalopathies make these tests less specific diagnostically, but they provide a valuable means of evaluating and following the more subtle deficits of such patients. Moreover, identification of specific areas of cognitive dysfunction is valuable in informing future cognitive rehabilitation efforts.

SUBSTANCES CAUSING TOXIC CORTICAL ENCEPHALOPATHIES

Solvents and Organic Compounds

Solvents comprise a heterogeneous group of substances with myriad uses in today's world. Common organic solvents may be classified according to chemical structure as aliphatic, aromatic, halogenated, or cyclic hydrocarbons; ketones; amines; alcohols; aldehydes; and ethers. They are commonly found in degreasing agents and cleaning solutions, as well as paints, inks, lacquers, varnishes, and adhesives. Moreover, most of these substances contain combinations of two or more neurotoxic solvent molecules.

In general, the neurological sequelae of toxicity from solvents are similar and consist of fatigue, headache, emotional instability, diminished impulse control, and impaired mental function. The World Health Organization has devised a classification system for the encephalopathies induced by solvents as a whole. This system is based on the severity of symptoms and employs labels of organic affective syndrome, mild chronic toxic encephalopathy, and severe chronic toxic encephalopathy.[2]

Chronic low-level exposures to fumes from paints, lacquers, fuels, and solvents may occur in occupational settings. Whether years of such low-level exposure can result in a chronic encephalopathy remains a matter of some debate.[3–6] That moderate to high levels of exposure to these substances can have lasting effects on the CNS is more well established. Hormes et al.[7] reported on the long-term sequelae of exposure in 20 solvent abusers, finding cognitive deficits including attention and memory deficits, executive dysfunction, and visuospatial disturbance in 60%. Half of the patients displayed motor disorders, and 45% had cerebellar dysfunction.

Several of the more common neurotoxic solvents are discussed individually in this section. It should be kept in mind that exposures to solvent compounds often involve more than one neurotoxic agent and that the effects of each are amplified by the others. The commonly encountered neurotoxic vapor CO is included in this section.

Toluene

Toluene, an aromatic alkylbenzene hydrocarbon compound is often present in paints, lacquers, glues, and solvents. Gasoline, containing up to 7% toluene by weight, represents the most significant source of toluene used in this country.[8] Myriad accounts of cases of acute and chronic toluene-induced encephalopathy exist and occur in the setting of accidental or intentional inhalation. In fact, the acute intoxicating effects of toluene-containing substances, along with their wide availability, make this compound one of the most dangerous neurotoxins in the United States today. Recreational use of glues, gasoline, and paints for their intoxicating effects is likely underestimated by many.

Acute toluene toxicity results in lightheadedness and euphoria. Incoordination, disequilibrium, confusion, and cognitive and memory deficits accompany these symptoms. Inappropriate behavior, mood fluctuations, and nystagmus are also common. With higher levels of exposure, unconsciousness, coma, and death may occur. The acute CNS effects of toluene reverse quickly after cessation of the exposure. Repeated exposures, however, can lead to chronic symptoms of intention tremor, motor incoordination, and cognitive deficits. Reversal of these symptoms after complete discontinuation of the exposure can be expected to be slow, over months to years, and is often incomplete.[9,10]

Its chemical structure makes toluene highly lipid soluble. It readily crosses the blood–brain barrier (BBB) and has an affinity for white matter. There is evidence that toluene causes not only myelin breakdown but also neural cell death. The mechanism of neural toxicity has not been fully established; it is unclear whether this is a direct effect or is secondary to the production of free radicals. Some evidence shows toluene may also alter neuronal response to certain neurotransmitters.[6,7]

The American Conference of Governmental Industrial Hygienists (ACGIH) has established exposure indices for workers at risk of toluene exposure. Urine hippuric acid levels are recommended at the end of shifts as a means of monitoring levels. Blood toluene levels may also be used. Neuroimaging studies typically reveal diffuse atrophy and decreased gray–white differentiation. Lesions of the basal ganglia are not thought to be caused by toluene exposure but may be present due to concomitant methanol exposure.[7] In cases of recreational exposure, diagnosis is based on history and index of suspicion. The clinician must often ask directly about such exposure, as the recreational user is often reluctant to volunteer this history. Aside from removal of the toxic source, no direct treatment exists for toluene toxicity and care is supportive only.

Trichloroethylene

Trichloroethylene (TCE) is an unsaturated chlorinated hydrocarbon used commercially as a degreasing agent. It is also present in insecticides, in cleaning solutions, and as a vehicle for paints, solvents, and glues. The release of TCE into the atmosphere by factories and into soil and water by improper waste disposal have been the cause of public exposure via air, water, and food products.[11–13] Recommended exposure limits established by the U.S. Environmental Protection Agency are based on the carcinogenic rather than neurotoxic properties of

TCE. Exposure limits for the CNS effects are not well established.[8]

Occupational exposure via inhalation is the most commonly reported means of acute TCE toxicity, whereas ingestion of TCE-contaminated drinking water has been a source of chronic exposure in entire communities.[8,13,14] Symptoms of acute toxicity include nausea, headache, dizziness, disorientation, stupor, and occasionally coma.

Trigeminal neuropathy with or without other cranial nerve dysfunction may be a prominent symptom of TCE toxicity and should raise the index of suspicion for this exposure. Peripheral neuropathy may also occur.[14]

Prognosis for complete recovery over hours to days is good if the exposure time is limited. Long-term deficits from more prolonged exposures include cranial nerve palsies and chronic encephalopathy. Short-term memory and attentional deficits, impaired visuospatial performance, depressed mood, and apathy commonly persist as well. Slow improvement of these encephalopathic features can occur over months.[15–19] With chronic low-level exposure, behavioral and mood changes are often the first signs. Fatigue, dizziness, and headache often follow and may be what bring the patient to medical attention.[14,20]

In addition to preventive measures, the ACGIH recommends laboratory monitoring for exposures in high-risk industrial settings. Blood levels of the TCE metabolite trichloroethanol are suggested.[21] Neuroimaging may be normal or may show varying degrees of bilateral cortical atrophy with or without accompanying atrophy of the cerebellar vermis.[7] Treatment for acute inhalational exposure consists of removing the victim from the fumes and providing fresh air or oxygen, if available. For acute ingestion, gastric lavage should be considered. The potential for cardiac arrhythmias and acute renal failure warrants close monitoring for these signs. The potential for victims of TCE toxicity to become sensitized to this substance should be recognized, and future avoidance of even low-level exposures is recommended.[8]

Perchlorethylene

Perchlorethylene (PCE), also known as tetrachloroethylene is used as a degreasing agent in industrial settings. Its previous medicinal use as an anesthetic and an antihelminthic agent has been documented.[7] Today, it is used most extensively in the dry-cleaning industry due to its ability to dissolve grease, wax, and oils without harming fabrics. Dry-cleaning workers have relatively high rates of exposure due to their handling of clothing saturated with PCE. Users of coin-operated dry-cleaning machines have also been victims of acute PCE intoxication.[7,22] PCE contamination of soil, groundwater, and food may lead to oral exposure, but the neurotoxicity of such exposure is not clear. Most reported cases of PCE toxicity occur by way of inhalation in the occupational setting.[23]

High-level exposure to PCE produces an acute encephalopathy, which is typically fully reversible after cessation of the exposure. Symptoms include headache, dizziness, and confusion. More prolonged exposure to high levels of TCE has been reported to result in persistent personality change, irritability, and outbursts of rage.[7] Chronic inhalation exposure more typically results in prominent memory impairment, chronic dizziness, drowsiness, and frequent fainting spells. Decreased tolerance to alcohol and multiple other chemicals has also been reported.[24,25]

Recommended limits for PCE in air and water have been proposed by various agencies, including the U.S. Occupational Safety and Health Administration (OSHA) and the ACGIH. These levels, however, are based on the carcinogenic properties rather than on risk of neurotoxicity. Available laboratory testing for PCE exposure includes levels in exhaled air or in blood. Urine testing of the PCE metabolite trichloroacetic acid may also be used. Trichloroacetic acid is also a metabolite of other solvents, including TCE, making this test less specific.[23] Neuroimaging is often normal, but bilateral cortical atrophy may be seen in cases of severe or prolonged exposure.[7]

Treatment of acute PCE encephalopathy is similar to that for TCE. Evacuating the victim from the source and providing fresh air and oxygen are the primary concerns when exposure is inhalational. Gastric lavage should be considered for oral ingestion, and supportive care should be provided. The victim should be closely monitored for cardiac arrhythmias, acute renal failure, and pulmonary edema.[8]

Carbon Disulfide

Carbon disulfide is used industrially in the manufacture of perfumes, cellophane, rayon, and some types of rubber. It is also present in varnish, solvents, and insecticides. Inhalation in an occupational setting is the most common source of toxicity, although transdermal absorption is also a danger. Carbon disulfide has an affinity for both gray and white matter, and symptoms of acute inhalational exposures above 3 to 4 ppm include tinnitus, dizziness, headache, and confusion. Lasting effects such as insomnia, intense irritability, and headaches may persist for months, but prognosis for significant recovery is good.[7,26] The chronic encephalopathy presents gradually and may be subtle at first. With higher levels or longer duration of exposure, the symptoms begin to resemble those described for acute exposure. Nightmares, sleep disturbance, irritability, and memory disturbance are common. Additional complaints that should raise suspicion for carbon disulfide toxicity include symptoms of peripheral neuropathy, parkinsonism, and retinopathy.[26,27]

No specific treatment has been found to reduce the effects of carbon disulfide once it has entered the body.

Early recognition and avoidance of ongoing exposure is therefore essential. Due to varied rates of absorption, air-level monitoring is an unreliable indicator and blood or urine levels should be used. Urine levels of the metabolite 2-thio-thiazolidine-4-carboxylic acid may also be used.[8] With higher levels of exposure, neuroimaging typically reveals cortical and subcortical atrophy with frontal lobe predominance. In addition, lesions in the globus pallidus and putamen have been reported.[7]

Carbon Monoxide

CO is a common byproduct of the burning of many substances. It is present in exhaust from automobiles and in cigarette smoke. CO exerts its neurotoxic effects by causing tissue hypoxia and free radical production.[28,29] It competes with oxygen for binding to hemoglobin in the blood, thus robbing the brain of its oxygen source. It has also been shown to exert direct neurotoxic effects at the cellular level and causes white matter destruction via lipid peroxidation.[30]

Headache, dizziness, and blurred vision are early signs of CO exposure. Overt cognitive deficits may be absent early on. Systemic signs that may alert the clinician to the diagnosis are nausea, abdominal pain, and generalized weakness.[28] An estimated 30% of CO-affected patients experience a delayed onset of encephalopathy after apparent full recovery. Cognitive deficits, personality change, parkinsonism, and psychosis may begin days or even months following the toxic event. The mechanism for this delayed syndrome is not well understood, but full to near-full recovery occurs in 50% to 75% within a year.[31,32]

CO levels in exhaled air can be measured at the time of exposure. Blood level testing of carboxyhemoglobin is more sensitive; however, it should be kept in mind that smokers have an elevated baseline level of carboxyhemoglobin.[28] Blood should be drawn as quickly as possible following exposure, as levels begin to drop rapidly when fresh air and oxygen are introduced. Fresh air and oxygen should be provided immediately on discovery of exposure. Hyperbaric oxygen also greatly enhances early recovery, although it is unclear whether it decreases the likelihood of the delayed neuropsychiatric syndrome. Once the victim is medically stable, neuropsychiatric testing is recommended. The Carbon Monoxide Neuropsychological Screening Battery was developed specifically for this purpose and provides an objective means of following the patient's clinical course.[33] Hyperbaric oxygen therapy is recommended if the victim has an abnormal score on the battery, has a carboxyhemoglobin level greater than 40%, or had loss of consciousness with the exposure.[28]

Following CO exposure, neuroimaging classically shows bilateral lesions of the globus pallidi (Figure 7-2). Lesions of the internal capsule and hippocampi are also often present. There may be a delay in appearance of

abnormalities on computerized tomography (CT) scan, and a normal CT scan in the emergency room should be followed by repeat imaging sometime in the next week.[7]

Benzene, Xylene, and Styrene

Benzene is one of most extensively used molecules in the United States today. It is used in the manufacture of explosives, rubber, lubricants, paints and dyes, detergents, pesticides, and many other common products. Its use as an additive to gasoline has greatly declined since the 1990s.[8] In addition to its neurotoxic effects, benzene is well known for its carcinogenic properties and hematopoietic effects. Findings of bone marrow suppression, anemia, leucopenia, or thrombocytopenia can be clues to the diagnosis of chronic benzene exposure.[34] Xylene is found in a multitude of solvents, paints, and varnishes and is present in various industrial settings. Styrene is a common ingredient in waxes, paints, varnishes, auto body putty, and polishes. It is often used in the manufacture of fiberglass-reinforced plastics.

Benzene, xylene, and styrene are structurally similar to toluene, and each produces an encephalopathy similar to that of toluene in the acute setting. Chronic CNS dysfunction also occurs but tends to be less severe, and chances of full recovery are better. Subjective complaints of memory and cognitive deficits, headache, fatigue, and irritability may, nonetheless, persist for weeks to months.[35–41]

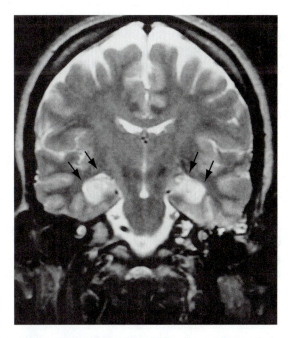

Figure 7-2. Neuroimaging classically shows bilateral lesions of the globus pallidi following carbon monoxide exposure. (Reprinted with permission from Grossman and Yousem. Neuroradiology: The Requisites, 2nd ed. Philadelphia: Mosby, an Imprint of Elsevier, 2003.)

Neuroimaging in cases of styrene exposure reveals a variable mix of atrophy of cortical and subcortical areas. Pathology studies show gliosis specifically in hippocampi and the sensorimotor cortex. Animal studies suggest derangements in the dopamine system following styrene intoxication; this finding may inform the choice of treatment for long-term symptoms.[7]

Ethanol

Ethyl alcohol or ethanol (EtOH) is the most common organic solvent to which Americans are exposed. Its acute effects are well recognized and obviously occur most often in the setting of recreational ingestion of beer, wine, or spirits. EtOH is also present in many household products, pharmaceuticals, and industrial solvents. The acute encephalopathy of EtOH toxicity is identical to that of other organic solvents and may range from euphoria to stupor and coma. It should be noted that EtOH exposure amplifies the toxicity of other solvents in the acute setting. This interaction is especially dangerous in the setting of recreational solvent inhalation, where concomitant EtOH consumption is common and can dramatically increase the chance of lethal outcome. Frequent EtOH ingestion can, on the other hand, reduce the acute effects of solvent exposure due to induction of the hepatic CYP2E1 enzymes that metabolizes both.[5,22]

EtOH exerts its effects on the CNS by binding nonspecifically to several neurotransmitter and neuromodulating receptors. It facilitates the γ-aminobutyric acid type A receptor and inhibits glutamate N-methyl-d-aspartate receptors.[42,43] Chronic use of EtOH can cause long-term memory and cognitive deficits. In many cases, long-term chronic alcohol abuse is combined with nutritional deficits, electrolyte disturbances, and exposure to other potentially neurotoxic substances, making it difficult to separate the effects of EtOH alone. There is evidence, however, that alcohol exerts direct toxic effects on neural tissues. Pathology studies on animals show that EtOH causes cortical changes even when nutrition and other factors are kept stable. Specifically, neurons in the basal forebrain and hippocampus are lost. Imaging and pathology studies indicate that these areas are also especially vulnerable in humans.[44]

The symptoms of chronic alcohol-induced encephalopathy are varied and no reliable factors, apart from specific vitamin deficiencies, have been identified as predictive of which set of symptoms is likely to occur. The amount and duration of abuse before onset of symptoms also differs markedly from person to person. Alcoholic dementia consists of widespread cognitive dysfunction and is probably due to direct neurotoxicity by EtOH. It is distinct from Wernicke-Korsakoff syndrome, but the exact pathophysiology behind it is not well understood. Increased ventricle size and diffuse atrophy of the cerebral hemispheres are seen on neuroimaging. The amount of atrophy, however, does not tend to correlate well with the degree of dementia.[44] Perceptual disturbances including visual illusions and visual, auditory, olfactory, or tactile hallucinations occur in about 25% of chronic alcohol abusers. These distortions seem to occur as a separate issue from the cognitive dysfunction. They are usually brief and episodic but rarely can progress to frank and unremitting psychosis.[45] Cerebellar degeneration also occurs, either alone or in combination with diffuse cerebral atrophy in the alcoholic population. Selective atrophy of the anterior and superior cerebellar vermis with relative sparing of the cerebellar hemispheres results in marked truncal ataxia with much milder limb ataxia (Figure 7-3).

Wernicke-Korsakoff Syndrome

Wernicke's and Korsakoff's syndromes are actually two clinically separate entities. They are linked causally to thiamine deficiency and often occur together in the alcoholic population. Wernicke's syndrome is an acute encephalopathy. Symptoms progress over days to weeks and consist of lethargy, ophthalmoplegia, impaired memory, decreased attention, and perceptual disturbances. If untreated, these symptoms can progress to stupor and coma (Figures 7-4 and 7-5). If treated, the symptoms may remit or may evolve into Korsakoff's syndrome. The major impairment in Korsakoff's syndrome involves memory, although other more subtle cognitive deficits may be present. Alertness and attention are notably preserved, and the individual appears behaviorally normal. A marked anterograde amnesia with inability to retain new information is the hallmark. This is often accompanied by a more patchy and variable retrograde amnesia.[42,45] Pathological changes in

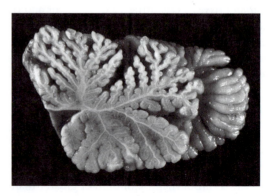

Figure 7-3. Chronic ethanol cerebellar degeneration. (Reprinted with permission from Gray F, De Girolami U, Poirier J. Escourolle and Poirier Manual of Basic Neuropathology, 4th edition. Philadelphia: Butterworth-Heinemann, an Imprint of Elsevier, 2004.)

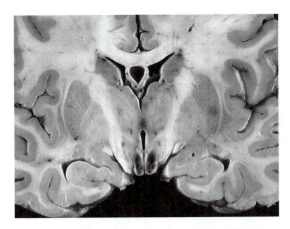

Figure 7-4. Acute Wernicke's encephalopathy. (Reprinted with permission from Gray F, De Girolami U, Poirier J. Escourolle and Poirier Manual of Basic Neuropathology, 4th edition. Philadelphia: Butterworth-Heinemann, an Imprint of Elsevier, 2004.)

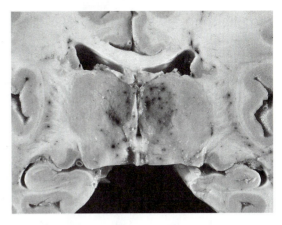

Figure 7-6. Pathological changes in Korsakoff's syndrome. (Reprinted with permission from Gray F, De Girolami U, Poirier J. Escourolle and Poirier Manual of Basic Neuropathology, 4th edition. Philadelphia: Butterworth-Heinemann, an Imprint of Elsevier, 2004.)

Korsakoff's syndrome are most notable in the hypothalamus, medial thalamus, mammillary bodies, and periaquiductal gray matter (Figure 7-6).[44]

Methanol poisoning may result from oral intake when used as a substitute for EtOH. Neurotoxicity results from methanol, as well as from its metabolites formaldehyde and formic acid, which block the process of cellular respiration. This may result in a diffuse and fairly nonspecific encephalopathy directly or as a result of ensuing metabolic acidosis. Methanol intoxication results in cerebral edema and necrosis of white matter and in retrolaminar myelin loss (Figure 7-7). Blindness is often an early indicator of methanol toxicity and results from optic nerve edema and necrosis.

THERAPEUTIC AGENTS

At high-enough doses, many medications have the potential to cause an acute and transient encephalopathy. However, some therapeutic agents cause encephalopathy

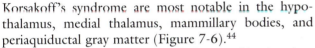

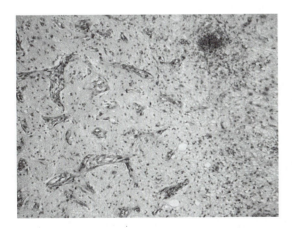

Figure 7-5. Microscopic appearance of the mammillary bodies from a patient with Wernicke's encephalopathy. (Reprinted with permission from Gray F, De Girolami U, Poirier J. Escourolle and Poirier Manual of Basic Neuropathology, 4th edition. Philadelphia: Butterworth-Heinemann, an Imprint of Elsevier, 2004.)

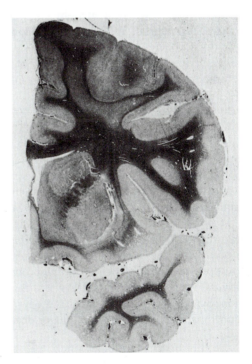

Figure 7-7. Methanol intoxication results in cerebral edema and necrosis of white matter and in retrolaminar myelin loss. (Reprinted with permission from Gray F, De Girolami U, Poirier J. Escourolle and Poirier Manual of Basic Neuropathology, 4th edition. Philadelphia: Butterworth-Heinemann, an Imprint of Elsevier, 2004.)

at therapeutic doses. Many such agents are used in the treatment of cancer.

Methotrexate

Methotrexate inhibits dihydrofolate reductase. It is used to treat breast cancer, lymphomas, leukemias, choriocarcinoma, and leptomeningeal metastases from various cancers. Its neurotoxic effects can be acute, subacute, or chronic. Acutely, about 10% of patients receiving intrathecal methotrexate develop an aseptic meningitis with headache, lethargy, nausea, vomiting, stiff neck, and fever. These symptoms generally resolve fully within 1 to 3 days.[46,47] A subacute syndrome consisting of behavioral changes, hemiparesis, aphasia, dysarthria, and seizures can occur within weeks to months of moderate- or high-dose administration. The symptoms present abruptly but generally resolve completely over days and do not tend to recur with further treatment. CT scans are normal but electroencephalograms (EEGs) typically show focal or generalized slowing.[46–49] The chronic encephalopathy associated with methotrexate usually develops more than 6 months after treatment. It is primarily a leukoencephalopathy with symptoms of decreased memory, concentration, hemiparesis, ataxia, and urinary incontinence. Magnetic resonance imaging (MRI) shows prominent nonenhancing white matter lesions in the cerebral hemispheres. Cortical atrophy and enlarged ventricles are also typical. Pathology specimens reveal loss of oligodendrocytes and fibrinoid necrosis of small blood vessels.[47] In general, the neurotoxicity of methotrexate is amplified by the effects of radiation therapy.[46]

Ifosfamide

Ifosfamide is an analogue of cyclophosphamide used in the treatment of several tumors, including sarcomas, testicular carcinoma, and lymphoma. It causes symptoms of CNS toxicity in 20% to 30% of treated patients. The most common CNS effect is encephalopathy with decreased attention and sometimes agitation. Hallucinations, seizures, cerebellar signs, or extrapyramidal signs can also occur. The seizures may be nonconvulsive and tend to respond to diazepam. Onset of symptoms tends to be fairly immediate, beginning during or within hours of infusion. Symptoms typically last 1 to 4 days. Rarely, the encephalopathy can progress to coma or death.[50,51]

Mechlorethamine

Mechlorethamine, also known as nitrogen mustard, HN2, or Mustargen, is used to treat Hodgkin's disease. Within days of administration, it can cause an encephalopathy, which is often accompanied by headache and lethargy. Other early symptoms can include hallucina-

tions, vertigo, hearing loss, and seizures.[46] Delayed-onset encephalopathy with personality change and seizures may occur months after infusion.[52]

Cytarabine

Cytarabine (cytosine arabinoside, Ara-C) is a pyrimidine analogue that inhibits DNA replication. It has been given intravenously for leukemias and lymphomas and intrathecally for leptomeningeal metastases.[46] Neurotoxicity is related to the route, as well as the dose administered. High-dose regimens carry a significant risk of neurotoxicity, with up to 30% developing symptoms. Encephalopathy, somnolence, and cerebellar ataxia usually present within 24 hours. MRI shows white matter changes and loss of cerebellar Purkinje cells in patients with ataxia. Neurological recovery may be incomplete and occurs over days to weeks following discontinuation of the medicine.[53–55]

BCNU

BCNU (carmustine) is the prototypical nitrosourea. It is highly lipid soluble and readily crosses the BBB. It is used in the treatment of gliomas, melanoma, and lymphoma and in preconditioning for bone marrow transplants. BCNU does not cause neurotoxicity at conventional doses, but at high doses it can cause a significant encephalopathy and myelopathy. When given intra-arterially, BCNU results in a progressive subacute encephalopathy in 10% of patients. The course is typically marked by progressive confusion, seizures, and hemiparesis contralateral to the side of infusion. The symptoms do not respond to steroids.[46]

L-Asparaginase

L-Asparaginase is an enzyme that converts asparagines to aspartic acid. It is used in the treatment of acute lymphoblastic leukemia. The primary CNS complication of L-asparaginase is its tendency to cause cerebrovascular events. Encephalopathy was previously common when higher doses were used but was probably secondary to hepatotoxicity and elevations in ammonia. The encephalopathy typically reversed over a few days as ammonia levels normalized.[47]

Fludarabine

Fludarabine is a purine analogue used in the treatment of chronic lymphocytic leukemia. At the high doses (more than 50 mg/m^2/day) used in early studies, delayed neurotoxicity was more common. A diffuse leukoencephalopathy became apparent 4 to 8 weeks after treatment and often progressed to coma and death. Current doses of less than 25 mg/m^2/day less often result in symptoms of neurotoxicity, and these symptoms, including somnolence, blurred vision, and hemiparesis, tend to be reversible.[46,55,56] Fludarabine may also increase the risk of progressive multifocal leukoencephalopathy, a condition to which chronic lymphocytic leukemia patients are already prone.[57]

5-Fluorouracil

5-Fluorouracil is an analogue of the pyrimidine uracil. It is used in the treatment of head and neck cancers and colorectal adenocarcinoma. Neurotoxic effects of 5-fluorouracil include encephalopathy and cerebellar symptoms of horizontal nystagmus and limb and gait ataxia. In most cases, these symptoms are fairly mild; however, patients with a deficiency of dihydropyrimidine dehydrogenase (an enzyme needed to metabolize 5-fluorouracil) may develop a profound encephalopathy and seizures.[58] Treatment regimens for colorectal adenocarcinoma may employ the combination of 5-fluorouracil and levamisole. This combination may result in a multifocal inflammatory leukoencephalopathy. The symptoms tend to respond to steroids and remit after discontinuation of the medications.[46,59]

Cisplatin

The platinating agent cisplatin is among the most commonly used chemotherapy agents. It is employed in the treatment of lung, ovarian, and gastrointestinal (GI) cancers. CNS toxicity with this agent is fairly uncommon. When infused intra-arterially for head and neck or brain tumors, a transient encephalopathy or, less often, a permanent leukoencephalopathy can occur.[47,60]

Interferon-α

Interferon-α is a naturally occurring cytokine with antiviral and immune-modulating effects. It is used in low doses in the treatment of melanoma, multiple myeloma, hairy cell leukemia, Kaposi's sarcoma, renal cell carcinoma, non-Hodgkin's lymphoma, and chronic myelogenous leukemia. Neurotoxicity is dose related, with higher doses producing lethargy, somnolence, and encephalopathy in a significant percentage of patients. Headaches commonly accompany the encephalopathy, and hallucinations and seizures may occur. MRI suggests a vasogenic edema in some cases. Electroencephalography generally reveals diffuse slowing, although occasionally generalized sharp-wave discharges are seen.[61,62] Most patients have complete recovery after discontinuation of treatment, but permanent deficits have been reported.[63]

Interleukin-2

Interleukin-2 is a naturally occurring cytokine with immune-modulating and antineoplastic effects. It is used in the treatment of metastatic melanoma and renal-cell carcinoma. Neuropsychiatric symptoms of encephalopathy, depression, hallucinations, and delusions occur in 30% to 50% of patients.[47] These symptoms tend to be dose dependent but usually remit after treatment is stopped. Rarely, administration of interleukin-2 leads to a severe encephalopathy with MRI evidence of lesions in gray and white matter. Focal neurological deficits may accompany the encephalopathy. Symptoms remit in most cases after discontinuation of therapy, but progression and death have been reported.[64–66]

PESTICIDES

Organophosphates

Organophosphates (OPs) are present in nearly 40% of all pesticides used in this country. They are highly lipid soluble and are easily absorbed through the skin and respiratory tract. Toxic exposures occur commonly in farmers, gardeners, crop dusters, and pesticide handlers. OPs are also readily absorbed through the GI tract. Accidental ingestion by children and intentional ingestion in suicide attempts represent an unfortunately high number of exposures annually. Their ability to produce paralysis of smooth and striated muscles has made them useful as agents of chemical warfare.[8]

OPs produce their toxic effects by binding to acetylcholinesterase (AChE). Inhibition of this important enzyme results in excess acetylcholine at neuromuscular junctions and at certain locations in the brain. The peripheral nervous system effects, including excessive salivation, lacrimation, sweating, and diarrhea, are widely recognized as signs of OP toxicity. The acute CNS effects may be mild and are often overshadowed by the peripheral effects at lower levels of exposure. With increased exposure levels, however, encephalopathy, dizziness, and hallucinations become more apparent. Severe encephalopathy, seizures, coma, and death may occur in cases of high levels of exposure. Different OP compounds may result in varied CNS effects, reflecting the distribution of different types of AChE throughout the brain.[8,67]

The delayed effects of OP toxicity on the peripheral nervous system can be debilitating and have been the focus of much attention in the literature. Prolonged CNS dysfunction is also a matter for concern. Studies indicate that cholinesterase inhibitors can cause changes in the mediation of cholinergic neurotransmission in the brain. Victims of high levels of OP exposure later score worse on mood inventories and on tests of sustained visual attention than their nonexposed counterparts.[68,69] Case reports suggest that executive function, memory, and certain learning domains may be impaired for prolonged periods in some individuals, but slow recovery of most functions is the trend.[70–73] Further studies are needed before conclusions can be drawn with regard to long-term brain dysfunction in the setting of chronic, low-level OP exposure.

Given the ease of absorption through the skin and respiratory tract, use of protective masks, gloves, and proper clothing is paramount to preventing toxic OP exposure. OPs should be kept well out of the reach of children and should be stored in well-marked containers. The ACGIH suggests monitoring of OP exposure in high-risk settings. Plasma cholinesterase activity levels are more sensitive to low-level exposure, but erythrocyte AChE activity is a better indicator of neuronal AChE inhibition.[8]

In the event of skin exposure, the skin should be immediately and thoroughly cleansed with soap and water. Any saturated clothing should be removed. In cases of OP ingestion, immediate gastric lavage is warranted to remove as much of the toxin as possible before absorption is complete. Cathartics should also be considered. When given early, oximes such as pralidoxime or obidoxime chloride are useful in minimizing subsequent peripheral neuropathy. These agents do not readily cross the BBB and are therefore less effective in reversing CNS toxicity. Atropine may be used to counteract the muscarinic effects of OPs, but it will not reverse the nicotinic effects and muscle weakness will therefore not improve. Atropine should be administered in small doses (0.5 to 1.0 mg) at 15-minute intervals until signs of OP reversal are apparent. Cessation of sweating and salivation, facial flushing, and papillary dilation signal effective reversal of toxicity. Due to the tendency for OPs to be stored in fatty tissues, continued observation and less frequent dosing of IV atropine (1 to 2 mg every hour) may be needed.[8,74] It should be noted that when seizures occur as a result of OP exposure, the mechanism is increased neuronal stimulation by excessive acetylcholine. These seizures do not respond robustly to dilantin or other antiepileptics and should be treated with atropine.[75]

Carbamates

Carbamates are also used extensively as pesticides. Their mechanism of action, like that of OPs, is inhibition of AChE. The toxicity of the carbamate compounds varies with the molecular structure, but in general the AChE inhibition is of shorter duration than that of OPs. The severity and duration of toxicity are accordingly less. Some carbamates such as disulfiram (Antabuse) and pyridostigmine are even mild enough to be used medically.[76]

Acute toxicity from carbamate exposure produces symptoms identical to OP toxicity. Symptoms of CNS toxicity, while often mild in adults, may be significant in children, and seizures, coma, and death can occur.[77] Encephalopathy, headaches, photophobia, dizziness, and irritability following high-dose exposure have been reported. Slow improvement seems to be the rule, but symptoms can last for years.[78,79] Case reports suggest that a chronic encephalopathy may result from long-term exposure to low doses of carbamates as well.[80] Objective evidence of CNS damage in such cases is lacking.

As with OPs, measures of erythrocyte AChE activity are suggested for monitoring carbamate exposure. Treatment of acute carbamate toxicity is also similar to that for OPs. Due to the shorter duration of action of carbamates, a higher level of caution is warranted in the administration of atropine. Continued use of atropine after reversal of carbamate binding can result in unwanted anticholinergic side effects.[8,76]

METALS

The toxic metals represent a diverse group of elements with a range of toxic effects on neuronal function. In small amounts, many of these metals are necessary to support biological functions. In larger quantities, however, they have deleterious effects on the CNS.

Lead

Lead occurs naturally in trace amounts in soil, rocks, and water. Hundreds of years of mining and smelting of lead for uses in ordinary household items, plumbing, paints, and gasoline have resulted in lead becoming one of the most dangerous neurotoxins in today's world. Environmental and occupational regulations imposed over the last 2 to 3 decades have substantially reduced the incidence of lead intoxication. Measures such as removal of lead from gasoline, residential plumbing, and house paints and reduction of the use of lead-soldered cans for food and beverages have resulted in a dramatic decrease in blood lead levels in the United States.[81,82]

Major sources of potential lead exposure today include lead mining and smelting plants, lead pipes, lead-based paint in older buildings, ceramic glazes, and lead shot. Lead continues to be encountered in the manufacture and recycling of storage batteries, in crystal glass manufacturing, and in certain compounds for auto body repair and manufacturing.[8] In addition, lead contaminates in the air, soil, and water can reach dangerous levels in areas around lead smelters and other industrial plants.[83–85]

Skin absorption of inorganic lead is limited, whereas organic lead such as that found in leaded gasoline is readily absorbed by this route. Inorganic lead is better absorbed through the GI or respiratory tracts. In industrial settings, the respiratory system is the most common route of intoxication as workers inadvertently inhale lead dust. In nonindustrial settings, GI absorption tends to be more common. Ingestion of contaminated water can raise blood lead levels of entire communities. Children are particularly susceptible to the effects of lead poisoning, and permanent neurological impairment is associated with exposures in utero and in early childhood. Small children may ingest contaminated soil or paint chips in older buildings. The susceptibility of children is further amplified because up to 50% of ingested lead is absorbed by the GI tract in children, compared to less than 20% in adults.[8]

Once absorbed, lead binds to erythrocytes and is distributed throughout the body. It is incorporated into the brain and soft tissues, where it may remain for weeks to months. Approximately half of absorbed lead becomes incorporated in the bone matrix, where it may remain for decades.[85] Lead is able to cross the placenta, where damage to the developing fetal nervous system can be particularly devastating. There are several known mechanisms by which lead damages the nervous system. It alters neural migration during CNS development, interferes with neural cell adhesion molecules, and impairs the timed programming of cell-to-cell interactions. Lead also interferes directly with certain neurotransmitter functions.[86]

Acute lead encephalopathy is most commonly seen in occupationally exposed adults or in children following ingestion of lead-containing paints or other items. Children tend to present with lethargy, confusion, ataxia and impaired motor functions, and irritability. Adults may display similar symptoms but more often complain of headache and fatigue. Hallucinations, seizures, and coma can occur in adults and children. Cerebral edema occurs with higher levels of exposure and can mimic a mass lesion with papilledema, positive Babinski sign, and even focal or lateralizing deficits.[87,88] GI complaints such as anorexia, abdominal cramping, and constipation may alert the practitioner to the possibility of lead exposure. In adults, the acute symptoms subside after cessation of the exposure and decline of blood lead levels. Neurological sequelae are more persistent in children, with the most profound effect on intelligence quotient levels.[8]

Repeated acute exposures or chronic low-level exposures lead to more persistent neurological dysfunction. Chronic lead encephalopathy in the adult manifests as decreased memory and slowed cognition. Fatigue, irritability, and headaches may be the focus of the victim's complaints. Often, the symptoms of encephalopathy present so gradually that they are overlooked for some time by victims and their family. Accompanying symptoms of poor sleep, arthralgias, myalgias, and paresthesias, anorexia, and abdominal discomfort are common.[85]

Neuroimaging in cases of lead exposure is often normal but can show diffuse or localized areas of edema. Electroencephalography typically shows diffuse slowing. Paroxysmal abnormalities can be present as well. Laboratory studies consistent with lead encephalopathy include anemia, elevated blood lead levels, decreased blood δ-aminolevulinic acid, and basophilic stippling on peripheral smear. In general, symptoms of encephalopathy appear with blood lead levels between 30 and 100 μg/dL.[8,89]

In the setting of acute lead exposure, chelation therapy should be initiated immediately. Removal of lead before it can be incorporated into the tissues is the goal. Due to increased absorption and higher-sensitivity exposures significant enough to cause an encephalopathy, a high mortality rate is seen in children. Even with chelation therapy, the mortality rate is as high as 25% to 38% with ethylenediaminetetraacetic acid or 2,3-dimercaptopropanol (dimercaprol, British anti-Lewisite) alone. When used in combination, however, some evidence suggests the two agents may reduce mortality further.[90] The oral chelating agent dimercaptosuccinic acid has been licensed by the U.S. Food and Drug Administration for reduction of blood lead levels of 45 μg/dL or higher. Animal studies, however, indicate that it does not significantly reduce brain lead levels.[8]

Mercury

Mercury exists in elemental, organic, and inorganic forms. It is found in thermometers, barometers, batteries, dental amalgams, electronic equipment, disinfectants, and antibacterial and antifungal agents. It is employed as a preservative in latex paints and in treated wood, and it is used in photography and in the manufacture of felt.[90] Mercury occurs naturally in rock and sediment and may leach into the water supply from these sources. More dangerous, however, is water contaminated by improper disposal of industrial waste. Once introduced into the water, mercury becomes methylated by microorganisms. These microorganisms are then ingested by aquatic species, resulting in increased concentrations of toxin. Levels of methylmercury, thus bioamplified, cause toxicity to humans who ingest the affected seafood. A tragic example of this process occurred in the 1950s in Minamata Bay, Japan. As a result of industrial dumping, more than 2000 people were exposed to toxic levels of mercury via ingestion of affected seafood.[91]

Neurological manifestations of methylmercury toxicity range from mild paresthesias and tremor to severe ataxia, spasticity, and visual and hearing loss. Encephalopathy may be a prominent feature and in severe cases may progress to coma and death.[90] The ability of the various forms of mercury to cause encephalopathy depends on the rate of peripheral metabolism and their ability to cross the BBB. Mercury salts, for example, are not highly lipid soluble and therefore do not easily cross into the CNS. Phenylmercury, on the other hand, easily penetrates the BBB but is quickly metabolized by the liver, which greatly decreases the number of toxic molecules that reach the brain.[8,92] Methylmercury is metabolized slowly and is actively transported across the BBB. Once inside the brain, mercury preferentially affects gray matter. Autopsy studies show that neuronal toxicity results in focal necrosis followed by phagocytosis and gliosis. Changes in the visual cortex and insula tend to be especially prominent.[93,94]

Chronic exposure to low levels of mercury is also known to directly affect cortical function. Chronic inhalation of mercury vapor is the mechanism behind the so-called mad hatter syndrome. This historical illness affected individuals employed in the manufacture of felt hats. It consists of a fairly well-defined set of features, including tremor, memory and cognitive decline, social withdrawal, and emotional lability. Specifically, the combination of tremor, gingivitis, and emotional excitability has been touted as the classic triad of long-term mercury exposure.[95–97]

Blood mercury levels can be used to measure exposure to inorganic or elemental mercury. Random urine levels do not accurately predict the severity of exposure, but serial urine samples can be useful in tracking exposure in an individual worker across time. Hair mercury levels reflect the sum of inorganic plus organic sources and can be useful in detecting exposure weeks to months after the event. Neuroimaging in methylmercury-exposed individuals shows varying degrees of atrophy of the occipital lobes and cerebellum, and pathology specimens show significant cell loss deep within the calcarine (visual) cortex. Within the cerebellum there is sparing of Purkinje cells with diffuse granular cell loss.[8]

Treatment of acute mercury intoxication has focused on facilitating elimination of the metal and provision of supportive care. Dimercaprol should be avoided as it can result in redistribution of mercury from peripheral tissues into the CNS. Some limited data suggest that unithion and succimer more safely facilitate the clearance of elemental mercury from the body and that these two agents and N-acetylcysteine may be useful in speeding the clearance of methylmercury.[85] More evidence is needed before conclusions can be drawn regarding the impact of these agents on long-term neurological outcomes.

Arsenic

Arsenic is used most extensively in this country as an ingredient in wood preservatives. It is also used in pesticides and herbicides and in the production of glass, electronics, and computer microchips. It exists naturally in varying levels in soil and plants. Most cases of acute arsenic poisoning are due to accidental ingestion of pesticides or inhalation in industrial settings. Arsenic may enter the body through the respiratory system or the GI system or via dermal absorption. Pulmonary absorption occurs with arsine gas or arsine dust. This route is commonly involved in industrial exposures. The efficiency of GI absorption depends on the type and solubility of the particular arsenic compound ingested, but several of the more commonly encountered compounds are almost completely absorbed. Certain arsenic compounds such as sodium arsenate are also absorbed fairly efficiently through the skin.[8]

Arsenic exerts its toxic effects on biological systems by inhibiting mitochondrial function. It binds to sulfhydryl groups of many proteins and interferes with several steps of oxidative metabolism in neurons and other cells.[90] Arsenic has a much higher affinity for white matter than for gray matter in the brain. The slow clearance of this toxin from brain tissues can result in a profound leukoencephalopathy following either acute or chronic exposures.

Following acute arsenic exposure, GI symptoms such as nausea, vomiting, abdominal pain, and bloody diarrhea tend to dominate early. Acute encephalopathy primarily manifests as confusion, with headache initially. In the hours to days following, delirium, hallucinations, and seizures may occur. Systemic symptoms in this time frame include hematuria, proteinuria, and jaundice. Mees' lines on the fingernails and sensorimotor neuropathy generally take 3 to 4 weeks to appear. Around this time, alopecia, hyperkeratosis, and renal failure become apparent. Diffuse encephalopathy at may be profound as well.[98]

Chronic arsenic exposure in the United States usually occurs in occupational settings. Groundwater contaminated by the leaching of arsenic into groundwater from natural sources has caused toxic exposure to entire communities in Bangladesh and West Bengal India.[99,100] Contamination of water, soil, and air via industrial pollutants has caused unnecessary exposure to still other communities.[101] Chronic encephalopathy is more commonly caused by exposure to organic than inorganic arsenic. Careful questioning and neuropsychiatric testing, however, reveal that subtle cognitive and personality disturbances do occur following exposure to inorganic arsenic.[102–104] Chronic arsenic encephalopathy generally manifests with confusion and irritability. Paranoid delusions and auditory or visual hallucinations can occur.[104,105] Although persistent deficits have been reported, arsenic encephalopathy, whether acute or chronic, generally improves following removal of the exposure.[101,105]

The appropriate laboratory investigation in cases of suspected arsenic toxicity depends on the time from exposure. The metal is detectable in the blood for only

2 to 4 hours; the methylated metabolites monomethyl-arsenic acid and dimethylarsenic acid may be detected for up to 24 hours. Inorganic arsenic is present in urine for up to 30 hours, while the metabolites may remain for 1 to 3 weeks. Organic arsenic, on the other hand, is completely excreted within 24 to 48 hours. Arsenic levels remain detectable in nails and hair for months.

EEGs of arsenic-exposed patients are usually normal, although in some severe cases mild background slowing may be seen. Neuroimaging in most cases of acute exposure is also normal. However, in very high levels of exposure, studies may show evidence of brain swelling or areas of hemorrhage or demyelination. Pathology examinations show petechial hemorrhages due to arteriolar occlusion and areas of demyelination and white matter necrosis throughout the brain.[8]

Treatment for arsenic toxicity consists of gastric lavage and use of cathartics in cases of ingestion. Administration of dimercaprol or British anti-Lewisite is recommended. The oral chelating agent dimercaptosuccinic acid may be given if the patient does not have vomiting and diarrhea. d-Penicillamine is believed to be less effective but may be used if dimercaptosuccinic acid is unavailable.[85,106] Aggressive supportive care and careful monitoring for renal and cardiac failure are also essential. Hemodialysis may be necessary when renal failure occurs.

Manganese

Manganese (Mn), an essential element, is present in all living organisms. In the human body, it functions as a cofactor for several enzymatic reactions. The primary source of this element is food; fruits, nuts, grains, and vegetables are all rich in Mn.[107]

Mn has replaced lead as a fuel additive and is used in fertilizers and in the manufacture of fireworks. It is used in iron and steel manufacturing, in metal-finishing operations, and as an alloy in welding.[90,108] The most common setting of toxic Mn exposure is occupational. Chronic exposures occur in mining, steel mills, and chemical industries. Mn may be absorbed through the respiratory tract, although the extent of absorption varies with particle size and valence of the Mn element. GI absorption is less than 5%.[8] Once absorbed, Mn is transported throughout the body and concentrates in mitochondria. Organic Mn crosses the BBB by passive diffusion. The remaining organic Mn is metabolized to inorganic Mn and is transported across the BBB by transferrin. Individuals with poor hepatic function are at increased risk of Mn toxicity due to decreased excretion of the metal.[109] Once in the brain, it accumulates in gray matter. The highest concentrations in normal brains are found in the melanin-rich globus pallidus and striatum.[110,111] The neurotoxicity of Mn is thought to result from potentiation of free radical production and apoptosis.[90,112]

The classic and most prominent manifestation of Mn toxicity is parkinsonism, but encephalopathy also occurs with both acute and chronic exposures. Acute toxicity can cause frank psychosis, with visual and auditory hallucinations, euphoria, and compulsive behaviors. Headache, irritability, and memory disturbance can be seen with acute or chronic Mn encephalopathy. These symptoms may be subtle early in chronic toxicity and may go unrecognized for some time. With continued exposure, behavioral changes progress. Emotional lability, compulsive laughter, and hallucinations may all present before the appearance of the typical motor features. Tremor, dysarthria, increased tone, and gait disturbance occur relatively late in the process.[110,112,113]

Recovery from toxicity depends somewhat on the duration and form of exposure but tends to be slow and minimal. Chronic inhalation exposure appears to have a poor prognosis from the standpoint of the encephalopathy and motor symptoms, but tremor does tend to improve some. Case reports of shorter exposures and of prolonged ingestion via drinking water indicate a somewhat-better prognosis in adults. In young children, however, even limited exposures have been shown to produce long-term developmental delays.[113–116]

EEG studies are typically normal in cases of Mn poisoning. CT scans are not useful diagnostically, but MRI reveals increased signal on T_1-weighted images within the basal ganglia. Neuropathological findings include cell loss in the globus pallidus, putamen, caudate, and substantia nigra.[8]

Rapid elimination from the blood limits the usefulness of serum Mn levels in diagnosis. Urine or stool levels provide better means of assessing potential toxic exposure. Treatment is generally limited to removal of the toxic source, but chelation with calcium–ethylenediaminetetraacetic acid has shown some benefit in cases of acute exposure. When significant levels of acute exposure occur, dialysis may also be used.[8]

Aluminum

Aluminum is abundant in the natural environment and is used extensively in construction, food packaging, cooking utensils, and pharmaceuticals. It is poorly absorbed following inhalation or ingestion, but toxicity can occur in circumstances of high levels or prolonged exposure. Encephalopathy is a primary feature of acute or chronic aluminum toxicity. The syndrome historically known as *potroom palsy* occurs via occupational exposure in aluminum smelter workers or in other industrial settings. Motor incoordination, poor memory, impaired cognition, and depression are the hallmark symptoms.[117–119] Dialysis-induced encephalopathy, also known as dialysis dementia, previously resulted more often due to the toxic effects of aluminum in dialysis fluid and in the phosphate binders used in dialysis patients. This syndrome occurs in patients after 2 to 7 years of dialysis. Often presenting initially with isolated speech abnormalities, neurological symptoms progress at varying rates and include episodic confusion, behavioral changes, myoclonus, seizures, and frank dementia.[90,120] Deionization of the dialysate and avoidance of aluminum-containing phosphate binders have dramatically reduced the incidence of this disorder.

EEG abnormalities seen in aluminum-exposed patients include background slowing, triphasic waves, and occasionally bilateral spike and wave morphologies. In cases of dialysis-induced encephalopathy, it is important to keep in mind that uremia can produce similar findings. CT and MRI scans typically show only cortical atrophy and enlarged ventricles, but cases of increased signal in white matter areas on T_2-weighted images have been reported with higher levels of exposure.[8]

Blood levels can be used to evaluate patients with potential aluminum toxicity. Normal blood levels are less than 10 µg/L. Concentrations greater than 60 µg/L may warrant chelation therapy. Seizures occurring from aluminum toxicity generally respond to antiepileptics.[8]

Tin

Tin is used extensively in canning, soldering, and electronics. It is used in the manufacture of some plastics and has multiple applications in chemical laboratories. Exposure to inorganic particulate or gas does not cause neurotoxicity. Organic tins, specifically trimethyltin (TMT) and triethyltin (TET), have serious effects on the CNS. They can cause a severe encephalopathy with predominant headache, memory loss, and apathy. Hallucinations, seizures, coma, and death often ensue.[121,122] A limbic–cerebellar syndrome with abnormal eye movements, ataxia, hyperphagia, and hypersexual behavior has been described following high-level exposures to TMT.[123]

EEG abnormalities are common in cases of tin toxicity. Background slowing with bursts of high-amplitude θ- and δ-activity are seen in both TMT and TET exposure. Findings of paroxysmal temporal θ-activity are especially common with TMT exposure, while abnormalities secondary to TET tend to be more diffuse. TET toxicity is associated with brain edema, which may be evident on MRI, whereas neuroimaging in TMT exposure is generally normal.

Urine levels of tin peak between 4 and 10 days and are the most reliable measure to assess tin toxicity. Urine absorption spectrometry may also be used.[122] Information is limited regarding the use of chelating agents in tin toxicity, but there is some evidence that plasmapheresis and d-penicillamine may be of benefit.[123]

Thallium

Thallium is used as a pesticide. It has also been used medicinally for fungal and other infections and cosmetically in depilatory agents. The most common source of toxic exposure is via ingestion of pesticides, or pesticide-contaminated food. Cases of exposure by depilatory agents and by contaminants in illicit drugs have also been reported.[124–126]

Peripheral neuropathy appears over the first week or two after acute exposure. A debilitating encephalopathy can develop during the first 2 to 3 weeks. Symptoms include cognitive impairment, ataxia, headache, and hallucinations. Behavioral changes, paranoia, sleep disturbances, and depression occur as well. Case reports indicate that cognitive and neuropsychological deficits tend to persist long after an acute exposure.[124,125]

Due to fairly rapid uptake in peripheral tissues, blood thallium levels are unreliable. Urine or saliva thallium levels can be useful. For more distant exposure (weeks to months), hair analysis should be used.[8] Nonspecific slowing may be seen on EEGs during the acute intoxication, and mild abnormalities sometimes persist in severe cases. Neuroimaging studies are typically normal.

Absorption and distribution of thallium take up to 24 hours, and gastric lavage and cathartics within this time frame may help reduce toxicity. Absorption from the GI tract may also be inhibited by administration of activated charcoal or Prussian blue (potassium ferric hexacyanoferrocyanate III). Potassium chloride also enhances elimination of thallium.[106,126,127]

BIOLOGICAL NEUROTOXINS

Many living organisms produce toxic chemicals as part of their natural defenses. The more potent of these can compromise the body's support systems, resulting in an indirect encephalopathy. This section is limited to those natural neurotoxins that directly affect the CNS and in which encephalopathy is a prominent part of the clinical syndrome.

Plant Toxins

Many plants have long been recognized for their mind altering potential. *Cannabis sativa* (marijuana) and *Lophophora williamsii,* from which mescaline is derived, are well known for the pleasant encephalopathy they produce. *Lobelia inflata* (lobelia) and *Argemone mexicana* (prickly poppy) are euphoriants. *Nicotiana* (tobacco) species, *Passiflora incarnata* (passion flower), and *Catha edulis* (khat) are strong CNS stimulants that can, at higher doses, produce an acute encephalopathic state marked by agitation, confusion, and decreased attention.[128] *Juniperus macropoda* (juniper), *Nepeta cataria* (catnip), *Piper methysticum* (kava), *Mandragora officinarum* (mandrake), and *Catharanthus roseus* (Madagascar periwinkle) have hallucinogenic properties and can all be found in herbal supplements. Benign at low doses, they can each produce an acute encephalopathy at higher doses. The widely used kitchen spice nutmeg (*Myristica fragrans*) also has hallucinogenic properties at high doses.[129] *Artemisia absinthium* (wormwood), *Valeriana officinalis* (valerian), and *Rauwolfia serpentina* (snakeroot) have sedative properties and produce an encephalopathic state at moderate to high doses.[128] Scopolamine is a plant alkaloid that is active in the CNS. It is present in varying quantities in plants belonging to the *Datura* genus. Among the most notable are *D. stramonium* (jimsonweed) and *D. snaveolus* (angel's trumpet). "Datura tea," brewed from the leaves of some *Datura* plants, has been used as a home remedy for decades and has been a source of acute CNS toxicity. Symptoms of confusion, abnormal behavior, and hallucinations result.[130]

The direct neurotoxic effects of these plants are generally fully reversible, and full recovery from acute encephalopathy is expected if effects from systemic compromise do not cause permanent CNS damage. The potential for long-term effects after repeated exposures to some of these agents remains under debate.

Mushrooms

Of nearly 5000 mushroom species in the United States, about 100 are toxic. Mushrooms that predominantly affect the nervous system generally produce an immediate response following ingestion. *Amanita muscaria, A. panthirina,* and mushrooms in the *Psilocybe* genus are among the more neuroactive mushrooms. Hallucinations and euphoria are primary symptoms of acute mushroom encephalopathy.[131]

Most toxic mushroom exposures occur in the setting of intentional recreational use, although occasionally accidental ingestion does occur. The mechanism of neurotoxicity of *A. muscaria* and *A. panthirina* is attributable to the presence of ibotenic acid. Ibotenic acid and its metabolite muscimol mimic the activity of the excitatory neurotransmitter glutamate. Resulting symptoms of neural excitation include agitation, ataxia, hallucinations, and mental status changes. Frank psychosis and seizures can occur. Activity on the peripheral nervous system is anticholinergic, producing muscle fasciculations, flushing, mydriasis, and urinary retention.[130,132] The activity of the *Psilocybe* genus of mushrooms is caused by the chemical psilocybin and its more potent metabolite psilocin. Both are indolealkylamines with chemical structures similar to that of the neurotransmitter serotonin. They bind to serotonin receptors throughout the brain and produce an lysergic acid diethylamide (LSD)–like effect. Symptoms include euphoria, visual illusions, vivid hallucinations, and reckless behavior. Anxiety, agitation, and decreased mental status also commonly occur. Peripheral effects include tachycardia, hypertension, and hyperthermia. Fortunately, the acute neurotoxic effects of mushrooms generally resolve completely.[128,132]

Marine Toxins

Most marine toxins target the peripheral nervous system but do not significantly affect the CNS. Domoic acid is an exception. Domoic acid is produced by the green algae *Chondria armata* and by the protozoa *Nitchia pungens*. The toxin is ingested and accumulates in mussels feeding on these organisms; humans in turn become exposed by ingesting the mussels. The toxicity of domoic is attributable to its chemical structure. It acts as an excitatory amino acid similar to but up to 30 times more powerful than glutamic acid. The excessive stimulation of susceptible neurons can lead to neuronal death.[130,133] The acute symptoms of domoic acid poisoning include GI distress, headache, confusion, and seizures. Cases of hemiparesis have been described. Recovery is slow, taking weeks to months. In many cases, recovery is complete, but prolonged sensory neuronopathy and significant memory deficits can occur.[134] Development of temporal lobe epilepsy has also been reported.[135]

Pathology findings on one victim of domoic acid poisoning revealed extensive neuronal loss in the hippocampi and patchy neuronal loss in the amygdale. These findings correlate with the memory deficit and susceptibility to seizures. It is thought that domoic acid binds to kainic acid receptors in these regions, causing cell death by overexcitation.[135]

Treatment of domoic acid toxicity is symptomatic. The seizures tend to respond to antiepileptic agents; however, limited case reports suggest that diazepam and phenobarbital may be superior to phenytoin in breaking seizures in this population.[133]

Spiders

Spider venoms are generally quite complex and contain multiple elements that are potentially toxic. Few spider species have large enough and strong enough fangs to make them a threat to adult humans, but young children can be vulnerable to their bites. The venom of the *Latrodectus* (widow) spiders contain a neurotoxin with high concentrations of leucine and isoleucine, as well as lower concentrations of tyrosine. While its primary target is the peripheral nervous system, there is evidence of CNS activity, and varying degrees of headache, dizziness, and restlessness occur acutely.[136]

Scorpions

Most scorpions encountered in the United States have relatively benign venoms with no neurotoxic effects. Exceptions can be found in some members of the *Centruroides* genus encountered in the western and southwestern United States. Specifically, *C. sculpturatus* and *C. exilicauda* have neurotoxic potential. In general, the effects are limited to the peripheral nervous system. However, the resulting motor restlessness, random movements of the head and neck, and roving eye movements can be misinterpreted as an encephalopathic state. This is especially true in children due to their tendency to react more strongly to the venom combined with poorer communication skills and immature psychological reactions. However, it should be noted that true changes in cognition, memory, and executive functions have not been reliably documented in victims of scorpion stings.[137] Other than scorpion antivenom, no drugs of proven value can reverse the acute effects of envenomation. Care is otherwise supportive. In the event of seizures, IV phenobarbital or diazepam are suggested.[136]

Snakes

Snakes venoms are complex and contain numerous compounds with varied sites of action. Several species of snake produce neuromuscular blocking agents, but few snake venoms have been found to be centrally active. Coral snake venom does cause euphoria and drowsiness, along with cranial nerve deficits. The extent to which the encephalopathic symptoms can be attributed direct action in the CNS is unclear. Whether or not encephalopathy occurs, treatment is the same. Administration of antivenom, if available, and supportive care for the systemic manifestations are the focus. Reversal of the CNS effects is expected to follow recovery of these systems.[138]

CONCLUSION

In today's industrialized society, there exist myriad substances with potentially toxic effects on the human brain. Symptoms of such toxicity are varied and often nonspecific. Moreover, the acuity with which they present differs widely depending on the substance and dose of exposure, making awareness and prevention essential in both work and home environments. Despite preventive efforts by numerous health organizations, the occurrence of CNS damage by environmental and industrial toxins is an all-too-common occurrence and physicians and care givers must remain vigilant for such events. While an exhaustive knowledge of all possible CNS toxins is an unattainable goal for most, a basic understanding of typical signs and symptoms of toxic encephalopathy is essential and, when combined with an appropriate level of vigilance, will aid in the timely identification of such exposures. Once suspicion is raised, the appropriate history, examination, and laboratory evaluations can narrow the list of potential toxins, making elimination and treatment possible.

References

1. Ginsberg MD. Carbon monoxide. In: Spencer PS, Schaumberg HH, eds. *Experimental and Clinical Neurotoxicology.* Baltimore: Williams & Wilkins; 1980:374.
2. National Institute for Occupational Safety and Health. Organic Solvent Neurotoxicity: NIOSH Current Intelligence Bulletin, No. 48. Cincinnati, Ohio: NIOSH; 1987.
3. Cherry N, Hutchins H, Pace T, et al. Neurobehavioral effects of repeated occupational exposure to toluene and paint solvents. *Br J Ind Med.* 1985;42:291–300.
4. Arlien-Soborg P, Bruhn P, Gyldensted P, et al. Chronic painters' syndrome: chronic toxic encephalopathy in house painters. *Acta Neurol Scand.* 1979;60:149–156.
5. Schaumberg HH, Spencer PS. Organic solvent mixtures. In: Spencer PS, Schaumberg HH, eds. *Experimental and Clinical Neurotoxicology.* 2nd ed. New York: Oxford University Press; 2000:894–897.
6. Brackner JV, Warren DA. Toxic effects of solvents and vapors. In: Klaassen CD, ed. *Casarett and Doull's Toxicology: The Basic Science of Poisons.* New York: McGraw-Hill; 2001:869–916.
7. Hormes J, Filey C, Rosenberg N. Neurological sequelae of chronic solvent vapor abuse. *Neurology.* 1986;36:689–702.
8. Feldman RG. *Approach to Diagnosis: Occupational and Environmental Neurotoxicology.* Philadelphia: Lippincott-Raven; 1999.
9. Lee BK, Lee SH, Lee KM, et al. Dose-dependent increase in subjective symptom prevalence among toluene-exposed workers. *Ind Health.* 1988;26:11–23.
10. Lazer RB, Ho Su, Melen O, et al. Multifocal central nervous system damage caused by toluene abuse. *Neurology.* 1983;33:1337–1340.
11. Fan AM. Trichloroethylene: water contamination and health risk assessment. *Rev Environ Contam Toxicol.* 1988;101:55–92.
12. Entz RC, Diachenko GW. Residues of volatile halocarbons in margarines. *Food Addit Contam.* 1988;5:267–276.
13. Burmaster DE. The new pollution: groundwater contamination. *Environment.* 1982;24:7–36.
14. Bernad PG, Newell S, Spyker DA. Neurotoxicity and behavior abnormalities in a cohort chronically exposed to trichloroethylene. *Vet Hum Toxicol.* 1987;29:475.
15. Perbellini L, Olivato D, Zedde A, et al. Acute trichloroethylene poisoning by ingestion: clinical and pharmacokinetic aspects. *Int Care Med.* 1991;17:234–235.
16. Feldman RG, White RF, Currie JN, et al. Long-term follow-up after single toxic exposure to trichloroethylene. *Am J Ind Med.* 1985;8:119–126.
17. Lawrence WH, Partyka EK. Chronic dysphagia and trigeminal anesthesia after trichloroethylene exposure. *Ann Intern Med.* 1981;95:710.
18. Leandri M, Schizzi R, Scielzo C, et al. Electrophysiological evidence of trigeminal root damage after trichloroethylene exposure. *Muscle Nerve.* 1995;18:467–468.

19. Szlatenyi CS, Wang RY. Encephalopathy and cranial nerve palsies caused by intentional trichloroethylene inhalation. *Am J Emerg Med.* 1996;14:464–467.

20. Burg JR, Gist GL, Alldred SL, et al. The national exposure registry: morbidity analysis of noncancer outcomes from trichloroethylene subregistry baseline data. *Int J Occup Med Toxicol.* 1995;4:237–257.

21. American Conference of Governmental Industrial Hygienists. Threshold Limit Values (TLVs) for Chemical Substances and Physical Agents and Biological Exposure Indices (BEIs). Cincinnati, Ohio: ACGIH; 1995.

22. Garnier R, Bedouin J, Pepin G, et al. Coin-operated dry cleaning machines may be responsible for acute tetrachloroethylene poisoning: reports of 26 cases including one death. *Clin Toxicol.* 1996;34:191–197.

23. Eicher T, Avery E. Toxic encephalopathies. *Neurol Clin.* 2005;23:353–376.

24. Freed DM, Kandel E. Long-term occupational exposure and the diagnosis of dementia. *Neurotoxicology.* 1988;9:391–400.

25. White RF. Differential diagnosis of probable Alzheimer's disease and solvent encephalopathy in older workers. *Clin Neuropsychol.* 1987;1:153–160.

26. Cassitto MG, Camerino D, Imbriani M, et al. Carbon disulfide and the central nervous system: a 15-year neurobehavioral surveillance of an exposed population. *Environ Res.* 1993;63:252–263.

27. Huang CC, Chu CC, Chen RS, et al. Chronic carbon disulfide encephalopathy. *Environ Neurol.* 1996;36:364–368.

28. Ernst A, Zibrak JD. Carbon monoxide poisoning. *N Engl J Med.* 1998;339:1603–1608.

29. Thom SR. Leukocytes in carbon monoxide–mediated brain oxidative injury. *Toxicol Appl Pharmacol.* 1993;123:234–247.

30. Thom SR. Carbon monoxide–mediated brain lipid peroxidation in the rat. *J Appl Phys.* 1990;68:997–1003.

31. Choi IS. Delayed neurologic sequelae in carbon monoxide intoxication. *Arch Neurol.* 1983;40:433–435.

32. Min SK. A brain syndrome associated with delayed neuropsychiatric sequelae following acute carbon monoxide intoxication. *Acta Psychiatr Scand.* 1986;73:80–86.

33. Messiers LD, Myers RAM. A neuropsychological screening battery for emergent assessment of carbon monoxide–poisoned patients. *J Clin Psychol.* 1991;47:675–684.

34. Agency for Toxic Substances and Disease Registry. Toxicological Profile for Benzene. Atlanta: U.S. Public Health Service, U.S. Department of Health and Human Services; 1997.

35. Bakinson MA, Jones RD. Gassings due to methylene chloride, xylene, toluene, and styrene reported to Her Majesty's Factory Inspectorate, 1961–1980. *Br J Ind Med.* 1985;42:181–190.

36. Klaucke DN, Johansen M, Vogt RL. An outbreak of xylene intoxication in a hospital. *Am J Ind Med.* 1982;3:173–178.

37. Ruitjen MWMM, Hooisma J. Brons JT, et al. Neurobehavioral effects of long-term exposure to xylene and mixed organic solvents in shipyard painters. *Neurotoxicology.* 1994;15:613–620.

38. Uchida Y, Nakatsuka H, Ukai H, et al. Symptoms and signs in workers exposed predominantly to xylenes. *Int Arch Occup Environ Health.* 1993;64:597–605.

39. Bond J. Review of the toxicology of styrene. *Crit Rev Toxicol.* 1989;19:227–249.

40. Edling C, Anundi H, Johansson G, Nilsson K. Increase in neuropsychiatric symptoms after occupational exposure to low levels of styrene. *Br J Ind Med.* 1993;50:843–850.

41. Crandall MS, Hartle RW. An analysis of exposure to styrene in the reinforced plastic boat-making industry. *Am J Ind Med.* 1985;8:183–192.

42. Nestler EJ, Self DW. Neuropsychiatric aspects of ethanol and other chemical dependencies. In: Yudofsky SC, Hales RE, ed. *The American Psychiatric Publishing Textbook of Neuropsychiatry and Clinical Neurosciences.* 4th ed. Washington, DC: American Psychiatric Publishing; 2002:899–921.

43. Kumari M, Ticku MK. Regulation of NMDA receptors by ethanol. *Prog Drug Res.* 2000;54:152–189.

44. Brust JCM. Persistent cognitive impairment in substance abuse. *Continuum.* 2004;5(10):144–150.

45. Brust JCM. Alcoholism. In: Rowland LP, ed. *Merritt's Neurology.* 10th ed. Philadelphia: Lippincott Williams & Wilkins; 2000:921–929.

46. Plotkin SR, Wen PY. Neurologic complications of cancer therapy. *Neurol Clin.* 2003;21:279–318.

47. Schiff D, Wen P. Central nervous system toxicity from cancer therapies. *Hematol Oncol Clin North Am.* 2006;20:1377–1398.

48. Martino RL, Benson AB, Merritt JA, Brown JJ, Lesser JR. Transient neurologic dysfunction following moderate-dose methotrexate for undifferentiated lymphoma. *Cancer.* 1984;54:2003–2005.

49. Walker RW, Allen JC, Rosen G, Caparros B. Transient cerebral dysfunction secondary to high-dose methotrexate. *J Clin Oncol.* 1986;4:1845–1850.

50. Gonzalez-Angulo AM, Orzano JA, Davila E. Ifosfamide-induced encephalopathy. *South Med J.* 2002;95(10):1215–1217.

51. Simonian NA, Gilliam FG, Chiappa KH. Ifosfamide causes a diazepam-sensitive encephalopathy. *Neurology.* 1993;43:2700–2702.

52. Sullivan KM, Storb R, Shulman HM, et al. Immediate and delayed neurotoxicity after mechlorethamine preparation for bone marrow transplantation. *Ann Intern Med.* 1982;97:182–189.

53. Winkelman MD, Hines JD. Cerebellar degeneration caused by high-dose cytosine arabinoside: a clinicopathological study. *Ann Neurol.* 1983;14:520–527.

54. Hwang TL, Yung WK, Estey EH, Fields WS. Central nervous system toxicity with high-dose Ara-C. *Neurology.* 1985;35:1475–1479.

55. Cheson BD, Vena DA, Foss FM, Sorensen JM. Neurotoxicity of purine analogs: a review. *J Clin Oncol.* 1994;12:2216–2228.

56. Cohen RB, Abdallah JM, Gray JR, Foss F. Reversible neurologic toxicity in patients treated with standard-dose fludarabine phosphate for mycosis fungoides and chronic lymphocytic leukemia. *Ann Intern Med.* 1993;118:114–116.

57. Cid J, Revilla M, Cervera A, et al. Progressive multifocal leukoencephalopathy following oral fludarabine treatment of chronic lymphocytic leukemia. *Ann Hematol.* 2000;79:392–395.

58. Takimoto CH, Lu ZH, Zhang R, et al. Severe neurotoxicity following 5-fluorouracil-based chemotherapy in a patient with dihydropyrimidine dehydrogenase deficiency. *Clin Cancer Res.* 1996;2:477–481.

59. Hook CC, Kummel DW, Kvolts LK, et al. Multifocal inflammatory leukoencephalopathy with 5-fluorouracil and levamisole. *Ann Neurol.* 1992;31:262–267.

60. Lyass O, Lossos A, Hubert A, Gips M, Peretz T. Cisplatin-induced non-convulsive encephalopathy. *Anticancer Drugs.* 1998;9:100–104.

61. Rohatiner AZ, Prior PF, Burton AC, Smith AT, Balkwill FR, Lister TA. Central nervous system toxicity of interferon. *Br J Cancer.* 1983;47:419–422.

62. Suter CC, Westmoreland BF, Sharbrough FW, Hermann RC Jr. Electroencephalographic abnormalities in interferon encephalopathy: a preliminary report. *Mayo Clin Proc.* 1984;59:847–850.

63. Meyers CA, Scheibel RS, Forman AD. Persistent neurotoxicity of systemically administered interferon-α. *Neurology.* 1991;41:672–676.

64. Karp BI, Yang JC, Khorsand M, Wood R, Merigan TC. Multiple cerebral lesions complicating therapy with interleukin-2. *Neurology.* 1996;47:417–424.

65. Vecht CJ, Keohane C, Menon RS, Punt CJ, Stoter G. Acute fatal leukoencephalopathy after interleukin-2 therapy. *N Engl J Med.* 1990;323:1146–1147.

66. Bernard JT, Ameriso S, Kempf RA, Rosen P, Mitchell MS, Fisher M. Transient focal neurologic deficits complicating interleukin-2 therapy. *Neurology.* 1990;40:154–155.

67. Finkelstein Y, Wolff M, Biegon A. Brain acetylcholinesterase after acute parathion poisoning: a comparative quantitative histochemical analysis postmortem. *Ann Neurol.* 1988;24:252–257.

68. Steenland K, Jenkins B, Ames RG, et al. Chronic neurologic sequelae to organophosphate pesticide poisoning. *Am J Pub Health.* 1994;84(5):731–736.

69. Rosenstock L, Keifer M, Daniell W, et al. Chronic central nervous system effects of acute organophosphate pesticide intoxication. *Lancet.* 1991;338:223–227.

70. Ames RG, Steenland K, Jenkins B, et al. Chronic neurologic sequelae to cholinesterase inhibition among agricultural pesticide applicators. *Arch Environ Health.* 1995;50:440–444.

71. Fiedler N, Kipen H, Kelly-McNeil K, et al. Long-term use of organophosphates and neuropsychological performance. *Am J Ind Med.* 1997;32:487–496.

72. Gershon S, Shaw FH. Psychiatric sequelae of chronic exposure to organophosphorus insecticides. *Lancet.* 1961;1:1371–1374.

73. Namba T, Nolte CT, Jackrel J, et al. Poisoning due to organophosphate insecticides: acute and chronic manifestations. *Am J Med.* 1971;50:475–492.

74. Ecobichon DJ. Toxic effects of pesticides. In: Klaassen CD, ed. *Casarett and Doull's Toxicology: The Basic Science of Poisons.* 5th ed. New York: McGraw-Hill; 1996:643–689.

75. Thiermann H, Mast U, Kimmeck R, et al. Cholinesterase status, pharmacokinetics and laboratory findings during obidoxime therapy in organophosphate poisoned patients. *Hum Exp Toxicol.* 1997;16:473–480.

76. Taylor P. Anticholinesterase agents. In: Goodman JC, Gilman A, Rall TW, et al., eds. *Goodman and Gilman's the Pharmacological Basis of Therapeutics.* 8th ed. Elmsford, NY: Pergamon Press; 1990:131–149.

77. Lifshitz M, Shahak E, Bolotin A, et al. Carbamate poisoning in early childhood and in adults. *Clin Toxicol.* 1997;53(1):25–27.

78. O'Malley M. Clinical evaluation of pesticide exposure and poisonings. *Lancet.* 1997;349:1161–1166.

79. Grendon J, Frost F, Baum L. Chronic health effects among sheep and humans surviving an aldicarb poisoning incident. *Vet Hum Toxicol.* 1994;36:218–223.

80. Branch RA, Jacqz E. Subacute neurotoxicity following long-term exposure to carbaryl. *Am J Med.* 1986;80:741–745.

81. Centers for Disease Control and Prevention. Second National Report on Exposure to Environmental Chemicals: Lead. Available at: http://www.cdc.govexposurereport/metals/pdf/lead.pdf. Accessed June 24, 2007.

82. Pinkle JL, Brody DJ, Ganter EW, et al. The decline in blood lead levels in the United States. *JAMA.* 1994;272:284–291.

83. Landrigan PF, Baker EL, Feldman RG, et al. Increased lead absorption with anemia and slowed nerve conduction in children near a lead smelter. *J Pediatr.* 1976;89:904–910.

84. Kenter M, Fischer T, Richter G. Changes in external and internal lead load in different working areas of a starter battery production plant in the period 1982–1991. *Int Arch Occup Environ Health.* 1994;66:23–31.

85. Kosnett MJ. Heavy metal intoxication and chelators. In: Katzung BG, ed. *Basic and Clinical Pharmacology.* 9th ed. New York: McGraw-Hill; 1998:970–981.

86. Goyer RA. Results of lead research: prenatal exposure and neurological consequences. *Environ Health Perspect.* 1996;104:1050–1054.

87. Pappas CL, Quisling RG, Ballinger WE, Love LC. Lead encephalopathy: symptoms of cerebellar mass lesion and obstructive hydrocephalus. *Surg Neurol.* 1986;26:391–394.

88. Perelman S, Hertz-Pannier L, Hassan M, Bourrillon A. Case report: lead encephalopathy mimicking a cerebellar tumor. *Acta Pediatr.* 1993;82:423–425.

89. Seppalainen AM. Electrophysiological evaluation of central and peripheral neural effects of lead exposure. *Neurotoxicology.* 1984;5:43–52.

90. Goyer RA, Clarkson TW. Toxic effects of metals. In: Klaassen CD, ed. *Casarett and Doull's Toxicology: The Basic Science of Poisons.* 6th ed. New York: McGraw-Hill; 2001:811–867.

91. Eyl TB. Organic-mercury food poisoning. *N Engl J Med.* 1971;284:706–709.

92. Gutknecht J. Inorganic mercury (Hg^{2+}) transport through lipid bilayer membranes. *J Membr Biol.* 1981;61:61–66.

93. Takeuchi T. Neuropathology of Minamata disease in Kumamoto, especially at the chronic stage. In: Roisin L, Shiaki H, Greeric N, eds. *Neurotoxicology.* New York: Raven Press; 1977:235–246.

94. Eto K. Pathology of Minamata disease. *Toxicol Pathol.* 1997;25:614–623.

95. Rowland LP. Occupational and environmental neurotoxicology. In: Rowland LP, ed. *Merritt's Neurology.* 10th ed. Philadelphia: Lippincott Williams & Wilkins; 2000:940–948.

96. Albers JW, Kallenbach LR, Fine LJ, et al. Neurologic abnormalities and remote occupational elemental mercury exposure. *Ann Neurol.* 1988;24:651–659.

97. Hunter D, Bomford RR, Russell DS. Poisoning by methyl mercury compounds. *QJM.* 1940;9:193–197.

98. Aminoff MS. Effects of occupational toxins on the nervous system. In: Bradley WG, Daroff RB, Fenichel GM, et al., eds. *Neurology in Clinical Practice.* 3rd ed. Boston: Butterworth-Heinemann; 2000:1511–1519.

99. Ratnaike RN. Acute and chronic arsenic toxicity. *Postgrad Med J.* 2003;79:391–396.

100. Chowdhury UK, Biswas BK, Chowdhury TR, et al. Groundwater arsenic contamination in Bangladesh and West Bengal, India. *Environ Health Perspect.* 2000;108:393–397.

101. Hotta N. Clinical aspects of chronic arsenic poisonings due to environmental and occupational pollution in and around a small refining spot. *Jpn J Const Med.* 1989;53:49–69.

102. Abernathy CO, Lin YP, Longfellow D, et al. Arsenic: health effects, mechanisms of actions, and research issues. *Environ Health Perpect.* 1999;107:593–597.

103. White RF, Proctor SP. Clinico-neuropsychological assessment methods in behavioral toxicology. In: Chang LW, Slikker W, eds. *Neurotoxicology: Approaches and Methods.* New York: Academic Press; 1995:711–726.

104. Bolla-Wilson K, Bleeker ML. Neuropsychological impairment following inorganic arsenic exposure. *J Occup Med.* 1987;29:500–503.

105. Morton WE, Caron GA. Encephalopathy: an uncommon manifestation of workplace arsenic poisoning? *Am J Ind Med.* 1989;15:1–5.

106. Sasser SM. Rodenticides. In: Viccellio P, ed. *Emergency Toxicology.* 2nd ed. Philadelphia: Lippincott-Raven; 1998:425–436.

107. Prohaska JR. Functions of trace elements in brain metabolism. *Physiol Rev.* 1987;67:858–910.

108. Mergler D. Manganese: the controversial metal. At what levels can deleterious effects occur? *Can J Neurol Sci.* 1996;23:93–94.

109. Layrargues GP, Shapcott D, Spahr L, Butterworth RF. Accumulation of manganese and copper in pallidum of cirrhotic patients: role in the pathogenesis of hepatic encephalopathy. *Metab Brain Dis.* 1995;10:353–356.

110. Swartz HM, Sarna T, Zecca L. Modulation by neuromelanin of the availability and reactivity of metal ions. *Ann Neurol.* 1992;32:569–575.

111. Huang C, Chu N, Lu C, et al. Chronic manganese intoxication. *Arch Neurol.* 1989;46:1104–1106.

112. Fuller GN, Goodman JC. *Central Nervous System Toxic and Metabolic Disorders: Practical Review of Neuropathology.* Philadelphia: Lippincott Williams & Wilkins; 2001.

113. Mena I, Marin O, Fuenzalida S, et al. Chronic manganese poisoning: clinical picture and manganese turnover. *Neurology.* 1967;17:128–136.

114. Bencko V, Cikrt M. Manganese: a review of occupational and environmental toxicology. *J Hyg Epidemiol Microbiol Immunol.* 1984;28:139–148.

115. Zhang G, Liu D, He P. Effects of manganese on learning abilities in school children. *Chin J Prevent Med.* 1995;29:156–158.

116. Bronstein AC, Kadushin FS, Riddle MW, et al. Oral manganese ingestion and atypical organic brain syndrome and autistic behavior. *Vet Hum Toxicol.* 1988;30:346.

117. Murray JC, Tanner CM, Sprague SM. Aluminum neurotoxicity: a reevaluation. *Clin Neuropharmacol.* 1991;14:179–185.

118. Longstreth WT, Rosenstock L, Heyer NJ. Potroom palsy? Neurologic disorder in three aluminum smelter workers. *Arch Intern Med.* 1985;145:1972–1975.

119. White DM, Longstreth WT, Rosenstock L, et al. Neurologic syndrome in 25 workers from an aluminum smelting plant. *Arch Intern Med.* 1992;152:1443–1448.

120. Alfrey AC, LeGendre GR, Kaehy WD. The dialysis encephalopathy syndrome: possible aluminum intoxication. *N Engl J Med.* 1976;294:184–188.

121. Feldman RG, White RF, Eriator II. Trimethyltin encephalopathy. *Arch Neurol.* 1993;50:1320–1324.

122. Aldridge WN, Brown AW, Brierley JB, et al. Brain damage due to trimethyltin compounds. *Lancet.* 1981;2:692–693.

123. Besser R, Kramer G, Thumler R, et al. Acute trimethyltin limbic-cerebellar syndrome. *Neurology.* 1987;37:945–950.

124. Thompson C, Dent J, Saxby P. Effects of thallium poisoning on intellectual function. *Br J Psychol.* 1988;153:396–399.

125. McMillan TM, Jacobson RR, Gross M. Neuropsychology of thallium poisoning. *J Neurol Neurosurg Psychiatr.* 1997;63:247–250.

126. Insley BM, Grufferman S, Ayleffe A. Thallium poisoning in cocaine abusers. *Am J Emerg Med.* 1986;4:545–548.

127. Thompson DF. Management of thallium poisoning. *Clin Toxicol.* 1981;18:979–990.

128. Doctor SV. Neuropsychiatric aspects of poisons and toxins. In: Ydofsk SC, Hales RE, eds. *The American Psychiatric Publishing Textbook of Neuropsychiatry and Clinical Neurosciences.* 4th ed. Washington, DC: American Psychiatric Publishing; 2002:891–898.

129. Farnsworth NR. Hallucinogenic plants. *Science.* 1986;162:1086–1092.

130. Norton S. Toxic effects of plants. In: Klaassen CD, ed. *Casarett and Doull's Toxicology: The Basic Science of Poisons.* 5th ed. New York: McGraw-Hill; 1996:841–853.

131. Shih RD. Mushroom poisoning. In: Viccellio P, ed. *Emergency Toxicology.* 2nd ed. Philadelphia: Lippincott-Raven; 1998:1081–1086.

132. Norton S. Toxic effects of plants. In: Klaassen CD, ed. *Casarett and Doull's Toxicology: The Basic Science of Poisons.* 6th ed. New York: McGraw-Hill; 2001:965–976.

133. So YT. Effects of toxins and physical agents on the nervous system: marine toxins. In: Bradley WG, Daroff RB, Finichel GM, et al., eds. *Neurology in Clinical Practice.* 3rd ed. Boston: Butterworth-Heinemann; 2000:1535–1539.

134. Teitelbaum JS, Zatorre RJ, Carpenter S, et al. Neurological sequelae of domoic acid intoxication due to the ingestion of contaminated mussels. *N Engl J Med.* 1990;322:1781–1787.

135. Cendes F, Andermann F, Carpenter S, et al. Temporal lobe epilepsy caused by domoic acid intoxication: evidence for glutamate receptor–mediated excitotoxicity in humans. *Ann Neurol.* 1995;37:123–126.

136. Findlay ER. Toxic effects of animal toxins. In: Klaassen CD, ed. *Casarett and Doull's Toxicology: The Basic Science of Poisons.* 5th ed. New York: McGraw-Hill; 1996:801–839.

137. Findlay ER. Toxic effects of terrestrial animal venoms and poisons. In: Klaassen CD, ed. *Casarett and Doull's Toxicology: The Basic Science of Poisons.* 6th ed. New York: McGraw-Hill; 2001:945–964.

138. Garcia-Prats VM. Reptilian envenomation. In: Viccellio P, ed. *Emergency Toxicology.* 2nd ed. Philadelphia: Lippincott-Raven; 1998:1035–1048.

CHAPTER 8

Toxic Encephalopathies II: Leukoencephalopathies

Maria K. Houtchens

INTRODUCTION

Neurotoxicity is an effect of toxins and chemicals that disrupts normal nervous system function. Some of the toxins act directly on neural cells and axons, while others interfere with blood supply and metabolism, both of which are critical for normal nervous system operations. Chemicals and toxins that impair cerebral function can be naturally occurring or synthetic. Depending on their level of potency and predilection toward a particular nervous system cell type, or structure, they cause a range of clinical syndromes. The majority of toxic encephalopathies involve cortical and/or subcortical neuronal function. Isolated encephalopathies primarily involving subcortical white matter are less common but are important to recognize. We specifically address neurotoxic conditions preferentially impairing cerebral white matter, or leukoencephalopathies.

Cerebral white matter has been identified as a distinct anatomic structure since the early 16th century. White matter plays a critical role in movement, sensation, and vision. Cognitive processing and emotional state also depend on white matter integrity due to its important long association tracts connecting the frontal lobe with the rest of the brain and its commissural tracts providing interlobar connections throughout the hemispheres.

Various diseases can affect integrity and function of the white matter, including genetic, infectious, demyelinating, inflammatory, vascular, and toxic–metabolic (Table 1). Leukoencephalopathy, therefore, warrants a careful consideration of a broad differential diagnosis.

Toxic leukoencephalopathy should be suspected in any patient who presents with acute or chronic behavioral deficits and who has a known or potential exposure to neurotoxic agents. Damage to the white matter tends to be diffuse; the clinical picture often parallels the severity and the extent of the fiber involvement and ranges from mild confusional states to severe dementia, stupor, and coma. In general, from a clinical perspective, neurobehavioral function tends to be the most affected in toxic leukoencephalopathies.[1]

WHITE MATTER TOXINS

Cranial Radiation

Cranial radiation is a well-established modality for the treatment of primary or metastatic brain tumors. Radiation can cause significant damage to the brain and may result in clinical symptoms as devastating as the sequelae of the tumor itself. Three types of injury can be seen as a result of radiation therapy to the brain: acute,

Table 1: Diseases of the White Matter

Genetic	Infectious	Demyelinating	Metabolic	Inflammatory	Toxic	Vascular
LEUKODYSTROPHIES	AIDS dementia	Multiple sclerosis	Vitamin B$_{12}$ deficiency	Systemic lupus	Cranial radiation	Binswanger dementia
Metachromatic leukodystrophy	Progressive multifocal leukoencephalopathy	Acute disseminated encephalomyelitis	Folate deficiency	Sjögren's disease	Chemotherapy	CADASIL
Krabbe's disease	Subacute sclerosing panencephalitis	Schilder's disease	Central pontine myelinolysis	Temporal arteritis	Toluene	Leukoariosis
Adrenoleukodystrophy	VZV encephalitis	Marburg variant	Hypertensive encephalopathy	Scleroderma	Ethanol	Cerebral amyloid angiopathy
Canavan's disease	CMV encephalitis	Balò's concentric sclerosis	Eclampsia	Primary CNS vasculitis	Heroin	
NEUROCUTANEOUS SYNDROMES	Lyme encephalopathy	Devic's disease	High-altitude cerebral edema	Sarcoidosis	Cocaine	
Neurofibromatosis type 1				Polyarteritis nodosa	Carbon monoxide	
Tuberous sclerosis					Other toxic substances	

AIDS, acquired immune deficiency syndrome; CADASIL, cerebral autosomal dominant arteriopathy with subcortical infarcts and leukoencephalopathy; CMV, cytomegalovirus; CNS, central nervous system; VZV, varicella zoster virus.

early delayed, and late delayed leukoencephalopathy. The dose of radiation that can induce leukoencephalopathy has been greater than 50 Gy in adults and 35 Gy in children, although individual variations can change susceptibility.

Acute reaction occurs at the time of treatment and likely results from cerebral edema. The symptoms may include transient confusion and temporary worsening of preexisting focal neurological symptoms. This process is self-limiting and may respond to steroid treatment. *Early delayed reaction* (Figure 8-1) can be seen within weeks to several months after cessation of treatment and is thought to arise from demyelination. Confusion and somnolence are common, and near-complete recovery is usually seen.[1,2] *Late delayed reaction* is seen within 6 months to 2 years after discontinuation of therapy, but reports of new symptoms attributable to this, starting as late as 20 years after completion of radiation therapy, can be found in the literature.[3] It is the most serious complication of cranial radiation and is thought to result from severe demyelination and necrosis. Death or serious disability can be the unfortunate outcome. Neurological symptoms may include dementia, personality change, progressive confusional states in adults, and severe learning impairment in children. Magnetic resonance imaging (MRI) shows a diffuse and confluent T2 hyperintense signal throughout the cerebral white matter (Figure 8-2).[3] Incontinence and gait disorder associated with ventriculomegaly are sometimes observed, suggesting that hydrocephalus may play a role in clinical symptoms in postradiation leukoencephalopathy patients. Cerebrospinal fluid (CSF) ventriculoperitoneal shunting was shown to offer mild clinical improvement in a retrospective study.[4] Hyperbaric oxygen therapy has also been used in adults and children with postradiation leukoencephalopathy. This treatment modality is safe and well tolerated. Its efficacy remains questionable.[5]

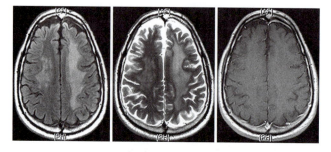

Figure 8-1. Magnetic resonance imaging (MRI) of an early delayed postradiation leukoencephalopathy. A 61-year-old man with radiation-induced encephalopathy, after 13 treatment cycles for management of primary central nervous system lymphoma. MRI shows nonenhancing diffuse white matter T2 and fluid-attenuated inversion recovery hyperintensities.

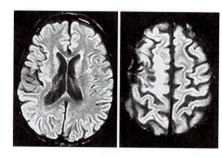

Figure 8-2. Magnetic resonance imaging (MRI) of a late delayed postradiation leukoencephalopathy. Fluid-attenuated inversion recovery images demonstrate asymmetrical white matter hyperintensities and predominant right-sided ventricular enlargement diagnosed as late delayed postradiation leukoencephalopathy 20 years after cranial radiation for a low-grade glioma. There was no evidence of tumor recurrence clinically or on MRI. (Duffey P, Chari G, Shaw P, et al. Progressive deterioration of intellect and motor function occurring several decades after cranial irradiation: a new facet in the clinical spectrum of radiation encephalopathy. Arch Neurol. 1996;53[8]:814–818.)

CHEMOTHERAPEUTIC AND IMMUNOSUPPRESSIVE AGENTS

Central nervous system (CNS) white matter is a target of some pharmaceutical (cyclosporine, tacrolimus, methotrexate) and occupational (triethyl tin) agents. Exposure to these may cause acute encephalopathy syndrome. Some agents have predilection toward occipital or parietal white matter (posterior leukoencephalopathy); delirium is accompanied by early visual impairment and spasticity in this condition.

Methotrexate (MTX) is a synthetic antimetabolite (antifolate), a weak organic acid, exhibiting its cytotoxic effects by inhibiting the enzyme dihydrofolate reductase, thus blocking purine biosynthesis. It is used in various cancer treatment regimens (trophoblastic tumors, non-Hodgkin's lymphoma, acute lymphoblastic leukemia, breast cancer, osteogenic sarcoma, primary CNS lymphoma, meningeal carcinomatosis). As an oral formulation, it is also beneficial as an adjunctive therapy in treatment of refractory rheumatological, dermatological, or neurological autoimmune conditions such as rheumatoid arthritis, psoriasis, and multiple sclerosis.

In humans, MTX administered orally of intravenously in low doses (30 to 60 mg/m^2) is not associated with significant neurotoxicity. Treatments with doses of 1 g/m^2 or higher produce acute or subacute encephalopathy in 20% of exposed patients.[6] Symptoms include headache, confusion, somnolence, and rarely, seizures and focal neurological deficits. Exact toxic mechanism is not known, but positron emission tomography studies show reduced cerebral glucose metabolism and evidence of blood–brain barrier impairment. This syndrome tends to be reversible, usually, without treatment. It does not always recur with repeated dosing of MTX.[7]

Following intrathecal or intraventricular MTX administration, two major leukoencephalopathy syndromes have been described: chronic leukoencephalopathy (usually following postradiation MTX administration) and localized white matter changes with edema and focal necrosis in proximity to intraventricular catheter sites.

The risk of progressive chronic leukoencephalopathy increases with younger age (<5), with associated preceding or concurrent cranial radiation, with presence of leptomeningeal disease, and with known obstruction of CSF flow. Symptoms may appear at the time of treatment or as late as 8 months following cessation of treatment and initially include subtle personality changes, decreased memory and intellectual function, and effortful speech. Overtime, abnormal gait, ataxia, sphincter dysfunction, and myoclonus (characteristically involving pharyngeal and peripheral muscles) ensue. CSF studies show elevated protein with lymphocytic pleocytosis. MRI shows extensive and severe fluid-attenuated inversion recovery (FLAIR) and T2 abnormalities in periventricular white matter (Figure 8-3; see also the Case Study in this chapter). A pathological study of the brain shows coagulation necrosis in the white matter in a perivascular pattern. White matter nerve fibers show damage with axonal swelling. This condition often results in death within several months of symptom onset.[8]

Patients with intraventricular catheters may develop focal areas of necrotizing encephalopathy similar to diffuse encephalopathic changes but focally, around the catheter tip, or alongside the shaft of the catheter. In these cases, clinical presentation is specific to the affected site. MRI usually reveals pericatheter T2 hyper-

densities. This pathology is thought to be a result of CSF backflow around the catheter, causing significantly elevated MTX concentrations in focal brain tissue.[9]

Nitrosoureas (BCNU, carmustine) are active lipid-soluble compounds in wide use for treatment of brain tumors. Their ability to readily cross the blood–brain barrier via passive diffusion is beneficial in neuro-oncology. The mechanism of neurotoxicity may include a direct drug-induced toxic effect on CNS and drug-induced metabolic encephalopathy. Leukoencephalopathy may follow high dose (600 to 800 mg/m²) intravenous or intra-arterial administration and may manifest in confusion, disorientation, occasional seizures, and white matter T2 hyperintensities on MRI that appear similar to postradiation abnormalities. Pathologically, changes include spongiform degeneration and reactive gliosis in the white matter.[10]

Cisplatin or carboplatin is an antitumor platinum-based compound, used alone or in combination for treatment of gynecological malignancies and testicular cancers. Most prominent neurotoxicity involves symmetrical sensory neuropathy, but CNS toxicity has rarely been described and includes several cases of necrotizing leukoencephalopathy.[11,12]

Cyclosporin A is a fungal-derived selective inhibitor of adaptive T- and B-cell responses widely used in postorgan transplantation immunosuppression and in treatment of refractory autoimmune diseases. It can cause non-dose-dependent, acute, diffuse leukoencephalopathy. Symptoms include headaches, confusion, disorientation, anxiety, visual disturbances, spasticity, and seizures. MRI shows white matter edema and T2 hyperintensities with a predilection toward posterior lobes akin to changes of hypertensive posterior leukoencephalopathy[19] (Figure 8-4). While the exact pathology of this process is not known, it is thought to be similar to acute, hypertensive encephalopathy and eclampsia, resulting from areas of focal vascular constriction and vasodilation. This causes a breakdown of blood–brain barrier and transudation of fluid into

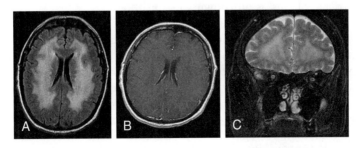

Figure 8-3. Methotrexate-induced leukoencephalopathy. *A,* fluid-attenuated inversion recovery T2 sequence showing a diffusely abnormal, confluent hyperintensity consistent with toxic leukoencephalopathy. *B,* Gadolinium-enhanced, T1 sequence showing absence of an abnormally enhancing signal corresponding to fluid-attenuated inversion recovery sequence hyperintensity. *C,* Coronal T2 sequence showing a confluent, abnormal signal in the cerebral white matter consistent with toxic leukoencephalopathy.

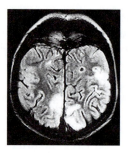

Figure 8-4. Magnetic resonance imaging (MRI) of cyclosporin A toxicity. MRI fluid-attenuated inversion recovery image showing an abnormal signal throughout the occipitoparietal cortex and cerebral white matter in a 9-year-old patient treated with cyclosporin A. (Tweddle DA, Windebank KP, Hewson QC, et al. Drug points: cyclosporin neurotoxicity after chemotherapy. *BMJ.* 1999;318:1113.)

cerebral white matter. Treatment cessation usually results in resolution of clinical syndrome and MRI changes within weeks to months.[14,15]

Tacrolimus (FK-506) is a macrolide antibiotic derived from soil organism *Streptomyces*. It is a T-cell and B-cell immunosuppressant used in treatment of posttransplant patients undergoing liver, pancreatic, renal, and cardiac transplantation. It is also used in organ and allogeneic hematopoietic stem cell transplantation. FK-506 therapy can be associated with serious leukoencephalopathy. In contrast to cyclosporin A–induced encephalopathy, high plasma levels of FK-506 are usually found in patients on this treatment who present with a change in level of consciousness (somnolence to coma), generalized, focal motor, or complex partial seizures, dysarthria, dysphasia, visual disturbances, and emotional changes. However, normal plasma levels have also been associated with FK-506-induced leukoencephalopathy.[16]

MRI of the brain is the most sensitive diagnostic study. MRI findings of predominantly posterior occipitoparietal subcortical white matter lesions in FLAIR and T2-weighted images were characteristic of those reported in the literature.[17]

Neurotoxic mechanism of tacrolimus is unknown. Pathologically, there is nonspecific patchy or diffuse demyelination, with an occasional report of astrocytosis, CNS phlebitis, and necrotizing angiopathy.[18,19] As with cyclosporin A, withholding or discontinuing treatment usually results in resolution of symptoms.

Isolated reports of toxic leukoencephalopathy have been seen with the other antineoplastic agents such as cytosine arabinoside, a combination regimen of 5-fluorouracil, and levamisole, fludarabine, thiotepa, interleukin-2, and interferon-α. These are infrequent, and detailed discussion of each substance is not offered in this chapter as these are described in more detail in Chapter 8.

LEUKOENCEPHALOPATHIES COMPLICATING SUBSTANCE ABUSE

Toluene (Methylbenzene)

Toluene (methylbenzene) is a natural substance of gasoline and crude oil. It is also used for synthesis of benzene and other chemicals, including graphic pigments, paints, and solvents. It is a highly lipophilic white matter toxin resulting in loss of myelin in cerebral and cerebellar white matter, as well as in diffuse cerebral and cerebellar atrophy.[20,21] Intentional abuse occurs through inhalation of toluene vapors from a rag soaked in paint or from a paper bag filled with paint or lacquer thinners, which contain toluene as principle component. While the prevalence of toluene abuse in the United States is unknown, it is estimated that 10% to 15% of people have used the inhalant.[22] Prolonged exposure to toluene vapors may result in multifocal leukoencephalopathy, with primary clinical manifestations of dementia, ataxia, brain-stem dysfunction, and corticospinal weakness. Dementia is the most disabling aspect of the syndrome, characterized by apathy, memory loss, visuospatial deficits, and preserved language function. Leukoencephalopathy of toluene abuse is evident on MRI scans and on postmortem examinations.[23]

In advanced cases, the pattern of multifocal white matter disease can suggest a diagnosis of multiple sclerosis in a young adult, if abuse history is not obtained.[24] Diagnosis, however, is usually clear and is based, in an acute setting, on solvent-smelling breath, perioral "huffer's" rash, and appropriate history. Toxicological screening can detect toluene in the blood; hippuric acid analysis of urine is also helpful.

Prolonged, low-level occupational exposures to pure toluene are rare; most industrial exposures include solvent mixtures and cause a so-called solvent syndrome, resulting in change in personality and progressing to permanent cognitive impairment.

Ethanol

Alcohol has been available to humans for thousands of years. The distillation process invented by the Arabs introduced more concentrated ethanol products to Europe in the Middle Ages. Over the subsequent centuries, ethanol abuse became a worldwide public health problem. In the United States, approximately 5% of total yearly mortality is a consequence of complications of ethanol abuse.[25]

Alcohol is a CNS depressant causing the euphoria and hyperactivity in early intoxication and sedation in later stages. Ethanol intoxication, either acute or chronic, may be associated with many toxic syndromes in the CNS or peripheral nervous system. Some of these syndromes are discussed in more detail elsewhere in this book. Here, we focus primarily on alcohol effects on white matter damage, considering a rather controversial condition of "alcoholic dementia" and Marchiafava-Bignami disease (MBD).

Loss of cognitive capacity in chronic heavy drinkers is, at times, unexplained by nutritional deficiency, head injury, liver failure, anoxia, or any other cause.

The term *alcoholic dementia* is appropriate when one is presented with a demented patient with a history of chronic alcohol abuse who is not deficient in thiamine and who has clinical cognitive disorder that exceeds isolated amnesia.[26] Alcoholics often have cognitive impairment that does not fit the pattern of typical Wernicke-Korsakoff's syndrome. The onset is gradual, and typical neurological features of Wernicke's encephalopathy are absent.[27] Pathological studies have been controversial, and reports of cerebral atrophy and ventricular enlargement and sulcal widening have been inconsistent among investigators.[28,29] Subsequent studies showed a disproportionate loss of cerebral white matter in chronic alcoholics and a significant burden of white matter lesions in alcoholics who had no other neurological complications of alcoholism.[30,31]

MBD or Marchiafava–Bignami disease is a primary degeneration of the corpus callosum associated with chronic alcohol consumption.[32] It was first described by two Italian pathologists who identified callosal demyelination in three chronic alcoholics presenting with seizures and subsequent coma. The diagnosis of MBD mainly rests on the evidence of central demyelination of the corpus callosum rather than on the variable clinical features. Demyelination usually starts medially and spreads rostrally and caudally, sparing the dorsal and ventral rims. Extension into the cerebral white matter involving anterior and posterior commissures, subcortical frontal lobes (Figure 8-5), (Figure 8-6), and the middle cerebellar peduncles has been described.[33–35] The symptoms of MBD may include psychiatric abnormalities, such as mania, paranoia, depression, cognitive dysfunction, and dementia. In later stages, seizures, hemiparesis, aphasia, dysarthria, and chorea have been seen. The symptoms of hemispheric disconnection can also be present and may include unilateral apraxia and agraphia without aphasia.[36]

It is generally accepted that the disease is mainly due to a deficiency in the vitamin B complex, and although many patients improve following administration of these compounds, others do not; some die from the disease.[37]

Heroin

Heroin is synthesized from morphine, a natural alkaloid contained in seed capsules of the poppy plant. Heroin crosses the blood–brain barrier faster than

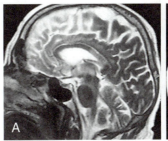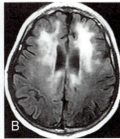

Figure 8-5. Marchiafava-Bignami disease: callosal and frontal white matter involvement. *A,* Midsagittal magnetic resonance imaging (MRI) T2-weighted image showing increased signal intensity in the posterior body of the corpus callosum without any mass effect. There is atrophy of the cerebellar vermis, particularly its superior aspects. *B,* Axial MRI fluid-attenuated inversion recovery image showing increased signal intensity in the frontal white matter and in the periventricular areas. (Arbelaez A, Pajon A, Castillo M. Acute Marchiafava-Bignami disease: MR findings in two patients. AJNR. 2003;24: 1955–1957.)

morphine and is metabolized to 6-acetylmorphine and morphine.[25]

Heroin pyrolysate, a form of heroin produced by heating heroin on tinfoil, is associated with spongiform leukoencephalopathy. Reports of such encephalopathy are coming from Europe and describe clinical syndrome of abnormal behavior, ataxia, quadriparesis, chorea, and myoclonus. Some cases have resulted in death.[38]

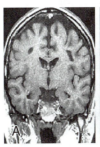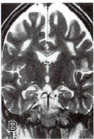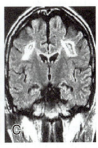

Figure 8-6. Symmetrical corpus callosum lesions in Marchiafava-Bignami disease. Fast spin echo T1-weighted *(A)* and T2-weighted *(B)* magnetic resonance images. The lesion of the corpus callosum shows the same signal intensity as the symmetrical lesions in the periventricular white matter (hypointensities in T1-weighted images, hyperintensities in T2-weighted images). In the fluid attenuated inversion recovery magnetic resonance image *(C),* the corpus callosum still shows a high-intensity signal area, whereas the lesions in the centrum semiovale appear slightly hypointense centrally and hyperintense peripherally. (Ferracci F, Conte F, Gentile M. Marchiafava-Bignami disease: computed tomograghic scan, 99mTc HMPAO-SPECT, and FLAIR MRI findings in a patient with subcortical aphasia, alexia, bilateral agraphia, and left-handed deficit of constructional ability. Arch Neurol. 1999;56:107–110.)

ENVIRONMENTAL TOXINS

Carbon Monoxide

Carbon monoxide (CO) is produced by fuel combustion in vehicles and is a byproduct of home and industrial energy consumption. CO intoxication is the most common fatal accidental poisoning in the United States. Mortality from acute exposure can be as high as 30%, and a similar number of victims can be left with permanent neurological sequelae.[39]

Cortical gray matter, especially the hippocampus, the basal ganglia, and the cerebellum are usually affected and are thought to be related to cerebral hypoxia due to CO binding to the ferrous iron complex of protoporphyrin IX in the hemoglobin molecule and reduction in tissue oxygen transport capacity of this protein. This syndrome is described elsewhere in the book. However, a delayed and widespread cerebral demyelination has also been described.

An initial report of delayed CO encephalopathy was published in 1926 and described a patient with abulia, akinetic mutism, dementia, and parkinsonian features.[40] Upon pathological examination of the patient's brain, diffuse cerebral demyelination with a variable degree of axonal loss was the most prominent feature. Similar cases were described subsequently; the predominant pathological feature in all of these cases was demyelination of centrum semiovale and the periventricular zones, with relative sparing of the corpus callosum, fornix, and anterior commissure.[41] No specific predictors of development of delayed encephalopathy have been identified, although some suggest that age greater than 50 years and severe coma at the onset of acute CO intoxication may predispose to delayed demyelination.

Similar leukoencephalopathy can follow other hypoxic–ischemic insults, such as postsurgical and postanesthesia complications, drug overdoses, anaphylactic reactions, prolonged seizures, and strangulation. Hemispheric white matter may be especially vulnerable to prolonged states of hypoxemia due to its reliance on deep penetrating arteries or due to reperfusion injury to myelin.[42]

Hyperbaric oxygen therapy has been used to treat delayed postischemic leukoencephalopathy with variable success.

Arsenic

Arsenic is a group Vb metal. It is uncommon in nature and is rarely a source of industrial or occupational human exposure. In the past, organic arsenicals were used in treatment of neurosyphilis. They were used as diuretics before development of the thiazides in 1950s. Inorganic arsenic salts are produced in the copper- and lead-smelting industry and were used in pesticides and rodenticides until 1960s.[43,44] Suicide and homicide have been attempted by ingestion of arsenic.[45]

Arsenic compounds are large, charged particles that do not readily cross the blood–brain barrier. Transient CNS impairment can be seen either in a form of "acute hemorrhagic encephalitis" or as "prolonged encephalopathy," with pathological correlates of multiple areas of necrosis and hemorrhage in the cerebral white matter. However, peripheral neuropathy is the best known neurotoxicity.[46]

OTHER COMPOUNDS

Triethylin (TET) belongs to a group of compounds known as *organotins*. It is a colorless, water-insoluble liquid that has been used in industrial chemicals and biocides. An epidemic of human TET intoxication was seen in France in 1950s, when a therapeutic medication was inadvertently contaminated with this compound. At that time, 102 people died, and another 100 were permanently disabled. Symptoms appeared within 4 days from exposure and included headache, nausea, vomiting, vertigo, signs of meningeal irritation, seizures, papilledema, and transient or permanent paralysis. Pathological studies revealed diffuse edema of the white matter.[47]

Hexachlorophene is a poorly soluble white powder with limited historical use as an antimicrobial and a cosmetic preservative. It had efficacy against gram-positive bacteria and had various uses in topical antibacterial ointments and soaps. It is absorbed through the skin, gut, and mucous membranes and is toxic to the brain and peripheral nerves, where it causes vacuolar myelinopathy.[48]

Clinical experience stems from accidental poisoning of 224 children in France following the use of contaminated talcum powder. Clinically, the children exhibited signs of increased intracranial pressure, seizures, paresis, and confusion. Pathologically, cerebral white matter had signs of extensive vacuolar demyelination, primarily in reticular formation and in the heavily demyelinated tracts of brainstem.[49]

Fumonisin B_1 is a mycotoxin detected in maize products worldwide. Leukoencephalopathy in livestock has been described with this compound.

Cycloleucine was originally developed as an anticancer drug in 1960s. It showed disappointing results in advanced solid tumor patients and severe neurotoxicity, which limited its use. The brain, spinal cord, and peripheral nerves are the primary targets for cycloleucine toxicity. It severely depletes an important component of myelin synthesis, resulting in vacuolar myelinopathy of the white matter. This compound is currently used only experimentally.[50]

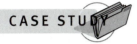

CASE STUDY

JH is a 51-year-old physician who initially presented to neurological attention with complaints of blurred vision. On examination, he was found to have bilateral uveitis. Upon identification of abnormal cells in the vitreous, the diagnosis of vitreal lymphoma was suspected, and it was confirmed following bilateral vitrectomy. He received six cycles of chemotherapy with MTX, which eventually had to be discontinued due to the patient's cognitive decline and changes on brain MRI consistent with MTX-induced leukoencephalopathy (see Figure 8-3).

Neuropsychological testing showed impairment in multiple cognitive domains relative to premorbid functioning. On many measures administered, the patient's performance fell in the below-average range. Tests included measures of verbal comprehension, perceptual organization, confrontation naming, verbal fluency, executive functioning, processing speed, and most measures of memory. JH was also described as depressed and withdrawn. He became permanently disabled due to his cognitive status despite discontinuation of chemotherapy treatment and prolonged remission of lymphoma.

REFERENCES

1. Filley CM. Toxic leukoencephalopathy. *Clin Neuropharmacol.* 1999;22(5):249–260.
2. Schultheiss TE, Kun LF, Ang KK, et al. Radiation response of the central nervous system. *Int J Radiation Oncology Biol Phys.* 1995;31:1093–1112.
3. Duffey P, Chari G, Shaw P, et al. Progressive deterioration of intellect and motor function occurring several decades after cranial irradiation: a new facet in the clinical spectrum of radiation encephalopathy. *Arch Neurol.* 1996;53(8):814–818.
4. Thiessen B, DeAngelis L. Hydrocephalus in radiation leukoencephalopathy: results of ventriculoperitoneal shunting. *Arch Neurol.* 1998;55(5):705–710.
5. Ashmalla HL, Thom SR, Goldwein JW. Hyperbaric oxygen therapy for the treatment of radiation-induced sequelae in children: the University of Pennsylvania experience. *Cancer.* 1996;77(1):2407–2412.
6. Spencer PS, Schaumburg HH, eds. *Experimental and Clinical Neurotoxicology.* 2nd ed. New York: Oxford University Press; 2000.
7. Phillips PC, Dhawan V, Strother SC, et al. Reduced cerebral glucose metabolism and increased brain capillary permeability following high-dose methotrexate chemotherapy: a PET study. *Ann Neurol.* 1987;21:59–62.
8. Schilsky RL. Antimetabolites. In: Perry MC, ed. *Chemotherapy Source Book.* Baltimore: Williams & Wilkins; 1992.
9. Lemann W, Wiley RG, Posner JB. Leukoencephalopathy complicating intraventricular catheters: clinical, radiographic and pathologic study of 10 cases. *J Neuroonc.* 1988;6:67–73.
10. Burger PC, Kamenar E, Schold SC, et al. Encephalomyelopathy following high dose BCNU therapy. *Cancer.* 1981;48:1318–1327.
11. Bruck W, Heise E, Friede RL. Leukoencephalopathy after cisplatin therapy. *Clin Neuropathol.* 1989;8:263–265.
12. Berman IJ, Mann MP. Seizures and transient cortical blindness associated with cis-platinum (II) diammine dichloride (PDD) therapy in a thirty-year-old man. *Cancer.* 1980;45:764–766.
13. Tweddle DA, Windebank KP, Hewson QC, et al. Drug points: cyclosporine neurotoxicity after chemotherapy. *BMJ.* 1999;318:1113.
14. Truwit CL, Denaro CP, Lake JR, et al. MR imaging of reversible cyclosporin A–induced neurotoxicity. *AJNR.* 1991;12:651–659.
15. Garg RK. Posterior leukoencephalopathy syndrome. *Postgrad Med J.* 2001;77(903):24–28.
16. Wong R, Beguelin G, De Lima, M, et al. Tacrolimus-associated posterior reversible encephalopathy syndrome after allogeneic haematopoietic stem cell transplantation. *Br J Haematol.* 2003; 122(1):128–134.
17. Bartynski WS, Zeigler Z, Spearman MP, et al. Etiology of cortical and white matter lesions in cyclosporin A and FK-506 neurotoxicity. *AJNR.* 2001;22:1901–1914.
18. Eidelman BH, Abu-Elmagd K, Wilson J, et al. Neurologic complications of FK-506. *Transplant Proc.* 1991;23:3175–3178.
19. Frank B, Perdrizer GA, White HM, et al. Neurotoxicity of FK-506 in liver transplant recipients. *Transplant Proc.* 1993;25:1887–1888.
20. Kornefeld M, Moser AB, Moser HW. Solvent vapor abuse leukoencephalopathy: comparison to adrenoleukodystrophy. *J Neuropathol Exp Neurol.* 1994;53:389–398.
21. Lazar RB, Ho SU, Melen O, et al. Multifocal central nervous system damage caused by toluene abuse. *Neurology.* 1983;33: 1337–1340.
22. Hornes JT, Filley CM, Rosenberg NL. Neurologic sequelae of chronic solvent vapor abuse. *Neurology.* 1986;36:698–702.
23. Rosenberg NL, Spitz MC, Filley CM, et al. Central nervous system effects of chronic toluene abuse: clinical, brainstem evoked response and magnetic resonance imaging studies. *Neurotoxicol Teratol.* 1988;10:489–495.
24. Davies MB, Weatherby SJ, Haq N, et al. A multiple sclerosis–like syndrome associated with glue-sniffing. *J R Soc Med.* 2000;93(6): 313–314.
25. Brust JCM. *Neurological Aspects of Substance Abuse.* Boston, Mass: Butterworth-Heinemann; 1993.
26. Lishman WA. Cerebral disorder in alcoholism: syndromes of impairment. *Brain* 1981;104:1–20.
27. Nicolas JM, Estruch R, Salamero M, et al. Brain impairment in well-nourished chronic alcoholics is related to ethanol intake. *Ann Neurol.* 1997;41:590–598.
28. Joyce EM. Aetiology of alcoholic brain damage: alcoholic neurotoxicity or thiamine malnutrition? *Brit Med Bull.* 1994;50:99–114.
29. Wang GJ, Volkow ND, Roque CT, et al. Functional importance of ventricular enlargement and cortical atrophy in healthy subjects and alcoholics as assessed with PET, MR imaging, and neuropsychologic testing. *Radiology.* 1993;186:59–65.
30. De la Monte SM. Disproportionate atrophy of cerebral white matter in chronic alcoholics. *Arch Neurol.* 1988;45:900–902.
31. Gallucci M, Amicarelli I, Rossi A, et al. MR imaging of white matter lesions in uncomplicated chronic alcoholism. *J Comput Assist Tomogr.* 1989;13:395–398.

32. Navarro JF, Noriega S. Marchiafava-Bignami disease. *Rev Neurol.* 1999;28:519–523.

33. Arbelaez A, Pajon A, Castillo M. Acute Marchiafava-Bignami disease: MR findings in two patients. *AJNR.* 2003;24: 1955–1957.

34. Ferracci F, Conte F, Gentile M. Marchiafava-Bignami disease: computed tomograghic scan, ^{99m}Tc HMPAO-SPECT, and FLAIR MRI findings in a patient with subcortical aphasia, alexia, bilateral agraphia, and left-handed deficit of constructional ability. *Arch Neurol.* 1999;56:107–110.

35. Baron R, Heuser K, Marioth G. Marchiafava-Bignami disease with recovery diagnosed by CT and MRI: demyelination affects several CNS structures. *J Neurol.* 1989;236:364–366.

36. Rosa A, Demiati M, Cartz L, et al. Marchiafava-Bignami disease, syndrome of interhemispheric disconnection, and right-handed agraphia in a left-hander. *Arch Neurol.* 1991;48:986–988.

37. Victor M. Persistent altered mentation due to ethanol. *Neurol Clin.* 1993;11:639–661.

38. Wolters ECH, Van Winjungaarden GK, Stam FC, et al. Leukoencephalopathy after inhaling "heroin pyrolysate." *Lancet.* 1982;2: 1233–1237.

39. Gorman DF, Clayton D, Gilligan JE, et al. A longitudinal study of 100 consecutive admissions for carbon monoxide poisoning to the Royal Adelaide Hospital. *Anaesth Intensive Care.* 1992;20: 311–316.

40. Grinker RR. Parkinsonism following carbon monoxide poisoning. *J Nerv Ment Dis.* 1926;64:18–25.

41. LaPresle J, Fardeau M. 1967. The central nervous system and carbon monoxide poisoning: II. Anatomical study of brain lesions following intoxication with carbon monoxide (22 cases). *Prog Brain Res.* 1967;24:31–74.

42. Ginsberg MD. Delayed neurological deterioration following hypoxia. *Adv Neurol.* 1979;26:21–47.

43. Beckett WS, Moore JI, Keogh JP, et al. Acute encephalopathy due to occupational exposure to arsenic. *Br J Ind Med.* 1986;43: 66–67.

44. Freeman JW, Couch JR. Prolonged encephalopathy with arsenic poisoning. *Neurology.* 1978;28:853–855.

45. Fincher RF, Koerker RM. Long-term survival in acute arsenic encephalopathy. *Ann J Med.* 1987;82:549–552.

46. Dong HQ, Wang KL, Ma YJ, et al. A clinical analysis of 117 cases of acute arsenic poisoning. *Chung Hua Nei Ko Tsa Chih.* 1993;32:813–815.

47. Georg J Krinke. Triethyltin. In: Spencer PS, Schaumburg HH, eds. *Experimental and Clinical Neurotoxicology.* Baltimore: Williams & Wilkins; 2000.

48. Steinschneider M. Hexachlorophene. In: Spencer PS, Schaumburg HH, eds. *Experimental and Clinical Neurotoxicology.* Baltimore: Williams & Wilkins; 2000.

49. Shuman RM, Leech RW, Alvord EC Jr. Neurotoxicity of hexachlorophene in the human: a clinico-pathologic study of 248 children. *Pediatrics.* 1974;54:689–695.

50. Powell HC. Cycloleucine. In: Spencer PS, Schaumburg HH, eds. *Experimental and Clinical Neurotoxicology.* Baltimore: Williams & Wilkins; 2000.

Toxic Optic Neuropathies

Jane W. Chan

Nutritional and toxic optic neuropathies are discussed in this chapter because of their overlap of clinical presentation and course. It is not always possible to distinguish between the two etiologies, such as in tobacco–alcohol amblyopia. Drugs, poisonous substances, and radiation can cause toxic optic neuropathies without underlying nutritional deficiencies.

NUTRITIONAL AND TOXIC OPTIC NEUROPATHIES

Symptoms

The symptoms and signs of nutritional and toxic optic neuropathies are similar in that they usually present simultaneously and bilaterally. Symptoms are progressive, with bilateral, symmetrical visual loss without pain. Some patients may initially only observe dyschromatopsia, such that certain colors, such as red, are not as bright. Usually only one eye may be involved in the early stages before the other becomes symptomatic. But if one eye is severely affected while the other eye has normal findings, then the diagnosis of nutritional or toxic optic neuropathy is questionable. A gradual progressive blurriness and then cloudiness often forms at the point of fixation.[1]

Signs

Visual acuity then declines rapidly or slowly to any level. Nutritional optic neuropathies usually result in visual acuity of 20/200 or better. A visual acuity of 20/400 or better is often seen in toxic optic neuropathies, except in methanol toxicity, which causes complete or nearly complete blindness. As visual acuity decreases, a protan defect develops. Because of the symmetrical and bilateral visual impairment, a relative afferent pupillary defect is not often present. The pupillary light response may be bilaterally sluggish or absent. The pupils are often dilated in completely or nearly blind patients. The most common visual field defects seen in nutritional or toxic optic neuropathies are central and cecocentral scotomas. In nutritional optic neuropathies, the optic disc may be normal or mildly hyperemic in the early stages. Splinter hemorrhages may occasionally be seen on or off the hyperemic disc. Over several months to years, papillomacular bundle atrophy and temporal disc pallor are followed by optic atrophy. In the early stages of toxic optic neuropathies, the optic discs usually appear normal. Disc edema and hyperemia is seen more often in acute intoxications. The severity and course of development of papillomacular bundle and temporal disc atrophy varies according to the type of toxin. For example, optic discs initially appear normal in ethambutol toxicity and then become atrophic if the drug is continued, whereas optic disc edema and flame-shaped hemorrhages are the initial presentation in amiodarone toxicity.[1]

Evaluation of a Nutritional or Toxic Optic Neuropathy

Evaluation of any patient suspected of having a nutritional or toxic optic neuropathy should include a detailed history of when a drug or toxin was ingested, family history, and dietary history. In toxic optic neuropathies, the visual loss may be acute or chronic. The onset of visual symptoms occurring during or immediately after exposure to the specific toxin and the occurrence of similar illnesses in coworkers or others exposed to the same drug or chemical may help establish the etiology of the visual loss.[1]

In addition to the history and examination, magnetic resonance imaging (MRI) of the brain and orbits with contrast is required to rule out compressive and ischemic lesions, as bilateral central vision loss can occur from bilateral occipital lesions. MRI of the optic nerves and optic chiasm with and without gadolinium and diffusion tensor imaging may be needed to assess for signs of inflammation, demyelination, or both.[1-3] Visual field testing by static or kinetic techniques is essential. Although central or cecocentral scotomas are more common in affected patients, bitemporal defects or peripheral field constriction may occasionally occur in patients with ethambutol or amiodarone toxicity, respectively. In any patient with bilateral central scotomas, laboratory investigation for vitamin B_{12} deficiency and folate deficiency must be performed.[1]

In diagnosing vitamin B_{12} (cobalamin) deficiency, serum B_{12} levels may be misleading because vitamin B_{12} may bind to transcobalamins that may lead to falsely normal serum B_{12} levels, such as in hepatic disorders. Falsely low serum levels may be seen in folate deficiency or during pregnancy. When the serum B_{12} level does not definitely demonstrate deficiency, serum methylmalonate and homocysteine levels should be measured. These precursors of the cobalamin-dependent pathway are elevated in a least 85% of patients with vitamin B_{12} deficiency. Although these elevated levels of metabolites are not specific for vitamin B_{12} deficiency, they are useful in establishing the diagnosis of vitamin B_{12} deficiency when the serum B_{12} level is in the low to normal range (200 to 350 pg/mL).[4]

To determine the cause of the vitamin B_{12} deficiency, antiparietal cell antibodies, which are present in about 85% of patients with autoimmune atrophic gastritis, and anti-intrinsic factor antibodies, which are more specific than sensitive, for should be measured. A Schilling test to look for vitamin B_{12} malabsorption syndrome should also be performed by a gastroenterologist.[4]

A complete blood cell count and examination of the peripheral blood smear for any macrocytosis, macroovalocytes, and hypersegmented neutrophils is also required to establish the diagnosis of megaloblastic anemia, since vitamin B_{12} deficiency is associated with this disorder.[4]

Other laboratory tests in the workup of nutritional or toxic optic neuropathy include red blood cell folate levels; Venereal Disease Research Laboratory; vitamin assays; serum protein concentrations; serum chemistry; urinalysis; heavy metal screening, especially for lead, thallium, and mercury; and Leber's hereditary optic neuropathy (LHON) genetic testing. Identification of the suspected toxin and its metabolite should be performed in the serum and urine (Table 1 and Table 2).[4]

NUTRITIONAL OPTIC NEUROPATHY

Vitamin deficiencies are now rare in the United States and in Western Europe. They are most likely to occur associated with general malnutrition; as a complication of another disease, such as malabsorption or alcoholism; as a consequence of therapy, such as hemodialysis or total parenteral nutrition; or as a result of an inborn error of metabolism. The vitamin deficiencies, including vitamin B_{12}, vitamin B_1, vitamin B_2, and folic acid, cause central vision loss, dyschromatopsia, cecocentral scotomas, and a selective loss of the papillomacular bundle.[5]

Vitamin B_{12} Deficiency Optic Neuropathy

Vitamin B_{12} deficiency is the underlying cause of several syndromes of nutritional optic neuropathy. The optic neuropathy may be the initial manifestation in a patient when no other neurological signs of vitamin B_{12} deficiency, such peripheral neuropathy and dementia, are evident. Males comprise 80% of affected patients.[6]

Vitamin B_{12} deficiency and its complications are more often seen in pernicious anemia, an autoimmune disorder resulting from antiparietal cell antibodies and anti-intrinsic factor antibodies that inhibit the production of intrinsic factor, which is required for absorption of vitamin B_{12} in the ileum. Pernicious anemia most often occurs in middle-aged and elderly white people. Optic neuropathy may be the initial feature of pernicious anemia, preceding the development of megaloblastic anemia and even lower cervical and upper thoracic posterior column demyelination and leukoencephalopathy. Patients with pernicious anemia and no visual symptoms may have abnormal visual evoked potentials (VEPs), suggestive of subclinical optic nerve lesions, optic chiasm lesions, or both.[1]

Vitamin B_{12} deficiency leads to elevated levels of methylmalonyl coenzyme A (CoA) that interferes with fatty acid synthesis, resulting in abnormal myelin formation.[7,8] This subclinical optic neuropathy can be detected

Table 1:	Drugs, Nutritional Deficiencies, and Toxins Associated with Toxic Optic Neuropathy
DRUGS	
Antimicrobials	Chloramphenicol, chloroquine, clioquinol, dapsone, ethambutol, iodochlor-hydroxyquinoline, isoniazide, linezolid, streptomycin
Immunomodulators or immunosuppressives	Cyclosporine, interferon-α, tacrolimus (FK-506)
Chemotherapeutics	Carboplatin, chlorambucil, cisplatin, 5-fluorouracil, methotrexate, nitrosourea (carmustine [BCNU], lomustine [CCNU], nimustine [ACNU]), paclitaxel, tamoxifen, 5-vincristine, cytosine arabinoside, purine analogs, procarbazine, cyclophosphamide, vinca alkaloids
Other drugs	Amiodarone, amantidine amoproxen, cafergot, chlorpropamide, cimetidine, clomiphene citrate, deferoxamine, disulfiram, emetine, infliximab, pheniprazine, quinine, sildenafil
NUTRITIONAL DEFICIENCIES	Vitamin B_1 (thiamin), vitamin B_2 (riboflavin), vitamin B_{12} (cobalamin), folate
TOXINS	Alcohol, arsacetin, carbon monoxide, carbon disulfide, carbon tetrachloride, cobalt chloride, ethchorvynol, ethylene glycol, hexachlorophene, iodoform, lead, mercury, methanol, methylacetate, methylbromide, octamoxin, organic solvents, perchloroethylene, pheniprazine, plasmocid, styrene, thallium, trichloroethylene, triethyl tin, tobacco, toluene, unshielded radiation exposure of more than 3000 rads

Adapted from Miller NR, Newman NJ, eds. *Walsh and Hoyt's Clinical Neuro-ophthalmology: The Essentials.* 5th ed. Baltimore: Williams & Wilkins; 1998.

by delayed P100 latencies. Vitamin B_{12} deficiency is also postulated to alter oxidative metabolism. It causes decreased levels of succinyl CoA, an integral component of Kreb's cycle. It is thought that impaired oxidative metabolism leads to elevated levels of methyltetrahydrofolate (MTHF), required for converting homocysteine to methionine. As a kainate receptor agonist, MTHF causes excessive depolarization[9,10] and depletion of adenosine triphosphate (ATP).[11,12]

Since the parvoretinal ganglion cells[13] of the papillomacular bundle have a higher energy demand than the magnoganglion cells,[14] the papillomacular bundle would be most affected by ATP deficiency secondary to vitamin B_{12} deficiency. This vulnerability may explain the development of a cecocentral scotoma in vitamin B_{12} deficiency optic neuropathy. ATP deficiency may also explain the onset of optic neuropathy when no other neurological signs are evident. Furthermore, ATP deficiency may be a possible mechanism to explain LHON, tobacco–alcohol amblyopia, and other toxic optic neuropathies.[5]

The diagnostic evaluation of suspected vitamin B_{12} deficiency consists of checking the serum cobalamin level and the serum methylmalonate and homocysteine levels. Although not specific for cobalamin deficiency, the metabolites, methylmalonate and homocysteine, can help establish a diagnosis of cobalamin deficiency when the serum cobalamin level is in the low to normal range (200 to 350 pg/mL).[4] Vitamin B_{12} levels below 100 pg/mL often produce neurological manifestations. Antiparietal cell antibodies, which are more sensitive, and anti-intrinsic factor antibodies, which are more specific, may both be used to identify patients with autoimmune atrophic gastritis. The cause of the vitamin B_{12} deficiency should then be evaluated by the Schilling test to determine the degree of cobalamin malabsorption. Because cobalamin deficiency is associated with megaloblastic anemia, a complete blood cell count and an examination of a peripheral blood smear should be performed to look for macrocytosis with macro-ovalocytes and hypersegmented neutrophils.[4]

The treatment of vitamin B_{12} deficiency is cyanocobalamin 1000 μg IM three times weekly for the first 2 weeks, followed by maintenance therapy of 500 to 1000 μg IM monthly. This replacement therapy is lifelong in most circumstances. Some patients who discontinue maintenance therapy may experience recurrence of neurological symptoms. Reversal of symptoms and signs is greater with early and aggressive therapy. High-dose

Table 2: Differential Diagnosis of Nutritional and Toxic Optic Neuropathies

- Arteritic ischemic optic neuropathy (giant cell arteritis)
- Nonarteritic ischemic optic neuropathy
- Infiltrative optic neuropathy (sarcoidosis)
- Infectious optic neuropathy (syphilis, Lyme, toxoplasmosis, herpes zoster)
- Optic neuritis from demyelinating disease
- Postradiation optic neuropathy
- Hereditary optic neuropathy (Leber's hereditary optic neuropathy, dominant optic neuropathy)
- Compressive optic neuropathy (orbital pseudo-tumor, thyroid eye disease)
- Autoimmune optic neuropathy (lupus)

Adapted from Miller NR, Newman NJ, eds. *Walsh and Hoyt's Clinical Neuro-ophthalmology: The Essentials.* 5th ed. Baltimore: Williams & Wilkins; 1998.

folate therapy corrects the megaloblastic anemia caused by cobalamin deficiency, but it does not improve and may even worsen the neurological disease.[4]

COMBINED NUTRITIONAL AND TOXIC OPTIC NEUROPATHIES

Cuban Epidemic of Optic Neuropathy

From 1991 to 1993, approximately 50,000 cases of nutritional optic neuropathy were reported during food shortages in Cuba. Most were adult men and women ranging from 25 to 60 years of age. Sadun et al.[15] studied the Cuban epidemic of optic neuropathy and defined diagnostic criteria for this syndrome. According to these criteria, the nerve fiber layer in the papillomacular bundle must be present with three of the five following symptoms or signs: (1) subacute bilateral visual loss, (2) dyschromatopsia, (3) cogwheel smooth pursuit, (4) central or cecocentral scotomas, or (5) impairment of contrast sensitivity.

In a study by Roman,[16] the 50,862 reported cases were analyzed further to reveal not only optic neuropathy but also sensorineural deafness, peripheral painful sensory neuropathy, and dorsolateral myeloneuropathy.

These clinical features were consistent with Strachan's syndrome and beriberi, disorders resulting from a deficiency of micronutrients.[17,18] Most Cubans significantly improved after multi-B vitamin and folate supplements. Less than 0.1% of them had any sequelae.

Vitamin B_{12} and folate deficiencies and environmental factors, such as chronic methanol ingestion and cyanide exposure, probably contributed to this syndrome. It was thought that formate accumulation from folic acid deficiency and methanol ingestion could cause oxidative phosphorylation defects.[19] In a study by Gay et al. of 34 affected Cubans with 65 controls,[19] dietary factors were associated with the occurrence of epidemic neuropathy in Cuba. Smoking and alcohol consumption augmented the adverse effects of dietary deficiencies. The Cubans had a diet consisting of low caloric energy, protein, fat, and micronutrients with a disproportionate excess of sugar.

The acquired mitochondrial dysfunction from dietary-related ATP deficiency could also lead to this Cuban epidemic. Some reports have even shown the presence of LHON mutations, which could have further predisposed some Cubans to develop optic neuropathy. In a report by Johns et al.,[20] mitochondrial DNA mutations in two of nine Cubans with optic neuropathy and peripheral neuropathy had LHON mutation at nucleotide position 9438 and a novel mutation at nucleotide position 9738 in the cytochrome-*c* oxidase subunit III gene. The stresses of poor diet, smoking, alcohol, and other environmental factors could have precipitated the clinical manifestation of LHON in these patients. LHON should be carefully distinguished from Cuban epidemic optic neuropathy.[21]

The affected Cubans in this epidemic who were treated with cyanocobalamine 3 mg/day and folate 250 mg/day within 3 months of onset of symptoms experienced visual recovery. In a study of 20 patients, average visual acuity recovered from 20/400 to 20/50 and average color vision on American Optical Color test plates improved from 2/8 to 7/8.[15]

Tobacco–Alcohol Amblyopia

The nutritional optic neuropathy in Cuba was also influenced by other environmental factors. Lincoff et al.[22] and Tucker and Hedges[23] described a clinical syndrome involving thiamine- and vitamin B_{12}–deficient optic neuropathy, glossitis, cheilitis, and cheilosis associated with cigarette smoking and alcohol consumption. This combined nutritional and toxic optic neuropathy is often called tobacco–alcohol amblyopia. It usually affects middle-aged men who are heavy smokers and alcoholics.[24] Subacute progressive, symmetrical, painless bilateral visual loss, dyschromatopsia, and central or cecocentral scotomas are characteristic symptoms.[25–27] Tortuous small retinal vessels may be seen. The optic discs initially appear normal and become pale later.[27]

The mechanism by which tobacco causes optic nerve toxicity is unclear, but it is believed that vitamin B_{12} deficiency and the cyanide in tobacco may play a role in optic nerve damage, possibly by demyelination.[28] Despite little change in current tobacco consumption in Western countries, new cases of tobacco–alcohol amblyopia have decreased, suggesting that nutritional deficiencies have an important role in this disorder. Other cases with no nutritional deficiencies detected have been associated with tobacco toxicity.[29] Cyanide and free radicals from the tobacco have been shown to decrease mitochondrial respiratory activity,[30] damage mitochondrial DNA,[31] and even cause changes in mitochondrial morphology.[32]

The treatment for tobacco–alcohol amblyopia is cessation of smoking and drinking. Visual recovery may be seen within a few weeks of treatment with hydroxycobalamin injections.[15]

Although only a few Cubans were affected by nutritional optic neuropathy, no specific genetic predisposition was identified in those who were affected. Some clinical features of tobacco alcohol amblyopia were similar to those of LHON, but the prodromal symptoms of weight loss, polyuria, fatigue, and other neurological manifestations, such as myelopathy and peripheral neuropathy appeared more consistently in Cubans with tobacco–alcohol amblyopia. Cogwheel smooth pursuit and visual recovery with vitamin supplementation also distinguished this epidemic disorder from LHON.[33]

Other Epidemics of Combined Nutritional and Toxic Optic Neuropathies

Similar epidemics of nutritional optic neuropathy have been studied in other parts of the world. Prisoners of war from Thailand[34] in 1945 and prisoners during the Korean War[35,36] developed nutritional amblyopia. With vitamin B complex supplementation, they recovered some vision as early as 2 weeks after therapy was initiated.

In Jamaica, Strachan's syndrome is associated with poor nutrition.[37] Bilateral visual loss with central or cecocentral scotomas and temporal disc pallor was associated with a painful sensory ataxic peripheral neuropathy and muscle atrophy. Gastric achlorhydria and malabsorption of vitamin B_{12} was found in most affected people. Treatment with vitamin B after many years of visual loss did not promote recovery.

A Strachan-like syndrome was also discovered in Nigeria in the 1970s by Osuntokun and Osuntokun.[38] The 360 Nigerians with tropical amblyopia presented with gradual or rapid visual loss, color defects, and peripheral constriction in 84% of affected people, rather than central scotomas. It was hypothesized that peripheral retinal damage may have contributed to the peripherally constricted visual fields, but 41% of affected people had marked bilateral temporal disc pallor, similar to that

seen in nutritional amblyopia. Cyanide from cassava beans, a staple food in Nigeria, was thought to have contributed to this disorder. Elevated levels of cyanocobalamin, plasma thiocyanate, cyanide, and urinary thiocyanate were all suggestive of cyanide exposure. A balance diet helped improve vision, and a return to the cassava diet worsened vision.

Removal of the toxin may lead to some reversal of the optic neuropathy. Oral maintenance replacement therapy of thiamine at 100 mg/day, folic acid at 1 mg/day, and vitamin B_{12} at 1000 mg/day may be appropriate for those with additional folate deficiency. Folate treatment itself only reverses the megaloblastic anemia caused by cobalamin deficiency and does not improve the optic neuropathy. Discontinuation of smoking and alcohol, along with a well-balanced diet emphasizing green vegetables and fruit, is critical for recovery in nutritional optic neuropathy.[4]

Folic Acid Deficiency Optic Neuropathy

Like vitamin B_{12}, folate is involved in methionine metabolism. Folate, in the form of MTHF, donates a methyl group to homocysteine to form methionine and tetrahydrofolate. Tetrahydrofolate helps metabolize formate. Folate deficiency leads to the accumulation of formate, which is also a toxic metabolite from methanol, causing optic neuropathy.[39] Folic acid deficiency causes other neurological manifestations, such as polyneuropathy and even subacute combined degeneration of the spinal cord. Although folate deficiency often occurs with other nutrient deficiencies, isolated folic acid deficiency was shown to cause optic neuropathy in a study by Golnik and Schaible[40] and in another study by Hsu et al.[41] The six patients with low folate levels but normal vitamin B_{12} levels developed bilateral visual loss, color defects, and central or cecocentral scotomas with optic discs that were normal or had temporal disc pallor. Measurement of erythrocyte folate, rather than serum folate, was found to be more sensitive in the early diagnosis of this disorder. With folate replacement therapy, their vision improved within 4 to 12 weeks of symptom onset.

Thiamine or Vitamin B_1 Deficiency Optic Neuropathy

Several studies have shown that isolated thiamine deficiency can cause optic neuropathy. Children maintained on a ketogenic diet for seizure control[42] developed bilateral visual loss with cecocentral scotomas and low serum transketolase (an indication of thiamine deficiency) with normal vitamin B_{12} and folate levels. After replacement therapy, their vision recovered. Five patients with tobacco amblyopia who were treated with thiamine and an inadequate diet recovered vision within

6 weeks of onset of symptoms.[8] In another case report of a patient with ulcerative colitis who developed no light perception and oculomotor palsy, thiamine replacement therapy resulted in visual recovery within a few days.[43]

Vitamin E Deficiency Optic Neuropathy

Vitamin E deficiency causes progressive ataxia, arreflexia, ophthalmoplegia, and pigmentary retinopathy. Optic neuropathy has been reported in a patient with cholestatic liver disease[44] and vitamin E deficiency with normal vitamin B$_{12}$ and folate levels. The patient developed optic disc pallor and pigmentary retinopathy. VEPs were bilaterally extinguished, and the electroretinogram was abnormal.

Zinc Deficiency Optic Neuropathy

Zinc is required for the metabolism of vitamin A in the eye.[45,46] Zinc plays an important role in stabilizing microtubules for axonal transport. Zinc deficiency causes defective rapid axonal transport in vitro and therefore may contribute to the development of optic neuropathy.

Although zinc deficiency may cause abnormal rod function, it has been associated with optic neuropathy in acrodermatitis enteropathica, an autosomal recessive defect in intestinal zinc absorption. Six patients with acrodermatitis enteropathica have been documented with optic atrophy.[47]

Further evidence linking zinc deficiency with optic neuropathy has indirectly been shown in the chelation of zinc by ethambutol, which may cause optic neuritis. In a study of 84 patients with ethambutol toxicity, those with lower zinc levels (less than 0.7 mg/L) had a higher incidence of optic neuritis than those with serum levels greater than 1 mg/L.[48]

Iatrogenic Malabsorption Syndrome–related Optic Neuropathy

A biliopancreatic bypass surgery to induce a malabsorption syndrome to treat morbid obesity can be complicated by hypocalcemia with metabolic bone disease, a marked steatorrhea and protein malnutrition[49] to cause a combined vitamin A deficiency and nutritional optic neuropathy. Visual function retuned to normal after oral vitamin and mineral supplementation.

TOXIC OPTIC NEUROPATHY

Tobacco-related Optic Neuropathy

See the Tobacco–Alcohol Amblyopia section.

Methanol-associated Optic Neuropathy

Methanol, used as an industrial solvent and in automotive antifreeze, is one of the most common causes of toxic optic neuropathy. Formic acid, its metabolite, blocks mitochondrial pathways in the retina and optic nerve.[50] The symptoms of methanol intoxication are usually delayed for 12 to 18 hours. During this latent period, methanol is oxidized to the more toxic formate, which then causes a metabolic acidosis, a hallmark of methanol intoxication. The degree of acidosis is an approximation of the severity of the intoxication. Drowsiness, headache, nausea, vomiting abdominal pain, and blurry vision are the common presenting symptoms and may be followed by blindness, coma, and cardiac arrest if intoxication is severe.[51] Permanent visual loss may occur within hours to days after ingestion of methanol.

Patients intoxicated with methanol may present with varying levels of visual loss, even with total permanent blindness. Central and cecocentral scotomas are usually present in patients with partial visual loss. In the early stages, the optic discs may be edematous and hyperemic with peripapillary retinal edema. Pupillary responses are often sluggish, and no response to light is indicative of a poor prognosis. Recovery of vision usually begins within a week, but in some cases vision may worsen again after several weeks of improvement. The optic discs become pale with glaucomatous-like cupping, and retinal arteries may appear attenuated.[1]

A serum methanol level greater than 20 mg/dL with a large anion gap, a high serum formate level, and a decreased serum bicarbonate level confirms the diagnosis of methanol intoxication. Administration of ethanol to interfere with the metabolism of methanol should be given, along with hemodialysis to remove the toxin and bicarbonate to restore acid–base balance. If treatment is delayed beyond the first several hours of ingestion of methanol, permanent visual damage may occur.[1]

Ethylene Glycol–associated Optic Neuropathy

Ingestion of ethylene glycol, an active ingredient in automobile antifreeze, causes toxic symptoms similar to those of methanol, such as nausea, vomiting, abdominal pain, coma, and cardiac arrest. Unlike the complications of methanol intoxication, renal failure occurs more often from ethylene glycol poisoning and the frequency of visual loss is lower.[52] The optic discs may initially appear normal followed by optic atrophy. Unlike the visual findings in methanol toxicity, papilledema from increased intracranial pressure may be associated with nystagmus and ophthalmoplegia.[1]

The presence of oxalate crystals in the urine confirms the diagnosis of ethylene glycol intoxication. Glycolate, a metabolite of ethylene glycol, causes a metabolic acidosis and large anion gap. Therefore, treatment is similar to that for methanol intoxication, which includes bicarbonate, ethanol, and hemodialysis.[52]

Methanol-induced Optic Neuropathy

Methanol intoxication may cause partial visual loss to irreversible blindness. In less severe cases, central and centrocecal scotomas predominate. Hyperemic disc swelling and some edema of the peripapillary retina may be seen. No pupillary reaction indicative of a poor visual prognosis. Vision may improve within a week of discontinuation of methanol. Vision occasionally may worsen weeks after first improving. The optic disc gradually become pale and may acquire cupping that mimics that in glaucoma. Retinal arteries may also be attenuated.

Methanol toxicity is mediated by formic acid, a metabolite. Methanol is catabolized to formaldehyde in the liver by alcohol dehydrogenase and catalase. Formaldehyde is then metabolized to formic acid by the liver and red blood cell aldehyde dehydrogenases.[53] Formate may block ATP production by inhibiting cytochrome-c oxidase,[54] which then can cause impaired axonal transport and loss of membrane polarity and conduction.[55] The disrupted salutatory conduction could lead to visual loss, and the axonal compression from retrobulbar disc swelling could obstruct anterograde axoplasmic flow.

Postmortem histopathological findings from four patients revealed that formate toxicity was selective for the retrolaminar optic nerve and the centrum semiovale.[56] Since cytochrome-c oxidase activity is lower in white matter than in gray matter,[57] oligodendroglia of the optic nerve and cerebral white matter could be more vulnerable to formate toxicity than could neurons of the retina or cerebral cortex.[57]

The diagnosis of methanol intoxication is based on a serum methanol level of greater than 20 mg/dL, a large anion gap, a high serum formate level, and a reduced serum bicarbonate level.

Treatment of methanol toxicity includes administration of ethanol, which interferes with the metabolism of methanol; administration of bicarbonate to correct the metabolic acidosis; and hemodialysis to eliminate the toxin.[4]

Toluene-associated Optic Neuropathy

Toluene inhalation can lead to a toxic optic neuropathy. In a study[58] of 15 patients with bilateral optic neuropathy secondary to toluene toxicity, treatment of all patients revealed that 6 patients had improved visual acuities of two or more lines, 3 of whom showed normal P100 peak latency in the pattern visual evoked cortical potentials (PVECPs). The visual prognosis and the PVECP changes were identical in both eyes of all patients. Changes in visual field defects were not mentioned in the study. The PVECP abnormalities in these patients suggest that prolonged exposure to toluene can cause optic nerve damage.

Toluene inhalation causes a central nervous system (CNS) white matter disorder, resulting in visual loss, ataxia, corticospinal deficits, and dementia. Unlike demyelination, toxicity results in an increase in very long chain fatty acids. Axonal swelling and thinning of the myelin sheath of peripheral nerves have been demonstrated on histopathological studies.[59]

Amiodarone- and Digoxin-associated Optic Neuropathy

Amiodarone, a diiodinated benzofuran derivative for the treatment of cardiac arrhythmias, has been hypothesized to be a cause optic neuropathy. Unilateral and bilateral anterior ischemic optic neuropathies (AIONs) have been reported in patients using amiodarone. Since these patients have similar risk factors of cardiovascular disease and crowded optic discs, it is difficult to distinguish whether their AION is a manifestation of a vascular occlusive disorder or amiodarone.[60] However, the incidence of optic neuropathy appears to be higher in patients on amiodarone, ranging from 1.3% to 1.79%, compared with the age-matched incidence of AIONs of 0.3%.[61,62] Some patients who need to take amiodarone may have worse underlying cardiovascular risk factors than the population and may already be at risk of developing an AION.

Evidence for the association of amiodarone and optic nerve damage is still inconclusive. The toxic optic neuropathy does not develop simultaneously with the toxic peripheral neuropathy. The optic neuropathy is not dose related, reversible, and demyelinating like the peripheral neuropathy. No dose-related or temporally related evidence for an increased frequency of toxic optic neuropathy exists like that for the development of corneal deposits and peripheral neuropathy.[63]

Colored halos around lights are the most common ocular symptoms during amiodarone treatment. In amiodarone-related optic neuropathy, patients have mild or no visual complaints. Unlike nonarteritic ischemic optic neuropathy (NAION), in which the onset of visual loss occurs from days to weeks, visual symptoms are slowly progressive and may begin 1 to 72 months after the initiation of amiodarone. Unlike NAION, in which the visual loss is rarely bilateral and simultaneous, amiodarone-induced optic neuropathy is characterized by bilateral, simultaneous, insidious loss of visual acuity up to 20/200 with bilateral disc edema persisting for months. Field defects are typically mild and peripheral (Table 3).[64,65]

In a review of 55 patients with amiodarone–optic neuropathy, Johnson et al.[65] found that only 65% of patients presented with painless bilateral simultaneous

Table 3: A Comparison of Neuro-Ophthalmic Features Between NAION and Amiodarone-Related Optic Neuropathy

Features	NAION	Amiodarone Optic Neuropathy
Medication use	Absent	Within 12 months of initiating amiodarone (median of 4 months)
Gender preference	Male = female	Male > female
Incidence	2.3–10.2 per 100,000 and >50 years of age	About 2% in patients treated with amiodarone
Ocular laterality at presentation	Unilateral	65% bilateral, 35% unilateral
Visual acuity on presentation	20/20; no light perception	20/20–20/200
Optic nerve cup-to-disc ratio	Small (<0.2) cup-to-disc ratio	Any cup-to-disc ratio
Increased intracranial pressure	Absent	Occasional
Duration of disc edema after a NAION attack or drug withdrawal	2–4 weeks	1–8 months (median of 3 months)

Adapted from Johnson LN, Krohel GB, Thomas ER. The clinical spectrum of amiodarone-associated optic neuropathy. *J Natl Med Assoc.* 2004;96(11):1477–1491.
NAION, nonarteritic ischemic optic neuropathy.

optic disc edema and 35% of patients had acute unilateral disc edema. The spectrum of amiodarone-associated optic neuropathy was categorized as follows: (1) insidious, (2) acute onset, (3) delayed progressive, and (4) presence or absence of optic disc edema. The most common form of amiodarone-associated optic neuropathy presents insidiously in about 40% of patients. The second most common type presents with an acute unilateral or bilateral visual loss in about 30% of patients. About 15% of patients presented with a retrobulbar optic neuropathy, in which the visual loss can be insidious or acute and in one or both eyes simultaneously. About 10% of patients taking amiodarone develop increased intracranial pressure greater than 200 mm H_2O. In 10% of patients, amiodarone-associated optic neuropathy has a delayed progressive onset. These patients may report visual loss before any appearance of optic disc edema and may develop disc edema days to weeks after amiodarone is withdrawn because of the long half-life of amiodarone of up to 110 days.[66–68]

In this same study, nearly 20% with amiodarone-associated optic neuropathy had 20/200 or worse on presentation. While 40% experienced some improvement in visual acuity, most patients had no change in visual acuity after stopping the drug. After drug withdrawal, 10% even had worsening of their visual acuity.

Optic atrophy was the common end stage for all patients with corresponding persistent field defects, similar to those in NAION.[65] The final outcome of visual acuity in patients with amiodarone-associated optic neuropathy was 20/30 compared to 20/60 in patients with NAION. This comparison may not be accurate because the visual acuity from 50 patients with amiodarone optic neuropathy was compared with that from 420 patients with NAION in the Ischemic Optic Neuropathy Decompression Trial.[69]

The exact pathophysiology of amiodarone-induced optic neuropathy is unclear. Amiodarone, like other amphiphilic drugs, binds to polar lipids and accumulates within lysosomes.[70] According to Garrett et al.,[70] fenestrated peripapillary choroidal capillaries are permeable to amiodarone. The choroidal interstitial fluid containing amiodarone may allow drug-induced phospholipidosis, in which membrane-bound bodies with multilamellar inclusion bodies accumulate in astrocytes and ganglion axons. Histopathological studies have shown intracytoplasmic lamellar inclusions in large axons.[71] The accumulation of these inclusions may impair axoplasmic flow to cause optic disc edema.

Amiodarone toxicity to the optic nerve is dose related, varying in range from 200 to 1200 mg/day. Decreasing the dose of amiodarone may improve the optic disc edema, and discontinuation of the drug allows gradual recovery. Since the half-life of amiodarone is up to 100 days, amiodarone-related optic disc edema lasts months—unlike the disc edema of NAION, which resolves within weeks. Unlike the persistent field defects in NAION, the mild peripheral field defects may improve in amiodarone-related optic neuropathy. Concurrent use of digoxin with amiodarone may increase the known side effects of digoxin, such as dyschromatopsia, visual disturbances, and visual field defects. Since the association of amiodarone and optic neuropathy remain controversial in some cases, the decision to discontinue amiodarone in the treatment of life-threatening cardiac arrhythmias is best made by the cardiologist.[65–67]

Disulfiram-associated Optic Neuropathy

Disulfiram, used in the treatment of chronic alcoholism, interferes with the metabolism of acetaldehyde, a metabolite of ethanol. Optic neuropathy may occur in patients who have abstained from alcohol and have continued to take disulfiram. The mechanism of toxicity on the optic nerve is unknown. Visual loss is usually subacute or chronic and symmetrical, with central or cecocentral scotomas. The optic discs are often normal initially and later become pale. The optic neuropathy usually recovers completely 1 to 5 months after discontinuing disulfiram.[1]

Ethambutol-associated Optic Neuropathy

Ethambutol, used in the treatment of *Mycobacterium tuberculosis,* is metabolized to a chelating agent that may impair the function of metal-containing mitochondrial enzymes, such as the copper-containing cytochrome-*c* oxidase of complex IV and the iron-containing NADH: Q oxidoreductase of complex I. This damage to the mitochondrial respiratory chain may lead to the development of optic neuropathy. Zinc may also play an important role in ethambutol toxicity of retinal ganglion cells.[72] Based on one postmortem study, demyelination of the optic chiasm was noted.[73]

Ethambutol toxicity to the optic nerve is dose dependent. Visual loss occurs more often in patients receiving 25 mg/kg/day or more. Visual loss does not develop until after treatment for at least 1.5 months and most often around 5 months. Visual loss can occur as late as 12 months after initiation of therapy.[74] More severe visual impairment may be seen in patients with impaired renal function because ethambutol is excreted by the kidneys.

Blue–yellow defects, more commonly than red–green defects, may be the initial presentation. Decrease in visual acuity is insidious and bilaterally symmetrical. Visual field typically show central scotomas or bitemporal defects and, less commonly, peripheral constriction. Optic discs are

initially normal but may develop mild temporal disc pallor if ethambutol is continued. Early diagnosis and prompt cessation of the ethambutol leads to a more favorable prognosis, as visual loss is usually irreversible.[75]

Chloramphenicol-associated Optic Neuropathy

Chloramphenicol was used to treat cystic fibrosis in children until 1970 when it was recognized that it caused a toxic optic neuropathy.[76] Children developed sudden onset bilateral central visual loss with cecocentral scotomas. Selective damage to the papillomacular bundle and tortuous retinal vessels were often seen. Histopathology revealed retinal ganglion cell loss and demyelination of the optic nerve, affecting mainly the papillomacular bundle.[76] Discontinuation of the drug and vitamin B complex treatment usually led to a recovery of visual function.

Linezolid-associated Optic Neuropathy

Linezolid disrupts RNA translation by binding to the 23S ribosomal RNA of the 50S ribosome subunit to interfere with ribosome assembly. It is used in the treatment of methicillin-resistant *Staphylococcus,* vancomycin-resistant *Enterococcus,* nosocomial pneumonia, and complicated skin infections.[77] Linezolid has been associated with toxic optic neuropathy in which patients present with decreased visual acuity, dyschromatopsia, and cecocentral scotomas. Early discontinuation of the antibiotic results in gradual but not full visual recovery. Most reports of linezolid toxic optic neuropathy described patients with initial visual acuity of 20/200 or worse improving to 20/30 or better after discontinuation of the drug. Color defects, visual field defects, and optic disc pallor also improve.[78–82]

Linezolid-related optic neuropathy may be associated with the duration of linezolid therapy. During randomized clinical trials of this drug, the monitoring of adverse effects of linezolid continued up to day 28 of treatment.[83] Several reports suggest that patients developed linezolid-related optic neuropathy after approximately 8 to 10 months of the standard dosage of 600 mg/day.[78,84] It is recommended that if patients will be receiving this antibiotic for more than 28 days they should be monitored with baseline and monthly eye examinations thereafter. Visual acuity, visual field, color vision, and dilated fundoscopy should be performed.

Interferon-α-associated Optic Neuropathy

Interferon-α (IFN-α), a glycoprotein secreted by the immune system in response to viral infections, serves as intracellular signaling to enhance expression of specific genes, enhance and induce lymphocytes to kill target cells, and inhibit virus replication in infected cells.[85] Since IFN-α has anticytokine, antiviral, immunomodulatory, and antiproliferative activities, it has been used to treat chronic hepatitis B and C, cancer, and essential thrombocytosis.[85] It has been postulated that IFN-α can produce autoantibodies and subsequently case deposition of immune complexes in the small arteries of the optic nerve. IFN-α can stimulate other cytokines that may lead to an inflammatory reaction of the blood vessels that might subsequently induce ischemia.[86–88]

AION is an uncommon complication of IFN-α treatment.[87] Two patients undergoing treatment with IFN-α developed bilateral simultaneous optic neuropathy within 3 months of starting this medication.[89] The bilateral optic disc edema and nerve fiber layer hemorrhages were associated with inferior nerve fiber bundle defects. Despite treatment with aspirin at 300 mg/day after cessation of IFN-α in one patient, visual acuities and field defects remained unchanged. In the other patient who was treated with IV methylprednisolone at 1 g/day for 3 days with prednisone taper after IFN-α was discontinued, visual acuities improved but field defects persisted. NAION may occur within 1 week to 3 months of starting after IFN-α treatment in patients who do not have underlying vasculopathic risk factors for NAION.[89–91] The two patients reported by Purvin[87] developed sudden bilateral, sequential visual loss with disc-related field defects and segmental optic disc edema, all features characteristic of AION. The degree of disc pallor may depend on the severity of ischemia. Underlying anemia may decrease perfusion to the optic nerve to cause pallid optic disc edema.[89] Only one patient improved after discontinuation of IFN-α treatment.[92]

Infliximab-associated Optic Neuropathy

Infliximab is a chimeric antibody of the immunoglobulin G class that inhibits tumor necrosis factor-α (TNF-α) and is given intravenously for the treatment of rheumatoid arthritis and Crohn's disease.[93] The inhibition of TNF-α has been associated, in rare instances, with the exacerbation of underlying demyelinating diseases, such as multiple sclerosis (MS).[86] High TNF-α levels have been found in MS plaques and mononuclear cells of patients with MS.[90] It has also been shown that the infusion of TNF-α in animal models of MS leads to worsening of their demyelinating disease.[92] Infliximab has been associated with the development of retrobulbar optic neuritis.[94,95] In a study by Foroozan et al.,[94] two women in their 5th decade developed retrobulbar optic neuritis after treatment with infliximab for rheumatoid arthritis, Crohn's disease, or both. Their vision improved to baseline after discontinuation of the drug.[94,95] Although these patients did not have underlying MS, it was postulated that TNF-α inhibition may have increased their risk for a demyelinating event.

Treatment with infliximab may also be complicated by a toxic optic neuropathy. After receiving three doses of infliximab for rheumatoid arthritis, three patients in their 5th and 6th decade developed acute bilateral disc edema with central, cecocentral scotomas, or inferior defects. Despite high-dose steroids, their vision did not improve. It was thought that the three cumulative doses of infliximab contributed to the development of their bilateral toxic optic neuropathy.[96]

Clomiphene Citrate–associated Optic Neuropathy

Hormonal agents such as clomiphene citrate are often used in the treatment of infertility and can increase the risk of hypercoagulable complications. Visual disturbances occur approximately 5% to 10%[97] of patients treated with clomiphene citrate. Optic neuritis has been reported during treatment with clomiphene.[98] They may develop transient blurry vision or "spots" in their vision. AION has been reported in a 31-year-old woman with primary infertility after receiving a 5-day course of clomiphene citrate at 50 mg taken orally each morning.[99] She developed acute right visual loss upon awakening with 20/200, a right relative afferent defect, decreased red saturation, and an inferior altitudinal defect in the right eye. The right optic disc was edematous and hyperemic with venous dilation and splinter hemorrhages. Two months later, her right visual acuity was 20/50 (−2) and she had right optic disc pallor.

Tamoxifen-associated Optic Neuropathy

Tamoxifen modulates estrogen receptor activity and is often used as either an adjuvant or a monotherapy in cancer treatment. The overall incidence of ocular toxicity is about 12%. Bilateral optic neuropathy rarely occurs, and early detection may help prevent permanent damage.[100] In a prospective study of 65 women with breast cancer who had a normal baseline eye examination and were started on oral tamoxifen of 20 mg/day,[100] 12% developed ocular toxicity in which 7 had a keratopathy, 3 had bilateral pigmentary retinopathy, and 1 had bilateral optic neuritis. The patient with optic nerve involvement had residual optic nerve pallor and decreased vision. The keratopathic changes were reversible with discontinuation of the drug. Yearly eye examinations were recommended for patients on long-term tamoxifen.

Sildenafil- and Tadalafil-associated Optic Neuropathy

Sildenafil is indicated for the treatment of erectile dysfunction in men, but has been shown to be associated with the development of NAION. A selective phosphodiesterase-5

(PDE5) inhibitor facilitates the nitric oxide–cyclic guanosine monophosphate pathway to relax smooth muscle in the corpus cavernosum, allowing inflow of blood during sexual stimulation. It is also hypothesized that its partial inhibition of phosphodiesterase 6 on the outer retinal photoreceptors causes a transient bluish tinge or haze to the vision and increased light sensitivity.[101]

At least seven men have been reported to have NAION from sildenafil so far in the literature.[102,103] In the reported cases of sildenafil associated with NAION by Pomeranz et al.,[102] the patients ranged from 42 to 49 years old and three of the five men had no cardiovascular risk factors. Two were taking aspirin daily, but the dose was not specified. Four of the men experienced acute loss of visual acuity approximately 45 minutes to 12 hours after drug intake. The dose of sildenafil ranged from 50 mg to 100 mg. One man had taken 50 mg of sildenafil each week, and his visual fields gradually worsened over the 15-month period. The visual disturbances occurred after the first dose in one patient and after two or three doses in another patient. Two of the men had been using sildenafil irregularly for about 2 years. The duration of treatment was not reported in the fifth patient. Visual changes often occurred unilaterally and were accompanied by headache in one patient and by intraocular pain in another. All of these men had small cup-to-disc ratios. After about 2 to 9 months of follow-up in four of the men, all had permanent peripheral constriction and three men had persistent reduction in visual acuity. In another report by Akash et al.,[104] a 54-year-old man developed permanent blindness in his left eye from NAION combined with a cilioretinal artery obstruction after an overdose of Viagra.

Structural features of the optic disc in patients affected by sildenafil may increase the risk of developing NAION. Small physiological cups are more common in patients with NAION, and it is believed that the crowding of nerve fibers through a small scleral canal are more susceptible to ischemic damage.[105–107] The close temporal relationship between use of sildenafil and NAION in patients with small cup-to-disc ratio in the unaffected eye and no vascular risk factors also suggests a possible causal relationship.[102,108–111]

Nitric oxide generated by sildenafil may be a possible toxic agent to the optic nerve and retinal ganglion cells. It has been shown that inhibition of nitric oxide synthetase decreased retinal ganglion cell damage in animals with glaucomatous optic neuropathy.[112] Nitric oxide is also a potent vasodilator and may interfere with autoregulation of blood flow to the optic nerve head.[113] Alteration in the perfusion of branches of the posterior ciliary artery that supply the optic nerve head has been implicated in NAION. Based upon Hayreh's theory that nocturnal hypotension could lead to ischemia in patients with a small cup-to-disc ratio, sildenafil could accentuate physiological nocturnal hypotension enough to decrease the perfusion pressure in posterior ciliary arteries.[109] In a study of 15 young, health males with a mean age of 39 years who underwent ocular blood flow measurements after oral ingestion of sildenafil at 100 mg, none developed permanent or transient visual loss, and no significant change in the optic nerve rim or foveolar choroidal blood flow was observed after treatment with sildenafil.[114] The exact pathophysiology of sildenafil in NAION remains uncertain.

Tadalafil, another related drug for erectile dysfunction specific for cyclic guanosine monophosphate PDE5 inhibitor has been associated with NAION.[115–117] Bollinger and Lee[115] reported a 67-year-old man with hypercholesterolemia who experienced an episode of transient, inferior blurring of the visual field within 2 hours after each of the four doses of tadalafil taken several days apart. Three days later, he took the fifth dose and developed a permanent right inferior visual field defect. He had right optic disc edema, and his normal left optic disc had a small cup-to-disc ratio. The visual field loss after repeated ingestion of tadalafil suggested that PDE5 inhibitors could be a risk factor for the development of NAION.

Vardenafil, another PDE5 inhibitor for erectile dysfunction, may also have the potential to cause NAION, but there have been no reports yet.

Radiation-induced Optic Neuropathy

Radiation-induced optic neuropathy is an ischemic process, usually presenting as a posterior ischemic optic neuropathy, about 18 months after radiotherapy and after cumulative doses of radiation greater than 50 Gy or single doses greater than 10 Gy. It is often seen as a complication of radiation therapy in the paranasal sinus and skull base regions and postoperatively for pituitary adenomas, parasellar meningiomas, frontal and temporal gliomas, craniopharyngiomas, and intraocular tumors.[118–123] The range of between safe and unsafe radiation doses may vary depending on individual tolerance. Previous or concurrent treatment with chemotherapy, such as methotrexate, ara-C, vincristine, and other multiple drug combinations can increase the risk of developing radiation-induced optic neuropathy. Radiation may alter cellular structures, such as the blood–brain barrier permeability, or arachnoid granulations to change the pharmacokinetics of drug distribution and clearance. For example, methotrexate administered concurrently or postradiation therapy is more toxic than when it is given before radiation treatment. Radiation is thought to increase blood–brain barrier permeability so that more methotrexate enters the CNS.[124,125] Therefore, the toxic effects of these chemotherapeutic drugs can potentiate the adverse effects of radiation, and vice versa.[126,127]

Radiation dose per fraction, total dose, total duration of treatment, volume of tissue irradiated, and type of radiation (proton, electron, or neutron) can also affect the risk of developing radiation-induced optic neuropathy.[128] When the total dose, fraction size, or volume increases, the frequency of complications increases but the latency to the onset of complications decreases.[128–130]

Preexisting medical disorders, such as diabetes and endocrinological disturbances from Cushing's syndrome and growth hormone–producing tumors, are additional risk factors.

Radiation-induced optic neuropathy is a form of late delayed radiation neurotoxicity that affects the white matter months to years after exposure of the anterior visual pathways to ionizing radiaton.[131] It is thought that radiation damages the DNA of normal tissues to initiate free radical–mediated damage of the vascular endothelium and glial cells in the white matter.[132–144] The number of vascular endothelial cells are reduced in experimentally radiated rat brains depending on the dose and the time of exposure.[135] In a case-controlled study by Levin et al.,[136] histological features were studied in optic nerves of 16 enucleated eyes from patients with uveal melanoma treated with proton beam irradiation, 6 from normal eyes, and 5 from eyes with nonradiated uveal melanomas. An increase in radiation dosage to the optic nerve was associated with a decrease in the number of endothelial cells. Endothelial cell counts did not correlate with age, gender, visual acuity, or interval after radiation treatment. In another study of 34 patients with late delayed radiation-induced injury using proton magnetic resonance spectroscopy,[137] N-acetyl aspartate–to–creatine and NAA–to–choline ratios decreased in areas with worsening brain injury. Since choline was not elevated in areas of mild to moderate brain injury, demyelination or glial hyperplasia was not a likely primary mechanism of late delayed radiation-induced injury. Unlike other types of ischemia, the ischemia in radiation-induced optic neuropathy involves a gradual decrease in oxygen gradient from normal tissue to damaged tissue. This gradual oxygen gradient is not conducive to cellular repair. On histology, radiation-injured optic nerves show obliterative endarteritis, endothelial hyperplasia, and fibrinoid necrosis replacing axonal and myelin loss.[138,139]

Radiation-induced optic neuropathy presents with acute, progressive visual loss in one eye or both eyes over weeks to months. Bilateral sequential visual loss is more common, and it is usually painless. Rarely is the interval between optic disc involvement as long as 7 months, according to Lessell.[140] Transient visual loss may be a premonitory symptom before radiation-induced optic neuropathy is diagnosed several weeks later.[141] Visual symptoms usually develop about 18 months after treatment is completed, but the latency is variable.[119,141,142] Visual loss is irreversible, but spontaneous improvement has occasionally been reported in patients who have radiation papillitis.[143]

The final visual acuity in most patients with radiation-induced optic neuropathy is 20/200 or worse.[144] The visual field may show altitudinal defects or central scotomas. If the distal optic nerve is affected, then a junctional syndrome with an optic neuropathy and a contralateral temporal hemianopsia may be seen.[145] A retrobulbar optic neuropathy is most common. The optic disc may initially appear normal and then become pale over 4 to 6 weeks.[119] After orbital or intraocular radiation, radiation papillopathy, affecting the anterior disc, may be seen. Optic disc edema is associated with subretinal fluid, peripapillary exudates, and cotton wool spots.[119] The optic disc then gradually becomes pale.

The differential diagnosis of radiation-induced optic neuropathy includes recurrence of the primary malignancy, arachnoiditis, a new radiation-induced parasellar tumor, and secondary empty sella syndrome with optic nerve and chiasmal prolapse.[146–148]

MRI of the brain and orbits with gadolinium and T1-weighted fat saturation of the orbits is the diagnostic procedure of choice to differentiate tumor recurrence from radiation-induced optic neuropathy.[149–151] On T1-weighted enhanced images, the injured optic nerves may occasionally enhance, and this enhancement usually resolves in several months. Radiation injury to the anterior visual pathways cannot always be detected in the early stages. In a postmortem study[152] of a 38-year-old man who was treated with interstitial brachytherapy (iridium-192 at 47 Gy) followed by limited-field irradiation of 45 Gy, the extent of injury[140] measured by MRI scan underestimated the damage seen on histology. Furthermore, MRI findings of radiation injury can even be occasionally seen before the neuro-ophthalmological manifestions.[140]

Treatment for radiation-induced optic neuropathy has been controversial. Corticosteroids and anticoagulants have offered limited success. Corticosteroids may not be the ideal treatment because radiation injury does not involve vasogenic edema or inflammation. Heparin and warfarin have been shown to be effective in increasing cerebral blood flow in five of eight patients with cerebral radionecrosis who experienced neurological improvement. But these drugs have not been shown to be beneficial in improving vision of patients with radiation optic neuropathy.[153] In a report by Barbosa et al.,[154] anticoagulation treatment in a patient with bilateral radiation-induced optic neuropathy resulted in no visual improvement. Radiation optic neuropathy has also been reported to occur despite being on anticoagulation during radiation treatment and during the time of visual loss.[155,156]

Evidence now shows that hyperbaric oxygen therapy appears to be a more effective therapy for radiation-induced optic neuropathy. It alters the oxygen gradient so that capillary angiogenesis is possible.[157] In a review by Borruat et al.,[158] patients receiving hyperbaric oxygen therapy with greater than or equal to 2.4 atmospheres experienced the best visual outcome compared to those who received no treatment and to those who received 2.0 atmospheres. Further review of data from previous cases suggested that hyperbaric oxygen therapy should be started as early as possible after the onset of visual loss. Treatment should consist of 30 sessions of 90 minutes each so that patients are breathing 100% oxygen at a minimum pressure of 2.4 atmospheres.

Based upon the experience and data of various treatments, some management strategies have evolved to help improve visual outcome. If one eye has been affected, serial eye exams must be done over the 10- to 20-month period after treatment to monitor for any signs of recurrence in the fellow eye, since bilateral

sequential involvement is not uncommon. Serial MRI of the brain and orbits should be performed over the 20-month period after radiation therapy is completed. Subclinical evidence of radiation necrosis on MRI should be treated with prophylactic hyperbaric oxygen therapy.[140] VEP may also play a role in detecting early radiation-induced optic neuropathy when the eye exam is normal. In a prospective study of 28 patients who underwent radiation therapy for uveal melanomas,[159] 18% of patients had no clinical signs of optic neuropathy but 50% developed abnormal VEPs, suggesting that subclinical radiation optic neuropathy had developed in some patients. Radiation-induced optic nerve injury may be more frequent than clinically expected.

CASE STUDY

A 46-year-old man presented with a 6-month history of bilateral blurry vision and photophobia. His blurry vision was constant, and he was diagnosed and treated for presbyopia. He also noted that colors were dim (Figure 9-1; see color plate). His past medical history was significant for hypertension. His family history was unremarkable. He did not take any medications, but he had been

smoking six cigars a day and drinking five alcoholic beverages a day for the past several years.

On examination, his visual acuity was 20/60 in both eyes (Figure 9-2). He had no relative afferent pupillary defect. Extraocular motility examination was normal. He had a red–green defect. Intraocular pressures were 17 mm Hg in the right eye and 15 mm Hg in the left eye.

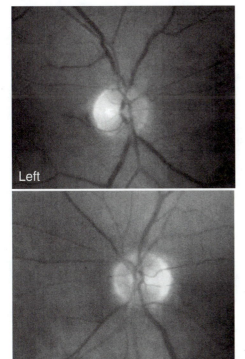

Figure 9-1. The optic nerves have mild temporal pallor (right optic disc, *left;* left optic disc, *right;* see color plate).

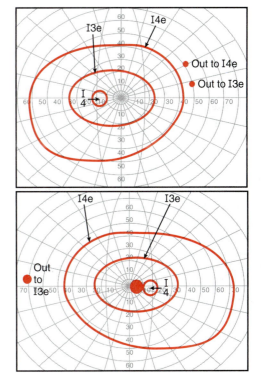

Figure 9-2. Goldmann visual field testing revealed bilateral cecocentral scotomas (left visual field, *left;* right visual field, *right*).

Laboratory tests revealed the following: hemoglobin, 13.5 g/dL (low); hematocrit, 39.4%

Continued

CASE STUDY—cont'd

(low); white cells, 10.1 (normal); rapid plasma reagin, nonreactive vitamin B_{12}, 466 pg/mL (normal); folic acid, 7.4 ng/mL (normal), mitochondrial DNA mutations for LHON, negative.

Tobacco amblyopia typically occurs in patients who are pipe and cigar smokers, and the etiology is unknown. There has been a marked decline in the incidence of tobacco amblyopia since the advent of genetic testing for LHON as it was felt that many patients were initially misdiagnosed. There is a large differential in patients with bilateral cecocentral scotomas, including nutritional optic neuropathy (vitamin B_{12} deficiency), LHON, Kjer's dominant optic atrophy, cilioretinal artery occlusion, infectious optic neuropathy such in syphilis, and psychogenic loss. A multifactorial etiology is postulated since only a minority of patients who smoke develop this disease and no dose-dependent correlation has been confirmed. Cyanide toxicity from cigarette smoke and relative malabsorption of vitamin B_{12} from the gut have been postulated as mechanisms but have not been proved.[160] Alcohol has also been postulated to be a cofactor in this disease process; however, alcohol alone has not been proved to be toxic to the visual pathways. Low serum vitamin B_{12} levels have been suspected as one factor.[161] Patients with tobacco amblyopia can have any level of visual acuity. It presents as a painless, progressive bilateral optic neuropathy with visual loss, dyschromatopsia, and cecocentral scotomas on visual field testing. Nystagmus, ptosis, and ophthalmoplegia can be present if the patient is experiencing Wernicke's encephalopathy. The optic nerve appears pale, and the rest of the fundus usually appears normal. An evanescent peripapillary retinopathy characterized by hemorrhages and dilated, tortuous vessels in the nerve fiber layer has been described in a case series.[162] Treatment consists of hydroxycobalamin injections or oral replacement therapy and cessation of smoking. Nonetheless, patients such as the one presented here who have continued to smoke and who receive vitamin B_{12} do improve. Previous studies have shown that hydroxycobalamin is superior to cobalamin alone in the treatment of these patients. Administration of the medications with an internist and close follow up with visual field testing is recommended when following these patients.

This patient was started on hydroxycobalamin injections once a week. Follow-up examinations revealed visual acuity of 16/15 in both eyes and resolutions of the central scotomas and dyschromatopsia in both eyes.

REFERENCES

1. Miller NR, Newman NJ, eds. *Walsh and Hoyt's Clinical Neuro-Ophthalmology.* vol 1. 5th ed. Baltimore: Williams & Wilkins; 1998.
2. Knox DL, Chen MF, Guilarte TR, Dang CV, Burnette J. Nutritional amblyopia: folic acid, vitamin B-12, and other vitamins. *Retina.* 1982;2(4):288–293.
3. Biousse V, Newman NJ. Neuro-ophthalmology of mitochondrial diseases. *Curr Opin Neurol.* 2003;16(1):35–43.
4. Johnnson RT, Griffin JW, McArthur JC, eds. *Current Therapy in Neurologic Disease.* 6th ed. St. Louis: Mosby; 2002:363–365.
5. Carelli V, Ross-Cisneros FN, Sadun AA. Optic nerve degeneration and mitochondrial dysfunction: genetic and acquired optic neuropathies. *Neurochem Int.* 2002;40(6):573–584.
6. Healton EB, Savage DG, Brust JC, Garrett TJ, Lindenbaum J. Neurologic aspects of cobalamin deficiency. *Medicine (Baltimore).* 1991;70(4):229–245.
7. Agamanolis DP, Chester EM, Victor M, Kark JA, Hines JD, Harris JW. Neuropathology of experimental vitamin B_{12} deficiency in monkeys. *Neurology.* 1976;26(10):905–914.
8. Dang CV. Tobacco–alcohol amblyopia: a proposed biochemical basis for pathogenesis. *Med Hypotheses.* 1981;7(11):1317–1328.
9. Choi DW. Glutamate neurotoxicity and diseases of the nervous system. *Neuron.* 1988;1(8):623–634.
10. Hampton CK, Garcia C, Redburn DA. Localization of kainic acid–sensitive cells in mammalian retina. *J Neurosci Res.* 1981;6(1):99–111.
11. Ingvar M. Cerebral blood flow and metabolic rate during seizures: relationship to epileptic brain damage. *Ann NY Acad Sci.* 1986;462:194–206.
12. Raley-Susman KM, Miller KR, Owicki JC, Sapolsky RM. Effects of excitotoxin exposure on metabolic rate of primary hippocampal cultures: application of silicon microphysiometry to neurobiology. *J Neurosci.* 1992;12(3):773–780.
13. Schiller PH, Logothetis NK, Charles ER. Functions of the colour-opponent and broad-band channels of the visual system. *Nature.* 1990;343(6253):68–70.
14. Cleland BG, Levick WR, Sanderson KJ. Properties of sustained and transient ganglion cells in the cat retina. *J Physiol.* 1973;228(3):649–680.
15. Sadun AA, Martone JF, Muci-Mendoza R, et al. Epidemic optic neuropathy in Cuba: eye findings. *Arch Ophthalmol.* 1994;112(5):691–699.
16. Roman GC. An epidemic in Cuba of optic neuropathy, sensorineural deafness, peripheral sensory neuropathy and dorsolateral myeloneuropathy. *J Neurol Sci.* 1994;127(1):11–28.
17. Macias-Matos C, Rodriguez-Ojea A, Chi N, Jimenez S, Zulueta D, Bates CJ. Biochemical evidence of thiamine depletion during the Cuban neuropathy epidemic, 1992–1993. *Am J Clin Nutr.* 1996;64(3):347–353.
18. Thomas PK, Plant GT, Baxter P, Bates C, Santiago Luis R. An epidemic of optic neuropathy and painful sensory neuropathy in Cuba: clinical aspects. *J Neurol.* 1995;242(10):629–638.
19. Gay J, Porrata C, Hernandez M, et al. Dietary factors in epidemic neuropathy on the Isle of Youth, Cuba. *Bull Pan Am Health Organ.* 1995;29(1):25–36.
20. Johns DR, Neufeld MJ, Hedges TR III. Mitochondrial DNA mutations in Cuban optic and peripheral neuropathy. *J Neuroophthalmol.* 1994;14(3):135–140.
21. Mojon DS, Kaufmann P, Odel JG, et al. Clinical course of a cohort in the Cuban epidemic optic and peripheral neuropathy. *Neurology.* 1997;48(1):19–22.
22. Lincoff NS, Odel JG, Hirano M. "Outbreak" of optic and peripheral neuropathy in Cuba? *JAMA.* 1993;270(4):511–518.

23. Tucker K, Hedges TR. Food shortages and an epidemic of optic and peripheral neuropathy in Cuba. *Nutr Rev.* 1993;51(12): 349–357.

24. Solberg Y, Rosner M, Belkin M. The association between cigarette smoking and ocular diseases. *Surv Ophthalmol.* 1998;42(6): 535–547.

25. Dunphy EB. Alcohol and tobacco amblyopia: a historical survey. XXXI DeSchweinitz lecture. *Am J Ophthalmol.* 1969;68(4): 569–578.

26. Pearce JM. Neurological aspects of alcoholism. *Br J Hosp Med.* 1977;18(2):132,134,136–137.

27. Samples JR, Younge BR. Tobacco–alcohol amblyopia. *J Clin Neuro Ophthalmol.* 1981;1:213–218.

28. Smiddy WE, Green WR. Nutritional amblyopia: a histopathologic study with retrospective clinical correlation. *Graefes Arch Clin Exp Ophthalmol.* 1987;225(5):321–324.

29. Rizzo JF 3rd, Lessell S. Tobacco amblyopia. *Am J Ophthalmol.* 1993;116(1):84–87.

30. Pryor WA. Biological effects of cigarette smoke, wood smoke, and the smoke from plastics:the use of electron spin resonance. *Free Radic Biol Med.* 1992;13(6):659–676.

31. Ballinger SW, Bouder TG, Davis GS, Judice SA, Nicklas JA, Albertini RJ. Mitochondrial genome damage associated with cigarette smoking. *Cancer Res.* 1996;56(24):5692–5697.

32. Kennedy JR, Elliot AM. Cigarette smoke: the effect of residue on mitochondrial structure. *Science.* 1970;168:1097–1098.

33. Newman NJ, Torroni A, Brown MD, Lott MT, Fernandez MM, Wallace DC. Epidemic neuropathy in Cuba not associated with mitochondrial DNA mutations found in Leber's hereditary optic neuropathy patients. Cuba Neuropathy Field Investigation Team. *Am J Ophthalmol.* 1994;118(2):158–168.

34. Gill GV, Bell DR. Persisting nutritional neuropathy amongst former war prisoners. *J Neurol Neurosurg Psychiatry.* 1982;45(10):861–865.

35. Carroll FD. Nutritional amblyopia. *Arch Ophthalmol.* 1966;76(3):406–411.

36. King JH Jr, Passmore JW. Nutritional amblyopia: a study of American prisoners of war in Korea. *Am J Ophthalmol.* 1955;39(4, Pt 2):173–186.

37. Montgomery RD, Cruickshank EK, Robertson WB, McNemeney WH. Clinical and pathological observations on Jamaican neuropathy: a report on 206 cases. *Brain.* 1964;87:425–462.

38. Osuntokun BO, Osuntokun O. Tropical amblyopia in Nigerians. *Am J Ophthalmol.* 1971;72(4):708–716.

39. McMartin KE, Ambre JJ, Tephly TR. Methanol poisoning in human subjects: role for formic acid accumulation in the metabolic acidosis. *Am J Med.* 1980;68(3):414–418.

40. Golnik KC, Schaible ER. Folate-responsive optic neuropathy. *J Neuroophthalmol.* 1994;14(3):163–169.

41. Hsu CT, Miller NR, Wray ML. Optic neuropathy from folic acid deficiency without alcohol abuse. *Ophthalmologica.* 2002;216(1):65–67.

42. Lessell S. Nutritional disorders: ophthalmological aspects. *Bull Soc Belge Ophtalmol.* 1983;208(Pt 1):469–472.

43. van Noort BA, Bos PJ, Klopping C, Wilmink JM. Optic neuropathy from thiamine deficiency in a patient with ulcerative colitis. *Doc Ophthalmol.* 1987;67(1–2):45–51.

44. Larsen PD, Mock DM, O'Connor PS. Vitamin E deficiency associated with vision loss and bulbar weakness. *Ann Neurol.* 1985;18(6):725–727.

45. Solomons NW, Russell RM. The interaction of vitamin A and zinc: implications for human nutrition. *Am J Clin Nutr.* 1980;33(9):2031–2040.

46. Russell RM, Cox ME, Solomons N. Zinc and the special senses. *Ann Intern Med.* 1983;99(2):227–239.

47. Karcioglu ZA. Zinc in the eye. *Surv Ophthalmol.* 1982;27(2): 114–122.

48. De Palma P, Franco F, Bragliani G, et al. The incidence of optic neuropathy in 84 patients treated with ethambutol. *Metab Pediatr Syst Ophthalmol.* 1989;12(1–3):80–82.

49. Scopinaro N, Gianetta E, Civalleri D, Bonalumi U, Bachi V. Two years of clinical experience with biliopancreatic bypass for obesity. *Am J Clin Nutr.* 1980;33 (2 Suppl):506–514.

50. Eells JT, Henry MM, Lewandowski MF, Seme MT, Murray TG. Development and characterization of a rodent model of methanol-induced retinal and optic nerve toxicity. *Neurotoxicology.* 2000;21(3):321–330.

51. Hsu HH, Chen CY, Chen FH, Lee CC, Chou TY, Zimmerman RA. Optic atrophy and cerebral infarcts caused by methanol intoxication: MRI. *Neuroradiology.* 1997;39(3):192–194.

52. Jacobsen D, McMartin KE. Methanol and ethylene glycol poisonings: mechanism of toxicity, clinical course, diagnosis and treatment. *Med Toxicol.* 1986;1(5):309–334.

53. Tephly TR, Makar AB, McMartin KE. Methanol: its metabolism and toxicity. In: Majchrowicz E, Noble EP, eds. *Biochemistry and Pharmacology of Ethanol.* vol 1. New York: Plenum; 1979: 145–162.

54. Nicholls P. Formate as an inhibitor of cytochrome-*c* oxidase. *Biochem Biophys Res Commun.* 1975;67(2):610–616.

55. Guyton AC. *Textbook of Medical Physiology.* Philadelphia: WB Saunders; 1981.

56. Sharpe JA, Hostovsky M, Bilbao JM, Rewcastle NB. Methanol optic neuropathy: a histopathological study. *Neurology.* 1982;32(10):1093–1100.

57. Wyndham RA. Experimental demyelination of the central nervous system: II. Respiratory enzyme systems of the brain in poisoning with cyanide and with azide. *Aust J Exp Biol Med Sci.* 1941;19:243–248.

58. Kiyokawa M, Mizota A, Takasoh M, Adachi-Usami E. Pattern visual evoked cortical potentials in patients with toxic optic neuropathy caused by toluene abuse. *Jpn J Ophthalmol.* 1999;43(5):438–442.

59. Hormes JT, Filley CM, Rosenberg NL. Neurologic sequelae of chronic solvent vapor abuse. *Neurology.* 1986;36(5):698–702.

60. Verslegers W, De Deyn PP. Visual impairment due to optic neuropathy in 2 patients on amiodarone, and ethambutol and isoniazide therapy, respectively. *Ned Tijdschr Geneeskd.* 2001;145(38):1872.

61. Feiner LA, Younge BR, Kazmier FJ, Stricker BH, Fraunfelder FT. Optic neuropathy and amiodarone therapy. *Mayo Clin Proc.* 1987;62(8):702–717.

62. Gittinger JW Jr, Asdourian GK. Papillopathy caused by amiodarone. *Arch Ophthalmol.* 1987;105(3):349–351.

63. Mindel JS. Amiodarone toxic optic neuropathy: reasons for doubting its existence [lecture]. North American Neuro-Ophthalmology Society Annual Meeting, Feb 25–Mar 2, 2006, JW Marriott Starr Pass Resort and Spa, Tucson, Arizona.

64. Chen D, Hedges TR. Amiodarone optic neuropathy: review. *Semin Ophthalmol.* 2003;18(4):169–173.

65. Johnson LN, Krohel GB, Thomas ER. The clinical spectrum of amiodarone-associated optic neuropathy. *J Natl Med Assoc.* 2004;96(11):1477–1491.

66. Pollak PT, Bouillon T, Shafer SL. Population pharmacokinetics of long-term oral amiodarone therapy. *Clin Pharmacol Ther.* 2000;67(6):642–652.

67. Singh BN. Amiodarone: the expanding antiarrhythmic role and how to follow a patient on chronic therapy. *Clin Cardiol.* 1997;20(7):608–618.

68. Somani P. Basic and clinical pharmacology of amiodarone: relationship of antiarrhythmic effects, dose and drug concentrations

to intracellular inclusion bodies. *J Clin Pharmacol.* 1989;29(5): 405–412.

69. Characteristics of patients with nonarteritic anterior ischemic optic neuropathy eligible for the Ischemic Optic Neuropathy Decompression Trial. *Arch Ophthalmol.* 1996;114(11):1366–1374.

70. Garrett SN, Kearney JJ, Schiffman JS. Amiodarone optic neuropathy. *J Clin Neuroophthalmol.* 1988;8:105–111.

71. Mansour AM, Puklin JE, O'Grady R. Optic nerve ultrastructure following amiodarone therapy. *J Clin Neuroophthalmol.* 1988;8(4):231–237.

72. Yoon YH, Jung KH, Sadun AA, Shin HC, Koh JY. Ethambutol-induced vacuolar changes and neuronal loss in rat retinal cell culture: mediation by endogenous zinc. *Toxicol Appl Pharmacol.* 2000;162(2):107–114.

73. Shiraki H. Neuropathy due to intoxication with anti-tuberculous drugs from neuropathological viewpoint. *Adv Neurol Sci.* 1973;17:120.

74. Melamud A, Kosmorsky GS, Lee MS. Ocular ethambutol toxicity. *Mayo Clin Proc.* 2003;78(11):1409–1411.

75. Fang JT, Chen YC, Chang MY. Ethambutol-induced optic neuritis in patients with end stage renal disease on hemodialysis: two case reports and literature review. *Ren Fail.* 2004;26(2):189–193.

76. Harley RD, Huang NN, Macri CH, Green WR. Optic neuritis and optic atrophy following chloramphenicol in cystic fibrosis patients. *Trans Am Acad Ophthalmol Otolaryngol.* 1970;74(5):1011–1031.

77. Linezolid. In: *Physicians' Desk Reference.* 5th ed. Montvale, NJ: Thomson PDR; 2004:2808–2815.

78. Lee E, Burger S, Shah J, et al. Linezolid-associated toxic optic neuropathy: a report of 2 cases. *Clin Infect Dis.* 2003;37(10):1389–1391.

79. Corallo CE, Paull AE. Linezolid-induced neuropathy. *Med J Aust.* 2002;177(6):332.

80. Rho JP, Sia IG, Crum BA, Dekutoski MB, Trousdale RT. Linezolid-associated peripheral neuropathy. *Mayo Clin Proc.* 2004;79(7):927–930.

81. Spellberg B, Yoo T, Bayer AS. Reversal of linezolid-associated cytopenias, but not peripheral neuropathy, by administration of vitamin B_6. *J Antimicrob Chemother.* 2004;54(4):832–835.

82. Frippiat F, Bergiers C, Michel C, Dujardin JP, Derue G. Severe bilateral optic neuritis associated with prolonged linezolid therapy. *J Antimicrob Chemother.* 2004;53(6):1114–1115.

83. Zyrox (linezolid) [package insert]. Rydaimere, New South Wales: Pharmacia Australia, 2002.

84. McKinley SH, Foroozan R. Optic neuropathy associated with linezolid treatment. *J Neuroophthalmol.* 2005;25(1):18–21.

85. Baron S, Tyring SK, Fleischmann WR Jr, et al. The interferons: mechanisms of action and clinical applications. *JAMA.* 1991;266(10):1375–1383.

86. Lohmann CP, Kroher G, Bogenrieder T, Spiegel D, Preuner J. Severe loss of vision during adjuvant interferon alfa-2b treatment for malignant melanoma. *Lancet.* 1999;353(9161):1326.

87. Purvin VA. Anterior ischemic optic neuropathy secondary to interferon alfa. *Arch Ophthalmol.* 1995;113(8):1041–1044.

88. Taylor JL, Grossberg SE. The effects of interferon-α on the production and action of other cytokines. *Semin Oncol.* 1998;25 (1 Suppl 1):23–29.

89. Foroozan R. Unilateral pallid optic disc swelling and anemia associated with interferon-α treatment. *J Neuroophthalmol.* 2004;24(1):98–99.

90. Gabler B, Kroher G, Bogenrieder T, Spiegel D, Preuner J, Lohmann CP. Severe, bilateral vision loss in malignant melanoma of the skin. Anterior ischemic optic neuropathy with irreversible vision and visual field loss in adjuvant interferon alfa-2b therapy. *Ophthalmologe.* 2001;98(7):672–673.

91. Vardizer Y, Linhart Y, Loewenstein A, Garzozi H, Mazawi N, Kesler A. Interferon-α-associated bilateral simultaneous ischemic optic neuropathy. *J Neuroophthalmol.* 2003;23(4):256–259.

92. Gupta R, Singh S, Tang R, Blackwell TA, Schiffman JS. Anterior ischemic optic neuropathy caused by interferon-α therapy. *Am J Med.* 2002;112(8):683–684.

93. Norcia F, Di Maria A, Prandini F, Redaelli C. Natural interferon therapy: optic nerve ischemic damage? *Ophthalmologica.* 1999;213(5):339–340.

94. Foroozan R, Buono LM, Sergott RC, Savino PJ. Retrobulbar optic neuritis associated with infliximab. *Arch Ophthalmol.* 2002;120(7):985–987.

95. Mejico LJ. Infliximab-associated retrobulbar optic neuritis. *Arch Ophthalmol.* 2004;122(5):793–794.

96. ten Tusscher MP, Jacobs PJ, Busch MJ, de Graaf L, Diemont WL. Bilateral anterior toxic optic neuropathy and the use of infliximab. *BMJ.* 2003;326(7389):579.

97. Roch LM II, Gordon DL, Barr AB, Paulsen CA. Visual changes associated with clomiphene citrate therapy. *Arch Ophthalmol.* 1967;77(1):14–17.

98. Padron Rivas VF, Sanchez A, Lerida Arias MT, Carvajal Garcia-Pardo A. Optic neuritis appearing during treatment with clomiphene. *Aten Primaria.* 1994;14(7):912–913.

99. Lawton AW. Optic neuropathy associated with clomiphene citrate therapy. *Fertil Steril.* 1994;61(2):390–391.

100. Noureddin BN, Seoud M, Bashshur Z, Salem Z, Shamseddin A, Khalil A. Ocular toxicity in low-dose tamoxifen: a prospective study. *Eye.* 1999;13 (Pt 6):729–733.

101. Goldstein I, Lue TF, Padma-Nathan H, Rosen RC, Steers WD, Wicker PA. Oral sildenafil in the treatment of erectile dysfunction: Sildenafil Study Group. *N Engl J Med.* 1998;338(20): 1397–1404. Erratum in: *N Engl J Med.* 1998;339(1):59.

102. Pomeranz HD, Smith KH, Hart WM Jr, Egan RA. Sildenafil-associated nonarteritic anterior ischemic optic neuropathy. *Ophthalmology.* 2002;109(3):584–587.

103. Pomeranz HD, Bhavsar AR. Nonarteritic ischemic optic neuropathy developing soon after use of sildenafil (viagra): a report of seven new cases. *J Neuroophthalmol.* 2005;25(1):9–13.

104. Akash R, Hrishikesh D, Amith P, Sabah S. Case report: association of combined nonarteritic anterior ischemic optic neuropathy (NAION) and obstruction of cilioretinal artery with overdose of Viagra. *J Ocul Pharmacol Ther.* 2005;21(4):315–317.

105. Beck RW, Servais GE, Hayreh SS. Anterior ischemic optic neuropathy: IX. Cup-to-disc ratio and its role in pathogenesis. *Ophthalmology.* 1987;94(11):1503–1508.

106. Burde RM. Optic disk risk factors for nonarteritic anterior ischemic optic neuropathy. *Am J Ophthalmol.* 1993;116(6): 759–764.

107. Doro S, Lessell S. Cup–disc ratio and ischemic optic neuropathy. *Arch Ophthalmol.* 1985;103(8):1143–1144.

108. Boshier A, Pambakian N, Shakir SA. A case of nonarteritic ischemic optic neuropathy (NAION) in a male patient taking sildenafil. *Int J Clin Pharmacol Ther.* 2002;40(9):422–423.

109. Cunningham AV, Smith KH. Anterior ischemic optic neuropathy associated with Viagra. *J Neuroophthalmol.* 2001;21(1):22–25.

110. Dheer S, Rekhi GS, Merlyn S. Sildenafil-associated anterior ischaemic optic neuropathy. *J Assoc Physicians India.* 2002;50:265.

111. Egan R, Pomeranz H. Sildenafil (Viagra)–associated anterior ischemic optic neuropathy. *Arch Ophthalmol.* 2000;118(2): 291–292.

112. Neufeld AH, Sawada A, Becker B. Inhibition of nitric-oxide synthase 2 by aminoguanidine provides neuroprotection of retinal ganglion cells in a rat model of chronic glaucoma. *Proc Natl Acad Sci USA.* 1999;96(17):9944–9948.

113. Sponsel WE, Paris G, Sandoval SS, et al. Sildenafil and ocular perfusion. *N Engl J Med.* 2000;342(22):1680.

114. Grunwald JE, Siu KK, Jacob SS, Dupont J. Effect of sildenafil citrate (Viagra) on the ocular circulation. *Am J Ophthalmol.* 2001;131(6):751–755.

115. Bollinger K, Lee MS. Recurrent visual field defect and ischemic optic neuropathy associated with tadalafil rechallenge. *Arch Ophthalmol.* 2005;123(3):400–401.

116. Escaravage GK Jr, Wright JD Jr, Givre SJ. Tadalafil associated with anterior ischemic optic neuropathy. *Arch Ophthalmol.* 2005;123(3):399–400.

117. Peter NM, Singh MV, Fox PD. Tadalafil-associated anterior ischaemic optic neuropathy. *Eye.* 2005;19(6):715–717.

118. Jiang GL, Tucker SL, Guttenberger R, et al. Radiation-induced injury to the visual pathway. *Radiother Oncol.* 1994;30(1):17–25.

119. Kline LB, Kim JY, Ceballos R. Radiation optic neuropathy. *Ophthalmology.* 1985;92(8):1118–1126.

120. Millar JL, Spry NA, Lamb DS, Delahunt J. Blindness in patients after external beam irradiation for pituitary adenomas: two cases occurring after small daily fractional doses. *Clin Oncol (R Coll Radiol).* 1991;3(5):291–294.

121. Regine WF, Kramer S. Pediatric craniopharyngiomas: long-term results of combined treatment with surgery and radiation. *Int J Radiat Oncol Biol Phys.* 1992;24(4):611–617.

122. Roden D, Bosley TM, Fowble B, et al. Delayed radiation injury to the retrobulbar optic nerves and chiasm: clinical syndrome and treatment with hyperbaric oxygen and corticosteroids. *Ophthalmology.* 1990;97(3):346–351.

123. Schoenthaler R, Albright NW, Wara WM, Phillips TL, Wilson CB, Larson DA. Re-irradiation of pituitary adenoma. *Int J Radiat Oncol Biol Phys.* 1992;24(2):307–314.

124. Geyer JR, Taylor EM, Milstein JM, et al. Radiation, methotrexate, and white matter necrosis: laboratory evidence for neural radioprotection with preirradiation methotrexate. *Int J Radiat Oncol Biol Phys.* 1988;15(2):373–375.

125. Balsom WR, Bleyer WA, Robison LL, et al. Intellectual function in long-term survivors of childhood acute lymphoblastic leukemia: protective effect of pre-irradiation methotrexate? A Children's Cancer Study Group study. *Med Pediatr Oncol.* 1991;19(6):486–492.

126. Fishman ML, Bean SC, Cogan DG. Optic atrophy following prophylactic chemotherapy and cranial radiation for acute lymphocytic leukemia. *Am J Ophthalmol.* 1976;82(4):571–576.

127. Marks LB, Spencer DP. The influence of volume on the tolerance of the brain to radiosurgery. *J Neurosurg.* 1991;75(2):177–180.

128. Marks JE, Wong J. The risk of cerebral radionecrosis in relation to dose, time and fractionation: a follow-up study. *Prog Exp Tumor Res.* 1985;29:210–218.

129. Safdari H, Fuentes JM, Dubois JB, Alirezai M, Castan P, Vlahovitch B. Radiation necrosis of the brain: time of onset and incidence related to total dose and fractionation of radiation. *Neuroradiology.* 1985;27(1):44–47.

130. Schultheiss TE, Higgins EM, El-Mahdi AM. The latent period in clinical radiation myelopathy. *Int J Radiat Oncol Biol Phys.* 1984;10(7):1109–1115.

131. Lampert PW, Davis RL. Delayed effects of radiation on the human central nervous system: "early" and "late" delayed reactions. *Neurology.* 1964;14:912–917.

132. Hopewell JW, van der Kogel AJ. Pathophysiological mechanisms leading to the development of late radiation-induced damage to the central nervous system. *Front Radiat Ther Oncol.* 1999;33:265–275.

133. Myers R, Rogers MA, Hornsey S. A reappraisal of the roles of glial and vascular elements in the development of white matter necrosis in irradiated rat spinal cord. *Br J Cancer Suppl.* 1986;7:221–223.

134. van der Kogel AJ. Radiation-induced damage in the central nervous system: an interpretation of target cell responses. *Br J Cancer Suppl.* 1986;7:207–217.

135. Omary RA, Berr SS, Kamiryo T, et al. 1995 AUR Memorial Award: γ-Knife irradiation-induced changes in the normal rat brain studied with 1H magnetic resonance spectroscopy and imaging. *Acad Radiol.* 1995;2(12):1043–1051.

136. Levin LA, Gragoudas ES, Lessell S. Endothelial cell loss in irradiated optic nerves. *Ophthalmology.* 2000;107(2):370–374.

137. Chan YL, Yeung DK, Leung SF, Cao G. Proton magnetic resonance spectroscopy of late delayed radiation-induced injury of the brain. *J Magn Reson Imaging.* 1999;10(2):130–137.

138. Crompton MR, Layton DD. Delayed radionecrosis of the brain following therapeutic x-radiation of the pituitary. *Brain.* 1961;84:85–101.

139. Ross HS, Rosenberg S, Friedman AH. Delayed radiation necrosis of the optic nerve. *Am J Ophthalmol.* 1973;76(5):683–686.

140. Lessell S. Friendly fire: neurogenic visual loss from radiation therapy. *J Neuroophthalmol.* 2004;24(3):243–250.

141. Borruat FX, Schatz NJ, Glaser JS. Postactinic retrobulbar optic neuropathy. *Klin Monatsbl Augenheilkd.* 1996;208(5):381–384.

142. Guy J, Schatz NJ. Hyperbaric oxygen in the treatment of radiation-induced optic neuropathy. *Ophthalmology.* 1986;93(8):1083–1088.

143. Brown GC, Shields JA, Sanborn G, Augsburger JJ, Savino PJ, Schatz NJ. Radiation optic neuropathy. *Ophthalmology.* 1982;89(12):1489–1493.

144. Arnold AC. Radiation optic neuropathy. Paper presented at the 21st Annual Meeting of the North American Neuro-Ophthalmology Society, February 23, 1995, Tucson, Arizona.

145. Borruat FX, Schatz NJ, Glaser JS, Feun LG, Matos L. Visual recovery from radiation-induced optic neuropathy: the role of hyperbaric oxygen therapy. *J Clin Neuro-ophthalmol.* 1993;13(2):98–101.

146. Kaufman M, Swartz BE, Mandelkern M, Ropchan J, Gee M, Blahd WH. Diagnosis of delayed cerebral radiation necrosis following proton beam therapy. *Arch Neurol.* 1990;47(4):474–476.

147. Spaziante R, de Divitiis E, Stella L, Cappabianca P, Genovese L. The empty sella. *Surg Neurol.* 1981;16(6):418–426.

148. Bernstein M, Laperriere N. Radiation-induced tumors of the nervous system. In: Gutin PH, Leibel SA, Sheline GE, eds. *Radiation Injury to the Central Nervous System.* New York: Raven Press; 1991.

148. Guy J, Mancuso A, Beck R, et al. Radiation-induced optic neuropathy: a magnetic resonance imaging study. *J Neurosurg.* 1991;74(3):426–432.

150. Hudgins PA, Newman NJ, Dillon WP, Hoffman JC Jr. Radiation-induced optic neuropathy: characteristic appearances on gadolinium-enhanced MR. *AJNR.* 1992;13(1):235–238.

151. McClellan RL, el Gammal T, Kline LB. Early bilateral radiation-induced optic neuropathy with follow-up MRI. *Neuroradiology.* 1995;37(2):131–133.

152. Oppenheimer JH, Levy ML, Sinha U, et al. Radionecrosis secondary to interstitial brachytherapy: correlation of magnetic resonance imaging and histopathology. *Neurosurgery.* 1992;31(2):336–343.

153. Glantz MJ, Burger PC, Friedman AH, Radtke RA, Massey EW, Schold SC Jr. Treatment of radiation-induced nervous system injury with heparin and warfarin. *Neurology.* 1994;44(11):2020–2027.

154. Barbosa AP, Carvalho D, Marques L, et al. Inefficiency of the anticoagulant therapy in the regression of the radiation-induced

optic neuropathy in Cushing's disease. *J Endocrinol Invest.* 1999;22(4):301–305.

155. Danesh-Meyer HV, Savino PJ, Sergott RC. Visual loss despite anticoagulation in radiation-induced optic neuropathy. *Clin Experiment Ophthalmol.* 2004;32(3):333–335.

156. Landau K, Killer HE. Radiation damage. *Neurology.* 1996;46(3):889.

157. Hammerlund C. The physiological effects of hyperbaric oxygen. In: Kindwall E, ed. *Hyperbaric Medicine Practice.* Flagstaff, Ariz: Best Publishing; 1995.

158. Borruat FX, Schatz NJ, Glaser JS, et al. Radiation optic neuropathy: report of cases, role of hyperbaric oxygen therapy, and literature review. *J Neuroophthalmol.* 1996;16:255–256.

159. Kellner U, Bornfeld N, Foerster MH. Radiation-induced optic neuropathy following brachytherapy of uveal melanomas. *Graefes Arch Clin Exp Ophthalmol.* 1993;231(5):267–270.

160. Freeman AG. Optic neuropathy and chronic cyanide intoxication: a review. *J Soc Med.* 1988;81:103.

161. Foulds WS, Chisholm IA, Bronte-Stewart JM, et al. Vitamin B_{12} absorption in tobacco amblyopia. *Br J Ophthalmol.* 1969;53:393.

162. Frisén L. Fundus changes in acute nutritional amblyopia. *Arch Ophthalmol.* 1983;101:577.

CHAPTER 10

Toxic Movement Disorders: The Approach to the Patient with a Movement Disorder of Toxic Origin

Alberto J. Espay

CHAPTER CONTENTS

INTRODUCTION

Movement disorders can arise within the context of toxic exposures. There is wide literature linking manganese to the development of parkinsonism and methylmercury to cerebellar toxicity. The best-known example of the connection between toxic exposures and movement disorders occurred in the early 1980s, when an analogue of meperidine intended to emulate the effects of heroin was synthesized by basement chemists without knowledge that one of its byproducts, 1-methyl-4-phenyl-1,2,3,6 tetrahydropyridine (MPTP), would trigger severe nonprogressive parkinsonism among its users.[1] MPTP is converted by monoamine oxidase to methyl-phenylpyridinium ion, a neurotoxin that directly targets nigral dopaminergic neurons and has since become a widely used animal model of Parkinson's disease. An earlier toxin, the pesticide rotenone, also demonstrated nigral neurotoxicity by affecting the complex I component of mitochondrial respiration.[2] However, MPTP has virtually disappeared as a source of clinical toxicity and studies have yet to definitely demonstrate that pesticide exposure is a risk for later development of Parkinson's disease.

Rather than an epidemiological focus, this chapter intends to provide a symptom-oriented approach to the potential toxic origin of movement disorders when these can be clearly demonstrated to result from such exposure. We do not, therefore, discuss the increased risks of parkinsonism among rural workers exposed to well water and pesticides, draw attention to the putative neuroprotective effects of smoking, or review the conflicting literature on the contribution of dental amalgams, if any, to the background population exposure to elemental mercury. Indeed, most clinically relevant knowledge regarding abnormalities of movement resulting from toxic exposures is contained in case reports and small case series rather than population-based studies.

A case study chosen for its relevance introduces each category of abnormal movement. Each of these and their causative exposures are summarized in Table 1, which is referenced throughout this chapter. Exposures of high relevance for clinicians, appropriately marked in Table 1, are expanded upon in the text. Table 2 focuses on the most common source for which a toxic movement disorders may be evaluated in the emergency room: iatrogenic acute dystonic reactions. Table 3 summarizes the key clinical findings that should raise

Table 1: Movement Disorders and Associated Toxic Exposures

Category	Organic Solvent	Gas	Pesticide (Insecticide)	Pharmaceutical Agent	Recreational Drug Abuse	Metal
Parkinsonism	Carbon disulfide[d]	Carbon monoxide[ac] Hydrogen sulfide[c]	Rotenone (affects complex I of the mitochondrial respiration and MPTP)	Metoclopramide[abce] Antipsychotics[ae] (not quetiapine or clozapine) Amphotericin B Pemoline Cinnarizine Flunarizine Tetrabenazine Methyldopa Reserpine	Methcathinone[a] ("ephedronic encephalopathy")	Manganese[ace]
Tremor	Toluene[d]		Organophosphates[d] Organochlorine Pyrethroids	Amiodarone[a] Lithium[ae] Valproate[a] Cimetidine Cyclosporine Methylxanthines (theophylline, caffeine) Phenothiazines Phenytoin Acyclovir SSRIs Tricyclics Tacrolimus	Ethanol[ae] Methadone Cocaine	Mercury vapor[d]
Ataxia	Toluene[d]	Nitrous oxide[ac] Nitrogen dioxide	Organophosphates[d]	Metronidazole[ab] Phenytoin[ab] Amiodarone Nitrous oxide[ac] Cytarabine Fludarabine Vidarabine 5-Fluorouracil	Chronic alcohol[ae] Heroin ("chasing the dragon")[ac] Ethylene glycol[c]	Methyl mercury[ace] Zinc[ac] Thallium[d]

Myoclonus	Bismuth[ace] Levodopa[a] Amantadine Opioids (morphine, hydromorphone, meperidine, fentanyl)[ab] Fentanyl withdrawal Tricyclics	GHB[ac] Alcoholic liver disease Cocaine[abd]	Bismuth[ace] Aluminum[c] Manganese (less common)
Chorea	Antipsychotics[ab] Birth control pills[a] Amphetamine[a] Phenytoin[a] Carbamazepine[b] Lithium Verapamil Tricyclics	Methadone[a] Heroin Cocaine[abd]	
Dystonia	Acute[b] Tardive[a]	Cocaine[abd] Heroin[b]	

Details in text [a], Table 2 [b], Table 3 [c], Table 4 [d], and Table 5 [e].
GHB, γ-hydroxybutyric acid; MPTP, 1-methyl-4-phenyl-1,2,3,6 tetrahydropyridine; SSRI, serotonin-specific reuptake inhibitor.

Table 2: Selected Pharmacological Causes of Acute Dystonic Reactions

NEUROLEPTICS
Butyrophenones (benperidol, haloperidol)
Phenothiazines (fluphenazine, perphenazine, prochlorperazine)
ANTIEMETICS
(metoclopramide, domperidone)
CALCIUM CHANNEL BLOCKERS
(diltiazem)
ANALGESICS
Opioids (fentanyl)
Antiarrhythmics (flecainide)
Anticonvulsants (carbamazepine, phenytoin)
ANTIDEPRESSANTS
Serotonin-specific reuptake inhibitors (fluvoxamine, paroxetine)
Tricyclics (amitriptyline, amoxapine)
Monoamine-oxidase inhibitors (phenelzine, tranylcypromine)
OTHERS
Sedatives (midazolam)
Stimulants (cocaine, heroin)
Methylphenidate poisoning

suspicion for specific toxic exposures. Table 4 provides a glimpse of movement abnormalities, not otherwise discussed, that are inconsistently present after a given toxic exposure or may be relatively less important compared to symptoms in other domains, which themselves are critical for appropriate diagnosis and steering of treatment. Finally, Table 5 is intended to highlight key therapeutic strategies for those relevant toxic exposures for which removal of the offending toxin is not sufficient for adequate resolution. When not otherwise stated, assume that the management of toxic-mediated movement disorders relies on the removal of the offending toxin with or without symptomatic treatment.

PARKINSONISM

Parkinsonism is the emblematic hypokinetic disorder, characterized by the presence of bradykinesia or slowness of movement and rigidity or stiffness, with or without tremor and walking or postural impairment. The phenomenology is believed to reflect impairment of nigrostriatal delivery of dopamine (e.g., MPTP parkinsonism), usually levodopa responsive, or a postsynaptic impairment of dopamine receptors (e.g., manganese parkinsonism), largely unresponsive to levodopa.

Manganese

Manganese intoxication may cause a levodopa-resistant tremorless parkinsonism with marked axial deficits in the form of dysarthria, dysphagia, and postural impairment.[5] This form of parkinsonism can be distinguished from Parkinson's disease by a predominant postural rather than resting tremor and symmetrical involvement with early oculomotor, speech, gait, and balance disturbances, particularly with a "cock walk" appearance due walking on

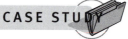

CASE STUDY

A 36-year-old man developed rapidly progressive sleepiness and slowness of movements followed by marked hypophonia, palilalia, micrographia, and impairment of walking and balance. He had difficulty with performance of fine motor tasks such as buttoning or using cutlery. Neurological exam demonstrated a symmetrical hypokinesia with mild axial rigidity, slowing and restriction in the range of saccadic vertical movements, decreased optokinetic nystagmus, short-stride and wide-based gait with arms held abducted from the sides, and falling on the pull test. His medical history was positive for hepatitis C virus. There was minimal elevation of aspartate and alanine aminotransferase levels. Brain magnetic resonance imaging (MRI) showed increased T1-weighted signal in the globus pallidus and substantia nigra. Blood and urine manganese levels were elevated. Treatment with levodopa at a dose of 600 mg/day was ineffective. He later admitted that, for at least 1 year, he had been intravenously injecting himself once or twice daily with a methcathinone solution prepared by combining 12 tablets containing 60 mg of pseudoephedrine hydrochloride with 0.3 g of potassium permanganate.

Table 3: Clinical Clues Suggesting a Specific Toxic Exposure

Key Deficit	Etiology
Ataxia and posterior cord sensory deficits with borderline cobalamin and high serum homocysteine	Nitrous oxide
Ataxia and posterior cord sensory deficits with low serum ceruloplasmin with or without a high serum zinc level	Copper-deficiency myelopathy due to chronic parenteral zinc in hemodialysis patients
Myoclonus and encephalopathy	GHB, heroin vapor ("chasing the dragon"), bismuth, aluminum-containing dialysates
Tremorless parkinsonism and a "cock walk"	Manganese
Ataxia with visual field constriction and circumoral paresthesias	Mercury
Parkinsonism and bilateral globus pallidum T2W hyperintensity (pallidal necrosis) as a delayed complication of a toxic encephalopathy	Carbon monoxide exposure
Same scenario but preceding toxic encephalopathy developed in an area with the "smell of rotten eggs," especially if near a petroleum refinery or paper mill	Hydrogen sulfide ("sewer gas") exposure
Postural tremor and "rabbit syndrome"	Metoclopramide (neuroleptic)–induced parkinsonism
Orobuccolinguomasticatory chorea	Neuroleptic-induced tardive dyskinesia
Multiple cranial neuropathies (bilateral facial palsy, dysarthria, dysphagia) and ataxia[3]	Ethylene glycol (ingestion of antifreeze, suicide attempt)

GHB, γ-hydroxybutyric acid.

toes with flexed arms and erect posture. Freezing and tendency to lean backward are common. The most important diagnostic finding is the presence of T1-weighted hyperintensity in the globus pallidus on brain MRI. Pathology studies emphasize the predilection of the internal segment of the globus pallidus with sparing of the substantia nigra pars compacta and the absence of Lewy bodies, a pattern precisely opposite to that of Parkinson's disease.[6] The case study illustrates a form of manganese toxicity resulting from the addictive use of methcathinone (also known as ephedrone), which can be synthesized from a common over-the-counter cold remedy, pseudoephedrine (Sudafed), using potassium permanganate as the catalyst.[7] Cases of this "ephedronic encephalopathy" were initially reported from Russia, Ukraine, and Estonia, where methcathinone use, to obtain amphetamine-like euphoria, has been pandemic.[8] Chelation therapy with ethylenediaminetetraacetic acid has resulted in mild to modest improvements, but permanent sequelae are likely.[9] Progression of deficits after cessation of exposure does not

appear to be the case, as it has been reported on other forms of manganism.[10]

Additional sources of manganese exposure include mining, welding, ferromanganese smelting, industrial and agricultural work, chronic liver failure with cirrhosis (acquired hepatolenticular degeneration), total parenteral nutrition, and ingestion of Chinese herbal pills. Sufficient exposure invariably results in pallidal T1-weighted brain MRI hyperintensity with normal T2-weighted signal, a specific biological marker of manganese accumulation,[11] although it is poorly correlated with serum manganese levels.[12] When both abnormal T1- and T2-weighted signals in the pallidum are present, the differential diagnosis moves away from manganese toxicity toward Wilson's disease, neurodegeneration with brain iron accumulation (formerly, Hallervorden-Spatz disease), melanoma, neurofibromatosis, calcification, hyperglycemia, blood products, and fat. Besides removal from the source of exposure, additional management suggestions for manganese toxicity are outlined in Table 5.

Table 4: Inconsistent or Secondary Toxic Movement Disorders

Movement	Primary Clues	Toxicity
Ataxia	Peripheral muscarinic (excessive salivation, tearing, urination, vomiting, diarrhea, wheezing) and nicotinic effects (fasciculation, cramps, weakness, tachycardia, hypertension); patients may have a characteristic garlic-like odor	Organophosphate toxicity
	Alopecia, optic neuropathy, and painful sensory neuropathy in the setting of renal, gastrointestinal, cardiovascular, and liver dysfunction	Thallium poisoning
	Repeated euphoria, muscle weakness, and renal failure developing with nystagmus, head titubation, intention tremor, and truncal ataxia	Toluene abuse (chronic "huffing" of gasoline, nail polishes, glues, and paint thinners)
Tremor	Gingivitis and erethism (excessive shyness intermixed with nervousness and irritability)	Mercury vapor (chronic occupational inhalation)
Parkinsonism	Demyelinating peripheral neuropathy, levodopa-unresponsive parkinsonism, psychiatric and sleep changes, and microangiopathic white matter lesions in the brain	Carbon disulfide (chronic occupational inhalation in manufacturing of rayon and vulcanized rubber)
Chorea	Rhabdomyolysis with or without myelopathic features; seizures are more common among first-time users	Cocaine overdose

Pharmaceutical Agents

Prochlorperazine and metoclopramide are two commonly used antiemetics and are often unsuspected sources of parkinsonism compared to antipsychotics. These agents have dopamine receptor blocking properties (for which they are termed *neuroleptics*) and are capable of inducing parkinsonism, as well as various other movement disorders.

Organized according to the order of appearance after drug initiation, the range of neuroleptic-induced movement disorders includes acute dystonic reactions, acute akathisia, parkinsonism, neuroleptic malignant syndrome, and tardive syndromes (including tardive dyskinesia, dystonia, tics, and akathisia). It is not uncommon for two or more drug-induced movement disorders (i.e., parkinsonism and tardive dyskinesia) to occur simultaneously in the same patient.[13] Drugs in the neuroleptic category include the phenothiazines fluphenazine and prochlorperazine, as well as the substituted benzamides metoclopramide, sulpiride, tiapride, and clebopride. The blockade of D2 receptors, largely in the striatum, is believed to account for acute dystonic reactions and especially drug-induced parkinsonism. Akathisia and neuroleptic malignant syndrome are likely due to more widespread dopamine antagonistic effects. The pathogenesis of tardive dyskinesia, which typically requires longer-term drug use, is not well understood but probably involves factors distinct from pure D2 receptor blockade. Drug-induced parkinsonism can be indistinguishable from idiopathic Parkinson's disease. A relatively prominent postural component of the tremor and the presence of low-frequency, high-amplitude facial tremor (rabbit syndrome) may raise suspicion as to the drug-related nature of the disorder.[14] Metoclopramide is more likely to cause parkinsonism among patients with renal failure and dose reduction or elimination is prudent in this setting.[15]

Abrupt withdrawal of chronically used neuroleptics may be associated with the emergence of a tardive dyskinetic syndrome. If these symptoms or a worsening of the tremor (in which case the term "tardive tremor" has been suggested[16]) become bothersome or disabling, it may be necessary to reintroduce the causative drug followed by a more gradual dose tapering. Patients with disabling iatrogenic parkinsonism may not improve sufficiently from withdrawal of the offending neuroleptic, and temporary symptomatic treatment with levodopa or a dopamine agonist is necessary.

More persistent symptoms suggest the possibility of an underlying primary parkinsonian disorder (possibly occult at drug initiation) that could have predisposed the patient to this complication. To avoid the parkinsonism of neuroleptic-type antiemetics, domperidone, a peripheral dopamine antagonist, or ondansetron, a selective serotonin 5-hydroxytryptamine (5-HT$_3$) receptor antagonist, are the drugs of choice for antiemetic control and motility

Table 5: Management of Selected Toxic Movement Disorders

Movement Disorder	Strategy
Manganese-induced parkinsonism	Chelation with EDTA Welders: Adequate ventilation and personal respiratory protection during welding Potassium permanganate poisoning: N-acetylcysteine may be used Liver cirrhosis: Liver transplantation TPN: Avoid manganese supplementation in excess of 0.018 μmol/kg/day Correct iron deficiency (increases gastric absorption of manganese)
Neuroleptic-induced parkinsonism	Abrupt drug withdrawal may trigger a tardive dyskinetic syndrome, which requires reintroduction and slow taper Levodopa or a dopamine agonist for symptom persistence despite drug discontinuation Domperidone is favored over metoclopramide or prochlorperazine when antiemesis is necessary
Alcohol withdrawal tremor	Benzodiazepines (diazepam or chlordiazepoxide) for 7 days Thiamine (vitamin B_1) supplementation Cautious use of beta-blockers (increase the risk of hallucinations)
Lithium-induced tremor	Correction of dehydration Management of diabetes insipidus Hemodialysis to increase elimination Beta-blockers (propranolol, atenolol [nadolol in liver failure patients]) Consider vitamin B_6 (900–1200 mg/day)[4] Avoid forced saline diuresis as it does not increase elimination and leads to hypernatremia
Mercury-induced ataxia	Succimer (DMSA) 10 mg/kg (350 mg/m²) orally every 8 hours for 5 days and then every 12 hours for 2 weeks Chelation with D-penicillamine or BAL (dimercaprol) Dialysis is of little benefit in methylmercury toxicity after neurotoxicity has developed
Bismuth-induced myoclonic encephalopathy	Drug discontinuation alone is sufficient. Avoid chelation therapy (clinical deterioration)

BAL, British anti-Lewisite; DSMA, dimercaptosuccinic acid; EDTA, ethylenediaminetetraacetic acid; TPN, total parenteral nutrition.

disorders of the upper gastrointestinal tract, especially in the elderly.[17] Other pharmacological agents associated with the induction of parkinsonism are listed in Table 1.

Gases

The most common mechanisms of carbon monoxide (CO) exposure are smoke inhalation from a parked and enclosed vehicle, gas from the kitchen stove, and a house's leaky gas heater. Although a period of pseudo-recovery follows an acute CO encephalopathy, parkinsonism typically develops after a latency of about 1 month, accompanied by cognitive impairment, psychotic behaviors, and incontinence.[18] Deficits include frontal release signs (glabellar and grasp reflexes), masked facies, axial-predominant rigidity, hypokinesia,

short-stepped gait, and retropulsion.[18] Bilateral pallidal necrosis is the typical imaging feature among survivors, manifested by sharp T2-weighted hyperintensity of the globus pallidus on brain MRI (Figure 10-1). The parkinsonism, however, may not be directly related to this abnormality but, rather, to the associated diffuse white matter hyperintensity.[19]

The CO-induced parkinsonism may remain stable or slowly improve. Chorea and dystonia as sequelae have been described,[20] but chorea, surprisingly, which appears with a median latency similar to that of the parkinsonian phenotype, tends to resolve within weeks.[21] Response to levodopa is suboptimal due to damage to postsynaptic nigrostriatal dopamine receptors. Atypical antipsychotics may improve the neuropsychiatric function.[22] No exposure-specific therapy is available.

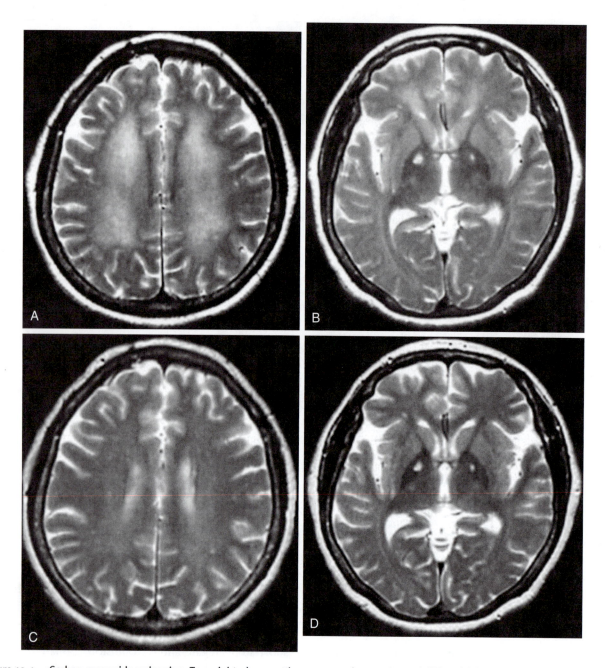

Figure 10-1. Carbon monoxide poisoning. T2-weighted magnetic resonance image showed diffuse high-signal changes in the white matter *(A)* and bilateral pallidal necrosis *(B)* at presentation, with nearly complete disappearance of the white matter abnormalities *(C)* with persistence of the pallidal necrosis at 14 months *(D)*.

Prevention of delayed parkinsonism from CO exposure may be achieved with hyperbaric oxygen administration shortly after the acute event and, still theoretically, with early treatment using noncompetitive *N*-methyl-d-aspartate receptor antagonists (e.g., ketamine), as shown in animal models.[23,24]

Another neurotoxic gas, hydrogen sulfide (Table 3), has rarely been associated with delayed-onset parkinsonism after patients survive an acute encephalopathy.

TREMOR

Tremor is an oscillatory abnormal movement that is rhythmic (e.g., essential and physiological), jerky, irregular, and posture dependent (e.g., dystonic), or slower and action dependent (e.g., cerebellar). It usually affects the upper limbs but may involve the head, voice, tongue, or legs. The latter distribution is often associated with

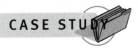

CASE STUDY

A 57-year-old man with posttraumatic complex partial seizures poorly responsive to carbamazepine and phenytoin was initiated on valproate. Shortly thereafter, he developed a moderately disabling postural and action tremor of the upper extremities. Acetazolamide at 8 mg/kg/day was started, advancing to 14 mg/kg/day in 5 days, which was followed by tremor improvement while maintaining seizure control.

parkinsonian disorders, discussed earlier, whereby the tremor is typically seen during rest. Tremor is the most common toxic, usually iatrogenic, movement disorder, and the list of well-established offending agents is shown in Table 1.

Pharmaceutical Agents

As valproic acid is widely used for epilepsy, migraine, and bipolar disorder, it has become the most common antiepileptic drug associated with tremor.[25] Unlike amiodarone and lithium (described later), among other drugs, the tremor induced by valproic acid more closely resembles essential tremor, with a slower frequency and a tendency to express at rest, suggesting parkinsonism. Although it usually appears at dosages greater than 750 mg/day, there is no clear correlation between tremor severity and plasma levels.[26] If withdrawal of valproate is not possible, as in the case study, acetazolamide has been suggested as a strategy to attenuate the drug-induced tremor while preserving its therapeutic benefit.[27]

The postural and action bilateral hand tremors induced by amiodarone and lithium tend to be of low amplitude and high frequency (6 to 10 Hz), unlike the large-amplitude, lower-frequency (4 to 8 Hz) expression of essential tremor. Lithium carbonate, mainly used as a mood stabilizer, is probably the most common cause of iatrogenic tremor. It has a narrow therapeutic range (0.6 to 1.2 mEq/L), and dose adjustments become critical in those with renal dysfunction or dehydration.[25,28] In addition to tremor with or without myoclonus, chronic lithium toxicity may be associated with nausea, somnolence, and in late stages, seizures and cardiac arrhythmias. Less common manifestations include nephrogenic diabetes insipidus and hypothyroidism. Interestingly, elimination of coffee in these patients can lead to tremor worsening, as caffeine increases lithium clearance and its elimination from the diet raises lithium levels.[29] Management of this toxicity is suggested in Table 5. Pindolol is the only beta-blocker that

may induce or exacerbate postural and action tremors and should be removed in the setting of otherwise unexplained tremor.[30,31]

Ethanol

A common feature of alcohol withdrawal is the development of postural tremor of variable amplitude and high frequency, usually above 8 Hz, affecting the hands but potentially extending to the legs, face, and tongue. Tremor is indeed a required element of the diagnostic criteria for alcohol withdrawal, besides anxiety, agitation, excessive sweating, altered consciousness, and hallucinations. Management is largely aimed at ensuring both seizure prophylaxis and tremor control with γ-aminobutyric acid (GABA)-ergic drugs such as benzodiazepines or γ-hydroxybutyric acid (GHB). Vitamin B$_1$ supplementation is recommended since thiamine deficiency is a frequent complication in alcoholic patients.[32] Intravenous administration of thiamine hydrochloride (100 mg) is preferable if patients have poor nutritional status or severe complications such as Wernicke's encephalopathy, a medical emergency.[33] Once alcoholic cerebellar degeneration has occurred (see the Ataxia section), chronic alcoholic patients develop a low-frequency (3 Hz) leg tremor best seen when the patient stands with feet together and knees half bent, which produced a slow "bobbing" of the body, or when the patient is recumbent with legs elevated and hips and knees are flexed, which causes a kicking movement.[32]

ATAXIA

Ataxia is loosely applied to the dysmetria of limb movements, represented partly as a wide-based, unsteady gait. Ataxia can result from vestibulo- and spinocerebellar causes, as well as toxic peripheral neuropathies, which lead to sensory ataxia from proprioceptive loss. Typical accompaniments of cerebellar ataxia are action tremor, dysarthria, and oculomotor abnormalities.

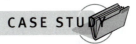

CASE STUDY

A 65-year-old woman complains of unsteadiness when walking. She has undergone extensive dental work over the last year. Her examination shows word-finding difficulty, poor delayed recall, position and vibratory loss in the legs and steppage, and mildly wide-based gait. Vitamin B$_{12}$ levels were low.

Gases

Sensory ataxia due to proprioceptive impairment can be a complication of cobalamin deficiency caused by nitrous oxide toxicity, an inorganic gas used as an inhalational anesthetic in surgical or dental procedures ("anesthesia paresthetica").[34,35] Chronic exposure to nitrous oxide can also be seen among adolescents from cartridges of this gas used as propellant for whipped-cream dispensers. Although chronic exposure is needed in normal individuals for the development of features suggestive of subacute combined degeneration of the spinal cord, shorter exposures (2 weeks to 2 months) among those with subclinical vitamin B_{12} deficiency may be sufficient for the myeloneuropathy illustrated by the case study to manifest. Initial reported clinical features are acral paresthesias and a "reverse" Lhermitte sign, which may correspond with examination findings of vibration and position sensory loss and hypo- or areflexia in the legs.[36] Later features may include distal leg weakness, hand clumsiness, erectile dysfunction, neurogenic bladder, and encephalopathy when hyperreflexia and Babinski signs, as well as more dense proprioceptive loss, may emerge. Nerve conduction studies show an axonal sensorimotor neuropathy. Serum B_{12} (cobalamin) levels may be normal or reduced. Other laboratory abnormalities may include elevated serum homocysteine and methylmalonate levels.[34] Most patients improve following elimination of the nitrous oxide exposure, but vitamin B_{12} and methionine supplementation may be used in those with residual deficits.

Recreational Drugs

Chronic alcohol abuse leads to progressive wide-based ataxia due to selective degeneration of the anterior and superior aspect of the cerebellar vermis. In these patients with truncal ataxia, the neurological examination may show no arm dysmetria and only mild clumsiness on heel to shin. However, tandem gait is disproportionally abnormal. Coexistent vitamin B_{12} deficiency may lead to a combined cerebellar and posterior cord–dependent sensory ataxia, adding a steppage gait component to the ataxia.

Among drug abusers, snorting or smoking heroin with the "chasing the dragon" technique (heating the drug on metal foil and "chasing" the resulting vapor with a tube or straw) causes gait ataxia, limb dysmetria, and dysarthria several weeks after exposure. The ataxia is slowly complicated by spastic quadriparesis as the T2-weighted and fluid-attenuated inversion recovery brain MRI begin to reveal diffuse symmetrical white matter hyperintensities in the posterior limb of the internal capsule, splenium of the corpus callosum, cerebellum, and brainstem.[37] In this progressive spongiform encephalopathy, chorea, myoclonus, blindness, and ultimately akinetic mutism, coma, and death have been reported.[38] Elevated lactate found on magnetic resonance spectroscopy has suggested the use of coenzyme Q as a treatment option, with variable response.

Metals

A similar picture to that of nitrous oxide toxicity that mimics the subacute combined degeneration seen in vitamin B_{12} deficiency can occur in copper deficiency myelopathy, which (in addition to postgastrectomy and other malabsorption states) can occur among patients in chronic hemodialysis undergoing repetitive parenteral zinc supplementation.[39,40] Spine MRI may show increased T2-weighted signal in the dorsal column. Low serum ceruloplasmin may be an initial clue to the diagnosis.[41] Oral copper supplementation prevents further neurological deterioration and may reverse some deficits.

Consumption of fish containing large amounts of methylmercury caused the Minamata Bay epidemic of ataxia, hypesthesia, and visual impairment in Kyushu Island, Japan, in the late 1950s.[42] Since methylmercury enters the aquatic food chain and reaches the highest concentration in long-living predatory seafood, lesser-scale organic mercury toxicity can occur with consumption of shark and swordfish from the oceans and pike and bass from freshwater. After latency from exposure measured in months, patients present with ataxia, tremors, dysarthria, visual field constriction, impaired hearing, and circumoral and acral paresthesias due to dorsal root and trigeminal sensory ganglion involvement.[43] Brain MRI demonstrates atrophy of the cerebellar vermis and hemispheres, with atrophy and hyperintense T2-weighted signal in the visual cortex.[44] To test for mercury exposure, and monitor response to chelation therapy, whole blood is required since organic mercury is mainly located in erythrocytes, whereas urinary excretion only accounts for less than 10% of methylmercury excretion. Urinary mercury concentrations correlate well with exposure to elemental or inorganic mercury, but this exposure, unlike that to methylmercury, is not associated with the development of abnormal movements.

Like chronic alcohol abuse, phenytoin treatment is associated with cortical cerebellar atrophy, usually affecting areas beyond the vermis and especially after repeated episodes of overdosing.[45,46]

DYSTONIA

Dystonia is a term applied to repetitive contraction of antagonistic sets of muscles, resulting in abnormal posturing, twisting, or repetitive jerky movements. The

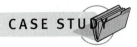

CASE STUDY

A 28-year-old woman presented to the emergency department with tightness and twitching across the facial muscles, upward rolling of the eyes with deviation of the head and gaze to the right, and stiffness of the neck muscles. The symptoms were associated with sweating and tachycardia at a rate of 130 beats/min. Further clinical examination and imaging were unremarkable. All blood tests were normal, including the electrolytes, C reactive protein, and white cell count. Ten days before her presentation, she had had colicky left flank pain with nausea and vomiting and had been prescribed ciprofloxacin for a presumed urinary tract infection. The tentative diagnosis was tetanus until it emerged that the patient had started taking metoclopramide the day before her presentation because of persistent nausea and a confirmation that a tetanus boost vaccination had been given the previous year. The patient's symptoms resolved 6 to 8 hours after onset.

overwhelming etiology of dystonia is iatrogenic, occurring either acutely after a specific exposure (acute dystonic reaction; Table 2) or delayed by months or years (tardive dystonia).

Pharmaceutical Agents

Acute dystonic reactions, exemplified by the case study,[47] are among the most common short-term motor complications of the use of neuroleptic drugs (see the Pharmaceutical Agents section under the

Parkinsonism section), although presumably less prevalent than later sequelae of such exposure, such as drug-induced parkinsonism and tardive dyskinesia. Acute dystonic reactions tend to occur within the first 5 days of exposure to the offending agent (Table 2). Typical deficits are oculogyric crises and dystonia, especially of the craniocervical region, with subtle dysarthria and dysphagia. In general, the face and neck are the most common areas affected, as suggested by "three Os" mnemonic: *oculogyric crisis, oculomandibular dystonia,* and *opisthotonos*.[48] These three elements were illustrated by the study. Blepharospasm, trismus, respiratory stridor, and limb dystonia can be accompanying features (Figure 10-2). The risk of acute dystonic reactions is increased 40-fold among those with a history of cocaine abuse,[49] suggesting that repeated cocaine exposure permanently alters dopamine function in the human brain. Although spontaneous resolution is expected, acute dystonic reactions are highly responsive to the anticholinergic action of benztropine or diphenhydramine, administered parenterally. Among those requiring neuroleptics, the incidence of acute dystonia may be reduced with prophylactic use of anticholinergic drugs.

Tardive dystonia results from chronic exposure to typical and some atypical (including olanzapine and risperidone) antipsychotic neuroleptics and far less commonly to the nonantipsychotic agents responsible for acute dystonia. Tardive dystonia can be focal, segmental, or generalized, and it commonly affects the face and neck followed by the arms and trunk.[50] The typical phenomenology consists of retrocollis, paroxysmal arching backward of the trunk, internal rotation of the arms, and flexion at the wrists (Figure 10-3). Reducing the dose of the offending agent, eliminating it altogether, or switching to quetiapine or clozapine might be helpful for both tardive dystonia and schizophrenia.[51,52]

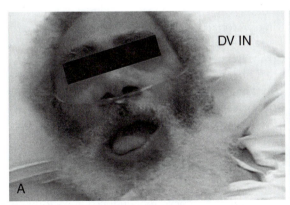
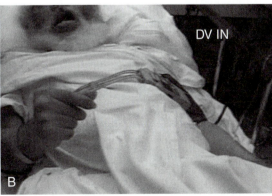

Figure 10-2. Acute dystonic reaction. Oculomandibular dystonia with primary tongue protrusion *(A)* and right-limb dystonia *(B)* as a presentation of acute dystonic reaction following exposure to a typical antipsychotic.

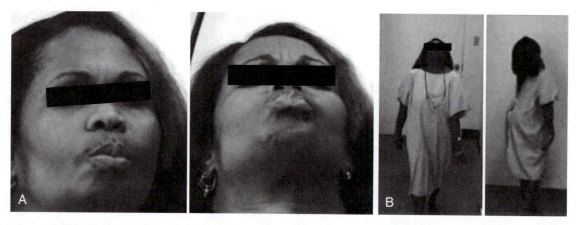

Figure 10-3. Tardive dystonia. Typical phenomenology of tardive dystonia: lower-face predominant involvement with paroxysmal retrocollis *(A)* associated with backward arching of the trunk, internal rotation of the arms, and wrist flexion when walking *(B)*.

MYOCLONUS

Myoclonus, defined as sudden, shocklike jerks, is among the most common movement disorders in encephalopathies. As such, a substantial number of toxic exposures that cause a depression of consciousness from drowsiness to coma may be accompanied by myoclonus. The term *myoclonic encephalopathy* is applied to progressive epileptic syndromes due to genetic or metabolic disorders, but myoclonus can occur due to pharmaceutical or recreational drug abuse.

Pharmaceutical Agents

The case study illustrates bismuth toxicity. The typical bismuth-induced encephalopathy presents with subacute changes in mental status and memory, psychosis, and

CASE STUDY

A 76-year-old woman had a rapidly progressive dementia with multifocal myoclonus, postural instability, and gait ataxia. When assessed at the hospital, she was restrained, disoriented, and spoke in a "word salad" with neologisms. She could not name her husband, recall a recent hospitalization, or name three common objects. Electroencephalography showed bihemispheric slowing. She had taken Pepto-Bismol for many years to control her irritable bowel syndrome. An elevated serum bismuth level established bismuth toxicity as the cause of the dementia. Elimination of Pepto-Bismol and slow reduction of serum bismuth levels was associated with clinical improvement.

depression with a prominent background of myoclonus and ataxia and occasionally electroencephalographic abnormalities exhibiting spike–wave or polyspike–wave complexes, with or without associated seizures. Patients have been misdiagnosed as Alzheimer's disease[53] and Creutzfeldt-Jacob disease.[54,55] Bismuth subsalicylate (Pepto-Bismol), used in the treatment of gastric ulcers, diarrhea, and *Helicobacter pylori* infection, is one of four medicinal bismuth compounds and belong to the heavy metal class of lead, mercury, gold, silver, and arsenic. A blood bismuth concentration during chronic therapy of 50 to 100 µg/mL is of concern, and a level greater than 100 µg/L should prompt cessation of therapy.[56] Hyperdensities in the basal ganglia and cerebral cortex may be seen on a head computerized tomography scan.[57] Although treatment with chelators like dimercapto–succinic acid and dimercapto–propanesulfonic acid has been proposed,[58] their use may aggravate the encephalopathy.[59] A similar myoclonic encephalopathy has been described as part of the so-called dialysis dementia (myoclonus associated with dysarthria, dysphasia, apraxia, personality changes, and occasionally, seizures) resulting from the use of aluminum hydroxide as a phosphate binder in patients undergoing prolonged dialysis, which has become rare.[60] Discontinuation of the bismuth intake or aluminum-containing dialysates should lead to slow but steady recovery.

Other pharmaceutical agents to consider as potential etiologies of myoclonus are drugs used in the treatment of Parkinson's disease and other parkinsonisms. Both levodopa and amantadine can induce reversible myoclonus. Since the motor benefits of levodopa would be expected to outweigh the myoclonic complication, addition of the serotonin antagonist methysergide may avoid the need for removal of levodopa.[61] This strategy rests on the assumption that levodopa-induced myoclonus is due to dysregulation of serotonin activity, with intermittent increases in its activity in the brain.

Finally, rapid escalation or relatively high doses of opioid may induce myoclonus, as is particularly well documented in the setting of acute or cancer-related pain[62,63] and in hemodialysis patients.[64] Proposed strategies to approach these patients include opioid dose reduction, opioid rotation, or use of benzodiazepines[65] or gabapentin[66] when the specific opioid is felt necessary, despite the induction of myoclonus. In addition to opioid-induced myoclonus, opioid-withdrawal myoclonus has been reported after removal of transdermal fentanyl[67] or meperidine in the setting of renal failure.[68] In all instances, the development of myoclonus is attributed to the neurotoxic effects of the accumulating metabolite normeperidine.[63]

Recreational Drugs

Overdose with GHB can cause myoclonus in the context of severe encephalopathy, seizures, respiratory depression, and bradycardia.[69] GHB, a $GABA_B$ receptor agonist, is formed by the dehydrogenation of one of its precursor 1,4-butanediols, a commercially available solvent contained in compact disc and printer cleaners and used to enhance the effects of alcohol at "rave" parties and, most notoriously, as a date-rape drug. When alcohol is ingested with large doses of 1,4-butanediol, a myoclonic encephalopathy with hallucinations and seizures (unlike what occurs with isolated alcohol toxicity) is followed by transient improvement as alcohol is metabolized, followed by a relapse once 1,4-butanediol is dehydrogenated to GHB. Treatment is supportive with benzodiazepines for seizures and atropine for bradycardia, as there is no specific antidote. Due to its short half-life, GHB toxicity usually resolves within 6 hours. It should be noted that, despite being a drug of abuse, GHB has found clinical use in the treatment of narcolepsy[70] and, paradoxically, alcoholism.[71] More intriguingly, Frucht and colleagues have successfully used GHB to treat alcohol-responsive drug-refractory posthypoxic myoclonus.[72]

Cocaine and amphetamine-like drugs, which more commonly induce chorea (described in the next section), may rarely be associated with limb or even ocular myoclonus.[73,74]

CHOREA

Chorea can be characterized as random, purposeless, dancelike movements that can affect any body part. In general, postsynaptic dopaminergic sensitivity is among the most accepted mechanisms unifying the various etiologies of chorea. As such, drugs that stimulate the dopamine system (e.g., methylphenidate and

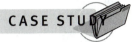

CASE STUDY

A 41-year-old woman with upper extremity pain due to complex regional pain syndrome type I (reflex sympathetic dystrophy) had failed to find relief from several drugs, including tricyclic antidepressants, anticonvulsants, and mexiletine. Significant pain relief was obtained after the introduction of 5 mg of methadone three times daily, with further improvement after a dose increase to 20 mg/day. One month after reaching this dose, the patient developed truncal choreiform movements, whose severity progressively increased to affect her speech and gait. A week after a direct switch to 60 mg/day of sustained-release oxycodone, with adequate pain relief, the chorea abated substantially, and 3 weeks later, it had disappeared.

cocaine) can cause hyperkinetic complications such as chorea or, less commonly, tics or myoclonus; drugs that inhibit this system (such as neuroleptics) are expected to generate a hypokinetic or parkinsonian syndrome.

Pharmaceutical Agents

Methadone can induce choreic movements involving the upper limbs, trunk, and speech, as the case study illustrates.[75] The association between methadone and chorea was first recognized in young men receiving methadone maintenance therapy for heroin addiction.[76] This complication is dose dependent and associated with rapid titration of the dose of methadone.[77] As a differential caveat, birth control pills are a well-established cause of chorea in women and should have been considered if the movements did not resolve with methadone substitution in the case study. Contraceptive-induced generalized chorea or hemichorea may appear acutely or subacutely within the first 5 weeks of exposure, more often among women with a history of Sydenham chorea, rheumatic fever, or cyanotic congenital heart disease.[78] Drug discontinuation reverses the chorea.

Buccolinguomasticatory or orofacial chorea, characterized by repetitive tongue twisting and protrusion and purposeless chewing, is the most common neuroleptic-induced abnormal movement in the elderly, tardive dyskinesias.[79] Movements may persist or worsen over time, despite, or sometimes because of, drug withdrawal. Displacement of older neuroleptics with the use of atypical antipsychotics, such as aripiprazole, clozapine, olanzapine, risperidone, quetiapine, and ziprasidone, may have reduced the incidence of tardive dyskinesias, but a careful epidemiological assessment is lacking.[80] The atypical neuroleptic risperidone has been used to improve tardive dyskinesia when discontinuation of the offending (usually typical) antipsychotic is insufficient.[81,82] Phenytoin can also induce orofacial chorea, among other movements, but concurrent use of other antiepileptics (especially lamotrigine) or preexistent lesions (thalamic infarctions) may be necessary for the chorea to develop.[83,84] Rare cases of choreic dyskinesias have been reported with carbamazepine.[85,86]

Recreational Drugs

Cocaine and amphetamine, through their enhancement of the dopamine transmission in the nigrostriatal and mesocorticolimbic circuit, may cause repetitive and stereotyped movements reminiscent of complex motor tics or stereotypies.[87] In particular, chewing and tooth-grinding were used in identifying abusers of amphetamine[88] and are expected to be observed among those abusing methamphetamine ("speed" or "ice"). Intermittent, slow limb movements, often associated with a sensation of restlessness or akathisia, can follow acute cocaine exposure for 2 to 6 days and are often referred to as "crack dancing" among addicts.[89] Although cocaine and amphetamine are well known to increase dopamine transmission in the nigrostriatal system by inhibiting neurotransmitter reuptake,[90] in turn leading to dose-dependent repetitive and stereotypical movements,[91] neither dopamine agonists nor blockers have proved useful in the treatment of substance abuse. Intriguingly, the amphetamine derivative 3,4-methylenedioxymethamphetamine (MDMA, Ecstasy) may also lead to chewing and tooth-grinding[92] despite its ability to reduce levodopa-induced dyskinesias in MPTP-treated animal models of Parkinson's disease, presumably through serotoninergic mechanisms.[93] Long-term MDMA administration, however, may be neurotoxic to dopamine nerve endings in mice, thus raising concerns about its therapeutic promise[94] (but supporting further investigation of serotoninergic agents in the treatment of levodopa-induced dyskinesia[95]). Finally, phencyclidine (PCP), which competitively inhibits dopamine, norepinephrine, and serotonin reuptake and blocks the N-methyl-d-aspartate receptor, is known to induce stereotypical movements and ataxia in animals, which are improved by neuroleptic agents.[96] Hallucinations are the overwhelming presentation in humans and likely overshadow the presence of abnormal movements in this intoxication.

REFERENCES

1. Ballard PA, Tetrud JW, Langston JW. Permanent human parkinsonism due to 1-methyl-4-phenyl-1,2,3,6-tetrahydropyridine (MPTP): seven cases. *Neurology.* 1985;35:949–956.
2. Greenamyre JT, Betarbet R, Sherer TB. The rotenone model of Parkinson's disease: genes, environment and mitochondria. *Parkinsonism Relat Disord.* 2003;9 (Suppl 2):S59–S64.
3. Spillane L, Roberts JR, Meyer AE. Multiple cranial nerve deficits after ethylene glycol poisoning. *Ann Emerg Med.* 1991;20:208–210.
4. Miodownik C, Witztum E, Lerner V. Lithium-induced tremor treated with vitamin B$_6$: a preliminary case series. *Int J Psychiatry Med.* 2002;32:103–108.
5. Cersosimo MG, Koller WC. The diagnosis of manganese-induced parkinsonism. *Neurotoxicology.* 2006;27:340–346.
6. Dierkes J, Westphal S, Luley C. The effect of fibrates and other lipid-lowering drugs on plasma homocysteine levels. *Expert Opin Drug Saf.* 2004;3:101–111.
7. de Bie RM, Gladstone RM, Strafella AP, Ko JH, Lang AE. Manganese-induced Parkinsonism associated with methcathinone (Ephedrone) abuse. *Arch Neurol.* 2007;64:886–889.
8. Sanotsky Y, Lesyk R, Fedoryshyn L, et al. Manganic encephalopathy due to "ephedrone" abuse. *Mov Disord.* 2007;22:1337–1343.
9. Levin OS. "Ephedron" encephalopathy. *Zh Nevrol Psikhiatr Im S S Korsakova.* 2005;105:12–20.
10. Huang CC, Chu NS, Lu CS, et al. The natural history of neurological manganism over 18 years. *Parkinsonism Relat Disord.* 2007;13:143–145.
11. Josephs KA, Ahlskog JE, Klos KJ, et al. Neurologic manifestations in welders with pallidal MRI T1 hyperintensity. *Neurology.* 2005;64:2033–2039.
12. Cook DG, Fahn S, Brait KA. Chronic manganese intoxication. *Arch Neurol.* 1974;30:59–64.
13. Grimes JD. Parkinsonism and tardive dyskinesia associated with long-term metoclopramide therapy. *N Engl J Med.* 1981;305:1417.
14. Wada Y, Yamaguchi N. The rabbit syndrome and antiparkinsonian medication in schizophrenic patients. *Neuropsychobiology.* 1992;25:149–152.
15. Sethi KD, Patel B, Meador KJ. Metoclopramide-induced parkinsonism. *South Med J.* 1989;82:1581–1582.
16. Tarsy D, Indorf G. Tardive tremor due to metoclopramide. *Mov Disord.* 2002;17:620–621.
17. Wilde MI, Markham A. Ondansetron: a review of its pharmacology and preliminary clinical findings in novel applications. *Drugs.* 1996;52:773–794.
18. Choi IS. Parkinsonism after carbon monoxide poisoning. *Eur Neurol.* 2002;48:30–33.
19. Sohn YH, Jeong Y, Kim HS, Im JH, Kim JS. The brain lesion responsible for parkinsonism after carbon monoxide poisoning. *Arch Neurol.* 2000;57:1214–1218.
20. Hsiao CL, Kuo HC, Huang CC. Delayed encephalopathy after carbon monoxide intoxication: long-term prognosis and correlation of clinical manifestations and neuroimages. *Acta Neurol Taiwan.* 2004;13:64–70.
21. Choi IS, Cheon HY. Delayed movement disorders after carbon monoxide poisoning. *Eur Neurol.* 1999;42:141–144.
22. Hu MC, Shiah IS, Yeh CB, Chen HK, Chen CK. Ziprasidone in the treatment of delayed carbon monoxide encephalopathy. *Prog Neuropsychopharmacol Biol Psychiatry.* 2006;30:755–757.
23. Thom SR, Fisher D, Zhang J, et al. Neuronal nitric oxide synthase and N-methyl-d-aspartate neurons in experimental carbon monoxide poisoning. *Toxicol Appl Pharmacol.* 2004;194:280–295.

24. Penney DG, Chen K. NMDA receptor–blocker ketamine protects during acute carbon monoxide poisoning, while calcium channel–blocker verapamil does not. *J Appl Toxicol.* 1996;16:297–304.

25. Morgan JC, Sethi KD. Drug-induced tremors. *Lancet Neurol.* 2005;4:866–876.

26. Karas BJ, Wilder BJ, Hammond EJ, Bauman AW. Valproate tremors. *Neurology.* 1982;32:428–432.

27. Lancman ME, Asconape JJ, Walker F. Acetazolamide appears effective in the management of valproate-induced tremor. *Mov Disord.* 1994;9:369.

28. Gelenberg AJ, Jefferson JW. Lithium tremor. *J Clin Psychiatry.* 1995;56:283–287.

29. Jefferson JW. Lithium tremor and caffeine intake: two cases of drinking less and shaking more. *J Clin Psychiatry.* 1988;49:72–73.

30. Koller W, Orebaugh C, Lawson L, Potempa K. Pindolol-induced tremor. *Clin Neuropharmacol.* 1987;10:449–452.

31. Teravainen H, Larsen A, Fogelholm R. Comparison between the effects of pindolol and propranolol on essential tremor. *Neurology.* 1977;27:439–442.

32. Neiman J, Lang AE, Fornazzari L, Carlen PL. Movement disorders in alcoholism: a review. *Neurology.* 1990;40:741–746.

33. Erstad BL, Cotugno CL. Management of alcohol withdrawal. *Am J Health Syst Pharm.* 1995;52:697–709.

34. Kinsella LJ, Green R. "Anesthesia paresthetica": nitrous oxide induced cobalamin deficiency. *Neurology.* 1995;45:1608–1610.

35. McMorrow AM, Adams RJ, Rubenstein MN. Combined system disease after nitrous oxide anesthesia: a case report. *Neurology.* 1995;45:1224–1225.

36. Layzer RB, Fishman RA, Schafer JA. Neuropathy following abuse of nitrous oxide. *Neurology.* 1978;28:504–506.

37. Bartlett E, Mikulis DJ. Chasing "chasing the dragon" with MRI: leukoencephalopathy in drug abuse. *Br J Radiol.* 2005;78:997–1004.

38. Kriegstein AR, Shungu DC, Millar WS, et al. Leukoencephalopathy and raised brain lactate from heroin vapor inhalation ("chasing the dragon"). *Neurology.* 1999;53:1765–1773.

39. Kumar N, Gross JB Jr, Ahlskog JE. Copper deficiency myelopathy produces a clinical picture like subacute combined degeneration. *Neurology.* 2004;63:33–39.

40. Yaldizli O, Johansson U, Gizewski ER, Maschke M. Copper deficiency myelopathy induced by repetitive parenteral zinc supplementation during chronic hemodialysis. *J Neurol.* 2006;253:1507–1509.

41. Kumar N, Crum B, Petersen RC, Vernino SA, Ahlskog JE. Copper deficiency myelopathy. *Arch Neurol.* 2004;61:762–766.

42. Harada M. Minamata disease: methylmercury poisoning in Japan caused by environmental pollution. *Crit Rev Toxicol.* 1995;25:1–24.

43. Uchino M, Okajima T, Eto K, et al. Neurologic features of chronic Minamata disease (organic mercury poisoning) certified at autopsy. *Intern Med.* 1995;34:744–747.

44. Korogi Y, Takahashi M, Okajima T, Eto K. MR findings of Minamata disease: organic mercury poisoning. *J Magn Reson Imaging.* 1998;8:308–316.

45. Luef G, Chemelli A, Birbamer G, Aichner F, Bauer G. Phenytoin overdosage and cerebellar atrophy in epileptic patients: clinical and MRI findings. *Eur Neurol.* 1994;34 (Suppl 1):79–81.

46. Kuruvilla T, Bharucha NE. Cerebellar atrophy after acute phenytoin intoxication. *Epilepsia.* 1997;38:500–502.

47. Dingli K, Morgan R, Leen C. Acute dystonic reaction caused by metoclopramide, versus tetanus. *BMJ.* 2007;334:899–900.

48. Pearce JMS, Clough CC. Drug-induced movement disorders. In: Shah NS, Donald AG, eds. *Movement Disorders.* New York: Plenum; 1986:343–364.

49. Hegarty AM, Lipton RB, Merriam AE, Freeman K. Cocaine as a risk factor for acute dystonic reactions. *Neurology.* 1991;41:1670–1672.

50. Fernandez HH, Friedman JH. Classification and treatment of tardive syndromes. *Neurologist.* 2003;9:16–27.

51. Charfi F, Cohen D, Houeto JL, Soubrie C, Mazet P. Tardive dystonia induced by atypical neuroleptics: a case report with olanzapine. *J Child Adolesc Psychopharmacol.* 2004;14:149–152.

52. Simpson GM. The treatment of tardive dyskinesia and tardive dystonia. *J Clin Psychiatry.* 2000;61 (Suppl 4):39–44.

53. Summers WK. Bismuth toxicity masquerading as Alzheimer's dementia. *J Alzheimers Dis.* 1998;1:57–59.

54. Von Bose MJ, Zaudig M. Encephalopathy resembling Creutzfeldt-Jakob disease following oral, prescribed doses of bismuth nitrate. *Br J Psychiatry.* 1991;158:278–280.

55. Gordon MF, Abrams RI, Rubin DB, Barr WB, Correa DD. Bismuth subsalicylate toxicity as a cause of prolonged encephalopathy with myoclonus. *Mov Disord.* 1995;10:220–222.

56. Serfontein WJ, Mekel R. Bismuth toxicity in man: II. Review of bismuth blood and urine levels in patients after administration of therapeutic bismuth formulations in relation to the problem of bismuth toxicity in man. *Res Commun Chem Pathol Pharmacol.* 1979;26:391–411.

57. Gardeur D, Buge A, Rancurel G, Dechy H, Metzger J. Bismuth encephalopathy and cerebral computed tomography *J Comput Assist Tomogr.* 1978;2:436–438.

58. Stevens PE, Moore DF, House IM, Volans GN, Rainford DJ. Significant elimination of bismuth by haemodialysis with a new heavy-metal chelating agent. *Nephrol Dial Transplant.* 1995;10:696–698.

59. Teepker M, Hamer HM, Knake S, et al. Myoclonic encephalopathy caused by chronic bismuth abuse. *Epileptic Disord.* 2002;4:229–233.

60. Alfrey AC, Mishell JM, Burks J, et al. Syndrome of dyspraxia and multifocal seizures associated with chronic hemodialysis. *Trans Am Soc Artif Intern Organs.* 1972;18:257.

61. Klawans HL, Goetz C, Bergen D. Levodopa-induced myoclonus. *Arch Neurol.* 1975;32:330–334.

62. Mercadante S. Pathophysiology and treatment of opioid-related myoclonus in cancer patients. *Pain.* 1998;74:5–9.

63. Kaiko RF, Foley KM, Grabinski PY, et al. Central nervous system excitatory effects of meperidine in cancer patients. *Ann Neurol.* 1983;13:180–185.

64. Hochman MS. Meperidine-associated myoclonus and seizures in long-term hemodialysis patients. *Ann Neurol.* 1983;14:593.

65. Eisele JH Jr, Grigsby EJ, Dea G. Clonazepam treatment of myoclonic contractions associated with high-dose opioids: case report. *Pain.* 1992;49:231–232.

66. Mercadante S, Villari P, Fulfaro F. Gabapentin for opioid-related myoclonus in cancer patients. *Support Care Cancer.* 2001;9:205–206.

67. Han PK, Arnold R, Bond G, Janson D, Abu-Elmagd K. Myoclonus secondary to withdrawal from transdermal fentanyl: case report and literature review. *J Pain Symptom Manage.* 2002;23:66–72.

68. Reutens DC, Stewart-Wynne EG. Norpethidine-induced myoclonus in a patient with renal failure. *J Neurol Neurosurg Psychiatry.* 1989;52:1450–1451.

69. Snead OC, III, Gibson KM. γ-Hydroxybutyric acid. *N Engl J Med.* 2005;352:2721–2732.

70. Fuller DE, Hornfeldt CS. From club drug to orphan drug: sodium oxybate (Xyrem) for the treatment of cataplexy. *Pharmacotherapy.* 2003;23:1205–1209.

71. Caputo F, Addolorato G, Lorenzini F, et al. γ-Hydroxybutyric acid versus naltrexone in maintaining alcohol abstinence: an open randomized comparative study. *Drug Alcohol Depend.* 2003;70:85–91.

72. Frucht SJ, Bordelon Y, Houghton WH. Marked amelioration of alcohol-responsive posthypoxic myoclonus by γ-hydroxybutyric acid (Xyrem). *Mov Disord*. 2005;20:745–751.

73. Hinkelbein J, Gabel A, Volz M, Ellinger K. Suicide attempt with high-dose Ecstasy. *Anaesthesist*. 2003;52:51–54.

74. Scharf D. Opsoclonus–myoclonus following the intranasal usage of cocaine. *J Neurol Neurosurg Psychiatry*. 1989;52:1447–1448.

75. Clark JD, Elliott J. A case of a methadone-induced movement disorder. *Clin J Pain*. 2001;17:375–377.

76. Wasserman S, Yahr MD. Choreic movements induced by the use of methadone. *Arch Neurol*. 1980;37:727–728.

77. Bonnet U, Banger M, Wolstein J, Gastpar M. Choreoathetoid movements associated with rapid adjustment to methadone. *Pharmacopsychiatry*. 1998;31:143–145.

78. Nausieda PA, Koller WC, Weiner WJ, Klawans HL. Chorea induced by oral contraceptives. *Neurology*. 1979;29:1605–1609.

79. Margolese HC, Chouinard G, Kolivakis TT, et al. Tardive dyskinesia in the era of typical and atypical antipsychotics: II. Incidence and management strategies in patients with schizophrenia. *Can J Psychiatry*. 2005;50:703–714.

80. Tarsy D, Baldessarini RJ. Epidemiology of tardive dyskinesia: is risk declining with modern antipsychotics? *Mov Disord*. 2006;21:589–598.

81. Chouinard G. Effects of risperidone in tardive dyskinesia: an analysis of the Canadian multicenter risperidone study. *J Clin Psychopharmacol*. 1995;15:36S–44S.

82. Bai YM, Yu SC, Lin CC. Risperidone for severe tardive dyskinesia: a 12-week randomized, double-blind, placebo-controlled study. *J Clin Psychiatry*. 2003;64:1342–1348.

83. Harrison MB, Lyons GR, Landow ER. Phenytoin and dyskinesias: a report of two cases and review of the literature. *Mov Disord*. 1993;8:19–27.

84. Zaatreh M, Tennison M, D'Cruz O, Beach RL. Anticonvulsants-induced chorea: a role for pharmacodynamic drug interaction? *Seizure*. 2001;10:596–599.

85. Bimpong-Buta K, Froescher W. Carbamazepine-induced choreo-athetoid dyskinesias. *J Neurol Neurosurg Psychiatry*. 1982;45:560.

86. Schwartzman MJ, Leppik IE. Carbamazepine-induced dyskinesia and ophthalmoplegia. *Cleve Clin J Med*. 1990;57:367–372.

87. Attig E, Amyot R, Botez T. Cocaine-induced chronic tics. *J Neurol Neurosurg Psychiatry*. 1994;57:1143–1144.

88. Ashcroft GW, Eccleston D, Waddell JL. Recognition of amphetamine addicts. *BMJ*. 2008;1:57.

89. Kamath S, Bajaj N. Crack dancing in the United Kingdom: apropos a video case presentation. *Mov Disord*. 2007;22:1190–1191.

90. Kuhar MJ, Ritz MC, Boja JW. The dopamine hypothesis of the reinforcing properties of cocaine. *Trends Neurosci*. 1991;14:299–302.

91. Canales JJ, Graybiel AM. A measure of striatal function predicts motor stereotypy. *Nat Neurosci*. 2000;3:377–383.

92. McGrath C, Chan B. Oral health sensations associated with illicit drug abuse. *Br Dent J*. 2005;198:159–162.

93. Iravani MM, Jackson MJ, Kuoppamaki M, Smith LA, Jenner P. 3,4-methylenedioxymethamphetamine (Ecstasy) inhibits dyskinesia expression and normalizes motor activity in 1-methyl-4-phenyl-1,2,3,6-tetrahydropyridine-treated primates. *J Neurosci*. 2003;23:9107–9115.

94. Green AR, Mechan AO, Elliott JM, O'Shea E, Colado MI. The pharmacology and clinical pharmacology of 3,4-methylenedioxymethamphetamine (MDMA, "Ecstasy"). *Pharmacol Rev*. 2003;55:463–508.

95. Goetz CG, Damier P, Hicking C, et al. Sarizotan as a treatment for dyskinesias in Parkinson's disease: a double-blind placebo-controlled trial. *Mov Disord*. 2007;22:179–186.

96. Sams-Dodd F. Effect of novel antipsychotic drugs on phencyclidine-induced stereotyped behaviour and social isolation in the rat social interaction test. *Behav Pharmacol*. 1997;8:196–215.

CHAPTER 11

Drug- and Toxin-Associated Seizures

Brandon Wills, Brett J. Theeler, and John P. Ney

INTRODUCTION

Seizures are the outward manifestation of abnormal electrical activity in the brain. Direct intoxication from known poisons or psychotropic drugs, withdrawal from medications or alcohol, or idiosyncratic reactions to pharmaceuticals may affect changes in brain chemistry that promote aberrant electrocerebral responses and, ultimately, seizures. Numerous poisons and medicines are associated with seizures, and awareness of these relationships is essential for the treating clinician. Drug- and toxin-associated seizures (DTSs) differ in etiology but may demonstrate distinct clinical features, which allow identification and treatment.

EPIDEMIOLOGY

The true incidence of DTSs from all sources is unknown, and epidemiological data are lacking. Estimates from poison control centers likely underrepresent true prevalence and may have a bias toward drug intoxication rather than withdrawal or adverse effects of inpatient treatment. Data from the California Poison Control System (CPCS) provide the most detailed analysis of DTS incidence and offending intoxicants. In 2003, 386 DTS cases from the CPCS were identified.[1] Of these, most were caused by prescription medications, particularly bupropion (23%), diphenhydramine (8.3%), and tricyclic antidepressants (TCAs; 7.7%). Only 15% were related to drugs of abuse. Most cases (68.6%) involved a single seizure, and less than 4% had associated status epilepticus. Of the 386 cases, 7 cases resulted in death.

Alcohol-withdrawal seizures have been reported to represent up to 49% of all emergency department–treated seizures and up to 25% of reported cases of status epilepticus.[2] Up to 9% of alcoholics have seizures,[3] but it is unclear whether these are alcohol-withdrawal seizures or they represent a higher incidence of epilepsy among alcoholics. The mortality rate for alcoholics with seizures is four times greater than that of the general population, but this could be due to multifactorial issues related to alcoholism rather than due to seizures alone.[4]

Attempts at characterizing the rate of iatrogenic DTSs in the hospital have been few. Wijdicks and Sharbrough[5] studied new onset seizures in the intensive care unit over 10 years and identified 18 cases of DTSs from iatrogenic drug withdrawal (opiates and midazolam) and 8 from iatrogenic drug toxicity. Another review of 3155 inpatient charts found only 18 cases of DTSs due to pharmaceuticals being taken as prescribed.[6]

SEMIOLOGY OF DRUG- AND TOXIN-ASSOCIATED SEIZURES

The study of epilepsy, genetic or acquired syndromes of unprovoked seizures, has created multiple classification systems for seizure types.[7] Most DTSs are generalized seizures,[8] described as tonic–clonic convulsions, referring to a state of generalized motor activation of both agonist and antagonist musculature, with initial rigid extension of arms and legs, and subsequent synchronous flexion–extension of arms, mimicking alternating decorticate and decerebrate posturing. Bowel and bladder voiding often takes place in the initial tonic phase of DTSs, and consciousness is lost. Eyelids are usually open.

A single seizure may go on for seconds or minutes and may proceed to status epilepticus, defined as continuous seizure activity for greater than a specified period (5 to 30 minutes), or provide for multiple seizures without intervening return to consciousness.[9] A postconvulsive quiescence in which the patient is confused or cannot be aroused is typical and referred to as the *postictal state*. In the DTS patient, this may be complicated by the effects of drugs or toxins on alertness. Likewise, the postictal state can be confused with ongoing electrical, subclinical status epileptics in which the brain continues to display electrical properties of seizure activity despite the abatement of convulsions. Although epileptics may have auras before generalized convulsions, auras are manifestations of partial onset seizures with subsequent secondary generalization and are unlikely in DTSs. Other features of partial seizures, such as lateralized gaze or head deviation, are uncommon in DTSs.

PATHOPHYSIOLOGY

Basic Principles

The active brain is a balance of excitatory and inhibitory influences on electrical activity. Excitatory stimuli are necessary for the transmission of neural impulses, from simple motor commands, to memory retrieval, to complex thought processes. Inhibition of electrical impulses prevents the spread of electrical activity beyond prescribed pathways for neural impulses. Action potentials are electrical events derived from the opening of sodium, calcium, chloride, and potassium ion channels in cell membranes, changing the electrical potential of the membrane relative to a threshold potential and facilitating impulse transmission along the length of a neuronal axon. At the termination of the axon, electrical activity continues along gap junctions or is propagated chemically across a synapse through the release of neurotransmitters. These latter are expelled from the axon terminal

and bind to postsynaptic receptors, inducing ion channel opening and activating G proteins and intracellular second messengers. The net effect of individual neurotransmitters on the postsynaptic membrane is excitatory or inhibitory, increasing or reducing the likelihood of action potential propagation.

In cortical neurons implicated in seizure activity, the most prominent neurotransmitters are glutamate and γ-aminobutyric acid (GABA). Glutamate mediates excitatory synapses through one of several postsynaptic receptors, which modulate calcium- or sodium-induced membrane depolarization. GABAergic synapses are inhibitory and thus responsible for opening chloride ion channels, which hyperpolarize the postsynaptic membrane, preventing the formation of action potentials.

Seizure activity is the result of excessive excitatory stimulation, failure of inhibition of aberrant electrical activity, or both. Far from being a manifestation of purely chaotic neuronal activity, seizures are notable on a macrocellular level for massive synchronous neuronal firing because of the activation of unchecked feedback loops. Inadequate inhibitory influences from $GABA_A$ receptor–mediated pathways have been implicated as the primary mechanism of seizure generation.[10] Without GABA inhibition, prolonged glutamate release results in calcium-related neurotoxicity and neuronal death.[11] A host of other neurochemicals are associated with seizure production and maintenance, and several animal models have been developed to describe the various mediators of seizure generation (Table 1).

Seizure Susceptibility

The *seizure threshold* is a concept that seeks to reconcile the balance of inhibitory and excitatory neuronal stimuli with individual predisposition to seizures. Each human has a tendency toward seizure activity based on genetics; the accumulation of acquired neuronal injuries, including hypoxia, trauma, and prior seizures; and the fluctuations of brain electrolytes and neural transmitters. Even the most genetically resistant brain can be tipped toward seizure activity by acute neuronal injury or severe metabolic or toxic disturbance. Conversely, someone with a family history of seizures, who may have had febrile seizures as a child or experienced a distant history of trauma or hypoxic brain injury, would likely have a greater seizure susceptibility than someone without those historical factors.

In animal models of epilepsy, "kindling" is invoked as an explanation of epileptogenesis. The "kindled" animal has experimentally applied electrical discharges (or local chemical infusion) to brain structures, which are not sufficient to cause convulsions.[12] After a latent period, the animal develops seizures in response to smaller amplitude electrical stimulations (or smaller chemical infusion)

Table 1: Some Prominent Neurochemicals Involved in Seizure Propagation and Prevention

Neurochemical	Mechanism	Net Effect (Receptor)	Experimental Models	Involved in Seizurogenic Toxins
GABA	↑Cl$^-$ influx	Inhibitory (GABA$_A$)	Bicuculline Pentylenetetrazole Picrotoxin	GHB withdrawal, benzodiazepine withdrawal, baclofen withdrawal, ethanol withdrawal
Glutamate	↑Na$^+$ influx ↑Ca^{++} influx	Excitatory (NMDA, AMPA)	NMDA AMPA Kainate	Ketamine (withdrawal), INH
Acetylcholine	↑Na$^+$ influx	Excitatory	Lithium–pilocarpine	Organophosphates, nerve agents
Adenosine	↑GABA ↓Glutamate	Inhibitory (A$_1$)	Aminophylline	Theophylline
Serotonin (5-HT)	↑GABA ↓Glutamate	Inhibitory (5-HT$_{1A}$)	5-HT$_{1A}$, 5-HT$_{2C}$ knockout mice	Ecstasy (MDMA), SSRI
Histamine	↑GABA ↓Glutamate ↓K$^+$ efflux	Inhibitory (H$_1$)	L-Histidine, metoprine	Antihistamine intoxication
Norepinephrine (NE)	↑GABA ↓Glutamate	Inhibitory	NE knockout mice	Amphetamines, TCAs, cocaine, ethanol withdrawal

5-HT, 5-hydroxytryptamine; AMPA, α-amino-3-hydroxy-5-methylisooxazole-propionate; GABA, γ-aminobutyric acid; GHB, γ-hydroxybutyric acid; INH, isoniazid; MDMA, 3,4-methylenedioxymethamphetamine; NMDA, N-methyl-d-aspartate; SSRI, serotonin-specific reuptake inhibitor; TCA, tricyclic antidepressant.

and eventually seizes spontaneously. The kindling process does not cause histopathological change to the brain regions stimulated, but subsequent seizure activity does.[13] Alcohol-withdrawal seizures and the development of a second focus in localization-related epilepsies have both been invoked as human correlates of kindling, but no direct evidence of kindling has been demonstrated in human clinical disease.[14]

Whether or not kindling occurs in humans, the kindling model highlights that the sum of exogenous incremental (even mild or subclinical) damage to neurons, acutely or remotely, increases seizure susceptibility. Status epilepticus de novo causes neuronal damage mimicking the pathology of temporal lobe epilepsy[15] and increases the likelihood of development of epilepsy by more than threefold relative to the risk from a single nonprolonged seizure.[16] Neonatal hypoxia, childhood hyperthermia, and traumatic brain injury are associated with alterations in glutamate and GABA receptor subtype function and expression with concomitant increases in seizure likelihood.[17] The latent period for spontaneous seizure development after these injuries may be years or even decades. For those who have a predisposition to seizures due to genetics or prior neuronal injury, the seizure threshold from toxic or metabolic insult is postulated to be lower.[18]

In addition to long-term effects from temporally distant neuronal damage, individual seizure susceptibility varies based on transient factors, particularly sleep deprivation, electrolyte disturbances, and intercurrent infections. Sleep deprivation has been shown to reduce the amount of current necessary to induce a generalized seizure in electroconvulsive therapy (ECT),[19] increase the likelihood of interictal epileptiform discharges on routine scalp-recorded electroencephalograms (EEGs),[20] and increase cortical excitability as measured by experimental transcranial magnetic stimulation.[21] High or low serum calcium and sodium, as well as hypomagnesemia, relative to physiological normal values can induce seizures, generally during rapid electrolyte shifts rather than chronic ion imbalance.[22] Both hyperglycemia[23] and hypoglycemia[24] are associated with seizures. Viral infections have been linked to increased seizure risk through direct central nervous system (CNS) involvement and hyperpyrexia leading to febrile seizures.[25] Nonfebrile seizures were the most common neurological complication of childhood influenza infection in one large study,[26] and respiratory and urinary tract infections have been found to worsen seizure frequency among epileptic children.[27]

Neurochemistry of Seizures

Given that the neuronal substrate for seizure propagation is variable based on the preceding factors, differing amounts of neurotoxins are capable of tipping the balance of excitation and inhibition to induce seizure activity. Still, the net effect is the same. In particular, inhibitors of GABAergic transmission are potent seizure generators, as are molecules that contribute to glutamate excitation. Neuroactive molecules that antagonize these mechanisms are effective anticonvulsants.

Adenosine has been demonstrated to inhibit glutamate release, accounting for a portion of its endogenous anticonvulsant effect.[28] Brain serotonin (5-hydroxytryptophan) at its most common receptors affects hyperpolarization (inhibition) of glutamatergic neurons and depolarization of GABAergic neurons, leading to net reduction in excitability in most neuronal networks.[29] Histamine also has strong anticonvulsant properties at the H_1 receptor, likely through similar mechanisms to serotonin.[30] The effects of norepinephrine and dopamine on brain neurons vary based on the receptor subtype but are largely inhibitory as well, as demonstrated by increased seizure susceptibility in catecholamine knockout mice.[31] Overdoses of biogenic amine agonists or reuptake inhibitors often induce seizures and may be a reflection of differential effects of acute and chronic treatment on receptor expression.[32]

Independent of glutamate or GABA, molecules that block the opening of voltage-gated calcium and sodium currents are generally anticonvulsant and inhibitory to the spread of action potentials.[33] However, many sodium channel blockers, including antiepileptic medications, can be proconvulsant at higher doses and in particular seizure types through mechanisms that have yet to be elucidated.[34]

Neuroanatomy of Generalized Seizures

Generalized seizures have long been thought to involve diffuse activation of the cerebral cortex without preference for anatomical region. However, recent neuroimaging studies in two models of epilepsy suggest that generalized seizure activity selectively activates some areas of the cortex, as well as areas of the subcortex, while sparing others during the ictal event. By tracking elevations in cerebral blood flow (CBF) markers via single-photon emission computed tomography (SPECT) and oxygenation levels in functional magnetic resonance imaging, the neuroanatomical networks involved in generalized seizure activity are being elucidated.

The use of ECT for the treatment of refractory depression has provided a human model for neuronal activation in generalized seizure activity. Bifrontal or bitemporal ECT induces generalized seizure activity in a controlled setting, allowing for SPECT imaging. Increases in CBF indicate increased metabolism through aberrant activation of neurons.[35] Tracking CBF with xenon or technetium markers during a bitemporal ECT-induced generalized seizure reveals focal hyperperfusion of frontal and temporal lobes, as well as distal parietal regions, with no changes to CBF in areas of intervening cortex. Subcortical regions, including the medial thalamus, and brainstem tegmentum also have increased CBF during ECT, suggesting that subcortical networks are involved in seizure propagation to distant cortex.[36]

Experimental models of generalized tonic–clonic seizures with rats using the GABA antagonist pentylenetetrazole (PTZ) also reveal neuroanatomical areas of focal activation. Using functional magnetic resonance imaging to image blood oxygen level–dependent signal intensity is an indicator of hypermetabolism and thus neuronal firing. The anterior thalamus, dentate gyrus of the hippocampus, and posterior midline retrosplenial cortex all show at least a twofold greater response to PTZ relative to other areas of the cerebrum in times just preceding and during generalized seizure activity.[37] These experiments again suggest that "generalized" seizures, likely including DTSs, are mediated by discrete cortical and subcortical regions.

Electrophysiology of Drug- and Toxin-associated Seizures

The electrical activity of the brain can be plotted using a scalp-recorded EEG. A scalp EEG is a map of potentials from leads on various regions of the scalp, which conform to underlying cortical electrical potentials. The potentials recorded at a given lead are compared to those of adjacent leads or to a reference potential (often the average of all recorded scalp potentials). The EEG provides temporal resolution because the changes in potential difference are graphed over time. Charting the resulting waveforms provides a basis for the clinical interpretation of the EEG. Rhythmic EEG activity is identified by its frequency and amplitude. Frequency measures fall into several ranges: the δ-range is less than 1 to 3 Hz, the ϑ-range is 4 to 7 Hz, the α-range is 8 to 13 Hz, and the β-range is 14 to 28 Hz.

The resting, wakeful EEG is highly organized with specific features.[38] There is typically a gradient of increasing amplitude and decreasing frequency from anterior to posterior leads. Frontal channels have lower-amplitude, β-frequency activity, and occipital channels are characterized by a higher-amplitude, resting α-frequency rhythm that attenuates with eye opening. Side-to-side differences are usually minor, and rhythms are generally synchronous in frequency and symmetrical in amplitude.

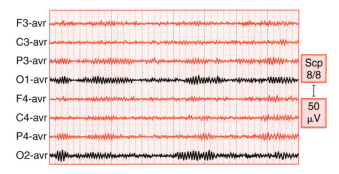

Figure 11-1. Electroencephalogram of normal, resting, wakeful, posterior-predominant α-rhythm.

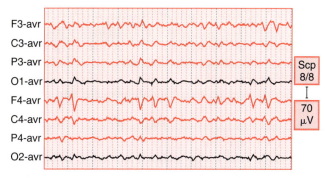

Figure 11-3. Electroencephalogram depicting diffuse δ-range slowing with sharply contoured bifrontal activity in an encephalopathic patient.

Drugs and toxins can alter the appearance of the EEG, even in the absence of seizures. (See also Chapter 17.) The effect of most neurotoxins is nonspecific, with posterior background or diffuse slowing and changes in amplitude. Certain toxins have characteristic effects on the EEG. For example, benzodiazepines and barbiturates increase β-frequency amplitude and distribution, often obscuring other waveforms.[39] At higher doses, these medications may result in diffuse slowing and, in the case of barbiturates, alternating bursts of high-amplitude activity followed by background suppression. Cocaine and amphetamines also increase β-activity at lower levels of intoxication, followed by diffuse slowing at higher blood concentrations.[40] Phencyclidine induces a pattern of unreactive ϑ-slowing with periodic bursts of δ-activity.[41]

The EEG recorded during most DTSs shows features of generalized seizures. During the seizure, typically diffuse, anterior-predominant, synchronous and symmetrical short-duration, and sharply contoured spikes and longer-duration slow waves are complexed and repeating in rhythmic fashion at 2 to 5 Hz, continuously, over the course of seconds or minutes.[42] Following this rhythmic activity, there may be amplitude suppression of background activity or slowing of the background frequencies, correlating with the postictal confusional state. The EEG may show epileptiform activity interictally (between seizures) in the absence of seizure activity,

including spikes or polyspikes, with some drug intoxications, particularly lithium and phenothiazines, or withdrawal states from alcohol,[43] benzodiazepines,[44] or barbiturates.[45] Figures 11-1 through 11-4 provide representative examples of various EEG recordings.

DISCUSSION OF ETIOLOGICAL AGENTS

Evaluation of the undifferentiated seizure patient is challenging, especially if there is clinical or historical suspicion of drug exposure or overdose. Many patients presenting with seizures do not have a clear etiology. History of a particular exposure is undoubtedly the most valuable information used to identify causal agents. Unfortunately, medical history and supplemental historians may not be present initially.

Several conditions can mimic or be mistaken for seizures. Psychogenic nonepileptic seizures and syncope can be mistaken for epileptic seizures.[46–48] Other conditions to consider in an acute setting include hypoglycemia, panic attacks, acute movement disorders,

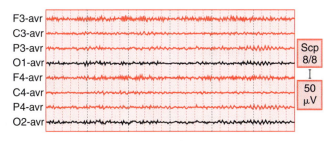

Figure 11-2. Electroencephalogram showing prominent anterior and diffuse β-activity following lorazepam administration.

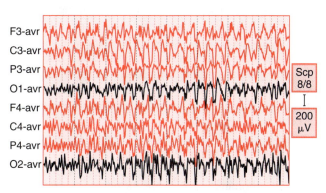

Figure 11-4. Electroencephalogram showing brainwaves during a generalized convulsive seizure, with high-amplitude, rhythmic, sharply contoured spikes and δ-activity and some overlying muscle artifact not fully filtered from the recording.

parasomnias, nonepileptic myoclonus, migraines, transient global amnesia, and rarely, transient ischemic attacks.[49-51] In children, the differential diagnosis is broader and includes other benign entities and movement disorders, such as nonepileptic staring spells, tics, shuddering attacks, breath-holding spells, and gastroesophageal reflux.[52-57]

Seizures can be provoked by many causes, including head injury, infection, medical illness, and toxic exposures. Additional history is often needed to help determine the underlying cause. Careful observation and description of the ictus may help determine a focal versus a generalized seizure onset. Focal features of the aura or of the seizure semiology prompt the need for urgent CNS imaging by computerized axial tomography or magnetic resonance imaging. Most seizures last a few seconds to a couple of minutes and abate without treatment with antiepileptics.[58] Seizures require treatment with anticonvulsants if protracted or repetitive.

Although some medications can produce seizures in therapeutic dosing, this section focuses on agents that often cause seizures in supratherapeutic dosing or overdose. Table 2 represents a robust yet far from complete list of xenobiotics associated with seizures. Table 3 is a shorter teaching aid that captures some classically described agents. Attempting to apply these large lists to the undifferentiated patient is of little utility given the lack of real-time confirmatory testing available. What may be of greater use to the clinician when historical information is lacking is to look for a constellation of symptoms and examination findings that can narrow the differential diagnosis and allow empirical therapy, if indicated. Furthermore, since many toxic seizures are treated similarly, the clinician should consider exposures that require specific and potentially lifesaving interventions. Therefore, etiological agents are discussed using a clinical presentation model. Toxidromes represent a constellation of vital signs and physical examination findings that can be used to classify types of intoxications. Similar to the use of toxidromes, identification of historical or clinical features may help narrow the differential diagnosis and allow empirical therapies. The following clinical presentation categories are not absolute or all-encompassing, especially in polypharmacy exposures. Consideration of toxic seizures should not obviate consideration of structural, infectious, metabolic, or other etiologies.

Sympathomimetic Presentation

The sympathomimetic toxidrome includes tachycardia, hypertension, mydriasis, diaphoresis, and psychomotor agitation. This presentation can be shared by many agents from different classes. Toxicity from stimulants such as cocaine, methamphetamine, and the various designer amphetamines

Table 2: Xenobiotics Associated with Seizures
ANALGESICS
Meperidine
Propoxyphene
Tramadol
Salicylates
ANTICONVULSANTS
Carbamazepine
Lamotrigine
Phenytoin
Tiagabine
Topiramate
CELLULAR ASPHYXIANTS
Azides
Carbon monoxide
Cyanide
Hydrogen sulfide
DRUGS OF ABUSE
Amphetamines
Cocaine
Phencyclidine
PLANTS, HERBS, OR NATURAL PRODUCTS
Ephedra
Gyromitra esculenta mushroom
Nicotine
Water hemlock
PSYCHIATRIC MEDICATIONS
Bupropion
Lithium
Olanzapine

Table 2: Xenobiotics Associated with Seizures—cont'd
Serotonin-specific reuptake inhibitors
Tricyclic antidepressants
Venlafaxine
WITHDRAWAL
Baclofen
Ethanol
Sedative—hypnotic
MISCELLANEOUS
Camphor
Diphenhydramine
Iron
Isoniazid
Lindane
Lidocaine and local anesthetics
Methylxanthines (theophylline, caffeine)
Organophosphates or carbamates
Quinine

Adapted with permission from Wills B, Erickson T. Drug- and toxin-associated seizures. *Med Clin N Am.* 2005;89(6):1297–1321.

Table 3: Agents that Cause Seizures
OTIS CAMPBELL*
Organophosphates
Tricyclic antidepressants
Isoniazid, insulin
Sympathomimetics
Camphor, cocaine
Amphetamines, anticholinergics
Methylxanthines (theophylline, caffeine)
Phencyclidine
Benzodiazepine withdrawal, botanicals (water hemlock), γ-hydroxybutyric acid
Ethanol withdrawal
Lithium, lidocaine
Lead, lindane

*The "town drunk" on *The Andy Griffith Show*.
Adapted with permission from Wills B, Erickson T. Drug- and toxin-associated seizures. *Med Clin N Am.* 2005;89(6):1297–1321.

(e.g., 3,4-methylenedioxymethamphetamine, or MDMA) can have similar presentations. Patients often exhibit tachycardia, hypertension, and psychomotor agitation. With more severe toxicity, hyperthermia, rhabdomyolysis, seizures, and obtundation may be seen.[59–64] Hyperthermia from severe cocaine and designer-amphetamine exposure is a sign of serious toxicity and should be identified and aggressively treated.[65–67] In addition to sympathomimetic effects, cocaine has a local anesthetic affect that may potentiate seizures and can result in myocardial fast sodium channel blockade. Similar to tricyclic antidepressants (TCAs), wide QRS tachycardia can be seen in severe cocaine toxicity and may be treated with bolus sodium bicarbonate therapy.[68] Sympathomimetics have also been associated with intracerebral hemorrhage and ischemic cerebral vascular accident; therefore, neuroimaging should

be considered before attributing seizures to purely pharmacological effects.[59,69–71]

Several drug-withdrawal syndromes have been described. Seizures and autonomic instability are typically seen with withdrawal from ethanol, sedatives (e.g., benzodiazepines and barbiturates), and baclofen. Ethanol withdrawal is a typical cause of DTSs seen in the emergency department. Patients experiencing withdrawal may exhibit tremor and visual hallucinations followed by generalized seizures and autonomic instability.[72] Seizures are typically brief, and status epilepticus is uncommon.[73] Withdrawal from sedative hypnotics is similar to ethanol withdrawal but may be more protracted due to the pharmacokinetics of these agents. Baclofen withdrawal may produce delirium, hallucinations, autonomic instability, hyperthermia, and seizures, which can be severe.[74–76] Intrathecal pump failure results in refractory symptoms and is difficult to treat due to challenges in achieving adequate CNS levels with administration of oral baclofen.[77–79]

Theophylline is a methylxanthine that has fallen out of favor over the last decade. National poison center data reported 4033 exposures in 1994 compared to 413 in 2006.[80–82] Of patients referred to a health-care facility, 1.4% resulted in fatalities in 1994 compared to 0.75% in 2006.[80,81] Despite a reduced prevalence of serious exposures, theophylline toxicity can be challenging to manage and deserves discussion. Acute overdoses typically present with vomiting and sympathomimetic signs, including agitation, tremor, tachycardia, and supraventricular dysrhythmias. Seizures are a common sequelae of toxicity. They are less likely to be observed with serum levels below 60 mg/L, are common with levels above 90 mg/L, and may occur at lower concentrations in chronic toxicity.[83,84] Supportive management for acute toxicity includes benzodiazepines for seizures and avoidance of phenytoin.[85] Enhanced elimination of theophylline should be considered for significant signs of toxicity or levels approaching 60 mg/L and can be achieved with multidose activated charcoal ("gut dialysis")[83,86] and hemodialysis or hemoperfusion for more severe cases or patients with contraindications to oral-activated charcoal.[83,87–89] Similar to salicylates and lithium, the threshold to initiate enhanced elimination modalities may be lower for chronic intoxication.

Tricyclic Antidepressants and Their Mimics

TCAs have multiple pharmacological effects, including amine reuptake inhibition and blockade of fast sodium channels, muscarinic, histamine, and peripheral α-receptors.[90,91] Patients presenting early after overdose may have a predominance of anticholinergic symptoms.[91] With moderate TCA overdose, progression of symptoms may include CNS depression, widened QRS tachycardia, and seizures. More severe cases may promptly develop ventricular dysrhythmias and shock, which can be rapidly fatal.[92] Electrocardiography can be a helpful tool to stratify the severity of intoxication and is a surrogate for the degree of fast sodium channel blockade. Patients with a QRS width greater than 100 msec (or >3 mm R wave in aVr) are at higher risk for seizures,[93–95] while those with a QRS width greater than 160 msec are at higher risk for ventricular dysrhythmias.[94] One study reported seizures and ventricular dysrhythmias in patients with a QRS width greater than 150 msec and none in patients with a QRS width less than 100 msec.[96] Patients who are alert with a QRS width less than 100 msec at 6 hours postingestion are unlikely to develop severe symptoms.[95] Several other pharmaceuticals may mimic TCA toxicity by causing widened QRS and seizures and are discussed in their corresponding sections (see also Table 4).

Opioids

The opioid toxidrome includes CNS depression, respiratory depression, and miosis. Several opioids have characteristics that result in variable effects on pupil size

Table 4: Drugs Potentially Causing a Wide QRS Interval and Seizures
Bupropion
Cocaine
Diphenhydramine
Lamotrigine
Propoxyphene
Quinine, quinidine, hydroxychloroquine
Tricyclic antidepressants
Venlafaxine
Adapted with permission from Wills B, Erickson T. Drug- and toxin-associated seizures. *Med Clin N Am.* 2005;89(6):1297–1321.

and exhibit other unique toxicities, including seizures. Propoxyphene is a synthetic opioid that in overdose can produce CNS depression, seizures, and cardiac conduction abnormalities,[97,98] making it a potential TCA mimic (see Table 4). Widened QRS seen on electrocardiography is likely due to fast sodium channel blockade and appears to be amenable to sodium bicarbonate or lidocaine therapy.[99,100] Meperidine is a narcotic analgesic that has fallen out of favor in many institutions due to the potential for drug–drug interactions. Most notably, meperidine was considered a contributing factor in the infamous Libby Zion case.[101] Normeperidine is a renally eliminated metabolite that can cause seizures when levels accumulate.[102,103] Tramadol is a newer analgesic that is a partial μ-agonist and monoamine reuptake inhibitor. One animal study suggested that high doses of tramadol produced seizures only in kindled rats.[104] Human experience suggests that seizures may occur in 8% to 54% of tramadol exposures[105,106] and may occasionally result in significant morbidity.[107]

The Psychiatric Patient

Suicidal patients attempting to overdose may have access to an array of over-the-counter and prescription medications and household products. Overdose patients with a known history of psychiatric illness may yield consideration of certain psychiatric medications. Diverse psychiatric medications from several classes reliably cause seizures in overdose. TCAs were discussed previously; other agents include non-TCAs, antipsychotics, and lithium.

Serotonin-specific reuptake inhibitors (SSRIs) appear to be relatively safer in overdose compared to TCAs and venlafaxine.[108] Generalized seizures are less common and tend to be brief and self-limited. Status epilepticus has been reported from SSRI overdose but is atypical.[109] One review of 469 SSRI overdoses reported seizures in 1.9%, signs of serotonin syndrome in 14%, and no deaths.[110] In this database, 80% of citalopram overdoses exhibited QTc intervals greater than 440 msec. In addition to seizures, citalopram has been associated with supraventricular tachycardia[111] and wide-complex tachycardia, which was responsive to sodium bicarbonate.[112] Another retrospective review of 225 "newer" antidepressant overdoses reported seizures in approximately 6% of citalopram and 8% of venlafaxine cases.[113] Venlafaxine is a serotonin–norepinephrine reuptake inhibitor, which has significant toxicity in overdose and can mimic TCAs by causing seizures and cardiotoxicity.[114] Animal data suggest that fast sodium channel blockade may be through a mechanism different than I_a antidysrhythmics and TCAs.[115] It is unknown whether there is a role for sodium bicarbonate in these patients.

Bupropion is a mixed amine reuptake inhibitor that is typically used as an antidepressant and smoking cessation aid. Seizures often occur with bupropion overdose and are typically brief and self-limited. Status epilepticus has been reported,[116] with overdose the incidence of seizures is approximately 15% to 19%.[117,118] Other reported symptoms included tachycardia, CNS depression, and hallucinations.[117,118] Electrocardiographical conduction delay is rare and does not typically result in dysrhythmias or seem to respond to sodium bicarbonate boluses.[117,119–121]

The antipsychotic medications, as a class, slightly increase the incidence of seizures in therapeutic dosing. Of the atypical antipsychotics, clozapine and olanzapine appear to have the highest potential to cause seizures from therapeutic dosing[122–124] or overdose.[125]

Lithium has been used for centuries for various psychiatric conditions, most notably bipolar disorder. Intoxication from lithium can be acute, chronic, or acute on chronic depending on clinical situation. Symptoms may include nausea, vomiting, tremor, and mental status alteration.[126] More severe toxicity results in coma, hyperreflexia, conduction disturbances, and seizures.[126] Unfortunately, lithium toxicity can result in chronic neurological dysfunction that is typically cerebellar in nature.[127] There is no antidote for lithium intoxication; therefore, the mainstay of therapy is to enhance elimination through administration of crystalloids and hemodialysis.[126]

The Epileptic Patient

Overdose of several different anticonvulsants can paradoxically precipitate seizures. Determining cause and effect for these cases can be challenging since this patient population is predisposed to having seizures at baseline. However, many cases of paradoxical seizures from antiepileptic overdose have been reported in patients with no known seizure disorder. Of the traditional antiepileptic drugs, phenytoin, carbamazepine, and vigabatrin have been implicated as having the potential to induce seizures in overdose.[128,129] Valproic acid toxicity typically results in various degrees of CNS depression, but paradoxical seizures are rare.[128,130,131] Newer antiepileptic drugs have found applications beyond treatment of seizures and may be used for mood stabilization, pain syndromes, or migraine prophylaxis. There is little experience regarding toxicity of these drugs; however, emerging data have identified several that have been associated with seizures in therapeutic use and overdose. Lamotrigine has been associated with seizures from therapeutic use,[132] high-dose usage,[133] and overdose.[134–137] Case reports suggest that lamotrigine may also produce QRS widening similar to TCA toxicity,[138,139] but risk for subsequent ventricular dysrhythmias is unknown. In one case, sodium loading appeared to reverse QRS widening.[139] Topiramate has been associated with CNS depression and status epilepticus in three cases of overdose.[140,141] These patients recovered after supportive therapy. Tiagabine overdose may result in various neurological symptoms, including CNS depression, coma, agitation, dystonia, seizures, status epilepticus, and hallucinations.[142–144] A U.S. poison center review of tiagabine exposures suggests that seizures and coma are more likely with doses greater than 224 mg and 270 mg, respectively.[142]

Refractory Seizures and Status Epilepticus

Although seizures from various xenobiotics are typically brief and self-limiting, occasionally they may produce status epilepticus or seizures refractory to traditional treatments. Some agents reliably produce severe, refractory seizures in overdose. Isoniazid (INH) is structurally similar to nicotinamide adenine dinucleotide and is used in the treatment of tuberculosis. INH is a hydrazine and is structurally similar to certain types of rocket fuel and toxins from *Gyromitra esculenta* mushrooms.[145,146] It causes a functional deficiency of pyridoxal 5-phosphate (activated vitamin B_6) through inhibition of pyridoxine phosphokinase. Since pyridoxal 5-phosphate is an essential cofactor for glutamic acid decarboxylase, GABA synthesis is suppressed, which likely leads to seizures. INH overdose is classically described as a triad of coma, severe lactic acidosis, and seizures that are refractory to standard therapy.[147,148] Doses of approximately 20 mg/kg can cause neurotoxicity[147]; however, 80 to 150 mg/kg doses are likely to result in seizures and severe toxicity.[149] The mainstay of treatment is administration of intravenous pyridoxine, which is discussed in greater detail in the Treatment section. Water hemlock *(Cicuta maculata)* is occasionally ingested after being mistaken for wild carrots, parsnips, or turnips.[150] Symptoms develop soon after even a small ingestion and can include delirium, salivation, severe seizures, and cardiac arrest.[150–152] Treatment is supportive; no specific antidote exists.

Tinnitus and Hearing Loss

Toxicity from various pharmaceuticals can result in tinnitus and ototoxicity. Tinnitus and hearing loss have been classically described with salicylate and quinine toxicity, the presence of which should be pursued with further evaluation. Absence of these findings unfortunately does not rule out significant exposures. In large overdoses, quinine can mimic TCA toxicity with associated QRS widening on electrocardiogram, dysrhythmias, and hypotension.[153,154] Seizures are uncommon but can occur in severe poisonings. Ocular toxicity is also well described, leading to acute blindness.[154,155] Quinine levels are not readily available, and treatment is supportive. Signs of cardiotoxicity may be amenable to sodium bicarbonate bolus therapy.[153,154] Enhancing the elimination of quinine may be possible through multiple doses of activated charcoal.[86,156] Salicylate intoxication can be acute or chronic. Acute poisoning typically results in initial gastrointestinal symptoms, hyperventilation, and tinnitus.[157] As toxicity progresses, patients exhibit worsening metabolic acidosis, tachycardia, diaphoresis, mental status changes, or agitation. Seizures are typically a late and ominous finding in severe salicylate intoxication and may precede cardiac arrest. Management of salicylate overdoses can be difficult since patients may present with relatively few symptoms and subsequently develop life-threatening toxicity. Salicylates often exhibit substantial delays in peak concentrations; therefore, serial levels must be obtained, in conjunction with acid–base status, to fully appreciate the progression of toxicity.[157] Urinary alkalinization is used to enhance salicylate elimination,[158] as well as to theoretically protect the CNS by reducing the proportion of nonionized serum salicylate. Hemodialysis is required for severe toxicity levels approaching 80 to 100 mg/dL, renal failure, pulmonary edema, cerebral edema, or refractory acidosis.[156,157]

INITIAL APPROACH TO EVALUATING DRUG- AND TOXIN-ASSOCIATED SEIZURES

The preceding discussion of specific etiological agents was intended to organize and summarize DTS agents into meaningful categories but did not include all potential causes. Many exposures not discussed are agents that are less likely to be clinically occult (e.g., iatrogenic intravenous bupivicaine injection and organophosphates) or those that do not have a clinically distinct presentation. Consultation with a clinical toxicologist can be helpful for assistance in management of DTS cases. A clinical toxicologist is available by consulting a regional poison control center and can be reached in all 50 states by calling (800) 222-1222.

The clinical evaluation of the undifferentiated DTS patient occurs in parallel to resuscitative interventions. Aggressive pursuit of historical information has the highest yield in determining likely etiologies and may include emergency medical service personnel, bystanders, family members, primary care physicians, and databases containing the patient's medication record. Initial priorities are management of the airway, supporting oxygenation, hemodynamic status, and initiation of empirical anticonvulsants. Patients should be placed on cardiac monitor and pulse oximeter, provided with supplemental oxygen, have a bedside glucose determination, and have intravenous catheter established. Initial laboratory studies for critically ill patients may include electrocardiography, chest x-ray, blood chemistry, lactate, liver function tests, or arterial blood gas. Obtaining serum concentrations of various drugs should be based on initial clinical and historical data. Table 5 lists drug levels that are typically available at many medical centers. Arbitrary screening of drug levels has low yield; however, acetaminophen and salicylate concentrations are often obtained in overdose patients due to the ubiquitous nature of these over-the-counter medications. Drug concentrations should be interpreted carefully since they are only a single data point in time. Drug levels need to be correlated to the time of ingestion, toxicokinetic profile, and clinical symptoms and often need to be obtained serially to safely and adequately prognosticate the significance of the exposure (e.g., salicylates and lithium). Results of urine drug screening should also be interpreted with caution. These qualitative assays suffer from many false negatives and false positives. Positive results only imply exposure; they do not confirm intoxication. Likewise, negative results do not exclude intoxication.

Gastrointestinal decontamination modalities include gastric lavage, oral-activated charcoal, and whole-bowel irrigation. Indications for each procedure are complex and vary based on patient status and clinician practices. Each procedure requires a cooperative patient with intact protective airway reflexes and no other contraindications. Patients who are actively seizing, anticipated to have seizures, or have significant CNS depression are at risk for complications including pulmonary aspiration. Consultation with a clinical toxicologist can be helpful in determining whether a decontamination

Table 5: Specific Laboratory Testing

Type of Test	Comments
GENERAL TESTING	
ECG	Wide QRS (see Table 3)
Chemistries, anion gap	Will identify hyponatremia, acid–base disorders
Lactate	Likely will be elevated from any seizure; will have marked elevations with INH overdose
Arterial blood gas, carboxyhemoglobin	
Creatine phosphokinase	
DRUG LEVELS TYPICALLY AVAILABLE	
Carbamazepine, phenytoin	
Lithium	
Lidocaine	
Salicylate	
Theophylline	
Tricyclic antidepressants	Generally not as helpful as ECG in predicting clinical course; levels greater than 1000 ng/mL may predict worse outcome
QUALITATIVE TESTING	
Cocaine, opioids	Only confirms exposure, toxidrome recognition may be more helpful; many false negatives with opioid screen (e.g., propoxyphene, methadone)
Amphetamines	Like opioids; many false positives and false negatives
LEVELS NOT READILY AVAILABLE	
Bupropion and other antidepressants	
Cholinesterase activity	May be useful for chronic exposures; not helpful for acute management
Diphenhydramine	
INH	
MDMA and other designer amphetamines	

ECG, electrocardiogram; INH, isoniazid; MDMA, 3,4-methylenedioxymethamphetamine.

Table 6: Agents that may Require Specific Therapy*

Therapy	Agent
Atropine or pralidoxime	Organophosphates, nerve agents
Dextrose	Insulin, sulfonylurea, other hypoglycemic agent
Hemodialysis	Lithium Theophylline Salicylates
Multidose activated charcoal	Carbamazepine with or without theophylline
Octreotide	Sulfonylurea
Pyridoxine	Isoniazid, *Gyromitra esculenta* mushrooms, monomethylhydrazine
Sodium therapy and serum alkalinization	Tricyclic antidepressants and other agents causing fast sodium channel blockade (see text and Table 3)
Urinary alkalinization	Salicylates

*Specific therapy in addition to anticonvulsant and resuscitative measures, not necessarily for discontinuation of seizure activity. Adapted with permission from Wills B, Erickson T. Drug- and toxin-associated seizures. *Med Clin N Am.* 2005;89(6):1297–1321.

procedure is warranted based on individual patient characteristics.

Enhanced elimination procedures include urinary alkalinization, multidose activated charcoal, and hemodialysis. Indications and utility of these interventions are discussed separately for individual agents in the preceding section and are listed in Table 6.

TREATMENT STRATEGIES

Initial Management

Initial resuscitation and supportive care are the mainstays for management of DTSs. Most patients maintain adequate respiratory function during seizures despite apneic periods. It is advisable to apply 100% oxygen and maintain a patent airway. Endotracheal intubation and hemodynamic support may be needed due to large doses of anticonvulsants or due to the overdose itself. Identification and treatment of associated medical complications of seizures such as hyperthermia, metabolic acidosis, rhabdomyolysis, cardiac dysrhythmias, and head, spinal, and orthopedic trauma may be necessary. Metabolic and medical complications can be the result of seizures, the underlying toxic profile of the exposure, or both.

DTSs are often self-limited and abate without requiring antiepileptics.[159–163] However, up to 15% of patients with drug-related seizures, particularly if related to overdose, may present with status epilepticus and thus require aggressive antiepileptic therapy.[6] Anticonvulsant guidelines have been developed for the treatment of status epilepticus, particularly with regard to the order and dosage of antiepileptic medications (Table 7).[164,165] Anticonvulsant therapy for protracted DTSs likely follows a similar treatment algorithm, with some important exceptions.

Treatment of Drug- and Toxin-related Status Epilepticus

Status epilepticus is a neurological emergency, considering a 17% to 23% mortality rate and that 10% to 23% of survivors suffering from persistent neurological disabilities.[165–168] Status epilepticus is classified into convulsive and nonconvulsive status epilepticus and generalized and partial status epilepticus based on the seizure semiology. Toxic–metabolic etiologies cause up to 19% of cases of status epilepticus.[169]

Benzodiazepines are generally first-line therapy for all causes of status epilepticus, including DTSs.[84,159–161,165,170,171] Benzodiazepines can be given intravenously and have a rapid onset of action, making them ideal for initial pharmacotherapy in status epilepticus.

Name	Loading Dose	Infusion Rate	Maintenance Dose	Half-Life
Lorazepam	0.05–0.1 mg/kg	2 mg/min	May repeat up to 10 mg	8–25 hours
Diazepam	0.15 mg/kg	<5 mg/min	May repeat up to 20 mg	28–54 hours
Phenytoin	20 mg/kg	50 mg/min	1.5 mg/kg q8h	24 hours
Fosphenytoin	20 PE/kg	150 mg/min	1.5 mg/kg q8h	24 hours
Phenobarbital	15–20 mg/kg	50 mg/min	0.5–1.0 mg/kg/hr	48–120 hours
Valproate	15–60 mg/kg	3–6 mg/kg/min	4–8 mg/kg/hr	15 hours
Midazolam	0.15–0.20 mg/kg to maximum loading dose of 2 mg/kg	0.1 mg/kg/hour	0.05 mg/kg/hour—2.9 mg/kg/hour	3 hours
Propofol	1-2 mg/kg* *Repeat 1-2 mg/kg boluses every 3 to 5 minutes until seizure stops to maximum loading dose of 10 mg/kg	Infusion rate: 2mg/kg/ hour (2 mg/kg/h)	*	2 hours
Pentobarbital	5–15 mg/kg	1 mg/kg/hour and titrate to EEG and vital signs	0.5–10 mg/kg/hr	15–60 hours
Thiopental	2–5 mg/kg	Titrate to EEG and vital signs	5 mg/kg/hr	12–36 hours
Levetiracetam	Undetermined	15 minutes	500–1500 mg q12h	6–8 hours

Table 7: Recommended Dosing of Antiepileptic and Anesthetic Agents Reported for Treatment of Refractory Status Epilepticus

PE, phenytoin equivalent.
*Do not exceed >5 mg/kg/h for >48 hours due to risk of propofol infusion syndrome

Benzodiazepine receptors in the brain are associated with and reside on $GABA_A$ receptor complexes. They potentiate the effect of GABA on $GABA_A$ receptors and increase neuronal inhibition by increasing chloride permeability, resulting in neuronal hyperpolarization.[172–174] Benzodiazepines also inhibit adenosine uptake, indirectly enhancing adenosine's activity at A_1 receptors, which may be an important mechanism in aborting seizures caused by adenosine antagonists such as theophylline.[172]

Intravenous lorazepam up to a total dose of 0.1 mg/kg is preferred among the benzodiazepines.[164,174] Lorazepam is preferred due to its favorable pharmacological profile and efficacy when compared with other benzodiazepines.[164,174] Lorazepam has an onset of action similar to diazepam, but lorazepam maintains its efficacy for hours and has no active metabolites.[164,174] Diazepam has a long half-life and is lipid soluble. This may theoretically result in rapid CNS penetration, but penetration is complicated by redistribution to peripheral fat stores, reducing efficacy and requiring repeated dosing. Lorazepam has been shown to be more effective than diazepam as first-line therapy in generalized convulsive status epilepticus; evidence suggests that patients treated with diazepam require intubation more often than those treated initially with lorazepam.[175–177] Other benzodiazepines, including midazolam, can be used as initial therapy. Like diazepam, midazolam is highly lipid soluble, with both a rapid onset of action and a short half-life, necessitating repeat dosing. When intravenous access cannot be obtained, diazepam can be given rectally and midazolam may be used in the intranasal, buccal, and intramuscular routes.

Benzodiazepines are particularly effective in DTSs, especially if the toxic mechanism of action involves a GABA mechanism. Direct and indirect $GABA_A$ antagonism results in seizures in clinical and laboratory settings.[172] Experimental convulsants used in animal models of epilepsy, such as picrotoxin and pentylenetetrazol, inhibit GABA at the $GABA_A$ receptor and can be aborted by benzodiazepines.[178,179] β-Lactam antibiotics, fluoroquinolones, and lindane are examples of agents with $GABA_A$ antagonism and are a clinical cause of drug-related seizures.[160,161,170,172,180] The use of benzodiazepines enhances GABAergic activity, making them an ideal treatment for DTSs caused by agents that antagonize GABA transmission at the $GABA_A$ receptor. Benzodiazepines may not be effective in some exposures, resulting in GABA depletion, such as INH toxicity.[171]

First-line therapy for non-DTS status epilepticus includes the use of phenytoin or the prodrug fosphenytoin.[164,165,181] Phenytoin or fosphenytoin is given after benzodiazepines for treatment of refractory status epilepticus. Phenytoin inhibits transmission at voltage-gated sodium channels, arresting seizure propagation.[174] Treatment with 18 to 20 mg/kg of phenytoin infused at 50 mg/min or 18 to 20 phenytoin equivalents (PEs) per kilogram of fosphenytoin infused at 150 fosphenytoin equivalents per minute is considered appropriate intravenous dosing. An additional 5 to 10 mg/kg of phenytoin or 5 to 10 PEs per kilogram of fosphenytoin can be given if initial dosing fails to control seizures.[165]

Despite phenytoin's and fosphenytoin's established roles in status epilepticus, several clinical situations limit use of these agents. Phenytoin has been reported to aggravate certain types of generalized seizures, particularly absence seizures and the myoclonus in juvenile myoclonic epilepsy.[128] Therefore, phenytoin and fosphenytoin may not be effective in treating absence or myolconic status epilepticus. With phenytoin, hypotension occurs in up to 50% of patients and cardiac arrhythmias in up to 2% of patients, particularly in the elderly and patients with heart disease.[164,165] Use of phenytoin is discouraged when status epilepticus is caused by drugs and toxins that have cardiovascular effects. Seizures and status epilepticus caused by some drugs and toxins may not respond or are worsened by phenytoin. For example, seizures related to theophylline, cocaine, cyclic antidepressants, and certain antimicrobials may not respond to phenytoin. Table 8 lists drugs and toxins that may not respond to phenytoin. The lack of efficacy of phenytoin in DTSs may be due to its lack of effect on the seizure threshold. Since DTSs are typically generalized, phenytoin's effect on sodium channels and seizure propagation may not be sufficient to abort this generalized seizure activity.

Phenobarbital is recommended as second-line therapy if status epilepticus is refractory to treatment with benzodiazepines and phenytoin or fosphenytoin.[164,165] Phenobarbital is often recommended after benzodiazepines for DTSs.[84,159,161,170,171] Phenobarbital is a barbiturate that acts mainly on the $GABA_A$ chloride channel and increases the inhibitory effect of GABA. Prolonged seizures caused by drugs and toxins with direct or indirect GABA antagonism are expected to respond to treatment with phenobarbital. Phenobarbital has a long plasma half-life, resulting in prolonged sedation, and can cause respiratory and myocardial depression. Recommended intravenous dosing for status epilepticus is 20 mg/kg at a rate of 50 to 75 mg/min.

Sodium valproate is the most widely prescribed antiepileptic drug in the world and is effective for all seizure types.[128] Valproate has multiple mechanisms of action, including increased GABA transmission, reduced release of excitatory amino acids such as glutamate, blockage of voltage-gated sodium channels, and serotonin and dopamine modulation.[128] Intravenous valproate is not approved by the U.S. Food and Drug Administration (FDA) for use in status epilepticus, but evidence increasingly demonstrates its effectiveness.[202,203] Intravenous valproate may be more effective than phenytoin against other types of status epilepticus, including absence and myoclonic status epilepticus.[204,205] Valproate can be

Table 8: Agents that may not Respond to Phenytoin

Agent	Comments	References
Isoniazid	May not respond to phenytoin; pyridoxine is preferred treatment	84,160,161,170,172,180,182–184
Gingko	Responds to pyridoxine; competitively inhibits toxic product in gingko seeds	84,160,161,170,172,180,182–184
Gyromitra esculenta mushrooms (monomethylhydrazine)	Responds to pyridoxine; mechanism similar to that for isoniazid toxicity	84,160,161,170,172,180,182–184
Penicillin	Benzodiazepines and phenobarbital may be more effective; phenytoin may not be effective	160,161,170,172,185,186
Carbapenems	Benzodiazepines and phenobarbital may be more effective	160,161,170,172,185,186
Cephalosporins	Benzodiazepines and phenobarbital may be more effective	160,161,170,172,185,186
Aztreonam	Benzodiazepines and phenobarbital may be more effective	160,161,170,172,185,186
Fluoroquinolones	Recommendations similar to those for penicillins based on mechanism of action	161,170,172
Lindane	Benzodiazepines and phenobarbital may be more effective	170,172,180
Lidocaine	Phenytoin may not be effective or may worsen seizures	161,171,187–189
Meperidine	Phenytoin and other antiepileptics may increase production of proconvulsant metabolite normeperidine	102,190
Theophylline	Phenytoin may not be effective or may worsen seizures; may respond to pyridoxine	160,161,171,191–196
Cocaine	Phenytoin may not be effective	159,197–199
Cyclic antidepressants	Phenytoin may not be effective	84,92,171,200,201

infused rapidly and safely administered to medically unstable patients, although hypotension with intravenous valproate has been reported.[204,206–208] Valproate has shown some anticonvulsant effect in some chemical models of seizures and status epilepticus. In an animal seizure model using 4-aminopyridine, valproate abolished ongoing status epilepticus while phenytoin did not.[178,209] The multiple mechanisms of action, decreased risk of cardiovascular side effects, and rapid intravenous dosing make it a reasonable choice as a third-line treatment for DTSs; however, this has not been systematically studied.

Levetiracetam is a newer antiepileptic medication with an oral and intravenous formulation that has been used for treatment of status epilepticus, although it also lacks approval by the U.S. FDA for this indication.[210–212] The exact mechanism of action is not known, although it binds to a specific synaptic vesicle protein, modulates calcium channels, and results in activation of GABA currents in the CNS.[210] No serious or life-threatening toxicities are known to be associated with levetiracetam, even with rapid intravenous infusion.[213] Levetiracetam is renally eliminated and does not induce hepatic enzymes or have significant interactions with other drugs. There is no published experience specific to DTSs and status epilepticus, but its favorable pharmacological profile may make it a safe option with failure of other therapies.

Status epilepticus occurs in three stages: a premonitory stage at 5 to 10 minutes, established status epilepticus at 10 to 30 minutes, and refractory status epilepticus at 30 to 60 minutes. It is known that ongoing seizure activity is a dynamic process with a gradual decrease in convulsive activity, sequential EEG changes, progressive neurochemical changes, neuronal damage, and increasing refractoriness to treatment. Status epilepticus is aborted with first-line medications in 80% of patients if these are started within the first 30 minutes, but this decreases to only 40% after 2 hours.[214] Refractory status epilepticus has been defined as generalized convulsive or nonconvulsive status epilepticus that continues after first- and second-line therapy or seizures persisting after 30 to 60 minutes of continuous treatment. Refractory status epilepticus has an increased rate of morbidity and mortality.[166,215,216]

The anesthetic agents midazolam and propofol have been widely used and are effective therapy for refractory status epilepticus.[169,217,218] Intubation and mechanical ventilation are typically required when using these agents. Midazolam is a lipophilic benzodiazepine with a rapid onset of action and short half-life. Propofol is a highly lipophilic anesthetic that is a GABA$_A$ agonist and may inhibit N-methyl-d-aspartate (NMDA) receptors and modulate certain calcium ion channels. Some suggest that these agents may have a role earlier in the treatment algorithm and should be considered after failure of first-line therapies. Evidence to support this recommendation is based on a large prospective randomized trial for treatment of status epilepticus.[177] The authors observed a poor response to phenytoin in patients refractory to lorazepam. The mechanism of these agents make them attractive for refractory DTSs and status epilepticus, although there is little published experience specific to DTSs outside of animal models.[219–222]

Ketamine is a unique anesthetic agent that has been used in cases of refractory status epilepticus.[223,224] Ketamine has a unique mechanism of action as an NMDA receptor antagonist. Ketamine has shown some efficacy and possible neuroprotective properties in a chemical model of seizures and in the setting of status epilepticus after nerve agent exposure.[225,226]

Barbiturate coma may be induced with pentobarbital or thiopental for refractory status epilepticus that have failed other therapies. Pentobarbital is the preferred agent,[164,165,169] and dosing is listed in Table 7. These medications are titrated to the EEG pattern, although the ideal titration and EEG pattern is controversial. It is not clear whether seizure termination, a burst-suppression pattern, or a flat EEG recording results in improved outcomes[164] Hypotension and gastrointestinal dysmotility are expected complications, and the use of these agents must be weighed against these risks. Most experts recommend continuing EEG suppression for 12 to 24 hours before beginning to taper.

Adjunctive Therapies

In addition to administering anticonvulsants, clinicians often are faced with the decision to initiate empirical adjunctive therapy without confirmation of the etiological agent. This practice is reasonable if there is the possibility of significant morbidity from the overdose and the risks of therapy are relatively low. For example, it is reasonable to administer sodium bicarbonate boluses when a patient presents with typical signs of severe TCA toxicity—without other confirmatory testing. The decision to initiate pyridoxine without a history of INH exposure may also be difficult; however, in the setting of refractory seizures, this therapy is safe and should be considered. Pyridoxine is typically given as a 5-g intravenous infusion or a dose equivalent to the ingested INH dose, if known. A newer antidote that is receiving significant attention is lipid rescue. Lipid emulsion is an emerging antidote that was originally investigated as treatment for bupivicaine cardiotoxicity. Lipid rescue may be effective for other seizure-causing lipid soluble pharmaceuticals, such as TCAs and bupropion.[227–229] Specific or adjunctive interventions are listed in Table 6.

CONCLUSION

Seizures as the result of drug or toxin exposures may occur for various agents. Evaluation of the undifferentiated DTS patient is best achieved through vigorous pursuit of historical data, a clinical presentation approach, and directed laboratory testing. Most DTSs require supportive care and benzodiazepines for seizures; however, some agents may need specific therapy.

REFERENCES

1. Thundiyil JG, Kearney TE, Olson KR. Evolving epidemiology of drug-induced seizures reported to a Poison Control Center System. *J Med Toxicol.* 2007;3(1):15–19.
2. Hillbom M, Pieninkeroinen I, Leone M. Seizures in alcohol-dependent patients: epidemiology, pathophysiology and management. *CNS Drugs.* 2003;17(14):1013–1030.
3. Chan AW. Alcoholism and epilepsy. *Epilepsia.* 1985;26(4):323–333.
4. Pieninkeroinen IP, Telakivi TM, Hillbom ME. Outcome in subjects with alcohol-provoked seizures. *Alcohol Clin Exp Res.* 1992;16(5):955–959.
5. Wijdicks EF, Sharbrough FW. New-onset seizures in critically ill patients. *Neurology.* 1993;43(5):1042–1044.
6. Messing RO, Closson RG, Simon RP. Drug-induced seizures: a 10-year experience. *Neurology.* 1984;34(12):1582–1586.
7. Engel J Jr. ILAE classification of epilepsy syndromes. *Epilepsy Res.* 2006;70 (Suppl 1):S5–S10.
8. Chang BS, Lowenstein DH. Epilepsy. *N Engl J Med.* 2003;349(13):1257–1266.
9. Lowenstein DH. Status epilepticus: an overview of the clinical problem. *Epilepsia.* 1999;40 (Suppl 1):S3–S8; discussion, S21–S22.
10. Murdoch D. Mechanisms of status epilepticus: an evidence-based review. *Curr Opin Neurol.* 2007;20(2):213–216.

11. Noe KH, Manno EM. Mechanisms underlying status epilepticus. *Drugs Today (Barc)*. 2005;41(4):257–266.

12. Majkowski J. Kindling: clinical relevance for epileptogenicity in humans. *Adv Neurol*. 1999;81:105–113.

13. Cavazos JE, Golarai G, Sutula TP. Mossy fiber synaptic reorganization induced by kindling: time course of development, progression, and permanence. *J Neurosci*. 1991;11(9):2795–2803.

14. Bertram E. The relevance of kindling for human epilepsy. *Epilepsia*. 2007;48 (Suppl 2):65–74.

15. DeGiorgio CM, Tomiyasu U, Gott PS, Treiman DM. Hippocampal pyramidal cell loss in human status epilepticus. *Epilepsia*. 1992;33(1):23–27.

16. Hesdorffer DC, Logroscino G, Cascino G, Annegers JF, Hauser WA. Risk of unprovoked seizure after acute symptomatic seizure: effect of status epilepticus. *Ann Neurol*. 1998;44(6):908–912.

17. Walker MC, White HS, Sander JW. Disease modification in partial epilepsy. *Brain*. 2002;125(Pt 9):1937–1950.

18. Aird RB, Gordon NS. Some excitatory and inhibitory factors involved in the epileptic state. *Brain Dev*. 1993;15(4):299–304.

19. Gilabert E, Rojo E, Vallejo J. Augmentation of electroconvulsive therapy seizures with sleep deprivation. *J Ect*. 2004;20(4):242–247.

20. Mendez OE, Brenner RP. Increasing the yield of EEG. *J Clin Neurophysiol*. 2006;23(4):282–293.

21. Scalise A, Desiato MT, Gigli GL, et al. Increasing cortical excitability: a possible explanation for the proconvulsant role of sleep deprivation. *Sleep*. 2006;29(12):1595–1598.

22. Castilla-Guerra L, del Carmen Fernandez-Moreno M, Lopez-Chozas JM, Fernandez-Bolanos R. Electrolytes disturbances and seizures. *Epilepsia*. 2006;47(12):1990–1998.

23. Tiamkao S, Pratipanawatr T, Tiamkao S, Nitinavakarn B, Chotmongkol V, Jitpimolmard S. Seizures in nonketotic hyperglycaemia. *Seizure*. 2003;12(6):409–410.

24. Frier B. Hypoglycaemia: clinical consequences and morbidity. *Int J Clin Pract Suppl*. 2000;(112):51–55.

25. Chung B, Wong V. Relationship between five common viruses and febrile seizure in children. *Arch Dis Child*. 2007;92(7):589–593.

26. Chung BH, Tsang AM, Wong VC. Neurologic complications in children hospitalized with influenza: comparison between USA and Hong Kong. *J Pediatr*. 2007;151(5):e17–18; author reply, e18–19.

27. Kazibutowska Z, Filipowicz A, Kudybka E. Effect of infections on the course and effectiveness of epilepsy treatment in children. *Neurol Neurochir Pol*. 1975;9(1):65–71.

28. Ribeiro JA, Sebastiao AM, de Mendonca A. Adenosine receptors in the nervous system: pathophysiological implications. *Prog Neurobiol*. 2002;68(6):377–392.

29. Bagdy G, Kecskemeti V, Riba P, Jakus R. Serotonin and epilepsy. *J Neurochem*. 2007;100(4):857–873.

30. Sangalli BC. Role of the central histaminergic neuronal system in the CNS toxicity of the first generation H1-antagonists. *Prog Neurobiol*. 1997;52(2):145–157.

31. Weinshenker D, Szot P. The role of catecholamines in seizure susceptibility: new results using genetically engineered mice. *Pharmacol Ther*. 2002;94(3):213–233.

32. Jobe PC, Browning RA. The serotonergic and noradrenergic effects of antidepressant drugs are anticonvulsant, not proconvulsant. *Epilepsy Behav*. 2005;7(4):602–619.

33. Holtkamp M, Meierkord H. Anticonvulsant, antiepileptogenic, and antiictogenic pharmacostrategies. *Cell Mol Life Sci*. 2007;64(15):2023–2041.

34. Sazgar M, Bourgeois BF. Aggravation of epilepsy by antiepileptic drugs. *Pediatr Neurol*. 2005;33(4):227–234.

35. Blumenfeld H, Westerveld M, Ostroff RB, et al. Selective frontal, parietal, and temporal networks in generalized seizures. *Neuroimage*. 2003;19(4):1556–1566.

36. McNally KA, Blumenfeld H. Focal network involvement in generalized seizures: new insights from electroconvulsive therapy. *Epilepsy Behav*. 2004;5(1):3–12.

37. Brevard ME, Kulkarni P, King JA, Ferris CF. Imaging the neural substrates involved in the genesis of pentylenetetrazol-induced seizures. *Epilepsia*. 2006;47(4):745–754.

38. Markand ON. Pearls, perils, and pitfalls in the use of the electroencephalogram. *Semin Neurol*. 2003;23(1):7–46.

39. Blume WT. Drug effects on EEG. *J Clin Neurophysiol*. 2006;23(4):306–311.

40. Holmes GL, Korteling F. Drug effects on the human EEG. *Am J EEG Technol*. 1993;33(1):1–26.

41. Stockard JJ, Werner SS, Aalbers JA, Chiappa KH. Electroencephalographic findings in phencyclidine intoxication. *Arch Neurol*. 1976;33(3):200–203.

42. Niedermeyer E. *Electroencephalography: Basic Principles, Clinical Applications, and Related Fields*. Baltimore: Williams & Wilkins; 1999.

43. Gerson IM, Karabell S. The use of the electroencephalogram in patients admitted for alcohol abuse with seizures. *Clin Electroencephalogr*. 1979;10(1):40–49.

44. Galimberti CA, Manni R, Parietti L, Marchioni E, Tartara A. Drug withdrawal in patients with epilepsy: prognostic value of the EEG. *Seizure*. 1993;2(3):213–220.

45. Essig CF, Fraser HF. Electroencephalographic changes in man during use and withdrawal of barbiturates in moderate dosage. *Electroencephalogr Clin Neurophysiol*. 1958;10(4):649–656.

46. Benbadis SR. A spell in the epilepsy clinic and a history of "chronic pain" or "fibromyalgia" independently predict a diagnosis of psychogenic seizures. *Epilepsy Behav*. 2005;6(2):264–265.

47. Eiris-Punal J, Rodriguez-Nunez A, Fernandez-Martinez N, Fuster M, Castro-Gago M, Martinon JM. Usefulness of the head-upright tilt test for distinguishing syncope and epilepsy in children. *Epilepsia*. 2001;42(6):709–713.

48. Zaidi A, Clough P, Cooper P, Scheepers B, Fitzpatrick AP. Misdiagnosis of epilepsy: many seizure-like attacks have a cardiovascular cause. *J Am Coll Cardiol*. 2000;36(1):181–184.

49. Cryer PE. Symptoms of hypoglycemia, thresholds for their occurrence, and hypoglycemia unawareness. *Endocrinol Metab Clin North Am*. 1999;28(3):495–500, v–vi.

50. Han SW, Kim SH, Kim JK, Park CH, Yun MJ, Heo JH. Hemodynamic changes in limb shaking TIA associated with anterior cerebral artery stenosis. *Neurology*. 2004;63(8):1519–1521.

51. Merritt TC. Recognition and acute management of patients with panic attacks in the emergency department. *Emerg Med Clin North Am*. 2000;18(2):289–300, ix.

52. Frankel EA, Shalaby TM, Orenstein SR. Sandifer syndrome posturing: relation to abdominal wall contractions, gastroesophageal reflux, and fundoplication. *Dig Dis Sci*. 2006;51(4):635–640.

53. Horrocks IA, Nechay A, Stephenson JB, Zuberi SM. Anoxic–epileptic seizures: observational study of epileptic seizures induced by syncopes. *Arch Dis Child*. 2005;90(12):1283–1287.

54. Kanazawa O. Shuddering attacks: report of four children. *Pediatr Neurol*. 2000;23(5):421–424.

55. Kotagal P, Costa M, Wyllie E, Wolgamuth B. Paroxysmal nonepileptic events in children and adolescents. *Pediatrics*. 2002;110(4):e46.

56. Rickards H. Tics and fits: the current status of Gilles de la Tourette syndrome and its relationship with epilepsy. *Seizure*. 1995;4(4):259–266.

57. Rosenow F, Wyllie E, Kotagal P, Mascha E, Wolgamuth BR, Hamer H. Staring spells in children: descriptive features distinguishing epileptic and nonepileptic events. *J Pediatr*. 1998;133(5):660–663.

58. Jenssen S, Gracely EJ, Sperling MR. How long do most seizures last? A systematic comparison of seizures recorded in the epilepsy monitoring unit. *Epilepsia*. 2006;47(9):1499–1503.

59. Spivey WH, Euerle B. Neurologic complications of cocaine abuse. *Ann Emerg Med.* 1990;19(12):1422–1428.

60. Ginsberg MD, Hertzman M, Schmidt-Nowara WW. Amphetamine intoxication with coagulopathy, hyperthermia, and reversible renal failure: a syndrome resembling heatstroke. *Ann Intern Med.* 1970;73(1):81–85.

61. Ramcharan S, Meenhorst PL, Otten JM, et al. Survival after massive Ecstasy overdose. *J Toxicol Clin Toxicol.* 1998;36(7):727–731.

62. Shannon M. Methylenedioxymethamphetamine (MDMA, "Ecstasy"). *Pediatr Emerg Care.* 2000;16(5):377–380.

63. Campkin NT, Davies UM. Another death from Ecstasy. *J R Soc Med.* 1992;85(1):61.

64. Henry JA, Jeffreys KJ, Dawling S. Toxicity and deaths from 3,4-methylenedioxymethamphetamine ("Ecstasy"). *Lancet.* 1992;340(8816):384–387.

65. Catravas JD, Waters IW. Acute cocaine intoxication in the conscious dog: studies on the mechanism of lethality. *J Pharmacol Exp Ther.* 1981;217(2):350–356.

66. Bordo DJ, Dorfman MA. Ecstasy overdose: rapid cooling leads to successful outcome. *Am J Emerg Med.* 2004;22(4):326–327.

67. Albertson TE, Derlet RW, Van Hoozen BE. Methamphetamine and the expanding complications of amphetamines. *West J Med.* 1999;170(4):214–219.

68. Hollander JE, Henry TD. Evaluation and management of the patient who has cocaine-associated chest pain. *Cardiol Clin.* 2006;24(1):103–114.

69. Hanyu S, Ikeguchi K, Imai H, Imai N, Yoshida M. Cerebral infarction associated with 3,4-methylenedioxymethamphetamine ("Ecstasy") abuse. *Eur Neurol.* 1995;35(3):173.

70. Gledhill JA, Moore DF, Bell D, Henry JA. Subarachnoid haemorrhage associated with MDMA abuse. *J Neurol Neurosurg Psychiatry.* 1993;56(9):1036–1037.

71. Manchanda S, Connolly MJ. Cerebral infarction in association with Ecstasy abuse. *Postgrad Med J.* 1993;69(817):874–875.

72. Victor M, Adams RD. The effect of alcohol on the nervous system. *Res Publ Assoc Res Nerv Ment Dis.* 1953;32:526–573.

73. Brust JC. Seizures and substance abuse: treatment considerations. *Neurology.* 2006;67 (12 Suppl 4):S45–S48.

74. Hyser CL, Drake ME Jr. Status epilepticus after baclofen withdrawal. *J Natl Med Assoc.* 1984;76(5):533, 537–538.

75. Peng CT, Ger J, Yang CC, Tsai WJ, Deng JF, Bullard MJ. Prolonged severe withdrawal symptoms after acute-on-chronic baclofen overdose. *J Toxicol Clin Toxicol.* 1998;36(4):359–363.

76. Kofler M, Arturo Leis A. Prolonged seizure activity after baclofen withdrawal. *Neurology.* 1992;42(3 Pt 1):697–698.

77. Greenberg MI, Hendrickson RG. Baclofen withdrawal following removal of an intrathecal baclofen pump despite oral baclofen replacement. *J Toxicol Clin Toxicol.* 2003;41(1):83–85.

78. Khorasani A, Peruzzi WT. Dantrolene treatment for abrupt intrathecal baclofen withdrawal. *Anesth Analg.* 1995;80(5):1054–1056.

79. Green LB, Nelson VS. Death after acute withdrawal of intrathecal baclofen: case report and literature review. *Arch Phys Med Rehabil.* 1999;80(12):1600–1604.

80. Litovitz TL, Felberg L, Soloway RA, Ford M, Geller R. 1994 annual report of the American Association of Poison Control Centers Toxic Exposure Surveillance System. *Am J Emerg Med.* 1995;13(5):551–597.

81. Bronstein AC, Spyker DA, Cantilena LR Jr, Green J, Rumack BH, Heard SE. 2006 Annual report of the American Association of Poison Control Centers' National Poison Data System (NPDS). *Clin Toxicol (Phila).* 2007;45(8):815–917.

82. American Association of Poison Control Centers. Toxic Exposure Surveillance System. Available at: http://www.aapcc.org. Accessed November 2007.

83. Paloucek FP, Rodvold KA. Evaluation of theophylline overdoses and toxicities. *Ann Emerg Med.* 1988;17(2):135–144.

84. Kunisaki TA, Augenstein WL. Drug- and toxin-induced seizures. *Emerg Med Clin North Am.* 1994;12(4):1027–1056.

85. Wills B, Erickson T. Drug- and toxin-associated seizures. *Med Clin North Am.* 2005;89(6):1297–1321.

86. American Academy of Clinical Toxicology; European Association of Poisons Centres and Clinical Toxicologists. Position statement and practice guidelines on the use of multi-dose activated charcoal in the treatment of acute poisoning. *J Toxicol Clin Toxicol.* 1999;37(6):731–751.

87. Bouffard J, Lardet G, Tissot S, Perrot D, Delafosse B, Motin J. Theophylline intoxication: toxicokinetic evaluation of hemodialysis. *Intensive Care Med.* 1993;19(2):122.

88. Gitomer JJ, Khan AM, Ferris ME. Treatment of severe theophylline toxicity with hemodialysis in a preterm neonate. *Pediatr Nephrol.* 2001;16(10):784–786.

89. Anderson JR, Poklis A, McQueen RC, Purtell JN, Slavin RG. Effects of hemodialysis on theophylline kinetics. *J Clin Pharmacol.* 1983;23(10):428–432.

90. Woolf AD, Erdman AR, Nelson LS, et al. Tricyclic antidepressant poisoning: an evidence-based consensus guideline for out-of-hospital management. *Clin Toxicol (Phila).* 2007;45(3):203–233.

91. Frommer DA, Kulig KW, Marx JA, Rumack B. Tricyclic antidepressant overdose: a review. *JAMA.* 1987;257(4):521–526.

92. Pimentel L, Trommer L. Cyclic antidepressant overdoses: a review. *Emerg Med Clin North Am.* 1994;12(2):533–547.

93. Liebelt EL, Francis PD, Woolf AD. ECG lead aVR versus QRS interval in predicting seizures and arrhythmias in acute tricyclic antidepressant toxicity. *Ann Emerg Med.* 1995;26(2):195–201.

94. Boehnert MT, Lovejoy FH Jr. Value of the QRS duration versus the serum drug level in predicting seizures and ventricular arrhythmias after an acute overdose of tricyclic antidepressants. *N Engl J Med.* 1985;313(8):474–479.

95. Hulten BA, Adams R, Askenasi R, et al. Predicting severity of tricyclic antidepressant overdose. *J Toxicol Clin Toxicol.* 1992;30(2):161–170.

96. Liebelt EL, Ulrich A, Francis PD, Woolf A. Serial electrocardiogram changes in acute tricyclic antidepressant overdoses. *Crit Care Med.* 1997;25(10):1721–1726.

97. Sloth Madsen P, Strom J, Reiz S, Bredgaard Sorensen M. Acute propoxyphene self-poisoning in 222 consecutive patients. *Acta Anaesthesiol Scand.* 1984;28(6):661–665.

98. Lawson AA, Northridge DB. Dextropropoxyphene overdose: epidemiology, clinical presentation and management. *Med Toxicol Adverse Drug Exp.* 1987;2(6):430–444.

99. Stork CM, Redd JT, Fine K, Hoffman RS. Propoxyphene-induced wide QRS complex dysrhythmia responsive to sodium bicarbonate: a case report. *J Toxicol Clin Toxicol.* 1995;33(2):179–183.

100. Whitcomb DC, Gilliam FR III, Starmer CF, Grant AO. Marked QRS complex abnormalities and sodium channel blockade by propoxyphene reversed with lidocaine. *J Clin Invest.* 1989;84(5):1629–1636.

101. Lowenstein J. Where have all the giants gone? Reconciling medical education and the traditions of patient care with limitations on resident work hours. *Perspect Biol Med.* 2003;46(2):273–282.

102. Armstrong PJ, Bersten A. Normeperidine toxicity. *Anesth Analg.* 1986;65(5):536–538.

103. Knight B, Thomson N, Perry G. Seizures due to norpethidine toxicity. *Aust NZ J Med.* 2000;30(4):513.

104. Potschka H, Friderichs E, Loscher W. Anticonvulsant and proconvulsant effects of tramadol, its enantiomers and its M1 metabolite in the rat kindling model of epilepsy. *Br J Pharmacol.* 2000;131(2):203–212.

105. Spiller HA, Gorman SE, Villalobos D, et al. Prospective multicenter evaluation of tramadol exposure. *J Toxicol Clin Toxicol.* 1997;35(4):361–364.

106. Jovanovic-Cupic V, Martinovic Z, Nesic N. Seizures associated with intoxication and abuse of tramadol. *Clin Toxicol (Phila)*. 2006;44(2):143–146.

107. Daubin C, Quentin C, Goulle JP, et al. Refractory shock and asystole related to tramadol overdose. *Clin Toxicol (Phila)*. 2007:1–4.

108. Whyte IM, Dawson AH, Buckley NA. Relative toxicity of venlafaxine and selective serotonin reuptake inhibitors in overdose compared to tricyclic antidepressants. *QJM*. 2003;96(5):369–374.

109. Wood DM, Rajalingam Y, Greene SL, et al. Status epilepticus following intentional overdose of fluvoxamine: a case report with serum fluvoxamine concentration. *Clin Toxicol (Phila)*. 2007;45(7):1–3.

110. Isbister GK, Bowe SJ, Dawson A, Whyte IM. Relative toxicity of selective serotonin reuptake inhibitors (SSRIs) in overdose. *J Toxicol Clin Toxicol*. 2004;42(3):277–285.

111. Cuenca PJ, Holt KR, Hoefle JD. Seizure secondary to citalopram overdose. *J Emerg Med*. 2004;26(2):177–181.

112. Engebretsen KM, Harris CR, Wood JE. Cardiotoxicity and late onset seizures with citalopram overdose. *J Emerg Med*. 2003;25(2):163–166.

113. Kelly CA, Dhaun N, Laing WJ, Strachan FE, Good AM, Bateman DN. Comparative toxicity of citalopram and the newer antidepressants after overdose. *J Toxicol Clin Toxicol*. 2004;42(1):67–71.

114. Blythe D, Hackett LP. Cardiovascular and neurological toxicity of venlafaxine. *Hum Exp Toxicol*. 1999;18(5):309–313.

115. Khalifa M, Daleau P, Turgeon J. Mechanism of sodium channel block by venlafaxine in guinea pig ventricular myocytes. *J Pharmacol Exp Ther*. 1999;291(1):280–284.

116. Morazin F, Lumbroso A, Harry P, et al. Cardiogenic shock and status epilepticus after massive bupropion overdose. *Clin Toxicol (Phila)*. 2007;45(7):794–797.

117. Belson MG, Kelley TR. Bupropion exposures: clinical manifestations and medical outcome. *J Emerg Med*. 2002;23(3):223–230.

118. Spiller HA, Ramoska EA, Krenzelok EP, et al. Bupropion overdose: a 3-year multi-center retrospective analysis. *Am J Emerg Med*. 1994;12(1):43–45.

119. Druteika D, Zed PJ. Cardiotoxicity following bupropion overdose. *Ann Pharmacother*. 2002;36(11):1791–1795.

120. Paris PA, Saucier JR. ECG conduction delays associated with massive bupropion overdose. *J Toxicol Clin Toxicol*. 1998;36(6):595–598.

121. Wills B, Zell-Kanter M, Aks S. QRS prolongation associated with bupropion ingestion. *J Toxicol Clin Toxicol*. 2004;42(5):724.

122. Hedges D, Jeppson K, Whitehead P. Antipsychotic medication and seizures: a review. *Drugs Today (Barc)*. 2003;39(7):551–557.

123. Lee JW, Crismon ML, Dorson PG. Seizure associated with olanzapine. *Ann Pharmacother*. 1999;33(5):554–556.

124. Amann BL, Pogarell O, Mergl R, et al. EEG abnormalities associated with antipsychotics: a comparison of quetiapine, olanzapine, haloperidol and healthy subjects. *Hum Psychopharmacol*. 2003;18(8):641–646.

125. Lennestal R, Asplund C, Nilsson M, Lakso HA, Mjorndal T, Hagg S. Serum levels of olanzapine in a non-fatal overdose. *J Anal Toxicol*. 2007;31(2):119–121.

126. Timmer RT, Sands JM. Lithium intoxication. *J Am Soc Nephrol*. 1999;10(3):666–674.

127. Kores B, Lader MH. Irreversible lithium neurotoxicity: an overview. *Clin Neuropharmacol*. 1997;20(4):283–299.

128. Perucca E, Gram L, Avanzini G, Dulac O. Antiepileptic drugs as a cause of worsening seizures. *Epilepsia*. 1998;39(1):5–17.

129. Spiller HA, Carlisle RD. Status epilepticus after massive carbamazepine overdose. *J Toxicol Clin Toxicol*. 2002;40(1):81–90.

130. Hirsch E, Genton P. Antiepileptic drug-induced pharmacodynamic aggravation of seizures: does valproate have a lower potential? *CNS Drugs*. 2003;17(9):633–640.

131. Sztajnkrycer MD. Valproic acid toxicity: overview and management. *J Toxicol Clin Toxicol*. 2002;40(6):789–801.

132. Trinka E, Dilitz E, Unterberger I, et al. Nonconvulsive status epilepticus after replacement of valproate with lamotrigine. *J Neurol*. 2002;249(10):1417–1422.

133. Guerrini R, Belmonte A, Parmeggiani L, Perucca E. Myoclonic status epilepticus following high-dosage lamotrigine therapy. *Brain Dev*. 1999;21(6):420–424.

134. Schwartz MD, Geller RJ. Seizures and altered mental status after lamotrigine overdose. *Ther Drug Monit*. 2007;29(6):843–844.

135. Dinnerstein E, Jobst BC, Williamson PD. Lamotrigine intoxication provoking status epilepticus in an adult with localization-related epilepsy. *Arch Neurol*. 2007;64(9):1344–1346.

136. Thundiyil JG, Anderson IB, Stewart PJ, Olson KR. Lamotrigine-induced seizures in a child: case report and literature review. *Clin Toxicol (Phila)*. 2007;45(2):169–172.

137. Braga AJ, Chidley K. Self-poisoning with lamotrigine and pregabalin. *Anaesthesia*. 2007;62(5):524–527.

138. Buckley NA, Whyte IM, Dawson AH. Self-poisoning with lamotrigine. *Lancet*. 1993;342(8886–8887):1552–1553.

139. Herold TJ. Lamotrigine as a possible cause of QRS prolongation in a patient with known seizure disorder. *CJEM*. 2006;8(5):361–364.

140. Anand JS, Chodorowski Z, Wisniewski M. Seizures induced by topiramate overdose. *Clin Toxicol (Phila)*. 2007;45(2):197.

141. Fakhoury T, Murray L, Seger D, McLean M, Abou-Khalil B. Topiramate overdose: clinical and laboratory features. *Epilepsy Behav*. 2002;3(2):185–189.

142. Spiller HA, Winter ML, Ryan M, et al. Retrospective evaluation of tiagabine overdose. *Clin Toxicol (Phila)*. 2005;43(7):855–859.

143. Kazzi ZN, Jones CC, Morgan BW. Seizures in a pediatric patient with a tiagabine overdose. *J Med Toxicol*. 2006;2(4):160–162.

144. Fulton JA, Hoffman RS, Nelson LS. Tiagabine overdose: a case of status epilepticus in a non-epileptic patient. *Clin Toxicol (Phila)*. 2005;43(7):869–871.

145. Michelot D, Toth B. Poisoning by *Gyromitra esculenta*: a review. *J Appl Toxicol*. 1991;11(4):235–243.

146. Karlson-Stiber C, Persson H. Cytotoxic fungi: an overview. *Toxicon*. 2003;42(4):339–349.

147. Maw G, Aitken P. Isoniazid overdose: a case series, literature review and survey of antidote availability. *Clin Drug Investig*. 2003;23(7):479–485.

148. Brent J, Vo N, Kulig K, Rumack BH. Reversal of prolonged isoniazid-induced coma by pyridoxine. *Arch Intern Med*. 1990;150(8):1751–1753.

149. Alvarez FG, Guntupalli KK. Isoniazid overdose: four case reports and review of the literature. *Intensive Care Med*. 1995;21(8):641–644.

150. Dyer S. Plant exposures: wilderness medicine. *Emerg Med Clin North Am*. 2004;22(2):299–313, vii.

151. Centers for Disease Control and Prevention. Water hemlock poisoning: Maine, 1992. *JAMA*. 1994;271(19):1475.

152. Heath KB. A fatal case of apparent water hemlock poisoning. *Vet Hum Toxicol*. 2001;43(1):35–36.

153. Wolf LR, Otten EJ, Spadafora MP. Cinchonism: two case reports and review of acute quinine toxicity and treatment. *J Emerg Med*. 1992;10(3):295–301.

154. Nordt SP, Clark RF. Acute blindness after severe quinine poisoning. *Am J Emerg Med*. 1998;16(2):214–215.

155. Hall AP, Williams SC, Rajkumar KN, Galloway NR. Quinine-induced blindness. *Br J Ophthalmol*. 1997;81(12):1029.

156. Erickson TB, Thompson TM, Lu JJ. The approach to the patient with an unknown overdose. *Emerg Med Clin North Am*. 2007;25(2):249–281; abstract, vii.

157. O'Malley GF. Emergency department management of the salicylate-poisoned patient. *Emerg Med Clin North Am.* 2007;25(2):333–346; abstract, viii.

158. Proudfoot AT, Krenzelok EP, Vale JA. Position paper on urine alkalinization. *J Toxicol Clin Toxicol.* 2004;42(1):1–26.

159. Earnest MP. Seizures. *Neurol Clin.* 1993;11(3):563–575.

160. Franson KL, Hay DP, Neppe V, et al. Drug-induced seizures in the elderly: causative agents and optimal management. *Drugs Aging.* 1995;7(1):38–48.

161. Garcia PA, Alldredge BK. Drug-induced seizures. *Neurol Clin.* 1994;12(1):85–99.

162. Olson KR, Kearney TE, Dyer JE, Benowitz NL, Blanc PD. Seizures associated with poisoning and drug overdose. *Am J Emerg Med.* 1994;12(3):392–395.

163. Wannamaker BB, Booker HE. *Epilepsy: A Comprehensive Textbook.* Philadelphia: Lippincott-Raven; 1997.

164. Gaitanis JN, Drislane FW. Status epilepticus: a review of different syndromes, their current evaluation, and treatment. *Neurologist.* 2003;9(2):61–76.

165. Lowenstein DH, Alldredge BK. Status epilepticus. *N Engl J Med.* 1998;338(14):970–976.

166. Claassen J, Lokin JK, Fitzsimmons BF, Mendelsohn FA, Mayer SA. Predictors of functional disability and mortality after status epilepticus. *Neurology.* 2002;58(1):139–142.

167. DeLorenzo RJ, Hauser WA, Towne AR, et al. A prospective, population-based epidemiologic study of status epilepticus in Richmond, Virginia. *Neurology.* 1996;46(4):1029–1035.

168. Logroscino G, Hesdorffer DC, Cascino G, Annegers JF, Hauser WA. Time trends in incidence, mortality, and case fatality after first episode of status epilepticus. *Epilepsia.* 2001;42(8):1031–1035.

169. Claassen J, Hirsch LJ, Emerson RG, Mayer SA. Treatment of refractory status epilepticus with pentobarbital, propofol, or midazolam: a systematic review. *Epilepsia.* 2002;43(2):146–153.

170. Wallace KL. Antibiotic-induced convulsions. *Crit Care Clin.* 1997;13(4):741–762.

171. Wills B, Erickson T. Chemically induced seizures. *Clin Lab Med.* 2006;26(1):185–209, ix.

172. Curry SC, Mills KC, Ruha AM. *Goldfrank's Toxicologic Emergencies.* 8th ed. New York: McGraw-Hill; 2006.

173. Macdonald RL, McLean MJ. Anticonvulsant drugs: mechanisms of action. *Adv Neurol.* 1986;44:713–736.

174. Morrell MJ. Antiepileptic medications for the treatment of epilepsy. *Semin Neurol.* 2002;22(3):247–258.

175. Chiulli DA, Terndrup TE, Kanter RK. The influence of diazepam or lorazepam on the frequency of endotracheal intubation in childhood status epilepticus. *J Emerg Med.* 1991;9(1–2):13–17.

176. Leppik IE, Derivan AT, Homan RW, Walker J, Ramsay RE, Patrick B. Double-blind study of lorazepam and diazepam in status epilepticus. *JAMA.* 18 1983;249(11):1452–1454.

177. Treiman DM, Meyers PD, Walton NY, et al. A comparison of four treatments for generalized convulsive status epilepticus: Veterans Affairs Status Epilepticus Cooperative Study Group. *N Engl J Med.* 1998;339(12):792–798.

178. De Deyn PP, D'Hooge R, Marescau B, Pei YQ. Chemical models of epilepsy with some reference to their applicability in the development of anticonvulsants. *Epilepsy Res.* 1992;12(2):87–110.

179. Fisher RS. Animal models of the epilepsies. *Brain Res Brain Res Rev.* 1989;14(3):245–278.

180. Shannon M, McElroy EA, Liebelt EL. Toxic seizures in children: case scenarios and treatment strategies. *Pediatr Emerg Care.* 2003;19(3):206–210.

181. Meierkord H, Boon P, Engelsen B, et al. EFNS guideline on the management of status epilepticus. *Eur J Neurol.* 2006;13(5):445–450.

182. Chin L, Sievers ML, Laird HE, Herrier RN, Picchioni AL. Evaluation of diazepam and pyridoxine as antidotes to isoniazid intoxication in rats and dogs. *Toxicol Appl Pharmacol.* 1978;45(3):713–722.

183. Miller J, Robinson A, Percy AK. Acute isoniazid poisoning in childhood. *Am J Dis Child.* 1980;134(3):290–292.

184. Morrow LE, Wear RE, Schuller D, Malesker M. Acute isoniazid toxicity and the need for adequate pyridoxine supplies. *Pharmacotherapy.* 2006;26(10):1529–1532.

185. Antoniadis A, Muller WE, Wollert U. Benzodiazepine receptor interactions may be involved in the neurotoxicity of various penicillin derivatives. *Ann Neurol.* 1980;8(1):71–73.

186. Gerald MC, Massey J, Spadaro DC. Comparative convulsant activity of various penicillins after intracerebral injection in mice. *J Pharm Pharmacol.* 1973;25(2):104–108.

187. DeToledo JC. Lidocaine and seizures. *Ther Drug Monit.* 2000;22(3):320–322.

188. DeToledo JC, Minagar A, Lowe MR. Lidocaine-induced seizures in patients with history of epilepsy: effect of antiepileptic drugs. *Anesthesiology.* 2002;97(3):737–739.

189. Sawaki K, Ohno K, Miyamoto K, Hirai S, Yazaki K, Kawaguchi M. Effects of anticonvulsants on local anaesthetic–induced neurotoxicity in rats. *Pharmacol Toxicol.* 2000;86(2):59–62.

190. Modica PA, Tempelhoff R, White PF. Pro- and anticonvulsant effects of anesthetics (Part I). *Anesth Analg.* 1990;70(3):303–315.

191. Commission on Classification and Terminology of the International League Against Epilepsy. Proposal for revised clinical and electroencephalographic classification of epileptic seizures. *Epilepsia.* 1981;22(4):489–501.

192. Bahls FH, Ma KK, Bird TD. Theophylline-associated seizures with "therapeutic" or low toxic serum concentrations: risk factors for serious outcome in adults. *Neurology.* 1991;41(8):1309–1312.

193. Blake KV, Massey KL, Hendeles L, Nickerson D, Neims A. Relative efficacy of phenytoin and phenobarbital for the prevention of theophylline-induced seizures in mice. *Ann Emerg Med.* 1988;17(10):1024–1028.

194. Hoffman A, Pinto E, Gilhar D. Effect of pretreatment with anticonvulsants on theophylline-induced seizures in the rat. *J Crit Care.* 1993;8(4):198–202.

195. Sugimoto T, Sugimoto M, Uchida I, Mashimo T, Okada S. Inhibitory effect of theophylline on recombinant $GABA_A$ receptor. *Neuroreport.* 2001;12(3):489–493.

196. Yoshikawa H. First-line therapy for theophylline-associated seizures. *Acta Neurol Scand Suppl.* 2007;186:57–61.

197. Derlet RW, Albertson TE. Anticonvulsant modification of cocaine-induced toxicity in the rat. *Neuropharmacology.* 1990;29(3):255–259.

198. Lason W. Neurochemical and pharmacological aspects of cocaine-induced seizures. *Pol J Pharmacol.* 2001;53(1):57–60.

199. Smith PE, McBride A. Illicit drugs and seizures. *Seizure.* 1999;8(8):441–443.

200. Callaham M, Schumaker H, Pentel P. Phenytoin prophylaxis of cardiotoxicity in experimental amitriptyline poisoning. *J Pharmacol Exp Ther.* 1988;245(1):216–220.

201. Citak A, Soysal DD, Ucsel R, Karabocuoglu M, Uzel N. Seizures associated with poisoning in children: tricyclic antidepressant intoxication. *Pediatr Int.* 2006;48(6):582–585.

202. Misra UK, Kalita J, Patel R. Sodium valproate vs phenytoin in status epilepticus: a pilot study. *Neurology.* 2006;67(2):340–342.

203. Trinka E. The use of valproate and new epileptic drugs in status epilepticus. *Epilepsia.* 2007;48 (Suppl 8):49–51.

204. Limdi NA, Shimpi AV, Faught E, Gomez CR, Burneo JG. Efficacy of rapid IV administration of valproic acid for status epilepticus. *Neurology.* 2005;64(2):353–355.

205. Peters CN, Pohlmann-Eden B. Intravenous valproate as an innovative therapy in seizure emergency situations including status epilepticus: experience in 102 adult patients. *Seizure*. 2005;14(3):164–169.

206. Kumar P, Vallis CJ, Hall CM. Intravenous valproate associated with circulatory collapse. *Ann Pharmacother*. 2003;37(12):1797–1799.

207. Sinha S, Naritoku DK. Intravenous valproate is well tolerated in unstable patients with status epilepticus. *Neurology*. 2000;55(5):722–724.

208. White JR, Santos CS. Intravenous valproate associated with significant hypotension in the treatment of status epilepticus. *J Child Neurol*. 1999;14(12):822–823.

209. Martin E, Pozo M. Valproate suppresses status epilepticus induced by 4-aminopyridine in CA1 hippocampus region. *Epilepsia*. 2003;44(11):1375–1379.

210. Bazil CW, Pedley TA. Clinical pharmacology of antiepileptic drugs. *Clin Neuropharmacol*. 2003;26(1):38–52.

211. Farooq MU, Naravetla B, Majid A, Gupta R, Pysh JJ, Kassab MY. IV levetiracetam in the management of non-convulsive status epilepticus. *Neurocrit Care*. 2007;7(1):36–39.

212. Rossetti AO, Bromfield EB. Levetiracetam in the treatment of status epilepticus in adults: a study of 13 episodes. *Eur Neurol*. 2005;54(1):34–38.

213. Ramael S, Daoust A, Otoul C, et al. Levetiracetam intravenous infusion: a randomized, placebo-controlled safety and pharma-cokinetic study. *Epilepsia*. 2006;47(7):1128–1135.

214. Lowenstein DH, Alldredge BK. Status epilepticus at an urban pub-lic hospital in the 1980s. *Neurology*. 1993;43(3 Pt 1):483–488.

215. DeLorenzo RJ, Garnett LK, Towne AR, et al. Comparison of status epilepticus with prolonged seizure episodes lasting from 10 to 29 minutes. *Epilepsia*. 1999;40(2):164–169.

216. Towne AR, Pellock JM, Ko D, DeLorenzo RJ. Determinants of mortality in status epilepticus. *Epilepsia*. 1994;35(1):27–34.

217. Fountain NB, Adams RE. Midazolam treatment of acute and refractory status epilepticus. *Clin Neuropharmacol*. 1999;22(5):261–267.

218. Rossetti AO, Reichhart MD, Schaller MD, Despland PA, Bogousslavsky J. Propofol treatment of refractory status epilepticus: a study of 31 episodes. *Epilepsia*. 2004;45(7):757–763.

219. Heavner JE, Arthur J, Zou J, McDaniel K, Tyman-Szram B, Rosenberg PH. Comparison of propofol with thiopentone for treatment of bupivacaine-induced seizures in rats. *Br J Anaesth*. 1993;71(5):715–719.

220. Momota Y, Artru AA, Powers KM, Mautz DS, Ueda Y. Posttreatment with propofol terminates lidocaine-induced epileptiform electroencephalogram activity in rabbits: effects on cerebrospinal fluid dynamics. *Anesth Analg*. 1998;87(4):900–906.

221. Peterson S, Purvis R, Griffith J. Propofol inhibition of lithium–pilocarpine–induced status epilepticus. *Epilepsia*. 2002;43 (Suppl 7):19.

222. Valiensi S, Martinez O, Reisin R, Granillo R, Christiansen S, Sottaro F. Effects of treatment with propofol with rats with pilocarpine-induced status epilepticus. *Epilepsia*. 2006;47 (Suppl 4):315.

223. Robakis TK, Hirsch LJ. Literature review, case report, and expert discussion of prolonged refractory status epilepticus. *Neurocrit Care*. 2006;4(1):35–46.

224. Sheth RD, Gidal BE. Refractory status epilepticus: response to ketamine. *Neurology*. 1998;51(6):1765–1766.

225. Hurley D. Ketamine plus diazepam reported to be neuroprotective against status epilepticus after nerve agent exposure. *Neurol Today*. 2007;7(13):19–20.

226. Schneider PG, Rodriguez de Lores AG. Bicuculline-induced seizures and muscarinic receptor changes are prevented by ketamine pretreatment. *J Neurochem*. 1999;73(Suppl):S180.

227. Harvey M, Cave G. Intralipid outperforms sodium bicarbonate in a rabbit model of clomipramine toxicity. *Ann Emerg Med*. 2007;49(2):178–185, 185.e1–4.

228. Picard J, Meek T, Weinberg G, Hertz P. Lipid emulsion for local anaesthetic toxicity. *Anaesthesia*. 2006;61(11):1116–1117.

229. Sirianni AJ, Osterhoudt KC, Calello DP, et al. Use of lipid emulsion in the resuscitation of a patient with prolonged cardiovascular collapse after overdose of bupropion and lamotrigine. *Ann Emerg Med*. 2008;51(4):412–415.

Toxic Causes of Stroke

Anand G. Vaishnav

INTRODUCTION

Stroke is defined as acute onset of focal neurological deficit caused by loss of vascular blood supply (ischemia) or rupture of blood vessels (hemorrhage). Stroke is the third leading cause of death in United States[1] and a leading cause of disability. Approximately 20% of survivors require institutional care after 3 months, and 15% to 30% are permanently disabled. It is estimated that there are approximately 700,000 strokes a year in United States.[2]

Ischemic Strokes

The majority (80%) of strokes are ischemic in nature, and effective prevention remains the best treatment. Prevention of stroke specifically targets modifiable risk factors such as hypertension, exposure to cigarette smoke, diabetes, atrial fibrillation, dyslipidemia, carotid artery stenosis, sickle cell disease, poor diet, physical inactivity, obesity, and alcohol abuse.[3]

Ischemic stroke is classified in several ways. One of the most popular classification systems, known as the TOAST classification, is based on the cause of stroke.[4] The TOAST classification defines five subtypes of ischemic stroke: (1) large-artery atherosclerosis, (2) cardioembolism, (3) small-vessel occlusion, (4) stroke of other determined etiology, and (5) stroke of undetermined etiology. Treatment for secondary stroke prevention is directed at risk factors and the cause of stroke according to the TOAST criteria. Toxic causes of stroke are classified as "stroke of other determined etiology."

Hemorrhagic Strokes

Hemorrhagic strokes are classified as intracerebral hemorrhage (ICH) and subarachnoid hemorrhage (SAH). Trauma and hypertension (uncontrolled sudden surge in blood pressure) are the most common causes of ICH. Rupture of an aneurysm is the most common cause of SAH.

Toxic Causes of Stroke

Toxic causes of stroke are rare because the central nervous system (CNS) is protected by the blood–brain barrier.[5] Furthermore, stroke is an acute event. In most cases, it is extremely difficult to identify a causal relationship between the exposure (a toxin) and the subsequent event (stroke) in an acute setting, especially in a disease that has multiple risk factors.

The most common toxic cause of stroke is substance abuse. The relationship between substance abuse and stroke is the main focus of this chapter. We make brief mention of other rare causes of stroke, such as infections, chemical agents, and snake venom. The chapter emphasizes toxic causes and not risk factors of stroke, such as cigarette smoking and heavy alcohol use. We have excluded global causes of ischemia, such as hypoxic ischemic encephalopathy and posterior reversible leukoencephalopathy syndrome, because they are not "focal" and do not fall under the classification of stroke.

Strokes from toxic causes usually occur in young populations, which have a higher proportion of illegal drug use and a lower instance of other traditional stroke risk factors. In populations younger than 50 years old, drug use may be noted in 12% to 34% of strokes.[6–9] Table 1 summarizes the toxic causes of stroke. Cocaine, amphetamines, and opiates are the most common causes of stroke. For practical purposes, we have classified toxic causes of stroke as common toxic causes of stroke, uncommon toxic causes of stroke, and miscellaneous toxic causes of stroke.

SUBSTANCE ABUSE AND MECHANISM OF ACTION

The mechanisms by which various substances produce strokes may be explained by their pharmacological effects on neurotransmitters.[10] Most act on plasma catecholamines. Amphetamines and over-the-counter sympathomimetics increase catecholamine release from central noradrenergic nerve terminals. Cocaine and phencyclidine (PCP) block reuptake of catecholamines

into nerve terminals. With the exception of opiates and lysergic acid diethylamide (LSD), all drugs of interest may produce mild to profound blood pressure elevation and heart rhythm disturbances. Cocaine and ethanol (more a risk factor of stroke when consumed in large amounts) also enhance platelet aggregability. Other known mechanisms include vasospasm, vasoconstriction, vasculitis, microaneurysm, and small- and large-vessel occlusions. Of importance is that in most cases either polydrug use or incomplete data prevent assigning cause and effect to a particular agent. Tables 2 and 3 summarize the major mechanisms of ischemic and hemorrhagic strokes caused by various agents.

CLINICAL PRESENTATION AND DIAGNOSIS

Most strokes caused by substance abuse and other toxins occur in a younger age group with significant male predominance.[10] Most of the men are in their second to fourth decades of life, and their presentation does not differ from other types of stroke: acute focal neurological deficits (numbness, weakness, speech difficulty, vertigo, double vision, loss of vision) and sometimes a severe headache. In cases of hemorrhage, headache occurs with or without focal neurological symptoms. Seizures or coma are rare. Symptoms may occur in the background of chronic drug abuse, overdose, or reexposure after prolonged abstinence. However, in most cases, symptoms occur either during or shortly after drug use by any route of administration. Symptoms may manifest within minutes or as long as 48 hours after drug use, with a strong association with drug use less than 6 hours before symptom onset.[6] It is important to note that in some cases blood pressure may be elevated, and cardiac arrhythmias are not uncommon. Physical stigmata such

Table 1: Toxic Causes of Stroke
COMMON CAUSES (SUBSTANCE ABUSE)
• Cocaine
• Opiates
• Amphetamines and associated stimulants
UNCOMMON CAUSES (SUBSTANCE ABUSE)
• Lysergic acid diethylamide
• Phencyclidine
• Sedatives
• Marijuana
MISCELLANEOUS CAUSES
• Central nervous system infections
• Snake venoms
• Inhalants

Table 2: Major Mechanisms of Ischemic Stroke	
• Vasoconstriction	Cocaine, amphetamines, LSD, PCP
• Embolism	Amphetamines, opiates, cocaine, CNS infections
• Vasculitis or arteritis	Cocaine, amphetamines, opiates, LSD, sedatives, CNS infections
• Enhancing coagulation	Cocaine

CNS, central nervous system; LSD, lysergic acid diethylamide; PCP, phencyclidine.

Table 3: Major Mechanisms of Cerebral Hemorrhage

• Hypertension	Cocaine, amphetamines, PCP
• Unmasking structural lesions	Cocaine, opiates
• Endocarditis	Cocaine, amphetamines
• Vasculitis	Cocaine, amphetamines, opiates, CNS infections
• Coagulopathy	Opiates, CNS infections, snake venoms

CNS, central nervous system; PCP, phencyclidine.

as needle marks, nasal septal perforations, or signs of infective endocarditis may be seen.[11]

There is a high index of suspicion for drug abuse in a stroke patient under 45 years of age in the absence of traditional stroke risk factors. History should be obtained not only from the patient but also from family members and relatives. A febrile illness, multiple sexual exposure, or travel history may indicate infection. The clinician should look out for physical stigmata that can heighten suspicion.

All patients should have urine and blood screens, and in select cases gastric juice analysis should be performed. Polydrug abuse is not uncommon. Workup to confirm the diagnosis is like that of any other stroke patient. A computerized tomography (CT) scan and magnetic resonance imaging (MRI) can visualize a stroke in most cases. Carotid duplex and transcranial duplex are done to rule out large-vessel atherosclerosis. Echocardiogram and electrocardiogram can detect cardioembolic cause and arrhythmias respectively. CT angiogram and MRI angiogram can help define vascular stenosis (narrowing), and cerebral angiogram is used in select cases to confirm the degree of stenosis or occlusion and to rule out vasculitis and aneurysms in cases with hemorrhage. In intravenous drug users, human immunodeficiency virus (HIV) testing should be considered. A brain biopsy may be needed in rare cases with evidence of vasculitis.

COMMON TOXIC CAUSES OF STROKE

Cocaine

Cocaine, a natural alkaloid, is extracted from leaves of an Andean shrub, *Erythroxylon coca*. It has been sold on the streets for many years as a water-soluble hydrochloride salt for nasal insufflation (snorting) or intravenous injection. It may be injected subcutaneously or intramuscularly, but these routes rarely are used because vasoconstriction slows absorption, and the drug is less likely to cause a "rush."[12]

Cocaine is a sympathomimetic agent that blocks reuptake of catecholamines into nerve terminals.[10] By blocking presynaptic reuptake of the neurotransmitters norepinephrine and dopamine, cocaine increases the quantity of neurotransmitters at the postsynaptic receptor sites. This reduction causes an acute rise in arterial pressure, tachycardia, and, besides stroke, can cause a predisposition to ventricular arrhythmias and seizures. There are approximately 2 million cocaine users in the United States, and since 1983, when the use of free-base cocaine known as crack was introduced, the number of cocaine-related strokes has increased constantly.[13–17] Westover et al. showed in a recent epidemiological study that cocaine users had twice the odds of experiencing from both hemorrhagic and ischemic stroke, accounting for all other risk factors of stroke.[18]

As stated earlier, cocaine can be taken intranasally, intravenously, or intramuscularly or it can be smoked as crack. It is striking that there is a high frequency of underlying aneurysm or vascular malformation in hemorrhagic strokes in cocaine users.[19] Cocaine hydrochloride is more often associated with hemorrhagic than occlusive stroke, whereas crack users experience hemorrhagic and occlusive strokes with roughly equal frequency.[20]

Parenteral cocaine users are at risk for stroke related to infection, including infective endocarditis, acquired immunodeficiency syndrome (AIDS), and hepatitis. In addition, cocaine-associated ischemic strokes are caused by vasoconstriction and disruption of cerebrovascular autoregulation in the presence of increased blood pressure.[10] Vasculitis as a cause of stroke is less common among cocaine users than among amphetamine users.[19] Cocaine-associated ischemic strokes have occurred in pregnant women and shortly after delivery in newborns whose mothers used cocaine.[14,21]

Brain hemorrhage usually occurs during or within hours of cocaine use, although delayed hemorrhages are also noted.[22,23] Nearly half of patients with cocaine-associated intracranial hemorrhage had saccular aneurysms or vascular malformation.[24] Parenchymal hemorrhages have been located in the cerebrum, brainstem, and cerebellum. There have been case reports of hemorrhages associated with superior sagittal sinus thrombosis, mycotic aneurysm rupture, dural arteriovenous fistula, and bleeding into embolic infarction or glioma.[25–27]

Opiates

Opiates are a common toxic cause of stroke. Heroin is the most widely used opiate. It can cause both ischemic and hemorrhagic strokes. Heroin is usually taken parenterally, and more than 2 million Americans have consumed heroin, with at least 1 million having a physical or psychical dependence.[28,29]

Infective endocarditis is common in heroin addicts because it is taken parenterally.[30–32] Strokes from infective endocarditis can be either ischemic or hemorrhagic. The most common mechanism for ischemic stroke is embolism after rupture of a septic (mycotic) aneurysm. The aortic, mitral, and tricuspid valves are usually affected by infective endocarditis, with *Staphylococcus aureus* and *Candida* being the most common sources of infection.[33]

Besides ischemic stroke caused by embolism secondary to infective endocarditis, there have been case reports of both large- and small-vessel arteritis, and a case has been reported in which small arteritis was associated with eosinophilia, serum hypergammaglobulinemia, and a positive Coombs test result.[10,34] There have also been cases of hypoxic ischemic encephalopathy, which suggests hypoventilation and hypotension produced by heroin.[35] While embolization of foreign material to the brain has not been reported with heroin, it has been reported at autopsy in abusers of other agents, including opiates. Pentazocine and tripelennamine were widely used in Midwestern cities in the 1970s. Tablets were crushed, suspended in water, passed through cotton or a cigarette filter, and injected intravenously. Cerebral infarct and hemorrhages were noted among users of these drugs.[36,37] Autopsies revealed talc and cellulose crystals in both pulmonary and cerebral vessels, and cerebral angiogram revealed a "beading" appearance, suggesting multiple emboli and vasculitic reaction to foreign material.[38–41] Rare cases of heroin abuse causing myelopathy have also been reported.[42,43]

Opiate-associated cerebral hemorrhage or SAH occurs after rupture of a septic aneurysm.[44–46] Patients with septic aneurysm present with insidious onset of neurological symptoms or progressive neurological symptoms. Such cases are unlike traditional SAH cases by rupture of berry aneurysm, where onset is sudden.[47] Septic aneurysm is associated with high mortality, and antibiotic therapy is rarely effective. These aneurysms can be surgically excised relatively successfully; thus, in patients with endocarditis, cerebral angiogram should be performed and mycotic aneurysm should be excised.[48] Heroin users can also have hemorrhagic strokes secondary to liver failure, hepatitis, and deranged clotting or secondary to heroin nephropathy with uremia or malignant hypertension.[10]

Amphetamines and Associated Stimulants

Amphetamines and associated stimulants can cause both hemorrhagic and ischemic strokes. Dextroamphetamine and methamphetamine are both abused intravenously. Overdose usually causes excitement, fever, and hypertension, which can be followed by coma, vascular collapse, and death.[49–51] Stroke cases are rare, with hemorrhages more common then ischemic strokes. The routes of amphetamine administration may be ingestion (oral), inhalation (smoke), or injection (intravenous). Oral use is associated with an approximately 1-hour lag time before onset of symptoms, whereas inhaled and intravenous methods yield effects within a few minutes.

There are numerous case reports of hemorrhages caused by amphetamine; most cases have been secondary to acute hypertension. Some cases related to cerebral vasculitis have also been noted.[52–56] Most cases occurred among chronic users of amphetamine, and most involved abuse of methamphetamine or dextroamphetamine; rare cases have been reported among users of pseudoephedrine and diethyproprion. Hemorrhages were both intracerebral and subarachnoid. In severe cases, cerebral angiogram showed a beading appearance suggestive of vasculitis.

Ischemic stroke secondary to amphetamine use has been most commonly associated with cerebral vasculitis; a few cases of multiple emboli have also been reported. In one report of polydrug abuse (amphetamine was used in all but two of the cases), necrotizing vasculitis similar to polyarteritis nodosa was noted.[57]

Phenylpropanolamine (PPA) was marketed in over-the-counter decongestants and diet pills. Users experienced acute hypertension, psychiatric symptoms, seizures, and hemorrhagic stroke.[58–61] There was also a reported case of cerebral arteritis causing ischemic stroke in a PPA user.[62] A large case–control study involving 43 U.S. hospitals found that appetite suppressants containing PPA increased the risk of SAH and ICH in women (OR, 16.58).[63] This finding led the U.S. Food and Drug Administration (FDA) to withdraw products containing PPA from the market.[64] While numerous case studies and case reports suggest an association between sympathomimetic cold remedies and stroke, controls were conspicuously lacking. A study comparing sympathomimetics containing PPA and other sympathomimetics would be ideal; however, with an FDA ban, such a study is unlikely to be undertaken.

Ephedrine and pseudoephedrine are present in over-the-counter decongestants and bronchodilators, and they have been associated with both ischemic and hemorrhagic stroke.[65–67] Ischemic and hemorrhagic strokes have also been reported with dietary supplements containing ephedra alkaloids,[68] and ischemic stroke has been reported with anorexiant phentermine and phendimetrazine.[69] Hemorrhagic stroke has been reported in association with the dietary supplements fenfluramine and phentermine.[70] A cohort study of subjects taking appetite suppressants found that dexfenfluramine, fenfluramine, and phentermine increased the risk of stroke (OR, 2.4).[71]

Ischemic stroke has also been reported with the use of 3,4-methylenedioxymethamphetamine (Ecstasy) and crushed methylphenidate.[72,73]

UNCOMMON TOXIC CAUSES OF STROKE

Lysergic Acid Diethylamide

LSD is an hallucinogen. Chemically, it is an ergot that can cause severe hypertension and lead to convulsions and coma.[74] Cases of ischemic stroke caused by use of LSD have been reported.[74,75] They can occur several days after ingestion of LSD, and cerebral angiogram has shown evidence of both a stenotic or occlusive disease and an intracranial vasculitic pattern (beading appearance). LSD is an uncommon toxic cause of stroke. Rare cases secondary to polydrug use (along with heroin) have been reported.[76,77]

Phencyclidine

PCP ("angel dust") can be smoked, eaten, or injected. It seems that a sudden increase in blood pressure is more likely, since case reports of stroke in PCP users have been mostly hemorrhages.[78,79] It blocks reuptake of catecholamines, causing increased blood pressure and vasoconstriction leading to both hemorrhagic and ischemic stroke.[80] It is important to note that hypertension can occur both early and late during intoxication.[81,82] A case of hypertensive encephalopathy has also been reported in a young woman with systemic lupus erythematosis who had consumed PCP and had a history of migraine.[83]

Sedatives

No cases have been reported of stroke exclusively related to use of sedatives (barbiturates, benzodiazepines); however, cases have occurred in association with use of other agents for which the underlying cause was cerebral vasculitis.[77,84] A single case of cerebral vasculitis in a barbiturate abuser has been reported; however, limited information was available on the amount and route of barbiturate consumed.[77] Sedatives usually cause hypotension-related global ischemic brain (hypoxic ischemic encephalopathy) but not focal (strokelike) symptoms.

Marijuana

While strokes have occurred in patients using marijuana, there is no evidence to suggest causality.[85,86] Marijuana is the illicit drug most widely used in the United States. There have been strokes in marijuana users; however, they had associated risk factors.[85,86] Thus, there is no clear cut evidence of marijuana causing strokes.

MISCELLANEOUS TOXIC CAUSES OF STROKE

Central Nervous System Infections

Strokes caused by CNS infections are secondary to complications of meningitis. There is inflammation of both large arteries and small perforating arteries secondary to local spread of infection to the vessel walls. Neurosyphilis, neurotuberculosis, and neurobrucellosis are common causes both in the presence and in the absence of AIDS caused by HIV infection. There is specifically an increase in both neurosyphilis and neurotuberculosis secondary to the AIDS epidemic.[87,88] Cerebrospinal fluid examination is usually diagnostic, and treatment is directed toward the underlying infection.

Ischemic and hemorrhagic strokes are rare but well-recognized complications of HIV infection. A review of 6 clinical and 11 autopsy cases revealed "stroke syndrome" in 1.3% with AIDS-related illnesses—compared to a general population risk of less than 0.1%.[89] Causes of stroke in AIDS patients include cardiac disease (myocarditis and nonbacterial endocarditis), cerebral vasculitis, CNS infection, and coagulopathy in non–drug-abusing, HIV-infected patients.[87,90] Parenteral drug abusers are at risk for infective endocarditis (embolic and rupture of mycotic aneurysm), vasculitis secondary to meningitis, and coagulopathy (hepatitis related) leading to hemorrhages.[87,90]

Tropical diseases cause stroke, mostly in developing countries. Most prevalent conditions causing cerebrovascular disease in the tropics include malaria, Chagas disease, cysticersosis, viral hemorrhagic fevers, gnathostomiasis, leptospirosis, and tuberculosis.[91] These conditions may cause cerebral infarcts or hemorrhages, in most instances related to either vascular damage secondary to angiitis or hemorrhagic diathesis with bleeding in other organs. There are estimated to be 500 million cases of malaria every year. Cerebral malaria can cause cerebral edema, diffuse or focal compromise of the subcortical white matter, and cortical, cerebellar, and pontine infarctions. Chagas disease is an independent risk factor for stroke in South America, where there are about 20 million chronic cases of the disease. Vascular complications of neurocysticercosis include transient ischemic attacks, ischemic strokes due to angiitis, and intracranial hemorrhages. The frequency of cerebral infarction associated with neurocysticercosis varies between 2% and 12%. Less common causes include gnathostomiasis (SAH) and viral hemorrhagic fevers due to arenavirus and flavivirus.

Snake Venom

All venoms of snakes of the Viperidae and Crotalidae families are hemotoxic.[92] A study by Mosquera et al. showed a prevalence of cerebrovascular complications, with stroke related to *Bothrops* spp. bites being 2.6%, the majority of them (7/8) cerebral hemorrhage and one ischemic stroke.[93]

Inhalants

Toluene, which is found in correction fluids, paint thinners, and some nail-polish removers, and trichloethylene, which is found in glues, sealants, and paints, are used to achieve euphoric intoxication. Ischemic strokes have been reported in glue sniffers (trichloethylene) and toluene abusers.[94,95] It is suggested that vasospasm is caused by sensitization of vessel receptors to circulating catecholamines.

CONCLUSION

Toxic causes of stroke are rare. However, a high index of suspicion is required when a young individual presents with stroke in the absence of traditional risk factors. The principles of management do not differ from the guidelines for acute ischemic and hemorrhagic stroke.[96,97] Specific attention should be directed toward sympathomimetic actions of drugs of abuse, such as hypertension and fever. Urinary acidification panels (PCP), urinary alkalization panels (amphetamines), and gastric lavage (PCP) should be performed in select cases. Secondary prevention of ischemic and hemorrhagic stroke is directed toward modifiable risk factors and avoidance of the causative agents.[3,98] Appropriate referral should be made for detoxification services in select cases.

ACKNOWLEDGEMENT

Supported by Building Interdisciplinary Research Careers in Women's Health Training Grant (NIH K-12 DA 14040-06). We thank Sherry Chandler Williams, ELS, for editing the manuscript and preparing the illustration.

REFERENCES

1. Centers for Disease Control and Prevention, Division of Heart Disease and Stroke Prevention. *MMWR Morb Mortal Wkly Rep.* 2008;57(18):481–485.
2. American Heart Association. Heart and Stroke Facts Statistics: 2004 Statistical Supplement. Dallas, American Heart Association, 2004. (http://www.americanheart.org/downloadable/heart/1072969766940HSStats2004Update.pdf)
3. Goldstein LB, Adams R, Alberts MJ, et al. Primary prevention of ischemic stroke: a guideline from the American Heart Association/ American Stroke Association Stroke Council. Co-sponsored by the Atherosclerotic Peripheral Vascular Disease Interdisciplinary Working Group; Cardiovascular Nursing Council; Clinical Cardiology Council; Nutrition, Physical Activity, and Metabolism Council; and the Quality of Care and Outcomes Research Interdisciplinary Working Group. *Stroke.* 2006;37:1583–1633.
4. Adams HP Jr, Bendixen BH, Kappelle LJ, et al. Classification of subtype of acute ischemic stroke: definitions for use in a multicenter clinical trial. TOAST: Trial of Org 1017. in Acute Stroke Treatment. *Stroke.* 1993;24:35–41.
5. Blain PG, Harris JB. *Medical Neurotoxicology: Occupational and Environmental Causes of Neurological Dysfunction.* New York: Oxford University Press; 1999.
6. Kaku DA, Lowenstein DH. Emergence of recreational drug abuse as a major risk factor for stroke in young adults. *Ann Intern Med.* 1990;113:821–827.
7. Sloan MA, Kittner SJ, Rigamonti D, Price TR. Occurrence of stroke associated with use/abuse of drugs. *Neurology.* 1991;41:1358–1364.
8. Sloan MA, Kittner SJ, Feeser BR, et al. Illicit drug-associated ischemic stroke in the Baltimore–Washington Young Stroke Study. *Neurology.* 1998;50:1688–1693.
9. Qureshi AI, Safdar K, Patel M, Janssen RS, Frankel MR. Stroke in young black patients: risk factors, subtypes, and prognosis. *Stroke.* 1995;26:1995–1998.
10. Sloan MA. Illicit drug use/abuse and stroke. In: Ginsberg MD, Bogousslavsky J, eds. *Cerebrovascular Disease: Pathophysiology, Diagnosis and Management.* Cambridge, Ma: Blackwell Science; 1998.
11. Brust JCM. *Neurological Aspects of Substance Abuse.* Boston: Butterworth-Heineman; 1993.
12. Levine SR, Brust JC, Futrell N, et al. Cerebrovascular complications of the use of the "crack" form of alkaloidal cocaine. *N Engl J Med.* 1990;323:699–704.
13. Cregler LL, Mark H. Medical complications of cocaine abuse. *N Engl J Med.* 1986;315:1495–1500.
14. Mody CK, Miller BL, McIntyre HB, Cobb SK, Goldberg MA. Neurologic complications of cocaine abuse. *Neurology.* 1988;38:1189–1193.
15. Golbe LI, Merkin MD. Cerebral infarction in a user of free-base cocaine ("crack"). *Neurology.* 1986;36:1602–1604.
16. Jacobs IG, Roszler MH, Kelly JK, Klein MA, Kling GA. Cocaine abuse: neurovascular complications. *Radiology.* 1989;170:223–227.
17. Klonoff DC, Andrews BT, Obana WG. Stroke associated with cocaine use. *Arch Neurol.* 1989;46:989–993.
18. Westover AN, McBride S, Haley RW. Stroke in young adults who abuse amphetamines or cocaine: a population-based study of hospitalized patients. *Arch Gen Psychiatry.* 2007;64:495–502.
19. Brust JC. Vasculitis owing to substance abuse. *Neurol Clin.* 1997;15:945–957.
20. Levine SR, Brust JC, Futrell N, et al. A comparative study of the cerebrovascular complications of cocaine: alkaloidal versus hydrochloride: a review. *Neurology.* 1991;41:1173–1177.
21. Chasnoff IJ, Bussey ME, Savich R, Stack CM. Perinatal cerebral infarction and maternal cocaine use. *J Pediatr.* 1986;108:456–459.
22. Davis GG, Swalwell CI. The incidence of acute cocaine or methamphetamine intoxication in deaths due to ruptured cerebral (berry) aneurysms. *J Forensic Sci.* 1996;41:626–628.
23. Kibayashi K, Mastri AR, Hirsch CS. Cocaine induced intracerebral hemorrhage: analysis of predisposing factors and mechanisms causing hemorrhagic strokes. *Hum Pathol.* 1995;26:659–663.
24. Simpson RK Jr, Fischer DK, Narayan RK, Cech DA, Robertson CS. Intravenous cocaine abuse and subarachnoid haemorrhage: effect on outcome. *Br J Neurosurg.* 1990;4:27–30.

25. Wojak JC, Flamm ES. Intracranial hemorrhage and cocaine use. *Stroke.* 1987;18:712–715.
26. Brown E, Prager J, Lee HY, Ramsey RG. CNS complications of cocaine abuse: prevalence, pathophysiology, and neuroradiology. *Am J Roentgenol.* 1992;159:137–147.
27. Keller TM, Chappell ET. Spontaneous acute subdural hematoma precipitated by cocaine abuse: case report. *Surg Neurol.* 1997;47:12–14; discussion, 14–15.
28. Halloway M. Rx for addiction. *Sci Am* 1991;264(3):94–103.
29. Kandel DB. Epidemiological trends and implications for understanding the nature of addiction. In: O'Brien CP, Jaffe JH, eds. *Addictive States. Res Publ Assoc Res Nerv Ment Dis* 1992;70:23.
30. Kokkinos J, Levine SR. Stroke. *Neurol Clin.* 1993;11:577–590.
31. Patel AN. Self-inflicted strokes. *Ann Intern Med.* 1972;76:823–824.
32. Brust JC. Stroke and drugs. In: Toole JF (ed): of *Handbook of Clinical Neurology.* rev series 2: Vascular Diseases, part 3. Amsterdam: Elsevier; 1989: p. 517.
33. Tuazon CU, Sheagren JN. Staphylococcal endocarditis in parenteral drug abusers: source of the organism. *Ann Intern Med.* 1975;82:788–790.
34. Brust JC, Richter RW. Stroke associated with addiction to heroin. *J Neurol Neurosurg Psychiatry.* 1976;39:194–199.
35. Ginsberg MD, Hedley-Whyte ET, Richardson EP Jr. Hypoxic-ischemic leukoencephalopathy in man. *Arch Neurol.* 1976;33:5–14.
36. Lahmeyer HW, Steingold RG. Pentazocine and tripelennamine: a drug abuse epidemic? *Int J Addict.* 1980;15:1219–1232.
37. Wadley C, Stillie GD. Pentazocine (Talwin) and tripelennamine (Pyribenzamine): a new drug abuse combination or just a revival? *Int J Addict.* 1980;15:1285–1290.
38. Caplan LR, Hier DB, Banks G. Current concepts of cerebrovascular disease stroke: stroke and drug abuse. *Stroke.* 1982;13:869–872.
39. Caplan LR, Thomas C, Banks G. Central nervous system complications of addiction to "T's and Blues." *Neurology.* 1982;32:623–628.
40. Houck RJ, Bailey GL, Daroca PJ Jr, et al. Pentazocine abuse: report of a case with pulmonary arterial cellulose granulomas and pulmonary hypertension. *Chest.* 1980;77:227–230.
41. Szwed JJ. Pulmonary angiothrombosis caused by "blue velvet" addiction. *Ann Intern Med.* 1970;73:771–774.
42. Lee MC, Randa DC, Gold LH. Transverse myelopathy following the use of heroin. *Minn Med.* 1976;59:82–83.
43. Richter RW, Rosenberg RN. Transverse myelitis associated with heroin addiction. *JAMA.* 1968;206:1255–1257.
44. Amine AR. Neurosurgical complications of heroin addiction: brain abscess and mycotic aneurysm. *Surg Neurol.* 1977;7:385–386.
45. Gilroy J, Andaya L, Thomas VJ. Intracranial mycotic aneurysms and subacute bacterial endocarditis in heroin addiction. *Neurology.* 1973;23:1193–1198.
46. Jara FM, Lewis JF Jr, Magilligan DJ Jr. Operative experience with infective endocarditis and intracerebral mycotic aneurysm. *J Thorac Cardiovasc Surg.* 1980;80:28–30.
47. Brust JC, Dickinson PC, Hughes JE, Holtzman RN. The diagnosis and treatment of cerebral mycotic aneurysms. *Ann Neurol.* 1990;27:238–446.
48. Frazee JG, Cahan LD, Winter J. Bacterial intracranial aneurysms. *J Neurosurg.* 1980;53:633–641.
49. Greenwood R, Peachey RS. Acute amphetamine poisoning; an account of 3 cases. *BMJ.* 1957;1:742–744.
50. Lewis E. Hyperpyrexia with antidepressant drugs. *BMJ.* 1965;1:1671–1672.
51. Zalis EG, Parmley LF Jr. Fatal amphetamine poisoning. *Arch Intern Med.* 1963;112:822–886.
52. Goodman SJ, Becker DP. Intracranial hemorrhage associated with amphetamine abuse. *JAMA.* 1970;212:480.
53. Chynn KY. Acute subarachnoid hemorrhage. *JAMA.* 1975;233:55–56.
54. Cahill DW, Knipp H, Mosser J. Intracranial hemorrhage with amphetamine abuse. *Neurology.* 1981;31:1058–1059.
55. Delaney P, Estes M. Intracranial hemorrhage with amphetamine abuse. *Neurology.* 1980;30:1125–1148.
56. D'Souza T, Shraberg D. Intracranial hemorrhage associated with amphetamine use. *Neurology.* 1981;31:922–923.
57. Citron BP, Halpern M, McCarron M, et al. Necrotizing angiitis associated with drug abuse. *N Engl J Med.* 1970;283:1003–1011.
58. Bernstein E, Diskant BM. Phenylpropanolamine: a potentially hazardous drug. *Ann Emerg Med.* 1982;11:311–315.
59. Forman HP, Levin S, Stewart B, Patel M, Feinstein S. Cerebral vasculitis and hemorrhage in an adolescent taking diet pills containing phenylpropanolamine: case report and review of literature. *Pediatrics.* 1989;83:737–741.
60. Kane FJ Jr, Green BQ. Psychotic episodes associated with the use of common proprietary decongestants. *Am J Psychiatry.* 1966;123:484–487.
61. Mueller SM, Muller J, Asdell SM. Cerebral hemorrhage associated with phenylpropanolamine in combination with caffeine. *Stroke.* 1984;15:119–123.
62. Ryu SJ, Lin SK. Cerebral arteritis associated with oral use of phenylpropanolamine: report of a case. *J Formos Med Assoc.* 1995;94:53–55.
63. Kernan WN, Viscoli CM, Brass LM, et al. Phenylpropanolamine and the risk of hemorrhagic stroke. *N Engl J Med.* 2000;343:1826–1832.
64. Fleming GA. The FDA, regulation, and the risk of stroke. *N Engl J Med.* 2000;343:1886–1887.
65. Pugh CR, Howie SM. Dependence on pseudoephedrine. *Br J Psychiatry.* 1986;149:798.
66. Wooten MR, Khangure MS, Murphy MJ. Intracerebral hemorrhage and vasculitis related to ephedrine abuse. *Ann Neurol.* 1983;13:337–340.
67. Loizou LA, Hamilton JG, Tsementzis SA. Intracranial haemorrhage in association with pseudoephedrine overdose. *J Neurol Neurosurg Psychiatry.* 1982;45:471–472.
68. Haller CA, Benowitz NL. Adverse cardiovascular and central nervous system events associated with dietary supplements containing ephedra alkaloids. *N Engl J Med.* 2000;343:1833–1838.
69. Kokkinos J, Levine SR. Possible association of ischemic stroke with phentermine. *Stroke.* 1993;24:310–313.
70. Wen PY, Feske SK, Teoh SK, Stieg PE. Cerebral hemorrhage in a patient taking fenfluramine and phentermine for obesity. *Neurology.* 1997;49:632–633.
71. Derby LE, Myers MW, and Jick H. Use of dexfenfluramine, fenfluramine and phentermine and the risk of stroke. *Br J Clin Pharmacol.* 1999;47(5):565–569.
72. Manchanda S, Connolly MJ. Cerebral infarction in association with Ecstasy abuse. *Postgrad Med J.* 1993;69:874–875.
73. Chillar RK, Jackson AL. Reversible hemiplegia after presumed intracarotid injection of Ritalin. *N Engl J Med.* 1981;304:1305.
74. Sobel J, Espinas OE, Friedman SA. Carotid artery obstruction following LSD capsule ingestion. *Arch Intern Med.* 1971;127:290–291.
75. Lieberman AN, Bloom W, Kishore PS, Lin JP. Carotid artery occlusion following ingestion of LSD. *Stroke.* 1974; 5:213–215.
76. Lignelli GJ, Buccheit WA. Angiitis in drug abusers. *N Engl J Med.* 1971;284:111–113.
77. Rumbaugh CL, Bergeron RT, Fang HC, McCormick R. Cerebral angiographic changes in the drug abuse patient. *Radiology.* 1971;101:335–344.
78. Eastman JW, Cohen SN. Hypertensive crisis and death associated with phencyclidine poisoning. *JAMA.* 1975;231:1270–1271.
79. Bessen HA. Intracranial hemorrhage associated with phencyclidine abuse. *JAMA.* 1982;248:585–586.

80. Ilett KF, Jarrott B, O'Donnell SR, Wanstall JC. Mechanism of cardiovascular actions of 1-(1-phenylcyclohexyl)piperidine hydrochloride (phencyclidine). *Br J Pharmacol Chemother*. 1966;28:73–83.

81. Crosley CJ, Binet EF. Cerebrovascular complications in phencyclidine intoxication. *J Pediatr*. 1979;94:316–318.

82. McCarron MM, Schulze BW, Thompson GA, Conder MC, Goetz WA. Acute phencyclidine intoxication: incidence of clinical findings in 1,000 cases. *Ann Emerg Med*. 1981;10:237–242.

83. Burns RS, Lerner SE. The effects of phencyclidine in man: A review. In: Domino EF, ed. *PCP (Phencyclidine): Historical and Current Perspectives*. Ann Arbor, Mich: NPP Books; 1981: p. 449.

84. Rumbaugh CL, Fang HC. The effects of drug abuse on the brain. *Med Times*. 1980;108:37s–41s, 45s–46s, 48s–49s passim.

85. Zachariah SB. Stroke after heavy marijuana smoking. *Stroke*. 1991;22:406–409.

86. Barnes D, Palace J, O'Brien MD. Stroke following marijuana smoking. *Stroke*. 1992;23:1381.

87. Berenguer, J, Moreno S, Laguna F, et al. Tuberculous meningitis in patients infected with the human immunodeficiency virus. *N Engl J Med*. 1992;326:668–672.

88. Tomberlin MG, Holtom PD, Owens JL, Larsen RA. Evaluation of neurosyphilis in human immunodeficiency virus–infected individuals. *Clin Infect Dis*. 1994;18:288–294.

89. al Deeb SM, Yaqub BA, Sharif HS, Phadke JG. Neurobrucellosis: clinical characteristics, diagnosis, and outcome. *Neurology*. 1989;39:498–501.

90. Paul, J, et al. Serological responses to brucellosis in HIV-seropositive patients. *Trans R Soc Trop Med Hyg*. 1995; 89:228–230.

91. Carod-Artal FJ. Strokes caused by infection in the tropics. *Rev Neurol*. 2007;44:755–763.

92. Merle H, Donnio A, Ayeboua L, et al. Occipital infarction revealed by quadranopsia following snakebite by *Bothrops lanceolatus*. *Am J Trop Med Hyg*. 2005;73:583–585.

93. Mosquera A, Idrovo LA, Tafur A, Del Brutto OH. Stroke following *Bothrops* spp. snakebite. *Neurology*. 2003;60:1577–1580.

94. Parker MJ, Tarlow MJ, Milne Anderson J. Glue sniffing and cerebral infarction. *Arch Dis Child*. 1984;59:675–677.

95. Lamont CM, Adams FG. Glue-sniffing as a cause of a positive radio-isotope brain scan. *Eur J Nucl Med*. 1982;7:387–388.

96. Adams HP Jr, del Zoppo G, Alberts MJ, et al. Guidelines for the early management of adults with ischemic stroke: a guideline from the American Heart Association/American Stroke Association Stroke Council, Clinical Cardiology Council, Cardiovascular Radiology and Intervention Council, and the Atherosclerotic Peripheral Vascular Disease and Quality of Care Outcomes in Research Interdisciplinary Working Groups. *Stroke*. 2007; 38:1655–1711.

97. Broderick J, Connolly S, Feldmann E, et al. Guidelines for the management of spontaneous intracerebral hemorrhage in adults: 2007 update. A guideline from the American Heart Association/American Stroke Association Stroke Council, High Blood Pressure Research Council, and the Quality of Care and Outcomes in Research Interdisciplinary Working Group. *Stroke*. 2007;38:2001–2023.

98. Sacco RL, Adams R, Albers G, et al. Guidelines for prevention of stroke in patients with ischemic stroke or transient ischemic attack: a statement for healthcare professionals from the American Heart Association/American Stroke Association Council on Stroke. Co-sponsored by the Council on Cardiovascular Radiology and Intervention. *Stroke*. 2006;37:577–617.

Toxic Myopathies

Hani A. Kushlaf

INTRODUCTION

This chapter discusses the general mechanisms by which toxic myopathies are produced and then describes in detail each toxin known to cause myopathy, including its clinical features, electrodiagnostic findings, and biopsy characteristics. Many of these drugs and toxins cause associated neuropathies and neuromuscular junction disorders, and some of them also cause cardiomyopathy.

Toxic myopathy should be considered in any patient who presents with weakness, myalgia or other muscular symptoms, elevated serum creatine kinase (CK), and rhabdomyolysis. Obtaining detailed medication history, including over-the-counter medications and herbal preparations or other supplements, is essential. Each drug on the medication list should be considered as the cause of myopathy as it may be a new adverse effect not previously identified (this is especially true of new drugs). In some patients, introduction of a drug or exposure to a myotoxic substance, in addition to low doses of other drugs already known to cause myopathy (e.g., 3-hydroxy-3-methylglutaryl–coenzyme A [HMG-CoA] reductase inhibitors, or *statins*), is associated with development of synergistic myotoxicity.

Removal of the offending agent usually results in resolution of the symptoms. Many reviews of toxic myopathies have been published.[1-4]

DIFFERENTIATING TOXIC MYOPATHY FROM OTHER CAUSES

In some cases, the myopathy is plainly toxic in origin, such as when there is a strong temporal relationship between the introduction of a novel medication and the later development of rhabdomyolysis, in addition to the absence of other contributing factors, and the lack of signs suggestive of another cause of myopathy (e.g., heliotrope rash or Gottron's papules in patients with dermatomyositis). Muscle biopsy findings are helpful in differentiating toxic myopathy from other causes, although it is important to recognize that toxic myopathy is still possible in patients with preexisting muscle disorders.

Several drugs have been reported to cause toxic myopathy, and it is helpful to confirm causation by following strict criteria:

1. A temporal relationship exists between exposure to an offending agent and development of myopathy.
2. No confounding variables can potentially act synergistically or can potentiate the effect of the agent in question.
3. Resolution, total or partial, of the symptoms occurs with withdrawal from exposure. If from a drug, rechallenging the patient with the same medication is not advised in these circumstances.

MECHANISMS OF TOXIC MYOPATHIES

A drug or toxin can cause muscle injury either directly by affecting myocytes or indirectly through an intermediary mechanism. Direct effects include mitochondrial injury and lysosomal injury (formation of autophagic vacuoles). Such direct effects can manifest as either localized or generalized processes. Indirect effects may be mediated by hypotension, prolonged immobility from loss of consciousness, hypokalemia, or induction of autoimmunity (Tables 1 and 2).

Factors that seem to play a role in the production of toxic myopathy include dose, duration of exposure, drug–drug interactions, individual susceptibility, and other factors that remain unknown. Conceivably, the higher the dose of the offending agent and the longer the duration of exposure, the more likely is toxic myopathy. These factors are mentioned where relevant in this chapter. Sometimes, more than one factor in a single patient causes toxic myopathy.

Asymptomatic CK Elevation

Asymptomatic serum CK elevation maybe the only sign of myotoxicity, as in the case of some patients with statin-induced myopathy. It is important to recognize because it can point to the development of necrotizing myopathy and rhabdomyolysis.

Focal Myopathy

Localized areas of muscle damage can occur with intramuscular drug injections secondary to needle insertion and due to toxic effects of the injected agent. Medications with a local myotoxic effect include opiates, paraldehyde, cephalothin, chloroquine, and chlorpromazine. Pathologically, dense focal fibrosis, scattered fiber necrosis, and variable inflammatory infiltration occur (Figure 13-1). A repeated muscular injection with pethidine has been reported as causing multiple contractures and fibrosis.[5]

Myalgia and Muscle Cramps

Manifestation of myalgia and muscle cramps might occur alone or with myotonia and asymptomatic elevation of serum CK. Drugs most commonly associated with myalgias and muscles cramps include HMG-CoA reductase inhibitors (statins), β-adrenoceptor agonists, succinylcholine, calcium channel blockers, diuretics, and chemotherapeutic agents. Stopping the offending agent typically results in immediate resolution of the symptoms.

Necrotizing Myopathies

In a necrotizing clinical syndrome, the patient presents with acute or subacute painful proximal myopathy developing over days to weeks, usually with preserved tendon reflexes.

Table 1:   Mechanisms of Toxin-Induced Muscle Damage
DIRECT TOXIC EFFECTS
Local
Diffuse
SECONDARY EFFECTS
Electrolyte disturbance
Immunological reaction
Compression (crush syndrome)
Ischemia
Neural activation
Adapted from Mastaglia FL, Argov Z. Toxic and iatrogenic myopathies. In: Mastaglia FL, Hilton-Jones D, eds. *Myopathies and Muscle Diseases*. London: Elsevier; 2007:P322.

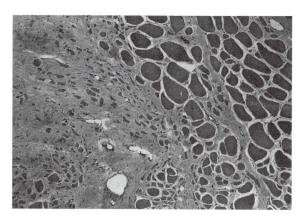

Figure 13-1. Typical pathology of focal myopathy, taken from an area of contracture. This biopsy was from a patient who repeatedly injected himself with pentazocine, an opiate derivative. The few remaining bundles of fibers show both atrophy and hypertrophy, and pronounced replacement of muscle with fibrous tissue can be seen. Little inflammatory response occurs in this chronic lesion (hematoxylin and eosin stain). (Dubowitz V, Sewry C. *Muscle Biopsy: A Practical Approach*. 3rd ed. London: Elsevier; 2007.)

Table 2:   Toxic Agent–Induced Myopathies

Pathogenic Classification	Agents	Clinical Features	Laboratory Features	Pathology
Necrotizing myopathy	Cholesterol-lowering agents Cyclosporine Labetalol Alcohol ε-Aminocaproic acid Organophosphates Snake venom	Acute or subacute onset; proximal weakness; with or without myalgias	Elevated serum CK EMG: Fibrillation potentials, myopathic MUAPs	Many necrotic muscle fibers; no evidence of endomysial inflammatory cell infiltrate invading non-necrotic muscle fibers or regeneration
Amphiphilic myopathy	Chloroquine Amiodarone Hydroxychloroquine Prehexiline	Acute or insidious onset; proximal and distal weakness; myalgias; sensorimotor neuropathy; hypothyroid (amiodarone)	Elevated serum CK EMG: Fibrillation potentials, myopathic MUAPs NCS: Axonal sensorimotor neuropathy	Autophagic vacuoles and inclusions apparent in some muscle fibers and in Schwann cells
Antimicrotubular myopathy	Vincristine Colchicine	Acute or insidious onset; proximal and distal weakness; myalgias; sensorimotor neuropathy	Normal or elevated CK EMG: Fibrillation potentials, myopathic MUAPs NCS: Axonal sensorimotor neuropathy	Autophagic vacuoles and inclusions evident in some muscle fibers; nerve biopsies demonstrating axonal degeneration
Mitochondrial myopathy	Zidovudine Germanium	Acute or insidious onset; proximal weakness; myalgias; rhabdomyolysis; painful sensory neuropathy	Normal or elevated CK EMG: Normal or myopathic NCS: Axonal sensory neuropathy or neuronopathy	Muscle biopsies revealing ragged red fibers or COX-negative fibers; also may see inflammatory cell infiltrates, cytoplasmic bodies, and nemaline rods
Inflammatory myopathy	D-penicillamine Interferon-α	Acute or insidious onset; proximal weakness; myalgias; with or without skin changes	Elevated serum CK EMG: Fibrillation potentials, myopathic MUAPs	Perivascular, perimysial, or endomysial inflammatory cell infiltrates
Hypokalemic myopathy	Amphotericin Toluene abuse Carbenoxolone Corticosteroids Alcohol abuse Lithium	Acute proximal or generalized weakness; myalgias	Elevated serum CK; low serum potassium	May see scattered necrotic laxatives fibers and vacuoles
Impaired protein synthesis	Emetine Ipecac syrup	Myalgia; proximal weakness; cardiomyopathy	Myopathic MUAPs	Focal mitochondrial loss; vacuoles
Critical illness myopathy	Corticosteroids Nondepolarizing neuromuscular blocking agents	Acute generalized weakness, including respiratory muscle	Serum CK normal or elevated NCS: Low-amplitude CMAP with relatively normal SNAP EMG: Fibrillation potentials, myopathic MUAPs or no voluntary MUAPs	Atrophy of muscle fibers; scattered necrotic fibers; fiber size variation; absence of myosin thick filaments

Continued

Table 2: Toxic Agent–Induced Myopathies—cont'd

Pathogenic Classification	Agents	Clinical Features	Laboratory Features	Pathology
Fasciitis	Toxic oil syndrome Eosinophilia–myalgia syndrome Macrophagic myofasciitis	Myalgia; skin changes; other systems involved	Eosinophilia	Vasculitis; connective tissue
Focal myopathy	Acute injection of IM drugs Chronic repeated IM injection	Acute: Pain, swelling, with or without abscess formation Chronic: Contracture	Acute: Elevated serum CK Chronic: Normal CK level	Acute: Focal necrosis Chronic: Fibrosis

CK, creatine kinase; CMAP, compound muscle action potential; COX, cytochrome C oxidase; EMG, electromyography; IM, intramuscular; MUAP, motor unit action potential; NCS, nerve conduction studies; SNAP, sensory nerve action potential.

Muscle biopsy shows necrosis and regeneration without inflammation. Serum CK is elevated variably, and there may be associated myoglobinuria.

Statin Drugs (HMG-CoA Reductase Inhibitors)

The statin group is used to treat hypercholesterolemia, and these agents work by inhibiting HMG-CoA reductase enzyme, the rate-limiting step in cholesterol synthesis. The mechanism by which these agents cause necrotizing myopathy remains to be elucidated.[6] Four types of presentations might occur in patients taking a statin. These include the following:

- Asymptomatic elevated serum CK
- Increased serum CK with exercise[7]
- Myalgia or cramps that may be associated with elevated serum CK; in some patients, withdrawal of the statin does not result in resolution of both[8,9]
- Rhabdomyolysis, which may be severe and even fatal; the incidence is 0.08% with simvastatin and lovastatin and 0.09% with pravastatin,[10] and the mortality rate is 7.8%[11]
- Myositis, which is rare with statin use[12]

The earliest ultrastructural changes in experimentally induced lovastatin myopathy involve the mitochondria and the sarcoplasmic reticulum. This suggests that the primary myotoxic effect of lovastatin is on the membranes of these organelles.[13] Fast-twitch muscles are apparently most vulnerable to lovastatin myopathy. A possible explanation for this is that the cholesterol content of a fast-twitch muscle is about 30% lower than that of a slow-twitch muscle. Therefore, fast-twitch muscles may be more vulnerable to damage caused by a decrease in cholesterol available for membrane biosynthesis.

Cerivastatin was withdrawn from the market because of the high risk of rhabdomyolysis[14] (16 to 80 times higher in comparison with other statins), and the issue was recently raised with rosuvastatin (the risk of rhabdomyolysis is 1.5 times more than with simvastatin).[15] Interestingly, when the results of randomized studies were evaluated, no significant difference was found in rates of myotoxicity and severe rhabdomyolysis between the control and the drug-treated groups; however, this seems not to be the case after the introduction of wide usage of these medications.[7]

Risk factors for statin-induced myopathy include advanced age (especially for patients older than 80 years), female gender, high statin doses, use of more than one cholesterol-lowering agent, renal insufficiency (especially if caused by diabetes), obstructive liver disease, and coadministration of drugs that inhibit or are metabolized by the CYP3A4 isoenzyme of the cytochrome P450 system.[16] These drugs include gemfibrozil and other fibrates, nicotinic acid, cyclosporin, azole antifungal agents, macrolide antibiotics, and niacin. Grapefruit juice, which contains the CYP3A4 inhibitor furanocoumarin, also increases the risk of developing myopathy.[17] Pravastatin is thought to carry a lower risk of inducing myopathy since it is not metabolized by the liver cytochrome P450 system.[18,19]

To reduce the risk of statin-associated myopathy, it is important to use the lowest drug dose to achieve the required level of cholesterol reduction, to avoid using multiple cholesterol-lowering agents whenever possible, and to use non-CYP3A4-metabolized statins (e.g., pravastatin) if possible when other medications that increase the risk of myopathy are being used.[20] The use of supplementary ubiquinone (coenzyme Q10) has not been proven to be protective.[21]

Controversy exists about the routine screening of CK levels before prescription of statins. I do recommend this to avoid having to stop the medication if any myalgic complaints appear and the CK level is then found to be elevated. Another debate is whether to stop statins in asymptomatic patients if a rise occurs in the CK level during treatment. It is not usually recommended to stop the statin if the CK rise is less than three to five times the normal upper limit.[9,22] Another controversy is whether to reintroduce a statin after an episode of rhabdomyolysis in patients who need the statin. Perhaps the safest options in this situation are either to commence another statin, such as pravastatin, with a lower risk of myotoxicity or to use ezetimibe, which inhibits intestinal absorption of cholesterol. However, recent reports indicate that ezetimibe may also cause myalgia and elevated serum CK when administered with a statin[23] (Figure 13-2).

Fibrates

Using fibrates for the treatment of hypercholesterolemia has been shown to cause necrotizing myopathy. The risk of the myopathy is six times greater in patients taking a statin.[24] The risk also increases in patients with renal failure, nephrotic syndrome, and hypothyroidism.

Nicotinic Acid

Nicotinic acid has been shown to cause reversible myopathy with pain and elevated serum CK that resolves with discontinuation.[25] The likelihood that nicotinic acid will cause rhabdomyolysis increases with statin coadministration.[26]

ε-Aminocaproic Acid

The mechanism by which ε-aminocaproic acid causes a myopathy is hypothesized to be related to lysine replacement in the sarcolemma, although it may also be related to interference with lysine involvement in carnitine synthesis.[27] Fibrin deposition may also be a mechanism since it has been shown in muscle biopsies in patients with this myopathy.[28] The myopathy ranges from a mild, self-limited condition to rhabdomyolysis (Figure 13-3).

Emetine

Emetine is used for the treatment of amebiasis and is a component of ipecac syrup. Emetine is both myotoxic and cardiotoxic. It has been shown to cause mitochondrial and myofibrillar change that can lead to myofiber necrosis. CK is usually elevated but can be normal in some patients with emetine-induced myopathy.[29] Muscle biopsies show myofiber necrosis and regeneration. Core target areas with loss of enzymatic activity and cytoplasmic bodies are also seen. After discontinuation of the emetine, it may take several weeks to months for the changes in muscle biopsy to resolve.

Cardiac Glycosides

Several reports from the Australian literature demonstrate that the cardiac glycosides scillarin A and B are causally related to necrotizing myopathy.[31] These glycosides are present in cough suppressants used by opiate addicts.

Organophosphates

Organophosphate insecticides more commonly cause neuropathy following acute or chronic exposure, but they have also been shown to cause a necrotizing myopathy that starts

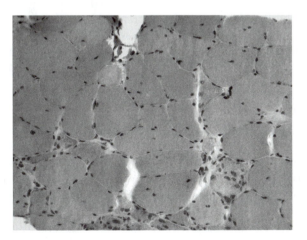

Figure 13-2. Quadriceps biopsy from a 71-year-old male showing necrosis and regeneration thought to have been induced by statins. The patient had a very high creatine kinase (20,000 IU/L) but very low sarcolemmal MHC class I, suggesting that he did not have a myositis (hematoxylin and eosin stain). (Dubowitz V, Sewry C. *Muscle Biopsy: A Practical Approach.* 3rd ed. London: Elsevier; 2007.)

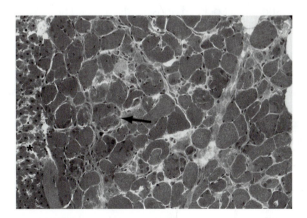

Figure 13-3. Acute necrotizing myopathy induced by ε-aminocaproic acid, showing multifocal fiber necrosis and macrophage activity, and marked regenerative response shown by many small basophilic areas around necrotic fibers (*arrows*). There is little lymphocytic infiltration, but macrophages are abundant (*, lymphocytic infiltration and macrophages; hematoxylin and eosin stain). (Dubowitz V, Sewry C. *Muscle Biopsy: A Practical Approach.* 3rd ed. London: Elsevier; 2007.)

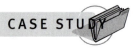

CASE STUDY

A 32-year-old female with anorexia nervosa and depression developed myalgia and increasing generalized weakness over several weeks, leading to inability to walk. She also had dysphagia and nasal regurgitation of liquids. She was not taking any regular medications. Sensation and reflexes were normal. The serum CK level was 15 times the normal level, and electromyography (EMG) supported a myopathic process. Muscle biopsy confirmed myopathy with cores and cytoplasmic bodies in muscle fibers. Urine screen for emetine was positive, and emetine myopathy was diagnosed. The patient subsequently admitted to purging with ipecac, which contains emetine. Her condition improved once she stopped this behavior.[30]

in the motor endpoint region.[32] Experimental evidence shows that the necrotizing myopathy can be prevented by prior denervation or by use of pyridine-2-aldoxime methiodide.[33]

Gasoline Sniffing

Gasoline sniffing has been shown in isolated reports to cause necrotizing myopathy with rhabdomyolysis that sometimes is associated with encephalopathy.[34,35]

Cyclosporine

Clinically evident disorders of muscle that are attributable to cyclosporine, an immunosuppressive cyclic peptide, are rare. The reported cases suggest two patterns of cyclosporine-associated muscle disorder. The first is a mild myopathy without evidence of rhabdomyolysis. Myalgia and muscle weakness develop weeks after the start of therapy. Some reported patients had been taking colchicines concomitantly.[36–38] Biopsies have revealed type II fiber atrophy, vacuole formation, and necrosis. Muscle symptoms can be expected to improve after dose reduction. The second pattern occurred in patients being treated concurrently with cyclosporine and an HMG-CoA reductase inhibitor (such as lovastatin or cerivastatin) and is characterized by rhabdomyolysis.[39,40] Seizures are a common side effect of cyclosporine therapy, especially in recipients of liver transplants. Some experimental findings suggest that cyclosporine may influence mitochondrial function.

Labetalol

A severe generalized myopathy may occur in patients treated with the antihypertensive alpha or beta blocker, labetalol. Willis and colleagues described two children who lost their ability to walk during labetalol therapy.[41] Serum CK was markedly elevated. Labetalol was discontinued, and muscle strength improved immediately. In an adult patient, muscle pain and serum CK elevation without weakness occurred. Light microscopy showed no abnormality, but electron microscopy demonstrated subsarcolemmal vacuoles and glycogen granules.[42]

Valproate

Valproic acid has been reported to cause rhabdomyolysis in a patient with carnitine palmitoyltransferase deficiency[43] and to cause myopathy in a patient with mitochondrial myopathy, encephalopathy, lactic acidosis, and stroke-like symptoms.[44]

Antipsychotic Agents

Some antipsychotic drugs, especially those with 5-hydroxytryptamine-2a (5-HT2a) receptor blockade, cause serum CK elevation in the absence of signs of neuroleptic malignant syndrome.[45,46] The magnitude of the elevation is up to 10% in patients treated with clozapine, risperidone, meperone, olanzapine, haloperidol, and loxapine.[47] The sarcolemma of muscle fibers contains 5-HT receptors and their blockade can cause serum CK to increase with the use of antipsychotic medications. The mechanism is hypothesized to be a compromise in the muscle fiber uptake of glucose secondary to serotonin receptor blockade, which might lead to changes in the sarcolemma associated with increase in its permeability to CK.[47]

Vitamin A Derivatives

Etretinate is used for the treatment of severe psoriasis. Only one case series documents a toxic myopathy secondary to etretinate. Three patients were described; all had proximal muscle weakness and tenderness, and CK levels were slightly increased. Muscle biopsy was done in one patient, and it showed segmental muscle necrosis.[48] Isotretinoin is used for treatment of severe acne. The use of isotretinoin is complicated rarely by increased serum CK level.[49]

Alcoholic Myopathy

Ethanol is well known for causing acute, subacute, and chronic forms of toxic myopathy. Experimental observations in humans and in animals have shown acute elevations in serum CK activity after administration of ethanol, with direct relationship between CK and blood alcohol levels.[50] Ultrastructural changes were found in muscle fibers in human volunteers after regular ingestion of large quantities of ethanol for 1 month.[51] Evidence from in vitro studies indicates that ethanol alters the configuration, fluidity, and Na/K-ATPase activity of cell membranes and inhibits calcium uptake by the sarcoplasmic reticulum.[52] Ethanol has also been shown to cause marked inhibition of oxidation of palmitic acid and glucose-6-phosphate, two of the major substrates for energy production in skeletal muscle.[53]

Several contributory factors may also be involved. Food deprivation, which is a common accompaniment of binge drinking, retards the metabolism of ethanol, allowing the development of high blood levels that may be toxic to skeletal muscle. This was demonstrated in the rat model of experimental alcoholic myopathy, where rhabdomyolysis was triggered by a period of food deprivation.[54]

Hypokalemia is present in some cases of alcohol withdrawal and may be severe enough to cause a hypokalemic myopathy.[55] Phosphate depletion, which may develop with chronic alcohol ingestion, may also contribute to the development of acute myopathy in some chronically malnourished alcoholics.

Acute Alcoholic Myopathy

The condition of acute alcoholic myopathy appears to be more common than generally appreciated since most patients seen in emergency rooms with alcohol intoxication or withdrawal have elevated serum CK.[52] This usually occurs in males following alcoholic binges, the condition varying from mild asymptomatic elevation of CK to acute rhabdomyolysis with tenderness in proximal and calf muscles, generalized weakness, myoglobinuria, acute tubular necrosis, and renal failure. Ethanol is considered to be the most important and most common cause of nontraumatic acute rhabdomyolysis.[56]

In some patients, the involvement is limited to calf muscles and the condition may mimic thrombophlebitis.[57] The prognosis is usually good with alcohol abstinence, but clinical recovery may take a few months to occur. Pathological changes in muscle biopsies consist of scattered myofiber necrosis, which is more prominent in cases with the severe form of acute rhabdomyolysis, and evidence of regeneration. Other changes include a mild mononuclear cell infiltrate in some cases and patchy loss of oxidative enzyme activity, especially in type I fibers.[58,59]

Chronic Alcoholic Myopathy

Chronic alcoholic myopathy is often subclinical, showing chronic progressive atrophy and weakness of shoulder and pelvic girdle muscles. These patients usually have associated liver cirrhosis, peripheral neuropathy, and evidence of cardiomyopathy. CK is usually normal. EMG shows myopathic and sometimes neuropathic potentials in proximal muscles. Muscle biopsy shows atrophy of type IIB fibers. Triglyceride also accumulates in muscle fibers,[60,61] and glycolytic and glycogenolytic enzyme activity is reduced,[62] accounting for the reduced lactic acid production during ischemic exercise in

alcoholics.[63] Type II fiber atrophy is also a common finding in biopsies from alcoholics without symptoms of muscle weakness, suggesting that, as in the case of acute alcoholic myopathy, chronic alcoholic myopathy is commonly subclinical.[64] In cases with an associated peripheral neuropathy, histological changes of denervation may also be found, even in the proximal lower limb muscles. Tubular aggregates may be present in some cases.[65] These patients usually improve with alcohol abstinence, and type IIB fiber atrophy has been shown to be reversible.[66]

Acute Rhabdomyolysis and Myoglobinuria

Rhabdomyolysis refers to severe damage of muscle fibers with resultant elevated serum CK and myoglobinuria. CK elevation is more than 10 times the normal level. Clinically, patients have generalized weakness and diffuse myalgias. Tendon reflexes are lost. Rhabdomyolysis can be complicated by compartment syndrome, hyperphosphatemia, hyperkalemia, hypocalcemia, and acute tubular necrosis.

The management of this syndrome is largely supportive, and resolution of the symptoms is expected to occur with appropriate management, although it has resulted in multiorgan failure and death. The list of causes of rhabdomyolysis is long, and at times more than one mechanism is operating to produce this clinical syndrome. Some medications are not inherently myotoxic, and other factors such as ischemia, compression, seizures,[67] and dystonia[68] may be contributory. These patients may develop a compartment syndrome, and as such they should be closely monitored in case they progress to needing fasciotomy. All agents mentioned earlier to cause necrotizing myopathy have the propensity to cause rhabdomyolysis.

Solvents

Toluene is present in paint sprays, lacquer thinners, and household glues and has been shown to cause rhabdomyolysis in intoxicated patients.[69]

Snake Venoms

Several snakes have been shown to cause rhabdomyolysis. These include the Australian tiger snake (*Notechis scutatus scutatus*), the taipan (*Oxyuranus scutellatus*), the mulga snake (*Pseudechis australis*), the sea snake (*Enhydrina schistose*), the coral snake (*Micrurus nigrocinctus*), the prairie rattlesnake (*Crotalus viridis viridis*), the Western diamondback rattlesnake (*Crotalus atrox*), the South American rattlesnake (*Crotalus durissus terrificus*), and the Costa Rican vipers (*Bothrops nummifer* and *Bothrops asper*).

These snakes produce venom that has peptides, phospholipases, or both that are specific to muscle membranes; hence, envenomation results in lysis of muscle cells.[70]

Spider Venom

Several spiders have been reported to cause rhabdomyolysis, including Arkansas and Honduran tarantulas (*Dugesiella hentzi* and *Aphonophelma* species), the brown recluse spider, and the redback spider.[71]

Wasp Venom: Hymenoptera

Two wasps have been reported to cause rhabdomyolysis—*Vespa cincta* and the hornet *Vespa affinis*. Envenomation by the African honeybee is also reported to cause rhabdomyolysis.[72]

Haff Disease

Haff in German means "lagoon." This disease was described in 1924 in a Baltic Sea area where people ate fish and within 24 hours developed myalgias, followed by rhabdomyolysis and myoglobinuria. The toxin causing the disease has never been identified. Recently, similar cases have been reported in the United States.[73]

Quail Disease

Quail disease has been reported in Mediterranean countries. It is rhabdomyolysis resulting from ingestion of quail. The toxin is derived from seeds containing hemlock *(Conium maculatum)* or hellebore (a veratrine alkaloid) ingested by the quail.[74]

Hypokalemic Myopathy

Disruption of water and electrolyte homeostasis can cause severe muscle damage. A reversible vacuolar myopathy may develop as a consequence of prolonged severe hypokalemia at a serum level below 2 mmol/L. Three syndromes of hypokalemic myopathy are recognized:

- A flaccid, transient, or persistent muscle weakness that affects mainly the proximal limb muscles. Tendon reflexes and sensation are preserved. In most cases, serum CK levels are markedly increased. Histological findings tend to be inconspicuous except for swelling and vacuolation of scattered muscle fibers. The vacuoles originate from T tubules. In more severe cases, evidence of fiber necrosis, phagocytosis, regeneration, and type II fiber atrophy may also be present.[75]
- A syndrome resembling familial periodic paralysis with areflexia.
- Severe muscle necrosis and myoglobinuria.

The clinical manifestations and morphological changes are quickly reversed by potassium repletion. The precise mechanism by which muscle is damaged in hypokalemia is unclear. At least three potentially harmful effects occur: abnormally low muscle blood flow with exercise, suppression of glycogen synthesis and storage, and deranged ion transport.

Even in asymptomatic hypokalemic injury, superimposition of any effort that demands expenditure of energy can precipitate frank myoglobinuria. The combined influence of exercise and fasting is a prime example. Prolonged hypokalemia may develop as a result of the injudicious use of laxatives.[76] It can also occur with thiazide diuretics,[77] treatment with mineralocorticoids, hyperaldosteronism, and lithium therapy.[78] Hypokalemic myopathy may also occur in compulsive licorice eaters[79] and has been observed during treatment with carbenoxolone.[80] Carbenoxolone is a derivative of glycyrrhizic acid, which occurs naturally in licorice root. It exhibits significant mineralocorticoid activity and was used for the treatment of peptic ulcers.

In addition, myopathy and myoglobinuria have been associated with severe hypokalemia from other causes. These include renal tubular acidosis from treatment with the antifungal drug amphotericin B,[81] renal damage due to toluene "sniffing," regional enteritis, *Giardia lamblia* infestation,[82] nasogastric suction plus parenteral hyperalimentation,[83] and chronic alcoholism.

Mitochondrial Myopathy

Zidovudine

Prolonged use of zidovudine (AZT) induces mitochondrial changes. Muscle biopsy shows ragged red fibers, abundance of cytochrome C oxidase negative fibers, and mitochondrial paracrystalline inclusions (Figure 13-4A–C).

Clinically, patients have proximal or generalized weakness, fatigue, and high serum CK levels. The myopathy improves with withdrawal of the medication.[84] The mechanism is shown to be due to inhibition of mitochondrial DNA replication and mitochondrial DNA depletion in muscle fibers.[85] Differentiation of zidovudine-induced myopathy from human immunodeficiency virus (HIV) myopathy is impossible at times, but in a case series of 48 HIV-infected patients,[86] no inflammatory changes were seen in patients with zidovudine-induced myopathy. On the other hand, in another series by Dalakas et al., inflammatory changes were seen with and without long-term zidovudine use.[87]

Germanium

Germanium is present in several elixirs and dietary supplements, and it has been shown to cause mitochondrial myopathy.[88] Germanium intoxication causes renal failure, anemia, and muscle weakness.

Statins

Statins have been shown to cause a mitochondrial myopathy that is different from the usual necrotizing myopathy. This rare myopathy is not associated with increases in CK levels, and the muscle biopsy shows mitochondrial changes.[89]

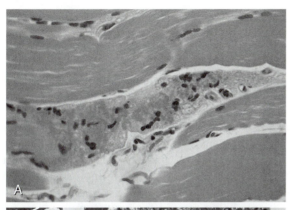

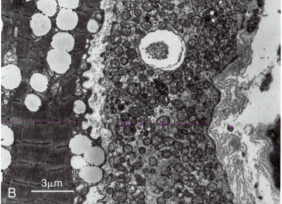

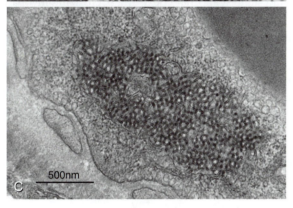

Figure 13-4. Zidovudine myopathy in human immunodeficiency virus infection showing a fiber section longitudinally undergoing degeneration (hematoxylin and eosin stain; (A) and electron micrographs of abnormal mitochondria (B) and tubuloreticular inclusions (C) in an endothelial cell. (Dubowitz V, Sewry C. *Muscle Biopsy: A Practical Approach.* 3rd ed. London: Elsevier; 2007.)

Inflammatory Myopathy

Interferon-α

Interferon-α is used for treatment of chronic viral hepatitis, as well as some forms of malignancy. It has been shown to induce polymyositis and dermatomyositis in some patients.[90–93]

Penicillamine-D

Penicillamine has been implicated in the development of polymyositis that is clinically and pathologically indistinguishable from the usual polymyositis. An association with HLA-B18, HLA-B35, and HLA-DR4 was reported in one series of cases, suggesting a genetic predisposition.[94] The dose associated with development of polymyositis is 600 mg/day on average but can be as low as 50 to 100 mg/day. The average latency to develop polymyositis is about 12 months.[95] In most cases prompt recovery follows penicillamine discontinuation, but in some patients a course of prednisolone is required.

Other medications that might cause inflammatory myopathy include procainamide, cimetidine, leuprolide, propylthiouracil, carbimazole, hydralazine, phenytoin, mesantoin, penicillin, and levodopa.

Eosinophilia–Myalgia Syndrome

An interstitial form of eosinophilic myositis and fasciitis was reported in the early 1990s in patients taking certain preparations containing the naturally occurring amino acid L-tryptophan.[96] More than 1500 cases of this syndrome occurred in the United States.[97] The syndrome was characterized by severe myalgia, muscle tenderness and hyperesthesia with edema and induration of the skin of the extremities resembling scleroderma, and a marked peripheral blood eosinophilia. In some cases, there was associated polyneuropathy and other systemic features. The bulk source of the tryptophan preparation in the American cases was traced to a single manufacturer, and the syndrome is now thought to have been due to a chemical contaminant.[98]

Toxic Oil Syndrome

In 1981, an epidemic of a new illness, now called *toxic oil syndrome,* occurred in Spain. Approximately 20,000 cases and 330 deaths were recorded in the first year of the epidemic.

The onset of the syndrome was usually acute, primarily with respiratory symptoms. Approximately 50% of patients developed an intermediate or chronic illness, with severe myalgia, eosinophilia, numbness of the extremities, and scleroderma-like skin lesions, among other findings. The basic pathological change in this disease is a vasculitis that affects mainly the intima of small arteries and veins. Skeletal muscle changes were most prominent during the third and fourth weeks of the illness. They consisted of an inflammatory infiltration involving particularly the perimysium and sheaths of intramuscular nerves and, to a lesser extent, the walls of veins and capillaries. These changes were followed by those of denervation atrophy secondary to a similar inflammatory involvement of the peripheral nerves.

Epidemiological and analytical chemical studies established a clear link between the syndrome and the ingestion of olive oil mixtures containing aniline-denatured rapeseed oil. However, the precise etiological agent has never been identified.[99] Aniline toxicity is quite distinct from that of toxic oil syndrome.

Macrophagic Myofasciitis

Macrophagic myofasciitis is an inflammatory myopathy of recent emergence in France and other Western countries, manifesting with diffuse arthromyalgias and fatigue. It is pathologically characterized by stereotypical accumulation of tightly packed, nonepitheloid macrophages in epi-, peri-, and endomysium (Figure 13-5). These macrophages show intracytoplasmic osmiophilic inclusions that represent aluminum hydroxide crystals corresponding to the adjuvant used in some vaccines administered intramuscularly. In the series from Gherardi and colleagues,[100] all 50 patients had received vaccines against hepatitis B (86%), hepatitis A virus (19%), or tetanus toxoid (58%) between 3 and 96 months before muscle biopsy. Some patients with macrophagic myofasciitis develop symptomatic demyelinating central nervous system involvement. Deltoid muscle biopsy searching for the characteristic pathological alterations of macrophagic myofasciitis should be considered in multiple sclerosis patients with diffuse myalgias.

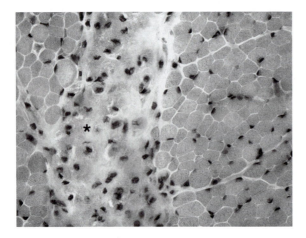

Figure 13-5. Macrophagic fasciitis induced by vaccination showing many macrophages in the perimysium (*). The muscle fibers show variation in size (range 5 to 25 μm), but there is no other pathological feature (child age 7 months at the time of the biopsy; hematoxylin and eosin stain). (Dubowitz V, Sewry C. *Muscle Biopsy: A Practical Approach.* 3rd ed. London: Elsevier; 2007.)

Corticosteroid Myopathy

Chronic Steroid Myopathy

Myopathy is a common complication of prolonged treatment with glucocorticoids. Doses typically associated with myopathy are more than 40 mg of prednisone per day, but even lower doses (more than 10 mg of prednisone or equivalent) are associated with myopathy if used for prolonged periods.[101] The risk of myopathy is greater with 9-α-fluorinated steroids (triamcinolone, betamethasone, and dexamethasone).

Patients being treated for brain tumor edema with dexamethasone and using phenytoin at the same time seem to have less risk of developing myopathy, probably secondary to increased hepatic metabolism of dexamethasone.[102]

The myopathy is proximal, clinically involving pelvic girdle muscles, and it is insidious in onset. Cranial nerve muscles are not involved except in patients using inhaled steroids who develop dysphonia.[103] It has also been reported that some asthmatic patients develop diaphragmatic weakness secondary to chronic steroid use.[101]

Serum CK is reduced or normal; if elevated, the level should suggest another coexisting necrotizing myopathy. EMG is normal or mildly abnormal in some cases, but typically it shows myopathic changes. Muscle biopsy shows decreased type II fibers, primarily type IIB, which are shown to be preferentially affected in experimental steroid myopathy.[104] The basis for this selective action is not known.

The basic cellular action of corticosteroids appears to be interference with messenger RNA synthesis and, in turn, muscle protein synthesis.[105] Denervated muscles are more sensitive to the effects of steroids than are normal muscles.[106]

Acute Quadriplegic Myopathy

Also known as critical illness myopathy, acute quadriplegic myopathy is different from chronic steroid myopathy but appears to be associated with the use of high-dose intravenous steroids in an intensive care unit setting.[107] The use of pancuronium and other nondepolarizing neuromuscular blockers also increases risk.

Clinically, patients have generalized weakness. Diaphragmatic weakness produces difficulty in weaning from mechanical ventilation. Serum CK levels are elevated or normal. Muscle biopsy shows selective loss of myosin filaments with preservation of Z bands on electron microscopy. Light microscopy demonstrates angulated fibers, fiber size variation, and atrophy of both fiber types (Figure 13-6A–C).

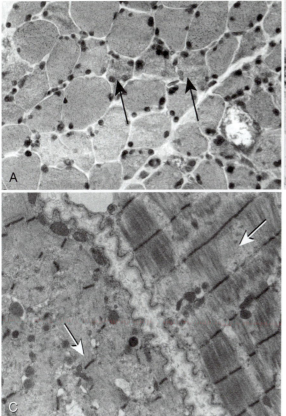
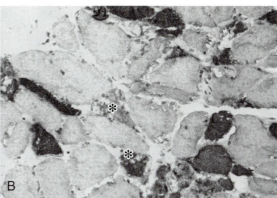

Figure 13-6. Critical illness myopathy showing several fibers with abnormal hematoxylin and eosin stain *(arrows; A)*; disruption of fast myosin immunolabeling (*; *B*), and electron micrograph showing varying degrees of selective A band loss *(arrows; C)*. (Dubowitz V, Sewry C. *Muscle Biopsy: A Practical Approach.* 3rd ed. London: Elsevier; 2007.)

EMG shows myopathic and neuropathic motor unit action potentials (MUAPs), in addition to spontaneous activity. Treatment is supportive.

Differentiating this syndrome from critical illness polyneuropathy may prove impossible because both often exist at the same time. The prognosis for critical illness myopathy is better than in patients with critical illness neuropathy, with most patients recovering either partially or fully, depending on the severity, in a few months.

Antimicrotubular Myopathy

Vincristine

Vincristine is a cell cycle–specific antineoplastic agent that interferes with RNA and protein synthesis and with polymerization of tubulin into microtubules. It commonly causes axonal peripheral neuropathy, and in some patients it is associated with a proximal myopathy.[108]

Electron microscopy shows formation of spheromembranous bodies thought to be derived from the sarcoplasmic reticulum and autophagic degeneration of muscle fibers.[109]

Colchicine

Like vincristine, the drug colchicine inhibits polymerization of tubulin into microtubules and causes a mitotic arrest. It is used for the treatment of gout and other conditions such as amyloidosis and familial Mediterranean fever. Colchicine use is associated with neuromyopathy that can occur with therapeutic dosing or overdose. Chronic renal insufficiency predisposes patients to this syndrome.[110] Reported patients have proximal weakness, distal sensory involvement, and areflexia. Stopping colchicine results in prompt recovery.[111]

Serum CK levels are usually elevated 10- to 20-fold. Muscle biopsy shows vacuolar myopathy and autophagic vacuoles without necrosis. The vacuoles react strongly with acid phosphatase. Some biopsies show central areas of altered staining on hematoxylin and eosin preparations with loss of enzyme activity resembling cores in histochemical preparations (Figure 13-7).

Autophagic Myopathy

A few medications that are amphiphilic cationic compounds interfere with lysosomal function and cause autophagic degeneration and accumulation of phospholipids

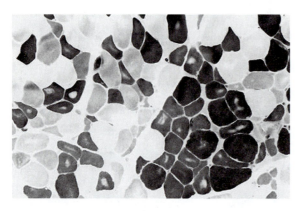

Figure 13-7. Myosin ATPase (pH 4.6) preparation showing central core formation in a case of colchicine myopathy. (Mastaglia FL, Hilton-Jones D, eds. Myopathies and muscle diseases. In: Aminoff MJ, Boller F, Swaab DF, series eds. *Handbook of Clinical Neurology*. London: Elsevier; 2007.)

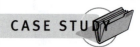

CASE STUDY

A 55-year-old female with systemic lupus erythematosus presented with a 1-month history of progressive limb weakness (more severe proximally), quadriceps atrophy, and absent ankle reflexes. She had been treated with prednisone 10 mg/day for 18 months and chloroquine phosphate for the last 5 months. The serum CK level was 170 IU/L (normal is less than 200 IU/L). EMG showed myopathic units with fibrillations and positive waves in multiple limb muscles. Nerve conduction studies indicated a sensorimotor peripheral neuropathy. A quadriceps muscle biopsy showed a vacuolar myopathy with numerous autophagic vacuoles in muscle fibers on electron microscopy. The biopsy findings were typical of chloroquine myopathy. She improved gradually over several months after stopping chloroquine.[113]

in lysosomes. Some of these drugs are also known to cause neuropathies. The class includes perhexiline, chloroquine, amiodarone, vincristine, and colchicine.[112]

Chloroquine

Chloroquine, a 4-aminoquinolone, is used in the treatment of malaria and many rheumatological diseases, such as systemic lupus erythematosus, rheumatoid arthritis, and scleroderma. Chloroquine causes neuromyopathy after treatment with doses of 250 to 750 mg/day for periods ranging from several weeks to 4 years.[113] Patients describe the insidious onset of painless proximal muscle weakness that is associated with atrophy in severe cases. Depression of deep tendon reflexes and mild sensory distal changes support an associated neuropathy.

CK levels are normal or slightly increased. EMG shows myopathic MUAPs and slowing on nerve conduction studies.[114] Light microscopy of muscle fibers shows autophagic vacuoles that preferentially affect type I muscle fibers, while electron microscopy shows myeloid bodies and curvilinear bodies (Figure 13-8A and B).

Experimental studies have shown a marked increase in lysosomal enzyme activity.[115] Accordingly, the lysosomal proteinase inhibitor ethyl(2s, 3s)-3([S]-3-methyl-l-[3-methylbutylcarbamoyl]methylbutylcarbamoyl)oxidrane-2-carboxylate (EST) is an effective treatment for chloroquine-induced myopathy in animals.[116]

Chloroquine can also cause cardiomyopathy in some cases.[117] The effects of chloroquine typically reverse slowly following discontinuation.

Hydroxychloroquine is a similar compound that causes biopsy changes similar to chloroquine.[118] Vacuolar changes are absent, but electron microscopy reveals accumulation of myeloid and curvilinear bodies. The changes are less numerous than in chloroquine-induced myopathy. Finally, quinacrine can cause muscle necrosis.

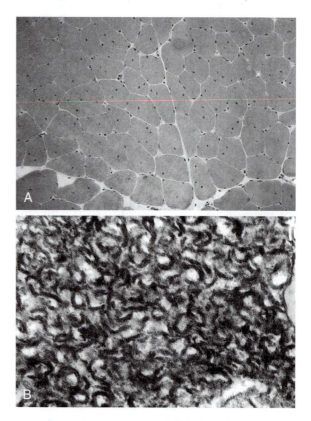

Figure 13-8. *A,* Pathological changes induced by chloroquine showing mild variation in fiber size and an increase in internal nuclei but no prominent vacuoles (hematoxylin and eosin stain). *B,* An electron micrograph from the same case shows curvilinear bodies. (Dubowitz V, Sewry C. *Muscle Biopsy: A Practical Approach.* 3rd ed. London: Elsevier; 2007.)

Amiodarone

The amphiphilic antiarrhythmic drug amiodarone commonly causes a demyelinating peripheral neuropathy. It also causes myopathy by two mechanisms. The first is by inducing hypothyroidism and subsequent proximal myopathy. The second is autophagic in nature and is usually seen in association with the neuropathy. Patients have both proximal and distal weakness. The legs are affected more often than the arms. EMG shows myopathic MUAPs in proximal muscles, while the MUAPs are neuropathic in distal muscles. Muscle biopsy shows autophagic vacuoles[119] and myofiber necrosis.[120] Similar changes are seen in nerve biopsies.

Perhexiline

Perhexiline has been used in the treatment of angina pectoris and is known to cause a demyelinating peripheral neuropathy in some patients. In some cases, patients have associated myopathy with myalgia and proximal muscle weakness. The myopathy can occur in isolation.[121] Electron microscopy of muscle biopsies shows membranous and granular inclusions of probable lysosomal origin.[122]

CONCLUSION

Toxic myopathy is common and should be considered in every patient with weakness, myalgia, and cramps. Risk factors include extremes of age and impairment in metabolism of myotoxic medications (e.g., renal or liver failure). A combination of more than one potentially myotoxic drug and alcohol intake increases the risk of toxic myopathy. Muscle biopsy findings can be of great help in identifying which drug, from a long list of medications, is causing myopathy. Drugs and other toxins can cause various myopathies, including necrotizing, microtubular, mitochondrial, and lysosomal storage, as well as inflammatory. The clinical spectrum is quite diverse, including asymptomatic elevated serum CK, myalgia and muscle cramps, proximal muscle weakness, generalized muscle weakness, and rhabdomyolysis with myoglobinuria. A search for a specific drug or toxic agent is important because discontinuation of exposure usually results in resolution of the symptoms.

Acknowledgments

The author of this chapter and the textbook editor would like to thank Dr. Andrew G. Engel, professor of neurology, Mayo Clinic, Rochester, Minnesota, for his review of this manuscript.

REFERENCES

1. Lane RJM, Mastaglia FL. Drug-induced myopathies in man. *Lancet.* 1978;2:562–565.
2. Khan MA. Effect of myotoxins on skeletal muscle fibers. *Prog Neurobiol.* 1995;46:541–560.
3. Guis S, Mattei JP, Liote F. Drug-induced and toxic myopathies. *Best Pract Res Clin Rheumatol.* 2003;17:877–907.
4. Sieb JP, Gillessen T. Iatrogenic and toxic myopathies. *Muscle Nerve.* 2003;27:142–156.
5. Mastaglia FL, Gardner-Medwin D, Hudgson P. Muscle fibrosis and contractures in a pethidine addict. *BMJ.* 1971;4:532–533.
6. Rosenson RS. Current overview of statin-induced myopathy. *Am J Med.* 2004;116:408–416.
7. Thompson PD, Nugent AM, Herbert PN. Increases in creatine kinase after exercise in patients treated with HMG-CoA reductase inhibitors. *JAMA.* 1990;264:2992.
8. Walravens PA, Greene C, Frerman FE. Lovastatin, isoprenes, and myopathy. *Lancet.* 1998;2:1097–1098.
9. Argov Z. Drug-induced myopathies. *Curr Opin Neurol.* 2000;13:541–545.
10. Pasternak RC, Smith SC Jr, Bairey-Merz CN, et al. ACC/AHA/NHLBI clinical advisory on the use and safety of statins. *J Am Coll Cardiol.* 2002;40:567–572.
11. Thompson PD, Clarkson P, Karas RH. Statin-associated myopathy. *JAMA.* 2003;289:1681–1690.
12. Goldman JA, Fishman AB, Lee JE, et al. The role of cholesterol-lowering agents in drug-induced rhabdomyolysis and polymyositis. *Arthritis Rheum.* 1989;32:358–359.
13. Waclawik AJ, Lindal S, Engel AG. Experimental lovastatin myopathy. *J Neuropathol Exp Neurol.* 1993;52:542–549.
14. Farmer JA. Learning from the cerivastatin experience. *Lancet.* 2001;358:1383–1385.
15. Alsheikh-Ali AA, Ambrose MS, Kuvin JT, et al. The safety of rosuvastatin as used in common clinical practice: a postmarketing analysis. *Circulation.* 2005;111:3051–3057.
16. Rosenson RS. Current overview of statin-induced myopathy. *Am J Med.* 2004;116:408–416.
17. Dreier JP, Endres M. Statin-associated rhabdomyolysis triggered by grapefruit consumption. *Neurology.* 2004;62:670.
18. Gadbut AP, Caruso AP, Galper JB. Differential sensitivity of C2–C12 striated muscle cells to lovastatin and pravastatin. *J Mol Cell Cardiol.* 1995;27:2397–2402.
19. Nakahara K, Kuriyama M, Sonoda Y, et al. Myopathy induced by HMG-CoA reductase inhibitors in rabbits: a pathological, electrophysiological, and biochemical study. *Toxicol Appl Pharmacol.* 1998;152:99–106.
20. Baker SK, Goodwin S, Sur M, et al. Cytoskeletal myotoxicity from simvastatin and colchicine. *Muscle Nerve.* 2004;30:799–802.
21. Ucar M, Mjorndal T, Dahlqvist R. HMG-CoA reductase inhibitors and myotoxicity. *Drug Saf.* 2000;22:441–457.
22. Pasternak RC, Smith SC Jr., Bairey-Merz CN, et al. ACC/AHA/NHLBI clinical advisory on the use and safety of statins. *J Am Coll Cardiol.* 2004;40:567–572.
23. Fux R, Morike K, Gundel UF, et al. Ezetimibe and statin-associated myopathy. *Ann Intern Med.* 2004;140:671–672.
24. Gaist D, Rodriguez LA, Huerta C, et al. Lipid-lowering drugs and risk of myopathy: a population-based follow-up study. *Epidemiology.* 2001;12:565–569.
25. Litin SC, Anderson CF. Nicotinic acid–associated myopathy: a report of three cases. *Am J Med.* 1989;86:481–483.
26. Reaven P, Witztum JL. Lovastatin, nicotinic acid, and rhabdomyolysis. *Ann Intern Med.* 1988;109:597–598.

27. Kane MJ, Silverman LR, Rand JH, et al. Myonecrosis as a complication of the use of ε-aminocaproic acid: a case report and review of the literature. *Am J Med.* 1988;85:861–863.

28. Mastaglia FL. Adverse effects of drugs on muscle. *Drugs.* 1982;24:304–321.

29. Duane DD, Engel AG. Emetine myopathy. *Neurology.* 1970;20:733–739.

30. Lacomis D. Case of the month, June 1996. anorexia nervosa. *Brain Pathol.* 1996;6:535–536.

31. Kennedy M. Cardiac glycoside toxicity: an unusual manifestation of drug addiction. *Med J Aust.* 1981;2:686, 688–689.

32. Karalliedde L, Henry JA. Effects of organophosphates on skeletal muscle. *Hum Exp Toxicol.* 1993;12:289–296.

33. Wecker L, Laskowski B, Dettbarn WD. Neuromuscular dysfunction induced by acetylcholinesterase inhibition. *Fed Proc.* 1978;37:2818–2822.

34. Kovanen J, Somer H, Schroeder P. Acute myopathy associated with gasoline sniffing. *Neurology.* 1983;33:629–631.

35. Streicher HZ, Gabow PA, Moss AH, et al. Syndromes of toluene sniffing in adults. *Ann Intern Med.* 1981;94:758–762.

36. Ducloux D, Schuller V, Bresson-Vautrin C, Chalopin JM. Colchicine myopathy in renal transplant recipients on cyclosporin. *Nephrol Dial Transplant.* 1997;12:2389–2392.

37. Gruberg L, Har-Zahav Y, Agranat O, Freimark D. Acute myopathy induced by colchicine in a cyclosporine treated heart transplant recipient: possible role of the multidrug resistance transporter. *Transplant Proc.* 1999;31:2157–2158.

38. Rana SS, Giuliani MJ, Oddis CV, Lacomis D. Acute onset of colchicine myoneuropathy in cardiac transplant recipients: case studies of three patients. *Clin Neurol Neurosurg.* 1997;99:266–270.

39. Mora C, Rodriguez ML, Navarro JF. Cerivastatin-induced rhabdomyolysis in a renal transplant on cyclosporin. *Transplantation.* 2001;72:551.

40. Omar MA, Wilson JP, Cox TS. Rhabdomyolysis and HMG-CoA reductase inhibitors. *Ann Pharmacother.* 2001;35:1096–1107.

41. Willis JK, Tilton AH, Harkin JC, Boineau FG. Reversible myopathy due to labetalol. *Pediatr Neurol.* 1990;6:275–276.

42. Teicher A, Rosenthal T, Kissin E, Sarova I. Labetalol-induced toxic myopathy. *BMJ.* 1981;282:1824–1825.

43. Kottlors M, Jaksch M, Ketelsen U-W, Weiner S, Glocker FX, Lücking C-H. Valproic acid triggers acute rhabdomyolysis in a patient with carnitine palmitoyltransferase type II deficiency. *Neuromuscul Disord.* 2001;11:757–759.

44. Lam CW, Lau CH, Williams JC, Chan YW, Wong LJC. Mitochondrial myopathy, encephalopathy, lactic acidosis and stroke-like episodes (MELAS) triggered by valproate therapy. *Eur J Pediatr.* 1997;156:562–564.

45. Boot E, de Haan L. Massive increase in serum creatine kinase during olanzapine and quetiapine treatment, not during treatment with clozapine. *Psychopharmacology (Berl).* 2000;150:347–348.

46. Meltzer HY, Cola PA, Parsa M. Marked elevations of serum creatine kinase activity associated with antipsychotic drug treatment. *Neuropsychopharmacology.* 1996;15:395–405.

47. Meltzer HY. Massive serum creatine kinase increases with atypical antipsychotic drugs: what is the mechanism and the message? *Psychopharmacology (Berl).* 2000;150:349–350.

48. Hodak E, David M, Gadoth N, Sandbank M. Etretinate induced skeletal muscle damage. *Br J Dermatol.* 1987;116:623–626.

49. Hodak E, Gadoth N, David M, Sandbank M. Muscle damage induced by isotretinoin. *BMJ.* 1986;293:425–426.

50. Haller RG, Drachman DB. Alcoholic rhabdomyolysis: an experimental model in the rat. *Science.* 1980;208:412–415.

51. Song SK, Rubin E. Ethanol produces muscle damage in human volunteers. *Science.* 1972;175:327–328.

52. Haller RG, Knochel JP. Skeletal muscle disease in alcoholism. *Med Clin North Am.* 1984;68:91–103.

53. Anderson TL, Torrance CA. Metabolic mechanisms of acute alcoholic myopathy. *Neurology.* 1984;34:81.

54. Haller RG. Experimental acute alcoholic myopathy: a histochemical study. *Muscle Nerve.* 1985;8:195–203.

55. Rubenstein AE, Wainapel SF. Acute hypokalemic myopathy in alcoholism: a clinical entity. *Arch Neurol.* 1977;34:553–555.

56. Urbano-Marquez A, Fernandez-Sola J. Effects of alcohol on skeletal and cardiac muscle. *Muscle Nerve.* 2004;30:689–707.

57. Walsh JC, Conomy AB. The effect of ethyl alcohol on striated muscle: some clinical and pathological observations. *Aust NZ J Med.* 1977;7:485–490.

58. Kahn LB, Meyer JS. Acute myopathy in chronic alcoholism: a study of 22 autopsy cases, with ultrastructural observations. *Am J Clin Pathol.* 1970;53:516–530.

59. Martinez AJ, Hooshmand H, Faris AA. Acute alcoholic myopathy: enzyme histochemistry and electron microscopic findings. *J Neurol Sci.* 1973;20:245–252.

60. Martin F, Ward K, Slavin G, et al. Alcoholic skeletal myopathy, a clinical and pathological study. *Q J Med.* 1985;55:233–251.

61. Sunnasy D, Cairns SR, Martin F, et al. Chronic alcoholic skeletal muscle myopathy: a clinical, histological and biochemical assessment of muscle lipid. *J Clin Pathol.* 1983;36:778–784.

62. Martin FC, Levi AJ, Slavin G, et al. Glycogen content and activities of key glycolytic enzymes in muscle biopsies from control subjects and patients with chronic alcoholic skeletal myopathy. *Clin Sci (Lond).* 1984;66:69–78.

63. Perkoff GT, Hardy P, Velez-Garcia E. Reversible acute muscular syndrome in chronic alcoholism. *N Engl J Med.* 1966;274: 1277–1285.

64. Martin FC, Slavin G, Levi AJ. Alcoholic muscle disease. *Br Med Bull.* 1982;38:53–56.

65. Chui LA, Neustein H, Munsat TL. Tubular aggregates in subclinical alcoholic myopathy. *Neurology.* 1975;25:405–412.

66. Slavin G, Martin F, Ward P, et al. Chronic alcohol excess is associated with selective but reversible injury to type 2B muscle fibres. *J Clin Pathol.* 1983;36:772–777.

67. Jennings AE, Levey AS, Harrington JT. Amoxapine associated acute renal failure. *Arch Intern Med.* 1983;143:1525–1527.

68. Cogen FC, Rigg G, Simmons JL, et al. Phencyclidine-associated acute rhabdomyolysis. *Ann Intern Med.* 1978;88:210–212.

69. Streicher HZ, Gabow PA, Moss AH, et al. Syndromes of toluene sniffing in adults. *Ann Intern Med.* 1981;94:758–762.

70. Mebs D, Ownby CL. Myotoxic components of snake venoms: their biochemical and biological activities. *Pharmacol Ther.* 1990;48:223–236.

71. Gabow PA, Kaehny WD, Kelleher SP. The spectrum of rhabdomyolysis. *Medicine (Baltimore).* 1982;61:141–152.

72. Franca FO, Benvenuti LA, Fan HW, et al. Severe and fatal mass attacks by "killer" bees (Africanized honey bees, *Apis mellifera scutellata*) in Brazil: clinicopathological studies with measurement of serum venom concentrations. *Q J Med.* 1994;87:269–282.

73. Buchholz U, Mouzin E, Dickey R, et al. Haff disease: from the Baltic Sea to the U.S. shore. *Emerg Infect Dis.* 2000;6:192–195.

74. Papadimitriou A, Hadjigeorgiou GM, Tsairis P, et al. Myoglobinuria due to quail poisoning. *Eur Neurol.* 1996;36:142–145.

75. Comi G, Testa D, Cornelio F, Comola M, Canal N. Potassium depletion myopathy: a clinical and morphological study of six cases. *Muscle Nerve.* 1985;8:17–21.

76. Basser LS. Purgatives and periodic paralysis. *Med J Aust.* 1979;1:47–48.

77. Jensen OB, Mosdal C, Reske-Nielsen E. Hypokalemic myopathy during treatment with diuretics. *Acta Neurol Scand.* 1977;55:465–482.

78. Chemali KR, Suarez JI, Katirji B. Acute hypokalemic paralysis associated with long-term lithium therapy. *Muscle Nerve.* 2001;24:297–298.

79. Famularo G, Corsi FM, Giacanelli M. Iatrogenic worsening of hypokalemia and neuromuscular paralysis associated with the use of glucose solutions for potassium replacement in a young woman with licorice intoxication and furosemide abuse. *Acad Emerg Med.* 1999;6:960–964.

80. Mohamed SD, Chapman RS, Crooks J. Hypokalaemia, flaccid quadriparesis, and myoglobinuria with carbenoxolone (biogastrone). *BMJ.* 1966;5503:1581–1582.

81. Drutz DJ, Fan JH, Tai TY, Cheng JT, Hsieh WC. Hypokalemic rhabdomyolysis and myoglobinuria following amphotericin B therapy. *JAMA.* 1970;211:824–826.

82. Cervello A, Alfaro A, Chumillas MJ. Hypokalemic myopathy induced by *Giardia lamblia.* *N Engl J Med.* 1993;329: 210–211.

83. Nadel SM, Jackson JW, Ploth DW. Hypokalemic rhabdomyolysis and acute renal failure: occurrence following total parenteral nutrition. *JAMA.* 1979;241:2294–2296.

84. Chalmers AC, Greco CM, Miller RG. Prognosis in AZT myopathy. *Neurology.* 1991;41:1181–1184.

85. Arnaudo E, Dalakas M, Shanske S, et al. Depletion of muscle mitochondrial DNA in AIDS patients with zidovudine-induced myopathy. *Lancet.* 1991;337:508–510.

86. Mhiri C, Baudrimont M, Bonne G, et al. Zidovudine myopathy: a distinctive disorder associated with mitochondrial dysfunction. *Ann Neurol.* 1991;29:606–614.

87. Dalakas MC, Illa I, Pezeshkpour GH, et al. Mitochondrial myopathy caused by long-term zidovudine therapy. *N Engl J Med.* 1990;322:1098–1105.

88. Higuchi I, Takahashi K, Nakahara K, et al. Experimental germanium myopathy. *Acta Neuropathol (Berl).* 1991;82:55–59.

89. England JD, Walsh JC, Stewart P, et al. Mitochondrial myopathy developing on treatment with the HMG-CoA reductase inhibitors: simvastatin and pravastatin. *Aust NZ J Med.* 1995;25:374–375.

90. Kälkner KM, Rönnblom L, Karlsson Parra AK, et al. Antibodies against double-stranded DNA and development of polymyositis during treatment with interferon. *QJM.* 1998;91:393–399.

91. Cirigliano G, Della Rossa A, Tavoni A, et al. Polymyositis occurring during α-interferon treatment for malignant melanoma: a case report and review of the literature. *Rheumatol Int.* 1999;19:65–67.

92. Dietrich LL, Bridges AJ, Albertini MR. Dermatomyositis after interferon-α treatment. *Med Oncol.* 2000;17:64–69.

93. Hengstman GJ, Vogels OJ, ter Laak HJ, et al. Myositis during long-term interferon-α treatment. *Neurology.* 2000;54:2186.

94. Carroll GJ, Will RK, Peter JB, et al. Penicillamine-induced polymyositis and dermatomyositis. *J Rheumatol.* 1987;14:995–1001.

95. Takahashi K, Ogita T, Okudaira H, et al. D-penicillamine-induced polymyositis in patients with rheumatoid arthritis. *Arthritis Rheum.* 1986;29:560–564.

96. Eidson M, Philen RM, Sewell CM, et al. L-tryptophan and eosinophilia–myalgia syndrome in New Mexico. *Lancet.* 1990;335:645–648.

97. Kaufman LD. Neuromuscular manifestations of the L-tryptophan-associated eosinophilia–myalgia syndrome. *Curr Opin Rheumatol.* 1990;2:896–900.

98. Belongia EA, Hedberg CW, Gleich GJ, et al. An investigation of the cause of the eosinophilia–myalgia syndrome associated with tryptophan use. *N Engl J Med.* 1990;323:357–365.

99. Posada DLP, Philen RM, Schurz H, et al. Epidemiologic evidence for a new class of compounds associated with toxic oil syndrome. *Epidemiology.* 1999;10:130–134.

100. Gherardi RK, Coquet M, Cherin P, et al. Macrophagic myofasciitis lesions assess long-term persistence of vaccine-derived aluminum hydroxide in muscle. *Brain.* 2001;124:1821–1831.

101. Bowyer SL, LaMothe MP, Hollister JR. Steroid myopathy: incidence and detection in a population with asthma. *J Allergy Clin Immunol.* 1985;76:234–242.

102. Dropcho EJ, Soong SJ. Steroid-induced weakness in patients with primary brain tumors. *Neurology.* 1991;41:1235–1239.

103. Williams AJ, Baghat MS, Stableforth DE, et al. Dysphonia caused by inhaled steroids: recognition of a characteristic laryngeal abnormality. *Thorax.* 1983;38:813–821.

104. Braunstein PW Jr, DeGirolami U. Experimental corticosteroid myopathy. *Acta Neuropathol (Berl).* 1981;55:167–172.

105. Rannels SR, Rannels DE, Pegg AE, et al. Glucocorticoid effects on peptide chain initiation in skeletal muscle and heart. *Am J Physiol.* 1978;235:E134–E139.

106. Livingstone I, Johnson MA, Mastaglia FL. Effects of dexamethasone on fibre subtypes in rat muscle. *Neuropathol Appl Neurobiol.* 1981;7:381–398.

107. Lacomis D, Zochodne DW, Bird SJ. Critical illness myopathy. *Muscle Nerve.* 2000;23:1785–1788.

108. Bradley WG, Lassman LP, Pearce GW, et al. The neuromyopathy of vincristine in man: clinical, electrophysiological and pathological studies. *J Neurol Sci.* 1970;10:107–131.

109. Anderson PJ, Song SK, Slotwiner P. The fine structure of spheromembranous degeneration of skeletal muscle induced by vincristine. *J Neuropathol Exp Neurol.* 1967;26:15–24.

110. Jagose JT, Bailey RR. Muscle weakness due to colchicines in a renal transplant recipient. *NZ Med J.* 1997;110:343.

111. Kuncl RW, Duncan G, Watson D, et al. Colchicine myopathy and neuropathy. *N Engl J Med.* 1987;316:1562–1568.

112. Drenckhahn D, Lullmann-Rauch R. Experimental myopathy induced by amphiphilic cationic compounds including several psychotropic drugs. *Neuroscience.* 1979;4:549–562.

113. Mastaglia FL, Papadimitriou JM, Dawkins RL, et al. Vacuolar myopathy associated with chloroquine, lupus erythematosus and thymoma: report of a case with unusual mitochondrial changes and lipid accumulation in muscle. *J Neurol Sci.* 1977;34:315–328.

114. Estes ML, Ewing-Wilson D, Chou SM, et al. Chloroquine neuromyotoxicity: clinical and pathologic perspective. *Am J Med.* 1987;82:447–455.

115. Eadie MJ, Ferrier TM. Chloroquine myopathy. *J Neurol Neurosurg Psychiatry.* 1966;29:331–337.

116. Stauber WT, Hedge AM, Trout JJ, et al. Inhibition of lysosomal function in red and white skeletal muscles by chloroquine. *Exp Neurol.* 1981;71:295–306.

117. Sugita H, Higuchi I, Sano M, Ishiura S. Trial of a cysteine proteinase inhibitor, EST, in experimental chloroquine myopathy in rats. *Muscle Nerve.* 1987;10:516–523.

118. Stein M, Bell MJ, Ang LC. Hydroxychloroquine neuromyotoxicity. *J Rheumatol.* 2000;27:2927–2931.

119. Meier C, Kauer B, Muller U, et al. Neuromyopathy during chronic amiodarone treatment: a case report. *J Neurol.* 1979;220:231–239.

120. Clouston PD, Donnelly PE. Acute necrotising myopathy associated with amiodarone therapy. *Aust NZ J Med.* 1989;19:483–485.

121. Tomlinson IW, Rosenthal FD. Proximal myopathy after perhexiline maleate treatment. *BMJ.* 1977;1:1319–1320.

122. Fardeau M, Tome FM, Simon P. Muscle and nerve changes induced by perhexiline maleate in man and mice. *Muscle Nerve.* 1979;2:24–36.

CHAPTER 14

Toxic Neuropathies

Patrick M. Grogan and Jonathan S. Katz

INTRODUCTION

Peripheral nerve dysfunction can result from exposure to various organic and nonorganic compounds. The incidence of toxic occupational exposures has steadily decreased over time because of a better understanding of various chemicals and their adverse effects on the body, a general appreciation of risk in society, and an improvement in occupational health safety laws. Other toxic exposures associated with the development of a polyneuropathy include ingestion of certain toxic plants and animals, uncommon encounters between man and nature, recreational substance abuse, and medications prescribed by health-care professionals. This chapter synthesizes the available published information on the various toxins and their effects on the peripheral nerve in an effort to keep physicians aware of their existence, clinical presentations, diagnosis, and treatments. Case studies are provided to emphasize aspects of certain toxins.

NEUROPATHY SECONDARY TO ALCOHOL AND DRUGS OF ABUSE

Alcohol

Chronic alcohol abuse is associated with a distal, symmetrical, primarily sensory polyneuropathy. These cases typically present with painful dysesthesias and sensory loss affecting the distal lower extremities and, in more severe cases, the hands.[1] Neurological examination reveals the distal sensory loss with hyporeflexia. There may be weakness in more advanced cases. Autonomic involvement usually accompanies the sensory features, resulting in distal skin atrophy, discoloration, and hair loss. Gait ataxia or other features of cerebellar involvement are present if there is concomitant alcoholic cerebellar degeneration. Other complications, including liver disease, poor nutrition, memory impairment, and social disorganization, are common since peripheral polyneuropathy is often only one component of more generalized manifestations of alcohol toxicity.

Laboratory studies in the patient with alcoholic neuropathy may detect a transaminitis with elevated γ-glutamyltransferase levels and elevated mean red blood cell corpuscular volume. Serological levels of thiamine and other B vitamins[2] are not reliable indicators of their intake in a patient's diet.[1] Electrodiagnostic studies typically reveal an axonal polyneuropathy marked by reduced amplitudes of sensory nerve action potentials to a greater degree than compound motor action potentials. These features may be noted even in the absence of strong clinical evidence for a peripheral neuropathy.[1-5] Some reports have identified significant conduction velocity slowing and F wave prolongation, either with[2,5,6] or without[7] amplitude reduction, suggesting a wider spectrum of electrodiagnostic characteristics. Pathological studies, however, have consistently reported axonal degeneration as the primary abnormality in alcoholic neuropathy.[1,2,4,5]

Some controversy exists as to whether the neuropathy observed in alcoholic patients is a direct toxic effect of alcohol or a secondary phenomenon related to nutritional deficiencies. Several observations have pointed to nutritional deficiency, specifically, in thiamine and the B vitamins. First, alcoholic neuropathy is clinically similar to the neuropathy observed in patients with thiamine deficiency,[8] and progression of the neuropathy stabilizes and may even improve with thiamine and other vitamin replacement.[9] Thiamine deficiency in the absence of alcohol use has also been shown experimentally to induce axonal damage in animals,[5,10] while alcohol use in nutritionally well-fed animals did not.[1] Finally, reduced blood levels of thiamine and other measurable B vitamins have been reported in patients with alcoholic neuropathy.[11]

In contrast, the major argument for a direct toxic effect of alcohol on peripheral nerve comes from the study by Behse and Buchthal in which patients with alcohol-related neuropathy were compared to postgastrectomy patients who developed neuropathy but had no history of alcoholism.[2] The neuropathies in these groups were clinically similar, but more than 60% of the alcoholic patients had no identifiable nutritional deficiency and the postgastrectomy patients displayed prominent conduction velocity slowing, suggesting a different type of neuropathy compared to the alcoholic group.[2] This study has been challenged, however, since nutritional deficiency was based on subjective weight loss and normal serological levels of thiamine, both of which are unreliable indicators of proper nutrition levels.[1] Moreover, the electrodiagnostic studies on postgastrectomy patients were based on only six patients, while varying degrees of conduction slowing can be present in alcoholic patients.[2,6,7]

The treatment of alcoholic neuropathy involves discontinuing alcohol consumption and resuming proper nutritional intake. Thiamine and B vitamin supplementation may have some beneficial effect as well.[9] Patients may hope for stabilization of the symptoms since, clearly, substantial improvement in these patients is uncommon and may relate to the typically chronic duration of the neuropathy and the irreversibility of ongoing axonal damage at the time of diagnosis. Studies looking at recovery patterns are limited.

Inhalants and Nitrous Oxide

Several neurological disorders are caused by vitamin B_{12} or cobalamin deficiency, including subacute combined degeneration of the spinal cord, encephalopathy, and a predominantly large-fiber, sensory polyneuropathy. Identical disorders have been reported in patients exposed to nitrous oxide through general anesthesia, or in inhalational abusers of nitrous oxide, due to its disruptive effects on vitamin B_{12}–dependent biochemical pathways. Nitrous oxide oxidizes cobalamin, thereby disrupting the cobalamin-dependent methionine synthase reaction necessary to create methionine, which is a substrate for myelin production.

Neuropathic symptoms include progressive distal sensory loss with paresthesias and pain, often beginning in the hands. Predominant vibratory and proprioceptive sensory loss occurs on examination secondary to the involvement of large-fiber sensory nerves and the dorsal columns of the spinal cord. A "reverse" Lhermitte sign, or a sharp electric sensation ascending from the toes with neck flexion, may also be seen.[12] Extremity weakness with spasticity and hyperreflexia indicates the additional presence of a myelopathy. Electrophysiological studies have demonstrated varying results, with generalized conduction slowing of motor and sensory fibers and preserved amplitudes seen in some cases[13] and a predominantly axonal polyneuropathy in others.[14,15] Replacement of vitamin B_{12} intramuscularly may be associated with improvement in the peripheral neuropathy,[14,16] although this is not a universal feature.[17]

Drugs of Abuse: Opiates, Sedatives, and Amphetamines:

Various peripheral nerve disorders have been reported in association with abuse and overdose of opiates, sedatives, and amphetamines, including mononeuropathies, brachial plexopathies, and Guillain-Barré syndrome.[18-22] In one study of 198 heroin users, 49% were reported to have developed a peripheral neuropathy.[21] The diagnosis was based on a patient questionnaire, and the symptoms reported were most consistent with transient mononeuropathies, which most likely developed secondary to prolonged limb compression that occurred during deep periods of unconsciousness. Such neuropathies are likely the most common peripheral nerve disorders encountered in patients abusing these drugs. After compressive neuropathies, it should be clear that data in this area comes primarily from case studies or series and definitive evidence of causation between drug use and any specific peripheral nerve disorder is generally lacking.

NEUROPATHY SECONDARY TO DRUGS OR IATROGENIC NEUROPATHY

Several medications may cause a peripheral neuropathy, most of which are consistent with a length-dependent, predominantly sensory axonopathy. A detailed review of each of these medications is not provided in this chapter, considering that several well-written publications on this subject are already available.[15,23–25] Table 1 provides a quick reference of those medications with strong evidence substantiating an association with neuropathy development, as well as a brief description of their clinical, electrophysiological, and histopathological characteristics.

NEUROPATHY SECONDARY TO HEAVY METALS

Arsenic

Exposure to potentially toxic levels of arsenic can occur from drinking contaminated groundwater, working in mining and ore smelting plants, accidental ingestion of pesticides, and most infamously, intentional suicidal or homicidal ingestions. The neuropathy is a painful, length-dependent, sensory-greater-than-motor, peripheral axonopathy affecting all extremities.[31] Initial symptoms begin 2 to 3 weeks following the initial exposure with pain in the distal lower extremities, which progresses to include sensory loss and weakness and eventually involvement of the distal upper extremities.[32,33] Examination reveals distal sensory loss, hypo- or areflexia, and normal to mildly weak distal musculature. Systemic abnormalities that may serve as important clues to the diagnosis include weight loss, severe alopecia, and white horizontal striations on the nails (Mees' lines). Reports of the electrodiagnostic abnormalities vary and range from mild motor conduction slowing[34] to an axonal neuropathy marked by low-amplitude sensory and motor action potentials with relatively preserved conduction velocities.[33] Higher levels of arsenic exposure are associated with a more severe, rapidly progressing polyneuropathy, with electrodiagnostic demyelination, which can appear clinically and electrodiagnostically similar to Guillain-Barré syndrome.[35] In its most extreme form, arsenic toxicity can progress to quadriparesis and ventilator dependence.[36]

Diagnosis can be confirmed by detecting elevated arsenic levels in blood, urine, hair, or nail clippings. Elimination of continued arsenic exposure and use of sulfur chelators, including dimercaptosuccinic acid or penicillamine, are the standard treatments.[33] Resolution of neuropathic complaints depends on the length and severity of arsenic exposure before initiation of therapy.

Lead

Lead toxicity may occur from occupational (metal soldering, ore smelters, battery manufacturers, industrial painters), and nonoccupational (accidental ingestion of leaded paint by children, leaded water and food containers, certain antibacterial ointments[37]) exposures. Fortunately, the

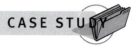

CASE STUDY

A 45-year-old woman living in a remote area of Alaska noted recurrent episodes of acute headache, nausea and vomiting, and a "swollen" sensation of her face, mouth, and throat. After 1 month of these symptoms, she noted slowly progressive, burning dysesthesias, pain, and numbness of her fingers and toes. The pain became excruciating after 1 to 2 weeks. On examination, she appeared ill and cachectic. Her hair appeared thin when compared to pictures taken only 2 months before, and she reported further loss of hair on her forearms and legs. Distal weakness and sensory loss was noted in all four extremities, more prominent in the legs. Reflexes were diffusely absent. A moderate to severe sensory ataxia was noted on gait examination. After several trips to a local physician, she was referred to a larger medical center for further evaluation. Electrodiagnostic studies demonstrated a diffuse, length-dependent, sensory-greater-than-motor axonopathy with only mild conduction slowing. F waves were unobtainable. Spinal fluid analysis was normal. Urine arsenic levels were obtained after an astute medical resident noted white lines on the nails of her fingers and toes; it returned 20× normal. Her husband was picked up by police for questioning after she reported several domestic disputes between them and that her favorite wine had recently "tasted funny." Although a bottle of wood cleaner containing arsenic was identified at the house, her husband was released from custody when the bottle was found unopened. High levels of arsenic were later identified in well water for their home. She had changed to drinking 2 to 3 glasses of water daily, as well as washing all her wine glasses, with water "from the tap" 2 to 3 months before symptom onset to save money, while her husband drank bottled water.

occurrence of lead toxicity has been greatly reduced due to improved public health. Peripheral neuropathy is one of the most common of the many effects that lead toxicity may have on the nervous system. Reports describe a pure motor neuropathy affecting the upper more than the lower extremities, presenting as symmetrical or asymmetrical wrist drop.[38] The weakness may involve other muscle groups of the distal upper extremities. Lower extremity involvement, including isolated foot drop, may also occur. A length-dependent, painful, predominantly sensory polyneuropathy has also been reported from lead exposure,[39,40] although the clinical and electrophysiological findings[39] from these reports leave open some questions as to the existence of this presentation. When sensory loss is noted by the patient or detected on clinical examination, it is usually minor in comparison to the motor abnormalities.[38] Abdominal pain, constipation, and microcytic, hypochromic anemia are characteristically present in lead poisoning and serve as critical clues to the diagnosis. The absence of these systemic features should raise doubts regarding the diagnosis.[38]

Electrodiagnostic studies in lead-induced neuropathy show that abnormalities of nerve conduction begin to occur with lead levels in blood above 70 μg/100 mL.[38] These studies reveal a range of electrophysiological abnormalities, from mild motor conduction slowing to axonal features with frank electromyographic denervation. Peripheral nerve pathology studies in lead intoxication show increased paranodal demyelination and internodal remyelination with low-level lead exposure, while advanced neuropathies demonstrate axonal degeneration.[38] Detecting elevated blood lead levels above 70 μg/100 mL, an established level below which peripheral neuropathy is unlikely to occur,[41] may further assist in the diagnosis.

Treatment of lead-induced neuropathy requires eliminating continued exposure and initiating therapy to enhance excretion with various chelating agents, such as ethylenediaminetetraacetic acid, penicillamine, and British anti-Lewisite. These agents are able to lower blood levels, but no conclusive evidence shows that this approach assists in the resolution of neuropathic symptoms.[33,38]

Thallium

Thallium toxicity has become rare since thallium was banned from use in pesticides in the 1970s. Currently, this neuropathy is only seen in unintentional ingestions, usually linked to attempted homicides. Neuropathic and systemic symptoms are similar to arsenic exposure with a painful, progressive, length-dependent, sensory-greater-than-motor axonopathy that develops within 1 to 2 weeks following exposure.[33] The pain and dysesthetic sensations in the limbs are severe and excruciating,[32] typically beyond that seen in common sensory neuropathies from other causes. Examination findings include distal sensory loss,

distal weakness, and hyporeflexia. Alopecia occurs similar to arsenic toxicity. A dark discoloration of the hair root under light microscopy also occurs because of gaseous inclusions induced by thallium, which cause light to diffract.[42] Electrodiagnostic and nerve biopsy findings are both consistent with axonal degeneration.[33] Diagnosis is made by thallium analysis in blood, urine, or hair samples. No specific therapy exists for the neuropathy, but gastric lavage, activated charcoal, hemodialysis, and Prussian blue all assist in blocking further absorption and accelerating removal of the toxin.[33]

NEUROPATHY SECONDARY TO ORGANIC CHEMICALS

Acrylamide

Chronic inhalation or skin exposure to acrylamide monomers, used in the creation of grouting agents, adhesives, and flocculators, may induce a length-dependent, sensorimotor, peripheral axonopathy.[33,43] Exposure has been generally limited to specific occupations, although recently, interest in acrylamide exposure has resurfaced with the discovery that it can be formed unintentionally by cooking certain foods at high temperatures (particularly French fries; Figure 14-1).[44] It is doubtful that consumption of such foods is likely to expose an individual to neurotoxic doses.

Distal sensory loss with ataxia, weakness, and hyporeflexia, initially starting in the lower extremities and gradually spreading to the arms, is characteristic of this neuropathy.[43] Autonomic dysfunction, with distal hyperhidrosis and cold skin temperature, are also often noted. Central nervous system effects, cerebellar dysfunction in particular, may accompany the neuropathy, accentuating the sensory ataxia. Electrophysiological studies reveal diffuse amplitude reduction of sensory nerve action potentials and minimal slowing of sensory and motor conduction velocities.[43] Histopathology studies have previously concluded the peripheral nerve injury is mediated by distal axonal degeneration affecting large myelinated axons most severely,[33] but more recent studies suggest impaired neurotransmitter release at the presynaptic terminal as the predominant mechanism of action.[45] Direct measurements of serum acrylamide levels are not commonly available.

Interest in acrylamide neuropathy has also surged because acrylamide neurotoxicity can be experimentally induced in rats. Experimental acrylamide neuropathy serves as a model of diffuse axonal polyneuropathy,[46] and its histochemical similarities to streptozotocin-induced diabetic neuropathy in rats have raised new theories regarding a possible common mechanism.[47] Several treatments, including the immunosuppressant FK-506 and

Table 1: Medications Causing Peripheral Neuropathy[15,23–30]

Drug Category	Drug Name	Neuropathy Phenotype		
		Motor	Sensory	Pain
Antineoplastic	Bortezomib*	+	+	+
	Misonidazole	−	+	+
	Platins (cisplatin* or oxaliplatin*)	−	+	+/−
	Suramin	+	+	+/−
	Taxols (paclitaxel or docetaxel)	+	+	+
	Thalidomide*	−	+	+
	Vinca alkaloids (vincristine*)	+	+	+/−
Immunosuppressant	Tacrolimus	+	+	−
Antibiotic, antimycobacterial, antiretroviral	Dapsone	+	+	+/−
	Dideoxynucleosides*	−	+	+
	Isoniazid	+	+	+/−
	Metronidazole	−	+	+/−
Antiarrhythmic	Amiodarone*	+	+	+/−
Other	Almitrine	−	+	+
	Disulfiram	−	+	+/−
	Perhexiline	+	+	+
	Phenytoin	−	+	+/−
	Pyridoxine	−	+	+

*indicates neuropathy is commonly associated with this medication.

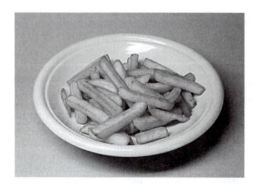

Figure 14-1. Acrylamide toxicity has been associated with consumption of starchy foods cooked at high temperatures, such as French fries.

the neurotrophic factor NT-3, have demonstrated promising results toward prevention of neuropathy progression in these experimental models.[44,46]

Carbon Disulfide

Chronic, low-level, inhalational exposure to carbon disulfide, used currently in rayon and cellophane production, in dry-cleaning, and as a component of certain insecticides for the conservation of grain, has been linked to the development of a distal sensorimotor axonopathy.[43,48] Fortunately, improvements in occupational health safety have reduced carbon disulfide levels in the workplace, and the current "safe" threshold limit value that may be measured serologically

Electrophysiological Characteristics	Pathology	Additional Characteristics
Axonal and demyelinating	—	Subjective improvement with lenalidomide salvage therapy
Axonal	Axonal degeneration	Infrequently used
Axonal	Axonal degeneration	Ototoxicity; possible prevention with calcium and magnesium
Axonal and demyelinating	Axonal degeneration	Electrophysiological conduction block
Axonal	Axonal degeneration	—
Axonal	Axonal degeneration	Dorsal root ganglion degeneration
Axonal	Axonal degeneration	Early autonomic features common
Axonal and demyelinating	—	Improvement with IVIG reported; protect versus acrylamide neuropathy
Axonal	Axonal degeneration	Pure motor variant reported
Axonal and demyelinating	Axonal degeneration and myelin splitting	—
—	Axonal degeneration	Responds to pyridoxine replacement
Axonal	Axonal degeneration	—
Axonal and demyelinating	Axonal degeneration and segmental demyelination	Optic neuropathy
Axonal	Axonal degeneration	Marked weight loss occasionally
Axonal	Axonal degeneration	Optic neuropathy
Demyelinating	Axonal degeneration and segmental demyelination	—
—	Axonal degeneration	—
Axonal	Axonal degeneration	—

has been established at less than 31 mg/m^3.[48,49] Even with these reductions, however, sensorimotor complaints and electrophysiological abnormalities have been reported in individuals with levels below this value.[48] Typical features of a distal neuropathy, including sensory loss, weakness, and hyporeflexia, are noted on examination. Electrophysiological studies demonstrate conduction velocity slowing in motor and sensory nerves[49] and fibrillations on electromyography of lower extremity muscles.[43] Nerve histopathology demonstrates predominantly large-fiber axonal and myelin degeneration.[50] Despite removal from exposure, sensory and motor complaints, as well as electrophysiological changes, may persist for years,[49] and there are no reported treatments.

Dioxin or Agent Orange

Agent Orange is the code name given to a particular herbicide that was used extensively during the Vietnam War from 1962 to 1971.[51] The herbicide contained an equal mixture of two phenoxy acids, one of which had an obligatory byproduct during its production, 2,3,7,8-tetrachlorodibenzo-p-dioxin, otherwise known as TCDD or dioxin. Various health issues among Vietnam War veterans became attributed, albeit with some controversy, to dioxin, including various cancers, birth defects in children fathered by veterans, cognitive or neuropsychiatric problems, and peripheral neuropathy.

Whether Agent Orange causes a neuropathy remains controversial. Neuropathic symptoms theoretically attributed to dioxin exposure are typically a distal sensory polyneuropathy affecting the lower extremities, with abnormal sensory findings and hyporeflexia on examination.[52] Most studies have noted that only individuals with higher exposures, characterized as those with dermatological changes ("chloracne") from direct contact with dioxin had any significant increase in risk for developing a polyneuropathy.[52,53] Experimentally, both electrodiagnostic and histological evidence for a toxic polyneuropathy has been observed in rats following an intraperitoneal injection of dioxin,[54,55] but it is unclear how this correlates with dioxin exposures reported in the Vietnam War or in particular occupations.

The National Academy of Sciences Institute of Medicine report on Agent Orange exposure concluded there was inadequate evidence to determine that exposure causes a peripheral neuropathy based on available Vietnam veteran studies.[51] The report included studies on veterans involved in Operation Ranch Hand who were responsive in varying capacities for aerial spraying of Agent Orange and likely had the highest levels of exposure. Subsequent to the Institute of Medicine report, two other reports on the association between dioxin and neuropathy in Vietnam veterans were published. The first concluded an increased odds ratio (2.5 to 5.8) of a "diagnosed" peripheral neuropathy in Operation Ranch Hand veterans with high serum dioxin levels.[56] This study is severely limited since no electrodiagnostic testing was employed, minimal objective evidence for a peripheral neuropathy was used, and a "diagnosed" neuropathy (their most conclusive definition for the presence of neuropathy) could be based purely on subjective sensory complaints. The second study assessed Korean military members who served in the Vietnam War and concluded that, in general, veterans were 2.39 times more likely to develop a peripheral neuropathy compared to non-Vietnam veterans.[57] It was unclear, however, what type of exposure any of their subjects had to Agent Orange, and no documentation showed what variables were used to make the diagnosis of a polyneuropathy, although it appears that nerve conduction studies were used. Thus, even taking these studies into account, there continues to be insufficient evidence to associate a peripheral polyneuropathy with prior Agent Orange exposure.

Ethylene Oxide

Ethylene oxide is a gas used for sterilization of medical equipment and has been implicated as a cause of an axonal polyneuropathy in medical personnel and hospital sterilizer workers.[43] It has also been implicated as a potential etiology for the neuropathy observed in patients on chronic dialysis.[58] The neuropathy reported is predominantly sensory, with or without objective sensory loss and hyporeflexia on examination. Mild motor and sensory conduction

slowing has been observed on electrophysiological testing in some studies, although others have found few abnormalities to suggest a peripheral neuropathy.[59] Nerve biopsy findings have ranged from relatively normal[59] to evidence of axonal degeneration.[43]

Hexane and Hexacarbons

Awareness of hexacarbon neuropathy related to n-hexane exposure developed in the 1960s when it was first reported.[60] N-hexane is a component of petroleum products, solvents, and glues and has been associated with occupational-related neuropathies in automobile mechanics,[60] shoemaking,[43,61] purse making,[62] furniture finishing,[43] and screen printing.[63] Recreational inhalant abuse has also been linked to n-hexane-associated neuropathy, i.e., "gasoline sniffer's neuropathy" and "glue-sniffer's neuropathy."[64,65]

The typical phenotype is a distal-predominant, sensorimotor polyneuropathy with sensory loss, distal weakness and atrophy, and hyporeflexia on examination.[43,66] A subacute, predominantly motor phenotype has also been reported; this may reflect a predisposition toward the development of focal, compressible neuropathies superimposed on a generalized polyneuropathy.[64,65] Weight loss, anorexia, cognitive slowing, and hallucinations can also be associated with the polyneuropathy, particularly in more severe cases. Electrophysiological testing may show decreased sensory amplitudes as the primary abnormality,[67] but several recent reports have documented multifocal motor conduction block with prominent conduction slowing in exposed patients.[61,62,64,65,68] The latter electrodiagnostic features appear more commonly in those patients reported with a predominantly motor phenotype. Nerve biopsy features range from normal findings in early or minimal exposure[65] to axonal loss with subperineurial edema, focal enlargement of axons, and paranodal myelin retraction.[64,68]

Treatment includes removal from exposure to n-hexane-containing compounds, although the neuropathy may still progress for several weeks and even months,[43,64] a phenomenon labeled in other cases of n-hexane neuropathy as "coasting."[65,69] This is typically followed by gradual spontaneous improvement over weeks to several years.[43,60] Claims of improvement with B-complex vitamin administration and Chinese traditional medicine have been reported,[66] but no formal studies support this.

Methyl Bromide

Peripheral neuropathy is an uncommon side effect of chronic exposure to methyl bromide. Exposure to methyl bromide may occur with use of soil fumigants,[70] but it is also used as a refrigerant and as a component in fire extinguishers. The development of neuropathic symptoms is usually associated with chronic, low-level exposure, typically resulting from inhalation, over several months,[71] but a more acute presentation, within 1 week of exposure through abraded skin, has also been reported.[70] A distal, sensorimotor axonal polyneuropathy occurs that is similar to other toxic neuropathies, both clinically and electrophysiologically.[43,70] With more acute exposures, the neuropathy can be accompanied by central nervous system deficits, including pyramidal signs, cerebellovestibular abnormalities, and encephalopathy.[33,71] The sensory loss and weakness following gradually resolve after removal of the exposure,[43] although minor sensory complaints may persist for several years.[71]

Organophosphorus Esters and Triorthocresyl Phosphate

While organophosphorus ester toxicity is most commonly remembered for its acetylcholinesterase blocking effects at cholinergic synapses (insecticides, biochemical weapons), awareness of its toxic effects on peripheral nerve is also important. Triorthocresyl phosphate (TOCP) is the most commonly reported cause of toxic neuropathies among the organophosphorus esters.[72–74] TOCP is used as a lubricant in the plastic industry and as an aircraft engine oil. The toxicity of TOCP and other organophosphorus in the peripheral nerve are due, at least partly, to their covalent modification of a neuronal protein known as neuropathy target esterase, resulting in axonal degeneration.[75,76]

The associated neuropathy manifests as a subacute, progressive, distal-predominant neuropathy affecting the lower extremities initially, followed within a few days by upper extremity involvement.[74] Symptom onset ranges from 8 days to 2 months following ingestion and may be limited to cramping of distal limb muscles.[72,74] Prominent distal weakness and atrophy, however, soon follows. Proximal extension is uncommon, but the distal weakness may be so severe that the patient is bedridden. Distal sensory loss may be present but is relatively mild in comparison to the motor involvement. Reflexes are universally reduced at the ankles but are typically retained elsewhere and may even be hyperactive several weeks to months after symptom onset.[72,74] There is no cranial nerve or respiratory involvement. Electrophysiological studies reveal diffuse amplitude reduction and mild to moderate conduction slowing of both motor and sensory nerves and neurogenic motor unit potentials, with abnormal spontaneous activity on electromyography in affected limbs.[72,74] Cerebrospinal fluid analysis may demonstrate mild elevations in protein but is otherwise normal.[72] No treatment can be offered, and the distal weakness is typically irreversible and severely disabling.

The notoriety of TOCP toxicity is most evident in past epidemics of individuals ingesting TOCP-contaminated substances. Significant historical epidemics have been documented in the United States during the Prohibition era of the 1920s and 1930s and in Calcutta, India, in the late 1980s. An estimated 15,000 individuals were afflicted with a "paralytic illness" following consumption of a patented "medicine" known as Jamaica ginger extract, colloquially known as "Jake"[73,77] (Figure 14-2). TOCP, a tasteless, colorless, odorless liquid, was added by bootleggers to alcohol-containing substances such as Jake to comply with U.S. Treasury Department regulations and chemical analysis during Prohibition.[77] The residual disability following Jake ingestion is evidenced in blues lyrics from the 1930s, including "Jake Walk Blues" by the Allen Brothers, and "Jake Liquor Blues" by Ishmon Bracey.[73,77] In 1988, a similar epidemic occurred in India, where approximately 500 individuals developed a "crippling illness." The neuropathy was eventually linked to ingestion of TOCP-contaminated rapeseed oil used in cooking.[72]

NEUROPATHY SECONDARY TO MARINE TOXINS

Ciguatera Neuropathy

Ciguatera was initially reported from eating snails, but it is now recognized that it may be associated with consumption of various tropical fish, including red snapper, grouper, and barracuda.[78,79] The causative agent, ciguatoxin, is produced by the dinoflagellate *Gambierdiscus toxicus* found in algae, which is eaten by smaller fish and then transmitted up the food chain.[80] Symptoms of nausea and vomiting develop within 3 to 12 hours of ingestion. The peripheral neuropathy is usually the most distressing neurological symptom,[78] although a spectrum of complaints, including myalgias, weakness, sensory abnormalities, headaches, tremor, and ataxia, commonly occur.

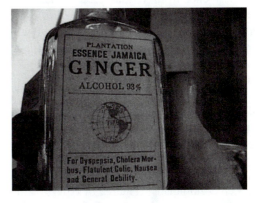

Figure 14-2. Bottle of Jamaica ginger extract, a substance often consumed during the Prohibition era and often contaminated with triorthocresyl phosphate. (From http://www.poppascountry.com/museum/museum07.jpg.)

The neuropathy from ciguatera toxin is marked by the onset of acral and perioral paresthesias, dysesthesias, and pruritus that develop 12 to 48 hours after ingestion of contaminated fish.[79–81] Paradoxical temperature reversal is a common complaint that is relatively specific to this neuropathy.[80,82] This reversal is marked by the experience of a warm, burning, and dysesthetic sensation when patients are exposed to cold temperatures on their skin. Less commonly, warm temperatures are perceived as normal or cold. Gross temperature perception using baths of varying water temperature is normal, but temperatures less than 25°C reliably produce severe burning and paresthesias that did not develop with exposure to warmer temperatures.[82] It has been suggested this phenomenon results from the toxins preferential activity on small, unmyelinated C-polymodal nociceptor fibers.[80,82,83]

Examination findings suggestive of a peripheral neuropathy are typically limited to reduced light touch, pain, and vibration sensation and hyporeflexia.[80–82] Although subjective weakness and myalgias are commonly reported, objective weakness is rarely found. Diagnosis is based on the clinical presentation and recognizing the temporal relation to fish ingestion. Electrophysiological studies have demonstrated a spectrum of characteristics, ranging from normal findings[80] to motor and sensory conduction slowing with preserved amplitudes.[81] Nerve biopsies show abnormalities of the myelin sheath, with prominent edema of the adaxonal Schwann cell cytoplasm in severe cases.[84] Bioassays are being developed to detect ciguatoxin levels in suspected fish tissues.[85]

Treatment of ciguatera is typically supportive, and symptoms usually resolve within days to weeks, although they can last for several months following exposure.[79,82] Recurrent sensory abnormalities may be noted with alcohol ingestion or exercise.[79] Infusions of hyperosmotic mannitol (10 mL/kg of 20% mannitol solution) have been reported to reduce the painful dysesthesias if administered within 48 hours of symptom onset, but this is based solely on empirical data from various case studies.[78] A study evaluating the effect of mannitol on nerves exposed to ciguatoxin in rats demonstrated no improvement in the electrophysiological abnormalities induced by the toxin.[86]

Tetrodotoxin-related Neuropathy

Tetrodotoxin is an exceptionally potent sodium channel blocker that is found in high concentrations in the skin and viscera of tetraodontiform fish, including puffer fish *(Fugu poecilonotus)* and porcupine fish *(Diodon hystrix),* as well as in blue-ringed octopus *(Hapalochlaena maculosa)* and certain amphibians (Figure 14-3).[87,88] The toxin is best recognized in tales of fatal poisonings following ingestion of improperly prepared fugu, an expensive Japanese delicacy of raw puffer fish that should only be eaten when prepared by a specially licensed chef.

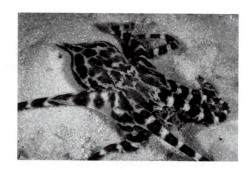

Figure 14-3.   The venom of the blue-ringed octopus contains tetrodotoxin, a potent sodium channel blocker. Human toxicity typically occurs due to accidental contact with it. (From the Barwon Bluff Marine Sanctuary Web site http://www.barwonbluff.com.au/bluff%20life/below%20waves/animals/inverts/molluscs/cephalods/pages/blue%20ring%20octopus.htm.)

Tetrodotoxin poisoning causes a rapidly progressive sensorimotor polyneuropathy that may affect bulbar and respiratory muscles. Acral and perioral paresthesias and sensory loss develop within minutes to hours of ingestion.[87,88] Limb weakness develops soon after and may result in flaccid quadriparesis.[88] Autonomic neuropathy symptoms, including hyperhydrosis, excessive salivation, hypotension, bradycardia, and temperature dysregulation, are common. Clinical severity depends on the amount of the toxin ingested, and it is recommended that the skin, liver, gonads, and intestines be avoided as these tissues contain the greatest concentrations of toxin.[89]

The underlying pathophysiology of tetrodotoxin poisoning relates to sodium channel blockade that impairs propagation of the nerve action potential. This conduction abnormality can be detected by electrophysiological studies that disclose evidence of profound sensorimotor conduction velocity slowing (less than 30 m/sec for upper extremities and less than 23 m/sec for lower extremities) without conduction block or temporal dispersion.[88] Prolonged terminal motor and F wave latencies are typically the most notable electrodiagnostic features.[88] Sensory nerve action potential amplitudes may be mildly reduced, but motor studies retain normal amplitudes and morphology. These abnormalities gradually resolve as the toxin clears.

Treatment is supportive, and recoveries may be dramatic. The literature contains examples of rapid improvements from a dense quadriparesis with respirator dependency back to normal, provided adequate supportive care is initiated early.[87,88]

Paralytic Shellfish Poisoning

Saxitoxin is a heat-stable, water-soluble compound found in various dinoflagellates that is concentrated in clams, mussels, and other shellfish that ingest the microorganisms. High concentrations of the dinoflagellates in water may discolor it black, pink, or red (i.e., red tide), during which times shellfish harvesting must be avoided.[89] Saxitoxin blocks sodium transport by binding to voltage-sensitive sodium channels of susceptible cell membranes.[90]

Ingestion of saxitoxin-contaminated shellfish may induce neuropathic complaints, which typically include numbness and paresthesias of the distal extremities and the perioral region.[91–93] Symptoms develop within 1 to 2 hours of ingestion and spontaneously resolve without residual abnormalities in 1 to 2 days. Subjective weakness has been reported in 30% to 70% of patients,[92,93] but reports of objective limb weakness are unusual. The term *paralytic* reflects the respiratory depression that can occur in severe poisonings. This has been attributed to blockade of diaphragmatic neurotransmission and has been demonstrated experimentally using diaphragmatic electromyography in rodents.[94] Electrophysiological testing shows moderately prolonged F wave latencies,[95] with prolonged motor and sensory latencies and slow conduction velocities in more severe intoxication.[96] The latter are similar to the electrodiagnostic changes seen with tetrodotoxin poisoning, which likely reflects the common effect on sodium channels.

Treatment for paralytic shellfish poisoning is supportive, with patients surviving even severe respiratory compromise if there is adequate ventilatory support. 4-Aminopyridine has shown promising benefits in rapidly reversing the diaphragmatic blockade experimentally, but no studies are available in humans.[94]

NEUROPATHY SECONDARY TO PLANT TOXINS

Amygdalin Neuropathy

The cyanogenic glycoside, amygdalin, is found in several plant sources, particularly in the seeds of apples, pears, and members of the *Prunus* species (apricots, plums, peaches, etc.).[97] Amygdalin is converted into hydrogen cyanide after ingestion and may induce cyanide toxicity. Reported neurological complications of cyanide toxicity include peripheral nerve demyelination, optic neuropathy, deafness, and parkinsonism.[97] Because these fruit seeds are uncommon in Western diets, clinical cyanide toxicity is rarely seen. The increased popularity of herbal medicines, however, may change this.

Recently, two cases were reported of a subacute polyneuropathy in young, otherwise healthy individuals who took no medications other than daily herbal "supplements"—apricot kernels in one and "taoren," or peach seeds, in the other.[98,99] Both noted gradual, slowly progressive sensory loss and mild weakness involving the distal extremities symmetrically several weeks after seed ingestion began. Burning dysesthesias were reported by one.[98] Deep tendon reflexes were diffusely reduced. Electrophysiological studies revealed a mixed sensorimotor polyneuropathy with diffusely reduced amplitudes. Conduction velocities were normal, but distal motor latencies were prolonged and the terminal latency index was reduced in one.[98] Laboratory workup for other causes of peripheral neuropathy was normal except for reduced vitamin B_{12} levels in one.[99] This latter finding was considered unrelated because no concomitant evidence of subacute combined degeneration or macrocytosis was present. Symptoms gradually improved after discontinuation of herbal supplements without residual neurological sequelae.

Buckthorn Neuropathy

Tullidora toxin is present in the seeds of a shrub of the buckthorn family, *Karwinskia humboldtiana*, which is found in southwestern Texas, New Mexico, California, and central and northern Mexico.[86] Ingestion of this toxin results in a subacute, progressive, symmetrical motor polyneuropathy similar to Guillain-Barré syndrome.[100–102] Symptoms of motor weakness may not be noticed until a few weeks following ingestion, but once they begin, they may progress rapidly to quadriplegia with respiratory or bulbar paralysis within a few days. Spinal fluid is typically normal and displays no evidence of the albuminocytological dissociation. Electrophysiological testing on cats experimentally exposed to tullidora reveals diffuse motor conduction slowing, typical of a demyelinating polyneuropathy.[102] Initial reports support "buckthorn neuropathy" as a primary demyelinating disease, with Schwann cell enlargement and degeneration of the myelin sheath.[100] More recent electron microscopy studies, however, reveal widened periaxonal spaces and redistribution of cytoskeletal elements in the axoplasm, suggesting axonal loss with secondary demyelination.[103] Treatment is generally supportive, and near-complete functional recovery is expected if patients survive the initial insult.

Neurolathyrism

A pure motor spastic paraplegia can occur from prolonged ingestion of *Lathyrus sativus*, commonly referred to as the grass or chickling pea.[104] This plant is common to southern Europe and central Asia, and increased reliance on it as a food source in times of famine have led to large numbers of cases. Clinical signs are usually limited to upper motor neuron involvement. Lower motor neuron involvement has been reported in 15% of patients[105] and a peripheral sensory polyneuropathy in 7%.[106] Electrophysiological studies in symptomatic patients have revealed primarily demyelinating abnormalities, including motor and sensory conduction slowing, prolonged distal motor latencies, and reduced motor unit recruitment on concentric needle electromyography.[104,106] Light and electron microscopy findings also support a demyelinating polyneuropathy, with irregular thickening, degeneration, and vesiculation of the myelin sheath in the paranodal regions.[106] Treatment is preventative, with discontinuation of further *Lathyrus* ingestion. Some patients notice mild improvement in spasticity over 1 to 3 months, although the neurological illness is typically irreversible.

Ergotism

Ergot intoxication secondary to excessive ingestion of rye contaminated by the fungus *Claviceps purpurea* has been linked to epidemics of limb ischemia and gangrene from the 9th to the 19th centuries.[107] Modern cases of ergotism are rare but have been reported in patients suffering from chronic migraines who use excessive doses of ergotamine tartrate. From this group, case reports of transient, isolated mononeuropathies, including bilateral peroneal and lateral popliteal neuropathies, have been

CASE STUDY

A 32-year-old man from Ethiopia developed diffuse cramping and progressive heaviness and weakness of his legs over 3 to 4 months. Drought conditions extending for several months prior had precipitated the increased use of *guaya*, or grass pea, in daily food consumption for his family and all other families nearby. As he was young and had a wife and three children to care for, he continued his daily job with the railway system near a large city that required extensive manual labor, despite the daily cramping and weakness sensations. He sought medical attention after he developed progressive stiffness in his legs that resulted in several falls. On examination, mild weakness was noted in all lower extremity muscles, slightly more noticeable in the proximal muscles. Prominent spasticity and hyperreflexia was noted in both legs. No significant weakness or alterations in muscle tone or bulk were found in his arms. His physician reported seeing similar cases in other individuals in local communities and had been recommending alternative food sources to avoid grass pea consumption. He followed the advice; 2 months afterward, he reported that the stiffness had lessened slightly but continued to cause limitations in ambulation and with climbing stairs.

reported.[107,108] It has been suggested the mononeuropathies are due to nerve ischemia, possibly secondary to diffuse vasoconstriction; however, the limited clinical and electrophysiological evidence documented does not provide convincing evidence to support this.

NEUROPATHY SECONDARY TO REPTILE AND INSECT TOXINS

Snakes

Snake envenomation following bites from cobras, kraits, coral snakes, pit vipers, and other snakes may produce clinical features related to neuromuscular junction dysfunction.[109] Commonly reported examination features include ptosis, bulbar and respiratory, and extremity weakness, all of which develop within 1 to 10 hours of exposure. Normal neuromuscular junction physiology may become disrupted at the presynaptic (α-bungarotoxin) or postsynaptic (β-bungarotoxin) nerve terminals.[109] Respiratory failure is the most serious and life-threatening consequence of snake envenomation, and aggressive respiratory support may be required. Isolated cases of distal sensory,[110] sensorimotor, and pure motor[111] polyneuropathies have been reported.

Ticks

A syndrome of rapidly progressive, pure motor weakness affecting limb, bulbar, respiratory, and ocular muscles occurs from exposure to certain tick species. Known as *tick paralysis*, the syndrome is caused by three tick varieties; *Dermacentor andersoni* (northwest United States), *Dermacentor variabilis* (southeast United States),[109] and *Ixodes holocyclus* (Australia).[112] The toxin from *I. holocyclus* has been shown to impair presynaptic release of acetylcholine,[112] which is also suspected in North American species; thus, tick paralysis is most consistent with a neuromuscular junction disorder, rather than a peripheral polyneuropathy.

The clinical syndrome is most commonly observed in children below the age of 9.[113,114] Symptoms of progressive, proximal-greater-than-distal limb weakness develop approximately 3 to 7 days after attachment of the female tick.[109,115] The weakness steadily progresses unless the tick is removed. Dysarthria, dysphagia, and respiratory compromise requiring assistive ventilation develop with involvement of bulbar muscles. Facial weakness and weakness of extraocular muscles may also be seen.[112,113,115] Hypo- or areflexia is common, but sensation is spared. Electrodiagnostic studies reveal a consistent pattern of reduced motor amplitudes with normal to minimally slowed conduction velocities with normal sensory studies.[112,114,115] One report described normal low- and high-frequency repetitive nerve stimulation.[114] Cerebrospinal fluid studies are unremarkable.[114,115]

Removal of the tick results in rapid resolution of clinical weakness over 1 to 2 days[113,115] with recovery of motor amplitudes on electrodiagnostic testing.[112,114,115] Case reports from Australia have noted slower clinical recovery than that seen in the United States, and mild worsening may even be observed 24 to 48 hours after tick removal. Respiratory support was required for more than 1 week following tick removal in certain cases.[112] It has, therefore, been suggested that antitoxin for *I. holocyclus* should be administered at the same time as tick removal to accelerate recovery.[112]

The polyradiculoneuritis, cranial neuropathies, and Guillain-Barré syndrome–like neuropathy associated with Lyme disease are other examples of neuropathic involvement related to tick exposure. As these are associated with the infectious organism, *Borrelia burgdorferi*, however, further descriptions of these entities are not provided in this chapter.

CONCLUSION

Several substances, both organic and manufactured, may induce peripheral nerve damage when people are exposed to them. The expected clinical phenotype is of a distal, sensory, or sensorimotor polyneuropathy, often painful, with axonal characteristics on electrodiagnostic and histopathological analysis. Treatment is limited, and often the only effective management is avoidance from or removal of the offending toxin and supportive care. Fortunately, most toxic neuropathies are self-limited and gradually improve following toxin elimination.

REFERENCES

1. Windebank AJ. Polyneuropathy due to nutritional deficiency and alcoholism. In: Dyck PJ, Thomas PK, eds. *Peripheral Neuropathy*. 3rd ed. Philadelphia: WB Saunders; 1993:1310–1321.
2. Behse F, Buchthal F. Alcoholic neuropathy: clinical, electrophysiologic, and biopsy findings. *Ann Neurol*. 1977;2:95–110.
3. Casey EB, Le Quesne PM. Electrophysiological evidence for a distal lesion in alcoholic neuropathy. *J Neurol Neurosurg Psychiatry*. 1972;35:624–630.
4. Blackstock E, Rushworth G, Gath D. Electrophysiologic studies in alcoholism. *J Neurol Neurosurg Psychiatry*. 1972;35:326–334.
5. Walsh JC, McLeod JG. Alcoholic neuropathy: an electrophysiological and histological study. *J Neurol Sci*. 1970;10:457–469.
6. D'Amour ML, Shahani BT, Young RR, Bird KT. The importance of studying sural nerve conduction and late responses in the evaluation of alcoholic subjects. *Neurology*. 1979;29:1600–1604.
7. Mawdsley C, Mayer RF. Nerve conduction in alcoholic polyneuropathy. *Brain*. 1965;88:335–356.
8. Shattuck GC. Relation of beriberi to polyneuritis from other causes. *Am J Trop Med Hyg*. 1928;8:539–543.
9. Victor M, Adams RD. On the etiology of the alcoholic neurologic diseases: with special references to the role of nutrition. *Am J Clin Nutr*. 1961;9:379–397.
10. North JD, Sinclair HM. Nutritional neuropathy: chronic thiamine deficiency in the rat. *AMA Arch Path*. 1956;62:341–353.
11. Fennelly J, Frank O, Baker H. Peripheral neuropathy of the alcoholic: I. Aetiological role of aneurin and other B-complex vitamins. *BMJ*. 1964;2:1290–1292.
12. Layzer RB, Fishman RA, Schafer JA. Neuropathy following abuse of nitrous oxide. *Neurology*. 1978;28:504–506.
13. Marie RM, Le Biez E, Busson P, Schaeffer S, Boiteau L, Dupuy B, et al. Nitrous oxide anesthesia-associated myelopathy. *Arch Neurol*. 2000;57:380–382.
14. Ogundipe O, Pearson MW, Slater NG, Adepegba T, Westerdale N. Sickle cell disease and nitrous oxide–induced neuropathy. *Clin Lab Haematol*. 1999;21:409–412.
15. Bosch EP, Smith BE. Disorders of peripheral nerves. In: Bradley WF, Daroff RB, Fenichel GM, Marsden CD, eds. *Neurology in Clinical Practice*. 3rd ed. Boston: Butterworth-Heinemann; 2000:2119.
16. Sesso RM, Iunes Y, Melo AC. Myeloneuropathy following nitrous oxide anesthaesia in a patient with macrocytic anaemia. *Neuroradiology*. 1999;41:588–590.
17. Stacy CB, Di Rocco A, Gould RJ. Methionine in the treatment of nitrous oxide–induced neuropathy and myeloneuropathy. *J Neurol*. 1992;239:401–403.
18. Shafer SQ. Disorders of spinal cord, nerve, and muscle. *Neurol Clin*. 1993;11:693–705.
19. Challenor YB, Richter RW, Bruun B, Pearson J. Nontraumatic plexitis and heroin addiction. *JAMA*. 1973;225:958–961.
20. Loizou LA, Boddie HG. Polyradiculoneuropathy associated with heroin abuse. *J Neurol Neurosurg Psychiatry*. 1978;41:855–857.
21. Warner-Smith M, Darke S, Day C. Morbidity associated with non-fatal heroin overdose. *Addiction*. 2002;97:963–967.
22. Sinsawaiwong S, Phanthumchinda K. Pentazocine-induced fibrous myopathy and localized neuropathy. *J Med Assoc Thai*. 1998;81:717–721.
23. LeQuesne, PM. Neuropathy due to drugs. In: Dyck PJ, Thomas PK, eds. *Peripheral Neuropathy*. 3rd ed. Philadelphia: WB Saunders; 1993:1571–1581.
24. Kannarkat G, Lasher EE, Schiff D. Neurologic complications of chemotherapy agents. *Curr Opin Neurol*. 2007;20:719–725.
25. Peltier AC, Russell JW. Recent advances in drug-induced neuropathies. *Curr Opin Neurol*. 2002;15:633–638.
26. Badros A, Goloubeva O, Dalal JS, et al. Neurotoxicity of bortezomib therapy in multiple myeloma: a single-center experience and review of the literature. *Cancer*. 2007;110:1042–1049.
27. Stubblefield MD, Slovin S, MacGregor-Cortelli B, et al. An electrodiagnostic evaluation of the effect of pre-existing peripheral nervous system disorders in patients treated with the novel proteasome inhibitor bortezomib. *Clin Oncol*. 2006; 18:410–418.
28. Filosto M, Rossi G, Pelizzari AM, et al. A high-dose bortezomib neuropathy with sensory ataxia and myelin involvement. *J Neurol Sci*. 2007;263(1–2):40–43.
29. Bhagavati S, Maccabee P, Muntean E, Sumrani NB. Chronic sensorimotor polyneuropathy associated with tacrolimus immunosuppression in renal transplant patients: case reports. *Transplant Proc*. 2007;39:3465–3467.
30. Muto O, Ando H, Ono T, et al. Reduction of oxaliplatin-related neurotoxicity by calcium and magnesium infusions. *Ganto-KagakuRyoho*. 2007;34:579–581.
31. Mukherjee SC, Rahman MM, Chowdhury UK, et al. Neuropathy in arsenic toxicity from groundwater arsenic contamination in

West Begal, India. *J Environ Sci Health Part A Tox Hazard Subst Environ Eng.* 2003;38:165–183.

32. Rusyniak DE, Furbee RB, Kirk MA. Thallium and arsenic poisoning in a small midwestern town. *Ann Emerg Med.* 2002; 39:307–311.

33. Aminoff MJ. Effects of occupational toxins on the nervous system. In: Bradley WF, Daroff RB, Fenichel GM, Marsden CD, eds. *Neurology in Clinical Practice.* 3rd ed. Boston: Butterworth-Heinemann; 2000:1511–1519.

34. Blom S, Lagerkvist B, Linderholm H. Arsenic exposure to smelter workers: clinical and neurophysiological studies. *Scand J Work Environ Health.* 1985;11:265–269.

35. Greenberg SA. Acute demyelinating polyneuropathy with arsenic ingestion. *Muscle Nerve.* 1996;19:1611–1613.

36. Wax PM, Thornton CA. Recovery from severe arsenic-induced peripheral neuropathy with 2,3-dimercapto-1-propanesulphonic acid. *J Toxicol Clin Toxicol.* 2000;38:777–780.

37. Fluri F, Lyrer P, Gratwohl A, Raetz-Bravo AE, Steck AJ. Lead poisoning from the beauty case: neurologic manifestations in an elderly woman. *Neurology.* 2007;69:929–930.

38. Windebank AJ. Metal neuropathy. In: Dyck PJ, Thomas PK, eds. *Peripheral Neuropathy.* 3rd ed. Philadelphia: WB Saunders; 1993:1549–1570.

39. Rubens O, Logina I, Kravale I, Eglite M, Donaghy M. Peripheral neuropathy in chronic occupational inorganic lead exposure: a clinical and electrophysiological study. *J Neurol Neurosurg Psychiatry.* 2001;71:200–204.

40. Mitchell CS, Shear MS, Bolla KI, Schwartz BS. Clinical evaluation of 58 organolead manufacturing workers. *J Occup Environ Med.* 1996;38:372–378.

41. Nielsen CJ, Nielsen VK, Kirkby H, Gyntelberg F. Absence of peripheral neuropathy in long-term lead-exposed subjects. *Acta Neurol Scand.* 1982;65:241–247.

42. Tromme I, Van Neste D, Dobbelaere F, et al. Skin signs in the diagnosis of thallium poisoning. *Br J Dermatol.* 1998;138: 321–325.

43. Schaumberg HH, Berger AR. Human toxic neuropathy due to industrial agents. In: Dyck PJ, Thomas PK, eds. *Peripheral Neuropathy.* 3rd ed. Philadelphia: WB Saunders; 1993: 1533–1548.

44. Gold BG, Voda J, Yu X, Gordon H. The immunosuppressant FK506 elicits a neuronal heat shock response and protects against acrylamide neuropathy. *Exp Neurol.* 2004;187:160–170.

45. Lopachin RM. Acrylamide neurotoxicity: neurological, morphological and molecular endpoints in animal models. *Adv Exp Med Biol.* 2005;561:21–37.

46. Pradat PF, Kennel P, Naimi-Sadaoui S, et al. Continuous delivery of neurotrophin 3 by gene therapy has a neuroprotective effect in experimental models of diabetic and acrylamide neuropathies. *Hum Gene Ther.* 2001;12:2237–2249.

47. Belai A, Burnstock G. Acrylamide-induced neuropathic changes in rat enteric nerves: similarities with effects of streptozotocin diabetes. *J Auton Nerv Syst.* 1996;58:56–62.

48. Godderis L, Braeckman L, Vanhoorne M, Viaene M. Neurobehavioral and clinical effects in workers exposed to CS2. *Int J Hyg Environ Health.* 2006;209:139–150.

49. Huang CC, Chu CC, Wu TN, Shih TS, Chu NS. Clinical course in patients with chronic carbon disulfide polyneuropathy. *Clin Neurol Neurosurg.* 2002;104:115–120.

50. Chu CC, Huang CC, Chu NS, Wu TN. Carbon disulfide induced polyneuropathy: sural nerve pathology, electrophysiology, and clinical correlation. *Acta Neurol Scand.* 1996;94:258–263.

51. Goetz CG, Bolla KI, Rogers SM. Neurologic health outcomes and Agent Orange: Institute of Medicine report. *Neurology.* 1994;44:801–809.

52. Thomke F, Jung D, Besser R, Roder R, Konietzko J, Hopf HC. Increased risk of sensory neuropathy in workers with chloracne after exposure to 2,3,7,8-polychlorinated dioxins and furans. *Acta Neurol Scand.* 1999;100:1–5.

53. Barbieri S, Pirovano C, Scarlato G, Tarchini P, Zappa A, Maranzana M. Long-term effects of 2,3,7,8-tetrachlorodibenzo-p-dioxin on the peripheral nervous system: clinical and neurophysiological controlled study on subjects with chloracne from the Seveso area. *Neuroepidemiology.* 1988;7:29–37.

54. Grehl H, Grahmann F, Claus D, Neundorfer B. Histologic evidence for a toxic polyneuropathy due to exposure to 2,3,7,8-tetrachlorodibenzo-p-dioxin (TCDD) in rats. *Acta Neurol Scand.* 1993;88:354–357.

55. Grahmann F, Claus D, Grehl H, Neundorfer B. Electrophysiologic evidence for a toxic polyneuropathy in rats after exposure to 2,3,7,8-tetrachlorodibenzo-p-dioxin (TCDD). *J Neurol Sci.* 1993;115:71–75.

56. Michalek JE, Akhtar FZ, Arezzo JC, Garabrant DH, Albers JW. Serum dioxin and peripheral neuropathy in veterans of Operation Ranch Hand. *Neurotoxicology.* 2001;22:479–490.

57. Kim JS, Lim HS, Cho SI, Cheong HK, Lim MK. Impact of Agent Orange exposure among Korean Vietnam veterans. *Ind Health.* 2003;41:149–157.

58. Windebank AJ, Blexrud MD. Residual ethylene oxide in hollow fiber hemodialysis units is neurotoxic in vitro. *Ann Neurol.* 1989;26:63–68.

59. Brashear A, Unverzagt FW, Farber MO, Bonnin JM, Garcia JG, Grober E. Ethylene oxide neurotoxicity: a cluster of 12 nurses with peripheral and central nervous system toxicity. *Neurology.* 1996;46:992–998.

60. Centers for Disease Control and Prevention. n-Hexane-related peripheral neuropathy among automotive technicians: California, 1999–2000. *MMWR.* 2001;50:1011–1013.

61. Pastore C, Izura V, Marhuenda D, Prieto MJ, Roel J, Cardona A. Partial conduction blocks in n-hexane neuropathy. *Muscle Nerve.* 2002;26:132–135.

62. Gluszcz-Zielinska A. Occupational n-hexane neuropathy: clinical and neurophysiological investigation. (in Polish.) *Med Pr.* 1999;50:31–36.

63. Puri V, Chaudry N, Tatke M. n-Hexane neuropathy in screen printers. *Electromyogr Clin Neurophysiol.* 2007;47:145–152.

64. Kuwabara S, Kai MR, Nagase H, Hattori T. n-Hexane neuropathy caused by addictive inhalation: clinical and electrophysiological features. *Eur Neurol.* 1999;41:163–167.

65. Burns TM, Shneker BF, Juel VC. Gasoline sniffing multifocal neuropathy. *Pediatr Neurol.* 2001;25:419–421.

66. Kuang S, Huang H, Liu H, Chen J, Kong L, Chen B. A clinical analysis of 102 cases of chronic n-hexane intoxication. (in Chinese.) *Zhonghua Nei Ke Za Zhi.* 2001;40:329–331.

67. Pastore C, Marhuenda D, Marti J, Cardona A. Early diagnosis of n-hexane-caused neuropathy. *Muscle Nerve.* 1994;17: 981–986.

68. Chang AP, England JD, Garcia CA, Sumner AJ. Focal conduction block in n-hexane polyneuropathy. *Muscle Nerve.* 1998;21:964–969.

69. Smith AG, Albers JW. n-Hexane neuropathy due to rubber cement sniffing. *Muscle Nerve.* 1997;20:1445–1450.

70. Lifshitz M, Gavrilov V. Central nervous system toxicity and early peripheral neuropathy following dermal exposure to methyl bromide. *J Toxicol Clin Toxicol.* 2000;38:799–801.

71. De Haro L, Gastaut JL, Jouglard J, Renacco E. Central and peripheral neurotoxic effects of chronic methyl bromide intoxication. *J Toxicol Clin Toxicol.* 1997;35:29–34.

72. Chakravarty A, Chatterjee S. Tri-ortho-cresyl phosphate neuropathy in India. *Prog Clin Neurosci.* 1989;365–373.

73. Morgan JP, Tulloss TC. The "Jake Walk Blues": a toxicologic tragedy mirrored in American popular music. *Ann Intern Med.* 1976;85:804–808.

74. Vasilescu C, Florescu A. Clinical and electrophysiological study of neuropathy after organophosphorous compounds poisoning. *Arch Toxicol.* 1980;43:305–315.

75. Johnson MK. The mechanism of delayed neuropathy caused by some organophosphorous esters: using the understanding to improve safety. *J Environ Sci Health B.* 1980;15:823–841.

76. Glynn P. Neuropathy target esterase. *Biochem J.* 1999;344: 625–631.

77. Baum D. Jake leg: how the blues diagnosed a medical mystery. *New Yorker.* 2003. Sept:50–57.

78. Pearn J. Neurology of ciguatera. *J Neurol Neurosurg Psychiatry.* 2001;70:4–8.

79. Lawrence DN, Enriquez MB, Lumish RM, Maceo A. Ciguatera fish poisoning in Miami. *JAMA.* 1980;244:254–258.

80. Butera R, Prockop LD, Buonocore M, Locatelli C, Gandini C, Manzo L. Mild ciguatera poisoning: case reports with neurophysiological evaluations. *Muscle Nerve.* 2000;23:1598–1603.

81. Cameron J, Flowers AE, Capra MF. Electrophysiological studies on ciguatera poisoning in man (part II). *J Neurol Sci.* 1991;101:93–97.

82. Cameron J, Capra MF. The basis of the paradoxical disturbance of temperature perception in ciguatera poisoning. *J Toxicol Clin Toxicol.* 1993;31:571–579.

83. Hamblin PA, McLachlan EM, Lewis RJ. Sub-nanomolar concentrations of ciguatoxin-1 excite preganglionic terminals in guinea pig sympathetic ganglia. *Naunyn Schmiedebergs Arch Pharmacol.* 1995;352:236–246.

84. Allsop JL, Martini L, Lebris H, Pollard J, Walsh J, Hodgkinson S. Neurologic manifestations of ciguatera: 3 cases with a neurophysiologic study and examination of one nerve biopsy. *Rev Neurol.* 1986;142:590–597.

85. Lewis RJ, Jones A, Vernoux JP. HPLC/tandem electrospray mass spectrometry for the determination of sub-ppb levels of Pacific and Caribbean ciguatoxins in crude extracts of fish. *Anal Chem.* 1999;71:247–250.

86. Purcell CE, Capra MF, Cameron J. Action of mannitol in ciguatoxin-intoxicated rats. *Toxicon.* 1999;37:67–76.

87. Trevett AJ, Mavo B, Warrell DA. Tetrodotoxic poisoning from ingestion of a porcupine fish *(Diodon hystrix)* in Papua New Guinea: nerve conduction studies. *Am J Trop Med Hyg.* 1997;56:30–32.

88. Oda K, Araki K, Totoki T, Shibasaki H. Nerve conduction study of human tetrodotoxication. *Neurology.* 1989;39:743–745.

89. Auerbach PS, Halstead BW. Hazardous aquatic life. In: Auerbach PS, Geehr E, eds. *Management of Wilderness and Environmental Allergies.* 2nd ed. St. Louis: CV Mosby; 1989:995–997.

90. Doyle DD, Guo Y, Lustig SL, Satin J, Rogart RB, Fozzard HA. Divalent cation competition with [^{3}H]saxitoxin binding to tetrodotoxin-resistant and -sensitive sodium channels: a two-site structural model of ion/toxin interaction. *J Gen Physiol.* 1993;101:153–182.

91. Centers for Disease Control and Prevention. Paralytic shellfish poisoning: Massachusetts and Alaska, 1990. *MMWR.* 1991;40:157–161.

92. Rodrigue DC, Etzel RA, Hall S, et al. Lethal paralytic shellfish poisoning in Guatemala. *Am J Trop Med Hyg.* 1990;42:267–271.

93. Gessner, BD, Middaugh JP. Paralytic shellfish poisoning in Alaska: a 20-year retrospective analysis. *Am J Epidemiol.* 1995;141:766–770.

94. Chang FC, Spriggs DL, Benton BJ, Keller SA, Capacio BR. 4-Aminopyridine reverses saxitoxin (STX)– and tetrodotoxin (TTX)–induced cardiorespiratory depression in chronically instrumented guinea pigs. *Fundam Appl Toxicol.* 1997;38:75–88.

95. De Carvalho M, Jacinto J, Ramos N, et al. Paralytic shellfish poisoning: clinical and electrophysiological observations. *J Neurol.* 1998;245:551–554.

96. Long RR, Sargent JC, Hammer K. Paralytic shellfish poisoning: a case report and serial electrophysiologic observations. *Neurology.* 1990;40:1310–1312.

97. Agency for Toxic Substances and Disease Registry. Cyanide toxicity. *Am Fam Physician.* 1993;48:107–114.

98. Garcia JR, Sripathi N, Newman DS. Thirty-nine-year-old male with distal paresthesias, cramps, and weakness. *J Clin Neuromuscul Dis.* 2008;9:6–7.

99. Chan TY. A probable case of amygdalin-induced peripheral neuropathy in a vegetarian with vitamin B$_{12}$ deficiency. *Ther Drug Monit.* 2006;28:140–141.

100. Calderon-Gonzalez R, Rizzi-Hernandez H. Buckthorn polyneuropathy. *N Engl J Med.* 1967;277:69–71.

101. Aoki K, Munoz-Martinez EJ. Quantitative changes in myelin proteins in a peripheral neuropathy caused by tullidora. *J Neurochem.* 1981;36:1–8.

102. Hernandez-Cruz A, Munoz-Martinez EJ. Tullidora *(Karwinskia humboldtiana)* toxin mainly affects fast-conducting axons. *Neuropathol Appl Neurobiol.* 1984;10:11–24.

103. Heath JW, Ueda S, Bornstein MB, Daves GD, Raine CS. Buckthorn neuropathy in vitro: evidence for a primary neuronal effect. *J Neuropathol Exp Neurol.* 1982;41:204–220.

104. Misra UK, Sharma VP. Peripheral and central conduction in neurolathyrism. *J Neurol Neurosurg Psychiatry.* 1994;57: 572–577.

105. Cohn DF, Striefler M. Human neurolathyrism: a follow-up study of 200 patients. *Arch Suisses Neurol Neurochir Psychiatrie.* 1981;128:151–156.

106. Cohn DF, Streifler M, Dabush S, Messer G. Peripheral nerve changes in chronic neurolathyrism. *Neurology India.* 1983;31:45–51.

107. Merhoff GC, Porter JM. Ergot intoxication: historical review and description of unusual clinical manifestations. *Ann Surg.* 1974;180:773–779.

108. Perkin GD. Ischaemic lateral popliteal nerve palsy due to ergot intoxication. *J Neurol Neurosurg Psychiatry.* 1974;37:1389–1391.

109. Harris JB, Goonetilleke A. Animal poisons and the nervous system: what the neurologist needs to know. *J Neurol Neurosurg Psychiatry.* 2004;75 (Suppl 3):iii40–iii46.

110. Seneviratne U, Dissanayake S. Neurological manifestations of snake bite in Sri Lanka. *J Postgrad Med.* 2002;48:275–278.

111. Kularatne SAM. Common krait *(Bungarus caeruleus)* bite in Anuradhapura, Sri Lanka: a prospective clinical study, 1996–98. *Postgrad Med J.* 2002;78:276–280.

112. Grattan-Smith PJ, Morris JG, Johnston HM, et al. Clinical and neurophysiological features of tick paralysis. *Brain.* 1997;120:1975–1987.

113. Dworkin MS, Shoemaker PC, Anderson DE. Tick paralysis: 33 human cases in Washington state, 1946–1996. *Clin Inf Dis.* 1999;29:1435–1439.

114. Venkataraman Vedanarayanan V, Evans OB, Subramony SH. Tick paralysis in children: electrophysiology and possibility of misdiagnosis. *Neurology.* 2002;59:1088–1090.

115. Felz MW, Davis-Smith C, Swift TR. A 6-year-old girl with tick paralysis. *N Engl J Med.* 2000;342:90–94.

CHAPTER 15

Psychiatric and Mental Health Aspects of Neurotoxic Exposures

Puneet Narang and Steven B. Lippmann

INTRODUCTION

The central nervous system effects of neurotoxic agents present a range of disturbances.[1] The most striking aspects may include changes in mood and personality. For example, exposure to neurotoxins like manganese or carbon disulfide can produce psychoses and suicidal tendencies. Exposure to solvents such as methylene chloride may result in delusions and hallucinations. Cognitive dysfunction manifests as lack of alertness, disorientation, reduced attention span, poor judgment, and memory loss, in addition to personality changes, after exposure to many neurotoxins, like carbon monoxide.

An undefined fraction of neurological and psychiatric illness could be caused or exacerbated by chronic, low-level contact with environmental neurointoxicants. Most reported incidences focus on high-dose exposures that are usually encountered during accidents or in occupational settings. The impact of low-dose, long-term exposure to neurotoxic agents is a less studied area; therefore, results from sporadic reports are often unclear. Neurotoxic sequelae range from devastating illnesses, such as parkinsonism and dementia, to subtle changes, like alterations in behavior or limitations in memory and cognition.

NEUROTOXICITY AND PSYCHIATRIC SEQUELAE

The ability to think, perceive, control emotions, plan, and function in daily routines can diminish drastically without pathology being detected by physical examination, laboratory studies, or neuroimaging.[2] There is a spectrum of psychological disturbances that can result from neurotoxic agents (Table 1).

Some important behavioral neurointoxicants encompass alkyltin pesticides like carbaryl, chlordane, heptachlor, malathion, and triadimefon; heavy metals such as aluminum, arsenic, cadmium, lead, manganese, and mercury; and organic solvents, as in carbon tetrachloride, dichloromethane, ethylene glycol, methanol, styrene, tetrachloroethylene, trichloroethylene, and tolu-

Table 1:	Neurotoxicity and Psychiatric Sequelae
AFFECTIVE SYMPTOMS: Apathy, languor, lassitude, lethargy, listlessness, excitability, irritability, nervousness, tension, restlessness, anger, antisocial, delinquent behavior	
COGNITIVE DEFICITS: Confusion, memory problems, reduced attention span, disorientation, intellectual deficits, learning problems	
PSYCHOTIC SYMPTOMS: Hallucinations, delusions	
OTHERS: Sleep disturbances, mental retardation	

ene. Others include industrial pollutants such as biphenyls and carbon disulfide, along with toxins commonly encountered in the food supply like dioxins, diethylhexylphthalate, n-hexane, and phenols. Heavy metals, organophosphates or other pesticides, agents of warfare, gases, solvents, substance abuses, and medications, including psychotropic drugs, are the neurotoxins that have received the most prominent, recent attention (Table 2).

Heavy Metals

Among the metals, mercury, lead, arsenic, aluminum, manganese, and cadmium are the most studied due to their major impact on public health. There has been controversy about dental-filling amalgams as an unlikely cause of mercury poisoning; however, the exposure is considered to be of a low level and unlikely to be associated with psychiatric sequelae. Emotional instability and cognitive impairments are the prominent changes noted in both organic and inorganic types of mercury exposure; however, these deficits are more characteristic of acute inorganic toxicity. Neuropsychological testing in acute inorganic toxic exposure cases has revealed pronounced impairments in frontal lobe domains.[3] Irritability, excitability, anxiety, insomnia, and social withdrawal are common presentations of mercury poisonings, which, when present as a symptom complex, is traditionally referred to as *erethism*.

A direct link between early lead exposure and extreme learning disability as sequelae of its neurotoxicity has been well confirmed. One study hypothesizes that lead exposure explains a large percentage of the variation in violent crime rates in the United States.[4] Another study, by the same author, claims a strong association between preschool blood levels of lead and subsequent crime rate trends over several decades and across nine countries.[5]

Aluminum neurotoxicity, although rarely seen, is classically associated with end-stage renal disease patients on hemodialysis with dialysate containing high levels of aluminum or in the primary management of hyperphosphatemia with aluminum-containing compounds. The characteristic clinical picture is one of chronic dementia and anemia that is resistant to erythropoietin, along with osteodystrophy unrelated to secondary hyperparathyroidism.[6]

Table 2:	Common Neurotoxic Agents and Associated Psychiatric Disorders				
Neurotoxin Disorder	**Lead**	**Mercury**	**Organophosphate**	**Carbon Monoxide**	**Solvent**
Anxiety	*1	*1	*1	*58	*60
Panic		*1	*1	*58	*60
Depression	*1	*1	*1	*58	*60
Bipolar	*1				
Posttraumatic stress			*55	*58	*60
Phobia		*1		*58	*61
Sleep	*53	*54	*56	*58	*60
Conduct	*1			*59	
Schizophrenia	*1				
Attention deficit	*1		*57		
* Indicates numbers in the Reference list.					

Pesticides

For decades, most research has focused on organophosphates, but evidence suggests that other types of pesticides, including organochlorines, carbamates, fungicides, and fumigants, are also neurotoxic. A paucity of evidence associates herbicides with changes in neurobehavioral performance, but herbicides have been implicated as risk factors for Parkinson's disease. It is critical to identify the specific agent associated with neurotoxicity; however, it is also essential to recognize that in the field, most workers are exposed to a blend of pesticides, which may contribute synergistically to neurotoxicity.

Organophosphate-induced neuropsychiatric disorders are commonly found after long-term organophosphate poisoning and are often described as chronic organophosphate-induced neuropsychiatric disorders. Such involvement may be caused by low-level exposures to organophosphates without acute cholinergic symptoms. The common clinical manifestations are impairments in memory, concentration, and learning. Anxiety, depression, psychoses, chronic fatigue, peripheral neuropathy, and autonomic dysfunction also occur.[7] Extrapyramidal symptoms, such as dystonia, resting tremor, bradykinesia, postural instability, and rigidity of facial musculature, in these cases, do not respond to levodopa.

Solvents

Cross-sectional epidemiological studies have documented higher frequencies of psychiatric complaints among solvent-exposed workers than among nonexposed personnel. The presence of such symptomatology has been reported in people exposed to solvents with no physical or mental complaints, but has also been noted in people presenting to a clinic with complaints of either a physical or a behavioral nature related to chronic long-term exposure or to an acute poisoning.[8,9] Complaints in individuals who experienced solvent exposure at work include concentration and memory deficits, diminished psychomotor speed, decreased mental flexibility, mood changes, altered personality, diffuse pain, and sleeping difficulties.[10]

Therapeutic Drugs

Pharmaceuticals often alter the function of nervous system either as a desirable effect or as an undesirable sequelae. Psychotropic drugs are an example wherein the various changes in brain are beneficial for the management of psychiatric disorders. Agents used to treat other illnesses (e.g., some anticancer drugs) may also have neurotoxic side effects. Often, such aspects are poorly documented or even undetected.

One of the major concerns is the possible effect of medications on the developing brain of a fetus. Teratogenicity of most prescription drugs has been subjected to limited testing. Over-the-counter drugs have even fewer studies on use during pregnancy. Physicians exert considerable caution in prescribing medications to pregnant women; indeed, avoiding iatrogenic toxicity to the unborn is stressed in medical practice.

The *Physicians' Desk Reference*[11] and similar publications illustrate that many prescription medications, including psychoactive ones, have neurotoxic effects of varying significance, some of which are an accepted consequence of the therapy. Proper testing of pharmaceuticals is required for the doctor and patient to make informed decisions about pharmacotherapy. However, neurotoxicity may be less fully assessed during drug evaluations, thus subjecting the public to greater risk. Controlled neurotoxicity assessments should be carried out before the safety of food additives or medicines can be established.

Autism and Neurotoxic Exposure

Thimerosal-containing vaccines have been the source of controversy surrounding the development of autism spectrum disorders and neurodevelopmental disorders in children exposed to them. These entities currently form a heterogeneous group of illnesses, which include Asperger's syndrome, Rett's syndrome, and generalized developmental disorder.[12] This issue was brought to prominence primarily as a result of the hypothesis that autism is a form of mercury poisoning.[13]

The Immunization Safety Review Committee[14] has concluded that the evidence was inadequate to either accept or reject an etiological relationship between thimerosal exposure from childhood vaccines and neurodevelopmental disorders of autism, attention deficit hyperactivity disorder, and speech or language delay.[14] Organophosphate and solvent exposure, too, have been associated with autism; however, they also lack evidence to prove any direct causal relationship.

Fluoride

The effect of fluoride on the central nervous system represents the newest area of research on its toxicity. Investigations have been spurred by the results from recent human studies conducted in China, India, Iran, and Mexico, which reported associations between elevated levels of fluoride exposure and intellectual deficits in children.[15] Data from animal and human research might suggest that fluoride at the levels found from drinking fluorinated water could be potentially harmful to the developing nervous system.[16] The increase in production of free radicals associated with fluorides raises the theoretical risk of developing Alzheimer's disease. Although final conclusions are not available, the concerns are provocative and of some public health interest.

Warfare Agents

Chemical exposures and stress are the leading cause of most cases of impaired neurobehavioral functioning during war or terrorist attacks. Chemical warfare agents commonly encountered include cyanide, chlorine, phosgene, mustard gas, arsenic compounds, Agent Orange, radiation, and organophosphates. Among the prominent examples where chemical weapons were used are World War I and II, the Vietnam War, and the Iran–Iraq War of the 1980s. Besides the other long-term health effects in exposed war veterans, various psychiatric symptoms have been reported. Gulf War syndrome refers to a nonspecific condition manifested by psychiatric and somatic symptoms purported to result from chemical exposures during that conflict in 1990 and 1991. Research performed since the war identified stress as the likely cause of Gulf War Syndrome, rather than chemical or biological exposures[17]; however, the finding that these veterans have elevated rates of neurological illness like amyotrophic lateral sclerosis emphasizes the need for clinicians to remain vigilant for neurological illness in Gulf War veterans.[18] The recognized mental effects of warfare agents include mood and perceptual abnormalities, with changes in behavior and cognition. The psychiatric management of victims of any potential or known toxic event should also include monitoring for mass hysteria or group-shared psychogenic illness.

Russians, during Russo-Japanese War, were the first ones to recognize stress as the cause of various behavioral oddities noted in soldiers at a war front and tried to propose a treatment plan for them. From 1914 to 1918, British doctors working in military bases recognized a range of behavioral symptoms in soldiers that compromised their fighting efficiency, and they termed the condition *shell shock*. Various reasons, ranging from direct injury to nerves to stress faced during war, were considered the cause of psychiatric illness in the soldiers. Recent research, however, favors a physical rather than a psychological basis for blast trauma.[19] The symptom complex identified as shell shock includes fatigue, slower reaction times, indecision, disconnection from one's surroundings, and inability to prioritize. Shell shock or combat stress reaction is considered a separate entity from acute stress disorder and posttraumatic stress disorder (PTSD). Since the days of its identification, there has been controversy regarding when to send affected soldiers back to a war front. An early return may result in long-term complications like PTSD, yet counseling, psychotropic medications, adequate food, and rest seem to serve the purpose of healing. A selected group of soldiers may need to be discharged from duty.

DIAGNOSIS

The CH^2OPD^2 (questionnaire including details about community, home and hobbies, occupation, personal habits, diet, and drugs) mnemonic, available from the Ontario College of Family Physicians Web site, is a valuable first-line exposure assessment tool for physicians. It provides a means of assessing exposure to toxic substances and may help diagnose the cause of medical problems or multiple symptoms in the absence of overt pathology.[20]

With the increasing awareness about the health sequelae attributable to toxic exposure from environmental sources, the role of neurotoxicology is expanding, but it is still in stages of infancy. Thus, the CH^2OPD^2 questionnaire is a valuable assessment tool to identify toxic exposures. Another well-recognized method of diagnosing an association between exposure and symptoms is "precautionary avoidance."[21] Although re-exposing the patient to a previous environment might be a way to strengthen the association between exposure and symptoms, it should be weighed against the odds of inducing PTSD in such situations.[22]

Long-term or low-dose exposures from environmental toxins usually go unrecognized by the victim. It then becomes the duty of physicians to consider environmental sources as the causative factor behind the unexplained symptoms. Psychotic features, including delusions, hallucinations, and paranoia, are observed in mercury, arsenic, and manganese poisoning. Suicidal depression resulting from poisoning with carbon disulfide has been well documented for more than a century.[23] Less severe changes in mood and energy levels have also been recognized in exposed populations; these may be the earliest clue to a neurotoxic exposure.[24] Keeping the affective changes in mind, questionnaires and symptom ratings are included in the assessment of individual cases and in epidemiological studies of involved populations. Thus, neuropsychological testing provides insight into the nature and extent of impairment. Among the tests used to strengthen the diagnosis of neurotoxic exposure, the Minnesota Multiphasic Personality Inventory (MMPI-R) may detect changes in psychological and personality functioning following neurotoxic exposure.[22] However, it has found little use in cross-sectional studies conducted on large groups as a result of its length and number of questions. Another clinical instrument that has been widely applied in cross-sectional analyses is the Profile of Mood States Questionnaire, which is a 65-item mood-rating scale.

Several questionnaires and rating scales help in obtaining information about subjective complaints from the exposed victim in a standardized manner. One commonly used instrument, the Q16 questionnaire, consists of 16 yes-or-no questions designed to gain information regarding symptoms from recent exposures.[25] Another rating scale that is popular for use in cross-sectional surveillance studies of occupationally exposed workers, as well as in the evaluation of suspected poisoning cases, is the Neurotoxic Symptom Checklist 60. It has 53 questions designed to gather information regarding mood, memory problems, sensory or motor disturbances, chest complaints, equilibrium disturbances, somatic problems, fatigue, and sleep disturbances, as well as 7 personality items.[26]

An analogue rating scale has been developed in Germany that has been evaluated in experimental poisoning studies for its ability to differentiate exposed from nonexposed individuals.[27] A relationship between age and exposure was detected; the oldest group and the highest exposed could be differentiated from others. However, the low exposure group could not be separated from the nonexposed, supporting the model of delayed neurotoxicity.[27]

The use of self-reports to identify subjective symptoms might be one way to recognize neurotoxicity at its early stages, but self-reports are subject to various reporting bias. Exposed victims seem to make answers fit what they believe to be the examiner's expectations; recall of objective events or subjective states may change over time. Gender and affiliation of the tester may also affect responses. To validate self-reports of subjective symptoms, structured clinical interviews, objective data collection, along with documented levels of exposure, should be used to eliminate bias.

Diagnostic Dilemma

For a considerable period, psychiatric disorders due to organic illness or exposure to toxic agents were ignored in psychiatry and considered an exclusive domain of neurology. The term "psycho-organic syndromes" was coined in an attempt to separate the psychiatric symptoms of endogenous illness and those due to general organic illness or related to toxic exposures.[28] The idea underlying the need to differentiate between functional and organic mental syndromes is to help establish diagnosis, treatment, and prognosis based upon the etiology.

Attempts to develop a classification system for neuropsychiatric disorders related to solvent exposure exemplify the enigma faced in distinguishing between psychological disorders and encephalopathies. It has remained a challenge to establish more specific criteria for the description of these disorders.[29] A review of the two manuals of psychiatric classification, the *Diagnostic and Statistical Manual of Mental Disorders* (DSM)[30] and the *International Classification of Diseases* (ICD),[31] reveals the dilemma faced by psychiatrists in developing criteria for classifying mental disorders resulting from organic illness or exposure to toxic agents.

In the DSM-IV, there is no specific code for encephalopathy. Diagnoses include dementia, delirium, amnestic disorder, other cognitive disorders, mental disorders due to a general medical condition, and substance-related disorders.[30] In the ICD-10 system, the neurotoxin-related encephalopathies can be diagnosed in the group of categories of organic mental disorders F00-F09 in Group V. The reference to neuropsychiatric disorders secondary to solvent exposure is described in Group VI, which defines the nervous system diseases and is labeled G92.1 for acute toxic encephalopathy and G92.2 for chronic toxic encephalopathy (CTE).[31]

The two most commonly used classification systems with diagnostic criteria for CTE are the one proposed by the World Health Organization (WHO)[32] and the other somewhat different one introduced by the Workshop on Neurobehavioral Effects of Solvents in Raleigh, North Carolina.[33] According to WHO, the CTE can be classified into three stages (organic affective syndrome, mild CTE, or severe CTE); the regimen proposed in Raleigh recognizes four stages (unspecific symptoms, changes in personality, impairment of intellectual function, or dementia).

In clinical practice, it is difficult to determine whether a patient's cognitive and behavioral symptoms are solvent induced. Usually the exposed has no significant neurological or neuropsychological impairment. Diagnosis of CTE is then made by exclusion from other causes, based on evaluation by a multidisciplinary diagnostic team. Neuropsychological testing is considered important for the diagnosis, but the differential diagnosis remains complicated, requiring an extensive diagnostic workup to rule out other causes. Depending on the etiology for the cognitive and behavioral symptoms, these may be irreversible changes that persist as cognitive deficits despite intervention. However, cognitive–behavioral therapy techniques focusing on changing illness manifestations and stimulating activity are useful for patients with CTE, especially in countering the fatigue-related problems of concentration and memory.

PSYCHIATRIC ISSUES

It is important to make a distinction between impairments and disabilities linked to psychiatric disorders, since this influences the prognosis and ability to rehabilitate.

Impairments are the cognitive and affective abnormalities associated with psychiatric disorders. Disability is defined as being unable to perform normal life activities to an extent that occupational functioning is compromised, along with disruption of social life.

From a significant proportion of people who are injured or become ill at work, only a small number remain permanently disabled. The severity of the disability and the individual adaptation to it are influenced by the person's understanding of the situation. Numerous other factors, including social or economic, determine the implications of the disability to the person. These issues clarify the dysfunction, define its consequences, and provide support for the degree of recovery versus chronicity.

Mild to severe depression is present in more than 90% of patients referred for psychiatric evaluation after a disabling injury. Depressive symptoms typically develop within approximately a year from the injury date. Anxiety and pain disorders sometimes appear as secondary reactions following depression. The cause of psychiatric dysfunction in a neurotoxin-subjected patient has been attributed to either an indirect pathway, as in a traumatic psychological reaction,[34] or a direct one resulting from neurological damage with a resultant affective disorder.[35] Alterations in frontotemporal brain metabolism following significant solvent poisoning are consistent with an underlying neurological disruption hypothesis.[36] This is also in agreement with research implicating frontotemporal pathology in cases of depression or anxiety.[37]

Psychiatrists may be a part of the disability management process, acting as either a treating clinician or an independent evaluator. Irrespective of the role, it is necessary to perform a comprehensive evaluation. Clinicians should not rely on prior assessments as guides to diagnosis or treatment. It is imperative that the psychiatrist avoid yielding to pressure to adopt the wishes of the employer, attorney, or governmental agency that made the referral. As a psychiatrist, the obligation is not only to provide the best care to the patient but also to maintain impartiality and to avoid favoring conclusions that suit the requesting entity.[38] Nevertheless, an evaluator physician remains an agent of the requesting body, rather than a personal advocate for the individual.

Multiple biopsychosocial issues are considered before assessment is completed. Each issue should be examined to allow an accurate assessment. A biopsychosocial approach to the assessment and treatment of a psychiatric disability helps the clinician understand the case, prevents the disability from developing into a chronic condition, and reduces the chances of relapse once treated. A comprehensive review of the condition, prognosis, and therapeutic requirements is always indicated.

Mood swings, along with impulsivity, are a common part of clinical picture seen in people exposed to neurotoxins. In the workplace, impulsivity can be dangerous.

The premorbid personality should be documented, since a prior presence of such a pattern would suggest a preexisting psychiatric condition, substance abuse, or both; its absence would raise the suspicion for a causal traumatic or toxic injury.

TREATMENT

Treating neurotoxicity is an interdisciplinary undertaking involving a psychiatrist, neurologist, and internist. Neurotoxic injury may be associated with adverse consequences, including psychological ones, as in an anxiety disorder,[39] other emotional symptoms,[40] and negative socioeconomic consequences. Effective strategies exist for psychological disorders, but access is often limited by the availability of specialists. Early, time-limited interventions, as in psychological debriefing, are indicated.[41] Management of a confirmed case of neurotoxicity should include these steps:

1. Remove from further exposure—This usually involves relocating the victim to another site with the help of the employer. It may become necessary to change jobs if exposure is to be avoided completely. Workers with significant impairment, psychological or physical, may find it hard to cope with a different assignment. Retirement on medical grounds may be required, but this, too, has potential stress factors.

2. Psychological interventions—These may include anxiety or stress reduction, anger management techniques, coping skills (including ways of compensating for a memory impairment), and provision of information about their problem. Facilitating understanding and support from all quarters, including employer, and family is also important. A treatment strategy for commonly encountered psychiatric disorders is described here:
   - Anxiety disorders—Treatment of anxiety varies depending on the nature of the disorder and person's characteristics. Therapies are conventional in type yet individualized to each case.
   - PTSD—Some promising studies suggest that early cognitive–behavioral interventions are an effective approach for management of PTSD.[42] An important aspect for effective treatment of PTSD is early diagnosis and fostering trauma victims to present for evaluation. However, it is advisable to wait 4 weeks after the trauma for follow-up assessments to establish whether adverse psychological effects persist. Unfortunately, the interface between times of an emergency and primary care visits is unsystematic; there is reluctance in routine cases to screen for PTSD following traumatic

193

events. Information booklets play an important role in prompting patients at risk for chronic PTSD to seek treatment, if initial psychological disturbances are not resolved during the early recovery period.

- Phobic anxiety—Sometimes phobic anxiety can lead to distress and lifestyle limitation of activities. Anxiety reduction techniques and the graded return to normal are often deemed helpful, but specific behavioral treatment may be required for full recovery.[43] Treating phobic anxiety includes record keeping of activity as a basis for monitoring, stress management of relaxation, distraction, cognitive procedures, and graded practice with a hierarchy of increasing activities. The therapeutic plan must not being overambitious but calls for consistent follow-up.

- Depression—Depression is one of the most common presenting symptoms associated with neurotoxic exposure. The chemicals that can result in affective disorders, including solvents, like chlorinated hydrocarbons; pesticides; and heavy metals, are the agents that cross the blood–brain barrier and have the potential to interfere with brain function. They act by up- or down-regulating neurotransmitter synthesis, blocking receptor sites, and poisoning essential enzymes of neuronal metabolism. Behavioral dysfunction from neurotoxic exposures may develop gradually and go unrecognized for years. However, there are times when the onset of environmentally triggered depression can be sudden—for example, after a pesticide application or new work in a solvent factory. Treatment of neurotoxin-related depression needs to be individualized and based upon the findings in the history, physical examination, laboratory testing, and knowledge about the offending agent. Start with avoidance, reduction, or removal of the toxins, as in chelation for removal of heavy metals or avoidance of associated drugs, when possible. Desensitization, counseling, and antidepressant medications are also applicable as needed.

- Antidepressant medicines—The most distressing psychiatric symptoms for the patient are hopelessness and suicidal thinking. Medications can be lifesaving; however, some people are sensitive to adverse effects of these drugs. Prescribing should be weighed by the risk-to-benefit ratio and should be closely followed.

- The suicidal patient—Suicidal thinking in exposed victims often tends to come on suddenly and abate quickly. Close professional observation and support are mandatory. Also effective are self-help groups, where suicidal crises can be calmed by others who have had similar experiences. Helpline call-in services are sometimes perceived as less useful, as they tend to focus on acute factors rather than on prevention. When active suicidal thinking is detected, the patient should be hospitalized, particularly if a comorbid mood disorder is present. While the typical picture is of brief, impulsive suicidal ideas, some people may become more persistently suicidal. In certain cases, those exposed suffer emotional and physical problems similar to those experienced by individuals with chronic, intractable pain; good support is especially important since some of these patients even consider "rational suicide," with calm preplanning, in view of their long-term poor prognosis for recovery.

THE FAMILY

Neurotoxicity affects not only the patient but also the patient's family. Usually, the ability to earn a living is dramatically compromised, reducing the family's financial circumstances. Mood swings, which are often the first sign of neurotoxic exposure, may have an adverse effect on the family, particularly on children. Agricultural exposures may induce direct toxic injuries on family members in contact with the primary victim, especially through clothing. The effects are most serious in younger people. Reports of behavioral oddities, poor school performance, and unusual physical symptoms should raise the diagnostic concern for neurotoxin exposure. A significant proportion of their problems may be related to disturbed family dynamics; however, direct toxicity should also be ruled out. This presentation requires collaborative attention by the psychiatrist and pediatrician.[44]

COMPENSATION

Financial and social consequences of trauma, either physical or mental, along with the blighting of ambitions, may be considerable and even unrecognized. Most victims of occupational injuries want recognition of their suffering, as well as financial compensation. Monetary issues, if not addressed, may impede progress. Innocent victims of trauma are generally slower to return to work than those who were to blame for their condition. Long, complex compensation procedures hinder treatment and rehabilitation. One of the most important aspects of timely compensation can be to allow interim payments and funding of care to treat complications and prevent chronic disability.

DISABILITY MANAGEMENT

The chances of an individual returning to former employment after an absence from work are determined by numerous factors beyond the nature and severity of the health problem.[45] Return to work among those emotionally affected is often slower than among those with physical injury. Liaison with the employer becomes essential in such cases. Factors affecting recovery and return to work include sociodemographical characteristics, job satisfaction, and referral to rehabilitation services. In an investigation of disability and return to work following occupational low back pain, a review concluded that the factors associated with protracted disability included poor workplace support, personal stress, shorter job tenure, prior episodes, heavier occupations with no available modifiable duties, delayed reporting, greater severity of pain, and more significant functional impairment.[46] Fault for an injury and management attitudes toward it plays a critical role in the speed and quality of recovery.

The following measures have been recommended to help physicians improve disability management: the use of standardized questionnaires, better communication between patients and employers, provision of specific return-to-work plans, early intervention, and applying behavioral approaches to pain and disability.[46] A systematic review undertaken to determine the effect on time lost from work of physical conditioning programs for workers with chronic pain demonstrated that physical conditioning programs that included a cognitive–behavioral component produce a clinically significant reduction in the number of sick days compared to conventional care.[47] Research on disability management and return-to-work factors related to anxiety disorders is important given their prevalence and the limited availability of treatment resources.[48] Workers receiving disability pensions for solvent exposure are at an increased risk of neuropsychiatric disability. Results differed with respect to type of solvent exposure and specific diagnostic entities.[49] The findings indicate that occupational solvent exposure may be the cause of mental and cognitive impairment that becomes chronic and disabling. In places where there is a high risk of traumatic events or neurotoxic exposures, good disability management and support is helpful for individuals with work-related injuries.[50]

CONCLUSION

An increasing spectrum of health sequelae are being attributed to toxic exposures. In the field of neurotoxicology, it is essential to assess exposure in known at-risk cases and for medical problems or symptoms in the absence of overt pathology. For occupational neurotoxic exposures, a preventive approach in the form of bioeffect monitoring seems to be a good strategy. Occupational toxicity causes complaints that are related to the level of the daily exposure, as well as to the cumulative degree.[51] Hence, monitoring complaints can be a first-line screening for exposed workers (primary prevention), as well as for those who already have developed a chronic solvent encephalopathy (disease screening).

Environmental monitoring, especially in short-term peak exposure measurements, is also needed as part of occupational hygiene. In practice, the "addition rule" to calculate exposure levels for chemical mixtures must be applied to the environmental monitoring data since exposure to subthreshold levels of different toxins raises the cumulative dose of toxin exposure risk.[52] Useful questionnaires for screening of chronic neurotoxic effects include the Q16 questionnaire[25] and the Neurotoxic Symptom Checklist 60.[26] As a first-line tool, the CH^2OPD^2 mnemonic is valuable for exposure assessment. A sound diagnosis requires a careful history and evaluation into occupational aspects and a comparison to known exposures. To arrive at the final diagnosis, always consider family and personal medical history, course of complaints, neurological assessment, general physical examination, routine laboratory analyses, electroencephalography, brain imaging, neuropsychological testing, and possibly a polysomnography.

Once a case of neurotoxic exposure is identified, an interdisciplinary approach involving the psychiatrist, neurologist, and internist is an effective strategy. Since no single effective therapy is cited for the exposed, depending upon the neurotoxic agent, a combination of cognitive–behavioral therapy, medication, and early personal counseling may be employed at regaining better socioeconomic function. If such individuals are not effectively treated, their psychiatric symptoms may prove extremely costly in health-care expenses, occupational absenteeism, and decreased workplace productivity.

REFERENCES

1. American Association on Intellectual and Developmental Disabilities. Mental Health Fact Sheet Linking Environmental Exposures with Psychological Disorders Fact Sheet. American Association on Intellectual and Developmental Disabilities; 2006.
2. Voller B, Benke T, Benedetto K, et al. Neuropsychological, MRI, and EEG findings after very mild traumatic brain injury. *Brain Inj.* 1999;13(10):821–827.
3. Haut MW, Morrow LA, Pool D, et al. Neurobehavioral effects of acute exposure to inorganic mercury vapor. *Appl Neuropsychol.* 1999;6(4):193–200.
4. Nevin R. How lead exposure relates to temporal changes in IQ, violent crime, and unwed pregnancy. *Environ Res.* 2000;83(1):1–22.

5. Nevin R. Understanding international crime trends: the legacy of preschool lead exposure. *Environ Res.* 2007;104(3):315–336.

6. Parkinson IS, Ward MK, Kerr DN. Dialysis encephalopathy, bone disease and anemia: the aluminum intoxication syndrome during regular hemodialysis. *J Clin Pathol.* 1981;34(11):1285–1294.

7. Ray DE, Richards PG. The potential for toxic effects of chronic, low-dose exposure to organophosphates. *Toxicol Teratol.* 2001;120:343–351.

8. Struwe G, Wennberg A. Psychiatric and neurological symptoms in workers occupationally exposed to organic solvents: results of a differential epidemiological study. *Acta Psychiatr Scand.* 1983;67:68–80.

9. Bolla KI, Schwartz BS, Agnew J, et al. Subclinical neuropsychiatric effects of chronic low-level solvent exposure in U.S. paint manufacturers. *J Occup Med.* 1990;32:671–677.

10. Ellingsen DG, Lorentzen P, Langård S. A neuropsychological study of patients exposed to organic solvents. *Int J Occup Environ Health.* 1997;3:177–183.

11. *Physicians' Desk Reference.* Oradel, NJ: Medical Economics; 1988.

12. Parker SK, Schwartz B, Todd J, et al. Thimerosal-containing vaccines and autistic spectrum disorder: a critical review of published original data. *Pediatrics.* 2004;114(3):793–804.

13. Bernard S, Enayati A, Redwood L, et al. Autism: a novel form of mercury poisoning. *Med Hypotheses.* 2001;56(4):462–471.

14. Institute of Medicine. *Thimerosal-containing Vaccines and Neurodevelopmental Disorders.* Washington DC: National Academy Press; 2001.

15. Xiang Q, Liang Y, et al. Effect of fluoride in drinking water on children's intelligence. *Fluoride.* 2003;36(2):84–94.

16. Schettler T. Known and suspected developmental neurotoxicants. In: *Harms Way: Toxic Threats to Child Development Greater Boston Physicians for Social Responsibility.* Cambridge, Ma. 2000:90–92. http://www.psr.org/site/PageServer?pagename=boston_ihw-report#ihwRptDwnld

17. Engel CC, Hyams KC, Scott K. Managing future Gulf War syndromes: international lessons and new models of care. *Philos Trans R Soc Lond B Biol Sci.* 2006;361(1468):707–720.

18. Horner RD, Kamins KG, Feussner JR, et al. Occurrence of amyotrophic lateral sclerosis among Gulf War veterans. *Neurology.* 2003;61(6):742–749.

19. Bhattacharjee Y. Shell shock revisited: solving the puzzle of blast trauma. *Science.* 2008;319(5862):406–408.

20. Marshall L, Weir E, Abelsohn A, Sanborn MD. Identifying and managing adverse environmental health effects: I. Taking an exposure history. *CMAJ.* 2002;166:1049–1055.

21. Marshall L, Weir E, et al. Occupational and environmental exposure. *CMAJ.* 2002;167:744–746.

22. Bolla KI, Roca R. Neuropsychiatric sequelae of occupational exposure to neurotoxins. In: Bleecker ML, ed. *Occupational Neurology and Clinical Neurotoxicology.* Baltimore: Williams & Wilkins; 1994:133–159.

23. Vigliani EC. Carbon disulphide poisoning in viscose rayon factories. *Br J Ind Med.* 1954;11(4):235–244.

24. White RF, Proctor SP. Clinico-neuropsychological assessment methods in behavioral neurotoxicology. In: Chang LW, Slikker W, ed. *Neurotoxicology: Approaches and Methods.* New York: Academic Press; 1995:711–726.

25. Lundberg I, Hogberg M, Michélsen H, et al. Evaluation of the Q16 questionnaire on neurotoxic symptoms and a review of its use. *Occup Environ Med.* 1997;54:343–350.

26. Hooisma J, Hänninen H, Emmen HH, Kulig BM. Symptoms indicative of the effects of organic solvent exposure in Dutch painters. *Neurotoxicol Teratol.* 1994;16:613–622.

27. Kiesswetter E, Sietmann B, Seeber A. Standardization of a questionnaire for neurotoxic symptoms. *Environ Res.* 1997;73(1–2):73–80.

28. Triebig G, Hallermann J. Survey of solvent related chronic encephalopathy as an occupational disease in European countries. *Occup Environ Med.* 2001;58:575–581.

29. Ramos AI, Jardim SRI, Filho FS. Solvent-related chronic toxic encephalopathy as a target in the worker's mental health research. *An Acad Bras Cienc.* 2004;76(4):757–769.

30. American Psychiatric Association. *Diagnostic and Statistical Manual of Mental Disorders.* 4th ed. Washington, DC: World Health Organization; 1992.

31. World Health Organization. *The ICD-10 Classification of Mental and Behavioural Disorders: Clinical Descriptions and Diagnostic Guidelines.* Geneva: WHO; 1992.

32. World Health Organization European Office. Chronic Effects of Organic Solvents on the Central Nervous System and Diagnostic Criteria. Copenhagen: WHO; 1985.

33. Proceedings of the Workshop on Neurobehavioral Effects of Solvents. October 13–16, 1985, Raleigh, North Carolina, USA. *Neurotoxicology.* 1986;7(4):1–95.

34. Schottenfeld RS, Cullen MR. Organic affective illness associated with lead intoxication. *Am J Psychiatry.* 1984;141:1423–1426.

35. Morrow LA, Ryan CM, Hodgson MJ, Robin N. Alterations in cognitive and psychological functioning after organic solvent exposure. *J Occup Med.* 1990;32:444–450.

36. Morrow L, Callender T, Lottenberg S, et al. PET and neurobehavioral evidence of tetrabromoethane encephalopathy. *J Neuropsychiatry Clin Neurosci.* 1990;2:431–435.

37. Robinson RG, Starkstein SE. Mood disorder following stroke: new findings and future directions. *J Geriatr Psychiatry.* 1989;22:1–15.

38. Williams CD, Yakima WA. Psychiatric disability in the workplace: An approach to understanding. *Academy of Organizational and Occupational Psychiatry, e-Bulletin.* 2000;8(3).

39. O'Donnell ML, Creamer M, Bryant RA, et al. Posttraumatic disorders following injury: an empirical and methodological review. *Clin Psychol Rev.* 2003;23:587–604.

40. Mason S, Wardrope J, Turpin G, Rowlands A. The psychological burden of injury: an eighteen month prospective cohort study. *Emerg Med J.* 2002:19:400–404.

41. Litz BT, Gray MJ, et al. Early intervention for trauma: current status and future directions. *Clin Psychol Sci Pract.* 2002;9:112–134.

42. Harvey AG, Bryant RA, Tarrier N. Cognitive behaviour therapy for posttraumatic stress disorder. *Clin Psychol Rev.* 2003, 23:501–522.

43. Mayou R, Farmer A. ABC of psychological medicine trauma. *BMJ.* 2002;325(7361):426–429.

44. Davies R, Ahmed G, Freer T. Psychiatric aspects of chronic exposure to organophosphates: diagnosis and management. *Adv Psychiatr Treat.* 2000;6:356–361.

45. Kenny D. Determinants of time lost from workplace injuries: the impact of the injury, the injured, the industry, the intervention and the insurer. *Int J Rehabil Res.* 1994;17(4):333–342.

46. Shaw WS, Pransky G, Fitzgerald TE. Early prognosis for low back disability: intervention strategies for health care providers. *Disabil Rehabil.* 2001;23(18):815–828.

47. Schonstein E, Kenny D, Keating J, et al. Physical conditioning programs for workers with back and neck pain: a Cochrane systematic review. *Spine.* 2003;28(19):E391–395.

48. Lepine, JP. The epidemiology of anxiety disorders: prevalence and societal costs. *J Clin Psychiatry.* 2002;63(14):4–8.

49. Mikkelsen S. Epidemiological update on solvent neurotoxicity. *Environ Res.* 1997;73(1–2):101–112.

50. Asmundson GJ, Norton GR, Allerdings MD, et al. Posttraumatic stress disorder and work-related injury. *J Anxiety Disord.* 1998;12(1):57–69.

51. Viaene MK, Pauwels W, Veulemans H, et al. Neurobehavioural changes and persistence of complaints in workers exposed to styrene in a polyester boat building plant: influence of exposure characteristics and microsomal epoxide hydrolase phenotype. *Occup Environ Med*. 2001;58:103–112.

52. American Conference of Governmental Industrial Hygienists. Threshold Limit Values for Chemical Substances Physical Agents and Biological Exposure Indices. Cincinnati, Ohio: American Conference of Governmental Industrial Hygienists, Technical Affairs Office; 1994–1995.

53. Pohl HR, Abadin HG, Risher JF. Neurotoxicity of cadmium, lead, and mercury. In: A Sigel, H Sigel, RKO Sigel, eds. *Neurodegenerative Diseases and Metal Ions*. ***: John Wiley & Sons; 2006:395–416.

54. Cordeiro Q Jr, Fráguas R Jr. Depression, insomnia, and memory loss in a patient with chronic intoxication by inorganic mercury. *J Neuropsychiatry Clin Neurosci*. 2003;15:457–458.

55. Hoffman A, Eisenkraft A, Finkelstein A, et al. A decade after the Tokyo sarin attack: a review of neurological follow-up of the victims. *Mil Med*. 2007;172(6):607–610.

56. Kamanyire R, Karalliedde L. Organophosphate toxicity and occupational exposure. *Occup Med*. 2004;54:69–75.

57. Eskenazi B, Marks AR, Bradman A, et al. Organophosphate pesticide exposure and neurodevelopment in young Mexican-American children. *Environ Health Perspect*. 2007;115(5): 792–798.

58. Hartman D. Missed diagnosis and misdiagnosis of environmental toxicant exposure: the psychiatry of toxic exposure and multiple chemical sensitivity. *Psychiatr Clin North Am*. 1998;21(3): 659–670.

59. Wakschlag LS, Pickett KE, Cook E Jr, et al. Maternal smoking during pregnancy and severe antisocial behavior in offspring: a review. *Am J Public Health*. 2002;92(6):966–974.

60. Viaene MK. Overview of the neurotoxic effects in solvent-exposed workers. *Arch Public Health*. 2002;60:217–232.

61. Dager SR, Holland JP, Cowley DS, Dunner DL. Panic disorder precipitated by exposure to organic solvents in the workplace. *Am J Psychiatry*. 1987;144:1056–1058.

NEUROTOXIC TESTING

CONTENTS

CHAPTER 16

Electrophysiological Evaluations

David G. Greer and Peter D. Donofrio

INTRODUCTION

When a clinician faces the dilemma of a patient with a condition of an unknown etiology, it is customary to go through a routine list of common systemic causes. These disorders likely account for the many of these complex cases, yet considering possible toxin exposure remains important because simple withdrawal of the agent may stop or reverse symptoms. The first step in determining whether toxicity is the main factor is obtaining a thorough history and physical examination. The interviewer should inquire about type of employment, access to chemicals, duration of the patient's occupation at a particular company, use of protective equipment and similar symptoms in coworkers. If the exposure occurred at home, the clinician should ask whether other family members are ill. If the history and physical examination support the possibility of a toxin-related condition, then appropriate testing is indicated.

This chapter does not address the vast amount of animal research into the neurological effects from toxicities but rather focuses on electrophysiological effects of exposures that are clinically relevant to humans. The following discussion is organized by test type and addresses pertinent clinical and electrographical findings correlating with certain toxin exposures.

ELECTROENCEPHALOGRAPHY

As a rule of thumb, the electroencephalogram (EEG) is often insensitive for the detection of chronic encephalopathies of mild severity. An EEG is useful in the evaluation of acute toxicity. Although the abnormalities observed are nonspecific, typically diffuse, and often symmetrical, focal and paroxysmal discharges may occur occasionally.

Table 1 lists medications and other chemicals that often produce abnormalities on an EEG when present in sufficient amounts. The categorization is divided into inorganic compounds, organic compounds, chemicals used in plastics manufacturing, organophosphates, commonly prescribed medications, and recreational drugs.

Lead poisoning can cause pathology in both children and adults. Adults may present with seizures, dementia, or a peripheral neuropathy (the latter is discussed later in this chapter). Children may develop mental retardation, increased intracranial pressure, headaches, seizures, optic

Table 1: Toxins and Medications that Cause EEG Abnormalities*

INORGANIC COMPOUNDS	MEDICATIONS
Aluminum	Aminophylline
Bismuth	Barbiturates
Lead	Benzodiazepines
Lithium	Bromides
Manganese	Carbamazepine
Mercury	Corticosteroids
Thallium	Isoniazid
Tin	Lamotrigine
	Metrizamide
ORGANIC COMPOUNDS	Neuroleptics
Carbon monoxide	Opiates
Chlorinated hydrocarbons	Penicillin
Cyanide	Salicylates
Ethanol	Tricyclic antidepressants
Methane	Vigabatrin
Methanol	Valproic acid
Toluene	
Trichloroethylene	RECREATIONAL DRUGS
	Amphetamine
PLASTICS-MANUFACTURING CHEMICALS	Cocaine
Acrylamide	Lysergic acid diethylamide
Hydrazines	Marijuana
Triorthocresylphosphate	Mescaline
	Methylphenidate
ORGANOPHOSPHATES	
Alkylphosphate	

EEG, electroencephalogram.
Data from Bauer G, Bauer R. EEG, drug effects, and central nervous system poisoning. In: Niedermeyer E, Lopes da Silva F, eds. *Electroencephalography: Basic Principles, Clinical Applications, and Related Fields.* 5th ed. Philadelphia: Lippincott Williams & Wilkins; 2005:701–716.

atrophy, and dystonia. The EEG usually shows diffuse slowing.[1] Paroxysmal discharges may occur, especially if the seizures are part of the clinical presentation. Fejerman and colleagues described a patient who presumably developed Lennox-Gastaut syndrome from lead poisoning.[2] Data from the Mexico City Prospective Lead Study suggest that lasting developmental effects from lead-induced increase in θ-activity may occur between 54 and 72 months of age and that quantitative θ-activity was correlated with the degree of serum lead level increase.[3]

Mercury is another heavy metal whose toxicity results in a range of neurological dysfunction, including peripheral neuropathy, cerebral and cerebellar atrophy, ataxia, dysarthria, and mental retardation. A classic triad of tremors, erethism, and gingivitis is sometimes seen. Mercurial erethism is characterized by behavioral and personality changes such as extreme shyness, excitability, loss of memory, and insomnia. An abnormal EEG by computerized analysis and impaired performance in neurobehavioral or neuropsychological tests may also be observed.[4] Photic driving has been shown to increase in those exposed to mercury and thus may function as a marker of central nervous system hyperexcitability from an early neurotoxic effect.[5] EEG findings usually consist of generalized slowing and epileptiform discharges.[1]

Manganese intoxication has been reported to cause status epilepticus in a child whose seizure resolved after treatment with chelation.[6] Although lower levels of manganese exposure may cause a parkinsonism-type illness as measured by diadochokinesometry, EEG and brainstem auditory evoked potential (BAEP) results in these patients were normal.[7] Because manganese is metabolized primarily through the hepatobiliary system, cholestatic liver disease may predispose to toxicity, particularly in those receiving parental nutrition.

Acute thallium poisoning may cause confusion, poor attention, and paranoid syndromes, particularly if the amount ingested is especially high. In cases from Tsai et al., central nervous system signs correlated with EEG changes of diffuse slow waves,[8] which may have to do with the predisposition of thallium to deposit in deep structures such as the corpus striatum, hypothalamus, and thalamus. Because toxicity can be reduced acutely with administration of Prussian blue, it is important to recognize thallium poisoning.

Several distinct neurological complications arise from alcohol abuse or the vitamin deficiencies that accompany excessive alcohol consumption. The EEG shows desynchronization and low amplitude in alcohol-withdrawal hallucinosis and delirium tremens.[1] Wernicke encephalopathy presents clinically as the triad of encephalopathy, ocular motility dysfunction, and ataxia. In this condition, the EEG may show periodic lateralizing epileptiform discharges.[9] EEG anormalities have also been described in fetal alcohol syndrome and after acute intoxication from alcohol.[1] Repeated EtOH withdrawal may produce a "kindling" effect for development of seizures unrelated to events of alcohol withdrawal.[10]

Poisoning with the chlorinated hydrocarbons may lead to myriad neurological signs, including imbalance, hyperirritability, ataxia, seizures, and neuropathy. In a cross-sectional study of 73 personnel working in the manufacture of DDT, 21% of the workers had EEG features of bitemporal sharp waves.[11] Trichloroethylene (TCE) "huffing" (voluntary inhalation) caused temporal lobe seizures and personality changes in one patient. TCE, a solvent for organic compounds, is also used as a degreaser in the metal industry.[12] Lindane, a powerful chlorinated hydrocarbon used as an insecticide and parasiticide, can cause seizures. Because of its high lipid solubility and consequent distribution in the brain, lindane is now considered a second-line agent.[13]

Organophosphate toxicity is well known to cause a defect in neuromuscular junction transmission and a delayed peripheral neuropathy (organophosphorus-induced delayed neuropathy). Nonspecific EEG slowing and paroxysmal discharges have been recorded in most organophosphate poisonings. The only exception is found in alkylphosphate poisoning in which fast rhythmic waveforms can be recorded in deep coma.[14] Terrorist attacks and mailborne anthrax earlier this decade spurred increasing awareness of possible future attacks with biological agents. Sarin is a powerful organophosphate nerve agent that inhibits acetylcholinesterase, producing a cholinergic reaction (i.e., miosis, nausea, vomiting, weakness, respiratory paralysis, and convulsions) designed to be incapacitating or lethal upon acute intoxication. Sarin gas–attack victims in Tokyo and Matsumoto subways in the mid-1990s underwent close follow-up. EEGs done in nine of the most severely affected individuals at Matsumoto all showed epileptiform discharges.[15] Two of these patients developed convulsions. Five years later, dementia and seizures were not seen in these patients and their EEGs were normal. On patient had a peripheral nerve lesion, and the other patients had normal neurological examinations. Similarly, in Tokyo, victims who did not die from cardiopulmonary arrest or develop anoxic brain injury recovered quickly to normal.[15] In contrast to the rapidly reversing effects of sarin, the organophosphorus (OP) compound soman is known to produce long-lasting epileptic seizure activity and associated brain damage. Nerve agent intoxication results in inhibition of acetylcholinesterase and a buildup of acetylcholine, leading to muscarinic receptor activation and eventually glutamate toxicity. δ-Activity measured in animal models has been correlated to pathologically damaged areas of the brain after soman-induced seizure.[16] The EEG has played an important role in the research to find reliable therapy for convulsions induced by agents used in biological warfare.[16]

When delivered in high doses, several therapeutic agents can cause EEG abnormalities. High-dose intravenous and intrathecal penicillin can result in generalized seizures, status epilepticus, and the expected EEG abnormalities they produce. Diffuse slowing can be seen in salicylate and corticosteroid toxicity. Aminophylline is commonly prescribed for the treatment of acute and chronic asthma and chronic obstructive pulmonary disease. Intoxication with aminophylline may produce status epilepticus or repetitive partial motor seizures that can be resistant to treatment. In these cases, the EEG may show periodic lateralizing epileptiform discharges.[17] In clinical trials, cefepime caused 0.2% of its patients to develop convulsions, most of whom had concurrent renal disease. Additional cases of cefepime-induced nonconvulsive status have since been reported.[18] Other agents shown to produce convulsions when used in excess include isoniazid and metrizamide.

Psychiatric agents' effects on EEG have been studied. Recently, mirtazapine has been shown to occasionally cause spike–wave complexes in patients with previously normal EEGs. Interestingly, these changes showed a right hemispheric predominance.[19] EEGs from schizophrenic inpatients placed on atypical antipsychotics, olanzapine, or amisulpride were compared to EEGs from those on haloperidol by Pogarell et al.; while no EEG abnormalities were seen in the haldol group, olanzepine and amisulpride users showed epileptiform discharges.[20] Amann et al. found that a disproportionate number of people treated with olanzepine had epileptiform changes on EEG when compared to seroquel or haloperidol.[21] Clozapine-induced stuttering and seizures has also been described.[22] Several quantitative electroencephalography studies on early predictors of treatment response to first-generation antipsychotics have produced consistent findings but have not influenced clinical management.[23]

Lithium toxicity typically manifests as tremor, myoclonus, or confusion. In addition to the expected abnormalities of diffuse slowing, the EEG may show periodic irritative discharges of short duration.[24] Marked change on EEG may help diagnose lithium intoxication when the serum level is only moderately elevated.[25]

Other agents often used by neurologists may cause changes on EEG. Valproic acid may lead to an encephalopathy, especially in older patients, manifested as triphasic waves and generalized slowing. Valproic acid also precipitates a hyperammonemic encephalopathy, with expected EEG findings of severe encephalopathy. Continuous generalized slowing, a predominance of θ- and δ-activity, occasional bursts of frontal intermittent rhythmic δ-activity, and triphasic waves may be present.[26] Tiagabine (Gabatril) has been associated with nonconvulsive status in patients with both generalized and partial epilepsies, as well as seizures in those without a prior seizure history.[27] Baclofen overdose can lead to a coma and seizures in which EEG shows suppression of background with semiperiodic sharp waves.[28]

Sevoflurane has been linked to epileptiform EEG changes, especially in the pediatric and elderly population.[29] EEG is now used intraoperatively to help monitor anesthesia depth.[30] Intraoperative electrophysiological monitoring is a rapidly growing field, and this brief review does not address this broad new area.

Certain recreational drugs produce EEG abnormalities, including lysergic acid diethylamide (LSD), mescaline, marijuana, cocaine, methylphenidate, and amphetamines.[31] LSD may produce acceleration of the dominant frequencies, decreased amplitude, and depression of slow waves.[31] The EEG is typically normal in subjects who use marijuana, yet mild slowing has been described. With chronic marijuana use, quantitative electroencephalography showed a persistent reduction in θ- and α-power that continued for 4 weeks of monitored abstinence. It has been hypothesized that these changes may contribute to cognitive alterations observed in marijuana abusers.[32] However, another study examining effect of 3,4-methylenedioxymethamphetamine (MDMA, or Ecstasy) use found the group that only used marijuana showed an increase in α2-power. This study[32] showed MDMA users had increased δ-activity centrally compared to both controls and those using marijuana and MDMA. Overall, however, most stimulants give rise to increasing β- and α-activity and a general reduction of EEG voltage.

QUANTITATIVE ELECTROENCEPHALOGRAPHY

Quantitative electroencephalography adds modern computer and statistical analyses to traditional EEG recordings and requires additional lead placements. Quantitative electroencephalography commenced more than 70 years ago when Dietsch[32a] applied Fourier analysis. Results are now often based on fast Fourier analysis and are compared to age-matched controls. Various uses for quantitative electroencephalography exist, such as identifying brain areas predominantly involved in psychopharmacological action. Extensive discussion about psychopharmacology is beyond the scope of this discussion about toxicology, yet ongoing work may prove useful to determine the most likely beneficial agent on an individual basis.

Quantitative electroencephalography studies in cocaine-dependent human patients show deficits in slow-wave brain activity, reflected in diminished EEG power in the δ- and θ-frequencies. Conversely, recently abstinent methamphetamine-dependent subjects demonstrate quantitative electroencephalography abnormalities that are consistent with a generalized encephalopathy.[33] This modality is also helping define outcomes in those with substance abuse history. The likelihood of rehabilitation based on quantitative electroencephalography differences has been demonstrated among cocaine-dependent subjects.[34]

Resting temporal and frontal EEG rhythms, and free copper levels, correlated across healthy, mildly cognitively impaired, and Alzheimer's disease subjects. Those with more advanced dementia showed more slowing in frontal and temporal areas and more free serum (unbound by ceruloplasmin) copper levels.[35]

Yoshimura et al. discussed a lock-and-key mechanism in schizophrenia and showed a reversal of the disease-induced change on EEG by haloperidol (supporting this theory), yet a reverse effect was seen after atypical antipsychotics were prescribed.[36] The authors hypothesize that this observation on EEG may further describe the difference in mechanism between typical and atypical antipsychotic agents.[36]

Effects of antiepileptic drugs have been studied using quantitative electroencephalography. Carbamazepine has shown higher likelihood to cause slowing, with a θ-increase and a decrease in α-mean frequency. Oxcarbazepine causes a decrease in α-mean frequency. Valproate did not decrease α-mean frequency, while lamotrigine increased it.[37] Given topiramate's relatively well-characterized effect on cognition, it was recently speculated that this agent would cause slowing on quantitative electroencephalography. However, data support no significant electroencephalographical differences between those on topiramate and those taking gabapentin or placebo.[38]

EVOKED POTENTIALS

Evoked potentials are defined as changes in voltage over time (waveforms) recorded over the cortex, spinal cord, or sensory ganglia produced by various peripheral stimuli, including those delivered to the eye (visual), ear (brainstem), or peripheral nervous system (somatosensory). Reference values for amplitudes and latencies have been determined for each technique based on specific stimulation and recording sites.

Compared to nerve conduction studies and electromyography, less information is available regarding evoked potential recording and its application in suspected neurotoxicity. Kokubun et al.[39] used somatosensory evoked potentials (SEPs) to measure the central conduction velocity in individuals with chronic alcoholism and polyneuropathy and spasticity. They showed that the average central latency (N21–P40) of the tibial SEP was increased by 10% in patients with spasticity, confirming the clinical suspicion of spinal cord or brainstem pathology.

Abnormalities in lower limb SEPs have been recorded in the myelo-opticoneuropathy associated with clioquinol intoxication.[40]

SEP latency delays also have been demonstrated in several workers exposed to inorganic mercury. Event-related auditory evoked potential (P300), BAEP, and diadochokinesometry were studied in people exposed to manganese. P300 and diadochokinesometry were affected, raising the likelihood that manganese exposure can cause parkinsonism.

One of the most feared adverse reactions to the treatment of tuberculosis is ethambutol toxicity. It results from the demyelination of the optic nerves, chiasm, and optic tracts. Both flash and pattern-reversal visual evoked potentials (VEPs) can uncover subclinical abnormalities in amplitude and latency weeks to months before the patient complains of changes in eyesight.[41] VEPs are particularly sensitive if the data are compared to results recorded before ethambutol prescription. VEP abnormalities have been reported in aluminum intoxication. Manesis et al. reported patients taking interferon alpha for hepatitis often developed increased P100 latency on VEP testing. Interestingly, those with hepatitis B were at higher risk than those with hepatitis C.[42]

Exposure polychlorinated biphenyls and methylmercury can be found in some fish species, and populations dependent on these fishes may be at higher risk of VEP delay. Levels of these chemicals in childhood were associated with subclinical VEP abnormalities, specifically latency of the N75 and the P100 components. Interestingly, intake of omega-3 polyunsaturated fatty acids was associated with a shorter latency of the P100, but an attempt at protection with selenium intake was associated with increased VEP abnormalities.[43]

In a case of attempted homicide by thallium poisoning, the patient's nerve conduction studies eventually normalized, yet the patient's abnormal VEP, showing axonal greater than demyelinating disease, did not improve 3 years after exposure.[44]

ELECTROMYOGRAPHY

Electromyography is an extremely effective tool for evaluating abnormalities in motor and sensory fibers of the peripheral nervous system. For the purpose of this chapter, electromyography is categorized into nerve conduction studies, repetitive stimulation, and needle examination. Blink reflex studies can be classified under nerve conduction studies and are discussed only briefly. Conventional nerve conduction studies measure the integrity of large myelinated motor and sensory fibers; consequently, they are insensitive for detecting small-fiber neuropathies. The four parameters measured in conventional nerve conduction studies are amplitude (microvolts in sensory nerves, millivolts in motor nerves), distal latency (msec), conduction velocity (m/sec), and F wave latencies (msec). Pathological processes primarily affecting the axon usually produce a reduction in amplitude and only minimal changes in conduction rate (latency and velocity) unless the disorder is advanced and the fastest conducting fibers are affected. Conversely, demyelinating and some membrane diseases produce impressive slowing of conduction velocity or other features suggestive of multifocal myelin loss, such as temporal dispersion or conduction block of proximal compound muscle action potentials (CMAPs). The latter presentation is suggestive of inflammatory neuropathies such as those seen in Guillain-Barré syndrome, chronic inflammatory demyelinating polyneuropathy, the neuropathies associated with monoclonal proteins, and rare toxic neuropathies.

The peripheral nervous system has a limited reaction to toxins. Schaumburg and Spencer[45] proposed that most toxins of the peripheral nervous system cause pathological reactions in one of four regions: (1) the distal sensory and motor axon (axonopathy); (2) the dorsal root ganglion; (3) the anterior horn cell, motor nerve, or both; or (4) the Schwann cell, resulting in a demyelinating neuropathy. Most toxic neuropathies can be grouped into one of the four categories on the basis of the primary neuroanatomical structure disrupted by the toxin. When applied clinically, this classification of toxic neuropathy sometimes becomes inexact and can be misleading because some toxic neuropathies cannot be neatly categorized into one group. In addition, some toxins produce disease in both the peripheral and the central nervous systems, particularly in the spinal cord, giving rise to confusing clinical abnormalities. Table 2 lists a classification of toxic polyneuropathies by anatomical site of pathology.

Most peripheral nerve toxins produce a distal axonopathy or a "dying-back neuropathy." The latter term may not be pathologically correct in some cases, but the concept makes for easier understanding of the expected clinical and electrophysiological abnormalities. The electrodiagnostic results typically parallel the abnormalities predicted by the clinical examination. In most cases, the first electrodiagnostic abnormality recorded in a toxic distal axonopathy is a reduction or absence of sensory nerve action potential (SNAP) amplitudes in the lower extremities. As the disease progresses, SNAP amplitudes diminish in the upper extremities, and a reduction is found in the lower extremity CMAP amplitudes, not necessarily in that order. Measures of conduction rate (conduction velocities, distal and F response latencies) remain normal until extensive axon loss ensues. When the latter occurs and there is loss of the fastest conducting fibers, conduction velocities drop below normal and distal latencies become prolonged—but only slightly and not to the extent seen in demyelinating conditions. In

Table 2: Toxic Polyneuropathy by Class of Agent and Anatomical Site of Pathology

PERIPHERAL AXON (INDUSTRIAL AGENTS)	PERIPHERAL AXON (THERAPEUTIC AGENTS)
Acrylamide	Amitriptyline
Arsenic (chronic exposure)	Chloramphenicol
Carbon disulfide	Chloroquine
Carbon monoxide	cis-Platinum
Cyanide	Colistin
Dichlorophenoxyacetic acid	Diphenylhydantoin
Ethylene oxide	Disulfiram
Glue sniffing	Ethambutol
Hexacarbons	Glutethimide
n-Hexane	Gold
Methyl bromide	Hydralazine
Methyl n-butyl ketone	Isoniazid
Organophosphates	Lithium
Polychlorinated biphenyl	Metronidazole
Sodium cyanate	Misonidazole
Styrene	Nitrofurantoin
Thallium	Nitrous oxide
Vacor	Phenytoin
	Podophyllin
DORSAL ROOT GANGLION	Statins
Adriamycin	Thalidomide
Methylmercury	Vinblastine
Paclitaxel (Taxol)	Vincristine
Pyridoxine poisoning	
	SCHWANN CELL (DEMYELINATING)
ANTERIOR HORN CELL	Amiodarone
Dapsone	Arsenic (acute exposure)
Lead	

some instances, the needle examination results may be the only indicator of abnormality, reflecting motor involvement before SNAP and CMAP amplitudes drop below accepted lower limits of normal for the control population. When abnormal, the needle examination typically shows changes consistent with axon loss in a distal gradient rather than a proximal pattern. This pattern of electrodiagnostic abnormality is observed in most toxin-related polyneuropathies and is well demonstrated in the toxicities associated with acrylamide, gold, nitrofurantoin, and vincristine exposure.

Thallium can lead to abdominal pain and dermatological and neurological symptoms. Alopecia, hyperkeratosis, and Mees' lines in nails may eventually be seen, but patients often present with dysesthesia, painful neuropathy, and muscle weakness.[8] In a case of attempted homicide by thallium, the patient showed progressive axonal abnormalities on a nerve conduction study until 3 months after exposure. F waves, which were initially absent, became normal at 3-year follow-up.[44]

Toxins that cause damage at the level of the dorsal root ganglia produce a clinical and electrodiagnostic picture quite different from the one observed in a distal axonopathy. The disorder begins insidiously yet can progress rapidly, leaving the patient in a state of relative deafferentation. Albin and colleagues[46] reported clinical and electrophysiological findings in two patients who developed a sensory ganglion neuronopathy after receiving massive doses of pyridoxine for the treatment of mushroom poisoning. Serial measurement of nerve conduction studies over 1 year identified complete loss of sensory potentials in the setting of relative preservation of CMAP amplitudes and measurements of motor conduction rate, an electrophysiological constellation suggestive of a sensory ganglionopathy. Similar electrodiagnostic findings can be seen or are anticipated after poisoning with adriamycin, methylmercury, and paclitaxel (Taxol). The latter causes a dose-dependent distal axonopathy that is sensory predominant and can be treated with glutamine. In a small study using high-dose paclitaxel chemotherapy, the group receiving glutamine showed less reduction in CMAP and SNAP amplitudes following treatment. Although the difference was not significant and the study was not placebo controlled, the glutamine group developed a less severe neuropathy.[47]

Selective toxicity to the anterior horn cell or motor nerve fibers is highly unusual. Both lead poisoning and treatment with dapsone can produce a clinical syndrome in which the anterior horn cells or motor nerves are affected exclusively.[48,49] In both situations, the upper extremities are more severely affected than the lower extremities, an unusual distribution for a toxic process. In lead toxicity, patients present with bilateral wrist drop; careful strength testing usually uncovers weakness also of the distal muscles innervated by the median and ulnar nerves.[49] If the lower extremities are weak, the patient usually has a foot drop, a finding more common in children than in adults. Electrophysiological studies usually demonstrate normal sensory potentials, reduced compound muscle action potential (CMAP) potentials, and near-normal conduction velocities in the upper extremity nerves.[49] These results are consistent with the electrodiagnostic abnormalities anticipated in an anterior horn cell disorder or a primarily motor axonopathy. At a blood lead concentration as low as 30 to 40 μg/dL, reduction in the nerve conduction velocity (NCV), prolongation of P300 latency, changes in postural balance, and changes in the R–R interval can be seen. Effects on latencies of somatosensory evoked potentials (SEP), visual evoked potential (VEP) and brainstem auditory evoked potentials (BAEP) occur at lead levels as low as 40 to 50 μg/dL.[50] Dapsone toxicity can produce a similar clinical and electrodiagnostic picture, although weakness is greater in median and ulnar innervated muscles compared to radial and peroneal innervated muscles.[48]

Most disorders of the peripheral Schwann cells arise from inflammatory, hereditary, or metabolic processes. Certain toxins, some in the form of medications, give rise to a demyelinating polyneuropathy, which can be confused with other diseases. For example, acute poisoning with large amounts of arsenic can produce a clinical presentation highly suggestive of Guillain-Barré syndrome.[51] The illness begins with complaints of abdominal pain, nausea, and vomiting, symptoms suggestive of a viral gastroenteritis. Approximately 7 to 10 days later, patients develop distal paresthesia and weakness, which quickly ascend the extremities. Over days, the patient's cranial nerves and respiratory system can be affected, an evolution further mimicking an acute inflammatory demyelinating polyneuropathy. The results of nerve conduction studies further confuse the distinction because, early in acute arsenic poisoning, features such as partial conduction block and temporal dispersion may be the only electrodiagnostic abnormalities.[51] Without laboratory verification of arsenic poisoning, the electrodiagnostic findings appear to substantiate the diagnosis of Guillain-Barré syndrome, leading to treatment with plasma exchange or intravenous immunoglobulin (IVIG) rather than penicillamine or British anti-Lewisite (BAL). As the disease progresses and serial nerve conduction studies are performed, the electrodiagnostic evolution of Guillain-Barré syndrome does not unfold. Serial testing in acute arsenic poisoning reveals evolutionary changes in amplitude, distal latency, and conduction velocity more in keeping with a dying-back axon-loss neuropathy. It has been hypothesized that massive poisoning with arsenic produces axon damage that manifests first as segmental demyelination and eventually as axon loss.

Amiodarone, a medication used to treat refractory ventricular arrhythmias, is associated with a chronic demyelinating neuropathy that can resemble chronic inflammatory demyelinating polyneuropathy.[52] If unrecognized by the treating physician, amiodarone withdrawal is delayed and the patient may be treated for CIPD with potentially toxic immunosuppressant agents or expensive therapies such as plasma exchange or IVIG. A similar drug toxicity can occur after treatment with perhexiline, an agent used in Europe for the treatment of coronary artery disease.[53] Tacrolimus, suramin, and chloroquine are also associated with demyelinating polyneuropathy. A tacrolimus-induced neuropathy that persists after drug withdrawal may respond to IVIG or plasma exchange. Suramin more commonly produces a sensory ganglionopathy of dorsal root neurons.[54]

L-Tryptophan is an over-the-counter preparation sometimes used to treat insomnia, depression, and premenstrual symptoms. In the late 1980s, an outbreak of a condition that came to be known as eosinophilia–myalgia syndrome occurred. Patients presented with myriad symptoms, including myalgia, arthralgia, rash, peripheral edema, cough, fever, alopecia, and a marked peripheral eosinophilia. Approximately 25% of patients developed a severe demyelinating peripheral neuropathy with electrodiagnostic features similar to those reported in acute arsenic poisoning and diphtheritic polyneuropathy.[55] Toxicologists eventually traced the disease to L-tryptophan manufactured by a single company and the accidental introduction of a contaminant, a d-L-tryptophan aminal of acetaldehyde.[55]

More recently, a controversy has ensued around the possible relationship between 3-hydroxy-3-methylglutaryl–coenzyme A (HMG-CoA) reductase inhibitors and peripheral neuropathy. This has led to much debate, given the broad use of these agents. Furthermore, it has been difficult to determine whether the individuals' neuropathy was due to the statin or an underlying metabolic abnormality, which often coexists with dyslipidemia, such as diabetes. Some data suggest statins can cause an axonal sensorimotor neuropathy or a purely small-fiber neuropathy,[54] but overall the incidence of statin neuropathy is felt to be rare. There is strong data connecting statin use to myopathy, which are discussed later in this chapter with other myopathies.

As multidrug therapy has prolonged the lives of human immunodeficiency virus (HIV) patients, more HIV-related and HIV treatment–related neuropathy is being seen. Nucleoside reverse transcriptase inhibitors cause a more abrupt, painful neuropathy than is seen normally from HIV infection.[54] Mechanistically, mitochondrial toxicity can be seen on nerve biopsy. Just as these medications compete for natural substrates in reverse transcriptase after being phosphorylated, they also affect mitochondrial DNA polymerase.[54] In a dose-dependent, subacute fashion, this causes an electrographical sensorimotor axonal neuropathy. The nucleoside reverse transcriptase inhibitors seem to be the most potent neurotoxic agents, notably staudine (d4T) and didanosine (ddI). Zalcitabine (ddC) also causes a distal sensory polyneuropathy (DSP), but this is usually seen at higher doses. The prevalence of DSP diagnosed by electrophysiology is 36% in a cohort of HIV-positive patients reported by Skopelitis et al. from the highly active antiretroviral therapy era.[56] Higher age, lower nadir of CD4 count, and combined use of neurotoxic antiretrovirals significantly elevated DSP prevalence. Most cases of DSP were subclinical, and only one-third presented clinically.[56]

Thalidomide, an agent used more recently for dermatological conditions and hematological malignancies such as multiple myeloma, can cause a painful, axonal sensorimotor neuropathy that continues after the agent is stopped.[54] A thalidomide derivative, lenalidomide, has recently been developed and has been approved by the U.S. Food and Drug Administration for treatment of myelodysplastic syndrome. It has not been shown to cause peripheral neuropathy.[57]

Some toxic neuropathies do not fit easily into the classification proposed by Schaumburg and Spencer in 1979.[45] In TCE toxicity, the trigeminal nerve is affected, often asymmetrically and in the absence of other cranial nerve or limb involvement.

Nitrous oxide is an example of a neurotoxin that causes dysfunction in both the central and the peripheral nervous systems. On examination, patients display a distal gradient loss of sensory function, hyperreflexia, increased tone, ataxia, and a Babinski sign.[58] As expected, the results of nerve conduction studies usually confirm the presence of a distal axonopathy.[58] Unmasking or exacerbation of underlying B_{12} deficiency or subacute combined degeneration can also be seen postoperatively when nitrous oxide is used in anesthesia.[59]

The neuropathy associated with diphtheria is unique because of its characteristic presentation of lower cranial nerve mononeuropathies followed by a delayed demyelinating polyneuropathy. Approximately 1 month after a throat infection with *Corynebacterium diphtheria,* patients develop a local pharyngeal–palatal neuropathy manifested by nasal speech and laryngeal weakness. After 4 to 8 weeks, a rapidly evolving motor and sensory neuropathy ensues. Several neurophysiological studies have demonstrated findings that imply a segmental demyelinating neuropathy with good preservation of axons. In a study of 11 patients reported by Kurdi and Abdulkader,[60] nerve conduction velocities in upper and lower extremity nerves were approximately 45% below the mean. Distal latencies varied between normal and markedly prolonged; median sensory responses were usually unobtainable. The authors did not comment on the presence or absence of conduction block or temporal dispersion, and F wave responses were not reported.[60] The electrophysiological abnormalities usually reached their peak by weeks 5 to 8, after

which recovery ensued. As observed in the other segmental demyelinating conditions, the electrodiagnostic findings did not parallel the clinical evolution. Early in the disease for one severely weak patient, normal nerve conduction results were recorded, yet several weeks later, the patient was improving and functioning close to the previous baseline in the setting of worsening or unimproved nerve conduction results.

In a case report, Solders et al.[61] described serial neurophysiological and autonomic function tests recorded over 1 year in a patient with diphtheritic neuropathy. Nerve conduction testing revealed slowing of the conduction velocities, prolonged F wave latencies, and multiple conduction blocks. The most marked changes were seen in the hands and feet 7 weeks after the onset of symptoms. In the first 3 to 5 weeks, prominent impairment of R–R variation and the Valsalva quotient was recorded, confirming involvement of the parasympathetic and sympathetic nervous systems in diphtheritic neuropathy. Surprisingly, galvanic skin responses were normal throughout the testing period. Fortunately, in both lower cranial mononeuropathies and diffuse polyneuropathy, recovery is rapid and is usually complete.

Myopathy is a known adverse effect of many therapeutic agents. Inflammatory myopathies generally show spontaneous activity upon needle insertion, indicating severe-enough disease to lead to effective denervation. Long-term corticosteroid use can cause a myopathy. Needle study shows minimal or no acute changes, but motor units usually show short amplitude and polyphasia.

Statins can also lead to a myopathy that can be associated with or without acute denervation. Advanced age, high dose, and concurrent renal disease are risk factors for developing statin-related myopathy.[62] Concurrent gemfibrizil use raises the risk of statin-induced rhabdomyolysis.[63] Proposed mechanisms of statin-related myopathy include reduction of coenzyme Q and cholesterol levels on the myocyte membrane. The most recent theory, however, involves reduced isoprenoids that result from the inhibited HMG-CoA reductase pathway. Through various mechanisms, the reduction of isoprenoids leads to increased intracellular calcium and subsequent caspase-3 activation, which triggers apoptosis.[63] Myopathy can be dose related, although most providers stop the drug for a while and switch to other nonstatin lipid-lowering drugs. Overall, given the obvious benefit and the relative rarity of this possible side effect, most physicians feel that the benefits of statin use easily outweigh the risks.[63]

Other agents that can cause myopathy include colchicine, which is a well-known precipitant of myopathy, as well as neuropathy.[64] d-Penicillamine, phenybutazone, and cimetidine are also linked to inflammatory myopathy.

REPETITIVE NERVE STIMULATION

The neurological conditions most commonly studied using repetitive nerve stimulation are myasthenia gravis and Lambert-Eaton mysthenic syndrome. Defects in neuromuscular junction transmission also have been described from toxicity to many medications, including antimicrobial agents, antirheumatic agents, anticonvulsant drugs, anticholinergic medications, calcium channel blockers, ocular products, birth control pills, lithium, phenothiazines, and radiocontrast media. Also known to interfere with the neuromuscular junction transmission are snake and insect venoms and electrolyte imbalances of calcium and magnesium.

Botulism can arise from an infected wound, a foodborne toxin, or a slow release of the toxin in the gut. The toxin blocks neurotransmitter release at peripheral cholinergic nerve terminals by cleaving docking proteins essential for exocytosis. This essentially prevents any substantial release of acetylcholine into the synaptic cleft. In adults, the disorder presents dramatically with gastrointestinal symptoms followed by dysphagia, diplopia, blurred vision, dysarthria, dry mouth, and rapid development of quadraparesis or quadriplegia and respiratory failure. Infantile botulism manifests as a failure to thrive, with a poor suck, weak cry, constipation, quadraparesis, hyperreflexia or areflexia, and respiratory failure.

In botulism, results of sensory conduction studies are normal, whereas motor conduction studies show reduced CMAPs and normal latencies and conduction velocities.[65] The diagnosis is usually confirmed on the basis of results of repetitive nerve stimulation, which shows a decremental response at low rates of stimulation and an incremental change at repetitive stimulation rates of 20 to 50 Hz.[65] The average increment is 73% (range 23% to 313%), a result not as impressive as that typically observed in Lambert-Eaton mysthenic syndrome (range 300% to 500%).[65] A further characteristic of the increment is its persistence for approximately 4 to 20 minutes after high rates of stimulation. This phenomenon can be followed serially using a single nerve stimulation and comparing the CMAP amplitude recorded at a specific time interval after activation to the amplitude recorded before activation. Fortunately, most patients with botulism recover well with supportive care. Antitoxin is effective only if infused within 24 hours of the toxin ingestion.

Organophosphates are highly toxic agents that are potent binders of acetylcholinesterase, thus producing competitive binding at the neuromuscular junction. Their primary uses are as nerve gases during war and as insecticides and pesticides. Clinically, patients present with symptoms reflective of muscarinic and nicotinic overstimulation because of uninhibited bombardment of the autonomic ganglia and neuromuscular junctions. Patients are observed to have miosis, wheezing, nausea, vomiting, abdominal cramping, sweating, increased salivation, bradycardia, hypotension, weakness, fatigue, and fasciculations.

Sensory nerve conduction study results are normal in organophosphate poisoning; reduced CMAPs are recorded in severe cases.[66] Unique to organophosphate toxicity are the results of repetitive nerve stimulation. After a single nerve stimulation, approximately 60% show multiple CMAPs of diminishing amplitude.[66] This phenomenon has been explained by the excessive prolongation of the suprathreshold excitatory postsynaptic potential beyond the muscle membrane's refractory period, thus producing a chemical repetitive stimulation of the postsynaptic receptor. Another unique phenomenon to OP poisoning is an intermediate syndrome when signs of the acute cholinergic syndrome (e.g., fasciculations and muscarinic signs) are no longer obvious. This is typically seen 2 to 4 days after exposure. An intermediate syndrome usually shows up as weakness in muscles of respiration (diaphragm, intercostal muscles, and accessory muscles, including neck muscles) and proximal limbs. Three characteristic phenomena are seen in OP poisoning: (1) repetitive firing following a single stimulus; (2) gradual reduction in twitch height or CMAP, followed by an increase after repetitive stimulation (the "decrement–increment response"); and (3) continued reduction in twitch height or CMAP after repetitive simulation ("decrementing response"). Of these, the decrementing response is the most common finding during the intermediate syndrome, while repetitive firing is more prominent during the acute cholinergic syndrome.[67]

BLINK REFLEX STUDIES

Blink reflex studies are useful for assessing the pathway from the trigeminal nerve through the brainstem to the facial muscles. In this technique, the trigeminal nerve is stimulated at the supraorbital notch and both ipsilateral and contralateral responses are recorded from the facial nerve. A comparison of the ipsilateral and contralateral latency periods can be used to infer disease localized to the trigeminal nerve, pons, medulla, or facial nerve. Before the development of brain magnetic resonance imaging, blink reflex results were often used to localize disorders of the posterior fossa, medulla, and central demyelinating conditions. Blink reflex testing can be used to evaluate patients with facial pain, although its sensitivity in trigeminal neuralgia is poor because of the infrequency of ophthalmic branch involvement. Blink reflex results can be abnormal in many peripheral demyelinating conditions, such as Guillain-Barré syndrome, diabetic neuropathy, chronic renal failure, and Charcot-Marie-Tooth disease, type I.

TCE is an organic solvent used by industry as a degreasing agent and as an inhalant anesthetic for brief operations and dental procedures. Because of its propensity to cause selective trigeminal neuropathy, TCE has been used in the past to treat trigeminal neuralgia.[68] Feldman et al. used blink reflex studies to test a group of workers who were occupationally exposed to TCE and compared their results to nonexposed employees.[68] Four patients with significant exposure to TCE showed prolonged R1 latencies that exceeded three standard deviations. None of the patients had abnormalities of nerve conduction in the limbs, changes that would have been expected had the neuropathy been generalized.[68]

AUTONOMIC TESTING

Simple bedside autonomic testing can be used to assess parasympathetic and sympathetic nervous system function. Sympathetic skin potentials are measured at the palm and the sole. They reflect the integrity of the small unmyelinated autonomic fibers, pathways not tested by routine nerve conduction studies of the motor and sensory nerves. Sinus arrhythmia testing assesses the function of the parasympathetic fibers to the sinoatrial node, whereas Valsalva ratio testing imparts information on the integrity of the sinoatrial node and the sympathetic nervous system.

Autonomic assessment has been performed on patients receiving botulinum toxin. Although botulinum toxin serotype B did cause significant decrease in saliva production compared to botulinum toxin serotype A, neither serotype caused any significant changes in other autonomic parameters.[69] Other than data from a single case of diphtheritic neuropathy, little data are available on the usefulness of autonomic testing for neurotoxicity.[61]

QUANTITATIVE SENSORY TESTING

Quantitative sensory testing (QST) has been available for more than 2 decades as a means to measure and document sensory thresholds using direct patient feedback. The modalities that can be tested include vibration, cold, warmth, heat pain, and cold pain. With regard to the fibers activated, vibration stimulates large myelinated fibers and the posterior column. Cold and warmth are mediated by separate small myelinated fibers. Heat pain and cold pain sensations are carried by small myelinated and unmyelinated fibers. In addition, cold pain can be propagated within special cold fibers.

QST should be considered complementary to nerve conduction studies and not as a substitute for nerve conduction studies. The fibers tested are different from those assessed using conventional nerve conduction studies. Furthermore, QST evaluates a longer pathway, from the sensory receptor to the peripheral nerve, spinal cord, and thalamus.

QST has been used to detect diffuse polyneuropathy in subjects exposed to industrial toxins. Halonen et al.[70] described 15 subjects exposed to industrial solvents who had abnormally high vibration thresholds (VTs) in the hands and feet. Most subjects with abnormal foot VTs also had abnormal nerve conduction study results. More than half of 41 workers exposed to acrylamide for 0.5 to 8 years had abnormal VTs in the hands and feet.[71] Measurement of VTs was considerably more sensitive than the bedside measurement of vibration using a tuning fork. Similar results have been found in workers exposed to xylene and toluene and in painters who used solvent-based paints. VTs have been used in hospitalized patients and personnel to detect early features of the polyneuropathy associated with ethylene oxide.[72] Ethylene oxide is used to sterilize heat-sensitive products and can produce a diffuse neuropathy after several months of daily exposure.

Measurements of VT, cold and warmth sensation, and heat pain sensation have been shown to be impaired in patients with chronic alcoholism. In the case of vibration testing, the threshold was abnormal regardless of age and duration of drinking.

QST can be useful in the early detection of the peripheral neuropathy associated with chemotherapy.[73] Elevated VT is an early sign of cisplatin-induced neuropathy. Some authors have reported abnormalities 6 weeks to 2 months before signs of neuropathy were discovered by other means. Abnormalities in QST also have been demonstrated in the neuropathies associated with vincristine and docetaxel use. QST has been used to quantify and confirm sensory neuropathy in patients receiving paclitaxel, but testing abnormalities did not precede symptoms or predict outcome.

Unlike acute arsenic poisoning, nerve conduction findings in chronic low-exposure arsenic toxicity are those expected in a distal axonopathy. In a study using QST in chronic arsenic exposure, Otto et al. found VTs were associated with urinary arsenic measures, and decreased pinprick sensitivity correlated with water arsenic concentration.[74] It was observed that the effects of arsenic occurred at concentrations well below the 1000 μg/L drinking water level specified by the U.S. National Research Council, and it was suggested that noncarcinogenic endpoints, such as VTs, be used in arsenic exposure risk assessment.[74]

Although QST has been beneficial in the diagnosis of some sensory neuropathies, its usefulness in diagnosing exposure to toxins has not been well established.

CONCLUSION

Properly chosen electrodiagnostic testing can be useful for identifying and confirming toxicity in the central and peripheral nervous systems. In some cases, the electrodiagnostic findings can detect disease before symptoms and signs become manifest. In other conditions, serial results can be used to document improvement or evolution of the neurological conditions.

REFERENCES

1. Niedermeyer E, Lopes da Silva FH. *Electroencephalography: Basic Principles, Clinical Applications and Related Fields*. Philadelphia: Lippincott Williams & Wilkins; 1999.
2. Fejerman N, Gimenez ER, Vallejo NE, Medina CS. Lennox's syndrome and lead intoxication. *Pediatrics*. 1973;52:227–234.
3. Poblano A, Rothenberg SJ, Schnaas L, Elias Y, Cruz ML. Spatial distribution of EEG θ-activity as a function of lifetime lead exposure in 9-year-old children. *Neurotoxicology*. 2001;22:439–446.
4. Satoh H. Occupational and environmental toxicology of mercury and its compounds. *Ind Health*. 2000;38:153–164.
5. Urban P, Nerudova J, Cabelkova Z, et al. EEG photic driving in workers exposed to mercury vapors. *Neurotoxicology*. 2003;24:23–33.
6. Herrero Hernandez E, Discalzi G, Dassi P, Jarre L, Pira E. Manganese intoxication: the cause of an inexplicable epileptic syndrome in a 3-year-old child. *Neurotoxicology*. 2003;24: 633–639.
7. Wennberg A, Hagman M, Johansson L. Preclinical neurophysiological signs of parkinsonism in occupational manganese exposure. *Neurotoxicology*. 1992;13:271–274.
8. Tsai YT, Huang CC, Kuo HC, et al. Central nervous system effects in acute thallium poisoning. *Neurotoxicology*. 2006;27:291–295.
9. Niedermeyer E, Freund G, Krumholz A. Sub-acute encephalopathy with seizures in alcoholics: a clinical–electroencephalographic study. *Clin Electroencephalogr*. 1981;12:113–129.
10. Gonzalez LP, Veatch LM, Ticku MK, Becker HC. Alcohol withdrawal kindling: mechanisms and implications for treatment. *Alcohol Clin Exp Res*. 2001;25:197S–201S.
11. Mayersdorf A, Israeli R. Toxic effects of chlorinated hydrocarbon insecticides: on human electroencephalogram. *Arch Environ Health*. 1974;28:159–163.
12. Mutez E, Le Rhun E, Perriol MP, et al. Trichloroethylene intoxication presenting with temporal seizures. *Rev Neurol (Paris)*. 2006;162:1248–1251.
13. Singal A, Thami GP. Lindane neurotoxicity in childhood. *Am J Ther*. 2006;13:277–280.
14. Okonek S RH. EEG veranderungen bei alkylphophatvergiftungen. *Z EEG*. 1975;6.
15. Yanagisawa N, Morita H, Nakajima T. Sarin experiences in Japan: acute toxicity and long-term effects. *J Neurol Sci*. 2006;249:76–85.
16. Carpentier P, Foquin-Tarricone A, Bodjarian N, et al. EEG changes caused by dimethoate treatment in three generations of rats. *Neurotoxicology*. 1994;15:731–734.
17. Jacobs MH, Senior RM. Theophylline toxicity due to impaired theophylline degradation. *Am Rev Respir Dis*. 1974;110:342–345.
18. Lam S, Gomolin IH. Cefepime neurotoxicity: case report, pharmacokinetic considerations, and literature review. *Pharmacotherapy*. 2006;26:1169–1174.
19. Juckel G, Schule C, Pogarell O, et al. Epileptiform EEG patterns induced by mirtazapine in both psychiatric patients and healthy volunteers. *J Clin Psychopharmacol*. 2003;23:421–422.
20. Pogarell O, Juckel G, Mulert C, et al. EEG abnormalities under treatment with atypical antipsychotics: effects of olanzapine and amisulpride as compared to haloperidol. *Pharmacopsychiatry*. 2004;37:304–305.
21. Amann BL, Pogarell O, Mergl R, Juckel G, Grunze H, Mulert C, Hegerl U. EEG abnormalities associated with antipsychotics: a comparison of quetiapine, olanzapine, haloperidol and healthy subjects. *Hum Psychopharmacol*. 2003;18:641–646.
22. Duggal HS, Jagadheesan K, Nizamie SH. Clozapine-induced stuttering and seizures. *Am J Psychiatry*. 2002;159:315.
23. Mucci A, Volpe U, Merlotti E, Bucci P, Galderisi S. Pharmaco-EEG in psychiatry. *Clin EEG Neurosci*. 2006;37:81–98.
24. Helmchen H, Kanowski S. EEG Changes during lithium therapy. *Nervenarzt* 1971;42:205–208.
25. Gallinat J, Boetsch T, Padberg F, et al. Is the EEC helpful in diagnosing and monitoring lithium intoxication? A case report and review of the literature. *Pharmacopsychiatry*. 2000;33:169–173.
26. Segura-Bruna N, Rodriguez-Campello A, Puente V, Roquer J. Valproate-induced hyperammonemic encephalopathy. *Acta Neurol Scand*. 2006;114:1–7.
27. Kellinghaus C, Dziewas R, Ludemann P. Tiagabine-related non-convulsive status epilepticus in partial epilepsy: three case reports and a review of the literature. *Seizure*. 2002;11:243–249.
28. Boutte C, Vercueil L, Durand M, Vincent F, Alvarez JC. EEG contribution to the diagnosis of baclofen overdose. *Neurophysiol Clin*. 2006;36:85–89.
29. Constant I, Seeman R, Murat I. Sevoflurane and epileptiform EEG changes. *Paediatr Anaesth*. 2005;15:266–274.
30. Riad W, Schreiber M, Saeed AB. Monitoring with EEG entropy decreases propofol requirement and maintains cardiovascular stability during induction of anaesthesia in elderly patients. *Eur J Anaesthesiol*. 2007;24:684–688.
31. Brown BB. Subjective and EEG responses to LSD in visualizer and non-visualizer subjects. *Electroencephalogr Clin Neurophysiol*. 1968;25:372–379.
32. Herning RI, Better W, Tate K, Cadet JL. EEG deficits in chronic marijuana abusers during monitored abstinence: preliminary findings. *Ann NY Acad Sci*. 2003;993:75–78.
32a. Dietsch G. Fourier-analyse von Elektrenkephalogrammer des Menschen. *Pfuger's Arch Ges Physiol*. 1932;230:106–112.
33. Newton TF, Kalechstein AD, Hardy DJ, et al. Association between quantitative EEG and neurocognition in methamphetamine-dependent volunteers. *Clin Neurophysiol*. 2004;115:194–198.
34. Prichep LS, Alper KR, Sverdlov L, et al. Outcome related electrophysiological subtypes of cocaine dependence. *Clin Electroencephalogr*. 2002;33:8–20.
35. Babiloni C, Squitti R, Del Percio C, et al. Free copper and resting temporal EEG rhythms correlate across healthy, mild cognitive impairment, and Alzheimer's disease subjects. *Clin Neurophysiol*. 2007;118:1244–1260.
36. Yoshimura M, Koenig T, Irisawa S, et al. A pharmaco-EEG study on antipsychotic drugs in healthy volunteers. *Psychopharmacology*. 2007;191:995–1004.
37. Clemens B, Menes A, Piros P, et al. Quantitative EEG effects of carbamazepine, oxycarbazepine, valproate, lamotrigine, and possible clinical relevance of the findings. *Epilepsy Res*. 2006;70:190–199.
38. Salinsky M, Storzbach D, Oken B, Spencer D. Topiramate effects on the EEG and alertness in healthy volunteers: a different

profile of antiepileptic drug neurotoxicity. *Epilepsy Behav.* 2007;10:463–469.

39. Kokubun Y, Oishi M, Takasu T, Sakamaki S. Somatosensory evoked potentials in chronic alcoholics with spasticity. *Arch Neurol.* 1988;45:318.

40. Shibasaki H, Kakigi R, Ohnishi A, Kuroiwa Y. Peripheral and central nerve conduction in sub-acute myelo-optico-neuropathy. *Neurology.* 1982;32:1186–1189.

41. Yiannikas C, Walsh JC, McLeod JG. Visual evoked potentials in the detection of subclinical optic toxic effects secondary to ethambutol. *Arch Neurol.* 1983;40:645–648.

42. Manesis EK, Moschos M, Brouzas D, et al. Neurovisual impairment: a frequent complication of α-interferon treatment in chronic viral hepatitis. *Hepatology.* 1998;27:1421–1427.

43. Saint-Amour D, Roy MS, Bastien C, et al. Alterations of visual evoked potentials in preschool Inuit children exposed to methylmercury and polychlorinated biphenyls from a marine diet. *Neurotoxicology.* 2006;27:567–578.

44. Kalita J, Misra UK. Sequelae of thallium poisoning: clinical and neurophysiological follow-up. *Eur Neurol.* 2006;56:253–255.

45. Schaumburg HH, Spencer PS. Toxic neuropathies. *Neurology.* 1979;29:429–431.

46. Albin RL, Albers JW, Greenberg HS, et al. Acute sensory neuropathy: neuronopathy from pyridoxine overdose. *Neurology.* 1987;37:1729–1732.

47. Stubblefield MD, Vahdat LT, Balmaceda CM, et al. Glutamine as a neuroprotective agent in high-dose paclitaxel-induced peripheral neuropathy: a clinical and electrophysiologic study. *Clinical Oncology.* 2005;17:271–276.

48. Gutmann L, Martin JD, Welton W. Dapsone motor neuropathy: axonal disease. *Neurology.* 26:514–516, 1976.

49. Windebank AJ. Metal neuropathy. In: Dyck PJ, Thomas PK, eds. *Peripheral Neuropathy.* 3rd ed. Philadelphia, PA.: W.B. Saunders, 1993:1549–1570.

50. Araki S, Sato H, Yokoyama K, Murata K. Subclinical neurophysiological effects of lead: a review on peripheral, central, and autonomic nervous system effects in lead workers. *Am J Ind Med.* 2000;37:193–204.

51. Donofrio PD, Wilbourn AJ, Albers JW, et al. Acute arsenic intoxication presenting as Guillain-Barré-like syndrome. *Muscle Nerve.* 1987;10:114–120.

52. Martinezarizala A, Sobol SM, McCarty GE, Nichols BR, Rakita L. Amiodarone neuropathy. *Neurology.* 1983;33:643–645.

53. Bousser MG, Bouche P, Brochard C, Herreman G. Peripheral neuropathies due to perhexilene maleate. *Coeur Med Interne.* 1976;15:181–188.

54. Peltier AC, Russell FW. Advances in understanding drug-induced neuropathies. *Drug Saf.* 2006;29:23–30.

55. Donofrio PD, Stanton C, Miller VS, et al. Demyelinating polyneuropathy in eosinophilia: myalgia syndrome. *Muscle Nerve.* 1992;15:796–805.

56. Skopelitis EE, Kokotis PI, Kontos AN, et al. Distal sensory polyneuropathy in HIV-positive patients in the HAART era: an entity underestimated by clinical examination. *Int J STD AIDS.* 2006;17:467–472.

57. Shah SR, Tran TM. Lenalidomide in myelodysplastic syndrome and multiple myeloma. *Drugs.* 2007;67:1869–1881.

58. Layzer RB, Fishman RA, Schafer JA. Neuropathy following abuse of nitrous-oxide. *Neurology.* 1978;28:504–506.

59. Otmani E. Postoperative dementia: toxicity of nitrous oxide. *Encephale.* 2007;33:95–97.

60. Kurdi A, Abdulkader M. Clinical and electro-physiological studies of diphtheritic neuritis in Jordan. *J Neurol Sci.* 1979;42:243–250.

61. Solders G, Nennesmo I, Persson A. Diphtheritic neuropathy: an analysis based on muscle and nerve biopsy and repeated neurophysiological and autonomic function tests. *J Neurol Neurosurg Psychiatry.* 1989;52:876–880.

62. Schech S, Graham D, Staffa J, et al. Risk factors for statin-associated rhabdomyolysis. *Pharmacoepidemiol Drug Saf.* 2007;16:352–358.

63. Harper CR, Jacobson TA. The broad spectrum of statin myopathy: from myalgia to rhabdomyolysis. *Curr Opin Lipidol.* 2007;18:401–408.

64. Duarte J, Cabezas C, Rodriguez F, Claveria LE, Palacin T. Colchicine-induced myopathy with myotonia. *Muscle Nerve.* 1998;21:550–551.

65. Cornblath DR, Sladky JT, Sumner AJ. Clinical electrophysiology of infantile botulism. *Muscle Nerve.* 1983;6:448–452.

66. Wadia RS, Chitra S, Amin RB, Kiwalkar RS, Sardesai HV. Electrophysiological studies in acute organophosphate poisoning. *J Neurol Neurosurg Psychiatry.* 1987;50:1442–1448.

67. Karalliedde L, Baker D, Marrs TC. Organophosphate-induced intermediate syndrome: aetiology and relationships with myopathy. *Toxicol Rev.* 2006;25:1–14.

68. Feldman RG, Niles C, Proctor SP, Jabre J. Blink reflex measurement of effects of trichloroethylene exposure on the trigeminal nerve. *Muscle Nerve.* 1992;15:490–495.

69. Tintner R, Gross R, Winzer UF, Smalky KA, Jankovic J. Autonomic function after botulinum toxin type A or B: a double-blind, randomized trial. *Neurology.* 2005;65:765–767.

70. Halonen P, Halonen JP, Lang HA, Karskela V. Vibratory perception thresholds in shipyard workers exposed to solvents. *Acta Neurol Scand.* 1986;73:561–565.

71. Deng H, He FS, Zhang SL, Calleman CJ, Costa LG. Quantitative measurements of vibration threshold in healthy-adults and acrylamide workers. *Int Arch Occup Environ Health.* 1993;65:53–56.

72. Bousser MG, Bouche P, Brochard C, Herreman G. Neuropathies périphériques au maléate de perhexiline. A propos de 7 observations. *Coeur Med Interne.* 1976;15(2):181–188.

73. Chaudhry V, Rowinsky EK, Sartorius SE, Donehower RC, Cornblath DR. Peripheral neuropathy from taxol and cisplatin combination chemotherapy: clinical and electrophysiological studies. *Ann Neurol.* 1994;35:304–311.

74. Otto D, Xia Y, Li Y, et al. Neurosensory effects of chronic human exposure to arsenic associated with body burden and environmental measures. *Hum Exp Toxicol.* 2007;26:169–177.

CHAPTER 17

Laboratory Assessment of Exposure to Neurotoxic Agents

Lawrence K. Oliver

INTRODUCTION

This chapter discusses some general principles of specimen collection for the measurement of toxic components, the methods usually employed for those measurements, and the analysis of specific neurotoxins. For each of the neurotoxins for which laboratory analysis is possible, the preferred method for analysis is given, along with guidelines for the interpretation of results and any analyte-specific cautions for using the laboratory data. Toxins not discussed in this chapter are ones for which no feasible laboratory analysis is available. These include most industrial organic toxins and those produced by the higher organisms—shellfish and envenomatoxins.

It is important to note that for any one analyte various methods may be used throughout the world for laboratory measurements. Many of these methods are old (even ancient) and lack sensitivity or specificity, and such methods are far too numerous to discuss here. Up-to-date laboratory practice uses methods like mass spectroscopy (in various forms) and immunoassays. In general terms, if your laboratory is using a colorimetric, spectrophotometric, or thin-layer procedure, treat results with considerable caution. These methods have a high likelihood of producing false-positive or false-negative results, particularly around the decision points related to limits found in normal people, largely because of interferences from other substances. It is wise to confirm results from such methods with the use of a reference procedure, even if it is a sendout test for your laboratory.

Methods for analysis of neurotoxins use general laboratory techniques in most cases. They are discussed thoroughly and in depth in various textbooks, two of which are listed at the end of this chapter and to which you should refer for more specific instrumentation details. Interpretive guidelines for laboratory testing results may be method specific. I refer to the procedures considered to be the optimum ones available commercially, and interpretive statements are based on those technologies and are derived directly from laboratory and general references listed in the References section. For many analytes, research laboratories have more esoteric methods available, but access is severely limited and use of those laboratories in routine medical care is not practical. The single exception is the analysis of acrylamide: it is currently not available commercially, but recent advances in the evaluation of acrylamide exposure indicate that commercialization is likely to occur in the near future, so I include that analyte in the Specific Analytes section.

First, I review the general principles of specimen collection for neurotoxin evaluation. While much of this section is developed from the criteria needed for assessment of metals, the differential diagnosis of many neurotoxic symptoms requires the measurement of one or more metals to rule out them as a possible source. Therefore, specimen collection must be done in a manner that prevents inadvertent contamination of the specimen with environmental sources of the toxin.

SPECIMEN COLLECTION

The phlebotomist assigned to collect blood, plasma, or serum for analysis of toxins must be especially careful to avoid contamination of the draw site. Special metal-free collection equipment and vials must be used when collecting blood for analysis for screening for environmental metal toxins. Contamination of the collection site can be avoided with careful cleaning with an alcohol swab. Iodine-containing disinfectants are to be avoided. Special metal-free collection tubes must be used for specimen transport. Any commercially available stainless steel needle or butterfly device is acceptable.

Follow the instructions of your laboratory to determine what specimen type to use. In general, ethylenediaminetetraacetic acid (EDTA) is the preferred anticoagulant, primarily because other agents are more likely to give microclotting over time, which can clog instrumentation and make processing difficult.

Urine must be collected into a container that does not use a metal cap for closure and does not have any glued inserts into the cap, since they contain sufficient metals to give falsely elevated results. Do not collect urine in the environment in which exposure is suspected. Never use a colored container for collection because of metal-containing dyes.

Most organic or protein-based neurotoxins are present in low levels in biological fluids, often have a short half-life, and are only marginally stable at ambient temperatures. It is highly recommended to keep a chart handy that outlines the specimen handling requirements for your laboratory so that time is not wasted in specimen collection or the sample is not compromised by delays after it is removed from the body.

GENERAL METHODOLOGIES USED FOR NEUROTOXINS

The analyses of metals, proteins, and small molecules have all changed dramatically over the past 10 years. Metals, for example, have evolved from colorimetric or spectrophotometric procedures, to atomic absorption, to flameless atomic absorption, to ICP-MS, with concomitant improvements in sensitivity and, most significantly, specificity. The time-honored procedures for measurement of

proteins—immunoassay—is still in common use, but the introduction of monoclonal antibodies has greatly improved the specificity and the long-term stability of the assays, with marginal improvements in sensitivity. Note that many proteins are neurotoxic at such low concentrations that current methods do not detect them in biological fluids. The measurement of small molecules such as in the street, or illicit, drugs is now best performed using one of the mass spectrometric methods. Immunoassays or older thin-layer procedures should be considered screening methods at best, and the clinician should require the more specific mass spectrometric procedure for confirmation, identification, and quantitation.

It is important to also note that virtually all organic molecules undergo metabolism once they are introduced into a physiological matrix. The metabolic pathways are often not defined, so even major metabolites of such molecules cannot be analyzed. In those cases, quantitative assessment of the levels, even for determining whether the suspected neurotoxin is the primary cause of the toxicity, is often not feasible from current commonly available technology. This is especially true for some reactive solvents (styrene, vinyl chloride), shellfish, and envenomatoxins.

Mass Spectroscopy

In mass spectroscopy, a biological sample is ionized, separated into individual molecules or fragments of molecules, and then accelerated into an ion beam using charged plates. The beam is directed toward an ion detector, and peaks representative of the ratio of mass to charge are quantified according to the number of particles at each ratio.

Mass spectroscopy is usually coupled with a separation technique such as chromatography to provide a cleaner sample for injection into the spectrometer. Gas and liquid chromatography front ends to mass spectrometric are in common use for the analysis of organic compounds.

Cautions

While all mass spectrometric techniques are specific, the application to the analysis of complex mixtures (such as screening for abused drugs) can occasionally give incorrect identifications because of structurally similar compounds being present.

Inductively Coupled Plasma Mass Spectroscopy

The most accurate and precise method for determination of metals is inductively coupled plasma mass spectrometry (ICP-MS). In this analysis, the specimens, calibrators, and controls are aspirated using a pneumatic nebulizer driven by high-pressure argon gas. The mixture is injected into a $6800°K$ argon gas discharge (plasma), which atomizes and ionizes the nebulized particles. The plasma is then directed into a mass spectrometer, which separates the ions by mass and quantitates them individually. The resolution is such that individual masses less than 1 D apart can be resolved. A known quantity of a metal rarely found in humans, such as rubidium or terbium, is added as an internal standard for quantitation.

One general caution for use of ICP-MS: Gadolinium (Gd) is in widespread use as a contrast agent and, when present in a sample of biological fluid, it is present at such high levels that it has a signal that overwhelms almost every other metal. If your patient is getting any Gd salt as part of a procedure, wait at least 48 hours (for a person with normal kidney function) before taking a sample for metal analysis. If your patient has impaired renal function, the half-life of Gd salts is longer and can lead to fibrosis due to the deposition of the salts in liver and skin. For patients with low glomerular filtration rate, less than 30 mL/min for every 1.73 m^2 body surface area, it is best to take the sample for metal analysis before administration of any Gd contrast agent.

Immunoassays

Analysis procedures that use an antibody to capture or label the targeted analyte rely on the specificity of that antibody to ensure that only the target analyte is being bound to the antibody. Cross-reactivity is the major problem with immunoassays, and it manifests itself in ways that are not easy for the laboratory to detect:

- Compounds with structural similarity to the target are detected and quantified but are not equivalently to the target.
- The matrix of the sample is critical to reliable processing of the antigen–antibody reaction. Changes in protein concentration, pH, and salt concentration can all affect performance.

If an immunoassay procedure is being used, make sure that your laboratory informs you of the exact specimen type (including anticoagulant, if appropriate: plasma from EDTA is not the same as plasma from heparin tubes, for example), the conditions under which the specimen is to be transported, and the cross-reactivity profile of their assay. The cross-reactivity profile ideally should include all compounds structurally similar to the target (amphetamine, methamphetamine, and 3,4-methylenedioxymethamphetamine, or MDMA, are considered structurally similar and cross-react with one another), as well as compounds that give similar clinical impressions.

Thin-Layer Chromatography

The acronym for thin-layer chromatography (TLC) is well chosen because it takes a great deal of "tender loving care" to obtain reproducible results with reliable clinical interpretation from this method. TLC involves highly operator-dependent methods. In the basic procedure, a gel is applied to a glass plate, plastic strip, or similar nonreactive support; the biological sample is spotted on one end of the support; and the device put into a chamber with a small amount of organic solvent in it. The solvent is wicked up the plate, carrying the substances in the fluid, along with the solvent, at rates dependent on several factors, including pH, polarity, and size. The organic substances are then visualized either using a spray (iodine is commonly used) or using charring, and the location of the bands thus visualized is used to identify the components. The technique is only crudely quantitative, and false identifications are common. It is a rapid procedure, however, and is often performed in smaller, local laboratories and hospitals. Negative results are generally more predictive than positive ones when obtained using TLC methods.

Screening Methods for Drugs, Including Immunoassays and Chromatographical Techniques

The common "comprehensive" screens for toxic drugs are usually limited to testing for pharmacologics and designer drugs that populate street use and street abuse. Therefore, many neurotoxins either are not detected or are detected but remain unidentified. Virtually none of the protein-based neurotoxins are detectable in drug screens.

The analysis of pharmacologics and the street drug modifications of them (e.g., MDMA and methamphetamine) is most commonly done using either an immunoassay or a chromatographical procedure. Immunoassays, such as for amphetamines, are designed to detect any member of a class of compounds, and the threshold level of detection varies for each member of that family. So, a "positive" result means only that one or more members of the class of compounds is present; identification of the particular member, and quantitation of the level of that compound, requires a more specific procedure such as gas or liquid chromatography. Gas and liquid chromatography methods are performed by adding a standard amount of a compound, similar to the one requested, to the sample and then putting the sample through a separation column and using a detector to indicate when and how much of each compound is eluted from the column. Detectors are of various types, and techniques include ionization, absorbance monitoring, redox, fluorescence, and thermal conductivity. The cautions to be aware of when a chromatographical technique is used include the following:

- Interference with either the internal standard or the compound itself. The laboratory usually recognizes that an interference exists and reports it to you. Ask your laboratory for lists of known interferences with its assay.

- Incorrect specimen type used. Laboratories assume that the specimen type submitted is the one requested, but their assay may not be valid for alternate types of biological fluids. Make sure your phlebotomist and specimen handlers are aware of the requirements. If there is any question about the appropriate specimen, include a note to the laboratory about what was actually collected.

24-HOUR URINE COLLECTIONS VERSUS RANDOM COLLECTIONS

Many substances have diurnal variability in their excretion patterns in urine. Consequently, the use of a random urine collection as a means of detecting toxicity is not as reliable as a 24-hour collection, which measures the integrated daily exposure to the substance. Regardless, a high concentration in a random urine collection can be indicative of significantly elevated body exposure. To approximate the 24-hour excretion from a random urine collection (ignoring the diurnal effect), consider 1500 mL as an average daily urinary output and correct accordingly.

HAIR–NAIL ANALYSIS

Hair and Nails

Properly done, hair analysis of the elements that bind to sulfhydryl groups in keratin is a useful, but problematic, means of approximating when the exposure occurred. The correlation between the hair or nail levels of a trace metal and the level in blood is variable and often confusing. A major part of the variability comes from the way the specimen is collected and processed before analysis. Consider the following:

- Washed versus unwashed hair—In general, use hair that has been washed to avoid environmental contamination on the surface of the hair. The useful metal levels are those combined with the keratin. A few shampoos contain some metal ions, but they (Mg, Na, K) are not neurotoxins. If you cannot get washed hair, notify your laboratory—most laboratories will wash the sample with a non-metal-containing detergent that also does not extract any metal from the structural component of the hair.
- Location—Hair that is closest to the scalp—the recent growth—correlates most closely with blood levels. Hair grows about 400 μm/day (1.0 cm/month). Hair keratin synthesized in the follicle takes approximately 1 week to extrude through the skin.[1] Pubic hair is acceptable.

- Nails—Take samples from all nails to give the best representative sample. Again, wash first to avoid environmental contamination.
- Hair color—Gray-reducing hair colorants often contain lead, and other coloring agents may contain other metals. Undyed hair is best. Differing natural hair colors appear to have some differing effects in the incorporation of various metals, but the effect is not reliable enough for interpretive differences.[2]
- Beards, razor clippings—Clippings from razors of facial or body hair generally are not acceptable.
- Submission—When sending hair or nails, do not apply tape to stick them to paper.

Hair–Nail Analytical Issues

Hair and nail samples are washed, dried, weighed, and then digested with concentrated nitric acid. The resulting solution is then analyzed, and the results are reported as micrograms of metal per gram of dry weight.

SPECIFIC ANALYTES

Mercury

Elemental mercury is nontoxic, but current methodologies do not distinguish between the elemental form and the +2 inorganic form or the organic forms, mostly trimethylmercury. Speciation methods will be available at reference laboratories in the near future and should be used when they become available. ICP-MS methods are used for measurement of mercury in all types of specimens.

Urine

The correlation between levels of excretion in the urine and clinical symptoms is considered poor—most mercury is excreted in the feces—but urinary mercury (Hg) is the most reliable way to assess exposure to inorganic mercury. Urine excretion of more than 20 μg/L indicates significant exposure.[3] Chelation therapy causes large increases in the amount of mercury found in the urine and is the preferred means for monitoring therapy. Clearance from neuronal tissue is slow compared to clearance from the circulation, however, and urine excretion is not a reliable means of ensuring that the neurotoxin is cleared.

Blood

Circulating organic mercury is mainly located in the red blood cells; thus, estimation of levels must be made on whole blood. The form of mercury bound to hemoglobin is the +2 state, and it binds to the sulfhydryl groups on many proteins. Hg+2 gets concentrated in the kidney, where the greatest toxicity occurs. Organic mercury, mostly trimethylmercury, is the most toxic of the forms of the element and is lipophilic, so it is bound to proteins in lipid-rich regions, such as the neuron, causing the neurotoxicity. Organic mercury is readily measured in assays for blood mercury but may not reflect the central nervous system load of the metal. Normal levels are less than 10 ng/mL, and toxicity is considered significant when the level is more than 50 ng/mL.

Hair and Nails

Send 0.5 g of hair (the length of the index finger and width of a pencil), or 0.5 g of nails from all 10 fingernails or toenails. Normal levels are less than 1.0 µg/g. The amount found approximates the severity of exposure.

Lead

Various methods are used for analysis of lead. ICP-MS is the reference procedure, although the Centers for Disease Control and Prevention programs have given a great deal of standardization across methods. Atomic absorption spectroscopy is widely used, and the results are comparable to ICP-MS, provided that the calibrator is in the same matrix as the specimen being analyzed. Voltammetry is now rarely used because of more complex sample preparation and increased risk of contamination.

Urine

Although bodily excretion of lead is slow, urinary lead increases in lead poisoning. Urinary excretion of up to about 125 µg every 24 hours is probably not associated with any evidence of lead poisoning. Most normals excrete less than 80 µg of lead per day.

Blood

The lead in blood is primarily in the erythrocytes, and blood levels have the strongest correlation with toxicity. The Centers for Disease Control has identified the blood lead test as the preferred test for detecting lead exposure in children. Chronic whole-blood lead of less than 10 µg/dL is normal in children. Chelation therapy is indicated when whole-blood lead concentration is greater than 45 µg/dL. Blood from finger sticks or earlobe sticks is also acceptable, provided that the skin is cleansed thoroughly before puncture.

Hair

Hair or nail analysis of lead can be used to corroborate blood analysis. If the hair is collected in a time sequence fashion (based on length from root), the approximate time of exposure can be assessed. Normally, hair lead content is less than 5 µg/g. Hair lead content of more than 25 µg/g indicates severe lead exposure.

Arsenic

Analysis of arsenic is best performed using ICP-MS. The toxic forms of arsenic are the inorganic species of As+3, As+5, and monomethyl and dimethyl arsine. The nontoxic organic forms are primarily arsenobetaine and arsenocholine. These latter forms are rapidly cleared in the urine and disappear within 48 hours after ingestion. The biological half-life of organic arsenic is 4 to 6 hours. Optimum use of the laboratory for assessing arsenic poisoning must rely on at least fractionation between the organic and the inorganic forms and, ultimately, speciation, the differentiation among the various oxidation states of the metal.

Urine

To assess toxicity, either use a method that fractionates the metal or wait for 48 hours after ingestion of seafood to clear the organic forms from the body. Screening methods that do not distinguish between the organic forms and the inorganic forms of arsenic should be used with great caution. Inorganic arsenic at concentrations of more than 25 µg every 24 hours (or approximately 20 µg/L for a spot urine collection) are considered toxic. While not recommended, the nonfractionated procedures are commonly used. For those methods, normal levels, usually quoted as less than 120 µg every 24 hours, greatly depend on consumption of such arsenic-containing foods as seafood, like crab or lobster. Toxicity interpretations are not reliable for screening methods until the reported concentration is more than 5000 µg every 24 hours. Arsenic may be elevated (up to 1000 µg every 24 hours) following ingestion of seafood such as crab, shrimp, and lobster. These foods contain trace amounts of other, nonorganic forms of arsenic, which is not considered to be a health problem. The urine arsenic concentration becomes normal within 3 days of abstinence if seafood ingestion is the only source of arsenic. If the urine arsenic concentration does not change significantly over 3 days, then an inorganic source of arsenic should be suspected. A urine excretion rate of more than 1000 µg every 24 hours indicates significant exposure. The highest level observed at the Mayo Clinic was 450,000 µg every 24 hours in a patient with severe symptoms of gastrointestinal distress, shallow breathing with classic "garlic breath," intermittent seizure activity, cardiac arrhythmias, and later onset of peripheral neuropathy.

Blood

Arsenic combines readily with proteins because of its great affinity for sulfhydryl groups. The affinity of arsenic for tissue proteins is responsible for the rapid removal of arsenic from blood. Arsenic becomes "normal" within 6 to 10 hours after exposure, so blood arsenic is not a good specimen for screening purposes. Blood arsenic is rarely fractionated into organic and inorganic portions, and the results reflect the total arsenic. Consequently, toxicity cannot be directly related to blood levels. Normal levels are less than 0.07 μg/mL. Use blood as the specimen type only when there is high confidence that the exposure is acute: within the past few hours at most. Otherwise, use urine or hair.

Hair

Hair is a natural repository for arsenic, since keratin contains many cysteine residues. Arsenic tends to be concentrated in hair. For purposes of timing exposure to metallic toxins, arsenic in hair is one of the more reliable measures, since the metal binds immediately and strongly. Levels greater than 0.1 μg/g indicate excessive exposure.

Thallium

The preferred method of analysis for thallium is ICP-MS. Blood, serum, plasma, urine, or hair and nails can be used for analysis, although the normal and toxic levels are best established for serum and urine. Normal levels for serum are less than 10 μg/mL, with observable toxic levels up to 50 ng/mL. Normal urine output is less than 10 μg every 24 hours. Toxic levels in the urine may go higher than 500 μg every 24 hours. The long-term sequelae from these elevated levels is poor.

Aluminum

Aluminum in serum collected using a metal-free vacutainer is analyzed by ICP-MS methods. Because many commercially available vacutainers use rubber caps that contain considerable amounts of aluminum, check with your laboratory for specific instructions on which tubes have been shown to be aluminum free. Never use wooden applicator sticks to break up the clot: they contain large amounts of aluminum. The samples are stable for several days at all temperatures. The reference range for all ages, both genders, is less than 6 ng/mL. Patients undergoing renal dialysis have higher levels, and aluminum is not removed during dialysis. Levels in these patients are usually less than 60 ng/mL, with toxic symptoms being evident at levels greater than 100 ng/mL.

Manganese

Graphite furnace atomic absorption spectroscopy is the preferred method for analysis of manganese in blood. Whole-blood levels are 10 times those in serum, and whole blood is the desired specimen type. Whole-blood levels above the upper limit of the normal range 18 ng/mL are indicative of likely manganism. Single values between one and two times the upper limit of normal may be due to differences in hematocrit and normal biological variation,

and these values should be interpreted with caution before concluding that hypermanganesemia is contributing to the disease process. Values greater than twice the upper limit of normal are more highly correlated with symptoms. For longitudinal monitoring, a sample of no more often than the half-life of the element (40 days) should be used.

Manganese in urine may also be used to monitor clearance of the metal upon treatment. A 24-hour collection is optimum, since excretion can be variable throughout the day. Collect in a metal-free container, with no preservatives added. Analysis is usually done using ICP-MS methods, with normal levels of up to 2 μg every 24 hours. Levels greater than 50 μg every 24 hour should be considered highly dangerous and require immediate action.

Amphetamines and 3,4-Methylenedioxymethamphetamine

See the earlier discussion on immunoassays and TLC.

Cocaine

The presence of cocaine, or its major metabolite, benzoylecgonine, indicates use within the past 4 days. Cocaine has a 6-hour half-life, so it is present in urine for 1 day after last use. Benzoylecgonine has a half-life of 12 hours, so it can be detected in urine up to 4 days after last use. Consequently, most assays are designed to detect benzoylecgonine, not cocaine itself. Quantitative results are sometime supplied by laboratories, but be aware that there is no correlation between concentration and pharmacological or toxic effects. Assays generally rely on the use of an antibody to detect the benzoylecgonine, but such antibodies are specific and there are no significant cross-reactants.

Ethanol and Other Alcohols

All such volatile alcohols are analyzed using headspace gas chromatography, a technique in which the alcohol is released from whole blood collected with a mixture of oxalate and fluoride added (to preserve the alcohol from oxidation) and then put through a gas chromatography instrument. All alcohols can be simultaneously determined using this procedure. An alternative, and popular method, for ethyl alcohol, is to use an enzymatic procedure requiring alcohol dehydrogenase to convert the alcohol to its aldehyde, producing the reduced form of nicotinamide adenine dinucleotide in the process, which is measured spectrophotometrically. The disadvantage to this method is that no other alcohols are measured, and simply asking the laboratory for an "alcohol level" without indicating a concern over methanol, isopropanol, or even ethylene glycol poisoning may lead to the incorrect test being performed. Toxic levels for most alcohols depend on use history. Methanol is generally considered toxic at levels greater than 100 µg/mL and isopropanol at levels greater than 500 µg/mL.

Nitrous Oxide

Nitrous oxide is not metabolized by the human body. While assays are available for nitrate and nitrite, those assays are useless in diagnosing or monitoring nitrous oxide poisoning. Other than the routine safety testing for tracking symptoms or certain severe consequences, such as megaloblastic hemopoiesis, no laboratory testing is available.

Organophosphates

Red cell acetylcholinesterase is most often used to detect past exposure to organophosphate insecticides with resultant inhibition of the enzyme. Both the pseudocholinesterase activity in serum and red cell acetylcholinesterase are inhibited by these insecticides, but they are dramatically different vis à vis the temporal aspect of the exposure. The half-life of the pseudoenzyme in serum is about 8 days, and the "true" cholinesterase (acetylcholinesterase) of red cells is more than 3 months (determined by erythropoietic activity). Prior exposure up to several weeks is determined by assay of the pseudoenzyme, and months after exposure is determined by measurement of the red cell enzyme.

Acetylcholinesterase Testing

For acetylcholinesterase testing, heparinized whole blood is required and must arrive at the laboratory within 72 hours of collection. If that is not possible, the erythrocytes should be washed at the collection site and submitted. To wash red blood cells:

1. Immediately centrifuge for 10 minutes at 650 × G.
2. Discard the plasma and buffy coat layers.
3. Add a cold 0.9% saline solution to the erythrocytes (about two times the volume of erythrocytes).
4. Mix gently by inversion and centrifuge again for 10 minutes at 650 × G.
5. Remove and discard the saline.
6. Repeat the wash steps (3 to 5) two more times.
7. After the final centrifugation, remove and discard the saline and a thin layer of the top cells.
8. Immediately freeze the washed, packed cells (red cell pellet from step 7), and send the specimen frozen in a plastic vial.

Methodology   Acetylcholinesterase is one of the few remaining reliable spectrophotometric tests. The substrate acetylthiocholine is split by acetylcholinesterase into thiocholine and acetate. The thiocholine then reacts with dithiobisnitrobenzoic acid (Ellman's reagent) to form the colored product thionitrobenzoic acid, which is measured at 405 nm.

Pseudocholinesterase Testing

For pseudocholinesterase testing, 1 mL of serum is usually required, and it can be either refrigerated or frozen. Stability at ambient temperatures is short and does not allow overnight specimen transport.

Methodology   The substrate, acetylthiocholine, is cleaved by propionylcholinesterase into acetate and thiocholine. The thiocholine reacts with dithiobisnitrobenzoic acid (Ellman's reagent) to form the yellow-colored 5-mercapto-2-nitrobenzoic acid, which is monitored at 405 nm. The rate of color formation is directly proportional to the propionylcholinesterase activity.

Reference Ranges and Interpretation   Acetylcholinesterase ranges are stated in relation to hemoglobin and are 26.7 to 49.2 U/g of hemoglobin. Pseudocholinesterase ranges are gender dependent:

Males

All ages: 3100 to 6500 U/L

Females

18 to 49 years: 1800 to 6600 U/L
≥ 50 years: 2550 to 6800 U/L

Children generally have lower levels of pseudocholinesterase activity than adults. At birth and for the weeks immediately following, the levels are approximately 50% of adult levels, and they climb until the child is about 6 years old, at which point they peak 10% to 15% above adult levels. The levels stabilize to adult levels by puberty.

Any acetylcholinesterase or pseudocholinesterase level below the bottom end of the range is considered evidence for exposure to toxic agents, but low acetylcholinesterase levels should be confirmed in a separate blood collection, since there are handling issues and short-term stability problems. Long-term monitoring of relief from exposure should be done using acetylcholine levels.

Another test for pseudocholinesterase uses inhibition by dibucaine to determine a "dibucaine number." This test is intended for detecting susceptibility to certain anesthetics and should not be used for neurotoxin exposure determination.

Carbon Monoxide

All common assays for carbon monoxide (CO) rely on the unique spectrophotometric qualities of the CO–hemoglobin complex. Blood is hemolyzed, then a spectrum is taken and absorbance is measured at several wavelengths. Laboratory reports usually include methemoglobin, oxyhemoglobin, and deoxyhemoglobin results. Carboxyhemoglobin diminishes at a rate of about 15% per hour when the patient is removed from the contaminated environment. Normal humans have a CO level of less than 1%, while smokers are around 7% and up to 15% for a heavy smoker. Toxic levels can start at 10% with tightness across the forehead, possible slight headache, and dilation of cutaneous blood vessels. Overt toxicity begins at 20%.

Cyanide

Cyanide is measured only in whole blood, is collected in EDTA or heparin, and can be sent to the laboratory at ambient, refrigerated, or frozen temperatures. In the laboratory, a strong acid is added to release the hydrogen cyanide gas, which is subsequently trapped in an adjacent chamber by bubbling through an alkaline mixture. Three chemicals, pyridine, barbituric acid, and chloramine-T, are added to produce a red color whose intensity is directly proportional to the amount of cyanide in the sample. Normal levels are less than 0.2 μg/mL, but concentrations of up to 2.0 μg/mL produce little or no side effects in most people. Neurotoxicity is evident at levels greater than 2.0 μg/mL, and lethality occurs at concentrations greater than 5 μg/mL.

Tetanus

Laboratory testing for exposure to tetanus is not the preferred means of diagnosis. Clinical observation is optimum. A positive wound culture for the agent, *Clostridium tetani*, is supportive but does not confirm the diagnosis. Subsequent to vaccination, a patient's immunological response may be assessed by determining the presence of tetanus toxoid antibody levels in the serum. An absence of antibody formation postvaccination may relate to immunodeficiency disorders—congenital, acquired, or iatrogenic—due to immunosuppressive drugs. Presence of an antibody titer immediately or shortly following suspected exposure to tetanus is evidence that the individual had an immune status against this agent, thus tending to rule out tetanus as the source. Similarly, development of a positive titer in a suspected individual over 1 to 3 months following exposure is evidence supporting tetanus as the toxic agent. Any result of at least 0.16 international units (IUs) per milliliter is indicative of an antibody response. Mild cases of tetanus have been observed, however, in patients with results in the range of 0.01 to 1.0 IU/mL.

Methodology

Immunoassays of the enzyme-linked immunoassay (ELISA) type are commonly used for this testing. A form of one or more antigens is attached to the bottom of a microtiter plate, the patient sample (serum) is added, and then a signaling agent, usually a second antibody directed toward human immunoglobulin G or immunoglobulin M and coupled with an enzyme, is added. The enzyme activity is then read out and interpreted in relation to a set of calibrators. Results are reported in units, or IUs per milliliter.

Diphtheria

Testing for antibodies against a diphtheria toxoid antigen provides information only about the immune status of the patient. Any positive results must be interpreted in relation to the time of exposure to determine whether antibodies were present before the exposure incident. If the patient is seronegative, monitoring the development of antibodies over 3 months can give information that may aid in the establishment of diphtheria as the neurotoxin.

Methodology

Immunoassays of the ELISA type are usually used for this testing. The diphtheria toxoid antigen is deposited on the base of wells of a microtiter plate, patient serum is added, and then a second antibody directed toward human immunoglobulin G is added. This second antibody has an enzyme coupled with it (commonly horseradish peroxidase or alkaline phosphatase), and the enzyme activity is measured in each well. Comparison to a set of calibrators gives a value that can be related to the amount of antibody to the toxoid in the patient. Results are reported in IUs per milliliter, with any result of at least 0.10 IU/mL indicative of antibodies present. Note that the antigen used in the assays is limited to the one used in the vaccines and it may not be identical to that found to be toxic. Therefore, exposure to diphtheria is not always accompanied by a positive analytical result.

Botulinum

Antibody tests for botulinum toxin are of limited availability, are similar in design and reporting to those described for tetanus and diphtheria, and suffer similar drawbacks. They are also of widely variable calibration, so results from one laboratory may differ substantially from those from another.

Thanks to the food industry and the use of botulinum in some medical products, standardized tests are available for the toxin itself. If a sample of the possible neurotoxic agent is available, you can contact the Center for Drug Evaluation Research at the U.S. Food and Drug Administration, which may be able to direct you to a laboratory doing such work. It is not routinely available. Other laboratory tests (e.g., edrophonium challenge and protein in spinal fluid) are used only to rule out other causes with similar symptoms.

Acrylamide

Metabolism of acrylamide begins immediately upon entry into the body, with production of an epoxide, glycidamide, that is purported to be genotoxic. Those two compounds can, in turn, combine with endogenous proteins to form molecular adducts,[4,5] or form mercapturic acid derivatives that are excreted in the urine.[6] Adduct formation with hemoglobin has been used as a measure of integrated exposure over time, since the erythrocyte lifetime of approximately 120 days allows capture of the acrylamide and glycidamide and retention of it tied to hemoglobin. In contrast, the mercapturic acid derivatives show up in urine within 24 hours and represent recent exposure. Smokers have been studied carefully, and urinary excretion levels of both mercapturic acid derivatives appear to be excellent biomarkers of smoking status.[7] The predominant method used for analysis is liquid chromatography–mass spectrometry tandem because that is the only procedure with the specificity and sensitivity to detect and quantitate any of these compounds. The assay is not routinely available in any commercial establishment, however, and may require collaboration with a specific researcher to get any results for clinical use. Twenty-four hour collections of urine are required, and because of analytical differences among laboratories, it is advised to collect a control urine from a known nonexposed person to be analyzed alongside the patient's sample. Mean urine levels in smokers are approximately six times normal, but there is a lot of overlap between the ranges. In general, hemoglobin adducts of acrylamide and glycidamide are increased in smokers and exposed people, but the overlap with the range in normal people is extensive, and interpretation within any individual could be problematic.

REFERENCES

1. Montagna W, Dobson LR. *Hair Growth*. Oxford: Pergamon Press; 1969:585.
2. Bertazzo A, Costa C, Biasiolo M, et al. Determination of copper and zinc levels in human hair. *Biol Trace Elem Res*. 1996;52(1):37-53.
3. Ewers U, Brockhaus A. Biologic monitoring of the pollutant burden of the human and its significance for the assessment of toxicological environmental factors.. *Off Gesundheitsw*. 1987;49:639–647.
4. Chevolleau S, Jacques C, Canlet C, et al. Analysis of adducts of acrylamide and glycidamide by liquid chromatography: electrospray ionization tandem mass spectrometry, as exposure biomarkers in French population. *J Chromatog*. 2007;1167:125–134.
5. Ogawa M, Oyama T, Isse T, et al. Hemoglobin adducts as a marker of exposure to chemical substances, especially PRTR Class I designated chemical substances. *J Occup Health*. 2006;48:314–328.
6. Bjellaas T, Stolen LH, Haugen M, et al. Urinary acrylamide metabolites as biomarkers for short-term dietary exposure to acrylamide. *Food and Chem Tox*. 2007;45:1020–1026.
7. Huang C, Li C, Wu C, et al. Analysis of urinary N-acetyl-S-(propionamide)-cysteine as a biomarker for the assessment of acrylamide exposure in smokers.. *Environ Res*. 2007;104:346–351.

ADDITIONAL READING

Methodologies used for neurotoxins, and the interpretive guidelines for many of them are covered extensively in several excellent textbooks and reference guides. Ones that are particularly thorough and current include the following:

Burtis CA, Ashwood ER, Bruns De, eds. *Tietz Fundamentals of Clinical Chemistry*. 6th ed. St. Louis: Saunders Elsevier; 2008.

Seiler HG, Sigel A, Sigel H, eds. *Handbook on Metals in Clinical and Analytical Chemistry*. New York: Marcel Dekker; 1994.

Baselt R. *Disposition of Toxic Drugs and Chemicals in Man*. 5th ed. Foster City, Calif: Chemical Toxicology Institute; 2000.

A broad-based reference book for interpretation of laboratory results is:

Mayo Medical Laboratories Interpretive Handbook. Rochester, Minn: Mayo Medical Laboratories; 2007–2008.

Cognitive Testing

Michael Hoffmann

INTRODUCTION

We all have the potential to be exposed to more than 50,000 substances distributed among commercial and industrial chemicals, cosmetics, food additives, pesticides, and of course medicinal drugs. Only a fraction of these (approximately 600) have standards set by U.S. Occupational Safety and Health Administration, and at the time of writing 201 had been regulated for neurotoxic effects.[1,2] In the broadest terms, neurotoxicology embraces numerous toxins, drugs, and chemical insults to the brain. The major categories include (1) heavy metals; (2) industrial toxins and solvents; (3) venom bites, stings, and plants poisons; (4) bacterial toxins; (5) addicting drugs such as opiates and synthetic analgesics; (6) sedative hypnotic drugs; (7) antidepressants and antipsychotic drugs; (8) psychoactive drugs and stimulants; and (9) antineoplastic and immunosuppressive drugs. The entire neuraxis is prone to chemical toxicity, with many areas of predilection documented. Some affect the central nervous system, some the peripheral nervous system, and some both. Without intending to incite paranoia, certain occupational activities are at particular risk. These include the occupations depicted in Table 1, with the common toxic agents responsible listed. Any of us may be given pharmacological agents such as antipsychotics, antidepressants, and even anti-nausea agents (promethazine) with the risk of potentially lethal syndromes such as neuroleptic malignant syndrome and malignant hyperthermia. Neuroleptic malignant syndrome carries with it a mortality rate of 15% to 30%, which underscores the need for keen vigilance.

The symptoms, signs, and syndromes whereby neurotoxicological agents may be identifiable in people range from asymptomatic to florid syndromes, coma, fulminating deterioration, and death. Because we may be asymptomatic, both the occupations at particular risk and screening questionnaires of possible exposure are of particular relevance. The U.S. Agency for Toxic Substances and Disease Registry has determined that heavy metals (lead, manganese, arsenic, cadmium, mercury, thallium, selenium, chromium, aluminum, cobalt, tin) are ranked first (lead), second (mercury), third (arsenic), and sixth (cadmium) according to their prevalence and severity of their toxicity.[3] The acute toxicity syndromes and agents usually pose less of a diagnostic problem and are not in need of neuropsychological or cognitive assessment. For example, nerve agents used in chemical warfare such as tabun, sarin, soman, and VX are similar in action to the insecticide malathion, being absorbed through the skin and merely more potent. These present with acetylcholine activity of hypersalivation, abdominal cramps, diarrhea, muscle paralysis, miosis, and respiratory arrest.

Table 1:   Occupations at Particular Risk for Neurotoxic Disease

Laboratory technicians	Ethylene oxide, solvents, mercury
Steel industry workers	Lead, manganese, copper, tin
Plastic industry workers	Styrene, formaldehydes
Electronic industry workers	Lead, Freon, arsine, tin, methylene chlorine
Automobile industry workers	Greasing agents, trichloroethylene
Transportation industry workers	Lead, solvents, carbon monoxide
Painters	Lead
Printing industry workers	Lead, solvents, methanol
Dry-cleaning personnel	Trichloroethylene, solvents
Hospital personnel	Ethylene oxide, anesthetics, alcohols
Agricultural workers	Pesticides, herbicides
Dentists, dental hygiene technicians	Mercury, anesthetic agents
Pharmaceutical and chemical industry workers	Array of substances

CLINICAL PRESENTATION OF NEUROTOXICITY

Neurotoxicity may present in two broad categories, cognitive–neuropsychiatric impairment and elementary neurological impairments. These may be considered in terms of the following components:

1. Cognitive and neuropsychiatric impairment
    Asymptomatic and identified by others (solvent)
    Encephalopathy
    Attentional disorders
    Memory impairment
    Concentration impairment
    Executive impairment
    Depression and anxiety
    Dementia
2. Elementary neurological presentations (motor weakness, sensory impairment, movement disorders, visual impairment)
    Toxic neuropathies
    Toxic myopathies
    Toxin-induced movement disorders (tremor, parkinsonism, myoclonus, dystonia chorea, ballismus, tics)

The focus of the chapter is therefore on the more chronic, covert, and subtle exposures to various neurotoxic substances where the acute and fulminant syndromes are less likely to manifest. In this context, a neurobehavioral approach follows a type of hierarchy of clinical, laboratory, and neuroradiological assessment. Firstly, screening questionnaires of possible exposure and of symptoms of exposure may be illuminating. Thereafter, a general examination follows that may reveal telltale signs such as the black line of lead sulfide in the gingival margins with lead poisoning or the characteristic transverse white lines 1 to 2 mm in width above the lunula of the fingernails with arsenic poisoning (Mees lines). A neurological examination may reveal characteristic movement disorders, such as the extremities, head, lips, and tongue tremor of mercury poisoning (Mad Hatter's disease). Many neuroradiological features have been reported with neurotoxic chemicals, such as the anatomical bithalamic changes with various solvents.[4] Paraclinical testing such as electroencephalography and evoked potentials may provide evidence that is missed by anatomical scanning. Magnetic resonance spectroscopy remains experimental at the time of writing but appears to have a promising future role in neurotoxic diagnosis.

Neurocognitive testing is an extension of the neurological examination. It should incorporate not only cognitive neurological testing but also neuropsychiatric testing because there is no distinction in the continuum of these disorders other than that imposed by the disciplines that have evolved, namely, neurology and psychiatry. In many instances, the cognitive impairment rendered by the toxic insult is at a neurochemical level, rather than disrupting fiber tracts or brain structure as is the case with other brain illness such as stroke, hemorrhage, brain tumor, trauma, and multiple sclerosis. This is not to say that both systems may be affected.

Concept of Channel- and State-dependent Systems

A basic tenet whereby substances may influence the brain demands an understanding of channel functions and state-dependent functions. Many brain illnesses are primarily due to neurochemical alterations (depression, anxiety, apathy, schizophrenia), and it is important to appreciate that neuroimaging even with sophisticated magnetic resonance modalities may not illuminate the deficit. We rely on accurate clinical assessment, and this includes cognitive assessment. Elementary neurological signs or so-called hard (versus soft) signs may also be absent even though an obvious cerebral deficiency exists. Axonal pathways that connect cortical areas in the cerebrum, whether cortical, subcortical, or subtentorial, are regarded as the point-to-point connectivity and substrate of channel functions.[5] The major pathways include the superior and inferior longitudinal fasciculus, arcuate fasciculus, uncinate fasciculus, corpus callosum, and insular-amygdaloid pathways. In addition to these channel pathways, all cortical regions receive so-called modulatory connections arising from brainstem neurons that innervate the cortex either directly or via the thalamus. These so-called state-dependent transmissions are responsible for attention, arousal, mood, and motivation and are subserved by six principal modulatory pathways. These allow rapid adjustments of information processing of the entire cerebral cortex (Table 2). Neurotoxicological insult may affect either system, and in the more subtle and covert instances a neurochemical alteration of the state-dependent system represents the neurological lesion, with deficits in attention, memory, frontal systems, and neuropsychiatric presentations particularly prominent.[5]

State-dependent Impairment: Neurochemistry of Neurotoxicity

Mercury, lead, and cadmium inhibit the glutamate uptake in human platelets, and several biochemical markers show parallel changes in the central nervous system and platelets.[6] Detection of biomarkers of exposure is advantageous in that it can be used to measure biomarkers soon after exposure, and hopefully

Table 2: Channel- and State-Dependent Networks of the Brain

CHANNEL-DEPENDENT SYSTEMS	
1. Perisylvian network for language	
2. Limbic network for memory and emotion	
3. Ventral occipitotemporal network for face and object recognition	
4. Dorsal parietofrontal network for spatial orientation	
5. Right hemisphere network for prosody, emotion, and attention	
6. Prefrontal network for executive function and comportment	
PRINCIPAL CHEMICAL PROJECTIONS TO THE CEREBRAL CORTEX FOR THE STATE-DEPENDENT SYSTEMS	
1. Cholinergic	Nucleus basalis of Meynert
2. Histaminergic	Hypothalamus
3. Dopaminergic	Ventral tegmental area
4. Serotonergic	Brainstem raphe nuclei
5. Noradrenergic	Locus ceruleus

before neurotoxic damage ensures, and allow appropriate prevention of further damage to the person. These may include combinations of biomarker and toxin, such as hemoglobin and carbon disulfide, prophyrins and metals, and mercapturates and styrene.[7,8] Peripheral biomarkers are a more effective means of measuring toxicity by sampling red blood cell, lymphocyte, and platelet receptors. Measurements of alterations in muscarinic, adrenergic, benzodiazepine, enzymes such as monamine oxidase B, acetylcholinesterase, serotonin uptake systems, and signal transduction systems (adenyl cyclase) is now possible.[9] The dopaminergic system is of particular interest in that it has been extensively studied and is prone to disruption by heavy metals and solvents, as well as an array of toxins that may affect dopamine β-hydroxylase activity, monamine oxidase activity, and dopamine transporter function. A specific example is "manganism," which is caused by manganese exposure; this, in turn, causes dopamine autoxidation, free radical formation, and neuron damage resulting in a syndrome similar to Parkinson's disease.[10]

SIGNATURE SYNDROMES PERTAINING TO PARTICULAR TOXINS, DRUGS, OR POISONS

Most patients with neurotoxicity present with impairments in three principal cognitive domains: concentration or attention impairment, executive function impairment, or memory impairment. This is due to the mechanism of injury or pathophysiology of the insult to the brain (Table 3). Tests for these are included in the Appendix as a semiquantitative assessment and in Table 4 for metric testing. However, some particular exceptions are of specific interest.

Solvent Exposure and Dementia of Alzheimer's Type Disease

Considerable evidence exists for a relationship between solvent exposure and a neurodegenerative disease such as Alzheimer's disease (AD) or an AD-like illness. Various definitions of solvent exposure have been used, with one example being measured as equal to 2000 workplace exposure hours.[16] With the aid of an industrial hygienist rating exposure scale, an increased risk of AD was correlated with years of solvent exposure for 89 AD patients and 89 controls in a case series and case–control study.[16] A community-based case–control study of solvent exposure (benzene, toluene, phenols, alcohols, ketones) and AD examined 139 people with AD and 243 controls, an odds ratio of 2.3 (95% confidence interval of 1.1 to 4.7); with men, the odds ratio was 6.0 (95% confidence interval of 2.1 to 17.2).[17] Butane inhalation is particularly toxic to the nervous system, presenting with an acute encephalopathy with prominent abulia. Magnetic resonance brain scanning is notable for severe bithalamic injury attributed to butane toxicity.[4]

Serotonin Syndrome

The serotonin syndrome is characterized by neuromuscular excitation (myoclonus, rigidity, hyperreflexia, hypertonicity), autonomic stimulation (flushing, tachycardia, hyperthermia, diaphoresis), and altered cognition

Table 4: Tests for Specific Cognitive Domains and Most Common Tests
APHASIAS, ALEXIAS, DYSGRAPHIAS, OR ACALCULIAS
1. Western Aphasia Battery II, revised
2. Boston Diagnostic Aphasia Examination, 3rd edition[11]
3. Boston Naming Test, version 2
FRONTAL NETWORK SYSTEMS
1. Wisconsin Card Sorting Test
2. Tower of London
3. Comprehensive Trail-making Test
4. Frontal Systems Behavioral Inventory
5. Rey Complex Figure Test[12]
6. Baron Emotional Intelligence Test
7. Stroop Neuropsychological Test[13]
MEMORY
1. Repeatable Battery for the Assessment of Neuropsychological Status
2. Rey Auditory Learning Verbal Test
3. Rey Complex Figure Test
4. Three Words–Three Shapes Test
5. Wide Range Assessment of Memory and Learning[14]
6. Wechsler Memory Scale III
COMPLEX VISUAL PROCESSING: SIMULTANAGNOSIA
1. Cookie Theft Picture Test, Boston Diagnostic Aphasia Examination, 2nd edition[11]
2. Visual Object and Space Perception Battery[15]

Table 3: The frontal network syndrome (frontal lobe syndrome) may be seen with the following lesions outside the frontal lobes:
1. Toxic encephalopathies (mercury, lead arsenic, bismuth, solvents)
2. Metabolic encephalopathies
3. Head of the caudate nucleus lesion, such as stroke
4. Dorsomedial thalamic nucleus lesions (tumor, stroke)
5. Multifocal white matter disease (subcortical vascular disease, multiple sclerosis)

Appendix: Bedside Cognitive Testing: A Semiquantitative Modified Method after Hoffmann[21]			
Neuropsychiatric (DSM-IV):			
Depression, anxiety, obsessive compulsive disorder, substance abuse			
A.	GENERAL ATTENTIONAL SYSTEMS		
	1.	Orientation of five items: Score 1 for each error; 0 is normal	
		Date and location: Name day, month, and year; day of week; and place (hospital or clinic)	/5
	2.	Attention and calculation: Score 1 for each error; 0 is normal	
		Calculation: Give five serial sevens; if unable, double to 128	/5
B.	LEFT HEMISPHERE NETWORK FOR LANGUAGE, GERSTMANN'S SYNDROME, AND ANGULAR GYRUS SYNDROME		
	3.	Speech and language	
		Naming: Name three objects (pen, watch, ID card) and name three colors; score 1 for each error; 0 is normal	/6
		Fluency: Grade as fluent (0), nonfluent (1), or mute (2)	/2
		Comprehension: Close your eyes and squeeze my hand; score 1 for each failure	/2
		Repetition: "Today is a sunny and windy day"; grade as no word (2), partial (1), or all words (0) repeated	/2
		Writing: Write a sentence to answer "What is your job?"; must contain subject and verb and make sense; score 1 for each failure	/3
		Reading: "Close your eyes"; grade as no words (2), partial (1), or all words (0) read	/2
	4.	Motor speech	
		Dysarthria: During interview, are words slurred?; grade as no (0), mild (1), or marked (2) slurring	/2
		Hypophonia: Grade as normal (0), voice softer than normal (1), or very low volume, barely audible (2)	/2
	5.	Praxis: Grade as impaired execution (1), unable to execute (2), or smooth execution (0)	
		Melokinetic: Thumb–finger opposition test; compare right + left (only if ≥4/5 power)	/2
		Buccolingual: Lick your lips and blow up your cheeks	/2
		Ideomotor apraxia: Clumsy action with pen or eating utensils	/2
		Ideational: Fold a piece of paper in half, write your name on it, and place it inside a file (or book)	/2
	6.	Right, left, and body part orientation: Score 1 for each error	
		Orientation: Place your left pointing finger on your right ear	/2
C.	HIPPOCAMPAL LIMBIC NETWORK FOR MEMORY AND EMOTION		
	7.	Memory: Score 1 for each error or omission; 0 is normal	
		Short-term memory: Register five words (orange, ocean, courage, rapid, building)	***

		Appendix: Bedside Cognitive Testing: A Semiquantitative Modified Method after Hoffmann[21]—cont'd	
		Test recall: Recall at 5 minutes	/5
		Remote memory: Recite the last three presidents or three important personal dates (graduations)	/3
	8.	Emotions: Grade as rarely (1), sometimes (2), frequently (3), or never (0)	
		Lability: Laughs or cries easily out of context	/3
D.		PREFRONTAL NETWORK OR SUBCORTICAL NETWORK FOR EXECUTIVE FUNCTION AND COMPORTMENT	
	9.	Serial motor programming: Score 1 for each error in the sequence	
		Luria motor sequence test (fist–palm–hand): Demonstrate sequence until the patient is able to replicate, and then do five cycles	/5
	10.	Word fluency: Grade as >15 (0), 13–15 (1), 10–12 (2), 7–9 (3), 4–6 (4), or 0–3 (5)	
		Say as many words starting with "s" as possible in 1 minute (no names or places)	/5
	11.	Environmental autonomy	
		Imitation behavior: Maintaining eye contact, pat the side of face, and then clap hands without suggesting the patient follow suit	
		Grade as copies all actions spontaneously (2), some actions (1), or no actions (0)	/2
		Utilization behavior: Place three objects in front of the patient (key, cell phone, pen)	
		Grade as unsolicited manipulation of one or two objects (1) or of all objects (2)	/2
	12.	Interference and inhibitory control: Score 1 for each incorrect response	
		Go–No–Go Paradigm: If the examiner taps once, raise your finger, but if the examiner taps twice, do not raise your finger; do three cycles: 1–1–2, 1–2–1, 2–2–1	/3
	13.	Abulia: Poverty of action and speech; grade as marked (2), somewhat (1), or none (0)	/2
	14.	Disinhibition: Comments or actions during interview; grade as occasional (1), frequent (2), or none (0)	/2
	15.	Impersistence: Discontinues Luria sequences, despite repeated coaxing three times; score 1 for any error	/1
	16.	Perseveration: During a Luria sequence test, duplicates same hand position; score 1 for any error	/1
E.		DORSAL RIGHT PARIETOFRONTAL NETWORK FOR VISUOSPATIAL FUNCTION, ATTENTION, EMOTION, AND PROSODY	
	17.	Visuospatial: Grade as impaired (1), marked (2), or none (0)	
		2D: Copy a 2D image of the examiner's drawn flower	/2
		3D: Copy a 3D representation of the examiner's cube	/2
	18.	Neglect syndromes: Score 1 for omission of one side	
		Tactile: Simultaneous stimulation of both arms	/1
		Auditory: Simultaneous stimulation of both ears	/1

Continued

Appendix: Bedside Cognitive Testing: A Semiquantitative Modified Method after Hoffmann[21]—cont'd

		Visual: Simultaneous stimulation of both fields	/1
		Motor neglect: Bisect a 10 cm line; score 1 for more than 1/4 (2.5 cm) distance from midline	/1
	19.	Anosognosia: Recognizes weakness (0), underestimation of (1), or complete denial of (2) deficit or illness	/2
	20.	Prosody: Score 1 if found; score 0 if not found	
		Speech: As per family, speech has become flat or monotone	/1
		Comprehension: Cannot comprehend different intonations (happy versus sad)	/1
		Repetition: Cannot repeat altered intonation (happy versus sad)	/1
F.		VENTRAL OCCIPITOTEMPORAL NETWORK FOR OBJECT AND FACE RECOGNITION	
	21.	Complex visual processing	
		Object agnosia: Cannot name three objects by visual inspection, but can by touch or sound; score 1 for each error	/3
		Achromatopsia: Cannot distinguish two hues or colors; score 1 for each error	/2
		Simultanagnosia: Using the Cookie Theft Picture Test, identify all three people or analog time telling (min/hr/sec); score 1 for each error	/3
		Optic ataxia: Touch the examiner's finger under visual guidance; score 1 for a miss	/1
		Optic apraxia: Look left, right, up or down to command; score 1 for any error	/1
		Prosopagnosia: Does not recognize family or friends by visual appearance; score 1 for any error	/1
		Line orientation: Draw 45-degree and 30-degree lines and match the two lines to a figure; score 1 for each error	/2
		Akinetopsia: Subjective report of impaired motion perception; score 1 if present	/1
		Astereopsis: Subjective report of depth perception impairment; score 1 if present	/1
		Hallucinations: Simple (colors, shapes), complex (scenes, people, animals), or experiential (out-of-body experience, autoscopy); score 1 if present	/1
		Illusions of shape or size: For example, macropsia or micropsia; score 1 if present	/1
		Denial of cortical blindness (Anton's syndrome): Score 1 if present	/1
G.		SYNDROMES WITH ILL-DEFINED NEURAL NETWORKS	
	22.	Disconnection syndromes: Score 1 if present, 0 if absent	
		Alien hand syndrome: The one hand interferes with the other during routine tasks	/1
		Alexia without agraphia: Can write but cannot read	/1
		Pure word deafness: Hears environmental sounds but not spoken speech.	/1

Appendix: Bedside Cognitive Testing: A Semiquantitative Modified Method after Hoffmann[21]—cont'd			
	23.	Delusional misidentification syndromes (incorrect identification of people or place): Score 1 if present	
		Reduplicative paramnesia: Person thinks that he or she is lying or geographically elsewhere	/1
		Capgras's or Fregoli's syndrome: Familiar people appear strange, or vice versa	/1
H.	MISCELLANEOUS SYNDROMES		
	24.	Amusia: May be receptive (poor appreciation of music) or expressive but no longer able to play or sing; score 1 if either is present	/1
	25.	Allesthesia: During neurological examination, transfers perceived tactile stimuli from left to the right; score 1 if present	/1
	26.	Autoscopy: During interview, reports out-of-body experience; score 1 if present	/1
	27.	Synesthesia: Activation of one sensory system induces perceived sensation in another; score 1 if present	/1
COGNITIVE SCORE TOTAL			—

DSM IV, *Diagnostic and Statistical Manual of Mental Disorders.* 4th ed.

(confusion, anxiety, obtundation, coma) and may vary from mild to severe presentations. The mild presentation forms in particular are challenging because they may not concern the patient yet are an important part of the differential in patients with mild cognitive changes, as well as coma. These have been described due to serotonin-specific reuptake inhibitors, monamine oxidase inhibitors, and atypical antipsychotic agents, often in combination. The pathophysiology is a hyperserotonergic state of the central, as well as the peripheral, nervous system.[18,19]

Posterior Reversible Encephalopathy Syndrome Due to Toxins, Drugs, and Diseases

Patients with posterior reversible encephalopathy syndrome present with cortical blindness, headaches, seizures, and other higher-order visual impairments, such as simultanagnosia and Balint's syndrome. As the name implies, it is a reversible syndrome, usually with a return to normality over days to weeks. Etiological factors include the following:

1. Illnesses
   Eclampsia
   Hypertensive crisis and urgency
2. Drugs
   Cyclosporin
   Tacrolimus
   Tacrolimus (FK-506)
   Methotrexate
   Interferon
   Cisplatin
   Cytarabine
   L-Asparaginase
   Intravenous immunoglobulin
   Erythropoietin
   Granulocyte colony-stimulating factor
3. Idiopathic
   Call Fleming syndrome

Clearly, the approach to cognitive deficit ascertainment with such a syndrome needs specific attention to the higher-order visual systems of the brain. This is readily appreciated after the screening cognitive evaluation. Metric tests such as the Visual Object and Space Perception Battery and Cookie Theft Picture Test of the Boston Diagnostic Aphasia Examination are appropriate to measure and monitor such patients neurologically.

NEUROBEHAVIORAL OR COGNITIVE ASSESSMENT FOR THE PATIENT WITH NEUROTOXICOLOGICAL SYNDROME

The major portions of the brain are concerned with secondary and tertiary association areas that subserve the protean cognitive functions that form the substrate of all behavior. Any lesion of the brain, to a greater or lesser extent, incurs cognitive impairment. As already noted, most patients present with problems in memory, executive functioning, and attention and concentration. This is similar to those with traumatic brain injury, diffuse white matter injury, and subcortical vascular disease (see Table 3). Hence, frontal executive functioning testing (Delis Kaplan Executive Function Systems Test), memory testing (Repeatable Battery for the Assessment of Neuropsychological Status), and sustained attention (Visual Search and Attention Test) are appropriate for most patients without unduly excessive testing time and commitment. However, a cognitive screening test should always be performed to screen for other networks that may be involved, such as the parieto-occipital in posterior reversible encephalopathy syndrome. This approach incorporates and synthesizes the different modes of information gleaned in this order from the following:

1. General medical history and examination
2. Neurological history and examination
3. Behavioral (cognitive) and neurological assessment
4. Neuropsychiatric assessment
5. Neuropsychological (metric) assessment
6. Multimodality magnetic resonance imaging lesion anatomy, dynamics, and in some, biochemistry
7. Functional neuroimaging (single-photon emission computed tomography, positron emission tomography, magnetic resonance perfusion scanning)

As with any cognitive evaluation in people, factors affecting interpretation and results include gender; age; educational level, usually measured in number of years (school, college, postgraduate, and other); race and ethnicity; concomitant neuropsychiatric conditions; and substance abuse.

Selection of Tests

Test selection is guided by the neurological and bedside neurobehavioral examination that appropriately selects the battery of psychometric tests focusing on the syndromes delineated. This avoids testing patients blindly, which is time consuming, expensive, and wasteful and excludes patients for whom testing is inappropriate (encephalopathy). This method also delineates syndromes requiring specific examination (dysphasic patients). The following cognitive domains are routinely screened for by bedside cognitive tests, with the first five done in specific order:

1. Level of consciousness
2. Attention
3. Aphasias and dysarthrias
4. Frontal network syndromes
5. Amnesias
6. Alexias

7. Anosognosias and neglect syndromes
8. Visuospatial dysfunction
9. Right–left orientation and body part naming
10. Appendicular and axial apraxias
11. Acalculias
12. Agraphias
13. Agnosias
14. Complex visual syndromes (simultanagnosia, prosopagnosia)
15. Achromatopsias
16. Visual illusions, hallucinations, and inquiry into content-specific delusions

The specific advantages of metric cognitive evaluation over bedside cognitive assessment include the following: administration and scoring are standardized, reliability and validity have been determined, normative values are available, and quantitative sequential testing over time is possible. Neither cause nor localization are inferred. This is also the view of the guidelines issued by the American Academy of Neurology, with the main indications for cognitive testing being for (1) questionable or subtle cognitive tests by bedside evaluation, (2) quantification of the deficit to enable tracking over time, and (3) determining the cognitive profile in terms of type and severity to guide rehabilitative effort.[20]

Mixture of Testing

Both a comprehensive cognitive, semiquantitative bedside battery (see the Appendix) and selected neuropsychological metric tests are recommended for optimum syndrome elicitation and heeding the constraints of patient cooperation, time, and cost. Metric tests are presented in a format corresponding to the specific cognitive domains, as well as the major network systems of the brain (Table 5). The reason for this presentation is that an aphasic presentation makes it obvious that the language domain requires evaluation, whereas at other times, a lesion seen on the magnetic resonance imaging scan requires the clinical or cognitive correlated to be ascertained according the major brain networks. Findings are reported in the context of clinical, investigative, and neuroradiological data and treatment recommendations (Table 6).

Examples of the More Commonly Employed and Newer Tests

Frontal Systems Behavioral Inventory[23]

With respect to frontal network syndromes, the quantifiable deficits on standardized tests often are unimpressive and may be normal. They may be too complex

Table 5: Cognitive Psychometric Assessment According to the Principal Networks of the Brain[5]

Neuropsychological tests that survey at least part of the five principal network systems:
FRONTAL SUBCORTICAL NETWORK
Wisconsin Card Sorting Test
Frontal Systems Behavioral Inventory
LEFT HEMISPHERE LANGUAGE NETWORK
Western Aphasia Battery coefficient
Boston Naming Test, version 3
RIGHT HEMISPHERE ATTENTIONAL AND VISUOSPATIAL NETWORK
Rey Complex Figure Test for the right hemisphere network
OCCIPITOTEMPORAL NETWORK
Visual Object and Space Perception Battery progressive silhouette subtest
HIPPOCAMPAL LIMBIC MEMORY NETWORK
Repeatable Battery for the Assessment of Neuropsychological Status memory subscales

Table 6: Reporting Findings in the Context of Clinical, Investigative, and Neuroradiological Data and Treatment Recommendations

DIAGNOSTIC CATEGORIES
1. History and neurological syndrome presentation
2. Elementary neurological examination
3. Cognitive screening neurological syndromes
4. Neuropsychiatric syndromes
5. Neuroradiological findings
6. Cognitive metric (neuropsychological) test findings
RECOMMENDATIONS
1. Recommendations: vocational
2. Recommendations: treatment (cognitive, pharmacotherapy)
3. Curtailing the primary disease process
4. Stimulant therapy (Modafinil, Amantadine, Bromocriptine, Adderall, Ritalin)
5. Cognitive therapy (Brain Age, versions 1 and 2)[22]
6. Psychiatric therapy
7. Antiseizure therapy

to test in the office, and performance in the office may not reflect daily behavior. Because of the paucity of objective signs, there is a risk of not diagnosing brain damage. Patients are most impaired in situations in which there is minimal external control of behavior. Hence, a neurobehavioral inventory is probably the most accurate and time-efficient way of assessing this.[5]

The Frontal Systems Behavioral Inventory consists of two, 46-item, hand-scored questions graded on a five-point Likert scale, which measures the three principal frontal syndromes of apathy, disinhibition, and impaired executive function, in addition to a total score. This is determined both before and after the illness or exposure and is scored by the patient, as well as a family member. Normative data are provided in T scores, where normal ranges from 50 to 60, with 60 to 65 as borderline. A graphical output system is provided, which facilitates monitoring and portrayal of the results to the family and colleagues.

Wisconsin Card Sorting Test (Computerized Version 4.0)[24]

The Wisconsin Card Sorting Test of frontal function or executive (metacognitive) function is scored according to nine categories. Before testing, color blindness needs to be excluded (e.g., by the Ishihara Plate Test) so that it does not influence the test result. The computer-administered 128-card (or 64-card) test is employed and the scoring includes the following:

Percentage errors (%)
Perseverative responses (%)
Perseverative errors (%)
Nonperseverative errors (%)
Conceptual level responses (%)
Categories completed
Trials to complete first category
Failure to maintain set
Learning to learn

Delis Kaplan Executive Function Systems Test[25]

Delis Kaplan is a new frontal test that derives most of its subtests from those known previously but standardizes them with normative data. The nine subtests include a trail-making test, verbal fluency tests, a design fluency test, color–word interference tests, a sorting test, a 20-questions test, a tower test, and proverb interpretation tests. This test is particularly advocated for formal executive or frontal network system assessment because it combines into one test most frontal tests we use separately, for example, the Tower of London or Hanoi tests, Stroop test, FAS test and trail-making test versions.

Emotional Intelligence Index[26]

Emotional intelligence is regarded as more important than cognitive intelligence or intelligence quotient and is important for performance in many aspects of everyday life. It also represents the repertoire an individual has of specific abilities, competencies, and skills to cope with life effectively. The test comprises of five principal areas and 15 subcategories (Table 7):

1. Intrapersonal emotional quotient
   Self-regard
   Self-awareness
   Assertiveness
   Independence
   Self-actualization
2. Interpersonal emotional quotient
   Empathy
   Social responsibility
   Interpersonal relationship
3. Stress management
   Stress tolerance
   Impulse control
4. Adaptability
   Reality testing
   Flexibility
   Problem solving
5. General mood
   Optimism
   Happiness

Comprehensive Trail-making Test[27]

Comprehensive trail-making tests attention, concentration, resistance to distraction, and cognitive flexibility or set shifting. It also tests visual search and sequencing demands of tasks, which is a timed test (in seconds) according to five levels of difficulty. The test is standardized for individuals age 11 to 74 and scored according to normalized T scores, with a mean of 50 and a standard deviation of 10. The raw score is in seconds to complete

Table 7: Interpretative Guidelines for Emotional Quotient Inventory Scores	
Interpretive Guideline	**Standard Score Range**
Markedly high: Atypically well-developed emotional capacity	>130
Very high: Extremely well-developed emotional capacity	120–129
High: Well-developed emotional capacity	110–119
Average: Adequate emotional capacity	90–109
Low: Underdeveloped emotional capacity	80–89
Very low: Extremely underdeveloped emotional capacity	70–79
Markedly low: Atypically impaired emotional capacity	<70

the task, and the typical testing time 10 minutes with interpretation.

Tower of London[28]

The Tower of London tests executive planning proficiency, incorporating delineation, organization, and integration of behaviors needed to achieve a goal. It has been shown to be sensitive to frontal lobe dysfunction due to both unilateral and bilateral disease.

Raw scores (total move scores) are converted into standard scores. The classification of abnormality includes two types of sequencing errors.

Visual Search and Attention Test[29]

Sustained attention is critical to information processing. The Visual Search and Attention Test is primarily an attention test and incorporates visual cancellation tasks to measure sustained attention, including a searching task for letters, symbols, and colors.

Wechsler Memory Scale[30]

The renowned Wechsler memory test focuses on the three clinically pertinent memory systems of immediate delayed and working memory. Each of these is tested in the visual and auditory (also called nonverbal) domains and in the two principal task formats of recall and recognition. This is the most comprehensive memory test, but it is also time consuming—at least 1 hour is required for administration and another half hour is needed for scoring.

Repeatable Battery for Assessment of Neuropsychological Status[31]

The Repeatable Battery for Assessment of Neuropsychological Status is a particularly easy-to-administer and popular memory test, although it measures other cognitive domains as well. After about 15 to 20 minutes of testing, a standardized score for immediate and delayed memory and attention is obtained. In addition, language and visuospatial and constructional abilities are measured in a standardized manner.

Three Words–Three Shapes Test[32]

A test of verbal and nonverbal memory, the Three Words–Three Shapes Test also measures incidental recall to distinguish from rote learning that most standard batteries test. The drilling procedure also enables testing of attentional deficits. The number of trials required to reach a criterion measures registration and acquisition, both sensitive to attention and motivational difficulties. The delayed recall at 5, 15, and 30 minutes measures retention of information over time. When free recall is impaired but multiple-choice recognition is normal, the predominant memory problem is one of retrieval.

Western Aphasia Battery[33]

A relatively quick and easy metric language evaluation, the Western Aphasia Battery gives important information. Eight aphasia subtypes (Broca's, Wernicke's, global, transcortical motor, transcortical sensory, transcortical mixed, anomic, conduction) may be diagnosed, and an aphasia quotient and a cortical quotient are obtained. The latter are particularly useful for monitoring improvement or deterioration over time.

Boston Naming Test[34]

The brief Boston Naming language test that can be accomplished in under 5 minutes. It basically tests the naming of 60 objects (line drawings) with progressive difficulty, although cultural influences are considerable with this test. The new second version also has a short form consisting of only 15 line drawings.

REFERENCES

1. Hartman DE. *Neuropsychological Toxicology*. New York: Pergamon Press; 1988:1–25.
2. Grandjean P, Landrigan PJ. Developmental neurotoxicity of industrial chemicals. *Lancet*. 2006;368:2167–2178.
3. Hu H. Poisoning, drug overdose and envenomation. In: *Harrison's Principles of Internal Medicine*. New York: McGraw-Hill; 2006: 2577–2580.
4. Kile SJ, Camilleri CC, Latchaw RE, Tharp BR. Bithalamic lesions of butane encephalopathy. *Pediatr Neurol*. 2006;35: 439–441.
5. Mesulam MM. *Principles of Behavioral Neurology*. London: Oxford University Press; 2002:1–120.
6. Borges VC, Santos FW, Rocha JB, Noqueira CW. Heavy metals modulate glutaminergic system in human platelets *Neurochem Res*. 2007;32:953–958.
7. Costa LG, Manzo L. Biochemical markers of neurotoxicity: research strategies and epidemiological applications. *Toxicol Lett*. 1995;77:137–144.
8. Manzo L, Castoldi AF, Coccini T. Assessing effects of neurotoxic pollutants by biochemical markers. *Environ Res Sect A*. 2001; 85:31–36.
9. Manzo L, Artigas F, Martinez M. Biochemical markers of neurotoxicity: basic issues and a review of mechanistic studies. *Hum Exp Toxicol*. 1996;15:20–35.
10. Smargiassi A, Mutti A. Peripheral biomarkers and exposure to manganese. *Neurotoxicology*. 1999;20:401–406.
11. Goodglass H, Kaplan E, Barresi B. *Boston Diagnostic Aphasia Examination*. 3rd ed. Philadelphia: Lippincott Williams & Wilkins; 2001.
12. Meyers JE, Meyers KR. *Rey Complex Figure*. Lutz, Fla: Psychological Assessment Resources; 2002.
13. Trennery MR, Crosson B, De Boe J. *Stroop Neuropsychological Test*. Lutz, Fla: Psychological Assessment Resources; 2007.
14. Sheslow D, Adams W. *Wide Range Assessment of Memory and Learning*. 2nd ed. Lutz, Fla: Psychological Assessment Resources; 2007.
15. Warrington EK, James M. *The Visual Object and Space Perception Battery*. London: Thames Valley Test Co., Harcourt Assessment, Psychological Corp.; 1991.
16. Freed DM, Kandel E. Long term occupational exposure and diagnosis of dementia. *Neurotoxicology*. 1988;9:391–400.
17. Kukall WA, Larson EB, Bowen JD. Solvent exposure as a risk factor for Alzheimer's disease: a case–control study. *Am J Epidemiol*. 1995;14:1059–1079.
18. Isbister GK, Buckley NA, Whyte IM. Serotonin toxicity: a practical approach to diagnosis and treatment. *Med J Aust*. 2007;187: 361–365.
19. Izchak K, Gordon ML, Manu P. Serotonin syndrome in elderly patients treated for psychotic depression with atypical antipsychotics and antidepressants: two case reports. *CNS Spectr*. 2007;12:596–598.
20. American Academy of Neurology, Therapeutics and Technology Assessment Subcommittee. Assessment: Neuropsychological Testing of Adults. Considerations for Neurologists: Report. Minneapolis, Minnesota: Therapeutics and Technology Assessment Subcommittee of the American Academy of Neurology; 1996.
21. Hoffmann M. Higher cortical function deficits after stroke: an analysis of 1000 patients from a dedicated cognitive stroke registry. *Neurorehabil Neural Repair*. 2001;15:113–127.
22. Brain Age. *Nintendo DS*. Redwood, Wash: Brain Age; 2007.
23. Grace J, Malloy PF. *Frontal Systems Behavior Scale*. Lutz, Fla: Psychological Assessment Resources; 2002.
24. Heaton R. *Wisconsin Card Sorting Test*. Computerized ver 4.0. Lutz, Fla: Psychological Assessment Resources; 2003.
25. Kaplan E. *Delis Kaplan Executive Function System*. San Antonio, Texas: Psychological Corp., Harcourt Assessment Co.; 2001.
26. Bar-On R. *EQI: BarOn Emotional Quotient Inventory*. Toronto: MHS; 1997.
27. Reynolds CR. *Visual Search and Attention Test*. Austin, Texas: Pro-ed; 2002.

233

28. Culbertson WC, Zillmer EA. *Tower of London*. New York: MHS (Drexel University); 2001.

29. Ternerry MR, Corsson B, DeBoe J, Leber WR. Lutz, Fla: Psychological Assessment Resources; 1990.

30. Wechsler D. *Wechsler Memory Scale (WAIS III)*. New York: Psychological Corp., Harcourt Brace; 1997.

31. Randolph C. *Repeatable Battery for the Assessment of Neuropsychological Status*. San Antonio: Psychological Corp., Harcourt Brace; 1998.

32. Weintraub S, Mesulam M-M. Mental state assessment of young and elderly adults in behavioral neurology. In: M-M Mesulam, ed. *Principles of Behavioral Neurology*. Philadelphia: FA Davis; 1985.

33. Kertesz A. *The Western Aphasia Battery Revised*. San Antonio, Texas: Psychological Corp., Harcourt Assessment Company; 2007.

34. Kaplan, E, Goodglass H, Barresi B. *Boston Naming Test,* 2nd ed. Philadelphia: Lippincott Williams & Wilkins: 2001.

CHAPTER 19

Neuroimaging in Neurotoxicology

Philippe Hantson and Thierry Philippe Jacques Duprez

INTRODUCTION

Until neuroimaging modalities emerged into routine clinical practice, knowledge about deleterious effect of toxins on brain came from neuropathological and biochemical studies.

With the availability of the computerized tomography (CT) scanner in clinical practice in the early 1970s, in vivo imaging completed the diagnostic armamentarium of neurotoxic conditions. Although the sensitivity to pathological brain changes using x-ray CT remained low, relevant workup of brain damage was enabled. Major changes observed on CT images were focal and global brain swelling and edema, resulting in decreased attenuation of x-rays (hypodensity), and hemorrhagic transformation, resulting in locally increased attenuation (hyperdensity). CT rapidly gained a key place in the workup of intoxicated patients because it triggered major therapeutic intervention such as surgical evacuation of blood collections, intracranial placement of catheters measuring pressure, or even decompressive craniectomy. It also allowed accurate monitoring of brain edema, thereby supporting dehydration strategies. Aside from its great clinical relevance, CT depicted in vivo the concept of selective vulnerability from neuropathological studies by demonstrating preferential involvement, e.g., the putamina in methanol poisoning.

Magnetic resonance imaging (MRI) entered clinical practice one decade later, in the early 1980s. The advantage of MRI over CT was obvious because of higher tissue contrast, allowing improved delineation of anatomical structures and more sensitive and conspicuous delineation of lesions due to toxic exposure. Only economic constraints, which are being solved in developed countries, have temporarily limited the use of MRI. Early after implementation in clinical practice, MRI has appeared to be the best-suited imaging modality in toxic conditions. Higher sensitivity to subtle changes in water content and lipid homeostasis allowed recognition of small diseased brain areas, which were far beyond the sensitivity of CT scan. However, despite being more dramatic, morphological MRI showed the same things as CT images: the preferential involvement of defined anatomical structures in some intoxications and focal or generalized cerebral edema as the main tissue in injured brain areas (Figure 19-1). Thus, there is no longer a reason to prefer CT to MRI in toxic conditions: the intravenous perfusion of the iodinated contrast agent revealing foci of breakdown of the so-called brain–blood barrier is of limited interest in toxic conditions; if needed, similar information can be obtained at MRI by a perfusing paramagnetic contrast agent, which enhances areas of disruption of the brain–blood barrier on T_1-weighted images. The concept that CT had superiority over MRI regarding

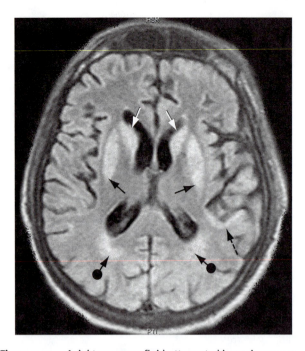

Figure 19-1. Axial transverse fluid-attenuated inversion recovery (FLAIR) magnetic resonance (MR) image in a case of severe hypoxic injury due to cardiac arrest featuring higher sensitivity of gray matter than white matter to oxygen deprivation. Putamina *(black arrows)* and caudate nuclei *(white arrows)* displayed bilaterally abnormal hypersignal intensity with homogeneous and symmetrical involvement. The cortical ribbon also exhibited areas of abnormally increased signal intensity, but only at a few places *(dotted arrows)*. Ultimately the deep periventricular parietal white matter was also involved in this very severe case *(ball-arrowheads)*. The cortical gray matter is involved in more severe cases. Involvement of the white matter is seen only in severe cases like this one. This variable susceptibility is thought to reflect variable demands in oxygen. Selective vulnerability of the deep gray matter is also observed in toxic conditions. (Adapted from Hantson P, Duprez T. The value of morphological neuroimaging after acute exposure to toxic substances. *Toxicol Rev.* 2006;25:87–98; and Hantson P, Duprez T, Mahieu P. Neurotoxicity to the basal ganglia shown by magnetic resonance imaging [MRI] following poisoning by methanol and other substances. *J Toxicol Clin Toxicol.* 1997;35:151–161.)

the detection of early extravased blood has become obsolete with the introduction of gradient-recalled techniques using the echoplanar imaging modality.

Crucial advantages of MRI are the capability of refining the anatomical substrate of toxic lesions by using a large palette of sequences for the morphological workup and the open investigational field of molecular, functional, and perfusion imaging.

Regarding morphological imaging, the comparative examination of T_1- and T_2-weighted images allows semiquantitative evaluation of the severity of edema. T_2-weighted images are most sensitive in delineating hyperintense edematous areas, but T_1-weighted images,

which are less sensitive, give additional information: the more severe the edema, the more visible the decrease in signal intensity of the same diseased areas. When considering the time course of hemoglobin degradation, the benefit of combining both weightings is also obvious: early deoxyhemoglobin and late hemosiderin appear hypointense on T_2-weighted images, and intermediate methemoglobin appears hyperintense on T_1-weighted images. In all cases of blood extravasation, the use of the gradient echo technique is beneficial because enhanced susceptibility effects generated by very small quantities of hemoglobin degradation product allow detection of micropetechiae. When available, the echoplanar imaging technique is best suited to this purpose.

The diffusion-weighted MRI has allowed major insights into the pathophysiology of cerebral edema. By measuring the diffusivity of free water within tissue voxels, the technique enables discrimination between the so-called vasogenic edema due to leakage of fluid from intravascular space to interstitial compartment with subsequent increase in water diffusivity resulting in increased calculated values for the apparent diffusion coefficient (ADC), and the so-called cytotoxic edema due to water inflow within cells because of failure of ATPase-dependant ionic pumps with subsequent cell swelling and reduction of interstitial space resulting in decreased ADC values reflecting lowered water diffusivity. At last, magnetic resonance spectroscopy gives molecular tissue information regarding, i.e., the neuronal density (N-acetyl aspartate), the membrane turnover (choline, or Cho), the lactate or amino acids concentration. Other parameters can be recorded and monitored, and we hope that more specific pathways directly involving toxic agents and their intermediate metabolites will be investigated.

In the following sections, we illustrate the value of neuroimaging techniques applied to specific intoxications.

ALCOHOLS AND SOLVENTS

Methanol

Methanol is a component of many solvents and antifreeze liquids. The main origin of accidental methanol poisoning is the illicit production of ethanol-like liquors. Methanol is poorly toxic by itself, but its biotransformation in the liver results in dramatically severe metabolic acidosis, leading to potentially life-threatening complications in intoxicated patients. The central nervous system (CNS) is a main target of methanol poisoning, mainly definite areas of the encephalon and the optic nerve (second cranial nerve). The severity of the CNS neurological involvement is directly related to the degree of metabolic acidosis due the accumulation of formic acid, which is the main toxic metabolite of methanol.[1] A delay, usually ranging from 12 to 24 hours, occurs before the appearance of clinical signs, radiological signs, or both of CNS involvement. This delay corresponds to the needed time for the biotransformation of methanol into formic acid, which inhibits the cytochrome oxidase of the mitochondrial respiratory cycle, thereby resulting in metabolic acidosis. Initial pathological studies in methanol-poisoned patients have indicated that the main feature in the condition was putaminal necrosis, usually complicated by hemorrhage (Figure 19-2). Preferential accumulation of formic acid in this specific area was demonstrated. The reasons the putamina exhibit exquisite sensitivity to methanol toxicity are unknown. However, putaminal damage is not fully specific to methanol poisoning and may be observed in other kinds of insults, like hypoxia or ischemia. Metabolic acidosis probably plays a prominent role in tissue toxicity in cases of methanol poisoning.[2] Methanol intoxication has been first investigated using CT imaging, which confirmed in vivo the preferential involvement of the putamina.[3] Abnormal hypodensity within the putamina appeared after a few days' delay in most cases, with poorly delineated margins corresponding to edema. Hemorrhagic transformation featured by secondarily appearing hyperdensity within initially hypodense damaged areas may occur. An incidence of 13.5% of hemorrhagic transformation has been reported in a series of 21 patients.[4] The potential role of heparin therapy in hemorrhagic transformation is debated since most patients have received

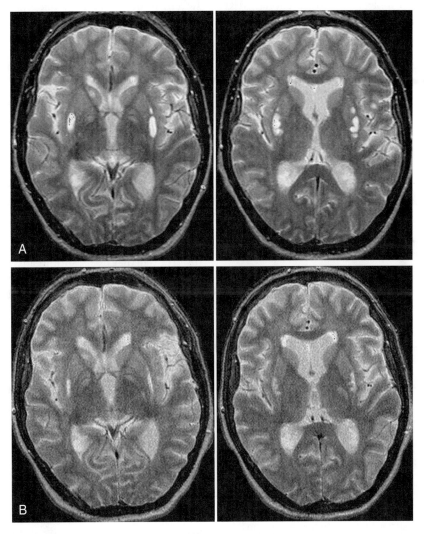

Figure 19-2. Magnetic resonance images in a 57-year-old woman admitted 24 hours after the ingestion of 250 mL of a methanol solution (initial blood methanol 170 mg/dL, arterial pH 7.18). *(A)* Axial transverse T$_2$-weighted magnetic resonance image 9 days after ingestion of antifreeze product, showing an abnormal hyperintense signal electively within both putamina. In this case of mild intoxication, the selective involvement of putamina excluding pallidi was obvious. *(B)* Similar view 20 days later showing partial subsidence of the lesions, which remained confined to the external margins of the putamina. (Adapted from Hantson P, Duprez T, Mahieu P. Neurotoxicity to the basal ganglia shown by magnetic resonance imaging [MRI] following poisoning by methanol and other substances. *J Toxicol Clin Toxicol.* 1997;35:151–161.)

systemic heparin therapy for hemodialysis. Later, imaging studies demonstrate delayed pseudocystic necrosis of the putamina. Patients with putaminal necrosis at imaging usually suffer visual sequelae, which are related not to putaminal injury but to the severity of the metabolic acidosis resulting in tissue damage to the anterior optical pathways.[5] Parkinsonism is paradoxically rare, even in the patients with extensive putaminal damage on CT–MRI scan.[6] In a patient who presented extrapyramidal symptoms within 8 days after the intoxication, investigation by 6-[18F]fluoro-L-dopa positron emission tomography (PET) performed after 3.5 months revealed symmetrical bilaterally impaired presynaptic dopaminergic activity in the striatum (Figure 19-3; see color plate).[7] Methanol-related brain injuries highly benefit from different "conventional" but also molecular and functional MRI modalities, which have become available for routine clinical use.[8] This particularly applies to the depiction of early cytotoxic versus vasogenic edematous or hemorrhagic changes. The "conventional" T_2-weighted sequences are sensitive to water content and allow a precise delineation of the extent of the brain vasogenic edema.[9] On the other hand, gradient echo T_2-weighted sequences are best suited for the detection of very small hemorrhagic foci because of the high sensitivity of the technique

to the susceptibility effect due to the deoxygenation of haemoglobin.[10] Later, when deoxyhemoglobin has been degraded into methemoglobin, the T_1-weighted images become more appropriate for blood depiction because of the paramagnetic effect of methemoglobin. The new information gained from most recent publications on MRI in methanol poisoning was that parenchymal edematous changes were not confined to the putamina but extended to lentiform nuclei, corona radiata, centrum semiovale, hippocampus, and cerebellum, which was unsuspected on previous CT studies (Figure 19-4).[11,12] Also, it is noteworthy that the subcortical white matter (and, to a lesser extent, the cortical gray matter ribbon) can be involved in the frontal and/or occipital lobes.[8,13] Only the subcortical associative fibers (U fibers) are almost always spared.[13] Recent publications have highlighted the interest of the diffusion-weighted sequences, which detect areas of restricted free-water diffusivity resulting in decrease in calculated ADC values within both putamina and white matter, with a possible additional involvement of the cerebral peduncles and of the splenium of the corpus callosum (Figure 19-5).[14,15] A possible explanation for diffusion abnormalities consistent with cytotoxic edema should be the inhibition of cytochrome oxidase and of the Na/K ATPase–dependent pump by formic acid. Additional hypoxic insult remains possible and can be superimposed to cytotoxic damage. As in subacute stroke, changes on diffusion-weighted images regress with time.

Ultimately, it has to be outlined that putaminal changes are not specific for methanol poisoning. The differential diagnosis should include Wilson's disease, Kearns-Sayre syndrome and Leigh's disease but also carbon monoxide and cyanide poisoning.[8]

Glycols

Ethylene glycol is a common antifreeze agent that can cause severe damage when ingested in overdose. Several metabolites are produced by hepatic biotransformation, and the accumulation of glycolic acid is usually regarded as the origin of the metabolic acidosis observed in the condition. Lethal outcomes are related to brain edema, which in turn is related to the severity of the metabolic acidosis. Ethylene glycol poisoning has been investigated less often by brain CT or MRI scans than has methanol. The usual CT feature in the condition is abnormal hypodensity within the central white matter, basal ganglia, thalami, midbrain, and upper pons, reflecting vasogenic brain edema that becomes detectable after a 24- to 48-hour delay.[16,17] Additional nonspecific cerebellar white matter abnormalities are also seen using brain MRI. Some patients develop delayed neuropsychological sequelae that do not seem to be directly related to MRI findings.[18] No specific cerebral MRI feature exists for glycol poisoning.

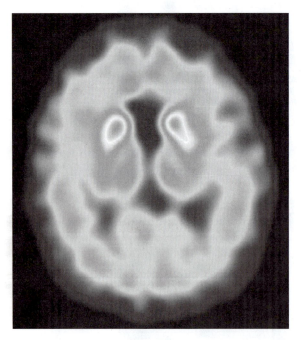

Figure 19-3. ^{18}F-dopa positron emission tomography scan performed 3.5 months after methanol poisoning in a patient who developed early extrapyramidal signs. Reduced uptake of the tracer occurs symmetrically in both putamina (*orange;* see color plate). (Adapted from Airas L, Paavilainen T, Marttila RJ, et al. Methanol intoxication-induced nigrostriatal dysfunction detected using 6-[18F]fluoro-L-dopa PET. *Neurotoxicology.* 2008;29:671–674.)

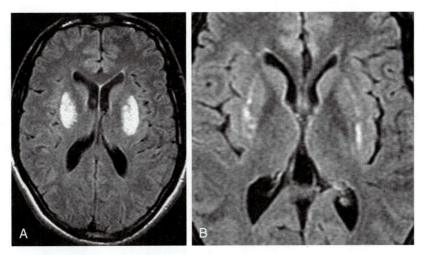

Figure 19-4. Magnetic resonance images in a 34-year-old man admitted with significant metabolic acidosis (pH 7.09) 12 hours after methanol ingestion. *(A)* Axial transverse fluid-attenuated inversion recovery magnetic resonance image 12 hours after ingestion of antifreeze product showing abnormal signal intensity within putamina and pallidi. In this severe case, initial lesions extended into the pallidi, thereby losing the specific pattern of elective putaminal involvement. *(B)* Similar image (magnified view) 19 days later showing complete recovery of lesions within pallidi and partial subsidence of the lesions within putamina, with a persistent thin, linear, abnormal hyperintense signal at the outer margins. The specificity of elective putaminal involvement, which was lost at the acute phase *(A)* (previous image), was restored on delayed examination *(B)*. (Adapted from Hantson P, Duprez T, Mahieu P. Neurotoxicity to the basal ganglia shown by magnetic resonance imaging [MRI] following poisoning by methanol and other substances. *J Toxicol Clin Toxicol.* 1997;35:151–161.)

Other Solvents

Chronic solvent-induced encephalopathy is characterized by mild or severe disturbances in attention and memory functions that may persist after the exposure to solvents has been interrupted. The underlying

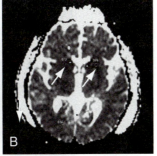

Figure 19-5. Diffusion-weighted imaging at magnetic resonance imaging investigation performed on day 3 in a 32-year-old man admitted with coma and severe metabolic acidosis following methanol ingestion. *(A)* Axial diffusion-weighted imaging (*b* factor = 1000 mm²/sec) showing increased signal in the bilateral caudate nuclei *(thin arrows)*, putamen *(asterisks)*, globus pallidus *(arrowheads)*, and splenium *(large arrow)*. *(B)* Axial ADC images. Low ADC values are seen in putamen *(arrows)* and caudate nuclei *(asterisks)*. (Adapted from Degirmenci B, Ela Y, Haktanir A, et al. Methanol intoxication: diffusion MR imaging findings. *Eur J Radiol Extra.* 2007;61:41–44.)

neurobiological mechanism of such disturbances is not fully elucidated. A relationship is probable between the duration and severity of exposure and the degree of memory and attention impairments. Inconclusive results have been obtained when analyzing brain CT or MRI scans. The main morphological changes observed in solvent-exposed workers with neurological signs were nonspecific diffuse brain atrophy and hypodense or T_2-hyperintense white matter changes suggesting demyelination.[19,20] Abnormal changes also involved thalami and other basal ganglia.

The authors demonstrated increased levels of Cho within the thalamus, basal ganglia, and parietal white matter using magnetic resonance spectroscopy. Others found reduced Cho levels in the frontal gray matter.[21,22] The changes in the dopaminergic pathway are more specifically investigated by single-photon emission computed tomography or PET imaging using appropriate tracers.

GASES

Carbon Monoxide

Carbon monoxide (CO) poisoning has been widely investigated using recent imaging modalities, mainly MRI. The pathophysiology of CO poisoning is still incompletely understood. It has been shown that CO produces anoxic brain injury by impairing the oxygen-carrying capabilities of hemoglobin. But CO is also able to interfere with many biochemical processes, including mitochondrial transport enzyme systems, lipid peroxidation, leukocyte adhesion to injured microvasculature, and nitric oxide release by vascular endothelium and blood platelets. The main pathological findings of edema, demyelination, and hemorrhagic necrosis at necropsy in fatal cases of CO exposure are not specific.

The clinical outcome after CO poisoning is uneasily predictable, mainly depending on type and duration of exposure. Only poor correlation between radiological findings and neurological outcome has been found. The delay between intoxication and imaging is crucial because some lesions may improve or worsen over time. In animal models, cerebral changes have been detected as early as 1 hour after acute CO exposure.[23]

It is empirically useful to separate lesions at acute phase from those appearing later, at the time of the delayed encephalopathy.

At the acute stage, MRI is the best imaging modality for demonstrating CO-related brain injury. In turn, CT examination is often unremarkable, thereby demonstrating lower sensitivity to early parenchymal injury. Lesions at the time are better characterized by using the full palette of magnetic resonance sequences, i.e., T_1-weighting for methemoglobin detection, T_2-weighting for vasogenic edema delineation, and diffusion-weighting for cytotoxic edema detection. As in many other toxic insults, basal ganglia are preferentially involved, mainly the globi pallidi (Figure 19-6).[24] Lesions are often symmetrical, typically with extension to the putamina, caudate nuclei, thalami and substantia nigra.[25,26] Hemorrhagic transformation and even necrosis are common findings in the globi pallidi. Parkinsonism occurs only in a minority of the patients with pallidal necrosis, probably because the damage to the nigrostriatal pathway is incomplete.[27]

The prevalence of the white matter lesions has been investigated in addition to deep gray matter damage.[28] Diffusion-weighted imaging may exhibit decreases in ADC values corresponding to cytotoxic edema as early as 12 hours after CO exposure.[29] Abnormally hyperintense areas within white matter may be seen on T_2-weighted images in a proportion ranging from 10 to 100% of the CO-poisoned patients according to the timing of imaging, patient selection, and type of exposure.[28] These changes may be observed in either superficial locations (subcortical white matter) or in a deeper location (border of lateral ventricles and centrum semiovale; Figure 19-7). They may correspond in variable proportions to myelin, axonal loss, or both. White matter changes are usually permanent but have limited reversibility over time, suggesting remyelination has been observed.[30,31]

Correlations between the extent of white matter damage and the severity of cognitive sequelae following CO

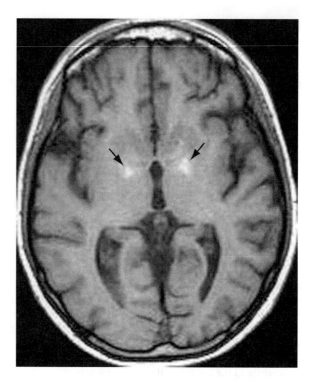

Figure 19-6. Carbon monoxide poisoning, acute phase. Unenhanced transverse T_1-weighted image showing hemorrhagic necrosis of both globi pallidi displaying an abnormal hyperintense signal due to the presence of hemoglobin degradation products. (Adapted from Hantson P, Duprez T. The value of morphological neuroimaging after acute exposure to toxic substances. *Toxicol Rev.* 2006;25:87–98.)

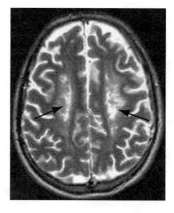

Figure 19-7. Carbon monoxide poisoning, chronic phase. T_2-weighted transverse imaging showing postanoxic encephalopathy with heterogenous areas of increased signal intensity of the white matter of both centrum semiovale corresponding to axonal loss and demyelination. (Images courtesy of Dr. D. Balériaux, Université ULB-Brussels; Adapted from Hantson P, Duprez T. The value of morphological neuroimaging after acute exposure to toxic substances. *Toxicol Rev.* 2006;25:87–98.).

poisoning remain a cornerstone question. In a prospective study, Parkinson et al. enrolled 73 consecutive CO-poisoned patients who had serial magnetic resonance and neurocognitive tests 1 day, 2 weeks, and 6 months after poisoning using a similar protocol at each timepoint. Of the patients, 32% had definite cognitive impairment and only 12% had increased white matter hyperintensities.[28]

Delayed encephalopathy after CO poisoning is defined by the recurrence of neurological or psychiatric signs after a transient symptom-free period following the acute phase. The free interval has a variable duration usually ranging from 2 to 3 weeks. Three topographical patterns of white matter damage have been described in the condition: (1) multifocal necrotic lesions prominently located within centrum semiovale and white matter tracts, (2) extensive necrotic areas in the periventricular white matter extending to the corpus callosum and the commissural tracts, and (3) patchy or extensive demyelination of the deep periventricular white matter.[32,33]

White matter changes are best investigated using fluid-attenuated inversion recovery (FLAIR) and diffusion-weighted sequences.[34–39] The former allows accurate delineation of hyperintense white matter lesions, thereby allowing the recognition of the topographical pattern. The abnormalities are usually symmetrical. The latter allows the calculation of ADC values, which are decreased at acute phase in the damaged areas when compared to normal ones. The prognostic value of low ADC values in white matter and their time course still has to be investigated, although a link between white matter demyelination and delayed neuropsychiatric impairment appears likely.

Cyanide

Cyanide exposure, either by inhalation or by ingestion, may result in irreversible brain damage. Like CO, cyanide demonstrates the highest affinity for the anatomical areas with very high oxygen demands. The lesions are therefore prominently located within putamina and globi pallidi. This was clearly seen initial brain CT studies showing reduced x-ray attenuation within these areas.[40,41] Highly oxygen-avid hippocampal gyri are paradoxically spared in most cases. Lesions are not immediately detectable but become visible after a variable delay, ranging from weeks to months. When persistence of lesions is observed at imaging, extrapyramidal signs usually develop, which are likely related to a progressive loss of nigrostriatal dopaminergic neurons. The hypothesis has been confirmed by PET studies showing a reduction of the uptake of labeled dopamine within striatum (putamina and caudate nuclei). MRI examinations in the condition have shown abnormal hyperintensities within putamina and globi pallidi on T_2-weighted images, which can be reversible.[42] In cases of severe edema, decreased intensity on corresponding areas

may be seen on T_1-weighted images. Extension of lesions to substantia nigra, subthalamic nucleus, and cerebellum has also been reported. Cortical necrosis, which has been described in neuropathological studies, may also be visible using MRI.[43,44]

Insulin

Patients having committed or undergone insulin overdose usually suffer from irreversible brain damage following deep hypoglycemia. Imaging studies of hypoglycemia in humans are obtained mostly from patients in hypoglycemic coma but rarely from patients with reversible focal neurological deficit. Cerebral hypoglycemic insult prominently affects the gray matter. Neurochemical changes in hypoglycemia significantly impair protein synthesis in many cerebral areas, with failure of ionic or energetic homeostasis, intracellular influx of calcium, and extracellular release of neuroactive amino acids. Excessive amounts of excitatory amino acids result in selective neuronal cell necrosis, prominently in the cortex, striatum, and hippocampus. Other structures, like the cerebellum, brainstem, and hypothalamus, have demonstrated resistance to hypoglycemia in a rat experimental model. CT examinations at the acute stage are often unremarkable. Depending on the severity and duration of hypoglycemia, decreased x-ray attenuation restricted to basal ganglia may be observed. Diffuse edematous swelling of brain parenchyma occurs in the most severe cases. In the chronic stage, CT findings of diffuse brain atrophy and subsequent enlargement of the ventricular system remain nonspecific. MRI studies have confirmed the preferential localization of the lesions to deep and cortical gray matter. After a delay of 7 to 14 days following the onset of the hypoglycemic coma, a strong bilateral T_2-hyperintensity and faint T_1-hypointensity due to increases in free water content are commonly observed within the caudate and lenticular nuclei, cerebral cortex, substantia nigra, and hippocampus (Figure 19-8).[45,46] The thalami are usually spared for unknown reasons. A possible explanation could be that hypoglycemia induces less severe energy failure than does ischemia. At the acute stage, increased T_2-signal intensity within gray matter may be observed on both FLAIR and diffusion-weighted images. Decreased ADC values in the injured areas are then obtained.[47–49] Thus far, diffusion-weighted imaging detects changes in water diffusivity not only resulting from oxygen deprivation, but also resulting from other metabolic changes. Like what happens in hypoglycemia, the diffusion-weighted hypersignal intensity reflecting decrease in water diffusivity and subsequently decrease in apparent diffusion coefficient (ADC) values due to cytotoxic edema with loss of transmembrane ionic homeostatis due to the failure of ATPase-dependant pumps, cell swelling, and interstitial space volume restriction. However, the topographical distribution and the temporal evolution of

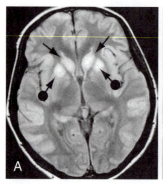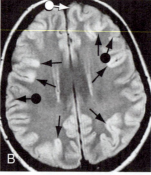

Figure 19-8. Acute insulin overdose in a 24-year-old woman who attempted suicide by injection of a vial containing 1000 units of insulin. *(A)* Slice through the central gray nuclei level showing hyperintensity within caudate nuclei *(arrows)* and anterior segment of the putamina *(ball arrowheads)*. *(B)* Slice through the roof of the upper part of the lateral ventricles: the cortex displays heterogeneity with areas of abnormally increased signal intensity *(arrows)*. (Adapted from Hantson P, Duprez T. The value of morphological neuroimaging after acute exposure to toxic substances. *Toxicol Rev.* 2006;25:87–98.)

hypoglycemic brain damage differ from that due to anoxia or ischemia. Monitoring of ADC changes can demonstrate the evolution from cell swelling with restricted water diffusivity at the acute stage to cell death with abnormally increased ADC values at chronic stages. A series of patients with reversible focal neurological deficits due to transient hypoglycemia has been investigated by diffusion-weighted imaging.[50–53] Transiently hyperintense lesions were seen bilaterally in internal capsules, in the corona radiate, and in the splenium of the corpus callosum. In conclusion, transient or definitive lesions can be observed using the different MRI techniques, according to the severity and duration of the hypoglycemia. The lesions are seen within cerebral cortex, hippocampus, and basal ganglia and are not specific to hypoglycemia. Differential diagnosis mainly includes ischemic injuries.

ILLICIT SUBSTANCES

Cocaine and Ecstasy

Both cocaine and 3,4-methylenedioxymethamphetamine (MDMA or Ecstasy) have drastic vasoconstrictive properties leading to increased risk for cerebrovascular events in chronic users. As seen in other ischemic or toxic insults, globi pallidi exhibit highest vulnerability. Pallidal necrosis is a prominent neuropathological finding at postmortem examinations of Ecstasy users.[54] It has been hypothesized that local release of serotonin induced by the intake of Ecstasy could result in prolonged vasospasm

with subsequent downstream ischemia. Conflicting results have been reported regarding the structural changes to cerebral gray matter after MDMA exposure. Authors found multiple areas of reduced gray matter density in the brainstem, cerebellum, and neocortex.[55] Others failed to confirm these observations. Also, functional MRI studies of neuronal activation led to divergent results concerning the effects of MDMA on brain activity patterns and cerebral areas, which are prominently affected in the condition.[56]

With the use of cocaine, abnormally increased signal intensity within hippocampi and globi pallidi have also been described using T_2- and diffusion-weighted MRI at acute phase (Figure 19-9).[57,58] Abnormal deep white matter T_2 and FLAIR hyperintensities have been regularly reported using brain MRI of chronic cocaine-dependent patients, but exceptionally in the acute phase of a single exposure (see Figure 19-9).[58] Intense vasoconstriction with subsequent demyelination has been hypothesized to explain parenchymal changes.[59] Cocaine-dependent subjects have reduced gray matter segmented volumes in the cerebellar hemispheres, as well as in the frontal and temporal cortex and in the thalamus.[60]

The chronic effects of cocaine use on the dopaminergic pathway are being investigated by functional MRI in animals and humans. Repeated exposure to cocaine could increase the density of the dopamine transporter in some brain subareas.

Heroin

Chronic inhalation of heroin has led to the description of a specific entity called "spongiform encephalopathy." At neuropathological examination, a spongiform white matter degeneration with multivacuolar degeneration of oligodendrocytes is observed.[61] The lesions mainly appear after repeated inhalation of heated heroin ("chasing the dragon") and more rarely after intravenous administration of pure heroin. A spongiform toxic leukoencephalopathy may also be observed in multiple drug abusers (e.g., combination of heroin and cocaine).[62,63] The main hypothesis to explain discrepancies in brain damage between inhalation and intravenous administration of heroin is that impurities liberated by heating and absorbed by sniffing are responsible for most brain damage. The patients usually develop progressive neurological and psychiatric disorders.[64] Only rarely has reversibility of clinical signs been reported. Limited reversibility in qualitative white matter changes has been described at MRI but with a significant loss of brain tissue cerebral volumetry. Symmetrical hyperintense areas within the white matter of the cerebellar hemispheres are seen on T_2-weighted and FLAIR images (Figure 19-10).[64–67] Cerebellar findings seem rather constant and specific in the condition.[64] Supratentorial changes are less constant. Periventricular and capsular deep

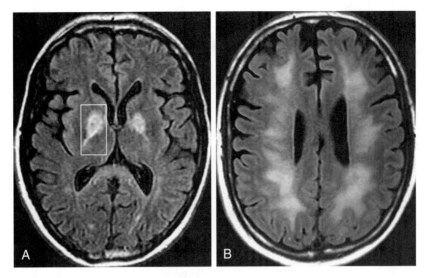

Figure 19-9. Acute exposure to cocaine in a 46-year-old man presenting with coma. *(A)* On magnetic resonance imaging performed on day 7, abnormally elevated signal intensity was seen within both pallidi and to a lesser degree within the splenium of the corpus callosum on the fluid-attenuated inversion recovery images. Both areas disclosed strong hyperintensity on diffusion-weighted images due to drastic reduction in apparent diffusion coefficient reflecting cytotoxic edema. *(B)* After 3 weeks *(right),* the pallidal damage evolved to liquefaction necrosis, together with the appearance of extensive supratentorial white matter changes. At 2 months clinical follow-up, the patient mainly suffered from akinetic mutism and mixed extrapyramidal and pyramidal spasticity. (Adapted from De Roock S, Hantson P, Laterre PF, et al. Extensive pallidal and white matter injury following cocaine overdose. *Intensive Care Med.* 2007;33:2030–2031.)

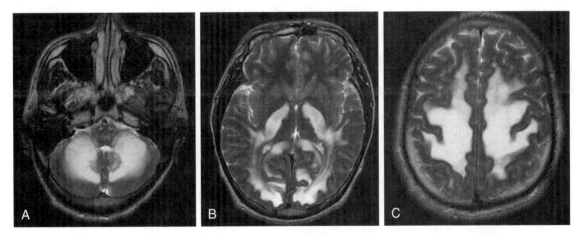

Figure 19-10. Axial transverse T_2-weighted magnetic resonance images at infra- *(A)* and supratentorial *(B, C)* levels in a case of severe heroin-induced leukoencephalopathy. Selective involvement of the white matter contrasting with the sparing of superficial and deep gray matter is obvious throughout brain. *(A)* Only a slightly abnormal increase in signal intensity is visible within the medulla oblongata involving pyramidal tracts, medial lemnisci, and posterior nucleus tractus solitarius. In turn, a strongly elevated hyperintense signal is present within the white matter of both cerebellar hemispheres. Superficial and deep cortical gray matter of the dentate nuclei are spared. *(B)* Abnormal signal intensity extends to the posterior limbs of internal capsules and temporal–occipital white matter. *(C)* Massive involvement of the white matter of the centrum semiovale encompassing pre- and postcentral gyri is obvious. (Adapted from Offiah C, Hall E. Heroin-induced leukoencephalopathy: characterization using MRI, diffusion-weighted imaging, and MR spectroscopy. *Clin Radiol.* 2008;63:146–152.)

white matter may be symmetrically affected. In severe cases, the subcortical white matter may also be involved, but the anterior limbs of the internal capsules are spared. Symmetrical lesions within globi pallidi have also been described. Relative sparing of the subcortical U fibers, which was seen using MRI, has been confirmed at brain biopsy.[68] Investigations by magnetic resonance spectroscopy may reveal unspecific reduction in N-acetyl aspartate and Cho levels, together with increased concentration of lactate within affected brain areas.[64] The reduction in N-acetyl aspartate levels reflects neuronal loss, and reduced Cho concentration is a sign of lower cell membrane turnover. In addition, the accumulation of lactate may be a marker for mitochondrial dysfunction matching the neuropathological findings of mitochondrial swelling within involved areas.

METALS

Manganese

Manganese overexposure in nonhuman primates and humans causes "neuromanganism," a neurodegenerative disorder presumably resulting from the accumulation of the metal in the basal ganglia, mainly the globi pallidi. Experimental models have shown that dopamine levels were reduced in these structures after manganese exposure. Manganese has paramagnetic properties and therefore can be detected in vivo on unenhanced T_1-weighted images because of shortening of the longitudinal relaxation time (T_1) of involved tissue. Manganese overexposure in humans and nonhuman primates therefore results in increased T_1-signal intensity of the basal ganglia, mainly the globi pallidi and substantia nigra.[69] Reversibility seems possible after interruption of exposure.[70] A parkinsonian syndrome has been recently described in methcathinone users in Russia and in the Baltic states.[71] Methcathinone is a psychostimulant that usually does not induce parkinsonism by oral use. The toxicity occurred after conditioning methcathinone for intravenous use, which was produced by oxidation of ephedrine or pseudoephedrine using potassium permanganate. Extrapyramidal symptoms appeared after a mean of 5.8 ± 4.5 years of intravenous methcathinone use. The T_1-weighted MRI showed symmetrical hyperintensity within the globi pallidi, substantia nigra, and substantia innominata in active methcathinone users. Some fading was found in the subjects who thereafter stopped the use of methcathinone.

Methylmercury

The neurotoxicity of methylmercury was particularly well documented by the disaster in Minamata. The main neurological signs were visual deficits, ataxia, and sensory disturbances. Some patients who had been exposed between 1955 and 1958 underwent MRI more than 30 years later. MRI showed atrophy of the visual and postcentral cortex and of the cerebellar vermis and hemispheres.[72] The visual cortex appeared slightly hypointense on T_1-weighted images and frankly hyperintense on T_2-weighted images. MRI also demonstrated lesions located in the calcarine area, cerebellum, and postcentral gyri, which well matched the main clinical triad featuring the syndrome: the constriction of the visual fields, ataxia, and sensory disturbance.

Lead

Occupational exposure to organic and inorganic lead may be associated with impairment in cognitive functions. Some studies have investigated the putative relationship between neurological disturbances and reduction of brain volumes calculated at MRI.[73]

Thallium

Abnormal signal intensity changes within corpus striatum (putamen + caudate) with asymmetrical distribution were observed in a single case.[75] Decrease in T1 signal intensity and increase in T2 signal intensity of diseased areas strongly suggested focal edema. Thallium poisoning is chiefly characterized by ascending paralysis, cranial nerve palsies, ataxia, tremor, convulsion, coma, and death. Rare neuropathological studies of the brain in the condition have shown chromatolytic changes in the motor cortex, globus pallidus, substantia nigra, and brainstem nuclei.[74] Only sparse neuroimaging data in thallium poisoning are available. Normal brain CT or MRI scans have been reported in patients with cognitive impairment following thallium poisoning. Asymmetrical changes in the corpus striatum (hypointense lesion on T_1-weighted images with corresponding hyperintensity on T_2-weighted images) compatible with edema were observed in a single case.[75] However, no clear correlation was found with clinical findings.

POSTERIOR REVERSIBLE ENCEPHALOPATHY SYNDROME

Posterior reversible encephalopathy syndrome (PRES) is a neurotoxic condition associated with vasogenic edema. Clinical presentation of PRES is featured by headaches, altered mental status, visual disturbance, and generalized seizures. Neuroimaging studies typically demonstrate focal and usually symmetrical areas of parenchymal edema.[76,77] The parietal and occipital

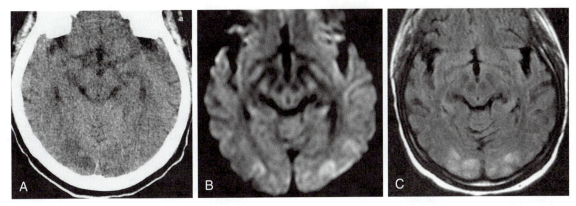

Figure 19-11. Imaging work-up including computerized tomography (CT) and magnetic resonance imaging (MRI) in a patient who developed posterior reversible encepahlopathy syndrome (PRES) after exposure to therapeutic doses of cyclosporine. *(A)* Unenhanced CT image showing decrease in x-ray attenuation (hypodensity) in the right medial occipital area. Preferential involvement of the subcortical white matter sparing the corresponding cortical ribbon and location suggested PRES. Similar changes were suspected in the mirror left-sided area but needed MRI examination for confirmation because bilaterality, if confirmed, would have strongly reinforced the diagnosis. *(B)* Fluid-attenuated inversion recovery (FLAIR) MRI in a similar slice location in the same patient confirming lesions on both medial areas. Observe involvement of both gray and white matter at this intermediate stage of the disease course, which reinforces the hypothesis. *(C)* Diffusion-weighted MRI in a corresponding slice location showing less extended bilateral occipital lesions with prominent involvement of the cortical ribbon. Both features of discrepancy between FLAIR and DW images regarding the lesions' extension and of concomitant presence of diseased areas with lowered and with increased ADC values were almost pathognomonic for PRES. Areas appearing hyperintense of FLAIR images but undetectable on DW images had vasogenic edema with increased ADC values (parametric ADC-mapped images not shown) and mainly involved sub-cortical areas. Areas appearing hyperintense on both modalities had cytotoxic edema and mainly involved the cortical ribbon.

lobes are most commonly affected, followed by the frontal lobes, the inferior temporal–occipital junction, and the cerebellum (Figure 19-11). Involvement of the basal ganglia, brainstem, or deep white matter is less common. Diffusion-weighted imaging has allowed insights into the pathophysiology of PRES by demonstrating prominent vasogenic edema with normal or slightly increased ADC values at an early stage of the disease course followed by a mixture of areas of vasogenic and cytotoxic edema (with decreased ADC values) at later stages. The primary mechanism of PRES seems to be a combination of systemic hypertension and dysregulation of autonomic innervation of the vessel walls, mainly in the posterior circulation. PRES has been described in association with various systemic conditions, including eclampsia, allogeneic bone marrow transplantation, and solid organ transplantation. Hypertension is absent in about 25% of patients. In these cases, the prominent mechanism seems to be the nervous autonomic dysregulation of arterial and arteriolar walls. Different antimitotic chemotherapeutic drugs known for autonomic neurotoxicity have been associated with PRES. It is a relatively common complication after solid organ transplantation in patients who concomitantly suffer systemic hypertension and receive either cyclosporine or tacrolimus for immunosuppression. Autonomic neurotoxicity of

both drugs is well established, but no direct correlation has been found between blood levels and neurotoxicity or PRES. Drug discontinuation and normalization of systemic tension synergistically result in clinical improvement.

REFERENCES

1. Hantson P, de Tourtchaninoff M, Simoens G, et al. Evoked potentials investigation of visual dysfunction after methanol poisoning. *Crit Care Med.* 1999;27:2707–2715.
2. Hantson P, Duprez T. The value of morphological neuroimaging after acute exposure to toxic substances. *Toxicol Rev.* 2006;25:87–98.
3. Aquilonius SM, Asmark H, Enoksson P, et al. Computerised tomography in severe methanol intoxication. *BMJ.* 1978;309:929–930.
4. Phang PT, Passerini L, Mielke B, et al. Brain hemorrhage associated with methanol poisoning. *Crit Care Med.* 1988;16:137–140.
5. Blanco M, Casado R, Vázquez F. CT and MR imaging findings in methanol intoxication. *Am J Neuroradiol.* 2006;27:452–454.
6. Fontenot AP, Pelak VS. Development of neurologic symptoms in a 26-year-old woman following recovery from methanol intoxication. *Chest.* 2002;122:1436–1439.
7. Airas L, Paavilainen T, Marttila RJ, et al. Methanol intoxication-induced nigrostriatal dysfunction detected using 6-[18F]fluoro-L-dopa PET. *Neurotoxicology.* 2008;29:671–674.

8. Hantson P, Duprez T, Mahieu P. Neurotoxicity to the basal ganglia shown by magnetic resonance imaging (MRI) following poisoning by methanol and other substances. *J Toxicol Clin Toxicol*. 1997;35:151–161.

9. Pelletier J, Habib MH, Khalil R, et al. Putaminal necrosis after methanol intoxication. *J Neurol Neurosurg Psychiatry*. 1992;55:234–235.

10. Bartoli JM, Laurent M, Moulin G, et al. Methanol intoxication: CT and MRI findings—report of two cases. *Ann Radiol (Paris)*. 1990;33:257–259.

11. Sefidbakht S, Rasekhi AR, Kamali K, et al. Methanol poisoning: acute MR and CT findings in nine patients. *Neuroradiology*. 2007;49:427–435.

12. Vara-Castrodeza A, Peréz-Castrillón, Duenas-Laita A. Magnetic resonance imaging in methanol poisoning. *Clin Toxicol*. 2007;45:429–430.

13. Rubinstein D, Escott E, Kelly JP. Methanol intoxication with putaminal and white matter necrosis: MR and CT findings. *Am J Neuroradiol*. 1995;16:1492–1494.

14. Degirmenci B, Ela Y, Haktanir A, et al. Methanol intoxication: diffusion MR imaging findings. *Eur J Radiol Extra*. 2007;61:41–44.

15. Peters AS, Schwarze B, Tomandl B, et al. Bilateral striatal hyperintensities on diffusion weighted MRI in acute methanol poisoning. *Eur J Neurol*. 2007;14:e1–e2.

16. Morgan BW, Ford MD, Follmer R. Ethylene glycol ingestion resulting in brainstem and midbrain dysfunction. *J Toxicol Clin Toxicol*. 2000;38:445–451.

17. Zeiss J, Velasco ME, McKann KM, et al. Cerebral CT of lethal ethylene glycol intoxication with pathologic correlation. *Am J Neuroradiol*. 1989;10:440–442.

18. Freilich BM, Altun Z, Ramesar C, et al. Neuropsychological sequelae of ethylene glycol intoxication: a case study. *Appl Neuropsychol*. 2007;14:56–61.

19. Ridgway P, Nixon TE, Leach JP. Occupational exposure to organic solvents and long-term nervous system damage detectable by brain imaging, neurophysiology or histopathology. *Food Chem Toxicol*. 2003;41:153–187.

20. Haut MW, Kuwara H, Ducatman AM, et al. Corpus callosum volume in railroad workers with chronic exposure to solvents. *J Occup Environ Med*. 2006;48:615–624.

21. Alkan A, Kutlu R, Hallac T, et al. Occupational prolonged organic solvent exposure in shoemakers: brain MR spectroscopy findings. *Magn Reson Imaging*. 2004;22:707–713.

22. Visser I, Lavini C, Booij J, et al. Cerebral impairment in chronic solvent-induced encephalopathy. *Ann Neurology*. 2008;63:572–580.

23. Jakular V, Penne D, Crowley M, et al. Magnetic resonance imaging of the rat brain following acute carbon monoxide poisoning. *J Appl Toxicol*. 1992;12:407–414.

24. O'Donnel P, Buxton PJ, Pitkin A, Jarvis LJ. The magnetic resonance imaging appearances of the brain in acute carbon monoxide poisoning. *Clin Radiol*. 2000;55:273–280.

25. Ferrier D, Wallace CJ, Fletcher WA, et al. Magnetic resonance features in carbon monoxide poisoning. *Can Assoc Radiol J*. 1994;45:466–468.

26. Kawanami T, Kato T, Kurita K, et al. The pallidoreticular pattern of brain damage on MRI in a patient with carbon monoxide poisoning. *J Neurol Neurosurg Psychiatry*. 1998;64:282.

27. Gandini C, Prockop LD, Butera R, et al. Pallidoreticular-rubral brain damage on magnetic resonance imaging after carbon monoxide poisoning. *J Neuroimaging*. 2002;12:102–103.

28. Parkinson RB, Hopkins RO, Cleavinger HB, et al. White matter hyperintensities and neuropsychological outcome following carbon monoxide poisoning. *Neurology*. 2002;58:1525–1532.

29. Sener RN. Acute carbon monoxide poisoning: diffusion MR imaging findings. *Am J Neuroradiol*. 2003;24:1475–1477.

30. Choi IS, Kim SK, Choi YC, et al. Evaluation of outcome after acute carbon monoxide poisoning by brain CT. *J Korean Med Sci*. 1993;8:78–83.

31. Yoshii F, Kozuma R, Takahashi W, et al. Magnetic resonance imaging and 11C-N-methylpiperone/positron emission tomography studies in a patient with the interval form of carbon monoxide poisoning. *J Neurol Sci*. 1998;160:87–91.

32. Ginsberg MD, Myers RE, McDonagh BF. Experimental carbon monoxide encephalopathy in the primate. II. Clinical aspects, neuropathology, and physiologic correlation. *Arch Neurol*. 1974;30:209–216.

33. Lapresle J, Fardeau M. The central nervous system and carbon monoxide poisoning. II. Anatomical study of the brain lesions following intoxication with carbon monoxide. *Prog Brain Res*. 1967;24:31–74.

34. Chu KC, Jung KH, Him HJ, et al. Diffusion-weighted MRI and 99m-Tc-HMPAO SPECT in delayed relapsing type of carbon monoxide poisoning: evidence of delayed cytotoxic edema. *Eur Neurol*. 2004;51:98–103.

35. Lo CP, Chen SY, Lee KW, et al. Brain injury after acute carbon monoxide poisoning: early and late complications. *Am J Roentgenol*. 2007;189:W205–W211.

36. Kinoshita T, Sugihara S, Matsusue E, et al. Pallidoreticular damage in acute carbon monoxide poisoning: diffusion-weighted MR imaging findings. *Am J Neuroradiol*. 2005;26:1845–1848.

37. Kim JH, Chang KH, Song IC, et al. *Am J Neuroradiol*. 2003;24:1592–1597.

38. Murata T, Kimura H, Kado H, et al. Neuronal damage in the interval form of CO poisoning determined by serial diffusion weighted magnetic resonance imaging plus ^{1}H-magnetic resonance spectroscopy. *J Neurol Neurosurg Psychiatry*. 2001;71:250–253.

39. Teksam M, Casey SO, Michel E, et al. Diffusion weighted MR imaging findings in carbon monoxide poisoning. *Neuroradiology*. 2002;44:109–113.

40. Grandas F, Artieda J, Obeso JA. Clinical and CT scan findings in a case of cyanide intoxication. *Mov Disord*. 1989;4:188–193.

41. Valenzuela R, Court J, Godoy J. Delayed cyanide induced dystonia. *J Neurol Neurosurg Psychiatry*. 1992;55:198–199.

42. Kasamo K, Okuhata Y, Satoh R, et al. Chronological changes of MRI findings on striatal damage after acute cyanide intoxication: pathogenesis of the damage and its selectivity, and prevention for neurological sequelae. A case report. *Eur Arch Psychiatry Clin Neurosci*. 1993;243:71–74.

43. Rachinger J, Fellner FA, Stieglbauer K, et al. MR changes after acute cyanide intoxication. *Am J Neuroradiol*. 2002;23:1398–1401.

44. Riudavets MA, Aronica-Pollak P, Troncoso JC. Pseudolaminar necrosis in cyanide intoxication: a neuropathology case report. *Am J Forensic Med Pathol*. 2005;26:189–191.

45. Fujioka M, Okuchi K, Hiramatsu LI, et al. Specific changes in human brain after hypoglycemic injury. *Stroke*. 1997;28:584–587.

46. Jung SL, Kim BS, Lee KS, et al. Magnetic resonance imaging and diffusion-weighted imaging changes after hypoglycemic coma. *J Neuroimaging*. 2005;15:193–196.

47. Shirayama H, Oshiro Y, Kinjo Y, et al. Acute brain injury in hypoglycaemia-induced hemiplegia. *Diabet Med*. 2004;21:623–624.

48. Maekawa S, Aibiki M, Kikuchi K, et al. Time-related changes in reversible MRI findings after prolonged hypoglycemia. *Clin Neurol Neurosurg*. 2005;108:511–513.

49. Hasegawa Y, Formato JE, Latour LL, et al. Severe transient hypoglycemia causes reversible change in the apparent diffusion coefficient of water. *Stroke*. 1996;27:1648–1655.

50. Albayram S, Ozer H, Gokdemir S, et al. Reversible reduction of apparent diffusion coefficient values in bilateral internal capsules in transient hypoglycemia-induced hemiparesis. *Am J Neuroradiol*. 2006;27:1760–1762.

51. Terakawa Y, Tsuyuguchi N, Nunomura K, et al. Reversible diffusion-weighted imaging changes in the splenium of the corpus callosum and internal capsule associated with hypoglycemia. *Neurol Med Chir (Tokyo)*. 2007;47:486–488.

52. Lo L, Than CHA, Umapathi T, et al. Diffusion-weighted MR imaging in early diagnosis and prognosis of hypoglycemia. *Am J Neuroradiol*. 2006;27:1222–1224.

53. Kim JH, Choi JY, Koh SB, et al. Reversible splenial abnormality in hypoglycemic encephalopathy. *Neuroradiology*. 2007;49:217–222.

54. Reneman L, Habraken JB, Majoie CB, et al. MDMA (Ecstasy) and its association with cerebrovascular accidents: preliminary findings. *Am J Neuroradiol*. 2000;21:1001–1007.

55. Cowan RL, Lyoo IK, Sung MS, et al. Reduced cortical gray matter density in human MDMA (Ecstasy) users: a voxel-based morphometry study. *Drug Alcohol Depend*. 2003;72:225–235.

56. Daumann J, Fishermann T, Pilatus U, et al. Proton magnetic resonance spectroscopy in Ecstasy (MDMA) users. *Neurosci Letters*. 2004;362:113–116.

57. Boulouri MR, Small GA. Neuroimaging of hypoxia and cocaine-induced hippocampal stroke. *J Neuroimaging*. 2004;14:290–291.

58. De Roock S, Hantson P, Laterre PF, et al. Extensive pallidal and white matter injury following cocaine overdose. *Intensive Care Med*. 2007;33:2030–2031.

59. Lyoo IK, Streeter CC, Ahn KH, et al. White matter hyperintensities in subjects with cocaine and opiate dependence and healthy comparison subjects. *Psychiatry Res*. 2004;131:135–145.

60. Sim ME, Lyoo IK, Streeter CC, et al. Cerebellar gray matter volume correlates with duration of cocaine use in cocaine-dependent subjects. *Neuropsychopharmacology*. 2007;10:2229–2237.

61. Hill MD, Cooper PW, Perry JR. Chasing the dragon: neurological toxicity associated with inhalation of heroin vapour. Case report. *CMAJ*. 2000;162:236–238.

62. Maschke M, Fehlings T, Kastrup O, et al. Toxic leukoencephalopathy after consumption of heroin and cocaine with unexpected clinical recovery. *J Neurol*. 1999;246:850–851.

63. Ryan A, Molloy FM, Farrell MA, et al. Fatal toxic leukoencephalopathy: clinical, radiological, and necropsy findings in two patients. *J Neurol Neurosurg Psychiatry*. 2005;76:1014–1016.

64. Offiah C, Hall E. Heroin-induced leukoencephalopathy: characterization using MRI, diffusion-weighted imaging, and MR spectroscopy. *Clin Radiol*. 2008;63:146–152.

65. Keogh CF, Andrews GT, Spacey SD, et al. Neuroimaging features of heroin inhalation toxicity: "chasing the dragon." *Am J Roentgenol*. 2003;180:847–850.

66. Bartlett E, Mikulis DJ. "Chasing the dragon" with MRI: leukoencephalopathy in drug abuse. *Br J Radiol*. 2005;78:997–1004.

67. Poen Tan T, Algra PR, Wolters EC. Toxic leukoencephalopathy after inhalation of poisoned heroin: MR findings. *Am J Neuroradiol*. 1994;15:175–178.

68. Kriegstein AR, Shungu DC, Millar WS, et al. Leukoencephalopathy and raised brain lactate from heroin vapour inhalation ("chasing the dragon"). *Neurology*. 1999;53:1765–1773.

69. Uchino A, Noguchi T, Nomiyama K, et al. Manganese accumulation in the brain: MR imaging. *Neuroradiology*. 2007;49:715–720.

70. Jiang Y, Zheng W, Long L, et al. Brain resonance magnetic imaging and manganese concentrations in red blood cells of smelting workers: search for biomarkers of manganese exposure. *Neurotoxicology*. 2007;28:126–135.

71. Stepens A, Logina I, Liguts V, et al. A Parkinsonian syndrome in methcathinone users and role of manganese. *N Engl J Med*. 2008;358:1009–1017.

72. Korogi Y, Takahashi M, Okajima T, et al. MR findings of Minamata disease: organic mercury poisoning. *J Magn Reson Imaging*. 1998;8:308–316.

73. Caffo B, Chen S, Stewart W, et al. Are brain volumes based on magnetic resonance imaging mediators of the associations of cumulative lead dose with cognitive function? *Am J Epidemiol*. 2008;167:429–437.

74. Insley BM, Grufferman S, Ayliffe HE. Thallium poisoning in cocaine abusers. *Am J Emerg Med*. 1986;4:545–548.

75. Tsai Y-T, Huang C-C, Kuo H-C, et al. Central nervous system effects in acute thallium poisoning. *Neurotoxicology*. 2006;27:291–295.

76. Bartynski WS. Posterior reversible encephalopathy syndrome: I. Fundamental imaging and clinical features. *Am J Neuroradiol*. 2008;29:1036–1042.

77. Bartynski WS, Boardman JF. Distinct imaging patterns and brain distribution in posterior reversible encephalopathy syndrome. *Am J Neuroradiol*. 2007;28:1320–1327.

SECTION 4

NEUROTOXIC SUBSTANCES

CONTENTS

CHAPTER 20 ••••

Clinical Aspects of Mercury Neurotoxicity

David R. Wallace, Elizabeth Lienemann, and Amber N. Hood

BACKGROUND

Chemistry of Mercury Action

A heavy, silvery, transition metal, mercury (Hg) is one of five elements that are liquid at or near room temperature. Mercury occurs in the Earth's crust, mainly in the form of sulfides. The red sulfide, cinnabar, is the main component of the mercury ores. Mercury is also released into the environment by human activities, for example, combustion of fossil fuels, waste disposal, and industrial activities. If heated, it is a colorless, odorless gas. Mercury, a known toxicant, is ubiquitous in the environment and naturally exists in three forms: elemental, inorganic, and organic.[1–2] Elemental mercury, also known as metallic mercury, has been used in thermometers and dental amalgams.[3–4] It has a melting point of $-39°C$, and although it is not absorbed well from the gastrointestinal tract, when the vapors are inhaled this form of mercury easily crosses into the circulatory system from the lungs.[1] Inorganic mercury salts ($HgCl_2$, for example) have had many uses in everyday life. A few of these uses include or included some medicines, skin-lightening creams, antibacterials, and explosive detonators.[1,3] This form of mercury has a low absorption rate when ingested (7% to 15%)[4]; however, extended exposure to mercury salts can lead to central nervous system (CNS) damage.[1] The third form of mercury, organic mercury,

is believed to be the most toxic of the three forms.[4] Two examples of organic mercury are ethylmercury, a component of thimerosal (used to preserve vaccines), and methylmercury.

Mercury in any of its three forms—elemental, inorganic, and organic—has a unique toxicity related to its differential accumulation in sensitive tissues. Mercury combines with other elements, such as chlorine, sulfur, or oxygen, to form inorganic mercury salts, which are usually white powders or crystals. Mercury also combines with carbon to make organic mercury compounds, such as methylmercury. The predominant source of methylmercury is atmospheric mercury deposited on the surfaces of bodies of water that is then biomethylated by microorganisms and subsequently biomagnified as it ascends the food chain. Metallic mercury is used to produce chlorine gas and caustic soda; it is also used in thermometers, dental fillings, and batteries. Mercury salts are sometimes used in skin-lightening creams and as antiseptic creams and ointments. Other products containing mercury include auto parts, fluorescent bulbs, medical products, vaccines, and thermostats. The biological half-life for inorganic mercury is about 40 days. For elemental mercury or mercury vapor, the biological half-life is linear, with a range of values from 35 to 90 days. The biological half-life is different for different organs. A fraction of the absorbed mercury remains in the body for a longer time, even years in the brain and bones.[5] It is biologically nonessential and toxic to all organisms.

History of Mercury Intoxication

The toxic effects of mercury have been observed over hundreds of years. During the Roman era, mercury intoxication was observed in the slaves mining quicksilver from the Almaden mine in Spain.[6] This mine is still one of the dominant mines, having produced 236 tons of mercury in 2000.[7] Mercury intoxication reportedly was experienced in the A.D. 752 by the builders of the giant bronze Buddha, which is coated with a mixture of gold, tin, and mercury.[6] Another group of working individuals, those in the fur and felt hat-making industries in the 17th century, also experienced mercury intoxication.[6]

More recent outbreaks of mercury toxicity occurred at Minamata Bay, Niigata, Japan, and Iraq, as well as along the Amazon River Basin. One of the worst industrial disasters in history was caused by the dumping of mercury compounds into Minamata Bay, Japan. The Chisso Corporation, a fertilizer and later petrochemical company, was found responsible for polluting the bay from 1932 to 1968. It is estimated that more than 3000 people suffered various deformities, severe mercury poisoning symptoms, or death from what became known as Minamata disease. The neurotoxic signs include ataxia, speech impairment, constriction of visual fields, hypoesthesia, dysarthria, hearing impairment, and sensory disturbances. These neurological problems persisted and were found in other areas of Japan as the mercury contamination spread.[8] Follow-up studies in the Minamata area 40 years after the spill and 30 years since a fishing ban was enacted revealed continued problems. In 1995, male residents of fishing villages in the area reported a significantly higher prevalence than town-resident controls for the following complaints: stiffness, dysesthesia, hand tremor, dizziness, loss of pain sensation, cramping, atrophy of the upper arm musculature, arthralgia, insomnia, and lumbago. In Iraq, mercury poisoning occurred after grain that had been treated with pesticide containing mercury was made into bread and eaten.[9] Mercury toxicity also occurs along the Amazon River Basin due to gold mining operations, deforestation, and damming of rivers.[6,10] All of these actions cause an increase in mercury levels in fish, which are then consumed by the indigenous people.[10]

ROUTE OF MERCURY EXPOSURE

Volcanic eruptions, erosion, occupations such as those in the thermometer and dry-cell battery industries, and dentistry are all routes of mercury exposure.[1-2] Individuals

may also be exposed to mercury through dental amalgams and a diet of fish that have been exposed to aquatic mercury sources.[2,11] Other populations that the Agency for Toxic Substances and Disease Registry consider to be at an increase risk of toxicity due to mercury exposure are those living close to a former mercury mining site, recycling facility, and municipal or medical incinerator.[4] Waste sites from industrial dumping and the burning of coal increases the environmental mercury content, which also increases the amount of exposure to the population.[2,4]

There are many more sources of mercury that could potentially cause harmful exposure to organisms (Table 1). Human exposure to inorganic mercury is mainly occupational, most commonly associated with mercury vapor. It is often related to specific working conditions, for example, mining, spillage of mercury compounds on work clothes or in the working environment, and handling of mercury salts in the chemical industry and laboratories.[12] Due to the health effects of mercury exposure, industrial and commercial uses are broadly regulated in Western countries. The World Health Organization, U.S. Occupational Safety and Health Administration, and U.S. National Institute for Occupational Safety and Health all agree that mercury is an occupational hazard and have established specific occupational exposure limits. Environmental releases and disposal of mercury is regulated in the United States, primarily by the Environmental Protection Agency. In recent years, governments have issued warnings that certain fish in excess quantities are unsafe due to methylmercury levels.

Table 1: Primary Sources of Elemental, Inorganic, and Organic Mercury Exposure

Elemental	Inorganic	Organic
Amalgam preparation	Disinfectant making	Bactericide preparation
Barometer manufacture	Dye making	Drug manufacture
Bronzing	Explosive production	Embalming or cremation
Dentistry	Fur processing	Farming
Photography	Laboratory research	Histology
Mercury refining	Tannery work	Insecticide production
Paint manufacture	Taxidermy	Seed handling

Such warnings especially target pregnant women because all forms of mercury cross the placenta to the fetus.

The risk of mercury to human health has been the subject of several reviews.[13–18] One of the most important points raised by these reviews is that the effect of chronic low-dose mercury exposure on humans is not known. The extent of absorption highly depends on the form of mercury to which the individual is exposed (Table 2). There are claims that long-term exposure to low concentrations of mercury vapor either cause or exacerbate degenerative diseases such as amyotrophic lateral sclerosis, Alzheimer's disease (AD), multiple sclerosis, and Parkinson's disease. Speculation has been most intense concerning AD after a report that mercury levels were higher in autopsy brains of AD patients than in brains of members of a control group.[19]

SIGNS AND SYMPTOMS OF MERCURY EXPOSURE

The symptoms and effects of mercury toxicity are vast and depend on the nature of metal, the route of administration, the length and dose of exposure, species type, gender, and age.[20–22] All symptoms that occur with mercury toxicity are too numerous to discuss in detail within this chapter; therefore, the focus is on the CNS. A partial list of these symptoms include tremor, insecurity, memory loss, fatigue, excitability, insomnia, hallucinations, and irritability.[2–3,23] Seizures, decreased strength, hearing loss, constricted visual field, and ataxia are other

CNS symptoms reported from mercury exposure.[2,9,23] The distribution of mercury and its effects on various organ systems is shown in Figure 20-1.

Mercury exposure has been associated with autoimmune disease,[24] scleroderma,[25] autism,[26] Alzheimer's disease, and Parkinson's disease.[20] While mercury may directly cause these diseases, it may also trigger or exacerbate current but unrecognized conditions, such as genetic factors.[26] It has been reported that autistic children have been exposed to elevated mercury and they have an atypical mercury metabolism.[22] The dysfunctions mercury causes in the immune, sensory, neurological, motor, and behavioral systems are similar to those found in autism.[26]

Mercury levels are found to be elevated in the blood of patients with Alzheimer's disease. In one study, mercury was found to be more than twofold higher in the blood of patients with Alzheimer's disease than in the control group.[27] Blood mercury levels of the individuals with Alzheimer's disease were found to be 2.64 ± 0.38 µg/L, while the control group that consisted of individuals without any psychiatric disorders levels was 1.09 ± 0.12 µg/L.[27] Postmortem brain tissue from patients with Alzheimer's disease shows elevated levels of mercury.[27–28]

Central Nervous System

The CNS is one of the main targets of mercury accumulation and damage. This metal's effects on the CNS are well known and numerous.[1,29] Some of these detrimental effects include disruption of neuronal migration,[1] neuronal degeneration,[9] and demyelination.[4] Mercury is capable of harming the blood–brain barrier by damaging the cerebral microvascular endothelial cells that compose this important barrier.[30] Ca^{2+} channels, neurotransmitter turnover, and nerve conduction are also affected by mercury.[30] High-dose mercury exposure can cause the cerebellum and limbic structures to undergo morphological and biochemical changes in both the adult and the developing CNS.[20,31] Lesions can be found in this area, as was seen in individuals diagnosed with Minamata disease.[31]

MECHANISM OF NEUROTOXICITY

Whether the primary cellular target of mercury is astrocytes or neurons, mercury can disturb cellular function through various mechanisms. Altering calcium ion homeostasis,[4,32] depleting antioxidants, especially glutathione,[33] and perturbing mitochondrial membrane potential[32] have all been reported upon mercury exposure. Disturbed glutamate activity[32] and enhanced

Table 2: Absorption of Elemental, Inorganic, and Organic Mercury Depending on Route of Contact

Form of Mercury	Extent of Absorption by Route of Contact		
	Ingestion	Dermal Contact	Inhalation
Elemental	Very low for liquid form	Moderate for vaporized form	High for vaporized form
Inorganic	Low to moderate (higher in infants and children)	Low to moderate	Low to moderate
Organic	High	Low to moderate	High

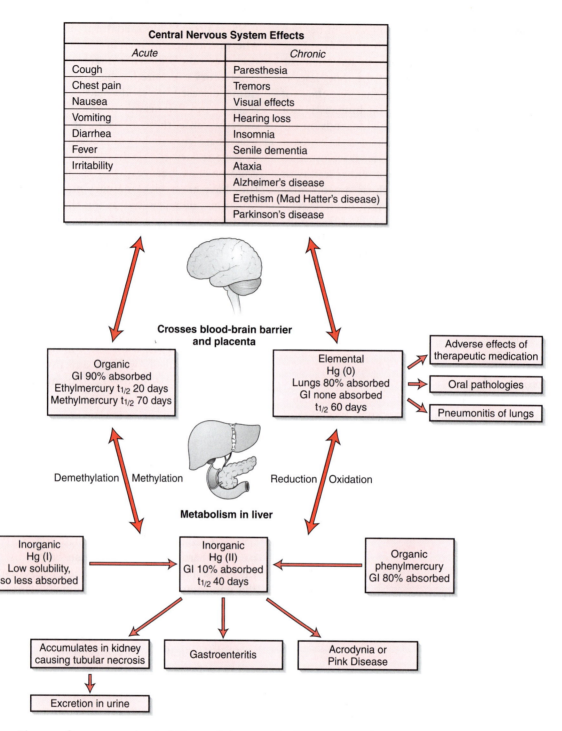

Figure 20-1. Diagram of exposure routes, toxicities, and pharmacokinetic parameters of mercury poisoning. Absorption of elemental, inorganic, and organic mercury depends on the route of exposure, as well as the chemical form of the metal. Central nervous system effects are separated by acute and chronic toxicities following elemental and organic exposure due to the ability of these mercury forms to cross the blood–brain barrier. Inorganic mercury is poorly absorbed from the gastrointestinal tract, and little inorganic mercury crosses the blood–brain barrier.

formation of reactive oxygen species (ROS)[34] are cellular effects of mercury toxicity. Mercury has been shown to inhibit $Na+ -K+ -Cl-$ cotransport[35] and to decrease adenosine triphosphate levels.[36] These effects, both individually and in combination, can lead to cell death through apoptosis, necrosis, or both (Figure 20-2).

In astrocytes, mercury inhibits the uptake of the excitatory neurotransmitters glutamate and aspartate.[11,37] Mercury further increases the extracellular levels of these amino acids by inducing their release from intracellular stores.[9,37] Such an increase in extracellular glutamate and aspartate can cause the N-methyl-d-aspartate receptors to overactivate, which could possibly cause the cell to enter into the excitotoxic cascade.[11,32] Neurodegeneration,[9] neuronal lesions,[11] and DNA damage[32] may be accelerated or develop in response to these excitotoxic effects. Due to the high affinity, approximately 10–15–10–23 of mercury for thiol groups, the major chemical reaction of mercury is with this group.[9,11] Glutathione levels in particular have been reported to be decreased due to mercury. This decrease of glutathione results in a reduced cellular defense against oxidative damage.[37] Decreased levels of glutathione also provide an opportunity for the formation and accumulation of ROS, along with the potential for an increase in damage done by other toxins from the environment.[20,37–38]

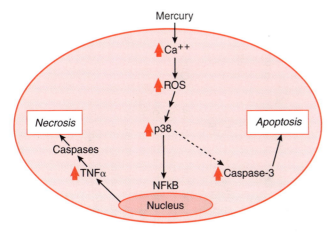

Figure 20-2. Cellular and intracellular effects of mercury involve multiple cascades. Mercury has been shown to increase intracellular calcium, which can increase the production of reactive oxygen species and p38. Elevations in p38 increase the activity of caspase-3, leading to apoptosis and nuclear factor-κB. Increased activity of tumor necrosis factor-α also increases the activity of various other caspases, resulting in cellular necrosis.

One action of ROS is to induce cell death, and at least one of mercury's effects, disrupting calcium homeostasis, can lead to an increased production of ROS.[39] Further depletion of glutathione[4] and enhanced lipid peroxidation and DNA damage[40] can occur due to ROS formation. Neuronal degeneration and cellular damage due to increased ROS production can lead to cell apoptosis, necrosis, or both (see Figure 20-2).[9,32,39]

Mercury in the nervous system can disrupt calcium homeostasis by causing an increase in intracellular calcium.[9,40] Depending on the mercury species, the resulting intracellular calcium concentrations may come from an influx from both extracellular spaces and intracellular stores.[29,40] Kim and Sharma[39] reported that this change in calcium homeostasis occurred before an increase in ROS production because ROS production could be eliminated by calcium antagonists. Mercury exposure results in a decrease in the membrane potential of mitochondria, an organelle that accumulates mercury.[39,41] This decreased membrane potential allows an efflux of Ca^{2+} out of the mitochondria, along with decreased Ca^{2+} uptake into the mitochondria.[42] This, together with the release of cytochrome c, results in the cell entering apoptosis.[39,41]

Peripheral Effects

Mercury exposure can have effects on many body systems. The renal, respiratory, cardiovascular, gastrointestinal, hepatic, immune, reproductive, and dermal systems have all been reported to have negative responses after mercury exposure. The renal system, particularly the epithelium cells of the proximal tubules, is one of the main mercury targets.[43–44] Signs of nephrotoxicity that have developed due to mercury exposure include reduced blood flow and glomerular filtration, as well as albuminuria.[38,45] The respiratory system is affected when mercury particles are inhaled. Mercury in the lungs can cause respiratory distress, pneumonitis,[23] and acute chemical bronchitis.[6] Another system affected by mercury is the cardiovascular system. Cardiovascular effects due to mercury exposure include decreased variability of heart rate, which is associated with heart failure,[46–47] and arterial hypertension caused by vascular smooth muscle contraction.[48] An increased risk for cardiovascular disease and progression of carotid atherosclerosis has been reported in individuals with mercury exposure.[4] Because mercury is corrosive to the mucous membranes, oral burning and stomatitis may occur when mercury is ingested.[23] Ulceration and hemorrhage can occur in the gastrointestinal tract with this route of mercury exposure.[35,40] Autoimmune abnormalities,[49] decreased fertility,[50] and dermatitis[2] have also been reported from exposure to mercury.

Table 3: Treatments for Mercury Intoxication Beyond Supportive Care

Chelating Agents

Drug Name	Description	Adult Dose	Pediatric Dose	Contraindications	Interactions	Preg. Class	Precautions
Dimercaprol (British anti-Lewisite)	DOC for acute Hg toxicity	3–5 mg/kg IM q4h/q2d, 2.5–3 mg/kg IM q6h/q2d, 2.5–3 mg/kg IM q12h/q7d	Same as adult	Hypersensitivity, peanut allergy, iron supplementation, methylmercury toxicity	Increase in toxicity in presence of selenium, iron, uranium, or cadmium	C	May be nephrotoxic—caution in oliguria or glucose-6-phosphate dehydrogenase deficiency; side effects include abdominal pain, bloating, headache, and increased blood pressure
Penicillamine (Cuprimine, Depen)	Complexes with Hg and excreted in urine	15–40 mg/kg/day—do not exceed 250–500 mg PO q6h ac; continue for 1 week	20–30 mg/kg/day PO every day or bid ac	Renal failure; previously documented penicillamine aplastic anemia	Increased effect of immunosuppressants or phenylbutazone; decreased digoxin effects	D	Thrombocytopenia, agranulocytosis and, aplastic anemia; GI disturbances
Succimer (Chemet)	DOC for chronic or mild Hg toxicity; also known as DMSA	10 mg/kg PO tid for 5 days, 10 mg/kg PO bid for 14 days	10 mg/kg or 350 mg/m² PO q8h–q5d, 10 mg/kg PO bid for 14 days	Hypersensitivity	Edetate calcium disodium or penicillamine	C	Caution in renal or hepatic dysfunction, mild GI irritation, strong sulfur odor; thrombocytosis, eosinophilia, and neutropenia subside when therapy is discontinued

Nonspecific Support Therapy

Drug Name	Mechanism of Action	Drug Name	Mechanism of Action
N-Acetyl cysteine	Regenerates glutathione, which is reduced in the presence of free radicals associated with Hg action	Vitamin E	Lipid-soluble vitamin that functions as a potent antioxidant
Selenium	Essential metal that is important in the function of selenoproteins (selenomethionine and selenocysteine) and functions as an antioxidant; higher concentrations of selenium can be toxic	Choline	Mainly investigational; has demonstrated some neuroprotective effects associated with glutamate and may have some neuroprotective properties following chronic exposure to methylmercury

DOC, drug of choice; DSMA, 2,3-dimercaptosuccinic acid, GI, gastrointestinal tract; Hg, mercury.

TREATMENT OF MERCURY INTOXICATION OR POISONING

Patients presenting in an emergency care environment must be given supportive care. The two major routes of exposure are via inhalation of elemental mercury and ingestion of caustic inorganic mercury. In these situations, the airway is checked to determine and remove obstructions as necessary, contaminated clothing is removed, and the sites of contact are irrigated with large amounts of water. Emesis should not be induced when inorganic mercury has been ingested. Gastric lavage is recommended for organic mercury ingestion, and activated charcoal can be administered to bind excess organic and inorganic mercury in the digestive tract. Chelating agents, which contain thiol groups, can be used if the patient is symptomatic. These agents compete with the thiol groups on proteins for the binding effects of mercury, thus removing mercury from the general circulation. These chelating agents can include the resin and polythiol, which is nonabsorbable and is efficacious for the removal of methylmercury from the digestive tract. In severe cases, hemodialysis can be used if renal function is significantly compromised. The addition of L-cysteine significantly improves the ability of hemodialysis to remove circulating mercury. A list of chelating agents, as well as some agents that have been proposed to be beneficial as nonspecific supportive agents, is found in Table 3.

CONCLUSION

Incidence of mercury exposure and intoxication has declined over the last few decades. In 2003, the annual report of the American Association of Poison Control Centers' Toxic Exposure Surveillance System reported just more than 3300 cases of mercury exposure. Less than one-fifth were children under the age of 6 years, and about half were older than 19. Less than 2% reported moderate to severe effects, and none of the individuals exposed died as a result of their exposure. Mercury compounds are highly potent but are nonspecific cellular poisons that influence many vital processes involving proteins. Mercury ions are protein precipitants and, as a result, cause severe necrosis on direct contact with tissue. They have affinity for several cellular components essential for the function and survival of the cell, such as enzymes, membrane proteins, antioxidants, nucleic acids, and mitotic apparatus. Toxicity is related to the covalent binding of mercury to sulfhydryl, carboxyl, amide, amine, and phosphoryl groups. There is still undoubtedly more to learn about the specific mechanisms of mercury-induced neurotoxicity.

REFERENCES

1. Tchounwou PB, Ayensu WK, Ninashvili N, et al. Environmental exposure to mercury and its toxicopathologic implications for public health. *Environ Toxicol.* 2003;18:149–175.
2. Saady JJ. Metals. In: Levine B, ed. *Principles in Forensic Toxicology.* Washington, DC: AACC Press; 2003:349–362.
3. Langford NJ, Ferner RE. Toxicity of mercury. *J Hum Hypertens.* 1999;13:651–656.
4. Patrick L. Mercury toxicity and antioxidants: I. Role of glutathione and alpha-lipoic acid in the treatment of mercury toxicity. *Altern Med Rev.* 2002;7:456–471.
5. International Programme on Chemical Safety. Environmental Health Criteria 118: Inorganic Mercury. Geneva: World Health Organization; 1991. Available at: http://www.inchem.org/documents/ehc/ehc/ehc118.htm. Accessed March 21, 2008.
6. Asano S, Eto K, Kurisaki E, et al. Acute inorganic mercury vapor inhalation poisoning. *Pathol Int.* 2000;50:169–174.
7. Hylander LD, Meili M. 500 years of mercury production: global annual inventory by region until 2000 and associated emissions. *Sci Total Environ.* 2003;304(1–3):13–27.
8. Ninomiya T, Ohmori H, Hashimoto K, et al. Expansion of methylmercury poisoning outside of Minamata: an epidemiological study on chronic methylmercury poisoning outside of Minamata. *Environ Res.* 1995;70:47–50.
9. Castoldi AF, Coccini T, Ceccatelli S, et al. Neurotoxicity and molecular effects of methylmercury. *Brain Res Bull.* 2001;55:197–203.
10. Gochfeld, M. Cases of mercury exposure, bioavailability, and absorption. *Ecotoxicol Environ Saf.* 2003;56:74–179.
11. Aschner M, Yao CP, Allen JW, et al. Methylmercury alters glutamate transport in astrocytes. *Neurochem Int.* 2000;37:199–206.
12. Bluhm RE, Bobbitt RG, Welch LW, et al. Elemental mercury vapor toxicity, treatment, and prognosis after acute, intensive exposure in chloralkali plant workers. I: History, neuropsychological findings and chelator effects. *Hum Exp Toxicol.* 1992;11:201–210.
13. Goering PL, Galloway WD, Clarkson TW, et al. Toxicity assessment of mercury vapor from dental amalgams. *Fund Appl Toxicol.* 1992;19:319–329.
14. Fung YK, Molvar MP. Toxicity of mercury from dental environment and from amalgam restorations. *J Toxicol Clin Toxicol.* 1992;30:49–61.
15. Enwonwu CO. Potential health hazard of use of mercury in dentistry: critical review of the literature. *Environ Res.* 1998;42:257–274.
16. Mjor IA. Side effects of dental materials. *BMJ (Clin Res Ed).* 1994;309:621–622.
17. Halbach S. Amalgam tooth fillings and man's mercury burden. *Hum Exp Toxicol.* 1994;13:496–501.
18. Aposhian HV, Maiorino RM, Rivera M, et al. Human studies with the chelating agents, DMPS and DMSA. *J Toxicol Clin Toxicol.* 1992;30:505–528.
19. Thompson CM, Markesbery WR, Ehmann WD, et al. Regional brain trace-element studies in Alzheimer's disease. *Neurotoxicology.* 1988;9:1–7.
20. Vicente E, Boer M, Netto C, et al. Hippocampal antioxidant system in neonates from methylmercury intoxicated rats. *Neurotoxicol Teratol.* 2004;26:817–823.
21. Bertossi M, Girolamo F, Errede M, et al. Effects of methylmercury on the microvasculature of the developing brain. *Neurotoxicology.* 2004;25:849–857.
22. Blaxill MF, Redwood L, Bernard S. Thimerosal and autism? A plausible hypothesis that should not be dismissed. *Med Hypotheses.* 2004;62:788–794.

23. Graeme KA, Pollack CV. Heavy metal toxicity: I. Arsenic and mercury. *J Emerg Med.* 1998;16:45–56.

24. McCabe MJ, Eckles KG, Langdon M, et al. Attenuation of CD95-induced apoptosis by inorganic mercury: caspase-3 is not a direct target of low levels of Hg2+. *Toxicol Lett.* 2005;155: 161–170.

25. Hess EV. Environmental chemicals and autoimmune disease: cause and effect. *Toxicology.* 2002;181–182:65–70.

26. Bernard S, Enayati A, Redwood L, et al. Autism: a novel form of mercury poisoning. *Med Hypotheses.* 2001;56:462–471.

27. Hock C, Drasch G, Golombowski S, et al. Increased blood mercury levels in patients with Alzheimer's disease. *J Neural Transm.* 1998;105:59–68.

28. Olivieri G, Brack C, Muller-Spahn F, et al. Mercury induces cell cytotoxicity and oxidative stress and increases β-amyloid secretion and tau phosphorylation in SHSY5Y neuroblastoma cells. *J Neurochem.* 2000;74:231–236.

29. Gasso S, Cristofol RM, Selema G, et al. Antioxidant compounds and Ca2+ pathway blockers differentially protect against methylmercury and mercuric chloride neurotoxicity. *J Neurosci Res.* 2001;66:135–145.

30. Papp A, Nagymajtenyi L, Vezer T. Subchronic mercury treatment of rats in different phases of ontogenesis: functional effects on the central and peripheral nervous system. *Food Chem Toxicol.* 2005;43:77–85.

31. Costa LG, Aschner M, Vitalone A, et al. Developmental neuropathology of environmental agents. *Ann Rev Pharmacol Toxicol.* 2004;44:87–110.

32. Juarez BI, Portillo-Salazar H, Gonzalez-Amaro R, et al. Participation of *N*-methyl-d-aspartate receptors on methylmercury-induced DNA damage in rat frontal cortex. *Toxicology.* 2005;207:223–229.

33. Bucio L, Garcia C, Souza V, et al. Uptake, cellular distribution and DNA damage produced by mercuric chloride in a human fetal hepatic cell line. *Mutat Res.* 1999;423:65–72.

34. Ercal N, Gurer-Orhan H, Aykin-Burns N. Toxic metals and oxidative stress: I. Mechanisms involved in metal-induced oxidative damage. *Curr Topics Med Chem.* 2001;1:529–539.

35. Jacoby SC, Gagnon E, Caron L, et al. Inhibition of Na+−K+−2Cl− cotransport by mercury. *Am J Physiol.* 1999;277:C684–692.

36. Fonfria E, Vilaro MT, Babot Z, et al. Mercury compounds disrupt neuronal glutamate transport in cultured mouse cerebellar granule cells. *J Neurosci Res.* 2005;79:545–553.

37. Shanker G, Aschner M. Identification and characterization of uptake systems for cystine and cysteine in cultured astrocytes and neurons: evidence for methylmercury-targeted disruption of astrocyte transport. *J Neurosci Res.* 2001;66:998–1002.

38. Crinnion WJ. Environmental medicine: III. Long-term effects of chronic low-dose mercury exposure. *Altern Med Rev.* 2000;5:209–223.

39. Kim SH, Sharma RP. Mercury-induced apoptosis and necrosis in murin macrophages: role of calcium-induced oxygen species and p38 mitogen-activated protein kinase signaling. *Toxicol Appl Pharmacol.* 2004;196:47–57.

40. Stohs SJ, Bagchi D. Oxidative mechanisms in the toxicity of metal ions. *Free Rad Biol Med.* 1995;18:321–336.

41. Toimela T, Tahti H. Mitochondrial viability and apoptosis induced by aluminum, mercuric mercury and methylmercury in cell lines of neural origin. *Archiv Fuer Toxikologie.* 2004;78: 565–574.

42. Atchinson WD, Hare MF. Mechanisms of methylmercury-induced neurotoxicity. *FASEB J.* 1994;8:622–629.

43. Carranza-Rosales P, Said-Fernandez S, Sepulveda-Saavedra J, et al. Morphologic and functional alterations induced by low doses of mercuric chloride in the kidney OK cell line: ultrastructural evidence for an apoptotic mechanism of damage. *Toxicology.* 2005;210:111–121.

44. Aleo MF, Morandini F, Bettoni F, et al. Endogenous thiols and MRP transporters contribute to Hg2+ efflux in HgCl2-treated tubular MDCK cells. *Toxicology.* 2005;206:137–154.

45. Van Vleet TR, Schnellmann RG. Toxic nephropathy: environmental chemicals. *Semin Nephrol.* 2003;23:500–508.

46. Grandjean P, Murata K, Budtz-Jorgensen E, et al. Cardiac autonomic activity in methylmercury neurotoxicity: 14-year follow-up of a Faroese birth cohort. *J Pediatr.* 2004;144:169–176.

47. De Jong MJ, Randall DC. Heart rate variability analysis in the assessment of autonomic function in heart failure. *J Cardiovasc Nurs.* 2005;20:186–195.

48. Golpon HA, Puchner A, Barth P, et al. Nitric oxide–dependent vasorelaxation and endothelial cell damage caused by mercury chloride. *Toxicology.* 2003;192:179–188.

49. Ben-Ozer EY, Rosenspire AJ, McCabe MJ Jr, et al. Mercuric chloride damages cellular DNA by a non-apoptotic mechanism. *Mutat Res.* 2000;470:19–27.

50. Horsted-Bindslev P. Amalgam toxicity: environmental and occupational hazards. *J Dentistry.* 2004;32:359–365.

Lead I: Epidemiology

Larry W. Figgs

INTRODUCTION

Epidemiology was not rigorously applied to plumbism until the later half of the 20th century, partly because modern epidemiological methods were not available until then. Lead is a prevalent environmental metal and a recognized neurological toxin.[1] Worldwide, prevalent lead exposure varies. Leaded gasoline combustion, indoor paint use in residential settings, and solder (tin cans) are common exposure vectors that account for much of the variability. Countries that restrict use of these vectors have populations with significantly lower blood lead levels (BLLs) than do countries that allow leaded gasoline, paints, and solder use. For example, after the United States banned the sale of leaded gasoline for automobiles, leaded paints for residential use, and leaded solder for tin can manufacture and plumbing during the 1970s, the proportion of children 1 to 5 years old with a BLL greater than or equal to 10 $\mu g/dL$ decreased from 88% before 1976 to approximately 3% in 2007.

CHILDREN

Among all newborn to 72-month-old children tested since 1997 in U.S. Centers for Disease Control and Prevention (CDC) state programs, the percentage of confirmed elevated BLL cases (i.e., BLL greater than 0 $\mu g/dL$) decreased from 7.6% in 1997 to 1.2% in 2006.[2,3] The estimated mean BLL is below 5 $\mu g/dL$. Lead's neurotoxic effects, at levels below 10 $\mu g/dL$, are associated with poor childhood cognitive function in a dose–response manner.[1] However, unlike some diseases that abate once the environmental toxin is removed, elevated BLLs affecting early brain development (in utero to 72 months) can lead to lifelong cognitive dysfunction. Consequently, clinically elevated BLLs in early life continue to be a major public health problem.

Federal agencies recommend action and intervention when a BLL is 10 $\mu g/dL$ or higher for children younger than 72 months old. States are free to determine the extent to which services are provided when BLLs exceed 10 $\mu g/dL$.

ADULTS

The CDC's Adult Blood Lead Epidemiology and Surveillance (ABLES) program in Atlanta, Georgia, tracks laboratory-reported BLLs among employed adults in the United States.[3] The ABLES program selected BLLs of at least 25 $\mu g/dL$ and BLLs of at least 40 $\mu g/dL$ as key action and intervention levels respectively, for adults. The first level, a BLL of at least 25 $\mu g/dL$, is based on the U.S. Health and Human Service's 2010 objective to reduce the prevalence of BLLs of at least 25 μg/dL among employed adults to 0 μg/dL.[4] The second level, a BLL of at least 40 μg/dL, is based on the level at which the U.S. Department of Labor's Occupational Safety and Health Administration requires workers to have an annual medical evaluation of health effects related to lead exposure.[5,6] ABLES data indicate that the incidence of an elevated BLL of at least 25 μg/dL declined from 2002 to 2004. However, projections using 1994 to 2004 ABLES data trends indicate that the national prevalence of adults with BLLs of at least 25 μg/dL will be approximately 5.7 per 100,000 employed adults in 2010.[7]

There is little evidence that BLLs below 30 μg/dL are neurotoxic in adult humans. Among subjects with BLLs at or above 40 μg/dL (1.2 cases per 100,000 employed 16- to 64-year-olds), a clinician might observe reduced nerve conduction velocities. Severe encephalopathy, risk drop, and peripheral neuritis are signs that appear when BLLs are at or above 100 μg/dL.

EXPOSURE VECTORS

Plumbism exists worldwide because many societies have not developed policies that regulate the manufacture, use, and disposal of lead and lead-base products. Even when production and use are regulated, some occupational tasks still carry significant lead exposure risk. Less common, but no less important, exposures occur among frequent travelers and populations experiencing significant immigration, especially if the immigrants are from countries where lead production and use of lead-based products are unregulated or poorly regulated. Less frequent exposure may occur among populations who routinely eat ethnic foods stored in lead-soldered tin cans or who use medicinal folk remedies containing lead.

U.S. exposure vectors may include leaded paints and lead-contaminated dust or soil, drinking water, occupations or hobbies, food, and food containers. Folk medicine vectors are also a concern.[8] Among U.S. children, indoor

Table 1: Industries Reporting Highest Number of Resident Workers 16 Years or Older with Elevated Blood Lead Levels (BLLs)[*†]

Industry	Total Workers with Elevated[‡] BLLs	Among All Workers with Elevated BLLs, % with BLLs ≥ 40 μg/dL
Storage batteries manufacturing (SIC 3691, NAICS 335911)	2499	6
Painting, paperhanging, and decorating (SIC 1721, NAICS 238320)	626	25
Lead ore mining (SIC 1031, NAICS 212231)	482	20
Secondary smelting (SIC 3341, NAICS 331492)	300	13
Bridge and tunnel construction (SIC 1622, NAICS 237310)	211	21
Primary battery manufacturing (SIC 3692, NAICS 335912)	210	19
Primary smelting (SIC 3339, NAICS 331419)	200	13
Lead paint removal (SIC 1799, NAICS 562910)	160	25
Copper foundries (SIC 3366, NAICS 331525)	114	18
Roll and draw nonferrous metals (SIC 3356, NAICS 331491)	90	18

[*]Adult Blood Lead Epidemiology and Surveillance program, Unites States, 2003–2004.
[‡]Elevated BLL ≥ 25 μg/dL.
[†]Based on Alaska, Arizona, California, Connecticut, Florida, Georgia, Hawaii, Illinois, Iowa, Kansas, Maine, Maryland, Massachusetts, Michigan, Minnesota, Missouri, Montana, Nebraska, New Hampshire, New Jersey, New Mexico, New York, North Carolina, Ohio, Oklahoma, Oregon, Pennsylvania, South Carolina, Texas, Utah, Washington, and Wisconsin.
NAICS = North American Industry Classification System; SIC = Standard Industrial Classification.
Adapted from Roscoe RJ, Graydon JR. Adult blood lead epidemiology and surveillance. *MMWR.* 2006;55:876.

and outdoor leaded paints, lead-contaminated dust or soil, and occupational clothing worn home by family members are the primary exposure vectors. The most frequently used strategies to prevent early childhood lead poisoning include identifying residences with lead paints (typically homes built before 1978), providing hazard mitigation strategies to at-risk populations, and providing risk mitigation education to lead-based industry employers and employees. A history of the child's current and past residential, preschool, and recreational sites often reveals the location of important exposure vectors. Removing the toxic vector from the environment is one of the key steps in treating diseases caused by this environmental neurotoxin.

The more common adult exposure vectors are occupational exposure (Table 1), leaded (indoor and outdoor) paints, and dust in the United States. However, unlike for children, occupation and hobby vectors play greater roles. Manufacturing, construction, and mining account for the highest annual averages. Shooting firearms, remodeling or renovation activities, hobbies (casting, ceramics, or stained glass), and gunshot wounds accounted for 23%, 13%, 11%, and 5%, respectively, of the important nonoccupational sources that produced annual BLL of at least 25 µg/dL (not shown in Table 1). Pica, ingesting lead-contaminated food or liquids, traditional or folk medicines, and retired workers accounted for 3% each. Interestingly, although we might expect a recall bias favoring an occupational exposure and some current or prospective health outcome, nonoccupational exposure from an unknown origin accounted for slightly more than a third, 36%, of the cases with an annual average BLL greater than 25 µg/dL. The specific industries with the highest frequencies were lead battery manufacturing; painting, paperhanging, and decorating; and lead ore mining.

A simple way to develop an exposure history is to consider where and how the exposure occurred: At home? Outdoors? At work? Combining the initial letters of each main word into the acronym HOW creates a simple memory tool to assess the location of potential exposure vectors (Figure 21-1).

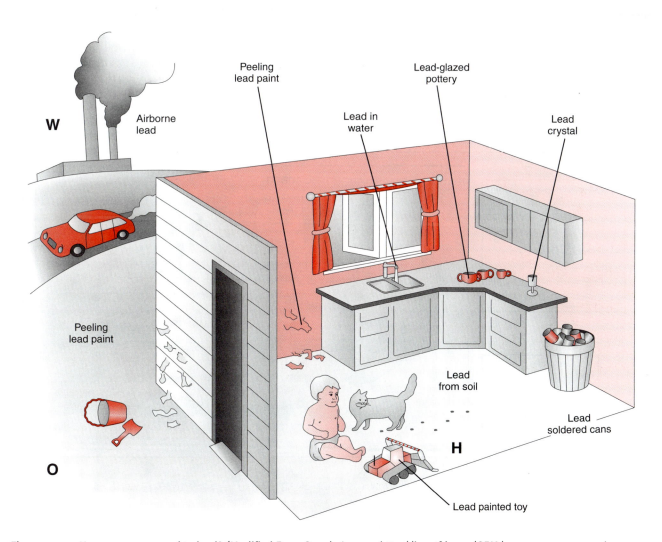

Figure 21-1. How are we exposed to lead? (Modified From Google Images http://img.tfd.com/GEM/gem_0003_0003_0_img0397.jpg. Accessed August 23, 2008.)

PREVALENCE

In 2005, the most recent year for which the CDC provided complete data on 37 of 50 states, the U.S. prevalence of BLLs greater than 25 μg/dL was approximately 7.4 cases per 100,000 employed workers 16 to 64 years old.[3] The U.S. prevalence in 2002, 2003, and 2004 was 9.2, 8.7, and 7.8 cases, respectively, per 100,000 employed workers of the same age group. The stratum-specific prevalence of BLLs elevated above 25 μg/dL, based on 37 reporting states, ranged from 0.5 cases per 100,000 workers 16 to 64 years old in Hawaii to 34 cases per 100,000 workers 16 to 64 years old in Kansas (including resident and nonresident workers). The three lowest prevalence estimates for employed workers 16 to 64 years old in 2005 were observed in Hawaii, New Mexico, and Arizona, with estimates of 0.5, 0.6, and 0.7 cases per 100,000 workers, respectively. The three highest prevalence estimates for employed workers 16 to 64 years old in 2005 were observed in Alabama, Missouri, and Kansas, with estimates of 29.6, 30.9, and 34.0 cases per 100,000 workers, respectively. Figure 21-2 illustrates the U.S. state-specific prevalence distribution for employed adults 16 to 64 years of age in 2005.

INCIDENCE

The 2005 U.S. incidence of BLLs greater than 25 μg/dL was approximately 4.4 cases per 100,000 employed workers 16 to 64 years old.[3] The U.S. incidence in 2002, 2003, and 2004 was 5.3, 5.4, and 4.9 cases, respectively, per 100,000 employed workers of the same age group. The stratum-specific incidence of BLLs elevated above 25 μg/dL, based on the same 37 reporting states from which the preceding prevalence data were derived, ranged from 0.3 cases per 100,000 workers 16 to 64 years old in Hawaii to 21.5 per 100,000 workers 16 to 64 years old in Kansas (including resident and nonresident workers). The three lowest incidence estimates for employed workers 16 to 64 years old in 2005 were observed in Hawaii, Arizona, and New Jersey, with estimates of 0.3, 0.4, and 0.5 cases per 100,000 workers, respectively. Using data from a 37-state sample,[3] the three highest incidence estimates of 15.3, 18.9, and 21.5 cases per 100,000 workers for employed workers 16 to 64 years old in 2005 were observed in Missouri, Pennsylvania, and Kansas, respectively. Figure 21-3 illustrates the U.S. state-specific incidence trends among employed adults 16 to 64 years of age in 2005.

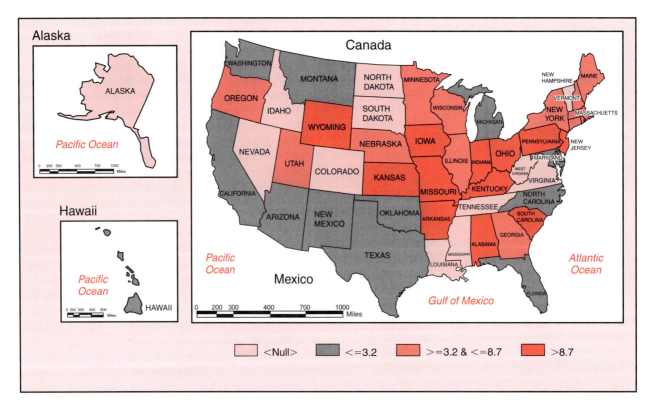

Figure 21-2. U.S. elevated blood lead level prevalence. The scale shows the number of new and existing cases with blood lead levels of at least 25 μg/dL among 100,000 employed adults 16 to 64 years old in 2005. Null category states did not report.

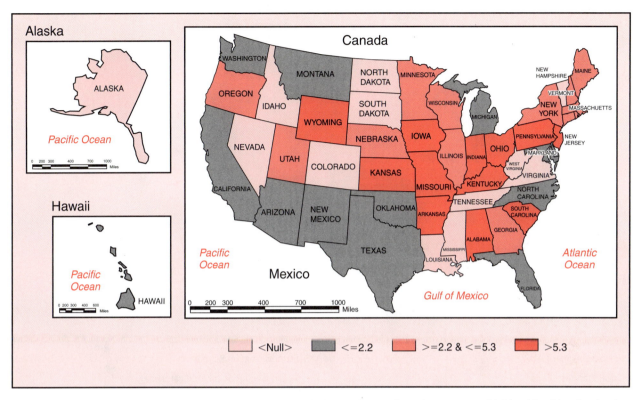

Figure 21-3. U.S. elevated blood lead level incidence. The scale shows the number of new cases with blood lead levels of at least 25 μg/dL that occurred among 100,000 employed adults 16 to 64 years old in 2005. Null category states did not report.

REFERENCES

1. Toscano CD, Guilarte TR. Lead neurotoxicity: from exposure to molecular effects. *Brain Res Brain Res Rev.* 2005;49: 529–554.
2. Centers for Disease Control and Prevention. Surveillance Data, 1997–2006: Tested and Confirmed Elevated Blood Lead Levels by State, Year, and Blood Lead Level Group for Children Less than 72 Months Old. Available at: http://www.cdc.gov/nceh/lead/surv/stats.htm. Accessed August 22, 2008.
3. Centers for Disease Control and Prevention, National Institute of Occupational Safety and Health. Adult Blood Lead Epidemiology and Surveillance (ABLES): Blood Lead Level Data: Reported from 2002 through 2005 CDC/NIOSH Adult Blood Lead Epidemiology and Surveillance Program. Available at: http://www.cdc.gov/niosh/topics/ABLES/2002-2005%20lead_data.xls. Accessed August 22, 2008.
4. U.S. Department of Health and Human Services. Healthy People 2010. Reduce the Number of Persons Who Have Elevated Blood Lead Concentrations from Work Exposures. Available at: http://www.healthypeople.gov/document/html/objectives/20-07.htm. Accessed August 22, 2008.
5. Occupational Safety and Health Administration, U.S. Department of Labor. Lead exposure in construction: interim rule. *Fed Regist.* 1993;58:26590–26649. [29 CFR § 1926.62].
6. Occupational Safety and Health Administration, U.S. Department Labor. Final: standard occupational exposure standard to lead. *Fed Regist.* 1978;43:52952–53014. [29 CFR § 1910.1025].
7. Roscoe RJ, Graydon JR. Adult blood lead epidemiology and surveillance. *MMWR.* 2006;55:876.
8. Karri SK, Saper RB, Kales SN. Lead encephalopathy due to traditional medicines. *Curr Drug Saf.* 2008;3:54–59.

Lead II: Neurotoxicity

Ray F. Garman

INTRODUCTION

Lead, a heavy (molecular weight 207.19) bluish–grayish metal, is found in the Earth, usually as a compound but occasionally as a metal (in four stable isotopes). It is the stable end state of decay of uranium, actinium, and thorium radioactivity. Easily molded, with a relatively low melting point (327.5°C); resistant to corrosion; a poor electrical conductor; and insoluble in water, it is widely used industrially, both as metal and as a compound. Certain uses have been dramatically reduced in recent years because of concerns outlined in this chapter. Major compounds are lead acetate (water repellant, mildew protection), lead chloride (brake linings), lead nitrate (matches, paper coating), and lead subacetate (sugar analysis), all of which are somewhat water soluble.

Numerous relatively insoluble compounds are also used. These include lead arsenate (insecticide, now generally not used), lead azide (explosives), lead chromate (pigment), lead oxide (rubber and plastics), and lead sulfate (photography). A host of other lead compounds have many other industrial uses. (See www.atsdr.cdc.gov/toxfag.html for related information from the Agency for Toxic Substances and Disease Registry, Public Health Service, CAS 7439-92-1.)

Lead is mined as an ore—galena, anglesite, or cerussite—and is often mixed with other metal ores. Most lead comes from Australia, China, the United States, Peru, Canada, and Mexico. Significant lead for industrial use now comes from scrap recycling, especially from lead-acid batteries.[1]

An earlier caution for lead phosphate and lead acetate, which were reasonably expected to be human carcinogens, has been widened to include lead compounds in general.[2] Organic lead compounds (such as tetraethyl lead) were in automotive gasoline until early 1996 and were source of much lead in the air before that time. This caused significant deposition of lead into the soil, but the level has since been dramatically reduced from this source.[1] (Some lead-added gasoline is still sold for aircraft as "100 low lead" and for automotive racing). Organic leads are significantly absorbed through the skin.

An estimate 6% of ingested lead is absorbed with a meal, but much more is absorbed if the individual has been fasting for 24 hours (60% to 80%); an estimated 50% is absorbed by children. Absorption is increased in iron-, calcium-, and vitamin D–deficient individuals. After several weeks, 94% of absorbed lead is in adult bones; 73% of absorbed lead is in children's bones. The estimated half-life in blood is 36 days.[1]

Excretion of absorbed lead is through urine (an estimated 75%) and bile (an estimated 15%), with the balance in saliva, sweat, nails and hair, and breast milk.[3]

DIAGNOSIS OF LEAD TOXICITY

There are many avenues of lead exposure, some obscure.

In Leipzig, over a 3- to 4-month period, 29 young patients were admitted with abdominal cramps, nausea, fatigue, and anemia. Most had headache, and some had additional neurological symptoms, including encephalopathy and extensor palsy in the forearm. Blood lead levels (BLLs) of up to 457 µg/dL were found. It took 8 weeks to discern that the source was street-purchased marijuana (sold by weight, with lead granules added to increase sale weight to unsuspecting purchasers). The heated lead was inhaled with the marijuana.[4]

In Newark, New Jersey, community athletic fields were found to have lead incorporated into nylon or nylon–polyethylene fibers (but not into polyethylene-only fibers). These fields, particularly if weathered or worn, had sufficiently high potential for lead exposure to pose a potential public health concern to the Centers for Disease Control and Prevention (CDC). The CDC recommended testing dust from such fields with nylon–nylon blend fibers and, and if dust contains more than 400 ppm lead, not allowing turf access to children younger than 6 years, ensuring protection of drinking containers from dust, and segregating playing clothes and shoes to ensure no spread of potential lead dust.[5]

Hobbyists may heat lead in stained glass work, use lead in ceramic glazes or incorporate it into homemade candles; and creators and downstream users of these products may be unaware of the lead hazard. "Flake white" oil paint used by artists contains lead carbonate (expressly *not* currently prohibited by the U.S. Consumer Product Safety Commission for this use).

The risks of older houses and lead-based paint are well known. Although lead was ordered removed from house paint in 1978, it is still widely extant.[1] Scraping or sanding of old paint may leave lead dust, creating a hazard in the soil around an older structure. Heating lead paint to facilitate removal increases the hazard of inhaled lead. Chipping of windowsills previously painted with lead paint may cause ingestion via pica (Box 1).

Other lead hazards in the home must be considered: a lead worker's clothes, shoes, and equipment may contaminate the house from outside environments, and previous hobby use of lead may be unknown to current inhabitants. Lead dust from paint

---

Box 1

Although lead was ordered removed from household paint in 1978, risk continues due to persistence of paint in houses. House paint produced before 1950 had higher concentrations of lead. Commercial lead test kits for surface and water lead content screening for home use are available (www.leadcheck.com) (Figure 22-1). These kits do not require technical expertise.

However, full assessment and remediation of a lead-contaminated structure or environment is a difficult task, and specialized knowledge and techniques are required to complete this successfully. Accordingly, reliance on a screening test kit alone is insufficient if risk history suggests lead contamination.

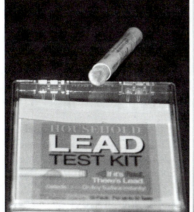 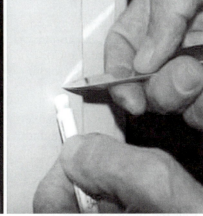

Figure 22-1. A positive result on a home test kit for lead *(left)*. The knife is scraping diagonally through several levels of paint to expose each level to the test wick *(right)*.

CASE STUDY

A self-employed contractor, who specialized in painting old houses, was seen in consultation after being hospitalized for evaluation of deterioration of judgment, irritability, confusion, and abdominal cramping. His family reported that he knew he should wear appropriate lead-protective respiratory gear but usually did not. Physical findings were nonspecific. He did not have peripheral motor neuropathy signs, discoloration of gums (Burton's lead line), or peripheral pallor—all classic signs of lead toxicity. Laboratory studies showed a BLL of 157 μg/dL and hemoglobin of 11.7 gm/dL. Basophilic stippling was not described, and a zinc protoporphyrin (ZPP) level was not reported. The BLL dropped to 24 μg/dL after succimer, rising to 43 μg/dL 1 month after succimer treatment. This latter level was considered fairly typical for someone with a high total body lead level, reflecting mobilization of body stores. He was asymptomatic at that time and was not retreated with succimer, although this was considered. He was instructed to change his work clothes usage, i.e., changing and bagging them for washing before leaving the work site; instructed in correct respirator mask usage; and taught to implement better worksite dust control. He continues to do well.

on vinyl miniblinds made before 1997 and lead dust from ammunition reloading are among other potential sources. Water service entrances of lead pipe, even if the internal household plumbing does not contain lead, are not uncommon. This may lead to elevated lead levels in a house's water supply. All such hazards, as they are identified, must be remediated to prevent lead reexposure.

Some natural remedies and botanical products contain significant lead. Ground galena (kohl) is a cosmetic used in many cultures and was brought into the United States for this purpose. (It is not supposed to be sold in the United States today.)

Of 230 medications tested, 20.7% traditional Indian ayurvedic medications were reported to have detectable lead, mercury, or arsenic in 2008.[6] Saper et al. found these 20.7% of metal-containing products exceeded at least one standard for lead, mercury, or arsenic medications. These were found in medications manufactured in both the United States and India from 37 manufacturers (one supplier refused to fill the order of 14 products after recognizing the authors had published a previous

study of ayurvedic medications). Lead was found in 20.9% of U.S.-manufactured products and 16.9% of Indian-manufactured products.[6] Medications designated as RASA Shastra are indicated as specifically containing heavy metals. Those with this designation had lead in 40.6% of them (median lead was 11.5 μg/g, range 2.5 to 25,590 μg/g). Medications considered non–RASA Shastra had lead in 15.2% of them (median lead was 7.0 μg/g, range 3.0 to 20.5 μg/g). The American National Standards Institute–National Sanitation Foundation International Dietary Supplement Standard 173 recommends that the lead ingestion limit should be 20 μg/day. A 1998 communication indicated 10% of 251 assayed Asian patent medicines contained lead, at a quantity of at least 10 ppm (median value was 29.8 ppm, range 10 to 319 ppm). Arsenic and mercury were also seen.[7]

All this suggests that the clinician must often be extraordinarily wide ranging in elucidating history, because a major premise in treatment is to insure that the treated patient does not resume exposure to a lead-contaminated environment (Box 2).

Avoidance of a return to a lead hazard environment is especially important in children, as they seem to be especially sensitive to the effects of lead. BLLs of 5 to 10 μg/dL have been associated with intellectual impairment.[8] Children are exposed, and retain, lead universally, as can be seen from BLLs around the world (Figure 22-2).[9]

Because BLLs of 5 to 10 μg/dL in children are suspect, lowering BLLs in children is meaningful. Lowering BLLs, and thus the total body burden of lead, may prevent the development of significantly less therapy-responsive neurological phenomena associated with lead toxicity, such as

Box 2

Mushak P. Lead remediation and changes in human lead exposure: some physiological and biokinetic dimensions. *Sci Total Environ.* 2003;303:35–50.

Office of Pollution Prevention and Toxics, U.S. Environmental Protection Agency. Testing Your Home for Lead in Paint, Dust, and Soil. EPA 2000; Publication 747-K-00-001. Available at: http://www.epa.gov/lead. Accessed July 26, 2008.

Office of Healthy Homes and Lead Hazard Control, U.S. Department of Housing and Urban Development/U.S. Environmental Protection Agency/Centers for Disease Control and Prevention. Paint Safety: A Field Guide for Painting, Home Maintenance, and Renovation Work. HUD 2001; Publication HUD-1779-LHC. Available at: http://www.hud.gov/offices/lead. Accessed July 6, 2008.

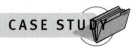

CASE STUDY

Two subcontractors in a battery plant were replacing exhaust ductwork, used for control of lead oxide dust. They were using dust masks over light beards, reportedly never having had respiratory fit testing. They were referred to my office after a local physician suspected lead toxicity due to headache, lethargy, and confusion. BLLs of 78 and 157 μg/dL were found, and succimer treatment was initiated. Symptoms responded slowly to chelation. Evaluation of the floorboards in the commuting truck and the back porch laundry of the employee driving to the job site showed significant lead dust, with remediation required for both areas.

diminished cognition.[10] The current CDC recommended maximum value for childhood BLL is 10 μg/dL (some think 5 μg/dL should be used because of evidence such as that reviewed earlier). Accordingly, stringent lead dust control in the child's environment, such as from work clothing and shoes and other household contamination, must be achieved in addition to specific treatment.

Treatment of children with elevated BLLs, after environmental remediation of lead contamination and potential of future contamination, is with chelation, plus insurance of good nutritional intake of calcium, iron, and zinc, as deficiencies of these minerals promote

retention of lead and perhaps increase intestinal absorption of lead.[1] Perhaps, however, the only truly effective measure is avoidance of lead exposure.

With continuing low-level accumulation, a transient higher lead exposure may elicit a previous clinically unapparent encephalopathy or neuropathy manifestation. Lead screening, which helps bring about reduction of the total body lead burden, may prevent these subclinical entities from progressing.

A telling indication of the ubiquity of lead exposure is the estimation of positive balance (retention) of 10 μg of lead daily lifelong.[11]

CLINICAL MANIFESTATIONS

Typical acute symptoms of lead toxicity are as follows:

- Headache
- Memory or behavioral deterioration
- Abdominal colic or vomiting
- Hematological changes
- Muscle or joint discomfort

More chronic exposure manifestations include the following:

- Muscle wasting
- Encephalopathy
- Peripheral neuropathy

Lead has been associated with cerebrovascular disease, a small increase in blood pressure, decreased glomerular filtration rate, hormonal changes, decreased vitamin D metabolism, and possibly changes in T-cell function and increased immunoglobulin E levels.[1]

Delayed Effects of Lead

Reports from White et al. suggest lead exposure was associated with poor performance on cognitive motor function tests in a group 50 years after childhood lead poisoning.[12] They quoted the Needleman study showed 14.2% of the lead-exposed subjects reported less than a 12th-grade education versus 3.1% of the control group (Lead exposure in this case measured from dentin concentrations in shed teeth).

Encephalopathy

The most severe manifestation of lead toxicity is lead encephalopathy, with symptoms of irritability, headache, lethargy, memory loss, and confusion being typical and the most severe symptoms being convulsions, delirium, and coma. Historically, this has been reported with a

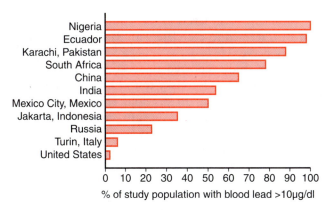

Figure 22-2. Prevalence of elevated blood lead in the United States and internationally. Elevated blood lead is considered a blood lead level greater than the current Centers for Disease Control and Prevention blood lead level of concern (more than 10 μg/dL). (From Toscano CD, Guilarte TR. Lead neurotoxicity: from exposure to molecular effects. *Brain Res Rev.* 2005;49:529–554.)

very high BLL (more than 300 µg/dL), but more recently encephalopathy has been reported at levels of 40 to 80 µg/dL. This has been reported with exposure to moonshine whiskey and has been reported as more common in older females.

The convulsions may be refractory to anticonvulsants. The headache and vomiting may be signs of associated brain edema. Irritability may be due to a lower threshold to stimuli.

Rapid treatment with a sequence of chelation and supportive care is indicated.[13]

Neurocognition

Schwartz et al. noted in a group of several hundred Korean lead workers with lead levels of 29 to 50 µg/dL that subclinical neurocognitive defects were present.[14]

A study in young adults after childhood exposure is detailed in the "Bunker Hill Experience."[15] In this epidemiological survey, approximately 280 individuals were managed with numerous studies, including peripheral nerve function and sensory and behavioral evaluations. They reported that decrements were seen in the sural sensory nerve, peroneal motor nerve, vibrotactile thresholds (fingers), and standing steadiness. More neuropsychiatric symptoms were seen in the lead-exposed group. The exposure group had poor performance on hand–eye coordination; simple reaction time; and simple digit, serial digit, learning wave, and progressive matrices in vocabulary tests. (The study's authors could not relate a significant association between neurological outcomes and tibial bone lead concentration.)[15] A study from Verona showed workers with BLLs of 45 to 60 µg/dL reported more physical symptoms and had poorer overall performance in perceptual and psychomotor tasks, such as a digital–symbol substitution test and picture completion, and in verbal ability, such as vocabulary and similarities, compared to matched workers with BLLs lower than 35 µg/dL and a group not exposed to lead.[16]

Stollery found that a detriment in process–response time was associated with a high lead group (41 to 80 µg/dL) but not with those with lower lead levels.[17]

Peripheral Neuropathy

Motor neuropathy of most active peripheral nerves is the classical finding. Chia et al. suggest that the median nerve is the most commonly affected, and this is supported by clinical experience.[18] This group has also suggested a BLL of 82.5 µg/dL is associated with abnormal nerve conduction velocity test results; a BLL of 29 µg/dL is not different from controls (posing the question of a 30- to 70-µg/dL range for an effect). The authors add that a nerve conduction velocity test is probably the wrong test (i.e., axonal deterioration found is not sensitive to this test).[18]

Lead Colic

Lead toxicity may present with abdominal cramps, nausea, and vomiting—a complex sometimes called lead colic. This toxicity is thought to typically occur at a high BLL (more than 100 µg/dL). However, some have reported these symptoms at a BLL as low as 40 µg/dL in adults.[19] An illustrative case report is that of a 47-year-old man who was hospitalized twice previously without correct diagnosis and presented with fatigue, diffuse abdominal cramps, constipation, and paresthesias of the upper extremities. He had a "lead line" (Burton's line) but apparently had not been asked about his work (battery recycling). His BLL was 148 µg/dL, and basophilic stippling was noted. Treated with 5-day cycles of ethylenediaminetetraacetic acid (EDTA; for three cycles) his BLL gradually dropped to 16 µg/dL.[20]

Middle Ear Effects

Lead is known to affect the middle ear. Experimental evidence shows damage to the Schwann cells of the auditory nerves. A group of 359 lead smelter workers with a mean BLL of 27.7 µg/dL (standard deviation 8.4, range 4.0 to 62 µg/dL) was studied. This group was on average 40.7 years old (standard deviation 9.08 years, range 20 to 63). Brainstem-evoked potentials were prolonged in those over 40 years of age. Bleecker et al. calculated an estimated cumulative lead dose over the working lifetime and found that conduction in the auditory canal, auditory pathway, and brainstem was inversely related to the cumulative lead levels in the study. They concluded that BLL seemed to correlate with damage to the distal auditory nerve.[21,22]

Another study reported on postural balance, gait, and the Bruininks-Oseretsky test of motor proficiency. This was a follow-up to previous studies suggesting that early childhood lead exposure was associated with increase of postural instability.[23] The authors concluded that there was possible damage to function of the vestibular or proprioception systems modulated by the cerebrum.

CONFIRMATION OF LEAD TOXICITY

The simple approach to confirmation of suspected lead-associated disorders is to test BLLs. Blood lead reflects the lead that is available from soft tissue and is more an indication of acute exposure and less an indication of the total body burden of lead. Of the total burden, 10% of lead is in blood, mostly in erythrocytes, and most of the balance is in bone. Bone deposition of lead is into cancellous bone and dense calcified bone. The former has more easily mobilized lead and might be considered an access site that is intermediate in accessibility to the total body lead burden. Blood heavy metal screening tests are readily available; a typical one tests for mercury, arsenic, and lead.

Bone has been suggested as a source of mobilized lead in pregnancy and lactation, as rises in BLLs from previous levels is often seen in pregnancy and in breast milk (thus the American Conference of Governmental Industrial Hygienists recommendation that BLL in pregnancy be no more than 10 µg/dL during pregnancy).[26]

Urine Tests

Urine screening tests for the three most familiar offenders—lead, mercury, and arsenic—are common, although cadmium copper and zinc excretion testing is also available. These should be screened in a 24-hour urine, with reference to creatinine excretion. An acceptable measure for urine lead levels is below 150 µg of lead per 1 g of creatinine for adults, according to the American Conference of Governmental Industrial Hygienists. Measuring urinary lead reflecting creatinine allows adjustment for renal damage from any source.[26]

Urine lead levels are also helpful as a reflection of mobilized lead. Urine lead excretion does vary with diet and renal function.

Radiographic Tests

Radiographic studies may reflect lead in multiple ways: plain films of the abdomen can demonstrate lead paint chips in children with pica or hewing of lead-painted windowsills. Long bones films may show metaphyseal bands, most commonly in knees and ankles.

Neurological Tests

Additional evidence for subtle or subclinical neurotoxicities may come from nerve conduction studies or neuropsychological testing,[24] but these are not recommended as screening studies because of lack of specificity.

Other Sites for Lead Analysis

Lead is also incorporated in hair, nails, and teeth (dentin), and these are markers of exposure. However, at this point, insufficient evidence exists to recommend these tests for clinical monitoring.

MONITORING OF LEAD EXPOSURE

In many U.S. industrial workplaces, monitoring of employees with lead exposure is required.[25] If a monitored employee in a workplace with a BLL of 60 µg/dL is found, regulations mandate immediate removal from the exposure workplace, with exclusion from lead exposure continuing until the BLL is 40 µg/dL. This lead worker surveillance program also requires a specified work history, worker counseling, physical examination, and blood analysis periodically; specific attention must be paid to BLL and ZPP levels.

This monitoring program is required for workers who are exposed to lead levels in air greater than 30 µg/m³ at a time-weighted average for 8 hours for more than 30 days/year. (This program is delineated later in this chapter.)

A more conservative guideline is from the American Conference of Governmental Industrial Hygienists, suggesting removal from work exposure at a BLL of 30 µg/dL in general and of 10 µg/dL during worker pregnancy.[26]

An even more conservative approach is suggested by the Association of Occupational and Environmental Clinics study group, which recommends removal from work exposure at a BLL of 10 µg/dL.[35]

TYPICAL WORKSITES

Of a group of 663 individuals in California identified as having BLLs of 25 µg/dL or greater from 2003 to 2005, 41% of these worked in the manufacturing of lead storage or battery industry and about 10% were each in painting (usually described as disturbing lead-based paint in older structures), in facilities that recycle lead batteries, or in heavy construction. Of the other individuals identified, 6% worked in firing ranges or in radiator repair shops and about 4% were each doing lead abatement, working in foundries using lead brass upon sheet metal work, or working with scrap material by cutting lead-covered waste material.[27]

The National Institute for Occupational Safety and Health has performed health hazard reviews on numerous firing ranges and raised specific concerns over findings of elevated lead levels in indoor facilities. In a detailed review, the institute offered clinical examples of these hazards.[29]

FEDERAL PROGRAM REGULATION

The Occupational Safety and Health Administration gives detailed indications for occupational lead exposure review under the regulatory guidance for lead (the final rule was promulgated in 1995).[25] Appendix C of the rule contains medical surveillance guidelines. This appendix gives a good outline and review of what is needed from the workplace standpoint. Significant points for this are outlined here.

The appendix has four sections: (1) monitoring procedures, (2) effects of lead poisoning, (3) a specific recommended medical evaluation, and (4) discussion of laboratory tests and their relative usefulness. This provides an appropriate approach to treatment of adult lead exposure and toxicity.

If workers are exposed to lead levels of 30 µg/m³ at a time-weighted average more than 30 days/year, they are required to be on a biological monitoring and medical surveillance program. BLLs must be determined every 6 months for people exposed to this action level. Employees to be assigned to an area with the ambient levels indicated earlier (30 µg/m³) must have this program. Frequency must be increased if through monitoring the level found is above 40 µg of lead per 100 g of whole blood. (This is now usually termed 40 µg/dL whole blood). Workers removed from lead due to an elevated blood level must have monthly BLLs and ZPP determinations.

If a person has a BLL at or above 40 µg/dL, an annual medical examination or consultation must be done. If signs and symptoms suggest lead toxicity; if the employee requests medical advice regarding lead exposure, lead effects on reproduction, or both; or if the employee has demonstrated difficulty with respirator fitting or use, examination is also required. This medical examination is also required when employees are removed from exposure to lead.

The medical evaluation is expected to include a detailed work history and environmental history to detail nonoccupational lead exposures.[25] The review suggests that neurological findings of irritability, insomnia, weakness, dizziness, loss of memory, confusion, hallucinations, lack of coordination, and ataxia, as well as diminished strength in hands or feet, disturbances in gait, difficulty in climbing stairs, or seizures, could be elicited. Requested in the examination is a neurological examination. The examination should also incorporate an adequate mental status evaluation, including a search for behavioral and psychological disturbances, memory testing, and evaluation for irritability, insomnia, hallucinations, and mental clouding. Gait, coordination, and tremor evaluation, as well as sensory motor function of peripheral nerves, is requested, with specific comment about strength testing of extensor muscle groups of all extremities. Other aspects of a general nonneurological physical examination are also detailed.

Under this regulation, removal from the workplace can occur if the medical provider so recommends based on medical expertise, but removal is mandated if the BLL is greater than 60 µg/dL or observed with a 6-month average of 50 µg/dL (return to work requires two consecutive BLLs of less than 40 µg/dL).[25] A return to work may include protective procedures appropriate for the individual employee. Provisions are supplied for second opinions of the employee's choice and, at times, a third opinion.

Special provisions for workers include a mandate that respirator protection cannot be used to avoid medical removal due to an elevated BLL or due to medical findings suggesting health impairment. The worker also, if medically removed, has earnings, seniority, and employment benefits protected for 18 months.

The employer must make available records of employee lead exposure to the physician evaluating the employee under these guidelines. The exposure record and medical surveillance records must be kept for 40 years, or 20 years after employment ends.

The discussion of neurological effects in appendix C indicates that the physician has the ability to order additional studies if clinically indicated. Electromyographic studies may be ordered, thus perhaps demonstrating slowing of nerve conduction, decreased number of action motor unit potentials, increased duration of motor unit potentials, and spontaneous fibrillation and fasciculations (at a BLL of 50 µg/dL).[25]

As part of this medical evaluation, laboratory studies of hemoglobin, hematocrit, and red cell, as well as red cell morphology determinations, are required, as are BLL and ZPP with blood urea nitrogen, serum creatinine, and routine urinalysis with microscopy. Additional laboratory testing deemed necessary, including nerve conduction studies, is allowed.

The California Department of Public Health also has less detailed information about lead in summarized form.[27] This includes a worksite evaluation form and a lead health evaluation form. The potentially exposed individual should be encouraged to use these with a personal physician.[27]

RECOMMENDATION FOR MEDICAL MANAGEMENT OF BLOOD LEAD LEVELS IN CHILDREN

The CDC reports that the newborn's BLL mostly reflects that of the mother; thereafter, the total body burden slowly rises during the individual's entire life. Decline in BLL, after removal from exposure, may be slow. The BLL should be maintained so that it is less than 10 µg/dL in children, and the CDC suggests that even at that level there may be significant deterioration of intellect. The CDC recommends targeted risk assessment in blood lead screening for children 1 and 2 years of age.[34]

Rogan et al. studied children who received succimer or placebo in an evaluation of chelation therapy on neuropsychological development.[31] In their study, 780 lead-exposed children had BLLs of 20 to 44 µg/dL. Reviews done before the study suggested that succimer could lower BLLs but might not improve scores on cognition, behavior, and neuropsychological function. The children were measured with the Bailey Scales of Infant Development II and the Wechsler Preschool and Primary Scale of Intelligence Revised for the Development of Neuropsychological Assessment, all as appropriate for age. Control children were also required to have BLLs between 20 and 44 µg/dL. Results suggested that succimer treatment was helpful in reducing BLL. The authors' conclusion with respect to psychological testing was that chelation did not significantly change these performance scores. Ultimately, they opined that patients had few clinical effects at levels of 20 to 44 µg/dL and concluded chelation did not need to be offered at these levels. They did note that the CDC gives "no specific recommendation" for chelation for children with BLLs 20 to 44 µg/dL, and their study did not suggest any change in this practice (i.e., lowering of the BLL for chelation). They stressed the need to implement environmental controls to prevent lead problems in children and to not depend on treatment, as treatment once neurotoxicity of lead is established may be relatively ineffective.[31]

Treatment with succimer (2,3-dimercaptosuccinic acid) was noted to give a mean BLL difference of 11 µg/dL 1 week after beginning of succimer treatment, with rebound (as is typically seen) 7 weeks later. Household environmental controls were instituted to the degree possible in this group and, over a study period of 36 months, BLL did slowly drop.[31]

Jusko et al found that a group of children followed from age 6 months to 6 years with measurement of peak and mean lead levels had an inverse relationship of low level BLL (mean lifetime 7.2 µg/dL) and full scale and performance IQ. They concluded that intellectual function in young children is impaired by BLL well below 10 µg/dL.[30]

CHELATION THERAPY

Before chelation therapy, prevention of lead exposure and clearance of any gastrointestinal lead should be confirmed. Avoidance of lead exposure should be continued for several weeks.[32]

Succimer, an oral preparation, is easy to use and effective. One recommended program is a dose of 10 mg/kg three times a day for 5 days and then twice daily for another 2 weeks. This may cause some gastrointestinal upset but is effective in lowering BLL and is easier than older chelating agents to use.

Older agents, calcium disodium EDTA (Versenate) and dimercaprol (British anti-Lewisite), should probably only be used with experienced assistance. Therapy may be complicated by cardiac arrhythmias and renal injury (tubular necrosis).

For children, an earlier publication from the American Academy of Pediatrics reviews detailed chelation guidelines (although updates should always be reviewed): chelation should be used if the BLL is greater than 45 µg/dL and at BLLs of 25 to 45 µg/dL in some situations (such as sustained levels even after lead abatement). If BLLs are 45 to 70 µg/dL, the pediatrician should treat with succimer if the clinical picture does not suggest encephalopathy (headache, persistent vomiting, and obtundation). The bowel must be clear of paint chips on x-ray.[1]

For severe lead toxicity or encephalopathy, dimercaprol (British anti-Lewisite) is used; one recommendation is 50 mg/m² IM every 4 hours for 5 days. This is a difficult therapy because of the injection requirement. (The product that is available may contain peanut oil. This allergy must be excluded before use.)[33] Alkalinizing urine during this treatment facilitates excretion.

Another chelating agent is calcium disodium EDTA (Versenate). For severe encephalopathy, this may be used with dimercaprol. The EDTA dose is 1 to 1.5 g/m² IV infusion daily for 5 days. IM dosing is possible. Adequate hydration and good renal flow is required when using this medication. This drug acts on a wider range of heavy metals than succimer, so the clinician should monitor urine for excess of other minerals removed and replace these as needed.

REFERENCES

1. U.S. Department of Health and Human Services, Public Health Service. Agency for Toxic Substances and Disease Registry: Toxicological Profile for Lead. Available at: http://www.atsdr.cdc.gov/toxfaq.html. Accessed August 30, 2008.
2. National Institute of Environmental Health. National Toxicology Program 2004. Eleventh Report on Carcinogens 2004. Available at: http://ntp-server.niehs.nih.gov/newhomeroc/roc11/Lead-Public.pdf. Accessed October 12, 2008.
3. Murthy G, Rhea U. Cadmium, copper, iron, lead, manganese, and zinc in evaporated milk, infant products, and human milk. *J Dairy Sci.* 1971;51:1001–1005.
4. Busse F, Omidi L, Timper K, et al. Lead poisoning due to adulterated marijuana. *N Engl J Med.* 2008;358:1641–1642 (correction, 2008;359:440).
5. CDC Health Advisory via Health Alert Network. Potential Exposure to Lead in Artificial Turf: Public Health Issues, Actions, and Recommendations. Available at: http://www.cdc.gov/CDCHAN-00275-08-06-18-ADV-N. Accessed June 26, 2008.

6. Saper R, Phillips R, Sehgal A, et al. Lead, mercury and arsenic in U.S.- and Indian-manufactured ayurvedic medicines sold via the Internet. *JAMA*. 2008;300:915–923.

7. Ko R. Adulterants in Asian patent medicines. *New Engl J Med*. 1998;339:847.

8. Canfield RL, Henderson CR, Cory-Slechta DA. Intellectual impairment in children with blood lead concentrations below 10 microg per deciliter. *N Engl J Med*. 2003;348:1517–1526.

9. Toscano C, Guilarte T. Lead neurotoxicity: from exposure to molecular effects. *Brain Res Rev*. 2005;49:529–554.

10. Ruff HA, Markowitz ME, Bijur PE, Rosen JF. Relationship among blood lead levels and cognitive development in two-year-old children. *Environ Health Perspect*. 1996;104:180–185.

11. Thompson JA. Balance between intake and output of lead in normal individuals. *Br J Ind Med*. 1971;28:189–194.

12. White R, Diamond R, Proctor S, et al. Residual cognitive defects 50 years after lead poisoning during childhood. *Brit J Ind Med*. 1993;50:613–622.

13. Holstege C, Huff J, Rowden A, et al. Lead Encephalopathy. Available at: http://www.emedicine.com/neuro/TOPIC185.HTM. Accessed September 3, 2008.

14. Schwartz D, Lee B, Lee G, et al. Association of blood levels dimer-captosuccinic acid-chelatable lead with neurobehavioral test scores in Korean lead workers. *Am J Epidemiol*. 2001;153:454–464.

15. Stokes L, Letz R, Gerr F, et al. Neurotoxicity in young adults 20 years after childhood exposure to lead: the Bunker Hill experience. *Occup Environ Med*. 1998;55:507–516.

16. Campara P, D'Andrea F, Micciolo R, et al. Psychological performance of workers with blood lead concentration below the current threshold limit value. *Int Arch Occup Environ Health*. 1984;53:233–246.

17. Stollery B. Reaction time changes in workers exposed to lead. *Neurotoxicol Teratol*. 1996;18:477–483.

18. Chia S, Chia K, Chia H, et al. Three-year follow-up of serial nerve conduction among lead exposed workers. *Scand J Work Environ Health*. 1996;22:374–380.

19. Rosenman K, Sims A, Luo Z, et al. Occurrence of lead-related symptoms below the current Occupational Health and Safety Act allowable blood lead levels. *J Occup Environ Med*. 2003;45:546–555.

20. Fonte R, Agosti A, Scafa F, et al. Anaemia and abdominal pain due to occupational lead. *Haematologica*. 2007;92:13–14.

21. Bleecker M, Ford D, Lindgren K, et al. Association of chronic and current measures of lead exposure with different components of brainstem auditory evoked potentials. *Neurotoxicology*. 2003;24:625–631.

22. Bleecker C, Lilienthal H, Ganzer U, et al. The effect of long-term subtoxical lead exposure on the inner ear. Available at: http://www.aro.org/archives/1999/620.html. Accessed August 26, 2008.

23. Bhattacharya A, Shukla R, Auyang E, et al. Effect of succimer chelation therapy on postural balance and gait outcomes in children with early exposure to environmental lead. *Neurotoxicology*. 2007;28:686–695.

24. Seppäläinen AM, Herberg S. Subclinical lead neuropathy. *Am J Ind Med*. 1980;1:413–420.

25. Occupational Safety and Health Administration, U.S. Department Labor. Final: Standard occupational exposure standard to lead. *Fed Regist*. 1978;43:52952–53014. [29 CFR § 1910.1025.]

26. American Conference of Governmental Industrial Hygienists. (2001, 2006). Lead and Inorganic Compounds-Documentation of the Threshold and Biological Exposure Indices, 7 ed. Available at http://www.acgih.org/store. Accessed August 30, 2008.

27. California Department of Public Health, Occupational Lead Poisoning Health Program. Workplace Hazard Alert: New Health Dangers from Lead. Available at: http://www.cdph.ca.gov/programs/olppp/documents/leadhazardrt.pdf. Accessed August 26, 2008.

28. Centers for Disease Control and Prevention, National Institute for Occupational Safety and Health. NIOSH Alert: Preventing Occupational Exposure to Lead and Noise at Indoor Firing Ranges. DHHS (NIOSH) 2007 Publication 2008. Accessed August 26, 2008.

29. California Department of Public Health, Occupational Lead Poisoning Health Program. California Industries with the Highest Number of Reported Cases of Lead Poisoning: 2005. Available at: http://www.cdph.ca.gov/programs/olppb/documents/topten.pdf. Accessed August 26, 2008.

30. Jusko T, Henderson C, Lanphar B, et al. Blood lead concentrations < 10 µg/dL and child intelligence at 6 years of age. *Environ Health Perspect*. 2008;116:243–248.

31. Rogan W, Dietrich K, Ware J, et al. The effect of chelation therapy with succimer on neuropsychological development in children exposed to lead. *N Eng J Med*. 2001;344:1421–1426.

32. Lidsky T, Schneider JS. Lead neurotoxicity in children: basic mechanisms and clinical correlates. *Brain*. 2003;126:5–19.

33. Woolf A. Recommendations for medical management of adult lead exposure. *Environ Health Perspect*. 2007;115:463–471.

34. Binns HJ, Campbell C, Brown MJ, et al. Interpreting and managing blood lead levels of less than 10 µ/dL in children and reducing childhood exposure to lead: recommendations of the Centers for Disease Control and Prevention Advisory Committee on Childhood Lead Poisoning Prevention. *Pediatrics*. 2007;120(5):e1285-1298. Accessed September 3, 2008.

35. Association of Occupational and Environmental Clinics. Medical management guidelines for lead-exposed adults. Revised 04/24/2007. Available at http://www.aoec.org/principles.htm. Accessed February 4, 2009.

Arsenic

Dominic B. Fee

INTRODUCTION

The toxicity of arsenic (As) is well known, largely because of its use as a homicidal–suicidal agent historically and in the entertainment industry. However, since arsenic is fairly ubiquitous, most individuals are unknowingly exposed to it. Despite being used for millennia, arsenic metabolism and pathophysiology has not been precisely defined, partially because each species processes this metalloid differently.

BACKGROUND AND SOURCES OF EXPOSURE

Historically, arsenic-containing compounds were used as pigments in cosmetics and paints and as pesticides.[1-3] Currently, arsenic is still widely used and is present in wood preservatives, fungicides, insecticides, pesticides, herbicides, paints, desiccants, chicken and other animal feeds as an essential element, semiconductors, transistors, chemotherapeutics, and "herbal" or "traditional" remedies (Table 1).[1-4] Most organic exposure in humans is from water-based organisms such as shellfish, fish, and seaweed.[1] Organic exposure is more common than inorganic.[1]

The oxidative state of arsenic and whether it is in an organic or inorganic form highly influence its toxicity to humans. Trivalent (arsenite) and pentavalent (arsenate) arsenic oxidative states are the most clinically relevant.[1,2] Inorganic arsenic is the predominate toxic form, with the trivalent state 60 times more toxic than the pentavalent.[1] Organic arsenic is considered nontoxic but could be toxic in high concentrations; furthermore, certain organic arsenic compounds generated during human metabolism of arsenic have been shown to be toxic.[2,5]

Most exposure to arsenic, both organic and inorganic forms, is through ingestion, with absorption in the small intestine; however, it can also occur via inhalation and transdermally.[2,3] Contaminated groundwater is the ultimate source for most exposures.[6-8] Mainly, this is geological; arsenic present in sedimentary rock can undergo reduction and subsequent release into aquifers,[9] and this contaminated water either is ingested directly (inorganic exposure) or enters the food chain and is then ingested (organic exposure).[10] Contamination can also occur because of industrial activity (e.g., mining, manufacturing, burning of arsenic-rich fossil fuels, and agricultural runoff).[2,11]

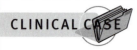

CLINICAL CASE

A 24-year-old female college student had progressive severe pain and loss of sensation of both feet for a couple of years. It began in her toes and progressed up to her ankles. She described specific instances of poor sensation, such as stepping on a piece of glass and not realizing it. At time of presentation, the loss of sensation had started to spread to her hands. She described severe burning and sharp pains of the hands and feet. Examination showed decreased sensation to light touch, pinprick, temperature, and position sense in the lower extremities in a "stocking" distribution, with the worse sensation at her toes. She also had a mild decrease to sensation in all modalities in her fingertips bilaterally. During her comprehensive, workup it was found that she had an elevated level of arsenic in her system (24-hour urine testing showed 135 µg/mL). Speciation demonstrated that it was inorganic arsenic. She had no idea how she was exposed and suspected no friends or family members. After moving to another town, her levels eventually decreased to normal and the neuropathy stabilized. However, she continued to have severe neuropathic pain even more than a year after levels had normalized. In the course of her case, multiple medications for pain relief, including gabapentin, tricyclics, and pregabalin, were tried. Ultimately, she received the most relief from pregabalin at 200 mg three times per day, along with hydrocodone or acetaminophen occasionally for breakthrough pain.

METABOLISM AND PATHOGENESIS

After absorption, arsenic is distributed to many organs, including liver, kidney, heart, lung, brain, and nerves.[2] Within cells, arsenic is protein bound to minimize immediate toxicity.[3] Elimination of arsenic has both hepatic and renal aspects and differs among species.[3,4] The pentavalent state is commonly reduced to the more toxic trivalent state.[3] Inorganic arsenic is methylated in the liver and potentially in other cells, to either mono- or dimethylated forms; in humans, methylated arsenic is rapidly excreted in the urine.[2,4,12] Recently, the methylated trivalent form has been shown to be toxic, suggesting that methylation may not be the primary detoxification pathway.[3,5] A small fraction of absorbed inorganic arsenic and many common organic arsenic compounds, such as arsenobetaine, are excreted unchanged in the urine.[4] In acute exposure, 50% of the absorbed arsenic is excreted in the urine over 3 to

5 days.[1] For weeks after an exposure, arsenic is retained in keratin-rich structures such as skin, nails, and hair.[1,13]

Arsenic has been shown to inactivate more than 200 enzymes, predominantly in pathways involving cellular energy, DNA replication and repair, and antioxidant systems.[1,3,4] It is thought that the trivalent state interacts with thiol groups and results in enzymatic inhibition by binding to sulfhydryl moieties, whereas the pentavalent state replaces phosphate in certain compounds.[1,14,15]

CLINICAL PRESENTATION

Clinical symptoms depend on whether there is a high-dose (acute), low-dose (chronic), or acute-on-chronic arsenic exposure. Most exposures, in both developed and developing countries, are chronic.[3]

Acute exposure, usually with urine concentrations greater than 50 to 100 µg in 24 hours or 35 to 50 µg/L in a random sample, results predominately in gastrointestinal symptoms, but other symptoms are common.[1] The gastrointestinal-based symptoms, including abdominal pain, vomiting, and diarrhea, are common and occur soon after exposure; in fact, arsenic toxicity mimics cholera so well that this contributed to its historical popularity as a poison.[3] Cardiopulmonary shock can develop with associated hypotension, pulmonary edema, and heart failure; renal failure and bone marrow suppression are often seen.[3] Neurologically, encephalopathy and a peripheral neuropathy can occur.[3] The encephalopathy is associated with impaired concentration, memory, and learning, as well as psychosis.[16,17] Interestingly, the onset of the polyneuropathy is delayed and can occur weeks after the exposure.[18] It can be a typical-appearing acquired, axonal polyneuropathy but can also resemble Guillain-Barré syndrome, a rapidly progressive, ascending demyelinating polyneuropathy associated with areflexia.[2,8,19,20] The polyneuropathy may take months to resolve, if ever.[3] The precise mechanism of these problems is not known; hypotheses include disruption of cytoskeletal structures, altered energy production, and free radical formation by disrupting oxidative phosphorylization, altered neurotransmitter levels, vascular compromise, or a combination of these.[2,3,21,22]

Chronic exposure is usually through ingesting low levels of arsenic; accumulation in organs is common, and tolerance can develop. Multisystem symptomatology is common, including gastrointestinal, cardiopulmonary, and neurological symptomatology similar to that seen in acute exposure but with a protracted onset.[1,8,23–25] Cutaneous symptoms are more prominent in chronic exposure and include hyperpigmentation, hyperkeratosis, Mees' lines on the nails (Figure 23-1), and increased incidence of squamous and basal cell carcinomas; other symptoms include anemia, hepatitis, peripheral vascular

Table 1: Common Arsenic Species, Usual Sources of Exposure, and Urinary Metabolites

Name	Chemical Formula	Usual Source of Exposure	Urinary Metabolite
Arsenic trioxide	As_2O_3 or As_4O_6	Smelting, industrial sources, naturally occurring in drinking water	As_2O_3 Monomethylarsonate Dimethylarsinate
Arsenic pentoxide	As_2O_5 or As_4O_{10}	Smelting, industrial sources, naturally occurring in drinking water	As_2O_3 and As_2O_5 Monomethylarsonate Dimethylarsinate
Arsine	AsH_3	Industrial applications, semiconductor manufacture, accidental formation	Monomethylarsonate Dimethylarsinate
Monomethylarsonate	$CH_3AsO(OH)_2$	Metabolic product of inorganic arsenic exposure	Mostly excreted unchanged as monomethylarsonate and some dimethylarsinate
Dimethylarsinate	$(CH_3)_2AsO(OH)$	Metabolic product of inorganic arsenic exposure	Mostly excreted unchanged as dimethylarsinate
Arsenobetaine	$(CH_3)_3AsCH_2COOH$	Common arsenical species found in certain seafood	Mostly excreted unchanged as arsenobetaine
Gallium arsenide	GaAs	Used in semiconductor manufacture	Not water soluble and poorly absorbed; mostly excreted in feces
Lewisite	$ClCH = CH-AsCl_2$	War gas (vesicant)	—
Valence states: +V arsenates +III arsenates 0 metallic arsenic			

Reprinted with permission from Franzblau A. Arsenic. In: Rosenstock et al., ed. *Textbook of Clinical Occupational and Environmental Medicine.* 2nd ed. Philadelphia: Saunders; 2004.

disease, altered taste, diabetes mellitus, and other cancers, such as bladder, kidney, and liver.[1,4,20,26–28] Children may be vulnerable to additional problems, such as decreased intelligence and hearing loss.[29–31]

DIAGNOSTIC TESTING

Arsenic toxicity is confirmed by demonstrating elevated concentrations of arsenic in the body. Assessing urine is the mainstay, with 24-hour collections better than spot urine testing; 24-hour urine levels greater than 50 to 100 μg or spot urine levels greater than 35 to 50 μg/L are consistent with acute arsenic toxicity.[1,3,20] Collection should be in a metal-free container to avoid contamination.[3] Blood can also be tested but is of limited usefulness because serum levels are cleared within a few hours.[20] Of note, most screening tests for arsenic do not differentiate between

organic and inorganic arsenic on initial reporting; therefore, it can be difficult to determine the significance of the total value reported. Nor does the testing routinely differentiate between the trivalent and the pentavalent states.

Since arsenic is rapidly cleared in acute exposure, hair or nails can be sent for analysis. Arsenic present in soaps and other products can, potentially, confound results; collecting pubic hair minimizes this concern. Hair sample arsenic levels of 1.0 to 3.0 mg/kg indicate acute exposure, and levels of 0.1 to 0.5 mg/kg indicate chronic exposure.[1] If concerned about intentional arsenic poisoning, then the clinician must maintain a "chain of custody" on the samples. The collection should be in front of a witness and then hand-carried to the laboratory; the clinician should document this appropriately in the chart.

Nerve conduction testing and electromyography may demonstrate distal symmetrical sensorimotor axonopathy or, in cases of acute exposure, conduction slowing similar to that seen in Guillain-Barré syndrome.[2,8,19,20]

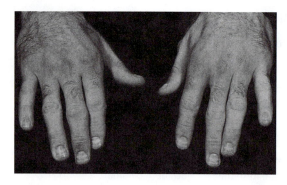

Figure 23-1. Arsenic poisoning and Mees' lines. (Courtesy of R. Pascuzzi, MD, Indianapolis, Indiana. From Ibrahim D, Froberg B, Wolf A, Rusyniak DE. Heavy metal poisoning: clinical presentations and pathophysiology. *Clin Lab Med.* 2006;26[1]:67–97, viii.)

TREATMENT

In acute exposure, initial treatment involves correcting dehydration and complications of organ failure.[3] Attempts can then be made to promote arsenic clearance. If the ingestion is recent, then activated charcoal with gastric lavage can be tried.[3] After arsenic has been absorbed, hemodialysis, chelation, or both are considerations, but they have not been rigorously studied.[3] The chelator, 2, 3-dimercapto-1-propanol, has been shown to be beneficial with acute exposure but not with chronic exposure.[20,32,33] As illustrated in this chapter's representative clinical case, chronic neuropathic pain may occur long after exposure to arsenic has ceased.

REFERENCES

1. Ratnaike RN. Acute and chronic arsenic toxicity. *Postgrad Med J.* 2003;79(933):391–396.
2. Rodriguez VM, Jimenez-Capdeville ME, Giordano M. The effects of arsenic exposure on the nervous system. *Toxicol Lett.* 2003;145(1):1–18.
3. Vahidnia A, van der Voet GB, de Wolff FA. Arsenic neurotoxicity: a review. *Hum Exp Toxicol.* 2007;26(10):823–832.
4. Abernathy CO, Liu YP, Longfellow D, et al. Arsenic: health effects, mechanisms of actions, and research issues. *Environ Health Perspect.* 1999;107(7):593–597.
5. Thomas DJ, Styblo M, Lin S. The cellular metabolism and systemic toxicity of arsenic. *Toxicol Appl Pharmacol.* 2001;176(2):127–144.
6. Matschullat J. Arsenic in the geosphere: a review. *Sci Total Environ.* 2000;249(1–3):297–312.
7. Gebel T. Confounding variables in the environmental toxicology of arsenic. *Toxicology.* 2000;144(1–3):155–162.
8. Mukherjee SC, Rahman MM, Chowdhury UK, et al. Neuropathy in arsenic toxicity from groundwater arsenic contamination in West Bengal, India. *J Environ Sci Health A Tox Hazard Subst Environ Eng.* 2003;38(1):165–183.
9. Nickson R, McArthur J, Burgess W, et al. Arsenic poisoning of Bangladesh groundwater. *Nature.* 1998;395(6700):338.
10. Chowdhury UK, Biswas BK, Chowdhury TR, et al. Groundwater arsenic contamination in Bangladesh and West Bengal, India. *Environ Health Perspect.* 2000;108(5):393–397.
11. Ayres RU. Toxic heavy metals: materials cycle optimization. *Proc Natl Acad Sci USA.* 1992;89(3):815–820.
12. Aposhian HV. Enzymatic methylation of arsenic species and other new approaches to arsenic toxicity. *Annu Rev Pharmacol Toxicol.* 1997;37:397–419.
13. Schoolmeester WL, White DR. Arsenic poisoning. *South Med J.* 1980;73(2):198–208.
14. Hughes MF. Arsenic toxicity and potential mechanisms of action. *Toxicol Lett.* 2002;133(1):1–16.
15. Aposhian HV, Zakharyan RA, Avram MD, et al. A review of the enzymology of arsenic metabolism and a new potential role of hydrogen peroxide in the detoxication of the trivalent arsenic species. *Toxicol Appl Pharmacol.* 2004;198(3):327–335.
16. Freeman JW, Couch JR. Prolonged encephalopathy with arsenic poisoning. *Neurology.* 1978;28(8):853–855.
17. Bolla-Wilson K, Bleecker ML. Neuropsychological impairment following inorganic arsenic exposure. *J Occup Med.* 1987;29(6):500–503.
18. Greenberg C, Davies S, McGowan T, et al. Acute respiratory failure following severe arsenic poisoning. *Chest.* 1979;76(5):596–598.
19. Greenberg SA. Acute demyelinating polyneuropathy with arsenic ingestion. *Muscle Nerve.* 1996;19(12):1611–1613.
20. London Z, Albers JW. Toxic neuropathies associated with pharmaceutic and industrial agents. *Neurol Clin.* 2007;25(1):257–276.
21. Chiou HY, Huang WI, Su CL, et al. Dose–response relationship between prevalence of cerebrovascular disease and ingested inorganic arsenic. *Stroke.* 1997;28(9):1717–1723.
22. Li W, Chou IN. Effects of sodium arsenite on the cytoskeleton and cellular glutathione levels in cultured cells. *Toxicol Appl Pharmacol.* 1992;114(1):132–139.
23. Santra A, Das Gupta J, De BK, et al. Hepatic manifestations in chronic arsenic toxicity. *Indian J Gastroenterol.* 1999;18(4):152–155.
24. Goddard MJ, Tanhehco JL, Dau PC. Chronic arsenic poisoning masquerading as Landry-Guillain-Barré syndrome. *Electromyogr Clin Neurophysiol.* 1992;32(9):419–423.
25. Gerr F, Letz R, Ryan PB, Green RC. Neurological effects of environmental exposure to arsenic in dust and soil among humans. *Neurotoxicology.* 2000;21(4):475–487.
26. Lewis DR, Southwick JW, Ouellet-Hellstrom R, et al. Drinking water arsenic in Utah: a cohort mortality study. *Environ Health Perspect.* 1999;107(5):359–365.
27. Mazumder DN, Haque R, Ghosh N, et al. Arsenic in drinking water and the prevalence of respiratory effects in West Bengal, India. *Int J Epidemiol.* 2000;29(6):1047–1052.
28. Rahman MM, Chowdhury UK, Mukherjee SC, et al. Chronic arsenic toxicity in Bangladesh and West Bengal, India: a review and commentary. *J Toxicol Clin Toxicol.* 2001;39(7):683–700.
29. Calderon J, Navarro ME, Jimenez-Capdeville ME, et al. Exposure to arsenic and lead and neuropsychological development in Mexican children. *Environ Res.* 2001;85(2):69–76.
30. Bencko V, Symon K, Chládek V, Pihrt J. Health aspects of burning coal with a high arsenic content: II. Hearing changes in exposed children. *Environ Res.* 1977;13(3):386–395.
31. Tsai SY, Chou HY, The HW, et al. The effects of chronic arsenic exposure from drinking water on the neurobehavioral development in adolescence. *Neurotoxicology.* 2003;24(4–5):747–753.
32. Wax PM, Thornton CA. Recovery from severe arsenic-induced peripheral neuropathy with 2,3-dimercapto-1-propanesulphonic acid. *J Toxicol Clin Toxicol.* 2000;38(7):777–780.
33. Vantroyen B, Heilier JF, Meulemans A, et al. Survival after a lethal dose of arsenic trioxide. *J Toxicol Clin Toxicol.* 2004;42(6):889–895.

Thallium

Daniel E. Rusyniak

INTRODUCTION

In 1861, Sir William Crookes heated a deposit from a sulfuric acid chamber and noted the transient spectrographic appearance of a bright green line. Crookes identified this line as a new heavy metal and named it thallium.[2] Although it has found use in several industrial processes and as a radiocontrast agent in medicine, thallium is best known for its toxicity.

Not long after its discovery, researchers discovered a unique property of thallium—it caused hair loss (alopecia).[3] This led to thallium being used to treat fungal infections of the scalp (i.e., ringworm) until reports of pediatric deaths resulted in it being clinically abandoned.[4] It was this recognition of thallium's toxicity, and its pharmacological properties, that led to its use as a rodenticide. As its use was widespread, outbreaks of accidental and criminal poisonings began to be reported. This led, in 1975, to thallium's removal from the U.S. market.[5-7] Thallium does continue to be used today in the manufacturing of optic lenses, semiconductors, and (in small doses) as a radiocontrast agent for the detection of cardiac disease. Despite its limited access to the public, thallium persists as a significant source of accidental and intentional poisonings in humans and animals.[1,8-14]

CELLULAR AND PHARMACOLOGICAL PROPERTIES OF THALLIUM

Thallium's pharmacological properties make its salts highly toxic. Of thallium's many pharmacological and physiological effects, four contribute the most to its toxicity: absorption, distribution, interruption of cellular processes, and elimination. In regard to thallium's absorption, its salts are tasteless, odorless, water soluble, and completely and rapidly absorbed by the GI tract. Within an hour of oral administration, a clinician can measure urine and fecal levels of thallium in poisoned animals.[15] Once absorbed, thallium is widely distributed throughout the body; the highest concentrations are found in the kidney and the lowest in the serum, fat, and central nervous system.[15] Once it enters tissues, thallium interrupts several critical metabolic enzymes. As both potassium and thallium are univalent cations with similar atomic radii, thallium interferes with K^+-dependent processes, including pyruvate kinase and sodium–potassium adenosine triphosphatase.[5,16,17] Another proposed mechanism for thallium's toxicity is its affinity for and inhibition of the following sulfhydryl-containing enzymes: pyruvate dehydrogenase complex, succinate dehydrogenase, hydrolases, oxidoreductases, and transferases.[5] Together,

CASE STUDY

After a weekend at work, a 58-year-old man developed severe pains in his feet and difficulty walking.[1] On a review of symptoms, he noted pains in his muscles and joints, pain on inspiration, and difficulty sleeping. He denied any gastrointestinal (GI) or other concurrent or precedent illnesses. His past medical history was unremarkable. He was on no medications, and his social history revealed him to be both a smoker and moderate drinker. His physical examination was remarkable for hypesthesia of the feet, decreased proprioception, and a wide gait. His laboratory evaluations were all normal, including the following: complete blood count; chemistry panels; thyroid tests; evaluation for connective tissue disorders; folate; and B_{12} levels. Magnetic resonance imaging of the brain revealed small, bilateral, subdural hygromas and generalized atrophy. Over the next week, his symptoms progressed in his feet and legs and now involved his hands; his pain became so severe that the weight of a bedsheet became intolerable. He was admitted to the hospital, and nerve conduction studies revealed a sensorimotor polyradiculoneuropathy—of the axonopathy type—affecting the distal nerves of the hands and feet. The patient's wife had also begun to notice that he was losing his hair—remarking that it could be painlessly pulled out in clumps. The man worked as an electrician for a local automotive company, and further investigation revealed that several of his coworkers complained of similar symptoms. Toxicological testing showed that this patient and eight of his coworkers had been poisoned with thallium; in total, five patients developed significant neuropathies and alopecia. Local Occupational Safety and Health Administration and police investigations suspected the source of thallium to be a breakroom coffeepot and the cause to be malicious—likely perpetrated by a disgruntled coworker.

the inhibition of potassium- and sulfhydryl-dependent processes decreases the breakdown of sugars and impairs energy production; if severe enough, this results in cell death.[5,18] Thallium has a unique means of elimination. Unlike many xenobiotics, it is not eliminated primarily in the urine; rather, it undergoes enterohepatic circulation, with fecal removal serving as the primary means of elimination.[15] As discussed later, this renders standard treatments (i.e., sulfhydryl chelators) for heavy metals useless.

CLINICAL SYMPTOMS OF THALLIUM POISONING

The clinical manifestations of thallium poisoning vary depending on the dose, the age of the victim, and whether the exposure is acute or chronic. In most cases, the presentation of a rapidly progressive peripheral neuropathy, combined with the development of alopecia, accurately describes acute thallium toxicity.

One of the earliest findings in thallium poisoning—typically occurring within 2 to 3 days of exposure—is the development of a rapidly progressive painful peripheral neuropathy.[6,14,19] Symptoms begin in the feet and legs and, if a large enough dose has been ingested, may progress to involve the hands. The pain of the neuropathy is described as "pins and needles" and may be excruciating—to the point where even the weight of a bedsheet is intolerable.[1,3,12,20] In the most severe cases, the neuropathy from thallium may rapidly ascend from the feet and legs and involve the respiratory muscles, necessitating the need for artificial respiration.[3,9,21] In these cases, the clinical picture can be misdiagnosed as Guillain-Barré syndrome.[20] Along with involvement of peripheral nerves, cranial neuropathies have been well reported.[3,9,19,20,22–24]

Perhaps the best-known complication of thallium poisoning is alopecia (Figure 24-1). Beginning around 5 to 14 days after exposure, victims describe losing their hair in clumps, often commenting that, if pulled, the hair comes out painlessly.[3] By 3 to 4 weeks, hair loss may be complete, resulting in near-total-body alopecia—including axillary

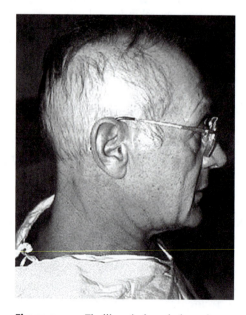

Figure 24-1. Thallium-induced alopecia.

hair, pubic hair, and lateral eyebrows.[25–28] One notable exception to the hair loss is the medial part of the eyebrow, which is typically spared; these hairs are typically in a resting nongrowth phase.[27,29] In survivors, hair regrowth typically begins by the fourth month after poisoning.[1] While the exact cause of alopecia is not known, either thallium's interruption of keratin synthesis or its interruption of metabolism in the hair matrix likely is responsible.[28,30] While alopecia is the most recognizable feature of thallium poisoning, peripheral neuropathies can occur, at lower doses, without the development hair loss.[1]

The central nervous system can also be affected in cases of severe thallium poisoning with all of the following having been reported: hallucinations, altered mental status, insomnia, psychosis, and coma.[3,6,9,19,23,31]

Along with the neurological and dermatological manifestations of thallium poisoning, less specific findings are reported. In some cases, the earliest symptoms of thallium poisoning—occurring within hours of exposure—are GI symptoms. Unlike arsenic, GI symptoms from thallium are not typically severe and do not dominate the early clinical picture. The GI symptoms most commonly reported are abdominal pain, vomiting, loose stool, and ultimately constipation or obstipation.[1,3,9,12,27] Other manifestations of thallium poisoning may include all of the following: diffuse myalgias, pleuritic chest pain, insomnia, hypertension, nonspecific ST–T wave changes, nail dystrophy (Mees' lines), hepatitis, and acute and chronic neuropsychiatric manifestations.[1,7,12,32]

DIAGNOSIS OF THALLIUM POISONING

Making the diagnosis of thallium poisoning early enough to institute effective therapy requires the following: (1) early recognition of symptoms, (2) neurological and clinical testing, and (3) analytical confirmation.

Making the diagnosis in thallium poisoning is notoriously difficult because it is uncommon and its symptoms may be attributed to other etiologies.[1] Further hampering the early diagnosis, alopecia—the most recognizable feature of thallium poisoning[11]—may not be evident for 5 to 14 days after the exposure.[28] Despite these difficulties, two readily available tests may aid in making the early diagnosis of thallium poisoning: nerve conduction studies and microscopic hair analysis.

Nerve conduction studies are useful in diagnosing and monitoring the recovery of patients with thallium poisoning.[1] They typically reveal a sensorimotor axonopathy, with the severity of neuropathy correlating with the severity of other symptoms and findings. In cases of severe poisoning, a nerve biopsy may reveal Wallerian degeneration with axonal destruction and secondary myelin loss.[19,33,34]

Once it has been established that patients have a neuropathy suspicious for thallium, the simple visual inspection of pulled hair—under a light microscope—may help make the diagnosis. When viewed under low power with a light microscope, the hair roots of thallium-poisoned patients appear darkened (Figure 24-2).[1,27] This finding has been reported as early as 4 days after poisoning.[27] The darkened roots are seen in the highest percentage in pulled hair from the scalp (95%), followed by hairs of the chest and legs (50% to 60%) and less commonly from eyebrows and eyelids (30%).[27] If repeated poisonings have occurred, several bands may be seen.[27] The blackened roots are not the accumulation of a pigment or the metal itself; rather, they represent an optical phenomenon: As the hair root matrix becomes disorganized from the interruption of cellular processes, it accumulates gaseous inclusions. These result in diffracting light and the appearance of a black stain.[25,28] When treated with acid or mechanical pressure gas, bubbles have been noted to escape the hair and the darkened strip disappears.[35]

Ultimately, the definitive diagnosis of thallium poisoning requires the identification of elevated concentrations of thallium in urine or hair. As with other metals, a 24-hour urine is considered the gold standard in thallium poisoning. In most people, levels should be at zero, but levels up to 20 μg/specimen may be considered normal. Hair also can be tested, with normal levels being less than 15 ng of thallium per gram of hair.[5] Hair analysis is not thought to be as reliable as urine analysis, and a negative hair test should not exclude the possibility of thallium poisoning. Along with hair and urine, postmortem tissues including paraffin tissue blocks and even

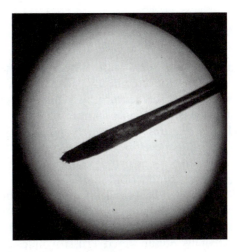

Figure 24-2. Blackened hair root in a thallium-poisoned patient under light microscopy.

cremated ashes have been used to confirm elevations of thallium in suspected criminal poisonings.[34,36]

TREATMENT OF THALLIUM POISONING

The primary objective in treating patients who are thallium poisoned is to increase its elimination and prevent further toxicity. The best-studied and most effective antidote for thallium poisoning is Prussian blue. Prussian blue is a complex of potassium hexacyanoferrate that was recently approved by the U.S. Food and Drug Administration for the treatment of cesium or thallium poisoning under the brand name Radiogardase. The manufacturer-recommended dose of Prussian blue is 3 g orally three times a day, but others have recommended 250 mg/kg/day.[23] Poorly absorbed, Prussian blue exchanges potassium for thallium in the gut, resulting in the fecal excretion of a thallium–Prussian blue complex. Numerous animal studies have shown Prussian blue to decrease mortality, to increase fecal elimination, and to decrease central nervous system thallium concentrations.[37–44] Although clinical trials are not possible for thallium poisoning, human case reports support the safety and efficacy of Prussian blue.[12,14,45] Based on thallium's affinity for sulfhydryl groups, several commonly used sulfur chelators have been studied in animal models of poisoning. None have been shown to be beneficial,[37,46–48] and some may actually increase brain concentrations and toxicity.[49] As some hospitals may not carry Prussian blue, activated charcoal may be used until Prussian blue is available.[1] In vitro studies demonstrate that activated charcoal effectively adsorbs thallium,[50,51] although its benefit in animal studies has been contradictory[40,48] and human data is anecdotal.[1]

CONCLUSION

Thallium represents a rare cause of heavy metal poisoning. It should be suspected in any patient with a rapidly progressive painful polyneuropathy. While hair loss represents the most identifiable feature, its onset can lag other clinical features and severely poisoned patents may die before its development. Detection of thallium poisoning requires its analytical confirmation in urine, but both nerve conduction studies and microscopic inspection of pulled hair can lend support to the diagnosis, facilitating early treatment. Treatment should begin as soon as the diagnosis is suspected and should consist of orally administered Prussian blue. Because thallium is not a common environmental or workplace contaminant and is not readily available to the public,

any thallium-poisoned patient should be considered a victim of a criminal act until proved otherwise.

REFERENCES

1. Rusyniak DE, Furbee RB, Kirk MS. Thallium and arsenic poisoning in a small Midwest town. *Ann Emerg Med*. 2002;39:307–311.
2. James FA. Of "Medals and Muddles," the context of the discovery of thallium: William Crookes's early spectro-chemical work. *Notes Rec R Soc Lond*. 1984;39:65–90.
3. Prick JJG, Sillevis Smitt WG, Muller L. *Thallium Poisoning*. Amsterdam: Elsevier; 1955.
4. Lynch GR, Lond MB. The toxicology of thallium. *Lancet*. 1930;Dec 20:1340–1344.
5. Mulkey JP, Oehme FW. A review of thallium toxicity. *Vet Hum Toxicol*. 1993;35:445–453.
6. Reed D, Crawley J, Faro SN, et al. Thallotoxicosis. *JAMA*. 1963;183:516–522.
7. Bank WJ, Pleasure DE, Suzuki K, et al. Thallium poisoning. *Arch Neurol*. 1972;26:456–464.
8. Insley BM, Grufferman S, Ayliffe HE. Thallium poisoning in cocaine abusers. *Am J Emerg Med*. 1986;4:545–548.
9. Desenclos JC, Wilder MH, Coppenger GW, et al. Thallium poisoning: an outbreak in Florida, 1988. *South Med J*. 1992;85:1203–1206.
10. Waters CB, Hawkins EC, Knapp DW. Acute thallium toxicosis in a dog. *J Am Vet Med Assoc*. 1992;201:883–885.
11. Moore D, House I, Dixon A. Thallium poisoning: diagnosis may be elusive but alopecia is the clue. *BMJ*. 1993;306:1527–1529.
12. Meggs WJ, Hoffman RS, Shih RD, et al. Thallium poisoning from maliciously contaminated food. *J Toxicol Clin Toxicol*. 1994;32:723–730.
13. Questel F, Dugarin J, Dally S. Thallium-contaminated heroin. *Ann Intern Med*. 1996;124:616.
14. Malbrain ML, Lambrecht GL, Zandijk E, et al. Treatment of severe thallium intoxication. *J Toxicol Clin Toxicol*. 1997;35:97–100.
15. Lund A. Distribution of thallium in the organism and its elimination. *Acta Pharmacol et Toxicol*. 1956;12:251–259.
16. Gehring PJ, Hammond PB. The interrelationship between thallium and potassium in animals. *J Pharmacol Exp Ther*. 1967;155:187–201.
17. Douglas KT, Bunni MA, Baindur SR. Thallium in biochemistry. *Int J Biochem*. 1990;22:429–438.
18. Melnick RL, Monti LG, Motzkin SM. Uncoupling of mitochondrial oxidative phosphorylation by thallium. *Biochem Biophy Res Commun*. 1976;69:68–73.
19. Davis LE, Standefer JC, Kornfeld M, et al. Acute thallium poisoning: toxicological and morphological studies of the nervous system. *Ann Neurol*. 1980;10:38–44.
20. Misra UK, Kalita J, Yadav RK, et al. Thallium poisoning: emphasis on early diagnosis and response to haemodialysis. *Postgrad Med J*. 2003;79:103–105.
21. Hologgitas J, Ullucci P, Driscoll J, et al. Thallium elimination kinetics in acute thallotoxicosis. *J Anal Toxicol*. 1980;4:68–75.
22. Cavanagh JB, Fuller NH, Johnson HRM. The effects of thallium salts, with particular reference to the nervous system changes: a report of three cases. *Q J Med*. 1974;170:293–319.
23. Hoffman RS. Thallium toxicity and the role of Prussian blue in therapy. *Toxicol Rev*. 2003;22:29–40.
24. Tabandeh H, Crowston JG, Thompson GM. Ophthalmologic features of thallium poisoning. *Am J Ophthalmol*. 1994;117:243–245.

25. Feldman J, Levisohn DR. Acute alopecia: clue to thallium toxicity. *Pediatr Dermatol.* 1993;10:29–31.

26. Heyl T, Barlow RJ. Thallium poisoning: a dermatological perspective. *Br J Dermatol.* 1989;121:787–791.

27. Moeschlin S. Thallium poisoning. *Clin Toxicol.* 1980;17:133–146.

28. Tromme I, Van Neste D, Dobbelaere F, et al. Skin signs in the diagnosis of thallium poisoning. *Br J Dermatol.* 1998;138: 321–325.

29. Koblenzer PJ, Weiner LB. Alopecia secondary to thallium intoxication. *Arch Dermatol.* 1969;99:777.

30. Cavanagh JB, Gregson M. Some effects of a thallium salt on the proliferation of hair follicle cells. *J Pathol.* 1978;125:179–191.

31. Saha A, Sadhu HG, Karnik AB, et al. Erosion of nails following thallium poisoning: a case report. *Occup Environ Med.* 2004;61:640–642.

32. McMillan TM, Jacobson RR, Gross M. Neuropsychology of thallium poisoning. *J Neurol Neurosurg Psychiatry.* 1997;63: 247–250.

33. Cavanagh JB. The "dying back" process: a common denominator in many naturally occurring and toxic neuropathies. *Arch Pathol Lab Med.* 1979;103:659–664.

34. Cavanagh JB. What have we learnt from Graham Frederick Young? Reflections on the mechanism of thallium neurotoxicity. *Neuropathol Appl Neurobiol.* 1991;17:3–9.

35. Metter D, Vock R. Structure of the hair in thallium poisoning. *Z Rechtsmed.* 1984;91:201–214.

36. Wecht C, Saitz G. *Mortal Evidence.* New York: Prometheus Books; 2007:324.

37. Rusyniak DE, Kao LW, Nanagas KA, et al. Dimercaptosuccinic acid and Prussian blue in the treatment of acute thallium poisoning in rats. *Clin Toxicol.* 2003;41:137–142.

38. Rauws AG. Thallium pharmacokinetics and its modification by Prussian blue. *Naunyn Schmiedebergs Arch Pharmacol.* 1974;284:295–306.

39. Kamerbeek HH, Rauws AG, Ham MT, et al. Prussian blue in therapy of thallotoxicosis: an experimental and clinical investigation. *Acta Med Scand.* 1971;189:321–324.

40. Heydlauf H. Ferric-cyanoferrate (II): an effective antidote in thallium poisoning. *Eur J Pharmacol.* 1969;6:340–344.

41. Manninen V, Malkonen M, Skulskii IA. Elimination of thallium in rats as influenced by Prussian blue and sodium chloride. *Acta Pharmacol Toxicol (Copenh).* 1976;39:256–261.

42. Barroso-Moguel R, Villeda-Hernandez J, Mendez-Armenta M, et al. Combined d-penicillamine and Prussian blue as antidotal treatment against thallotoxicosis in rats: evaluation of cerebellar lesions. *Toxicology.* 1994;89:15–24.

43. Rios C, Monroy-Noyola A. D-penicillamine and Prussian blue as antidotes against thallium intoxication in rats. *Toxicology.* 1992;74:69–76.

44. Meggs WJ, Cahill-Morasco R, Shih RD, et al. Effects of Prussian blue and N-acetylcysteine on thallium toxicity in mice. *Clin Toxicol.* 1997;35:163–166.

45. Pearce J. Studies of any toxicological effects of Prussian blue compounds in mammals: a review. *Food Chem Toxicol.* 1994;32:577–582.

46. Mulkey JP, Oehme FW. Are 2,3-dimercapto-1-propanesulfonic acid or Prussian blue beneficial in acute thallotoxicosis in rats? *Vet Hum Toxicol.* 2000;42:325–329.

47. Van der Stock J, Schepper J. The effect of Prussian blue and sodium-ethylenediaminetetraacetic acid on the faecal and urinary elimination of thallium by the dog. *Res Vet Sci.* 1978;25:337–342.

48. Lund A. The effect various substances on the excretion and the toxicity of thallium in the rat. *Acta Pharmacol et Toxicol.* 1956;12:260–268.

49. Kamerbeek HH, Rauws AG, Ham MT, et al. Dangerous redistribution of thallium by treatment with sodium diethyldithiocarbamate. *Acta Med Scand.* 1971;189:149–154.

50. Hoffman RS, Stringer JA, Feinberg RS, et al. Comparative efficacy of thallium adsorption by activated charcoal, Prussian blue, and sodium polystyrene sulfonate. *Clin Toxicol.* 1999;37:833–837.

51. Lehmann PA, Favari L. Parameters for the adsorption of thallium ions by activated charcoal and Prussian blue. *Clin Toxicol.* 1984;22:331–339.

CHAPTER 25

Aluminum

Gregory A. Jicha and Sarah A. Carr

INTRODUCTION

Neurological consequences of toxic aluminum exposure include encephalopathy, seizures, motor neuron degeneration, parkinsonism, and death.[1,2] Aluminum toxicity has been implicated in the development of Alzheimer's disease (AD), amyotrophic lateral sclerosis (ALS), Parkinson's disease (PD), and ALS–parkinsonism–dementia complex in Guam (ALS/PDC), but definitive evidence of a causal role for aluminum in the development of these degenerative disease states is debated.[1–23] Documented aluminum toxicity in humans is rare and occurs primarily through iatrogenic or occupational exposure, although simple environmental exposure may also play a role in the development of chronic aluminum toxicity.[1–5,7,10,11,24–32]

Aluminum, the third most abundant element and the most common metal in the Earth's crust (8.1% by weight), is ubiquitous in the environment in which we live.[33] Chronic exposure to aluminum is unavoidable. Fortunately, most aluminum-containing compounds are relatively insoluble at physiological pH, limiting absorption of aluminum through ingestion or inhalation (only 0.06% to 0.1% absorbed).[17,28–34] Aluminum toxicity therefore requires either chronic exposure to extremely high levels of aluminum-containing compounds or direct inoculation of aluminum via dialysates, parenteral nutrition, or implanted foreign materials, such as surgical cements.[25,26,32,35–39] Nonneurological consequences of aluminum toxicity, including renal osteodystrophy and hypochromic microcytic anemia, can be profound but are not discussed further in this chapter.[25,32,33]

Aluminum has no known physiological role.[33] The toxic consequences of aluminum exposure are thought to be related to dysregulation of other essential metals or ions; deposition of insoluble aluminum precipitates in vulnerable tissues; or protein, lipid, or nucleotide interactions resulting in conformational and structural alterations, aggregation, and functional alterations in essential cellular machinery and processes.[1,2,6,27,32,33,40–47] Much of what is known regarding aluminum toxicity has come from epidemiological, pathological, and animal studies.[1,40,47–49] Complete reversal of the neurotoxic effects of aluminum may not be possible once they occur, but some success has been achieved in the treatment of aluminum toxicity using metal chelators such as desferroxamine.[32,50–53]

The present chapter highlights our current understanding of aluminum neurotoxicity, focusing on animal studies, iatrogenic toxicity (including exposure via dialysis, parenteral nutrition, surgical cements, and current controversies regarding vaccine adjuvants, over-the-counter drugs, and antiperspirants), epidemiology of environmental and occupational exposure, and the potential relationship of aluminum toxicity with the development of neurodegenerative diseases such as AD, ALS, PD, and ALS/PDC.

ANIMAL STUDIES

Aluminum toxicity in animals was first described by Siem and Dollken in 1886,[52,53] but was popularized by the seminal experiments of Klatzo and colleagues in the mid-1960s.[54] Klatzo's initial discoveries stemmed from the observation of vacuolar degeneration in the spinal cords of animals receiving either diphterotoxin or control aluminum-based adjuvant injections. The toxic effects seen were eventually found to be related to the aluminum hydroxide in the adjuvant.

Further work by Terry and colleagues demonstrated neurofibrillary aggregates with the vacuoles, spurring interest in the role of aluminum in neurofibrillary degeneration (NFD) and established a putative link between aluminum toxicity and AD.[55,56] However, unlike the neurofibrillary tangles (NFTs) in AD, aluminum-induced NFD (Al-NFDs) exhibited distinct histochemical properties and ultrastructural appearance by electron microscopy. Al-NFDs, unlike NFTs, were not reactive with thioflavin-S and did not exhibit birefringence after staining with Congo red dye.[54] Ultrastructurally, Al-NFDs are composed of 10-nm straight filaments with a diameter of 2.0 nm, in contrast to the paired helical filaments of NFTs with a twisted helical appearance and diameter of 3.2 nm.[57,58] Pathologically, Al-NFDs are found in the proximal axon and perikaryon, whereas NFTs are more classically seen in the perikaryon and dendritic arbor (Figure 25-1).[2,20,21,44,54–56,58] Further immunohistochemical and biochemical studies revealed distinct

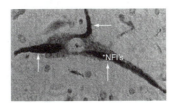

Figure 25-1. Neurofibrillary tangles in axons imaged in a single neuron from hippocampal region of aluminum-treated aged rabbits. (Walton JR. A longitudinal study of rats chronically exposed to aluminum at human dietary levels. *Neurosci Lett.* 2007;412[1]:29–33.)

differences in composition, with Al-NFDs largely composed of neurofilament proteins, in contrast with NFTs largely composed of the microtubule-associated protein τ.[1,2,20,58–60] Despite these important differences, many similarities between Al-NFDs and NFTs exist, and more recent evidence has demonstrated that Al-NFDs also contain the protein τ, β-amyloid, and ubiquitin similar to NFTs from AD (Figure 25-2).[61,62]

Aluminum-induced neurodegeneration in the rat affects similar anatomical regions that are involved in AD, including the hippocampus and diffuse cortical regions.[63] Aluminum administration in animal models has also been shown to result in widespread loss of cortical cholinergic innervation similar to that seen in AD.[64] Aluminum-treated animals also display deficits in learning and memory as assessed by various behavioral measures, including the Morris water maze, eye-blink conditioning, open field, and conditioned aversive avoidance tasks.[63,65–68] Animal models of aluminum toxicity recapitulate many biochemical changes (NFD, cholinergic loss, oxidative stress), patterns of neuroanatomical vulnerability, and behavioral alterations seen in AD (Figure 25-3).[2] Despite the development and widespread use of transgenic animal models of AD over the last decade, a continued usefulness and role for animal models of aluminum toxicity in AD research has been proposed.[69]

IATROGENIC TOXICITY

The first clear, undisputed evidence for aluminum neurotoxicity in humans emerged from the development and widespread use of hemodialysis in people with renal failure in the 1970s.[70–77] At that time, the widespread use of dialysates containing high levels of aluminum contaminants was common. Both neurotoxic and systemic effects of direct aluminum exposure that bypassed the barriers to aluminum absorption in the gastrointestinal (GI) tract and lungs became recognized. Dialysis encephalopathy, renal osteodystrophy, and hypochromic microcytic anemia were all identified as related to aluminum exposure, leading to reformulation of dialysate composition and removal of the harmful aluminum contaminants.[75,77] Dialysis encephalopathy is now quite rare, but cases of aluminum toxicity resulting in the syndrome of dialysis encephalopathy are still seen in this patient population as the result of chronic ingestion of aluminum-based phosphate binders and impaired renal clearance of aluminum absorbed through the GI and pulmonary systems, even in people not undergoing dialysis therapy.[25,26,76,77]

The clinical signs and symptoms of dialysis encephalopathy are directly related to plasma levels of aluminum resulting from exposure.[33] Low plasma levels of aluminum

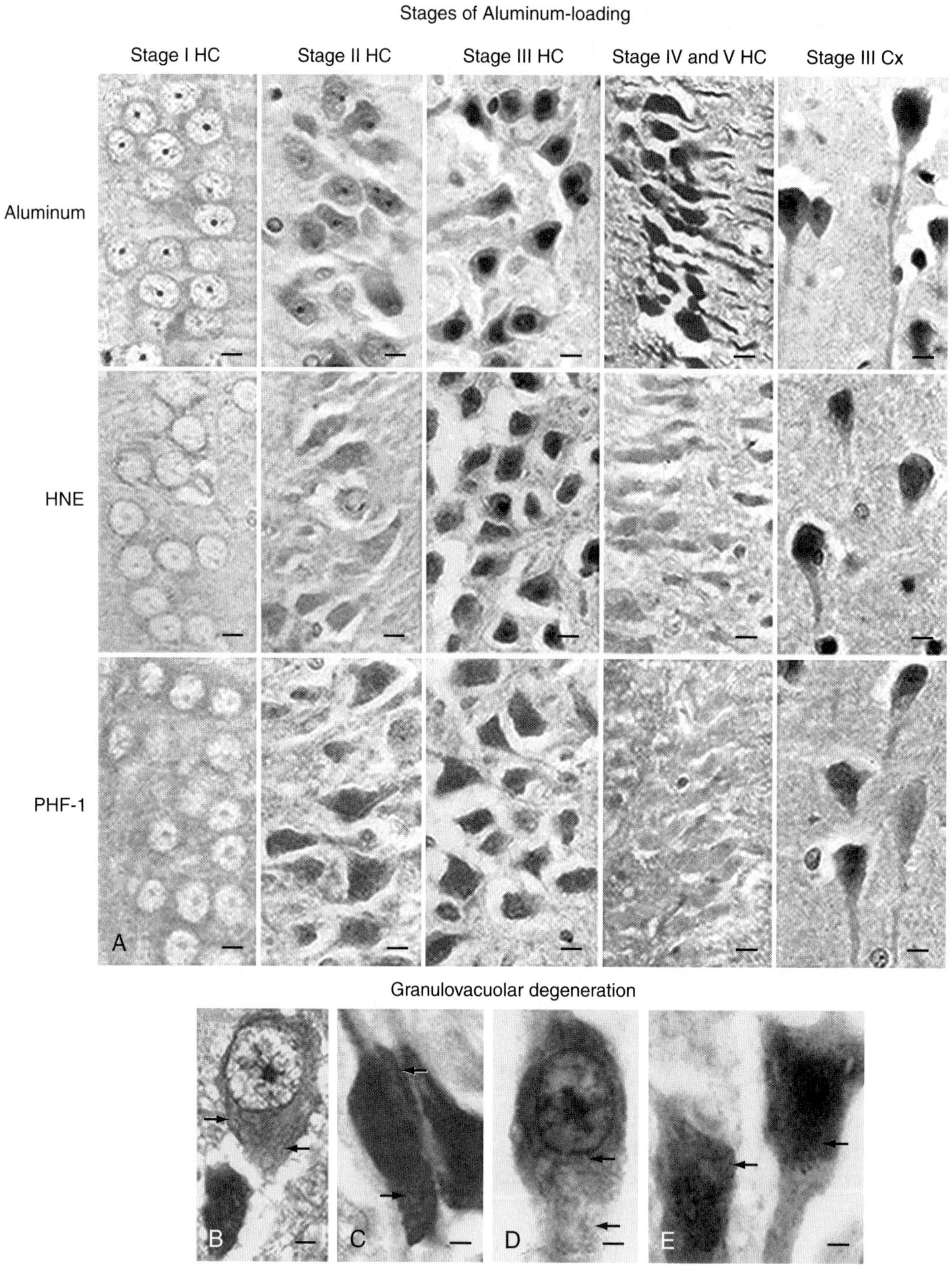

Stages of Aluminum-loading

Figure 25-2. *(A)* Stages of aluminum loading, oxidative damage, and the hyperphosphorylated protein τ in hippocampal (HC) neurons (columns 1–4) and layer V cortical (Cx) neurons (column 5). Row 1: neurons stained for aluminum at increasing stages of aluminum loading. In column 4, hippocampal neurons with Stage IV aluminum loading are recognizable by their magenta nuclei and blue cytoplasm (upper part of micrograph), whereas those at Stage V aluminum loading have a magenta nucleus and magenta cytoplasm (lower part of micrograph). Row 2: Immunostaining with 4-hydroxy-2-nonenal (HNE), a marker for oxidative damage. Row 3: Immunostaining with plant homeodomain finger protein 1 (PHF-1), a marker for the hyperphosphorylated protein τ. The micrographs in rows 2 and 3 illustrate equivalent cells in sections adjacent to those shown in row 1. Scale bars = 10 μm. *(B–E)* granulovacuolar degeneration (GVD) in hippocampal neurons from cognitively damaged rats. Arrows designate some vacuoles that contain visible GVD granules within the plane of focus: *(B)* Stained with hematoxylin and eosin; *(C)* Stained for aluminum; *(D)* Immunostained for HNE-associated oxidative damage; *(E)* Immunostained with PHF-1 for the hyperphosphorylated protein τ. Scale bars = 2 μm. (Walton JR. An aluminum-based rat model for Alzheimer's disease exhibits oxidative damage, inhibition of PP2A activity, hyperphosphorylated τ, and granulovacuolar degeneration. *J Inorg Biochem.* 2007;101[9]:1275–1284.)

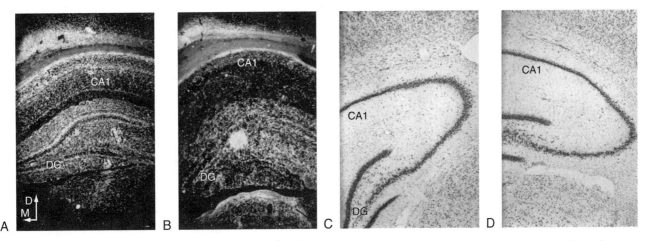

Figure 25-3. In the ipsilateral hippocampus, acetylcholinesterase (AChE) labeling was strongly depleted in CA1 and to a lesser extent in the dentate gyrus (DG) after aluminum infusion (B) compared to saline-injected controls (A). (C–D) The cresyl violet stain illustrates the lack of cellular disruption and the intact organization in both groups. Scale bars = 200 μm. (Platt B, Fiddler G, Riedel G, Henederson Z. Aluminum toxicity in the rat brain: histochemical and immunocytochemical evidence. *Brain Res Bull.* 2001;55[2]:257–267.)

(50 μg/L) result in mild cognitive slowing and electroencephalogram abnormalities, including diffuse slowing and emergence of epileptiform discharges.[71,78–80] At higher levels, progressive and irreversible development of encephalopathy, seizures, and myoclonus ensues. Untreated, the syndrome invariably leads to death within a year of the onset of symptoms. Elimination of aluminum exposure and the use of chelating agents, such as desferroxamine, at least partially reverse these signs and symptoms if instituted early in the course of disease.[81–85] Neuropathological examination of brain tissue from patients who have expired from dialysis encephalopathy has demonstrated changes similar to those in the animal models of aluminum toxicity, including the deposition of argyrophilic granular material in lysosomes, vacuolar degeneration, and glial inclusions.[86–88] These pathological features are distinct from those seen in AD or other degenerative disease states that have been linked to aluminum toxicity, casting doubt on the potential role aluminum exposure may play in these disease states.

Developmental delay and features of dialysis encephalopathy can also be seen in conjunction with prolonged parenteral nutrition, especially in premature infants.[36,74] Reductions in aluminum contaminants have reduced the occurrence of such iatrogenic exposure; however, isolated cases are still occasionally reported in the literature. Like dialysis encephalopathy in renal patients not undergoing dialysis, the occurrence of aluminum toxicity may again be related to suboptimal renal function as a result of prematurity or other medical complications.[36,74]

The use of aluminum-based cements in otoneurological surgery has also been implicated in a clinical syndrome indistinguishable from that seen in dialysis encephalopathy.[35,37–39] The surgical procedures implicated involve direct contact of the aluminum-containing cement with the cerebrospinal fluid (CSF) compartment, allowing direct access of aluminum to the central nervous system tissues. Six patients in total were affected, and following the publication of data implicating the cement as causal, the product was removed from the market and the company that manufactured it went bankrupt.[39]

A common theme in the preceding noted causes of aluminum toxicity in humans is the direct systemic inoculation of aluminum bypassing the barriers to GI and pulmonary absorption. While less dramatic than the preceding examples, chronic aluminum toxicity can occur through ingestion or inhalation and has caused great concern among toxicologists in regards to further instances of iatrogenic as well as occupational and environmental exposures to aluminum and aluminum-based compounds.

Antacids, buffered analgesics, adjuvants, and antiperspirants all contain significant levels of aluminum (up to 53% weight/weight by some estimates).[24,29,31,89] GI, dermatological, and pulmonary barriers may be inadequate to prevent aluminum toxicity, given chronic exposure to such high levels of aluminum-containing compounds.[29,31,33] Antacids when taken at the maximum daily dosage can increase aluminum intake by 277 to 3809 mg/day. Even with GI absorption limited at a range of 0.06% to 0.1% of dietary intake, possible systemic uptake of aluminum could theoretically reach 3.8 mg/day, enough to produce the clinical signs and symptoms seen in fulminate dialysis encephalopathy. Absorption in the GI system can also be enhanced by ingestion in acidic media, such as juice, soft drinks, and alcoholic beverages, suggesting that even greater systemic absorption can occur on the basis of dietary and other factors.[29,33] Different aluminum derivatives also have different solubilities at neutral pH, again potentially enhancing the systemic absorption of toxic quantities of aluminum.[29,33] In Europe, patient information leaflets warn against the use of aluminum-containing antacids by people with impaired renal function, during pregnancy, and during breastfeeding because of concerns about potential toxicity.[29]

Buffered analgesics such as aspirin, diclofenac, and ibuprofen contain aluminum-based buffers to enhance dissolution and absorption of the active agent. While nonsteroidal antiinflammatory drug (NSAID) ingestion in approved dosage regimens is unlikely to cause significant increases in aluminum absorption, NSAID overuse, abuse, or chronic administration within regulatory guidelines have raised concern regarding the potential for increased aluminum intake.[29]

Adjuvants used in routine vaccination, including diphtheria and tetanus toxoid vaccine, are often aluminum based, raising concerns about the safety of such vaccinations in vulnerable individuals.[89] The initial discoveries by Klatzo were based on observations of such toxicity in animals involving this route of exposure to aluminum-based compounds.[54] Despite this concern, it is widely appreciated that the low doses of aluminum included in such adjuvant preparations pose no immediate or chronic health risks to individuals undergoing routine vaccination procedures that incorporate the use of aluminum-based adjuvants.[89]

Antiperspirants often contain significant quantities of aluminum-based compounds, raising concern about their potential for promoting aluminum absorption and toxicity.[24] While intact skin is an efficient barrier to absorption of aluminum and aluminum salts used in standard antiperspirant preparations, breaches to the intact skin barrier as a result of culturally dependent shaving practices may allow direct systemic access of aluminum through this portal.[24,33] While no reports have surfaced that directly implicate antiperspirant use with aluminum neurotoxicity, this remains an important alternative route for systemic administration of toxic aluminum doses.

ENVIRONMENTAL AND OCCUPATIONAL EXPOSURE

Aluminum concentrations in public drinking water have been implicated in the potential consequences of aluminum toxicity including the development of AD for the last 20 years, yet no resolution of this debate has occurred.[1,2,7,34,90] Aluminum-containing compounds are commonly used in water purification processes, thus increasing levels of aluminum contamination in drinking water from industrialized nations. More than two-thirds of current epidemiological studies investigating aluminum levels in drinking water have reported an association of elevated aluminum levels with cognitive decline and dementia of the AD type.[2] Accidental environmental aluminum contamination of drinking water supplies, as occurred in England in 1988, when 20 tons of aluminum sulfate were accidentally emptied into the drinking water reservoir, has spurred the debate on possible risks of environmental exposure to aluminum.[91–95] Impaired attention and executive function demonstrated by performance on the digit–symbol subtest of the Wechsler Memory Scale, as well as abnormalities in visual evoked potentials, were noted in exposed individuals compared to nonexposed siblings. Despite these observations, no causal link between environmental exposure and neurological sequelae of aluminum toxicity has been definitively established. Individual variability in absorption kinetics and influence of dietary intake of modulators such as acidic compounds and competing metal ions create significant confounds in establishing such a causal link.

The risk of occupational exposure to aluminum has increased dramatically in recent years, concomitant with the increased worldwide demand for aluminum products. Typical occupational exposure results from smelting, welding, or electrolysis.[10,22,28,96,97] A recent meta-analysis of the neurobehavioral effects of occupational aluminum exposure concluded that there is a dose–response relationship between exposure and neurobehavioral deficits, primarily on the digit-symbol subtest of the Wechsler Memory Scale.[28] Similar selective neurocognitive deficits were seen in the accidental aluminum exposure in Camelford, England, described earlier.[92,98] The authors also commented on several limitations and caveats of their interpretation, including (1) effect sizes were less than those usually required to show significance in comparable studies; (2) significant heterogeneity was related to type and duration of occupational exposure for welders and longer exposure times, posing a greater risk for neurobehavioral decline; and (3) several confounding variables, including age and education, as an estimate of premorbid intelligence skewed the results by exaggerating the effect size.[28] Despite these caveats, the authors' conclusions strongly support the notion that occupational exposure to aluminum has deleterious effects on neurobehavioral function.

ALUMINUM AND NEURODEGENERATIVE DISEASE

Evidence linking aluminum exposure and human neurodegenerative diseases such as AD, ALS, PD, and ALS/PDC include examples of in vitro scientific plausibility, animal model observations, and epidemiological data.[2,15,48,90] Aluminum facilitates the proteinaceous aggregation of neurofilaments, α-synuclein, and microtubule-associated proteins, including τ- and β-amyloid that form the pathological hallmarks of AD, ALS, PD, and ALS/PDC.[2,43–46,58–61] Aluminum toxicity also leads to neurodegeneration and neuronal loss that is a hallmark of these human disease states.

A role for aluminum in the development of PD is suggested by studies demonstrating aluminum-induced conformational changes and subsequent enhanced aggregation of α-synuclein in vitro.[45,46] Of all studied metals, aluminum is most efficient at inducing Thioflavin T–positive α-synuclein polymerization in vitro.[46] Epidemiological studies have demonstrated an increased risk of PD with dietary and occupational exposure to aluminum.[3,10,22] Selective accumulation of aluminum in vulnerable neurons in the substantia nigra of PD has been documented, further supporting a putative role for aluminum toxicity in the development of PD.[12]

Aluminum-induced spinal motor neuron degeneration was first noted by Klatzo more than 40 years ago, drawing a link between aluminum toxicity and ALS.[54] While aluminum toxicity can cause widespread neuronal degeneration, spinal motor neurons are particularly susceptible to the toxic effects of aluminum exposure.[99] Axonal spheroids comprising aggregated neurofilament subunits are seen both in animal models of aluminum toxicity and in human ALS.[21,59,60,99] These pathological accumulations are close to identical in biochemical, anatomical, and ultrastructural detail.[59] Postmortem studies in humans have found evidence for elevated aluminum in the brain and spinal cord of people with ALS.[13] Epidemiological studies have also implicated aluminum exposure as a risk factor for the development of ALS.[4] Further suggestions of a relationship between ALS and aluminum toxicity come from studies investigating ALS/PDC of Guam.

Elevated aluminum content in drinking water from Guam has been suggested as a causative factor in the development of ALS/PDC. Focal accumulations of aluminum in degenerating neuronal perikarya, dendritic processes, and cerebral blood vessels have been detected by both histochemical (solochrome azurine) and x-ray microanalytical techniques.[8,9,18,19,23,100] Relative deficiencies of calcium and magnesium in drinking waters from endemic areas have been postulated to have enhanced the absorption of aluminum and other metals in these areas.[101] The introduction of water treatment plants in these areas has increased the content of available calcium and magnesium and reduced the levels of aluminum contaminants several fold, which in turn has been linked to the observed reduction in ALS/PDC incidence over the last several decades. Aluminum toxicity is only one of many environmental factors that have been implicated in ALS/PDC, and definitive evidence for a causal link is currently lacking.

While potentially causative links and associations between aluminum toxicity and development of neurodegenerative diseases such as PD, ALS, and ALS/PDC of Guam are intriguing, the links between development of AD and aluminum exposure were the first noted and have persisted in the literature to the present day. Despite the noted differences in biochemical composition in Al-NFDs and NFTs from AD brains, the observed lack of association of aluminum exposure with senile plaques of the AD type, the inconclusive results of epidemiological studies investigating aluminum exposure in AD, and the conflicting evidence of elevated aluminum content associated with the pathological lesions seen in AD brains, the aluminum hypothesis has survived and is still regarded by many as a plausible explanation for the development of AD.[1,2] Proponents of this hypothesis have conceded that aluminum exposure is not solely responsible for AD but maintain belief that aluminum exposure is at least an aggravating factor in some cases of AD. Aluminum staining can be seen in areas such as the hippocampus that undergo early degeneration in AD (Figure 25-4; see color plate).

Methods for detection of aluminum in AD brains that have led to contradictory results in the field are poorly understood. Confounds of such assessments include a poor understanding of and limited ability to account for aluminum speciation (different forms of aluminum-containing chemical compounds) and imprecision in detecting microneuroanatomical, cellular, and subcellular regions of focal aluminum accumulation.[33] More precise analytical techniques for the quantitation of aluminum using electron microscopy–based spectrometry and laser microprobe mass analysis have been developed and used for such studies, yet the results remain contradictory among studies and firm conclusions cannot be drawn.[33]

The contradictory results from epidemiological studies investigating the potential association of aluminum exposure to risk for AD have been suggested to be due to confounds of dietary intake, pH, other mineral contaminants (fluoride, silicon, magnesium, calcium, iron), age of exposed individuals, and even genetic polymorphisms that may influence aluminum absorption and passage through the blood–brain barrier.[1,2,7,29,31,33,49] Ingestion of aluminum-containing compounds in acidic media (fruit juice, soda, ethanol-containing beverages) greatly enhances aluminum absorption that would not occur otherwise. This confound has not been addressed in any existing epidemiological study. A complex interplay between other metal ions and molecular and cellular processes responsible for their physiological functions can greatly influence aluminum absorption to toxic levels given adequate exposure and can result in interference with normal physiological processes required to maintain cellular health and prevent degeneration.[6,41,42,102] Age is a major

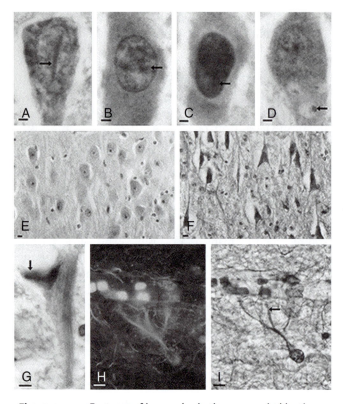

Figure 25-4. Features of human brain tissue revealed by the stain for aluminum. *(A–C)* Nuclei of neurons in transition between Stages III and IV have aluminum staining in the form of straight *(A, arrow)* or radiating *(B, arrow)* fibrils or as an amorphous substance *(C, arrow)*. Scale bar = 2.5 μm. *(D)* Granules (e.g., arrow) stain for aluminum in vacuoles of a Stage II neuron with early-stage granulovacuolar degeneration. Scale bar = 2.5 μm. *(E)* and *(F)* Extremes of aluminum staining in CA1 hippocampal neurons from aged human brain tissue. *(E)* Stage I neurons from a nondemented control brain exhibit minimal staining (nucleoli only) for aluminum. *(F)* Stage V neurons from an AD brain exhibit maximal staining for aluminum (nucleus and cytoplasm). Scale bar = 20 μm. *(G)* The nucleus (arrow) appears to be extruding from this neurofibrillary tangle–bearing neuron. Scale bar = 2.5 μm. Fluorescent image *(H)* and bright field image *(I)* of an astrocyte with processes containing aluminum that abuts a capillary containing erythrocytes that stain for aluminum. The arrow indicates an astrocyte process. Scale bar = 5 μm (see color plate). (Walton JR. Aluminum in hippocampal neurons from humans with Alzheimer's disease. *Neurotoxicology.* 2006;27[3]:385–394.)

these results are currently in dispute.[103,104] After review of published studies evaluating the link between environmental aluminum exposure and AD, a 1997 World Health Organization report concluded that a causal link between aluminum and AD could not be established.[105] This same report also concluded that the positive association between aluminum exposure and AD demonstrated in several epidemiological studies could not be completely dismissed.

Perhaps the most convincing arguments against the hypothesis that aluminum exposure may be causal in AD stem from the lack of evidence implicating aluminum in amyloidogenic pathways, which constitutes the prevailing hypothesis on the development of AD currently.[106,107] Neither animal models of aluminum toxicity nor documented human aluminum toxicity seen in dialysis encephalopathy are associated with the development of β-amyloid-associated senile or neuritic plaques.[26,40,48,69,87,88] While sporadic case reports and limited autopsy studies have suggested that such features can be present, they are not ubiquitous in cases of documented aluminum toxicity and their prevalence can be explained in light of the findings of such common pathological features in the brains of cognitively normal elderly subjects.[108–110]

Aluminum has not been identified as an integral component of β-amyloid plaques, despite the noted association of other metal ions such as copper, iron, and zinc with such pathological deposits.[1,2] Several in vitro studies of β-amyloid have suggested that aluminum induces conformational changes in this protein, leading to increased β-pleated sheet structure, and is capable of potentiating fibrillization and formation of toxic species of β-amyloid (Figure 25-5).[111–113] In vivo studies of the AD transgenic Tg2576 mouse have demonstrated that aluminum exposure increases both soluble and insoluble β-amyloid species and markers of oxidative such as F2 isoprostanes in hippocampal and cortical neurons, as seen in human AD.[114] While such lines of evidence are convincing to some, a clear link between human AD and aluminum exposure remains to be demonstrated.

CONCLUSION

Further research investigating the risks of environmental aluminum exposure, the molecular pathogenesis of aluminum toxicity in both animals and humans, and the potential association of chronic aluminum exposure to the development of degenerative disease is needed. While much debate exists regarding the relationship of aluminum toxicity to the development of degenerative disease such as AD, PD, ALS, and ALS/PDC in humans, iatrogenic and occupational exposures have been clearly linked to the development of fulminate neurological presentations of

factor that may influence the association of aluminum exposure with resultant toxicity through the influence of age-related subclinical impairment in renal function (allowing toxic levels of aluminum to accumulate) or through increased susceptibility of neuronal populations to undergo degeneration.[66] Still other studies have postulated links between polymorphisms in the transferrin gene that may alter aluminum absorption through biochemical pathways involved in iron homeostasis, although

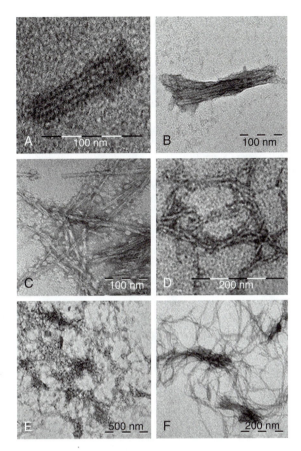

Figure 25-5. *(A–F)* Representative transmission electron microscopy images of ABri precipitated in the presence of no additional metal *(A;* scale bar = 100 nm); Al(III) *(B* and *C;* scale bars = 100 nm); Fe(III) *(D;* scale bar = 200 nm); Zn(II) *(E;* scale bar = 500 nm); and Cu(II) *(F;* scale bar = 200 nm). Magnifications are ×300K *(A* and *B);* ×200K *(C);* ×120K *(D* and *F);* and ×60K *(E).* (Khan A, Ashcroft AE, Korchazhkina OV, Exley C. Metal-mediated formation of fibrillar ABri amyloid. *J Inorg Biochem.* 2004;98[12]:2006–2010.)

aluminum toxicity. Human neurological signs and symptoms invariable include alterations in mental status that range from subtle neuropsychological deficits to severe encephalopathy and death. Continued efforts focused on reducing iatrogenic, occupational, and environmental exposure to aluminum are clearly warranted.

COMMENT

This case report highlights many of the challenges faced by medical practitioners when entertaining the diagnosis of aluminum toxicity. Clearly this patient had documented aluminum toxicity; however, the presentation was complicated by comorbid bismuth toxicity, which can also lead to neurocognitive sequelae similar to those

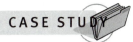

CASE STUDY

A 54-year-old man was brought by his family for evaluation in the Memory Disorders Clinic. He had been experiencing difficulties with his memory over the last 2 years that were characterized by inattentiveness, frequent repeating behaviors, misplacement of objects, and moderate difficulty operating his privately owned company. The family members that accompanied him were unsure whether the difficulties were progressive or static but did relate the onset of symptoms to his acquisition of a metal refinery for development and eventual resale. His past medical history was unremarkable. He was on no medication. His Folstein Mini-Mental State Examination (MMSE) score was 25, with 2 points lost on serial sevens and all 3 points lost on delayed recall. Neurological and physical examinations were otherwise unremarkable. Neuropsychological testing was performed, which showed evidence for mild to moderate impairment in attention, memory, and executive function, and was interpreted as consistent with a diagnosis of AD. Standard laboratory workup for reversible causes of dementia, including hemogram, comprehensive metabolic panel (electrolytes, hepatic and renal function), rapid plasma reagin test, thyroid function studies, folate, and vitamin B_{12} levels, showed all results were normal. Magnetic resonance imaging of the brain was normal for the patient's age. Heavy metal screen revealed elevated levels of aluminum and bismuth. Chelation therapy using ethylenediaminetetraacetic acid and desferroxamine resulted in normalization of the laboratory values at his next visit 6 months later.

Despite therapeutic intervention the patient continued to decline, and his MMSE was 22 at his 1-year follow-up. Neuropsychological evaluation at this time showed persistent amnesia, further progression of the attentional and executive deficits, and developing trouble with visuospatial dysfunction. Magnetic resonance imaging of his brain was repeated, which showed evidence for progressive atrophy of the entorhinal cortices and hippocampi. A positron emission tomography scan of the brain showed a pattern of hypometabolism consistent with a diagnosis of AD. Combination therapy with a cholinesterase inhibitor and *N*-methyl-d-aspartate antagonist was initiated, and the patient's diagnosis was changed from heavy metal–induced encephalopathy to AD.

seen in AD. Occupational and environmental exposures to heavy metals often involve concomitant exposure to multiple toxic moieties, leading to difficulties in interpreting the causal effects of an individual agent. In addition, the documented progression of cognitive decline after correction of heavy metal levels raises the question of an underlying degenerative disease (i.e., AD) and the possibility that the metal toxicity was an incidental finding unrelated to the patient's cognitive decline. No other cases of dementia were reported among his employees, who presumably had even greater exposure to the heavy metal contaminants. Nonetheless, it is interesting to speculate that his aluminum exposure may have triggered the onset of a degenerative process identical in phenotype to that seen in sporadic AD. A definitive diagnosis in this case must wait for autopsy, searching for the pathological hallmarks of AD and evidence for aluminum deposition in degenerating neurons of the central nervous system.

REFERENCES

1. Gupta VB, Anitha S, Hegde ML, et al. Aluminium in Alzheimer's disease: are we still at a crossroad? *Cell Mol Life Sci.* 2005;62(2):143–158.
2. Miu AC, Benga O. Aluminum and Alzheimer's disease: a new look. *J Alzheimers Dis.* 2006;10(2–3):179–201.
3. Altschuler E. Aluminum-containing antacids as a cause of idiopathic Parkinson's disease. *Med Hypotheses.* 1999;53(1):22–23.
4. Bergomi M, Vinceti M, Nacci G, et al. Environmental exposure to trace elements and risk of amyotrophic lateral sclerosis: a population-based case–control study. *Environ Res.* 2002;89(2):116–123.
5. Caban-Holt A, Mattingly M, Cooper G, Schmitt FA. Neurodegenerative memory disorders: a potential role of environmental toxins. *Neurol Clin.* 2005;23(2):485–521.
6. Deloncle R, Guillard O. Mechanism of Alzheimer's disease: arguments for a neurotransmitter–aluminium complex implication. *Neurochem Res.* 1990;15(12):1239–1245.
7. Flaten TP. Aluminium as a risk factor in Alzheimer's disease, with emphasis on drinking water. *Brain Res Bull.* 2001;55(2):187–196.
8. Garruto RM, Fukatsu R, Yanagihara R, Gajdusek DC, Hook G, Fiori CE. Imaging of calcium and aluminum in neurofibrillary tangle–bearing neurons in parkinsonism–dementia of Guam. *Proc Natl Acad Sci USA.* 1984;81(6):1875–1879.
9. Garruto RM, Swyt C, Yanagihara R, Fiori CE, Gajdusek DC. Intraneuronal co-localization of silicon with calcium and aluminum in amyotrophic lateral sclerosis and parkinsonism with dementia of Guam. *N Engl J Med.* 1986;315(11):711–712.
10. Gorell JM, Rybicki BA, Cole Johnson C, Peterson EL. Occupational metal exposures and the risk of Parkinson's disease. *Neuroepidemiology.* 1999;18(6):303–308.
11. Gresham LS, Molgaard CA, Golbeck AL, Smith R. Amyotrophic lateral sclerosis and occupational heavy metal exposure: a case–control study. *Neuroepidemiology.* 1986;5(1):29–38.
12. Hirsch EC, Brandel JP, Galle P, Javoy-Agid F, Agid Y. Iron and aluminum increase in the substantia nigra of patients with Parkinson's disease: an x-ray microanalysis. *J Neurochem.* 1991;56(2):446–451.
13. Kasarskis EJ, Tandon L, Lovell MA, Ehmann WD. Aluminum, calcium, and iron in the spinal cord of patients with sporadic amyotrophic lateral sclerosis using laser microprobe mass spectroscopy: a preliminary study. *J Neurol Sci.* 1995;130(2):203–208.
14. McLachlan DR. Aluminum and Alzheimer's disease. *Neurobiol Aging.* 1986;7(6):525–532.
15. McLachlan DR, Fraser PE, Dalton AJ. Aluminium and the pathogenesis of Alzheimer's disease: a summary of evidence. *Ciba Found Symp.* 1992;169:87–98; discussion, 99–108.
16. McLachlan DR, Lukiw WJ, Kruck TP. New evidence for an active role of aluminum in Alzheimer's disease. *Can J Neurol Sci.* 1989;16(4 Suppl):490–497.
17. Meiri H, Banin E, Roll M. Aluminum ingestion: is it related to dementia? *Rev Environ Health.* 1991;9(4):191–205.
18. Perl DP, Gajdusek DC, Garruto RM, Yanagihara RT, Gibbs CJ. Intraneuronal aluminum accumulation in amyotrophic lateral sclerosis and parkinsonism–dementia of Guam. *Science.* 1982;217(4564):1053–1055.
19. Piccardo P, Yanagihara R, Garruto RM, Gibbs CJ Jr, Gajdusek DC. Histochemical and x-ray microanalytical localization of aluminum in amyotrophic lateral sclerosis and parkinsonism–dementia of Guam. *Acta Neuropathol.* 1988;77(1):1–4.
20. Shin RW, Lee VM, Trojanowski JQ. Neurofibrillary pathology and aluminum in Alzheimer's disease. *Histol Histopathol.* 1995;10(4):969–978.
21. Tanridag T, Coskun T, Hurdag C, Arbak S, Aktan S, Yegen B. Motor neuron degeneration due to aluminium deposition in the spinal cord: a light microscopical study. *Acta Histochem.* 1999;101(2):193–201.
22. Wechsler LS, Checkoway H, Franklin GM, Costa LG. A pilot study of occupational and environmental risk factors for Parkinson's disease. *Neurotoxicology.* 1991;12(3):387–392.
23. Yasui M, Yase Y, Ota K, Mukoyama M, Adachi K. High aluminum deposition in the central nervous system of patients with amyotrophic lateral sclerosis from the Kii Peninsula, Japan: two case reports. *Neurotoxicology.* 1991;12(2):277–283.
24. Antiperspirant drug products for over-the-counter human use. Final monograph. Final rule. *Fed Regist.* 2003;68(110):34273–34293.
25. de Wolff FA. Toxicological aspects of aluminum poisoning in clinical nephrology. *Clin Nephrol.* 1985;24 (Suppl 1):S9–S14.
26. de Wolff FA, Berend K, van der Voet GB. Subacute fatal aluminum poisoning in dialyzed patients: postmortem toxicological findings. *Forensic Sci Int.* 2002;128(1–2):41–43.
27. Hewitt CD, Savory J, Wills MR. Aspects of aluminum toxicity. *Clin Lab Med.* 1990;10(2):403–422.
28. Meyer-Baron M, Schaper M, Knapp G, van Thriel C. Occupational aluminum exposure: evidence in support of its neurobehavioral impact. *Neurotoxicology.* 2007;28(6):1068–1078.
29. Reinke CM, Breitkreutz J, Leuenberger H. Aluminium in over-the-counter drugs: risks outweigh benefits? *Drug Saf.* 2003;26(14):1011–1025.
30. Soni MG, White SM, Flamm WG, Burdock GA. Safety evaluation of dietary aluminum. *Regul Toxicol Pharmacol.* 2001;33(1):66–79.
31. van der Voet GB, de Wolff FA. Intestinal absorption of aluminium from antacids: a comparison between hydrotalcite and algeldrate. *J Toxicol Clin Toxicol.* 1986;24(6):545–553.
32. Yokel RA, McNamara PJ. Aluminium toxicokinetics: an updated minireview. *Pharmacol Toxicol.* 2001;88(4):159–167.
33. Priest ND. The biological behaviour and bioavailability of aluminium in man, with special reference to studies employing aluminium-26 as a tracer: review and study update. *J Environ Monit.* 2004;6(5):375–403.

34. Priest ND, Talbot RJ, Newton D, Day JP, King SJ, Fifield LK. Uptake by man of aluminium in a public water supply. *Hum Exp Toxicol.* 1998;17(6):296–301.

35. Guillard O, Pineau A, Fauconneau B, et al. Biological levels of aluminium after use of aluminium-containing bone cement in post-otoneurosurgery. *J Trace Elem Med Biol.* 1997;11(1):53–56.

36. Gura KM, Puder M. Recent developments in aluminium contamination of products used in parenteral nutrition. *Curr Opin Clin Nutr Metab Care.* 2006;9(3):239–246.

37. Hantson P, Mahieu P, Gersdorff M, Sindic C, Lauwerys R. Fatal encephalopathy after otoneurosurgery procedure with an aluminum-containing biomaterial. *J Toxicol Clin Toxicol.* 1995;33(6):645–648.

38. Renard JL, Felten D, Bequet D. Post-otoneurosurgery aluminium encephalopathy. *Lancet.* 1994;344(8914):63–64.

39. Reusche E, Pilz P, Oberascher G, et al. Subacute fatal aluminum encephalopathy after reconstructive otoneurosurgery: a case report. *Hum Pathol.* 2001;32(10):1136–1140.

40. Carpenter DO. Effects of metals on the nervous system of humans and animals. *Int J Occup Med Environ Health.* 2001;14(3):209–218.

41. Mendez-Alvarez E, Soto-Otero R, Hermida-Ameijeiras A, Lopez-Real AM, Labandeira-Garcia JL. Effects of aluminum and zinc on the oxidative stress caused by 6-hydroxydopamine autoxidation: relevance for the pathogenesis of Parkinson's disease. *Biochim Biophys Acta.* 2002;1586(2):155–168.

42. Miu AC. The silicon link between aluminium and Alzheimer's disease. *J Alzheimers Dis.* 2006;10(1):39–42.

43. Muma NA, Singer SM. Aluminum-induced neuropathology: transient changes in microtubule-associated proteins. *Neurotoxicol Teratol.* 1996;18(6):679–690.

44. Perl DP, Pendlebury WW. Aluminum neurotoxicity: potential role in the pathogenesis of neurofibrillary tangle formation. *Can J Neurol Sci.* 1986;13(4 Suppl):441–445.

45. Uversky VN, Li J, Bower K, Fink AL. Synergistic effects of pesticides and metals on the fibrillation of (α-synuclein: implications for Parkinson's disease. *Neurotoxicology.* 2002;23(4–5):527–536.

46. Uversky VN, Li J, Fink AL. Metal-triggered structural transformations, aggregation, and fibrillation of human (α-synuclein: a possible molecular NK between Parkinson's disease and heavy metal exposure. *J Biol Chem.* 2001;276(47):44284–44296.

47. Yokel RA. The toxicology of aluminum in the brain: a review. *Neurotoxicology.* 2000;21(5):813–828.

48. Erasmus RT, Savory J, Wills MR, Herman MM. Aluminum neurotoxicity in experimental animals. *Ther Drug Monit.* 1993;15(6):588–592.

49. Rondeau V. A review of epidemiologic studies on aluminum and silica in relation to Alzheimer's disease and associated disorders. *Rev Environ Health.* 2002;17(2):107–121.

50. Coburn JW, Norris KC. Diagnosis of aluminum-related bone disease and treatment of aluminum toxicity with deferoxamine. *Semin Nephrol.* 1986;6(4 Suppl 1):12–21.

51. Porter JB, Huehns ER. The toxic effects of desferrioxamine. *Baillieres Clin Haematol.* 1989;2(2):459–474.

52. Asch W, Asch D. *The Silicates in Chemistry and Commerce.* London: Constable; 1918.

53. Dollken U. Ueber die wirkung des aluminum mit besondrer berucksichtigung der durch das aluminum verursachten lasionen im zentrlnerven system. *Naunyn Schmiedebergs Arch Exp Path Pharmac.* 1897;40:98–120.

54. Klatzo I, Wisniewski H, Streicher E. Experimental production of neurofibrillary degeneration: I. Light microscopic observations. *J Neuropathol Exp Neurol.* 1965;24:187–199.

55. Terry RD, Pena C. Experimental production of neurofibrillary degeneration: II. Electron microscopy, phosphatase histochemistry and electron probe analysis. *J Neuropathol Exp Neurol.* 1965;24:200–210.

56. Wisniewski H, Terry RD, Hirano A. Neurofibrillary pathology. *J Neuropathol Exp Neurol.* 1970;29(2):163–176.

57. Kidd M. Paired helical filaments in electron microscopy of Alzheimer's disease. *Nature.* 1963;197:192–193.

58. Kidd M. The history of the paired helical filaments. *J Alzheimers Dis.* 2006;9(3 Suppl):71–75.

59. Strong MJ. Aluminum neurotoxicity: an experimental approach to the induction of neurofilamentous inclusions. *J Neurol Sci.* 1994;124 (Suppl):20–26.

60. Wakayama I, Nerurkar VR, Strong MJ, Garruto RM. Comparative study of chronic aluminum-induced neurofilamentous aggregates with intracytoplasmic inclusions of amyotrophic lateral sclerosis. *Acta Neuropathol.* 1996;92(6):545–554.

61. Huang Y, Herman MM, Liu J, Katsetos CD, Wills MR, Savory J. Neurofibrillary lesions in experimental aluminum-induced encephalopathy and Alzheimer's disease share immunoreactivity for amyloid precursor protein, Aβ, α 1-antichymotrypsin and ubiquitin–protein conjugates. *Brain Res.* 1997;771(2):213–220.

62. Savory J, Huang Y, Herman MM, Reyes MR, Wills MR. (τ-Immunoreactivity associated with aluminum maltolate–induced neurofibrillary degeneration in rabbits. *Brain Res.* 1995;669(2):325–329.

63. Miu AC, Andreescu CE, Vasiu R, Olteanu AI. A behavioral and histological study of the effects of long-term exposure of adult rats to aluminum. *Int J Neurosci.* 2003;113(9):1197–1211.

64. Kumar S. Biphasic effect of aluminium on cholinergic enzyme of rat brain. *Neurosci Lett.* 1998;248(2):121–123.

65. Colomina MT, Roig JL, Sanchez DJ, Domingo JL. Influence of age on aluminum-induced neurobehavioral effects and morphological changes in rat brain. *Neurotoxicology.* 2002;23(6):775–781.

66. Miu AC, Olteanu AI, Miclea M. A behavioral and ultrastructural dissection of the interference of aluminum with aging. *J Alzheimers Dis.* 2004;6(3):315–328.

67. Rabe A, Lee MH, Shek J, Wisniewski HM. Learning deficit in immature rabbits with aluminum-induced neurofibrillary changes. *Exp Neurol.* 1982;76(2):441–446.

68. Roig JL, Fuentes S, Teresa Colomina M, Vicens P, Domingo JL. Aluminum, restraint stress and aging: behavioral effects in rats after 1 and 2 years of aluminum exposure. *Toxicology.* 2006;218 (2–3):112–124.

69. Bharathi, Shamasundar NM, Sathyanarayana Rao TS, Dhanunjaya Naidu M, Ravid R, Rao KS. A new insight on Al-maltolate-treated aged rabbit as Alzheimer's animal model. *Brain Res Rev.* 2006;52(2):275–292.

70. Alfrey AC. Dialysis encephalopathy syndrome. *Annu Rev Med.* 1978;29:93–98.

71. Alfrey AC. Dialysis encephalopathy. *Clin Nephrol.* 1985;24 (Suppl 1):S15–S19.

72. Arieff AI. Aluminum and the pathogenesis of dialysis encephalopathy. *Am J Kidney Dis.* 1985;6(5):317–321.

73. Flaten TP, Alfrey AC, Birchall JD, Savory J, Yokel RA. Status and future concerns of clinical and environmental aluminum toxicology. *J Toxicol Environ Health.* 1996;48(6):527–541.

74. Golub MS, Domingo JL. What we know and what we need to know about developmental aluminum toxicity. *J Toxicol Environ Health.* 1996;48(6):585–597.

75. Jack R, Rabin PL, McKinney TD. Dialysis encephalopathy: a review. *Int J Psychiatry Med.* 1983;13(4):309–326.

76. Loghman-Adham M. Safety of new phosphate binders for chronic renal failure. *Drug Saf.* 2003;26(15):1093–1115.

77. Tzamaloukas AH, Agaba EI. Neurological manifestations of uraemia and chronic dialysis. *Niger J Med.* 2004;13(2):98–105.

78. Hughes JR, Schreeder MT. EEG in dialysis encephalopathy. *Neurology.* 1980;30(11):1148–1154.

79. Luda E, Canavese C, Rocca G. The EEG in progressive dialysis encephalopathy: II. The EEG and clinical indices of PDE in cases treated with desferrioxamine. *Ital J Neurol Sci.* 1984;5(4): 375–380.

80. O'Hare JA, Callaghan NM, Murnaghan DJ. Dialysis encephalopathy: clinical, electroencephalographic and interventional aspects. *Medicine (Baltimore).* 1983;62(3):129–141.

81. Ackrill P, Ralston AJ, Day JP. Role of desferrioxamine in the treatment of dialysis encephalopathy. *Kidney Int Suppl.* 1986;18:S104–S107.

82. Arze RS, Parkinson IS, Cartlidge NE, Britton P, Ward MK. Reversal of aluminium dialysis encephalopathy after desferrioxamine treatment. *Lancet.* 1981;2(8255):1116.

83. Hernandez P, Johnson CA. Deferoxamine for aluminum toxicity in dialysis patients. *Anna J.* 1990;17(3):224–228.

84. Nakamura H, Rose PG, Blumer JL, Reed MD. Acute encephalopathy due to aluminum toxicity successfully treated by combined intravenous deferoxamine and hemodialysis. *J Clin Pharmacol.* 2000;40(3):296–300.

85. Sprague SM, Corwin HL, Wilson RS, Mayor GH, Tanner CM. Encephalopathy in chronic renal failure responsive to deferoxamine therapy: another manifestation of aluminum neurotoxicity. *Arch Intern Med.* 1986;146(10):2063–2064.

86. Reusche E. Argyrophilic inclusions distinct from Alzheimer neurofibrillary changes in one case of dialysis-associated encephalopathy. *Acta Neuropathol.* 1997;94(6):612–616.

87. Reusche E, Koch V, Lindner B, Harrison AP, Friedrich HJ. Alzheimer morphology is not increased in dialysis-associated encephalopathy and long-term hemodialysis. *Acta Neuropathol.* 2001;101(3):211–216.

88. Reusche E, Seydel U. Dialysis-associated encephalopathy: light and electron microscopic morphology and topography with evidence of aluminum by laser microprobe mass analysis. *Acta Neuropathol.* 1993;86(3):249–258.

89. Piyasirisilp S, Hemachudha T. Neurological adverse events associated with vaccination. *Curr Opin Neurol.* 2002;15(3):333–338.

90. Jansson ET. Aluminum exposure and Alzheimer's disease. *J Alzheimers Dis.* 2001;3(6):541–549.

91. Allen WM, Sansom BF. Accidental contamination of the public water supply at Lowermoor, Camelford: an assessment of the possible veterinary consequences. *Vet Rec.* 1989;124(18):479–482.

92. Altmann P, Cunningham J, Dhanesha U, Ballard M, Thompson J, Marsh F. Disturbance of cerebral function in people exposed to drinking water contaminated with aluminium sulphate: retrospective study of the Camelford water incident. *BMJ.* 1999;319(7213):807–811.

93. Altmann P, Cunningham J, Marsh F, Dhanesha U, Ballard M, Thompson J. Camelford water incident. *BMJ.* 2000;320(7248):1536.

94. Exley C, Esiri MM. Severe cerebral congophilic angiopathy coincident with increased brain aluminium in a resident of Camelford, Cornwall, UK. *J Neurol Neurosurg Psychiatry.* 2006;77(7):877–879.

95. Powell JJ, Greenfield SM, Thompson RP, et al. Assessment of toxic metal exposure following the Camelford water pollution incident: evidence of acute mobilization of lead into drinking water. *Analyst.* 1995;120(3):793–798.

96. Polizzi S, Pira E, Ferrara M, et al. Neurotoxic effects of aluminium among foundry workers and Alzheimer's disease. *Neurotoxicology.* 2002;23(6):761–774.

97. Rifat SL, Eastwood MR, McLachlan DR, Corey PN. Effect of exposure of miners to aluminium powder. *Lancet.* 1990;336(8724):1162–1165.

98. McMillan TM, Freemont AJ, Herxheimer A, et al. Camelford water poisoning accident: serial neuropsychological assessments and further observations on bone aluminium. *Hum Exp Toxicol.* 1993;12(1):37–42.

99. Kihira T, Yoshida S, Komoto J, Wakayama I, Yase Y. Aluminum-induced model of motor neuron degeneration: subperineurial injection of aluminum in rabbits. *Neurotoxicology.* 1995;16(3):413–424.

100. Garruto RM, Yanagihara R, Gajdusek DC. Disappearance of high-incidence amyotrophic lateral sclerosis and parkinsonism–dementia on Guam. *Neurology.* 1985;35(2):193–198.

101. Oyanagi K. The nature of the parkinsonism–dementia complex and amyotrophic lateral sclerosis of Guam and magnesium deficiency. *Parkinsonism Relat Disord.* 2005;11 (Suppl 1):S17–S23.

102. Gillette Guyonnet S, Andrieu S, Vellas B. The potential influence of silica present in drinking water on Alzheimer's disease and associated disorders. *J Nutr Health Aging.* 2007;11(2):119–124.

103. Farrar G, Altmann P, Welch S, et al. Defective gallium-transferrin binding in Alzheimer disease and Down syndrome: possible mechanism for accumulation of aluminium in brain. *Lancet.* 1990;335(8692):747–750.

104. Rondeau V, Iron A, Letenneur L, et al. Analysis of the effect of aluminum in drinking water and transferrin C2 allele on Alzheimer's disease. *Eur J Neurol.* 2006;13(9):1022–1025.

105. World Health Organization. *Aluminum.* Geneva: World Health Organization; 1997.

106. Eckman CB, Eckman EA. An update on the amyloid hypothesis. *Neurol Clin.* 2007;25(3):669–682, vi.

107. Hardy JA, Higgins GA. Alzheimer's disease: the amyloid cascade hypothesis. *Science.* 1992;256(5054):184–185.

108. Bennett DA, Schneider JA, Arvanitakis Z, et al. Neuropathology of older persons without cognitive impairment from two community-based studies. *Neurology.* 2006;66(12):1837–1844.

109. Knopman DS, Parisi JE, Salviati A, et al. Neuropathology of cognitively normal elderly. *J Neuropathol Exp Neurol.* 2003;62(11):1087–1095.

110. Schmitt FA, Davis DG, Wekstein DR, Smith CD, Ashford JW, Markesbery WR. "Preclinical" AD revisited: neuropathology of cognitively normal older adults. *Neurology.* 2000;55(3):370–376.

111. House E, Collingwood J, Khan A, Korchazkina O, Berthon G, Exley C. Aluminium, iron, zinc and copper influence the in vitro formation of amyloid fibrils of Aβ42 in a manner which may have consequences for metal chelation therapy in Alzheimer's disease. *J Alzheimers Dis.* 2004;6(3):291–301.

112. Kawahara M, Muramoto K, Kobayashi K, Mori H, Kuroda Y. Aluminum promotes the aggregation of Alzheimer's amyloid β-protein in vitro. *Biochem Biophys Res Commun.* 1994;198(2):531–535.

113. Mantyh PW, Ghilardi JR, Rogers S, et al. Aluminum, iron, and zinc ions promote aggregation of physiological concentrations of β-amyloid peptide. *J Neurochem.* 1993;61(3):1171–1174.

114. Pratico D, Uryu K, Sung S, Tang S, Trojanowski JQ, Lee VM. Aluminum modulates brain amyloidosis through oxidative stress in APP transgenic mice. *FASEB J.* 2002;16(9):1138–1140.

Manganese

Brent Furbee

INTRODUCTION

History of Manganism

Manganism was first described by John Couper in 1837 when two workers in Scotland involved in the grinding of manganese ore developed paraplegia. In both cases, the loss of motor activity was worse in the lower extremities and sensory activity was spared. Couper reported an absence of tremor or gastrointestinal symptoms. Upon removal from their work environment, symptoms did not further progress, but they did not improve. Subsequently, three other workers were noted to have a staggering gait. Suspecting that manganese (Mn) might be the cause, they were removed from the workplace and progression stopped. Of interest, Couper says, "As soon as the staggering, which is the first symptoms of the disease, was remarked, their employment was changed. In all of them the paralysis gradually diminished, and at the end of a few weeks was entirely gone."[1]

The conditions in which the grinders worked were far from hygienic. "The surface of their bodies is of course constantly covered with the manganese; the air which they breathe is loaded with it in the form of fine powder, and they are ever exposed from neglect of cleanliness, to swallow portions of it along with their food."[1]

As other authors added to the body of literature, a clearer clinical picture of manganism began to emerge. Rodier (1955) described 150 Moroccan manganese miners, all of whom worked underground. Most were drilling manganese, with a few helpers who worked in immediate proximity to the drilling. Rodier described prodromal, intermediate, and established phases.

In the *prodromal phase,* the earliest signs of problems were loss of appetite and declining strength to the point that even simple tasks required sustained effort. Victims became apathetic and nonconversant. Occasionally, they experienced an excitatory period that Rodier labeled "manganese psychosis." Their gait then became staggering, their speech grew incoherent, and some began to behave aggressively. Initial hypersexual behavior was followed by impotence. A period of somnolence was followed by increasing insomnia.

As the prodromal period transitioned into the *intermediate phase,* speech deteriorated and stuttering was common. A change in facies reflected a dazed appearance termed "masque manganique." While most patients were characterized as being "in a perpetual state of euphoria," spasmodic weeping was occasionally encountered.[2] Motor skills also deteriorated with marked slowing and clumsiness. This was associated with increasing accidents. Some workers began to have problems with eating and drinking.[2] Rodier listed the disorders of the intermediate period as shown in Table 1.[2]

The *established phase* was marked by muscular hypertonia in extension, particularly in the lower limbs and face. Muscle rigidity led to further gait disturbance, including a positioning on the balls of the feet with ankles extended, knees and elbows flexed. This gait was termed *pas du coq* because it reminded observers of a rooster's gait. Walking backward became impossible for these patients. It was in the latter part of this third stage that tremor was sometimes seen.[2]

In the early to mid-1900s, more reports of manganism surfaced. Interestingly, even in extremely poor hygienic conditions, the number of affected workers represented a small percentage of all exposed workers.[2,3] In fact, in a report on Egyptian miners by Abd el Naby and Hassanein, the authors noted, "Even if we make allowance for those patients who have been missed or wrongly diagnosed, it would appear that this type of poisoning is still a rarity in this country."[3] Among reports during that time, affected workers were exposed to manganese concentrations of 30 per cubic meter to hundreds of milligrams (Figures 26-1 and 26-2).[4]

By 1954, 200 cases of suspected manganism had been reported worldwide. Parnitzke and Peiffer[5] reviewed the six autopsy reports with histopathology available at that time in an attempt to better characterize the central nervous system target of manganism. The results identified the basal ganglia and, more specifically, the globus pallidus as that target. The caudate and putamen were also damaged.[5–7]

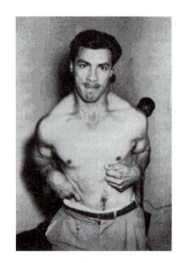

Figure 26-1. Facial grimace, elbows flexed upon standing, and wrist flexion are characteristics associated with manganism. (Mena I, Marin O, Fuenzalida S, et al. Chronic manganese poisoning: clinical picture and manganese turnover. *Neurology.* 1967;17:129–136.)

Clinical Presentation

More recently, medical advances have allowed better characterization of the clinical and pathological features of manganism and a more accurate way to distinguish it from non-manganese-related disorders. A report of smelter workers in Taiwan in 1989 helped researchers understand the characteristics of manganism and the exposure concentrations necessary to cause it. The workers had been exposed for 30 minutes each day, 7 days a week to concentrations of manganese exceeding 28.8 mg/m^3. The workers were grouped by exposure estimates from (1) office, designing, and packaging workers; (2) foundry,

Table 1: Symptoms and Signs of Manganism Reported by Rodier[2]

Symptom or Sign	Percentage (%)
Clumsiness of movement	82
Exaggeration of reflexes in lower limbs	74
Hyperemotionalism	71
Speech disorders	70
Masque manganique	65
Spasmodic laughter	47
Difficulty in certain movements	45
Spasmodic tears	32
Adiodokinesis	30

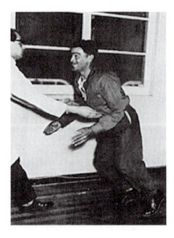

Figure 26-2. Patient after slight push from behind. Note flexion of arms and knees. (Mena I, Marin O, Fuenzalida S, et al. Chronic manganese poisoning: clinical picture and manganese turnover. *Neurology.* 1967;17:129–136.)

foundry-related, non-furnace workers, non-furnace maintenance workers, and metal cutters; (3) furnacemen; and (4) furnace foremen and maintenance workers. Cases only came from the fourth group (furnace foremen and maintenance workers), the group with the highest exposure. Of note, many workers were exposed to concentrations of more than 4.0 mg/m³ but did not develop symptoms.[8,8a]

When the ventilation system was fixed, the air concentration of manganese during electrode fixation and welding decreased to less than 4.4 mg/m³. No new cases were reported. These workers, like those in previous reports, demonstrated some findings that are similar to idiopathic Parkinson's disease (IPD), including generalized bradykinesia and rigidity.

Four of the patients received 6-fluorodopa (6-FD) and 18F-2-fluoro-2-deoxyglucose (FDG) positron emission tomography (PET) studies. Their results were compared with normal patients and those with Parkinson's disease. Magnetic resonance imaging (MRI) results were normal in three of the four manganism patients. The fourth had high signal intensity in the corona radiata and posterior limb of the left internal capsule. The 6-FD PET scans in manganism and normal subjects were normal, while subjects with Parkinson's disease had a significantly lower concentration. On FDG-PET, manganism patients demonstrated an overall decrease in local cerebral metabolic rate for glucose.[9]

Huang et al. reported, "There were parkinsonian clinical features with bradykinesia, rigidity, and clumsiness. It is of interest that the preliminary result of neuropsychological evaluation in our patients showed normal cognitive function except for visual perception, which is in contrast to the 'manganese madness' reported in miners. This difference may be dose dependent since our patients had relatively mild disease."[8]

In 1991, Hua and Huang reported a case–control study comparing the 4 manganism patients with 17 asymptomatic workers from the same ferromanganese plant, 8 patients with IPD, and 19 control subjects.[10] They concluded that neurobehavioral changes occurred only in the 4 patients demonstrating parkinsonism, not in the manganese-exposed nonparkinsonian subjects.[10]

By 1993, Huang et al. reported, "The order of occurrence of neurological symptoms in these six patients was determined. The most frequent initial symptom was gait disturbance. Patients tended to fall because of freezing in turning. Writing difficulty and hypophonia were the next initial symptoms in chronological order of onset. Fatigue and muscle cramps were also frequent."[11] They found that of 18 items tested muscle stiffness, sleep disturbance, fatigue, walking backward, freezing during turning, and writing tended to worsen; however, tremor showed some improvement. The authors observed that

in manganism the earliest signs are freezing during turns and difficulty walking backward. In IPD, however, a resting, pill-rolling tremor with a frequency of 3 to 7 Hz may worsen as the disease progresses. In patients with manganism, tremor is not prominent but is postural, and it exhibits high frequency and low amplitude. It tends to disappear as other deficits progress. Similar to Wilson's disease, foot dystonia, dystonic gait (cock's gait), and dystonic smile occur in manganism.[11] Levodopa therapy was not helpful for the four patients in whom it was tested.[12]

At 10-year follow-up, the most prominent progression of symptoms was associated with gait disturbance, rigidity, speed of foot tapping, and writing (Huang 1998). Approximately 15 years following the initial diagnosis, Huang et al. reported, "The neurological manifestations included micrographia, masked facies, hypophonia or stuttering speech, dystonia; gait en bloc, difficulty in walking especially backwards, postural instability, and rigidity. All patients did not have resting tremor except for patient 4, who had tongue tremor while stretching out his tongue."[13]

Huang et al. demonstrated that uptake of technetium 99m–TRODAT-1, a cocaine analogue that can specifically bind to the dopamine transporter sites at presynaptic dopamine neuron terminal was significantly higher in patients with chronic manganism than that in Parkinson's disease patients. The authors suggested that a technetium 99m–TRODAT-1 single-photon emission computed tomography (SPECT) scan may be a better tool for the differentiation of manganism from Parkinson's disease.[13]

Manganism may be distinguished from IPD by the presence of symmetry of symptoms, more frequent dystonia, a propensity to fall backward, and a gait with plantar–flexion and flexion of the elbows called "cock walk." The authors reported a continual deterioration of the patients' symptoms over the initial 5 to 10 years after termination of exposure that eventually plateaued.

The pathological and clinical features of manganism and IPD may be confused. The substantia nigra is the primary target of IPD, and decreased dopamine production is responsible for its clinical features. Manganism primarily targets the globus pallidus and has somewhat different clinical manifestations, among which is a poor response to treatment with levodopa. Those findings that tend to favor manganism include the following:

- Clinical presentation—Retropulsion, cock walk, symmetrical effects, infrequent tremor, facial grimacing.
- MRI—Hyperintensities of the globus pallidus on T1-weighted images, indicating increased manganese exposure but not toxicity (Figure 26-3).
- Response to levodopa—For some patients, initial improvement followed by decline. As opposed to

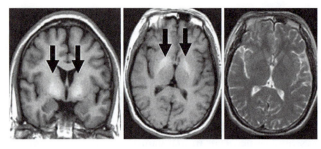

Figure 26-3. Hyperintensity of the globus pallidus (arrows) in a smelter worker exposed to low levels of airborne manganese. (Jiang Y, Zheng W, Long L, et al. Brain magnetic resonance imaging and manganese concentrations in red blood cells of smelting workers: search for biomarkers of manganese exposure. *Neurotoxicology.* 2007;28:126–135.)

IPD patients, levodopa-induced motor complications are not seen.

- FD-PET—Normal. IPD patients show decreased striatal uptake, especially in the posterior putamen.
- Pathology—Degeneration of neurons in the globus pallidus but an absence of Lewy bodies. IPD is associated with degeneration of neurons in the substantia nigra pars compacta and pars reticularis, locus ceruleus, dorsal motor nucleus of the vagus nerve, nucleus basalis of Meynert, cortex, spinal cord, and peripheral nervous system. In IPD, Lewy bodies are common.[14,15]

In most cases, it appears that onset of symptoms occurs during exposure. If the exposure is terminated when symptoms are initially seen, partial or complete recovery occurs. While several case reports have documented improvement or disappearance of symptoms following removal from exposure,[1,16,17] resolution does not always occur. Once symptoms become severe, recovery is unlikely.

Mechanism of Action

The exact mechanism by which manganese causes central nervous system damage continues to be under intense investigation. MRI studies of the human brain indicate that manganese accumulation is highest in the globus pallidus internus, striatum, and substantia nigra reticulata. In contrast to IPD, the substantia nigra pars compacta is spared. Thus, manganism is not a product of dopamine depletion. Numerous studies have identified possible mechanisms of toxicity, but they have been somewhat hindered because they were in vitro or animal studies. Still, they seem to indicate that the glial cells, particularly astrocytes, are targets for manganese toxicity.

Given the numerous effects proposed to occur at the cellular level, Fitsanakis et al. (2006) hypothesized that

manganese targets the globus pallidus, causing a decrease in release of γ-aminobutyric acid (GABA) to the subthalamic nucleus. This would result in disinhibition of the subthalamic nucleus and increased glutamate input into the substantia nigra, leading to chronic overstimulation (Figure 26-4). The authors point out the conflicting data exist regarding whether manganese increases or decreases GABA concentrations, suggesting that it may be dose dependent.

Energy Metabolism and Mitochondria

Glial cells appear to have the ability to incorporate up to 200 times the extracellular concentration of manganese, with up to 70% sequestered in the mitochondria.[18,19] In vitro animal studies indicate that manganese inhibits oxidative phosphorylation, leading to decreased adenosine triphosphate (ATP) production and increased lactate production.[20,21] This also increases the generation of reactive oxygen species, thereby inducing oxidation of membrane polyunsaturated fatty acids and producing lipid peroxidation products. It is believed that the reduction in ATP affects the mitochondrial permeability transition, leading to damage of the mitochondrial membranes.

Dopaminergic Neurotransmission

Kim et al. reported SPECT scans of brain after labeling dopamine transporters with (1r)-2β-carboxymethoxy-3β-(4-iodophenyl)-tropane, which demonstrated a decrease

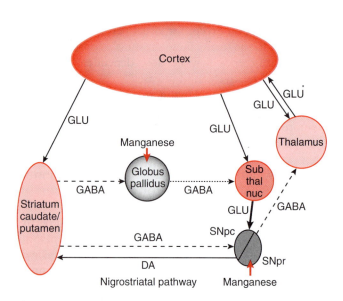

Figure 26-4. Manganese causes decreased output of γ-aminobutyric acid from the globus pallidus. In turn, the subthalamic nucleus increases glutamate output, resulting in overstimulation of the downstream targets and leading to excitotoxic damage. (Adapted from Fitsanakis 2006.)

in the number of transporters with the administration of manganese.[22] The authors assert that manganese causes parkinsonism by damaging output pathways downstream of the nigrostriatal dopaminergic pathway.[22] This is consistent with the hypothesis than manganese, by damaging the globus pallidus, decreases release of GABA, thereby reducing the inhibitory effect of this neurotransmitter on the subthalamic nucleus. This results in an increase of glutamate release and is consistent with the excitotoxicity observed in some animal studies.[20]

Glutaminergic Neurotransmission

Brouillet et al. injected $MnCl_2$ into the striatum of rats and found that ATP production dropped to 51% of that in controls.[20] They felt changes were consistent with N-methyl-d-aspartate (NMDA) excitotoxic lesions. NMDA agonist MK-801 blocked the damage.[20] Astrocytes are responsible for removal of glutamate (NMDA receptor agonist), and that activity appears to be decreased in the presence of manganese.[23] In a recent study, Erikson et al. observed an increase in glutamate transporters at low level exposures to inhaled $MnSO_4$, while larger concentrations caused them to decrease.[24]

Peripheral Benzodiazepine Receptors

Peripheral benzodiazepine receptors (PTBRs) are found on mitochondria in astrocytes. Treatment with manganese has been reported to up-regulate binding sites for a PTBR ligand. It has been proposed that this may cause conformational changes in DNA, adversely affecting gene transcription and ultimately expression.[25] PTBR receptors have also been associated with oxidative metabolism and mitochondrial proliferation.[26]

Glyceraldehyde-3-Phosphate Dehydrogenase

Some studies have suggested that chronic exposure of astrocytes to manganese leads to an increase in the expression and activity of glyceraldehyde-3-phosphate dehydrogenase. This has led to speculation that it may have some impact on apoptosis.

Reactive Oxygen Species

Increased uptake of L-arginine, a precursor of nitric oxide in manganese-exposed astrocytes, has led to the speculation that this increases free radical formation. This is consistent with the observation that manganese is bound to the mitochondrial inner membrane after uptake. That is the location of the electron transport system and site of production of oxygen free radicals.[23,25,26] Milatovic et al. proposed that oxidative stress and decreasing mitochondrial energy production lead to an opening of the mitochondrial permeability transition pore in the inner mitochondrial membrane, resulting in an influx of ions and other solutes, which destroys the inner membrane potential.[27] This leads to swelling of the mitochondrial matrix, movement of metabolites across the membrane, and disruption of oxidative phosphorylation. That would lead to cessation of ATP production and generation of reactive oxygen species, resulting in cellular demise.[27]

PHARMACOKINETICS

Absorption

Of the manganese passing through the gastrointestinal tract, 3% to 5% is absorbed. Grains, nuts, tea, and legumes serve as the main dietary source, which averages about 5 mg/kg/day[14] with a range of 2 to 6 mg.[28] People on strict vegetarian diets may ingest even more.[29] The recommended daily intake of manganese is 2 to 5 mg/day. Manganese is an essential element for humans. It is necessary for the formation of arginase and glutamine synthetase. Superoxide dismutase, an important antioxidant mitochondrial enzyme, requires manganese for its formation.

Inhalation is the most common form of manganese absorption in the workplace. Manganism has been most often observed in mining, smelting, and grinding of manganese. The risk in other occupations is a matter of great controversy and continued study. Occupations that have been associated with manganese exposure (but not necessarily manganism) are shown in Table 2.

Speciation, solubility, and particle size influence the amount of inhalational absorption. Speciation refers to different chemical, physical, or morphological states of metals.[30] Manganese combined with different elements behaves in distinctively different ways. Solubility is influenced by speciation. Manganese chloride is more soluble and thus more quickly absorbed than manganese dioxide, which is insoluble. Roels et al. demonstrated significantly less gastrointestinal absorption of MnO_2 compared to $MnCl_2$.[31] Particle size is also an important factor for inhalation absorption of manganese. Larger particles are deposited in the upper airways, where they are cleared and swallowed in sputum. Once in the gastrointestinal tract, only a small amount is absorbed. Kim demonstrated that about 80% of all inhaled small (0.1 to 2 μm) particles are cleared by exhalation.[32] Most particles greater than 1 μm tend to localize at or near the carina. Approximately 20% of respirable particles are deposited in the alveoli, and a significant portion of those are removed by macrophages. Manganese particles that are absorbed by macrophages are then carried out of the alveoli and bronchioles via the mucociliary escalator. From there they are coughed from the pulmonary tree

Table 2: Occupational and Environmental Sources of Manganese

| Mining |
| Ore sorting |
| Milling/bagging of manganese-containing ore |
| Refining |
| Ferromanganese or silicomanganese crushing, smelting |
| Production of high-carbon steel |
| Electric arc welding |
| Manufacturing of |

Amethyst glass	Algicides	Ceramics
Disinfectants	Dry-cell batteries	Fertilizer
Fireworks	Fruit or flower preservatives	Fungicide
Glass-bonding materials	Incendiaries	Livestock supplements
Matches	Porcelain	Varnishes

| Water purifiers |
| Illicit production of methcathinone (potassium permanganate exposure) |
| Some radiological contrast media |

Table 3: Workplace Standards for Manganese Fume (as Manganese)[33]*

OCCUPATIONAL SAFETY AND HEALTH ADMINISTRATION (OSHA)	
Permissible exposure limit[†]	5 mg/m³ ceiling
American Conference of Governmental Industrial Hygienists	0.2 mg/m³ TWA[‡]
NATIONAL INSTITUTE FOR OCCUPATIONAL SAFETY AND HEALTH (NIOSH)	
Recommended exposure limit[§]	1 mg/m³ TWA 3 mg/m³ STEL[‖]

*Immediately dangerous to life and health is any concentration of any substance that poses an immediate threat to life, would cause irreversible or delayed effects, or would interfere with an individual's ability to escape from a dangerous atmosphere.[34]
[†]A legal exposure limit established by OSHA for TWA exposures in any 8-hour work shift during a 40-hour workweek.
[‡]TWA, time-weighted average. Refers to the total exposure of a worker to contaminants in workroom air in a workday. Usually 8 hours.
[§]An exposure limit recommended by NIOSH for TWA exposures in any 10-hour work shift during a 40-hour workweek.
[‖]STEL, short-term exposure limit. A 15-minute TWA exposure limit established by OSHA that cannot be exceeded at any time during a workday.

and swallowed. In the gastrointestinal tract, a small amount may be absorbed, leaving most to be excreted in bile. For U.S. governmental workplace standards, see Table 3.

Distribution

Once absorbed, about 80% of manganese is bound to β-globulin and albumin. It is then distributed to tissue throughout the body, particularly to the liver and kidneys.[35] A small fraction is bound, in its trivalent form, to transferrin. The means by which manganese crosses the blood–brain barrier is debated. Proposed mechanisms include diffusion,[36] divalent metal transport-1, ZIP8, and transferrin.[37] It appears that diffusion is the most common route of transfer out of the brain.[38] Of note, some animal studies suggest that the mechanism by which manganese crosses the blood–brain barrier may be saturable.[39,40]

Elimination

Whether inhaled or ingested, manganese is eventually taken up by the liver and excreted in bile.[41] Inhaled manganese is largely removed from the bronchial tree by coughing or expiration. Particles smaller than 1 μm can advance to the alveoli. There, some ultrafine particles are simply exhaled. Remaining particles are scavenged by microphages, which remove metals, and are transported out via the mucociliary escalator. They are then coughed out and expectorated or swallowed to undergo gastrointestinal passage or absorption.

Manganese does not undergo metabolism. It exists in several oxidation states, and its valence states may vary within the body. It is taken up as Mn^{2+} or Mn^{4+} but exists as Mn^{3+} in most enzymes. Manganese is primarily excreted in bile. Urinary excretion of manganese accounts for less than 1% of its elimination.[28] The elimination half-life of manganese is about 40 days in humans. It appears to be longer in the brain. Excretion appears to increase with increasing exposure; therefore, half-life would decrease.[42,43]

POPULATIONS AT RISK

For more than 50 years, chronic liver disease has been associated with a form of parkinsonism originally known as *portal-systemic encephalopathy*.[44,45] In the early 1990s, MRI studies showed hyperintensities in the globus pallidus on T1-weighted images.[46] Hauser et al. demonstrated increased blood manganese levels in cirrhotic patients, with those MRI changes suggesting chronic hepatic disease impaired manganese excretion.[47] Klos et al. used postmortem tissue samples to confirm the presence of manganese in patients with liver failure who developed parkinsonism and had positive MRI results.[48]

Patients undergoing parenteral hyperalimentation have been shown rarely to have elevated serum manganese concentrations and MRI changes consistent with manganese exposure. Of those, a few have had neurological symptoms consistent with parkinsonism that improved after manganese exposure was terminated.[49,50]

TESTING FOR MANGANESE

Urine manganese levels in the general population range from 0 to 2 $\mu g/d$[51] but can vary somewhat among laboratories. Urine is considered a poor marker for exposure or toxicity.[52] Specimens collected following chelation can show a marked increase in excretion even in the absence of increased exposure.[53–55] Careful collection of specimens is essential for accurate determination of manganese concentrations.

Serum manganese levels are lower than blood levels because about 85% of manganese is bound to hemoglobin in erythrocytes. Reference ranges vary from laboratory to laboratory. Reported ranges are generally from 0.9 to 2.9 $\mu g/L$. Whole-blood manganese concentrations measured by atomic absorption spectrophotometry range from 3.9 to 15 $\mu g/L$.[56] Again, this range can shift depending on the reporting laboratory. Blood concentrations do not correlate with toxicity.

MRI has been used to demonstrate the presence of manganese in the brain. Hyperintensities of the globus pallidus on T1-weighted images can demonstrate exposure but do not indicate toxicity (see Figure 26-3). Dietz et al. found MRI, while correlating with MnO_2 exposure in 90 workers, did not predict neurological impairment when compared to controls.[57]

THERAPY

Chelation with calcium ethylenediaminetetraacetic acid (Ca-EDTA) has been used in patients with manganese exposure with mixed results. Herrero Hernandez et al. reported success in manganese-exposed patients with parkinsonism if started early in the course of their symptoms.[58] It has yet to be established as beneficial in manganese toxicity. The administration of chelating agents does increase metal excretion in patients. Because manganese exposure is ubiquitous, it is not surprising that urinary excretion of manganese and other metals follows administration of agents such as calcium EDTA. In fact, urinary excretion of manganese following calcium EDTA administration to patients without any exposure history has been shown to elevate urinary manganese many times over within a few hours of administration.[53–55]

Levodopa, a key therapy in the treatment of IPD, has been largely ineffective in the management of manganism. This is consistent with the theory that manganism is not due to dopamine depletion. Some patients have had initial improvement, only to lose any long-term benefit.[12] In fact, levodopa failure is a factor in differentiating manganism from IPD.

A few case reports regarding the use of para-aminosalicylic acid have touted remarkable improvement, but to date there are not sufficient data to determine the significance of that finding.[59,60]

CONCLUSION

Manganism is a devastating form of parkinsonism that is fortunately rare today. Its diagnosis is established primarily by clinical presentation, augmented by supporting historical, laboratory, and radiological data. No single diagnostic test exists, and no specific treatment has been determined effective. Prevention of high-dose exposure to manganese remains the most reliable means of avoiding potentially devastating neurological consequences.

REFERENCES

1. Couper J. On the effects of black oxide of manganese when inhaled into the lungs. *Br Ann Med Pharmacol.* 1837;I:41–42.
2. Rodier J. Manganese poisoning in Moroccan miners. *Br J Ind Med.* 1955;12:21–35.
3. Abd el Naby S, Hassanein M. Neuropsychiatric manifestations of chronic manganese poisoning. *J Neurol Neurosurg Psychiatry.* 1965;28:282.
4. Mena I, Marin O, Fuenzalida S, et al. Chronic manganese poisoning: clinical picture and manganese turnover. *Neurology.* 1967;17:129–136.

5. Parnitzke K, Peiffer J. On the characteristics and pathological anatomy of chronic manganese poisoning. *Arch Psych Neurol Disord (J Neurol Psychiatry)*. 1954;192:404–429.

6. Ashizawa R. Autopsy report on a case involving chronic manganese poisoning. *Japanese J Med Sci VII*. 1930;I:173–191.

7. Canavan M, Cobb S, Drinker C. Chronic manganese poisoning. *Arch Neurol*. 1934;32:501–513.

8. Huang CC, Chu NS, Lu CS, et al. Chronic manganese intoxication. *Arch Neurol*. 1989;46:1104–1106.

8a. Wang JD, Huang CC, Hwang Y-H, et al. Manganese induced parkinsonism: an outbreak due to an unrepaired ventilation control system in a ferromanganese smelter. *Brit J Ind Med*. 1989;46:856–859.

9. Wolters EC, Huang CC, Clark C, et al. Positron emission tomography in manganese intoxication [see comment]. *Ann Neurol*. 1989;26:647–651.

10. Hua MS, Huang CC. Chronic occupational exposure to manganese and neurobehavioral function. *J Clin Exp Neuropsychol*. 1991;13:495–507.

11. Huang CC, Lu CS, Chu NS, et al. Progression after chronic manganese exposure. *Neurology*. 1993;43:1479–1483.

12. Lu CS, Huang CC, Chu NS, et al. Levodopa failure in chronic manganism [see comment]. *Neurology*. 1994;44:1600–1602.

12a. Huang CC, Chu NS, Lu CS, et al. Long-term progression in chronic manganism: ten years follow-up. *Neurology*. 1998;50:698–700.

13. Huang CC, Weng YH, Lu CS, et al. Dopamine transporter binding in chronic manganese intoxication. *J Neurol*. 2003;250:1335–1339.

14. Jankovic J. Searching for a relationship between manganese and welding and Parkinson's disease [see comment]. *Neurology*. 2005;64:2021–2028.

15. Olanow CW. Manganese-induced parkinsonism and Parkinson's disease. *Ann NY Acad Sci*. 2004;1012:209–223.

16. Crump KS, Rousseau P. Results from eleven years of neurological health surveillance at a manganese oxide and salt producing plant. *Neurotoxicology*. 1999;20:273–286.

17. Flinn R, Neal P, Fulton W. Industrial manganese poisoning. *J Ind Hyg Toxicol*. 1941;23:874–887.

17a. Fitsanakis VA, Au C, Erikson KM. The effects of manganese on gglutamate, dopamine and γ-aminobutyric acid regulation. *Neurochem Int*. 2006;48:426–433.

18. Aschner M, Gannon M, Kimelberg HK. Manganese uptake and efflux in cultured rat astrocytes. *J Neurochem*. 1992;58:730–735.

19. Tholey G, Bloch S, Ledig M, et al. Chick brain glutamine synthetase and Mn2+–Mg2+ interactions. *Neurochem Res*. 1987;12:1041–1047.

20. Brouillet EP, Shinobu L, McGarvey U, et al. Manganese injection into the rat striatum produces excitotoxic lesions by impairing energy metabolism. *Exp Neurol*. 1993;120:89–94.

21. Gavin CE, Gunter KK, Gunter TE. Mn2+ sequestration by mitochondria and inhibition of oxidative phosphorylation. *Toxicol Appl Pharmacol*. 1992;115:1–5.

22. Kim Y, Kim JM, Kim JW, et al. Dopamine transporter density is decreased in parkinsonian patients with a history of manganese exposure: what does it mean? *Mov Disord*. 2002;17:568–575.

23. Chen C-J, Liao S-L. Oxidative stress involves in astrocytic alterations induced by manganese. *Exp Neurol*. 2002;175:216–225.

24. Erikson KM, Dorman DC, Lash LH, et al. Manganese inhalation by rhesus monkeys is associated with brain regional changes in biomarkers of neurotoxicity. *Toxicol Sci*. 2007;97:459–466.

25. Normandin L, Hazell AS. Manganese neurotoxicity: an update of pathophysiologic mechanisms. *Metab Brain Dis*. 2002;17:375–387.

26. Hazell AS. Astrocytes and manganese neurotoxicity. *Neurochem Int*. 2002;41:271–277.

27. Milatovic D, Yin Z, Gupta RC, et al. Manganese induces oxidative impairment in cultured rat astrocytes. *Toxicol Sci*. 2007;98:198–205.

28. Barceloux D. Manganese. *Clin Toxicol*. 1999;37:293–307.

29. Gibson R. Content and bioavailability of trace elements in vegetarian diets. *Am J Clin Nutr*. 1994;59:1223S–1232S.

30. Yokel RA, Lasley S, Dorman DC. The speciation of metals in mammals influences their toxicokinetics and toxicodynamics and therefore human health risk assessment. *J Toxicol Environ Health*. 2006;9:63–85.

31. Roels H, Meiers G, Delos M, et al. Influence of the route of administration and the chemical form (MnCl₂, MnO₂) on the absorption and cerebral distribution of manganese in rats. *Arch Toxicol*. 1997;71:223–230.

32. Kim C. Methods of calculating lung delivery and deposition of aerosol particles. *Respir Care*. 2000;45:695–711.

33. Occupational Safety and Health Administration. Safety and Health Topics: Manganese Fume (as Mn). Philadelphia: OSHA; 2007.

34. Van Ert M, Crutchfield C, Sullivan JJ. Principles of environmental and occupational hazard assessment. In: Sullivan JJ, Krieger G, eds. *Clinical Environmental Health and Toxic Exposures*. Philadelphia: Lippincott Williams & Wilkins; 2001:30–49.

35. Bush VJ, Moyer TP, Batts KP, et al. Essential and toxic element concentrations in fresh and formalin-fixed human autopsy tissues. *Clin Chem*. 1995;41:284–294.

36. Crossgrove JS, Yokel RA. Manganese distribution across the blood–brain barrier: IV. Evidence for brain influx through store-operated calcium channels. *Neurotoxicology*. 2005;26:297–307.

37. Aschner M, Guilarte TR, Schneider JS, et al. Manganese: recent advances in understanding its transport and neurotoxicity. *Toxicol Appl Pharmacol*. 2007;221:131–147.

38. Yokel RA, Crossgrove JS, Bukaveckas BL. Manganese distribution across the blood–brain barrier: II. Manganese efflux from the brain does not appear to be carrier mediated. *Neurotoxicology*. 2003;24:15–22.

39. Murphy VA, Wadhwani KC, Smith QR, et al. Saturable transport of manganese(II) across the rat blood–brain barrier. *J Neurochem*. 1991;57:948–954.

40. Wadhwani KC, Murphy VA, Smith QR, et al. Saturable transport of manganese(II) across blood–nerve barrier of rat peripheral nerve. *Am J Physiol*. 1992;262:R284–288.

41. Stopford W. *Welding and Exposures to Manganese Assessment of Neurological Adverse Effects*. Durham, NC: Duke University Medical Center; 2005:1–62.

42. Mahoney JP, Small WJ. Studies on manganese: III. The biological half-life of radiomanganese in man and factors which affect this half-life. *J Clin Invest*. 1968;47:643–653.

43. Mena I, Horiuchi K, Burke K, et al. Chronic manganese poisoning: individual susceptibility and absorption of iron. *Neurology*. 1969;19:1000–1006.

44. Sherlock S, Summerskill W, White L, et al. Portal-systemic encephalopathy: neurological complications of liver disease. *Lancet*. 1954;267:453–457.

45. Victor M, Adams R, Cole M. The acquired (non-Wilsonian) type of chronic hepatocerebral degeneration. *Medicine*. 1965;44:345–396.

46. Inoue E, Hori S, Narumi Y, et al. Portal-systemic encephalopathy: presence of basal ganglia lesions with high signal intensity on MR images. *Radiology*. 1991;179:551–555.

47. Hauser RA, Zesiewicz TA, Martinez C, et al. Blood manganese correlates with brain magnetic resonance imaging changes in patients with liver disease. *Can J Neurol Sci*. 1996;23:95–98.

48. Klos KJ, Ahlskog JE, Kumar N, et al. Brain metal concentrations in chronic liver failure patients with pallidal T1 MRI hyperintensity. *Neurology*. 2006;67:1984–1989.

49. Nagatomo S, Umehara F, Hanada K, et al. Manganese intoxication during total parenteral nutrition: report of two cases and review of the literature. *J Neurol Sci.* 1999;162:102–105.

50. Ono J, Harada K, Kodaka R, et al. Manganese deposition in the brain during long-term total parenteral nutrition. *JPEN J Parenter Enteral Nutr.* 1995;19:310–312.

51. ARUP Laboratories (Associated Regional Utah Pathologists) aruplab.com http://www.aruplab.com/guides/ug/tests/0025070.jsp. Accessed February 11, 2009.

51a. Mayo Medical Laboratories. http://www.aruplab.com/guides/ug/tests/0025070.jsp. Accessed February 11, 2009.

52. Myers JE, Thompson ML, Naik I, et al. The utility of biological monitoring for manganese in ferroalloy smelter workers in South Africa. *Neurotoxicology.* 2003;24:875–883.

53. Allain P, Mauras Y, Premel-Cabic A, et al. Effects of an EDTA infusion on the urinary elimination of several elements in healthy subjects. *Br J Clin Pharmacol.* 1991;31:347–349.

54. Cranton E, Liu Z, Smith I. Urinary trace and toxic elements and minerals in untimed urine specimens relative to urine creatinine: I. Concentrations of elements in fasting urine. *J Adv Med.* 1989;2:331–349.

55. Sata F, Araki S, Murata K, et al. Behavior of heavy metals in human urine and blood following calcium disodium ethylenediamine tetraacetate injection: observations in metal workers. *J Toxicol Environ Health A.* 1998;54:167–178.

56. Pleban PA, Pearson KH. Determination of manganese in whole blood and serum. *Clin Chem* 1979;25:1915–1918.

57. Dietz MC, Ihrig A, Wrazidlo W, et al. Results of magnetic resonance imaging in long-term manganese dioxide–exposed workers. *Environ Res.* 2001;85:37–40.

58. Herrero Hernandez E, Discalzi G, Valentini C, et al. Follow-up of patients affected by manganese-induced parkinsonism after treatment with CaNa2 EDTA. *Neurotoxicology.* 2006;27:333–339.

59. Jiang Y-M, Mo X-A, Du F-Q, et al. Effective treatment of manganese-induced occupational parkinsonism with p-aminosalicylic acid: a case of 17-year follow-up study. *J Occup Environ Med.* 2006;48:644–649.

60. Ky SQ, Deng HS, Xie PY, et al. A report of two cases of chronic serious manganese poisoning treated with sodium para-aminosalicylic acid. *Br J Ind Med.* 1992;49:66–69.

61. Jiang Y, Zheng W, Long L, et al. Brain magnetic resonance imaging and manganese concentrations in red blood cells of smelting workers: search for biomarkers of manganese exposure. *Neurotoxicology.* 2007;28:126–135.

CHAPTER 27 ····

Illicit Drugs I: Amphetamines

Bryan S. Judge and Daniel E. Rusyniak

INTRODUCTION

History of the Usage of Amphetamine and Its Analogues

In 1887, German chemist L. Edeleano synthesized β-phenylisopropylamine, commonly known as *amphetamine*. Little did he realize the impact that his newly created drug and its derivatives (referred to as *amphetamines* in this chapter) would have on society in the future. Largely forgotten for more than 30 years since it was initially produced, researchers in the mid-1920s took interest in amphetamine as a substitute for ephedrine, which had been the primary therapy for asthma and at the time was expensive due to a supply shortage.[1] The medicinal use of amphetamine went mainstream in the early 1930s, when it was marketed as a Benzedrine inhaler and used to treat asthma and nasal congestion. Soon after the introduction of Benzedrine, the powerful anorexiant and stimulant effects of amphetamine became widely recognized; these properties, combined with affordable and readily available inhalers, led to rampant abuse of the amphetamine-impregnated paper within the inhaler.[2] Methamphetamine (*d*-phenylisopropylmethylamine hydrochloride) was introduced in 1940 and marketed as Methedrine, and by the

early 1940s amphetamine and methamphetamine were used legally under numerous trade names for the treatment of alcohol abuse, depression, narcolepsy, Parkinson's disease, and weight loss.

Both amphetamine and methamphetamine were issued to Allied and Axis troops during World War II to combat fatigue and sleep. Even Winston Churchill and Adolf Hitler were prescribed amphetamine by their physicians, and it is thought that the führer's insomnia and tremor, among other symptoms, could have been attributable to his use of this substance.[3,4] The amphetamine abuse problem in the United States that had been ignited with Benzedrine was further fueled by the return of former GIs who had been exposed to the drug during the war. Japan faced a similar abuse problem with methamphetamine when supplies of the drug that had been allocated for soldiers were made available to the public at the end of the war.

In 1949, the manufacturer of Benzedrine—Smith, Kline, and French—halted production of the inhaler due to mounting concerns about its abuse and replaced it with Benzedrex; however, this inhaler containing the amphetamine-like compound, propylhexedrine, was also largely misused. Other companies continued to produce amphetamine inhalers and attempted to curtail abuse by marketing them with a deterrent that would prevent ingestion. Finally, in 1959 the U.S. Food and Drug Administration prohibited over-the-counter sales of amphetamine inhalers. Amphetamine was placed into Schedule II with the passage of the Controlled Substances Act of 1970. Although this legislation resulted in a steady decline in the abuse of amphetamine during the 1970s, a significant amount of the amphetamine that was still being abused originated from supplies that had been legally manufactured, prescribed, or shipped.[5]

Designer amphetamines became popular in the 1980s as a means of bypassing the regulatory controls set in place by the Controlled Substances Act.[6] Essentially any derivative of amphetamine or methamphetamine such as 3,4-methylenedioxyamphetamine (MDA, "love drug") or 3,4-methylenedioxymethamphetamine (MDMA, Ecstasy) could be sold legally because these derivatives were not officially recognized as illicit by the existing legal restrictions.[7] However, in 1986 the Anti-Drug Abuse Act closed this loophole by outlawing analogues of controlled substances.[8] Despite this amendment, many "designer drugs" continue to be widely abused, in particular MDMA.

Ecstasy (MDMA) has gained widespread popularity as a drug of abuse over the past several decades. Primary users include teenagers and young adults at mass-gathering dance parties known as *raves*.[9] Data from the National Survey on Drug Use and Health has demonstrated a substantial decline in first-time users of Ecstasy in the United States; first-time users of Ecstasy 12 years and older was 168,000 in 1993, peaked in 2000 at 1.9 million, and declined to 615,000 in 2005.[10,11] Despite the decline in first-time Ecstasy use over the past several years, the Drug Abuse Warning Network estimated that 10,752 U.S. emergency department visits were associated with Ecstasy use in 2005.[12]

Methamphetamine abuse and production escalated at an alarming rate in the United States during the 1990s and early years of the new millennium. Sold as "ice," "crank," or "stove top" on the street, it can be manufactured inexpensively and with relative ease from a few raw materials in clandestine laboratories. In 1994, self-reported use of methamphetamine among adults was less than 2%; however, by 2004, approximately 5% of adults reported using methamphetamine,[13] 318,000 individuals used methamphetamine for the first time,[10] and more than 17,000 clandestine methamphetamine laboratories were seized throughout the United States.[14] In response to the widespread methamphetamine problem, many states passed legislation restricting the sale of precursor chemicals (anhydrous ammonia, ephedrine, pseudoephedrine) used in the production of methamphetamine.[15] Limiting the availability of the raw materials necessary for the synthesis of methamphetamine appears to have had some impact on the production of methamphetamine as the number of clandestine laboratory incidents fell to 7347 in 2006.

Today, Edeleano's discovery and its analogues (dextroamphetamine, methamphetamine, methylphenidate, pemoline, phendimetrazine, and phetermine) are being used for a limited number of medical conditions that include attention-deficit/hyperactivity disorder, narcolepsy, and weight reduction. Despite their controlled status, the misuse of amphetamines continues to be problematic—substantiated by the recent surge in both Ecstasy and methamphetamine usage. Although abuse patterns for amphetamines have fluctuated over the past several decades, illicit use of these stimulants is anticipated to persist for years to come.

NEUROPHARMACOLOGY OF AMPHETAMINES

The principal pharmacological action of amphetamines—responsible for their behavioral and physiological effects—is the release of monoamines within the central nervous system. The mechanisms involved are complex and are not reviewed here; several thorough reviews are already available.[16,17] In vitro studies have shown amphetamine and methamphetamine to have low potency for releasing serotonin, but they are extremely effective at releasing norepinephrine and dopamine.[18,19] On the other hand, ring-substituted amphetamines such as MDMA cause the release of dopamine to a lesser degree yet are equally potent in releasing serotonin and norepinephrine.[18-21] In vivo models are in agreement with these findings, with the exception that MDMA results in the release of more dopamine in vivo than in vitro.[22,23] This difference may be explained partly by serotonin-mediated release of dopamine in vivo.[24,25] After central monoamines are released, many receptors are activated that subsequently mediate the complex physiological responses to amphetamines. In relationship to the development of hyperthermia—one of the more significant complications of amphetamine use—studies have suggested a role for $\alpha 1$,[26-28] dopamine-1,[29] dopamine-2,[30,31] and serotonin-2A receptors.[32,33] Regardless of which central receptors are primarily involved, the common mechanism underlying toxicity associated with amphetamines appears to be excessive stimulation of the sympathetic nervous system.

The case discussed here should impart some devastating and potentially lethal effects associated with the abuse of amphetamines. The clinical syndromes that patients can develop from the illicit use of amphet-

CASE STUDY

An 18-year-old male was brought to the emergency department by the police after throwing chairs and starting a fight at a party. He was handcuffed, agitated, hallucinating, and yelling profanities. A pacifier was found among his personal effects. Friends that accompanied him to the emergency department reported that he took something to get "up" for the party.

His vital signs were as follows: blood pressure at 150/84 mm Hg, oxygen saturation at 98% on room air, pulse at 160 beats/min, respiratory rate at 20 breaths/min, and temperature at 39.2°C. The patient appeared to be well developed and nourished. His physical examination was unremarkable with the exception of a few pertinent findings: his pupils were dilated to 7 mm bilaterally, and reacted slowly to light. He was profusely diaphoretic. The patient moved all of his extremities spontaneously, he had seven beats of clonus in his lower extremities, and muscle tone was increased in his lower extremities more than in his upper extremities. Immediate glucose testing revealed a concentration of 118 mg/dL. The patient was placed on a cardiac monitor, and an electrocardiogram revealed sinus tachycardia with a QRS duration of 92 msec and QTc interval of 402 msec. The patient was initially treated with a total of 15 mg of lorazepam over 30 minutes, which helped calm him. He received 1 L of normal saline over 60 minutes for hydration. His temperature had declined to 38°C within 1 hour of presentation. Initial laboratory studies were remarkable for alanine aminotransferase of 67 international units (IU) per liter, aspartate aminotransferase of 93 IU/L, bicarbonate of 17 mEq/L, creatine phosphokinase of 2884 IU/L, sodium of 117 mEq/L, and white blood cell count of 14,300 cells/mm³. A urine drugs of abuse screen was positive for amphetamines.

The patient was admitted to the intensive care unit, where therapy consisted of normal saline and lorazepam to control his neuropsychiatric symptoms. Twenty-four hours after presentation, his mental status was markedly improved, temperature normalized, creatine phosphokinase declined to 1756 IU/L, and sodium increased to 132 mEq/L. He subsequently admitted to taking several Ecstasy tablets while at the rave and was discharged without sequelae after 3 days in the hospital.

versus chronic), underlying comorbidities, and concomitant use of other pharmacological agents. The following sections provide a brief overview of several effects—with primary emphasis on neurological syndromes—that can be encountered in the clinical setting.

Cerebrovascular Anomalies

Amphetamine use has long been linked with acute stroke in young adults; most evidence, however, has come via case reports.[34] A few epidemiological studies support a causal role of amphetamines in the development of acute hemorrhagic stroke. In a population-based, retrospective, case–control study involving 347 women age 15 to 44 years, use of amphetamines was associated with a 3.8 times greater risk (95% confidence interval [CI] = 1.2 to 12.6) of developing either a hemorrhagic or an ischemic stroke.[35] This study was limited, however, by size: only 10 strokes were reported in users of amphetamines. In a large cross-sectional study using a statewide hospital database, amphetamine abuse was strongly associated (OR 4.95, 95% CI = 3.24 to 7.55) with the development of hemorrhagic but not ischemic stroke.[36] This study also demonstrated that increases in the prevalence of stroke related to amphetamine abuse paralleled statewide increases in reported methamphetamine abuse.

The use of phenylpropanolamine, a previously available over-the-counter agent that can be chemically reduced to amphetamine, has been associated with hemorrhagic stroke. In a multicenter case–control study of phenylpropanolamine and hemorrhagic stroke, women between the ages of 18 and 49 who used a phenylpropanolamine-containing product had twice the risk (95% CI = 1.0 to 3.9) of developing a hemorrhagic stroke; if they were using phenylpropanolamine as an appetite suppressant, they had a 16.6 times higher risk (95% CI = 1.51 to 182) of hemorrhagic stroke.[37] This same study found no increased risk among men using phenylpropanolamine, although no male subject was using it as an appetite suppressant. In a similar study, based in Korea, an increased risk (OR 3.6, 95% CI = 1.08 to 13.80) of hemorrhagic stroke was found in women, but not men, who were taking cough medicine containing phenylpropanolamine.[38]

The mechanism of hemorrhagic stroke induced by amphetamines is likely related to acute increases in blood pressure. Individuals harboring cerebral vascular malformations may be especially vulnerable to this complication.[39] Cerebral inflammatory vasculitis has been documented pathologically in association with amphetamines in a small number of cases and is another potential mechanism for hemorrhagic and ischemic stroke.[40]

amine and its analogues can be influenced by numerous factors, including the particular substance abused, the time frame in which the substance was used (acute

Dyskinesias and Stereotypies

The acute and chronic abuse of amphetamine-like compounds has been associated with movement disorders and repetitive behaviors. These effects most likely occur secondary to increased dopaminergic and glutamatergic activity and inhibition of γ-aminobutyric acid within the neostriatum.[41,42] Individuals may perform tasks repeatedly, such as cleaning their house, polishing their nails, or fidgeting with objects (e.g., a radio or watch).[43] Others may pick at their skin or grind their teeth (bruxism); users of Ecstasy often use pacifiers to alleviate the latter condition. Patients can develop choreoathetoid movements after the acute or chronic usage of amphetamines,[44,45] and the authors have cared for several children who developed dyskinesias after accidentally ingesting therapeutic doses of commonly prescribed stimulants, such as amphetamine or dextroamphetamine and methylphenidate. Normally, the movement disorders resolve with abstinence or when the drug effect has lessened; however, in some instances they may persist for years.[46]

Hyperthermia

Body temperature regulation requires the coordinated balance between systems producing heat and those dissipating it. As a result, any exogenously administered xenobiotic capable of increasing heat production or decreasing heat dissipation can cause hyperthermia. When taken in the appropriate setting, amphetamines can do both, resulting in the development of profound hyperthermia.

The mechanism of amphetamine-induced hyperthermia involves complex interactions between the environment in which it is taken and the drug-induced physiological changes. The effect of ambient temperature on changes in core body temperature induced by amphetamines has been well documented, with several animal studies demonstrating increased hyperthermia and toxicity when MDMA[47] and methamphetamine[48,49] are given at elevated ambient temperatures. This may have important implications for users of ring-substituted amphetamines like MDMA, a drug that is often taken in hot and crowded dance clubs.[9] Similar corollaries have been made with the stimulant cocaine, where deaths occur more often during months with elevated ambient temperatures.[50]

The physiological mechanisms by which amphetamines increase body temperature involve the combined effects of impairing heat dissipation and increasing heat generation. Impaired heat dissipation occurs through constriction of cutaneous vascular beds. This has been shown in rats with MDMA[51] and in humans with cocaine.[52] Heat generation occurs due to a combination of work- and non-work-related metabolism. Amphetamines increase locomotor activity in animals[53,54] and are commonly taken by humans to increase stamina while dancing at raves or participating in sporting events.[55] As motor activity elevates body temperature, supplies of adenosine triphosphate are exhausted; when amphetamines are added to this milieu, exaggerated body temperatures and toxicity can ensue.[56–58]

Amphetamines also boost heat production through non-work-related metabolism—referred to as *nonshivering thermogenesis*. Nonshivering thermogenesis occurs primarily by uncoupling oxidative phosphorylation and is mediated by a group of mitochondrial proteins known as *uncoupling proteins*. The stimulation of uncoupling protein-1 (UCP1) in brown adipose tissues represents the primary site of nonshivering thermogenesis in rodents[59] and has been shown to be involved in hyperthermia induced by amphetamines.[60,61] Although adult humans have little brown fat, another uncoupling protein, UCP3, has been detected in abundance in human skeletal muscle.[62] While the role of skeletal muscle uncoupling protein in human thermogenesis has been controversial, recent work suggests that it may have an integral role in methamphetamine and MDMA-induced hyperthermia; mice lacking UCP3 express a blunted hyperthermic response to MDMA and methamphetamine and are protected against subsequent mortality.[63–65]

Despite the similarity in symptoms, amphetamine-related hyperthermia is not a form of malignant hyperthermia. This distinction is crucial, as many authors have advocated the use of dantrolene to treat hyperthermia from amphetamines.[66,67] Despite one study demonstrating exaggerated responses to MDMA in swine that were genetically susceptible to malignant hyperthermia, no studies show that dantrolene reduced or prevented hyperthermia from MDMA.[66,68] Likewise, a difference in the mechanism of toxicity is found between the two disorders: amphetamine-induced hyperthermia is mediated by the central release of catecholamines, whereas malignant hyperthermia results from the uncontrolled release of calcium within the sarcoplasmic reticulum of skeletal muscle.[69] While dantrolene is unlikely to cause harm in patients with amphetamine-related hyperthermia, it is important that treatments are primarily targeted at decreasing central excitation; this can be accomplished through the judicious use of benzodiazepines or similar hyperpolarizing drugs.

Although typically mild and self-limited, hyperthermia from amphetamines can be profound and result in mortality.[70–72] Fatal intoxications usually produce a clinical picture characterized by the following: diaphoresis, tachycardia, muscle rigidity, rhabdomyolysis, metabolic acidosis, seizures, hyperkalemia, coagulopathy, and marked hyperpyrexia—with temperatures as high as 43.9°C being reported.[73] Mortality rates appear to correlate directly with the degree of hyperthermia; cases in which body temperature was reported to be greater than 41.5°C resulted in fatality two-thirds of the time.[74]

Metabolic Disturbances

The misuse of amphetamines can cause excessive adrenergic stimulation that may result in hyperglycemia, hypokalemia, leukocytosis, and metabolic acidosis.[75] The stimulation of β-adrenoreceptors by catecholamines results in an increase of intracellular cyclic adenosine monophosphate activity, which enhances Na^+K^+-ATPase and causes K^+ ions to shift inside cells. Excessive adrenergic stimulation also promotes the breakdown of fatty acids and glycogenolysis, resulting in metabolic acidosis and hyperglycemia, respectively. Clinicians should suspect poisoning with amphetamines or other agents (e.g., caffeine, cocaine, and phencyclidine) that cause hyperadrenergic stimulation in a patient who presents with a sympathomimetic toxidrome and the previously mentioned metabolic disturbances.

Parkinsonism

In both human and animal studies, methamphetamine has been shown to decrease concentrations of dopamine and markers of dopamine function within the basal ganglia.[76-83] This has led some authors to speculate that methamphetamine abuse may lead to the early development of Parkinson's disease.[81] However, only one case–control study has shown an association between remote amphetamine use and early onset of Parkinson's disease.[84] As methamphetamine abuse has dramatically increased in the last 5 years, future studies may be better suited to answer this question. Unlike methamphetamine, ring-substituted amphetamines such as MDMA result in the reduction of brain concentrations of serotonin but not dopamine.[20] Aside from a few contested case reports,[85,86] no long-term studies to date show an association between MDMA use and Parkinson's disease.

Washout Syndrome

One of the manifestations of stimulant abuse recognized by clinicians, but rarely reported, is the "washed-out" or "washout" syndrome. While only reported with cocaine,[87-89] it is reasonable to assume similar presentations can occur after amphetamine abuse. Briefly, this syndrome occurs after extended binges of stimulants such as cocaine, or presumably amphetamines, and is characterized by marked somnolence, mild hypotension, hyporeflexia, and dysconjugate gaze on physical examination. Patients may be sedated to the point of undergoing painful procedures without response. The proposed mechanism is depletion of central catecholamines; interestingly, this may be one potential explanation for reduced monoamine levels found at autopsy after amphetamine overdose.[79] Treatment for the washout syndrome is supportive, and the diagnosis

requires ruling out other potential life-threatening disorders first—intracerebral trauma or infection, for example.

Amphetamines and Thyroid Disorders

Amphetamines have been reported to increase serum T4 levels in rodents[26] and in humans.[90] While studies in animals demonstrate that the acute release of thyroid hormone is not involved in hyperthermia and toxicity from amphetamines,[91] animals or patients who are hyperthyroid can develop an exaggerated response, thereby increasing their risk for death.[92-95] Conversely, patients who are hypothyroid may be protected from amphetamine toxicity.[26,65,91,92] The practicality of this knowledge is that patients who develop hyperthermia and toxicity after using amphetamines may benefit from thyroid studies after a period of convalescence.

Psychosis

Seeking the ultimate high, abusers of amphetamines can go on binges for days to weeks at a time. These periods are characterized by minimal sleep, little need for food, and escalating usage of amphetamines due to acute tolerance.[96] During these binges users can present to the emergency department with numerous psychiatric manifestations, including agitation, aggressive behavior, anxiety, hallucinations, and psychosis.[97] Psychomotor agitation and hyperthermia can result in metabolic acidosis, rhabdomyolysis, renal failure, disseminated intravascular coagulation, cardiovascular collapse, and death.[98] Psychosis, resembling paranoid schizophrenia, can occur with chronic use, with large single doses, or during binges of amphetamines.[99,100] Typically, the psychosis abates a few days after drug cessation; however, in some cases it can last for weeks or recur despite abstinence.[101] While other stimulants such as cocaine can cause psychosis, it tends to occur more often with amphetamines, which is likely secondary to the more intense dopaminergic effects of amphetamines.[41]

Syndrome of Inappropriate Antidiuretic Hormone Secretion

Profound hyponatremia can be problematic with the use of MDMA resulting in seizures, coma, cerebral edema, and even death.[102-105] MDMA stimulates the release of vasopressin (antidiuretic hormone), which can induce a syndrome of inappropriate antidiuretic hormone secretion.[106] Consumption of large quantities of water and excessive sweating that can occur during raves may also contribute to the development of hyponatremia.[107,108] Interestingly, the frequency with which Ecstasy-associated hyponatremia develops appears to be related to differences in sex. A retrospective review found that women were four times more likely than men to have Ecstasy-associated hyponatremia and in those with hyponatremia, coma was common.[109] While not proved from their study, the authors postulated that women may develop Ecstasy-associated hyponatremia more often because estrogen stimulates the release of vasopressin.

Withdrawal from Amphetamines

Amphetamine withdrawal is a common problem among chronic abusers—about 9 out of every 10 experience symptoms after the abrupt discontinuation of amphetamines.[110] During withdrawal, patients can experience anxiety, agitation, fatigue, hypersomnia, increased appetite, intense drug craving, sadness or depression, suicidal ideations, and vivid or unpleasant dreams.[111] Although the symptoms associated with amphetamine withdrawal usually resolve in a few days, sometimes they may last for weeks to months.[112] Relapse is problematic because of intense craving that occurs during withdrawal. Treatment options for amphetamine withdrawal are limited. Previously, this condition had been treated with amineptine but was removed from the market due to a number of reports of abuse. Recently, reboxetine, a selective noradrenaline reuptake inhibitor, has been reported to be successful in the treatment of a limited number of cases of amphetamine withdrawal; however, further research is necessary to support the routine use of reboxetine in the treatment of amphetamine withdrawal.[113,114]

DIAGNOSTIC ANALYSIS

Diagnosis through history is often unreliable because many poisoned patients are incapable or reluctant to provide a precise history. Therefore, laboratory testing is necessary. Blood samples should be sent for a comprehensive metabolic panel, and a 12-lead electrocardiogram should be performed—both of which may assist with diagnosis and therapy and provide crucial information regarding end-organ toxicity. Creatinine phosphokinase should be monitored to evaluate for rhabdomyolysis or compartment syndrome in patients who are agitated, have muscular rigidity, or are found "down." Depending on the clinical presentation, other tests such as a complete blood count, coagulation profile, chest x-ray, computerized axial tomography of the head, and lumbar puncture may be indicated.

The routine use of serum and urine drug screens in the evaluation of patients suffering from the toxic effects of amphetamines is often not helpful and is advised against.

False-positive and false-negative results occur often with urine drug screens; many cold and over-the-counter medications contain ephedrine and pseudoephedrine and cross-react with amphetamines due to structural similarities.[115] False-negative results can occur because MDMA has been reported to be undetectable with certain urine assays.[116] On the other hand, while a true-positive result on the urine drug screen can establish exposure to amphetamines within in the past few days, it should not falsely reassure the clinician that amphetamines are responsible for the patient's clinical condition. In addition, the turnaround time for comprehensive toxicology testing is several hours, rendering it useless for acute management, and the results once obtained seldom affect either treatment or outcomes.[117–119] Rather, proper medical decision making is best achieved through routine diagnostic tests and methodically assessing and reassessing the patient's clinical condition.

TREATMENT OF ACUTE AMPHETAMINE INTOXICATION

Part of the problem with developing specific treatments for acute amphetamine toxicity has been the incomplete understanding of which central receptors are important in mediating toxicity. In treating patients who have used ring-substituted amphetamines, like MDMA, therapies have largely focused on the use of drugs to block central serotonin function or peripheral adrenergic receptors. In his original review on serotonin syndrome,[120] Sternbach made a case for the role of serotonin-1A receptors in the development and treatment of the disorder; serotonin syndrome has been associated with ring-substituted amphetamines. This recommendation was largely based on animal models of the serotonin-behavioral syndrome, which is caused by drugs that agonize serotonin-1A receptors.[121] However, drugs that are agonists at serotonin-1A receptors do not cause hyperthermia; rather, they cause hypothermia.[121–123] Recent studies have shown that activation of serotonin-1A receptors by MDMA is actually protective and that treatment with drugs that antagonize serotonin-1A receptors, such as propranolol, may actually worsen hyperthermia and toxicity.[124] Most studies involving MDMA have placed emphasis on serotonin-2A and dopamine-1 receptors in mediating hyperthermia.[29,125,126] These studies, however, typically employed pretreatment models, and although helpful in delineating mechanisms, they offer little in the way of support for clinical treatments.

To date, the authors know of only two animal studies in which clinically available agents have been employed after the establishment of MDMA-mediated hyperthermia. In one of these studies, the commonly used antipsychotic olanzapine reduced MDMA hyperthermia and cutaneous vasoconstriction; in the other, carvedilol reduced MDMA hyperthermia and rhabdomyolysis.[28,32] Olanzapine has effects on various receptor systems, including muscarinic, serotonin-2A, dopamine-1, and dopamine-α1 receptors.[127] Carvedilol is an antagonist of both α1– and β–adrenergic receptors. This makes it a more attractive treatment choice for amphetamine toxicity than other nonselective β-blockers, such as propranolol and nadolol that do not block α-receptors and can theoretically result in unopposed stimulation of α-receptors, leading to worse toxicity. With both of these studies, the agents were used at significantly larger doses than commonly used in humans and lack any clinical evidence as to their role in humans. In clinical practice, some have recommended cyproheptadine or chlorpromazine for the treatment of serotonin syndrome; both have serotonin-2A antagonist properties.[128–130] While both are reported to be beneficial, it is important to keep in mind that their utility is derived solely from case reports.

The role of antipsychotics in treating amphetamine intoxication has been controversial. Several animal models have shown benefit in reducing toxicity from amphetamines with the butyrophenone haloperidol[131,132] and, as mentioned earlier, the atypical antipsychotics olanzapine and clozapine.[32,127] There are, however, concerns with use of these drugs. Many new atypical antipsychotics are muscarinic antagonists (e.g., olanzapine and quetiapine).[133] Use of these drugs in large doses could result in impaired sweating, increases in heart rate, and central antimuscarinic toxicity. A recent study has raised new concerns about the use of antipsychotics in methamphetamine psychosis. Rats given haloperidol 2 days after a simulated methamphetamine binge developed damage to GABAergic neurons within the substantia nigra.[134] These findings, however, may not be relevant to clinicians, as the rats were given multiple high doses of methamphetamine without treatment followed by the administration of haloperidol 2 days later.

Due to similarities in the clinical presentation of serotonin syndrome and malignant hyperthermia, it has become tempting to speculate and even assume that the molecular underpinnings of anesthetic- and MDMA-induced hyperthermic syndromes are the same. However, both animal and human studies have shown mixed results, without convincing evidence to support the use of dantrolene in cases of serotonin syndrome.[67,136–139]

Because it is often not possible to clinically distinguish the cause of a patient's psychomotor agitation, perhaps the best choice for treatment are drugs that hyperpolarize neurons reducing centrally mediated catecholamine release, such as benzodiazepines and barbiturates.[139] Both benzodiazepines and barbiturates have been shown to decrease toxicity from amphetamines and serotonin syndrome in rats[140,141] and have been reported to be useful in humans.[142] The anticonvulsant and anxiolytic properties, safety and availability, various routes of administration, ability to titrate to effect, and lack of contraindication in other etiologies of drug-induced hyperthermia make benzodiazepines a reasonable treatment choice in cases of sympathomimetic and serotonin syndromes. Anecdotally, in cases of severe toxicity, we have found the use of propofol to be an effective agent at rapidly gaining control of the patient and in controlling the manifestations of excess adrenergic activation.

As hyperthermia represents one of the most serious complications of amphetamine intoxication, intuitively it makes sense that physicians seek to actively cool their patients. Few studies, however, have looked at the role of active cooling for amphetamine intoxication. In one of the studies evaluating this, dogs that were administered lethal doses of amphetamine and subsequently cooled through a femoral artery catheter had dramatically increased survival times.[143] While clinicians and researchers have largely ignored this simple treatment step, teenagers and young adults have employed this method of treatment in the form of chilled rooms available at raves, known as "chill out" rooms. No research, however, has been done in humans on this topic except in the setting of exertional and nonexertional heat stroke. With heat stroke, various means of external cooling, including cool water submersion and evaporative cooling with misting and fans, has shown rapid cooling of hyperthermic patients[144] and increased survival in animals.[145] Based on what is currently known, it would seem prudent to recommend similar methods of cooling for patients with life-threatening hyperthermia from serotonin syndrome.

CONCLUSION

Amphetamine abuse and its associated morbidity and mortality remain problematic throughout the United States. The neurological consequences of acute amphetamine intoxication are multiple and include dyskinesias, psychosis, serotonin syndrome, syndrome of inappropriate antidiuretic hormone, and stroke. Understanding the neuropharmacology and clinical presentations associated with amphetamines will aid the clinician in diagnosing and appropriately treating its toxicity.

REFERENCES

1. Rasmussen N. Making the first anti-depressant: amphetamine in American medicine, 1929–1950. *J Hist Med Allied Sci.* 2006;61:288–323.

2. Jackson CO. The amphetamine inhaler: a case study of medical abuse. *J Hist Med Allied Sci.* 1971;26:187–196.

3. Leavesley JH. Adolph Hitler. *Med J Aust.* 1985;142:687–688.

4. Lovell R. Lord Moran's prescriptions for Churchill. *BMJ.* 1995;310:1537–1538.

5. Streit F. Recommendations for demand reduction of amphetamines. *Chem Depend.* 1980;4:135–143.

6. Jerrard D. "Designer drugs": a current perspective. *J Emerg Med.* 1990;8:733–741.

7. Buchanan JF, Brown CR. "Designer drugs": a problem in clinical toxicology. *Med Toxicol.* 1988;3:1–17.

8. U.S. Drug Enforcement Administration. Controlled Substance Analogues. Available at: http://www.usdoj.gov/dea/pubs/abuse/1-csa.htm. Accessed August 4, 2007.

9. Schwartz RH, Miller NS. MDMA (Ecstasy) and the rave: a review. *Pediatrics.* 1997;100:705–708.

10. Substance Abuse and Mental Health Services Administration. Results from the 2005 National Survey on Drug Use and Health: National Findings (Office of Applied Studies, NSDUH Series H-30, DHHS Publication No. SMA 06-4194). Rockville, Md: SMA; 2006.

11. Substance Abuse and Mental Health Services Administration. Results from the 2002 National Survey on Drug Use and Health: National Findings (Office of Applied Studies, NHSDA Series H-22, DHHS Publication No. SMA 03-3836). Rockville, Md: SMA; 2003.

12. Substance Abuse and Mental Health Services Administration. Drug Abuse Warning Network, 2005. National Estimates of Drug-Related Emergency Department Visits. (Office of Applied Studies, DAWN Series D-29, DHHS Publication No. SMA 07-4256). Rockville, Md: SMA; 2007.

13. Hunt D, Kuck S, Truitt L. Methamphetamine Use: Lessons Learned. Final report to the National Institute of Justice, February 2006 (NCJ 209730). Available at: http://www.ncjrs.gov/pdffiles1/nij/grants/209730.pdf. Accessed August 5, 2007.

14. U.S. Drug Enforcement Administration. Maps of Methamphetamine Lab Incidents. Available at: http://www.usdoj.gov/dea/concern/map_lab_seizures.html. Accessed August 5, 2007.

15. Hunt D. Methamphetamine abuse: challenges for law enforcement and communities. *NIJ J.* 2006:24–27.

16. Fleckenstein AE, Volz TJ, Riddle EL, et al. New insights into the mechanism of action of amphetamines. *Annu Rev Pharmacol Toxicol.* 2007;47:681–698.

17. Seiden LS, Sabol KE, Ricaurte GA. Amphetamine: effects on catecholamine systems and behavior. *Annu Rev Pharmacol Toxicol.* 1993;33:639–677.

18. Fitzgerald JL, Reid JJ. Interactions of methylenedioxymethamphetamine with monoamine transmitter release mechanisms in rat brain slices. *Naunyn Schmiedebergs Arch Pharmacol.* 1993;347:313–323.

19. Rothman RB, Baumann MH, Dersch CM, et al. Amphetamine-type central nervous system stimulants release norepinephrine more potently than they release dopamine and serotonin. *Synapse.* 2001;39:32–41.

20. Baumann MH, Wang X, Rothman RB. 3,4-Methylenedioxymethamphetamine (MDMA) neurotoxicity in rats: a reappraisal of past and present findings. *Psychopharmacology (Berl).* 2007;189:407–424.

21. Fitzgerald JL, Reid JJ. Effects of methylenedioxymethamphetamine on the release of monoamines from rat brain slices. *Eur J Pharmacol.* 1990;191:217–220.

22. Gough B, Imam SZ, Blough B, et al. Comparative effects of substituted amphetamines (PMA, MDMA, and METH) on monoamines in rat caudate: a microdialysis study. *Ann NY Acad Sci.* 2002;965:410–420.

23. Yamamoto BK, Spanos LJ. The acute effects of methylenedioxymethamphetamine on dopamine release in the awake-behaving rat. *Eur J Pharmacol.* 1988;148:195–203.

24. Bankson MG, Cunningham KA. 3,4-Methylenedioxymethamphetamine (MDMA) as a unique model of serotonin receptor function and serotonin–dopamine interactions. *J Pharmacol Exp Ther.* 2001;297:846–852.

25. Koch S, Galloway MP. MDMA induced dopamine release in vivo: role of endogenous serotonin. *J Neural Transm.* 1997;104:135–146.

26. Sprague JE, Banks ML, Cook VJ, et al. Hypothalamic–pituitary–thyroid axis and sympathetic nervous system involvement in hyperthermia induced by 3,4-methylenedioxymethamphetamine (Ecstasy). *J Pharmacol Exp Ther.* 2003;305:159–166.

27. Sprague JE, Brutcher RE, Mills EM, et al. Attenuation of 3,4-methylenedioxymethamphetamine (MDMA, Ecstasy)–induced rhabdomyolysis with $\alpha1$- plus $\beta3$-adrenoreceptor antagonists. *Br J Pharmacol.* 2004;142:667–670.

28. Sprague JE, Moze P, Caden D, et al. Carvedilol reverses hyperthermia and attenuates rhabdomyolysis induced by 3,4-methylenedioxymethamphetamine (MDMA, Ecstasy) in an animal model. *Crit Care Med.* 2005;33:1311–1316.

29. Mechan AO, Esteban B, O'Shea E, et al. The pharmacology of the acute hyperthermic response that follows administration of 3,4-methylenedioxymethamphetamine (MDMA, "Ecstasy") to rats. *Br J Pharmacol.* 2002;135:170–180.

30. Aguirre N, Ballaz S, Lasheras B, et al. MDMA ("Ecstasy") enhances 5-HT$_{1A}$ receptor density and 8-OH-DPAT-induced hypothermia: blockade by drugs preventing 5-hydroxytryptamine depletion. *Eur J Pharmacol.* 1998;346:181–188.

31. Bowyer JF, Davies DL, Schmued L, et al. Further studies of the role of hyperthermia in methamphetamine neurotoxicity. *J Pharmacol Exp Ther.* 1994;268:1571–1580.

32. Blessing WW, Seaman B, Pedersen NP, et al. Clozapine reverses hyperthermia and sympathetically mediated cutaneous vasoconstriction induced by 3,4-methylenedioxymethamphetamine (Ecstasy) in rabbits and rats. *J Neurosci.* 2003;23:6385–6391.

33. Herin DV, Liu S, Ullrich T, et al. Role of the serotonin 5-HT$_{2A}$ receptor in the hyperlocomotive and hyperthermic effects of (+)-3,4-methylenedioxymethamphetamine. *Psychopharmacology (Berl).* 2005;178:505–513.

34. Buxton N, McConachie NS. Amphetamine abuse and intracranial haemorrhage. *J R Soc Med.* 2000;93:472–477.

35. Petitti DB, Sidney S, Quesenberry C, et al. Stroke and cocaine or amphetamine use. *Epidemiology.* 1998;9:596–600.

36. Westover AN, McBride S, Haley RW. Stroke in young adults who abuse amphetamines or cocaine: a population-based study of hospitalized patients. *Arch Gen Psychiatry.* 2007;64:495–502.

37. Kernan WN, Viscoli CM, Brass LM, et al. Phenylpropanolamine and the risk of hemorrhagic stroke. *N Engl J Med.* 2000;343:1826–1832.

38. Yoon BW, Bae HJ, Hong KS, et al. Phenylpropanolamine contained in cold remedies and risk of hemorrhagic stroke. *Neurology.* 2007;68:146–149.

39. Selmi F, Davies KG, Sharma RR, et al. Intracerebral haemorrhage due to amphetamine abuse: report of two cases with underlying arteriovenous malformations. *Br J Neurosurg.* 1995;9:93–96.

40. Harrington H, Heller HA, Dawson D, et al. Intracerebral hemorrhage and oral amphetamine. *Arch Neurol.* 1983;40:503–507.

41. Gold LH, Geyer MA, Koob GF. Neurochemical mechanisms involved in behavioral effects of amphetamines and related designer drugs. *NIDA Res Monogr.* 1989;94:101–126.

42. Karler R, Calder LD, Thai LH, et al. The dopaminergic, glutamatergic, GABAergic bases for the action of amphetamine and cocaine. *Brain Res.* 1995;671:100–104.

43. Rhee KJ, Albertson TE, Douglas JC. Choreoathetoid disorder associated with amphetamine-like drugs. *Am J Emerg Med.* 1988;6:131–133.

44. Mattson RH, Calverley JR. Dextroamphetamine-sulfate-induced dyskinesias. *JAMA.* 1968;204:400–402.

45. Klawans HL, Weiner WJ. The effect of d-amphetamine on choreiform movement disorders. *Neurology.* 1974;24:312–318.

46. Lundh H, Tunving K. An extrapyramidal choreiform syndrome caused by amphetamine addiction. *J Neurol Neurosurg Psychiatry.* 1981;44:728–730.

47. Malberg JE, Seiden LS. Small changes in ambient temperature cause large changes in 3,4-methylenedioxymethamphetamine (MDMA)–induced serotonin neurotoxicity and core body temperature in the rat. *J Neurosci.* 1998;18:5086–5094.

48. Ali SF, Newport GD, Holson RR, et al. Low environmental temperatures or pharmacologic agents that produce hypothermia decrease methamphetamine neurotoxicity in mice. *Brain Res.* 1994;658:33–38.

49. Miller DB, O'Callaghan JP. Elevated environmental temperature and methamphetamine neurotoxicity. *Environ Res.* 2003;92:48–53.

50. Marzuk PM, Tardiff K, Leon AC, et al. Ambient temperature and mortality from unintentional cocaine overdose. *JAMA.* 1998;279:1795–1800.

51. Pedersen NP, Blessing WW. Cutaneous vasoconstriction contributes to hyperthermia induced by 3,4-methylenedioxymethamphetamine (Ecstasy) in conscious rabbits. *J Neurosci.* 2001;21:8648–8654.

52. Crandall CG, Vongpatanasin W, Victor RG. Mechanism of cocaine-induced hyperthermia in humans. *Ann Intern Med.* 2002;136:785–791.

53. Milesi-Halle A, McMillan DE, Laurenzana EM, et al. Sex differences in (+)-amphetamine- and (+)-methamphetamine-induced behavioral response in male and female Sprague-Dawley rats. *Pharmacol Biochem Behav.* 2007;86:140–149.

54. Spanos LJ, Yamamoto BK. Acute and subchronic effects of methylenedioxymethamphetamine [(+/−)MDMA] on locomotion and serotonin syndrome behavior in the rat. *Pharmacol Biochem Behav.* 1989;32:835–840.

55. Avois L, Robinson N, Saudan C, et al. Central nervous system stimulants and sport practice. *Br J Sports Med.* 2006;40 (Suppl 1):i16–i20.

56. Duarte JA, Leao A, Magalhaes J, et al. Strenuous exercise aggravates MDMA-induced skeletal muscle damage in mice. *Toxicology.* 2005;206:349–358.

57. Harding M, Peterson DI. The effect of exercise and limitation of movement on amphetamine toxicity. *J Pharmacol Exp Ther.* 1963;145:47–51.

58. Rusyniak DE, Tandy SL, Hekmatyar SK, et al. The role of mitochondrial uncoupling in 3-4, methylenedioxymethamphetamine mediated skeletal muscle hyperthermia and rhabdomyolysis. *J Pharmacol Exp Ther.* 2005;312:629–639.

59. Nicholls DG, Locke RM. Thermogenic mechanisms in brown fat. *Physiol Rev.* 1984;64:1–64.

60. Blessing WW, Zilm A, Ootsuka Y. Clozapine reverses increased brown adipose tissue thermogenesis induced by 3,4-methylenedioxymethamphetamine and by cold exposure in conscious rats. *Neuroscience.* 2006;141:2067–2073.

61. Wellman PJ. Influence of amphetamine on brown adipose thermogenesis. *Res Commun Chem Pathol Pharmacol.* 1983;41:173–176.

62. Boss O, Samec S, Paoloni-Giacobino A, et al. Uncoupling protein-3: a new member of the mitochondrial carrier family with tissue-specific expression. *FEBS Letters.* 1997;408:39–42.

63. Mills EM, Rusyniak DE, Sprague JE. The role of the sympathetic nervous system and uncoupling proteins in the thermogenesis induced by 3,4-methylenedioxymethamphetamine. *J Mol Med.* 2004;82:787–799.

64. Mills EM, Banks ML, Sprague JE, et al. Uncoupling the agony from Ecstasy. *Nature.* 2003;426:403–404.

65. Sprague JE, Mallett NM, Rusyniak DE, et al. UCP3 and thyroid hormone involvement in methamphetamine-induced hyperthermia. *Biochem Pharmacol.* 2004;68:1339–1343.

66. Fiege M, Wappler F, Weisshorn R, et al. Induction of malignant hyperthermia in susceptible swine by 3,4-methylenedioxymethamphetamine ("Ecstasy"). *Anesthesiology.* 2003;99:1132–1136.

67. Hall AP, Henry JA. Acute toxic effects of "Ecstasy" (MDMA) and related compounds: overview of pathophysiology and clinical management. *Br J Anaesth.* 2006;96:678–685.

68. Rusyniak DE, Banks ML, Mills EM, et al. Dantrolene use in 3,4-methylenedioxymethamphetamine (Ecstasy)–mediated hyperthermia. *Anesthesiology.* 2004;101:263; author reply, 264.

69. Lister D, Hall GM, Lucke JN. Porcine malignant hyperthermia: III. Adrenergic blockade. *Br J Anaesth.* 1976;48:831–838.

70. Dar KJ, McBrien ME. MDMA induced hyperthermia: report of a fatality and review of current therapy. *Intensive Care Med.* 1996;22:995–996.

71. Ginsberg MD, Hertzman M, Schmidt-Nowara WW. Amphetamine intoxication with coagulopathy, hyperthermia, and reversible renal failure: a syndrome resembling heatstroke. *Ann Intern Med.* 1970;73:81–85.

72. Henry JA, Jeffreys KJ, Dawling S. Toxicity and deaths from 3,4-methylenedioxymethamphetamine ("Ecstasy"). *Lancet.* 1992;340:384–387.

73. Milroy CM, Clark JC, Forrest AR. Pathology of deaths associated with "Ecstasy" and "eve" misuse. *J Clin Pathol.* 1996;49:149–153.

74. Gowing LR, Henry-Edwards SM, Irvine RJ, et al. The health effects of Ecstasy: a literature review. *Drug Alcohol Rev.* 2002;21:53–63.

75. Judge BS. Differentiating the causes of metabolic acidosis in the poisoned patient. *Clin Lab Med.* 2006;26:31–48.

76. Volkow ND, Chang L, Wang GJ, et al. Loss of dopamine transporters in methamphetamine abusers recovers with protracted abstinence. *J Neurosci.* 2001;21:9414–9418.

77. Volkow ND, Chang L, Wang GJ, et al. Association of dopamine transporter reduction with psychomotor impairment in methamphetamine abusers. *Am J Psychiatry.* 2001;158:377–382.

78. Wilson JM, Kalasinsky KS, Levey AI, et al. Striatal dopamine nerve terminal markers in human, chronic methamphetamine users. *Nat Med.* 1996;2:699–703.

79. Moszczynska A, Fitzmaurice P, Ang L, et al. Why is parkinsonism not a feature of human methamphetamine users? *Brain.* 2004;127:363–370.

80. Bowyer JF, Holson RR. Methamphetamine and amphetamine neurotoxicity. In: Chang LW, Dyer RS, eds. *Handbook of Neurotoxicology.* New York: Marcel Dekker; 1995:845–870.

81. Guilarte TR. Is methamphetamine abuse a risk factor in parkinsonism? *Neurotoxicology.* 2001;22:725–731.

82. Hanson GR, Rau KS, Fleckenstein AE. The methamphetamine experience: a NIDA partnership. *Neuropharmacology.* 2004;47 (Suppl 1):92–100.

83. Seiden LS, Sabol KE. Neurotoxicity of methamphetamine-related drugs and cocaine. In: Chang LW, Dyer RS, eds. *Handbook of Neurotoxicology.* New York: Marcel Dekker; 1995:825–843.

84. Garwood ER, Bekele W, McCulloch CE, et al. Amphetamine exposure is elevated in Parkinson's disease. *Neurotoxicology.* 2006;27:1003–1006.

85. Kuniyoshi SM, Jankovic J. MDMA and parkinsonism. *N Engl J Med.* 2003;349:96–97.

86. Mintzer S, Hickenbottom S, Gilman S. Parkinsonism after taking Ecstasy. *N Engl J Med.* 1999;340:1443.

87. Roberts JR, Greenberg MI. Cocaine washout syndrome. *Ann Intern Med*. 2000;132:679–680.

88. Sporer KA, Lesser SH. Cocaine washed-out syndrome. *Ann Emerg Med*. 1992;21:112.

89. Trabulsy ME. Cocaine washed out syndrome in a patient with acute myocardial infarction. *Am J Emerg Med*. 1995;13:538–539.

90. Morley JE, Shafer RB, Elson MK, et al. Amphetamine-induced hyperthyroxinemia. *Ann Intern Med*. 1980;93:707–709.

91. Sprague JE, Yang X, Sommers J, et al. Roles of norepinephrine, free fatty acids, thyroid status, and skeletal muscle uncoupling protein 3 expression in sympathomimetic-induced thermogenesis. *J Pharmacol Exp Ther*. 2007;320:274–280.

92. Dolfini E, Kobayashi M. Studies with amphetamine in hyper- and hypothyroid rats. *Eur J Pharmacol*. 1967;2:65–66.

93. Halpern BN, Drudi-Baracco C, Bessirard D. Exaltation of toxicity of sympathomimetic amines by thyroxine. *Nature*. 1964;204:387–388.

94. Halpern BN, Drudi-Baracco C, Bessirard D. Potentiation of the absolute toxicity and group toxicity of L-ephedrine by thyroxine. *C R Seances Soc Biol Fil*. 1964;158:1284–1289.

95. Martin TL, Chiasson DA, Kish SJ. Does hyperthyroidism increase risk of death due to the ingestion of Ecstasy? *J Forensic Sci*. 2007;52:951–953.

96. Smith DE. An analysis of 310 cases of acute high-dose methamphetamine toxicity in Haight-Ashbury. *Clin Toxicol*. 1970;3:117–124.

97. Smets G, Bronselaer K, De Munnynck K, et al. Amphetamine toxicity in the emergency department. *Eur J Emerg Med*. 2005;12:193–197.

98. Henry JA. Metabolic consequences of drug misuse. *Br J Anaesth*. 2000;85:136–142.

99. Hart JB, Wallace J. The adverse effects of amphetamines. *Clin Toxicol*. 1975;8:179–190.

100. Dalmau A, Bergman B, Brismar B. Psychotic disorders among inpatients with abuse of cannabis, amphetamine and opiates: do dopaminergic stimulants facilitate psychiatric illness? *Eur Psychiatry*. 1999;14:366–371.

101. Yui K, Ishiguro T, Goto K, et al. Precipitating factors in spontaneous recurrence of methamphetamine psychosis. *Psychopharmacology*. 1997;134:303–308.

102. Sue YM, Lee YL, Huang JJ. Acute hyponatremia, seizure, and rhabdomyolysis after Ecstasy use. *J Toxicol Clin Toxicol*. 2002;40:931–940.

103. Kalantar-Zadeh K, Nguyen MK, Chang R, et al. Fatal hyponatremia in a young woman after Ecstasy ingestion. *Nat Clin Pract Nephrol*. 2006;2:283–288.

104. Satchell SC, Connaughton M. Inappropriate antidiuretic hormone secretion and extreme rises in serum creatinine kinase following MDMA ingestion. *Br J Hosp Med*. 1994;51:495.

105. Ajaelo I, Koenig K, Snoey E. Severe hyponatremia and inappropriate antidiuretic hormone secretion following Ecstasy use. *Acad Emerg Med*. 1998;5:839–840.

106. Wolff K, Tsapakis EM, Winstock AR, et al. Vasopressin and oxytocin secretion in response to the consumption of Ecstasy in a clubbing population. *J Psychopharmacol*. 2006;20:400–410.

107. Brvar M, Kozelj G, Osredkar J, et al. Polydipsia as another mechanism of hyponatremia after "Ecstasy" (3,4-methylenedioxymethamphetamine) ingestion. *Eur J Emerg Med*. 2004;11:302–304.

108. Kalant H. The pharmacology and toxicology of "Ecstasy" (MDMA) and related drugs. *CMAJ*. 2001;165:917–928.

109. Rosenson J, Smollin C, Sporer KA, et al. Patterns of Ecstasy-associated hyponatremia in California. *Ann Emerg Med*. 2007;49:164–171.

110. Srisurapanont M, Jarusuraisin N, Kittirattanapaiboon P. Treatment for amphetamine withdrawal. *Cochrane Database Syst Rev* 2001;(4):CD003021.

111. Lago JA, Kosten TR. Stimulant withdrawal. *Addiction*. 1994;89:1477–1481.

112. Watson R, Hartmann E, Schildkraut JJ. Amphetamine withdrawal: affective state, sleep patterns, and MHPG excretion. *Am J Psychiatry*. 1972;129:263–269.

113. Cox D, Bowers R, McBride A. Reboxetine may be helpful in the treatment of amphetamine withdrawal. *Br J Clin Pharmacol*. 2004;58:100–101.

114. Molina JD, de Pablo S, Lopez-Munoz F, et al. Monotherapy with reboxetine in amphetamine withdrawal syndrome. *Prog Neuropsychopharmacol Biol Psychiatry*. 2006;30:1353–1355.

115. Saito T, Mase H, Takeichi S, et al. Rapid simultaneous determination of ephedrines, amphetamines, cocaine, cocaine metabolites, and opiates in human urine by GC-MS. *J Pharm Biomed Anal*. 2007;43:358–363.

116. Cody JT, Schwarzhoff R. Fluorescence polarization immunoassay detection of amphetamine, methamphetamine, and illicit amphetamine analogues. *J Anal Toxicol*. 1993;17:23–33.

117. Brett AS. Implications of discordance between clinical impression and toxicology analysis in drug overdose. *Arch Intern Med*. 1988;148:437–441.

118. Kellerman AL, Fihh SD, LoGerfo JP, et al. Impact of drug screening in suspected overdose. *Ann Emerg Med*. 1987;16:1206–1216.

119. Sporer KA, Ernst AA. The effect of toxicologic screening on management of minimally symptomatic overdoses. *Am J Emerg Med*. 1992;10.

120. Sternbach H. The serotonin syndrome. *Am J Psychiatry*. 1991;148:705–713.

121. Isbister GK, Buckley NA. The pathophysiology of serotonin toxicity in animals and humans: implications for diagnosis and treatment. *Clin Neuropharmacol*. 2005;28:205–214.

122. Gudelsky GA, Koenig JI, Meltzer HY. Thermoregulatory responses to serotonin (5-HT) receptor stimulation in the rat: evidence for opposing roles of 5-HT$_2$ and 5-HT$_{1A}$ receptors. *Neuropharmacology*. 1986;25:1307–1313.

123. Hjorth S. Hypothermia in the rat induced by the potent serotonin-ergic agent 8-OH-DPAT. *J Neural Transm*. 1985;61:131–135.

124. Rusyniak DE, Zaretskaia MV, Zaretsky DV, et al. 3,4-Methylene-dioxymethamphetamine- and 8-hydroxy-2-di-n-propylamino-tetralin-induced hypothermia: role and location of 5-HT$_{1A}$ receptors. *J Pharmacol Exp Ther*. 2007;323:477–487.

125. Nisijima K, Yoshino T, Yui K, et al. Potent serotonin (5-HT)(2A) receptor antagonists completely prevent the development of hyperthermia in an animal model of the 5-HT syndrome. *Brain Res*. 2001;890:23–31.

126. Van Oekelen D, Megens A, Meert T, et al. Role of 5-HT(2) receptors in the tryptamine-induced 5-HT syndrome in rats. *Behav Pharmacol*. 2002;13:313–318.

127. Blessing WW. New treatment for Ecstasy-related hyperthermia. *Intern Med J*. 2003;33:555–556.

128. Graudins A, Stearman A, Chan B. Treatment of the serotonin syndrome with cyproheptadine. *J Emerg Med*. 1998;16:615–619.

129. Lappin RI, Auchincloss EL. Treatment of the serotonin syndrome with cyproheptadine. *N Engl J Med*. 1994;331:1021–1022.

130. Gillman PK. The serotonin syndrome and its treatment. *J Psychopharmacol (Oxf)*. 1999;13:100–109.

131. Catravas JD, Waters IW, Davis WM, et al. Letter: Haloperidol for acute amphetamine poisoning: a study in dogs. *JAMA*. 1975;231:1340–1341.

132. Derlet RW, Albertson TE, Rice P. Protection against d-amphetamine toxicity. *Am J Emerg Med*. 1990;8:105–108.

133. Burns MJ. The pharmacology and toxicology of atypical antipsychotic agents. *J Toxicol Clin Toxicol*. 2001;39:1–14.

134. Hatzipetros T, Raudensky JG, Soghomonian JJ, et al. Haloperidol treatment after high-dose methamphetamine administration

is excitotoxic to GABA cells in the substantia nigra pars reticulata. *J Neurosci.* 2007;27:5895–5902.

135. Makisumi T, Yoshida K, Watanabe T, et al. Sympatho-adrenal involvement in methamphetamine-induced hyperthermia through skeletal muscle hypermetabolism. *Eur J Pharmacol.* 1998;363:107–112.

136. Singarajah C, Lavies NG. An overdose of Ecstasy: a role for dantrolene. *Anaesthesia.* 1992;47:686–687.

137. Watson JD, Ferguson C, Hinds CJ, et al. Exertional heat stroke induced by amphetamine analogues: does dantrolene have a place? *Anaesthesia.* 1993;48:1057–1060.

138. Webb C, Williams V. Ecstasy intoxication: appreciation of complications and the role of dantrolene. *Anaesthesia.* 1993;48:542–543.

139. Vogel WH, Miller J, DeTurck KH, et al. Effects of psychoactive drugs on plasma catecholamines during stress in rats. *Neuropharmacology.* 1984;23:1105–1108.

140. Derlet RW, Albertson TE, Rice P. Antagonism of cocaine, amphetamine, and methamphetamine toxicity. *Pharmacol Biochem Behav.* 1990;36:745–749.

141. Nisijima K, Shioda K, Yoshino T, et al. Diazepam and chlormethiazole attenuate the development of hyperthermia in an animal model of the serotonin syndrome. *Neurochem Int.* 2003;43:155–164.

142. Derlet RW, Rice P, Horowitz BZ, et al. Amphetamine toxicity: experience with 127 cases. *J Emerg Med.* 1989;7:157–161.

143. Zalis EG, Lundberg GD, Kaplan G, et al. The effect of extracorporeal cooling on amphetamine toxicity. *Arch Int Pharmacodyn Ther.* 1966;159:189–195.

144. Hadad E, Rav-Acha M, Heled Y, et al. Heat stroke: a review of cooling methods. *Sports Med.* 2004;34:501–511.

145. Chou YT, Lai ST, Lee CC, et al. Hypothermia attenuates circulatory shock and cerebral ischemia in experimental heatstroke. *Shock.* 2003;19:388–393.

CHAPTER 28

Illicit Drugs II: Opioids, Cocaine, and Others

John C.M. Brust

INTRODUCTION

This chapter addresses possible or probable neurotoxic effects of drugs used recreationally. Ethanol is covered in Chapter 29, and psychostimulants other than cocaine are described in Chapter 27.

DEFINITIONS

There are two kinds of drug dependence.[1–3] Psychic dependence leads to craving and drug-seeking behavior. Physical dependence produces somatic withdrawal symptoms and signs. Different drugs produce different degrees of psychic dependence and different forms of physical dependence; psychic and physical dependence can coexist or occur alone. Addiction is psychic dependence. Tolerance is the need to take an increasing dose of a drug to achieve the desired effect or to avoid withdrawal. Tolerance may be the result of increased metabolism and decreased availability of the drug (metabolic or pharmacokinetic tolerance) or the result of adaptive changes in the brain (cellular or pharmacodynamic tolerance). The term *drug abuse* is a social judgment based on the perception that nonmedicinal use of a substance is harmful.

OPIOIDS

Acting variably at μ-, δ-, and κ-receptors, opioids include agonists, antagonists, and mixed agonist–antagonists (Table 1).[4] They differ in their degree of addiction liability. The agent most often abused is heroin (diacetyl-morphine), classified by the U.S. Food and Drug Administration as Schedule 1 (high potential for abuse, no accepted medical use).

Intended doses of opioid agonists produce drowsy euphoria, analgesia, and cough suppression, often accompanied by miosis, nausea, vomiting, sweating, pruritus, hypothermia, postural hypotension, constipation, and decreased libido. Injected or smoked, heroin produces a brief ecstatic "rush" usually followed by relaxed euphoria.

Table 1: Opioids Currently or Recently Available in the United States

AGONIST

Tincture of opium (laudanum)

Camphorated tincture of opium (paregoric)

Morphine (morphine sulfate injection; MS Contin, Oramorph)

Heroin (legally available only for investigational use)

Methadone (Dolophine)

Fentanyl (Sublimaze, in Innovar, Duragesic patch)

Sufentanil (Sufenta)

Alfentanil (Alfenta)

Oxymorphone (Numorphan)

Hydromorphone (Dilaudid)

Codeine

Oxycodone (Oxy-Contin; in mixtures, e.g., Percodan, Percocet, Tylox)

Hydrocodone (in mixtures, e.g., Hycodan, Lortab, Lorcet, Tussionex, Vicodin)

Levorphanol (Levo-Dromoran)

Meperidine (pethidine; Demerol, Pethadol)

Propoxyphene (Darvon; in Darvocet, Wygesic)

ANTAGONIST

Naloxone (Narcan)

Naltrexone (Trexan)

Nalmefene (Revex)

MIXED AGONIST–ANTAGONIST

Pentazocine (Talwin, Talwin Nx, in Talacen)

Butorphanol (Stadol)

Buprenorphine (Buprenex)

Overdose causes coma, respiratory depression, and pinpoint (but reactive) pupils.

Treatment of overdose includes ventilator support and naloxone in dosage titrated to severity of symptoms. Naloxone is short acting, so patients receiving it require close observation.[5,6] Heroin is often taken with other drugs, especially ethanol or cocaine, resulting in a confusing clinical picture. Street heroin preparations contain an array of adulterants, either pharmacologically inactive (lactose, baking soda, mannitol) or active (procaine, lidocaine, strychnine, quinine).[7]

Opioid withdrawal produces irritability, lacrimation, rhinorrhea, sweating, yawning, mydriasis, myalgia, muscle spasms, piloerection, nausea, vomiting, abdominal cramps, fever, hot flashes, tachycardia, hypertension, orgasm, and intense drug craving.[3] Seizures and delirium are not features of opioid withdrawal, which more resembles a severe flulike illness. An exception to the benign (albeit highly unpleasant) nature of opioid withdrawal is its occurrence in newborns, whose symptoms can include myoclonus or seizures, sometimes with fatal outcome. Opioid withdrawal can be prevented or treated with long-acting methadone. Paregoric is often used in neonates.[8]

Heroin addicts receiving long-term methadone maintenance therapy may be dysphoric between doses or experience decreased libido, but they display little or no cognitive or behavioral abnormality, even after many years.[9] Neurological complications of μ-receptor agonists are therefore more likely the result of indirect effects (e.g., infection, trauma, adulterants, and immune mechanisms) than direct neurotoxicity.

Indirect Effects

Stroke

Heroin users are prone to stroke unrelated to liver or kidney disease, endocarditis, or acquired immune deficiency syndrome (AIDS).[10–12] Patients with cerebral infarction sometimes have symptoms or laboratory evidence of hypersensitivity, including irregularity of cerebral vessels at angiography. (Angiographical "beading" is not specific for angiitis, however.) Another possible mechanism for stroke, embolism of foreign material to the brain, is best documented in injectors of pentazocine combined with the antihistamine tripelennamine ("Ts and blues").[13] Heroin myelopathy is possibly vascular, as well as immunological, in which paraparesis, sensory loss, and urinary retention follow ingestion, sometimes after a period of abstinence.[14]

Nerve and Muscle

Mononeuropathy and polyneuropathy occur in heroin users as a result of AIDS, antiretroviral therapy, ethanol abuse, malnutrition, injection into nerves, and pressure palsies. In the absence of such indirect effects, heroin users can develop sensorimotor polyneuropathy and brachial or lumbosacral plexopathy.[15] The mechanism is likely immunological, perhaps related to an adulterant.

Rhabdomyolysis with myoglobinurra in heroin users can follow overdose, suggesting direct muscle compression, or follow injection without loss of consciousness, suggesting hypersensitivity.[16,17]

Neurotoxicity

Optic Atrophy

Optic atrophy occurred in a heroin dealer whose mixture contained large amounts of quinine. When he removed quinine from the preparation, vision improved despite continued heroin use.[18]

Chasing the Dragon

"Chasing the dragon" refers to the practice of heating heroin on metal foil and then inhaling the vapor through a straw or tube. Spongiform encephalopathy affected 47 Dutch dragon chasers, whose symptoms included apathy, bradyphrenia, and cerebellar ataxia progressing to spastic quadriparesis, tremor, chorea, myoclonus, pseudobulbar palsy, fever, blindness, and in 11 cases, death.[19] Autopsy showed spongiform white matter degeneration affecting cerebrum, cerebellum, and spinal cord. Heroin samples included variable amounts of procaine, phenacetin, caffeine, antipyrene, strychnine, quinine, lidocaine, and diethylcarbonate, but the disorder could not be reproduced in animals, and the responsible toxin has never been identified. Subsequent cases have been reported from around the world. In two New York City dragon chasers, magnetic resonance spectroscopy showed elevated brain lactate, and clinical improvement followed treatment with antioxidants including coenzyme Q, suggesting mitochondrial dysfunction.[20]

1-Methyl-4-Phenyl-1,2,3,6-Tetrahydropyridine

During the early 1980s, parkinsonism began appearing in injectors of a meperidine analogue, 1-methyl-4-proprionoxypiperidine (MPPP), which was sold as "synthetic heroin."[21] The responsible toxin was an unintended byproduct of MPPP synthesis, 1-methyl-4-phenyl-1,2,3,6-tetrahydropyridine (MPTP). In these patients, bradykinesia and rigidity were severe and did not improve with abstinence, but there was no dementia and or autonomic impairment. Symptoms responded to levodopa and dopamine agonists, but typical side effects including dyskinesias, on–off phenomena, and psychiatric symptoms were prominent, and attempts to wean after years of dopaminergic therapy were unsuccessful. The toxin that directly destroys neurons in the substantia nigra is a metabolite of MPTP, 1-methyl-4-phenylpyridinium (MPP^+), which inhibits production of ATP and stimulates formation of superoxide radicals.[22] Metabolism of MPTP to MPP^+ is blocked by type B monoamine oxidase inhibitors such as deprenyl.

Seizures

In some animal models, opioid agonists lower seizure threshold, but their occurrence during heroin overdose is more likely the result of concomitant drug use (e.g., ethanol withdrawal or cocaine intoxication) than heroin toxicity. A case–control study found that heroin use, both past and present, was a risk factor for new onset seizures independent of overdose, head trauma, infection, ethanol, or other illicit drugs, and in none of the patients studied did a seizure occur in the setting of overdose.[23]

Meperidine　Although similar in action to morphine and heroin, meperidine (Demerol) produces a neurotoxic metabolite, normeperidine, that can cause tremor, agitation, delirium, hallucinations, myoclonus, and seizures.[24] The combination of meperidine with monoamine oxidase inhibitors exacerbates symptoms and can be fatal.

Pentazocine　Low doses of the mixed agonist–antagonist pentazocine produce euphoria, sedation, impotence, and anhidrosis; higher doses cause headache, nausea, blurred vision, diplopia, tachycardia, hypertension, urinary retention, depressed respiration, dysphoria, delusions, hallucinations, and seizures.[5] Subcutaneous or intramuscular injections of pentazocine cause severe focal skin and muscle fibrosis, the result of precipitation of the acidic drug.[25]

Uncertain Neurotoxicity

Fetal Effects

As with other drugs, determining the effects of fetal exposure to opioids is confounded by lack of prenatal care, exposure to other agents, especially ethanol and tobacco, and parenteral psychopathology or low intelligence. Infants exposed to heroin in utero are often of low birth weight and small for gestational age. Respiratory distress syndrome is common, and the frequency of sudden infant death is several times that of unexposed infants.[26,27] Studies of in utero–exposed rodents describe abnormal neuronal density, axonal branching, and dendritic arborization, but such studies have not been consistent.[28–30] Similarly inconsistent are human studies of intellectual function and behavior in children prenatally exposed to opioids.[31–34]

COCAINE

An alkaloid obtained from the South American shrub *Erythroxylon coca*, cocaine differs pharmacologically from amphetamine-like psychostimulants in at least two ways. Whereas amphetamines cause presynaptic release of neurotransmitters (principally dopamine, norepinephrine, and serotonin), cocaine's principal action is to block neurotransmitter reuptake.[35] Unlike the amphetamines, moreover, cocaine is a local anesthetic.

Cocaine hydrochloride can be taken intranasally or parenterally. Converted to alkaloidal cocaine (free base, "crack"), it can be smoked, allowing higher doses over prolonged periods.[36] Desired effects of cocaine are similar to those produced by amphetamine-like agents: alert euphoria with increased motor activity and physical endurance. Parenteral or smoked cocaine produces an ecstatic "rush" clearly distinguishable from that of opioids.[1] Repeated use results in stereotypic activity progressing to bruxism and dyskinesias and in paranoia progressing to hallucinatory psychosis.[37,38] Overdose, as with the amphetamines, causes headache, chest pain, flushing, sweating, delirium, cardiac arrhythmia, hypertensive crisis, myoclonus, seizures, myoglobinuria, shock, coma, and death.[39] Malignant hyperthermia and disseminated intravascular coagulation occur.[40] Treatment includes benzodiazepine sedation, oxygen, bicarbonate for acidosis, anticonvulsants, cooling, blood pressure control, respiratory support, and cardiac monitoring.[41]

In the presence of ethanol, cocaine is metabolized to cocaethylene, which binds to the dopamine transporter as avidly (or more so) than cocaine itself, with possibly synergistic toxicity.[42]

Cocaine withdrawal produces fatigue, depression, and hunger, but few measurable somatic signs. Suicidal depression may require hospitalization.[43]

Cocaine is intensely addictive. Rodents and monkeys self-administer the drug to the exclusion of food and water until they die.[44] The addictive liability of cocaine, as with other psychostimulants, is closely associated with the release of dopamine in the ventral tegmental area–nucleus accumbens pathway.[1]

Indirect Effects

Cocaine-associated Stroke

Cocaine users are at increased risk for coronary artery disease, cardiomyopathy, and both ischemic and hemorrhagic stroke.[1] Angina pectoris and acute myocardial infarction are the result of increased myocardial oxygen demand, combined with cocaine-induced coronary artery constriction. Cocaine also causes myocardial contraction band necrosis, myocarditis, dilated cardiomyopathy, and cardiac arrhythmia (including ventricular fibrillation).[45] Cocaine-related cardiac disease in turn increases the risk for cardioembolic stroke.[46] However, most strokes in cocaine users are not cardiogenic.

By 2002, more than 600 cocaine-related strokes had been reported, roughly half ischemic and half hemorrhagic. Ischemic strokes included transient ischemic attacks and infarction of cerebrum, thalamus, brainstem, spinal cord, and retina.[1,47] Although angiography sometimes showed irregular constrictions and dilations of cerebral vessels ("beading"), vasculitis was demonstrated histologically in only a few cases, and only one of these had vessel wall necrosis.[48] In both ischemic and hemorrhagic stroke, cerebral vessels were usually histologically normal. The major mechanism for ischemic stroke is direct vasoconstriction of cerebral vessels, which has been demonstrated in human volunteers receiving cocaine.[49] The cocaine metabolite, benzoylecgonine, which can be detected in urine of heavy users for days to weeks, is also vasoconstrictive, probably explaining strokes occurring days after drug exposure.[50] Cocaine also has prothrombotic effects on platelets, endothelin, protein C, and antithrombin III.[51]

Cocaine-related intracranial hemorrhages have been intraparenchymal, subarachnoid, and intraventricular.[52] Cerebral angiography often reveals saccular aneurysm or vascular malformation in such patients. The mechanism of hemorrhage is likely surges of hypertension during drug use, with particular vulnerability in subjects with preexisting vascular anomalies.

Neurotoxicity

Seizures

In contrast to users of amphetamine-like drugs, in whom seizures are usually accompanied by signs of overdose, cocaine often produces seizures without other evidence of toxicity.[53] Single tonic–clonic seizures are most common, but focal seizures occur, and status epilepticus can be refractory to anticonvulsant therapy. Pharmacologically active cocaine metabolites probably explain seizures occurring many hours after use. Cocaine-related seizures in animals display a kindling pattern: that is, seizure threshold decreases progressively with repeated drug exposure.[54] The reported incidence of seizures ranged from 1.4% among hospitalized cocaine users[55] to 9% among heavy crack users participating in a phone survey.[56] The degree to which cocaine's local anesthetic properties contribute to its epileptogenicity is uncertain.

Abnormal Movements

As noted, movement disorders are increasingly prevalent with repeated cocaine use. Dystonia and chorea usually last only minutes to days after use, but sometimes such movements can emerge during abstinence or can persist for weeks.[57] The mechanism is unclear but is more likely a toxic than a withdrawal effect.

Rhabdomyolysis

Rhabdomyolysis can occur in cocaine users in the absence of other symptoms.[58] It has been attributed to both muscle ischemia and direct muscle toxicity. Recurrences are common.

Uncertain Neurotoxicity

Cognitive Effects

Cocaine and amphetamine-like psychostimulants have different morphological effects on monoaminergic nerve terminals. Amphetamine damages brain dopaminergic nerve terminals, methylenedioxymethamphetamine (Ecstasy) damages serotonergic nerve terminals, and methamphetamine damages both.[59] By contrast, cocaine depletes nerve terminals of dopamine but does not cause morphological damage.[60] Controversial is whether chronic cocaine users develop lasting cognitive or behavioral abnormalities and, if so, by what mechanism.

Protracted depression in abstinent users has been attributed to permanent depletion of limbic dopamine. However, although severe depression can be a feature of acute withdrawal, many cocaine users have a history of depressive illness or bipolar disorder before drug use. Chronic cocaine use as a cause rather than a result of depression is biologically plausible but speculative.

Human studies using controls have demonstrated abnormalities in auditory recall, reaction time, attention, executive function, visuoperception, manual dexterity, and declarative memory in abstinent cocaine users.[61–64] As with other drugs, it is difficult to interpret such studies in the absence of pre–drug use comparisons. One study found worse neuropsychological performance among cocaine users who also consumed large amounts of ethanol, possibly related to the additive toxic effects of cocaethylene.[65] Another study described persistent schizophrenic symptoms emerging in long-term users.[66]

In a study that identified cognitive impairment and cerebral atrophy in chronic cocaine users, impaired cognition remained after adjustments for tobacco, ethanol, other drugs, nutrition, head injury, and human immunodeficiency virus (HIV), but cerebral atrophy did not.[67] A study using magnetic resonance imaging found accelerated loss of temporal lobe volume with age in chronic cocaine users, as well as abnormal white matter signals consistent with "subclinical vascular events."[68,69] Positron emission tomography and single-photon emission computed tomography studies showed decreased metabolic activity in the frontal lobes, inconsistently correlating with deficits on psychometric testing, especially executive function, organization, set maintenance, verbal learning, and concept attainment.[70–72] Magnetic resonance spectroscopy identified reduced N-acetyl aspartate (a neuronal or axonal marker) in the thalamus of chronic cocaine users,[73] and diffusion tensor imaging found "white matter microstructural abnormalities" in inferior brain regions.[74]

Case reports describe cognitive impairment in cocaine users in whom imaging reveals patchy abnormalities consistent with infarction. In one such report, cerebral angiography showed moyamoya-like collaterals, suggesting a progressive rather than an acute process.[75]

Evidence thus favors cognitive and behavioral impairment as a consequence of chronic cocaine use. The mechanism may be ischemic rather than directly neurotoxic.

Fetal Effects

During the American crack epidemic of the 1980s and 1990s, children exposed to cocaine in utero ("crack babies") received considerable media attention. Reports described increased spontaneous abortion, abruptio placentae, retarded fetal growth, decreased head circumference, and various congenital anomalies affecting the genitourinary system, skeletal system, gastrointestinal system, cardiovascular system, ocular system, and central nervous system (CNS).[76–78] Cocaine-exposed newborns often have tremor, irritability, and hypertonia.[79] Some have seizures that continue during the first weeks of life; such symptoms and signs are the result of acute toxicity, not withdrawal.[80] Ischemic and hemorrhagic strokes are often encountered in neonates exposed to cocaine in utero.[81]

A problem with such reports is that cocaine-using mothers tend to avoid prenatal care; to abuse other substances, including tobacco and ethanol; to underreport cocaine use; to have a high prevalence of sexually transmitted diseases, including HIV and syphilis; and to be socioeconomically impoverished. A study that found intrauterine growth retardation, small head circumference, and hypertonic tetraparesis among cocaine-exposed newborns compared to controls verified recent and remote cocaine exposure by employing maternal hair analysis but relied on self-report to determine tobacco exposure.[82] Another study attributed the same symptoms to tobacco exposure, relying on urine assays for the nicotine metabolite cotinine to verify tobacco exposure but using meconium levels of a cocaine metabolite to verify cocaine exposure.[83] Thus, the former study may have underestimated tobacco exposure and the latter may have underestimated cocaine exposure.

A review of 74 reports addressing the effects of prenatal cocaine exposure dismissed 38 on methodological grounds. Systematic analysis of the remaining 36 studies failed to identify a "consistent negative association between prenatal cocaine exposure and physical growth, developmental test scores, or receptive or expressive language" after controlling for tobacco, ethanol, marijuana, or the quality of the child's environment.[84] Other studies of children 4 to 9 years failed to find intelligence quotient (IQ) differences in those prenatally exposed to cocaine.[85–87] In another study, mild disturbances in executive function were accompanied by frontal lobe abnormalities detected on diffusion tensor imaging.[88]

Animal studies provide evidence that cocaine does damage fetuses. Reported abnormalities include skeletal anomalies, reduced fetal weight, intracranial hemorrhage, deficient conditioning to noxious stimuli, decreased exploratory behavior, delayed eye maturation, congenital hearing loss, enhanced susceptibility to cocaine-induced seizures later in life, and perinatal mortality.[89–94] Morphological abnormalities include hippocampal dysplasia and habenular degeneration.[95,96]

Cocaine decreases uterine and placental blood flow,[97] and it is uncertain whether the effects of prenatal cocaine exposure, to whatever degree they turn out to be, are the result of CNS hypoxia, direct neurotoxicity, or both; whether the damage occurs early in gestation, late in gestation, or both; and whether the damage involves cocaine's effects on dopamine, serotonin, or other neurotransmitters (which early in development act as trophic factors). Toxic effects of cocaine metabolites, e.g., norcocaine, might be contributory. It is also uncertain whether fetal cocaine-exposure might produce neurochemical effects not evident at birth or early childhood but emerging with maturity.

MARIJUANA

Marijuana consists of leaves and flowers of the hemp plant, *Cannabis sativa;* a more potent product, hashish, is made from a resin coating the plant and containing the psychoactive compound, Δ-9-tetrahydrocannabinol (Δ-9-THC). Stereospecific G protein–coupled receptors, termed CB1, are present on neurons of the central and peripheral nervous systems of all vertebrates, and two endogenous ligands, anandamide and 2-arachidonylglycerol, bind to them. Δ-9-THC also binds CB1 receptors, which are located on presynaptic nerve terminals, where they inhibit release of many neurotransmitters, including glutamate, γ-aminobutyric acid (GABA), acetylcholine, norepinephrine, dopamine, and serotonin.[98,99]

In the United States, marijuana is usually smoked, but it can be eaten. The desired effect is relaxed euphoria; associated symptoms include depersonalization, subjective time-slowing, impaired memory, impaired balance and hand steadiness, conjunctival injection, tachycardia, and postural hypotension.[100] High doses produce auditory or visual illusions or hallucinations, psychotic excitement, acute dysphoria, panic, and bradycardia. Fatal overdose has not been documented, however. Acute adverse reactions can last hours to a few days. "Flashbacks" consist of the spontaneous reappearance weeks to months after using marijuana of hallucinations or other symptoms associated with the original use. In humans, withdrawal symptoms are infrequent and subtle and include emotional lability, anxiety, insomnia, nausea, tremor, and headache. Drug craving is common, however. Marijuana is often taken with other drugs, including heroin, cocaine, and phencyclidine.

Uncertain Neurotoxicity

Cognitive Effects

Whether marijuana causes lasting mental abnormalities is controversial despite decades of study.[101] During the 1960s, reports of a marijuana "antimotivational syndrome," with apathy, decreased attentiveness, and memory impairment, led to reports from diverse countries, some describing cognitive abnormalities among cannabis users and others finding no association.[102,103] Confounding such studies is lack of information as to intellectual function before drug use and uncertainty as to the length of abstinence necessary to assure drug washout. A study of college undergraduates compared those who smoked marijuana nearly daily to those who smoked every several days; testing was performed after at least 19 hours of abstinence, and heavy users were more impaired on tests of attention and executive function, but the differences could plausibly be ascribed to residual acute drug effect, withdrawal, or neurotoxicity.[104] A study comparing current heavy marijuana users with former users and controls found cognitive impairment in heavy users at days 1 and 7 of abstinence, but by day 28 there were no differences between groups.[105]

Long-term marijuana users (mean 24 years) were significantly impaired on tests of attention and memory compared to short-term marijuana users (mean 10 years); testing followed at least 12 hours of abstinence, and the results were not affected by how recently the subjects had last used marijuana.[106] A potential confounder in that study is that nearly half of the long-term users also used ethanol or other drugs. A similar study found impaired visual scanning in adults who began marijuana use before age 15 but not in those who began use after age 15.[107] A study of adolescents and adults matched for age and IQ found a negative effect of heavy marijuana use on executive functioning and psychomotor speed; testing followed at least 28 days of abstinence, and subjects who used ethanol or other drugs or who had other psychiatric disorders were excluded.[108] This study, compared to others, provides the most convincing evidence that heavy marijuana use has long-term adverse effects on cognition.[109]

In rodents, Δ-9-THC caused impaired memory and learning that persisted after several months of abstinence.[110] Both Δ-9-THC and a synthetic CB1 receptor agonist caused morphological changes in the hippocampus.[111] Studies of Δ-9-THC effects on CB1 receptors have been inconsistent.[112]

Marijuana, Schizophrenia, and Depression

Marijuana use is common among patients with schizophrenia or depression; whether psychiatric disturbance is the cause of the drug use, or vice versa, is disputed.[113] Some studies found marijuana to be a risk factor for

319

depression among users with no depressive symptoms before use.[114–116] Marijuana use can aggravate symptoms in schizophrenia or trigger relapse, and some longitudinal studies of psychosis-free subjects found marijuana use to be a risk factor for development of schizophrenia.[117–119] On the other hand, schizophrenic subjects often use marijuana to counter distressing symptoms. It is more likely that marijuana use precipitates depressive or schizophrenic symptoms among vulnerable individuals than that it causes these disorders.[120]

Fetal Effects

Marijuana smoking during pregnancy is associated with decreased birth length and weight.[121] It is unclear whether the mechanism is direct toxicity or related to noncannabinoid effects, such as ventilation–perfusion abnormalities.[122] It is also unclear whether neurobehavioral abnormalities accompany these changes. One study described abnormal behavior in the first few weeks of life.[123] Another described normal behavior at 1 and 2 years of age but impaired learning and memory and impulsivity at 4 years.[124] A literature review concluded that in utero marijuana exposure resulted in impaired executive function, including attention and hypothesis testing.[125]

In a rodent study, maternal cannabis exposure was associated with abnormal neurodevelopment affecting nigrostriatal and mesolimbic dopaminergic neurons.[126] Several behavioral studies with animals using pair-fed controls and surrogate fostering failed to demonstrate long-term adverse effects of fetal marijuana exposure on learning or behavior.[127]

PHENCYCLIDINE

Arylcyclohexylamine compounds such as phencyclidine (PCP, "angel dust") are called "dissociative anesthetics" because of their electroencephalographic effects in animal models.[1] PCPs effects on neurotransmitter systems include binding to σ-receptors and blocking N-methyl-d-aspartate (NMDA) glutamate receptors.[128] Taken recreationally, PCP can be eaten, snorted, or injected, but it is most often smoked, and most users take additional drugs, especially marijuana, cocaine, and ethanol. The pharmacologically related anesthetic ketamine is also used recreationally.[129]

The desired effect of PCP is euphoria, but dysphoria and paranoia are common even with low doses. With increasing dosage there is subjective time-slowing, decreased sensory perception, altered body image, amnesia, agitation, analgesia, synesthesias, tachycardia, hypertension, sweating, ataxia, psychosis, hallucinations, dystonia, myoclonus, seizures, rhabdomyolysis, stupor or coma, respiratory depression, and shock.[130] A useful diagnostic sign is burstlike nystagmus. Fever may progress to malignant

hyperthermia. Analgesia can cause painless self-injury, and death is often the result of violence, including homicide, suicide, and accidents. Treatment of PCP overdose includes a calm environment, restraints for violent patients, forced diuresis, cooling, blood pressure control, anticonvulsants (although seizures are uncommon), and titered sedation with a benzodiazepine.[131] Neuroleptics should be avoided; they can lower seizure threshold, potentiate hypotension, aggravate dystonia, cause a neuroleptic malignant syndrome with myoglobinuria, and through their anticholinergic effects, aggravate psychosis or delirium.

PCP users infrequently experience withdrawal symptoms; some describe nervousness and tremor. Drug craving is common, however, and PCP is reinforcing in animals.[132]

Neurotoxicity

Phencyclidine and Schizophrenia

Whereas cocaine and amphetamine-like psychostimulants reproduce "positive" symptoms of schizophrenia (paranoia, agitation, delusions, hallucinations) but not "negative" symptoms (alogia, affective flattening, impaired attention, avolition), PCP produces the full spectrum of schizophrenia.[133] Volunteers receiving PCP displayed negativism, withdrawal, autism, bizarre responses to proverb interpretation and projective testing, impoverished speech and thinking, and catatonic posturing. Schizophrenic patients and PCP-intoxicated subjects—but not amphetamine-intoxicated subjects—have decreased frontal lobe metabolism. In rodents, PCP decreases dopaminergic neurotransmission in the prefrontal cortex and increases dopaminergic neurotransmission in mesolimbic circuits, similar to what is found in schizophrenia.[134] The mechanism of PCPs psychotomimetic properties is uncertain and might involve its ability to bind to σ-receptors rather than to its action at NDMA receptors.[128] Also unclear is whether chronic PCP use can cause persistent behavioral or cognitive abnormalities. As with other drugs, causality is difficult to establish. Preexisting schizophrenia might be aggravated by PCP exposure, but some subjects who were apparently normal before drug use reportedly developed long-lasting flattened affect, depersonalization, disordered thinking, and impaired memory.[135]

In rats, PCP and related compounds cause neuronal vacuolization in the cingulate gyrus and retrosplenial cortex. Effects are dose related and with low doses are reversible, but high doses cause irreversible neuronal necrosis.[136]

Fetal Effects

Infants exposed prenatally to PCP had abnormal behavior and irregular respirations during sleep, as well as anomalies of the heart, lungs, urinary and skeletal systems, cerebellum, corpus callosum, and optic chiasm.[137–139] As with other drugs, lack of prenatal care or additional substance abuse could confound the findings, but one study did adjust for such variables and found abnormalities of attention, tendon reflexes, and grasp and root reflexes.[140] A study of 12 prenatally exposed infants at 18 months of age found impaired language, behavior, and fine motor coordination.[141] Another study of 9 exposed infants found normal psychomotor development at 2 years of age.[142]

Animals prenatally exposed to PCP or ketamine have abnormal electroencephalographic activity, monoamine metabolism, hippocampal physiology, spatial learning, brain and body weight, myelination, dopamine receptor sensitivity, synaptic pruning, thalamic morphology, and neuronal migration.[143,144]

HALLUCINOGENS

In low doses, hallucinogenic compounds alter perception, thought, or mood while preserving alertness, attentiveness, memory, and orientation. Also known as psychedelics, most are indole-containing ergot derivatives. In North America, the agents most often used recreationally are mescaline (from peyote cactus), psilocin and psilocybin (from certain mushroom species), and the synthetic compound d-lysergic acid diethylamide (LSD).[1] Hallucinogenic effects appear to depend on binding to serotonin 5-hydroxytryptamine (5-HT$_2$) receptors.[145]

Taken orally, these agents produce similar effects, namely, perceptual (distortions, hallucinations), psychological (altered mood, depersonalization), and somatic (dizziness, paresthesias, tremor).[146] Visual illusions (micropsia, macropsia, altered body image, prolonged after image, synesthesia) progress to hallucinations, which can be formed and elaborately beautiful or grotesque. There is subjective time-slowing, derealization, and memory intrusion; trivial objects may seem profoundly significant. Adverse reactions, consisting of depression, paranoia, or panic, can lead to homicide, self-injury, or suicide.[147] Such symptoms can often be managed nonpharmacologically with calm reassurance; benzodiazepines may be used for agitation. Very high doses of LSD cause hypertension, respiratory depression, coma, and seizures, and hyperactivity during intoxication can produce severe hyperthermia.[148]

Flashbacks consist of spontaneous paroxysmal recurrence of symptoms without taking the drug; they tend to decrease in frequency over months.[149] "Posthallucinogen perceptual disorder" refers to visual disturbances that are continuous and last many years.[150]

Reports of chromosomal aberrations in leukocytes of LSD-users were not borne out in subsequent studies.[151] Anecdotal reports describe deformities in infants prenatally exposed to LSD[152,153] and LSD is teratogenic in animals.[154]

Animals do not self-administer mescaline, psilocybin, or LSD, and these agents do not appear to produce either physical or psychic dependence.

Controversial are anecdotal reports of permanent mental change in LSD users, including paranoia, depression, psychosis, impaired memory, passivity, and tangential thinking.[150] As with other drugs, causality is difficult to establish. The weight of evidence is against long-term cognitive or behavioral impairment.

INHALANTS

Various household and industrial products are inhaled recreationally for their intoxicating effects (Table 2).[155,156] Users are often children. Desired effects resemble ethanol intoxication, with relaxed euphoria, ataxia, diplopia, and slurred speech but sometimes impulsivity and violence. Higher doses cause toxic psychosis, sometimes with formed hallucinations, and there may be progression to coma and seizures. Death can be the result of vomiting and aspiration, suffocation by plastic bags containing the substance, accidents, violence, or cardiac arrhythmia.[157] Symptoms are short lived and, in the absence of cardiorespiratory complications, seldom require specific treatment.

Abrupt discontinuation in chronic users can produce mild symptoms resembling ethanol withdrawal. Psychic dependence (i.e., addiction) is common.

Neurotoxicity

Toluene

Chronic toluene exposure causes various persistent neurological symptoms and signs, especially cognitive impairment and cerebellar ataxia. Also reported are pyramidal signs and cranial neuropathies, including oculomotor disturbance, anosmia, sensorineural deafness, and optic atrophy.[158] Autopsies show cerebral and cerebellar atrophy, degeneration of white matter tracts, and histopathological findings similar to these found in adrenoleukodystrophy.[159] Toluene probably does not cause peripheral neuropathy.[160]

n-Hexane

Severe peripheral neuropathy affects sniffers of glues and lacquer thinners containing n-hexane.[161] Paresthesias and weakness in distal limbs progress to quadriplegia over a few weeks. Nerve biopsy reveals segmental distention of axons by masses of neurofilaments and secondary demyelination. Incomplete improvement occurs with abstinence, and the emergence of spasticity with recovery suggests CNS damage initially masked by the neuropathy. Responsible toxins are n-hexane and its metabolite 2,5-hexanedione.[162]

Table 2: Abused Inhalants and Their Contents

Products	Contents
Aerosols (refrigerants, cleaners, hair sprays, deodorants, antiseptics)	Aliphatic and halogenated hydrocarbons
Dry-cleaning fluids, furniture polish	Halogenated hydrocarbons, naphtha
Glues, cements	Toluene, acetone, benzene, xylene, n-hexane, trichloroethylene, butyl alcohol, methylethylketone, chloroform, triorthocesyl phosphate, ethanol
Paints, lacquers, paint and lacquer thinners	Toluene, methylene chloride, aliphatic acetates, ethanol
Lighter fluid	Aliphatic and aromatic hydrocarbons
Fire-extinguishing agents	Halogenated hydrocarbons
Nail-polish remover	Acetone, aliphatic acetates, benzene
Typewriter correction fluid	Trichloroethane, trichloroethylene
Marker pens	Toluene, xylene
Bottled fuel gas, natural gas	Butane, propane, methane, ethane
Mothballs	Naphthalene, paradichlorobenzene
Petroleum	Aromatic and aliphatic hydrocarbons, tetraethyl lead
Anesthetics	Nitrous oxide, diethyl ether, halothane, enflurane, trichloroethylene
Room odorizers	Amyl, butyl, and isobutyl nitrite

Nitrous Oxide

Sniffers of nitrous oxide, often obtained from whipped cream cartridges, develop myeloneuropathy that resembles combined systems disease secondary to cobalamin deficiency.[163] There are varying combinations of peripheral neuropathy, myelopathy, and altered mentation, but anemia is not a feature, and serum vitamin B_{12} levels are usually normal.[164] Nitrous oxide oxidizes cobalamin, inactivating the vitamin B_{12}–dependent enzymes methionine synthetase and methylmalonyl-CoA mutase. Treatment is with cyanocobalamin.

Nitrites

Amyl, butyl, and isobutyl nitrite, commercially available as room odorizers, are often taken with ethanol, marijuana, or sedatives. The euphoric high lasts only seconds to minutes, and cerebral vasodilation often causes increased intracranial pressure and headache.

Nitrite-induced methemoglobinemia causes tachycardia, dyspnea, lethargy, stupor, seizures, cardiac arrhythmia, hypotension, and sometimes death, even when treated with methylene blue.[165]

Gasoline

In addition to neurotoxic toluene, some gasolines contain lead, and anecdotal reports describe encephalopathy with altered mentation, chorea, and seizures, as well as peripheral neuropathy and myopathy.[166,167]

Trichloroethylene

Present in dry-cleaning fluids, trichloroethylene causes trigeminal neuropathy.[168]

Mothballs

Mothballs containing naphthalene cause headache, lethargy, vomiting, hemolysis, hyperkalemia, fever, hepatic and renal failure, seizures, and coma.[169]

Effects in Pregnancy

Animal studies demonstrate that some inhalants, especially toluene and trichloroethane, are teratogenic.[170] In humans an alleged "fetal solvent syndrome" includes microcephaly, craniofacial anomalies, and growth retardation. Case–control and cohort studies are inconsistent, however: some describe increased risk for CNS anomalies, and some do not. Children exposed in utero to toluene had delayed growth and development, including cognition, speech, and motor skills.[171,172]

SEDATIVES AND HYPNOTICS

Sedative and hypnotic agents include numerous barbiturates, benzodiazepines, and miscellaneous drugs, such as ethchlorvynol, methaqualone, and zolpidem (Table 3). They are often taken recreationally, although the abuse liability of barbiturates is considerably greater than that of benzodiazepines.[173] Barbiturates and benzodiazepines act in different ways at GABA receptors.[174] Barbiturate overdose causes coma and respiratory depression, and withdrawal resembles what is seen with ethanol, including seizures and delirium tremens. Benzodiazepine intoxication and withdrawal are milder; respiratory depression is unusual unless another agent (e.g., ethanol)

Table 3:	Sedatives or Hypnotics
Barbiturates (e.g., phenobarbital, amobarbital, pentobarbital, secobarbital)	
Benzodiazepines (e.g., alprazolam, diazepam, chlordiazepoxide, lorazepam, oxazepam, triazolam)	
Nonbarbiturate, nonbenzodiazepine agents	
Ethchlorvynol	
Glutethimide	
Hydroxyzine	
Meprobamate	
Methaqualone	
Zolpidem	
Zaleplon	
γ-Hydroxybutyric acid, γ-butyrolactone, 1,4-butanediol	

is taken,[175] but withdrawal seizures are not unusual following abrupt discontinuation.[176]

Certain sedative drugs have particular neurotoxicities. Methaqualone (banned in the United States and often combined with an antihistamine) reportedly causes delirium, hallucinations, myoclonus, and seizures in overdose.[177] Glutethimide (as a street drug often combined with codeine) produces anticholinergic signs, including fever and dilated unreactive pupils.[178,179] Ethchlorvynol, glutethimide, and methaqualone reportedly cause peripheral neuropathy.[180–182]

A special class of sedative includes γ-hydroxybutyric acid (GHB) and its precursors γ-butyrolactone and 1,4-butanediol.[183–186] GHB binds not only to GABA receptors but also to its own receptors in the brain. Notorious as a "date rape" drug, GHB is often taken with ethanol. Low doses produce euphoria and drowsiness, but higher doses can result in agitation, hallucinations, tremor, myoclonus, seizures, coma, respiratory depression, bradycardia, and hypotension. Treatment is supportive and may include benzodiazepines for seizures. GHB withdrawal resembles that of ethanol, and when ethanol has also been taken symptoms can be severe and protracted. Animals self-administer GHB, and human addiction occurs.

Neurotoxicity

Cognitive Impairment

Chronic barbiturate abuse is anecdotally associated with psychological and social deterioration, but as with other drugs neurotoxic effects on cognition and behavior are difficult to establish. Unlike ethanol, barbiturates do not appear to cause brain shrinkage.[187] Neuropsychological deficits described in subjects abstinent after chronic benzodiazepine use are difficult to separate from the effects of the resulting anxiety.[188,189] Other studies found no significant cognitive morbidity associated with long-term benzodiazepine use.[190] Data are lacking on long-term cognitive and behavioral effects of other sedatives and hypnotics.

Fetal Effects

Detrimental effects on IQ are described in adults exposed in utero to barbiturates, as well as in children taking barbiturates for febrile seizures.[191,192] Animal studies of fetal exposure describe impaired brain growth and learning, as well as morphological abnormalities of neurons in the cerebellum, hippocampus, and cerebral cortex.[193,194]

A report from Sweden described dysmorphism and mental retardation resembling fetal alcohol syndrome in children exposed in utero to benzodiazepines.[195] The observation awaits confirmation by further studies in humans and animals.

Data are lacking as to the effects of fetal exposure on other sedative or hypnotic agents.

REFERENCES

1. Brust JCM. *Neurological Aspects of Substance Abuse, 2e.* Boston: Butterworth-Heinemann; 2004.

2. Cami J, Farre M. Drug addiction. *N Engl J Med.* 2003;349:975–986.

3. Kosten TR, O'Connor PG. Management of drug and ethanol withdrawal. *N Engl J Med.* 2003;348:1786–1795.

4. Law P-Y, Wong YH, Loh HH. Molecular mechanisms and regulation of opioid receptor signaling. *Annu Rev Pharmacol Toxicol.* 2000;40:389–430.

5. Nelson LS. Opioids. In: Goldfrank LR, Flomenbaum NE, Lewin NA, et al., eds. *Goldfrank's Toxicologic Emergencies.* 6th ed. Stamford, Conn: Appleton & Lange; 1998:975.

6. Sporer KA. Acute heroin overdose. *Ann Intern Med.* 1999;130:584–590.

7. Hamid A. The heroin epidemic in New York City: current status and prognosis. *J Psychoactive Drugs.* 1977;29:375.

8. Osborn DA, Jeffrey HE, Cole MJ. Sedatives for opiate withdrawal in newborn infants. *Cochrane Database Syst Rev.* 2002;(3): CD002053.

9. Specka M, Finkbeiner T, Lodemann E, et al. Cognitive–motor performance of methadone-maintained patients. *Eur Addict Res.* 2000;6:8–19.

10. Brust JCM, Richter RW. Stroke associated with addiction to heroin. *J Neurol Neurosurg Psychiatry.* 1976;39:194.

11. Brust JCM. Stroke and substance abuse. In: Mohr JP, Choi DW, Grotta JC, et al., eds. *Stroke: Pathophysiology, Diagnosis, and Management.* 4th ed. Philadelphia: Churchill Livingstone; 2004:725–745.

12. Celius EG. Neurologic complications of substance abuse: illustrated by two unusual cases. *Tidsskr Nor Laegeforen.* 1997;117:356–357.

13. Caplan LR, Thomas C, Banks G. Central nervous system complications of addiction to "T's and blues." *Neurology.* 1982;32:623–628.

14. McCreary M, Emerman C, Hanna J, Simon J. Acute myelopathy following intranasal insufflation of heroin: case report. *Neurology.* 2000;55:316–317.

15. Dabby R, Djaldetti R, Gilad R, et al. Acute heroin-related neuropathy. *J Periph Nerv Syst.* 2006;11:304–309.

16. Richards JR. Rhabdomyolysis and drugs of abuse. *Am J Emerg Med.* 2000;19:51–56.

17. Rice EK, Isbel NM, Becker GJ, et al. Heroin overdose and myoglobinuric acute renal failure. *Clin Nephrol.* 2000;54:449–454.

18. Brust JCM, Richter RW. Quinine amblyopia related to heroin addiction. *Ann Intern Med.* 1971;74:84–88.

19. Wolters EC, Van Winjungaarden GK, Stam FC, et al. Leukoencephalopathy after inhaling "heroin pyrolysate." *Lancet.* 1982;2:1233–1237.

20. Kriegstein AR, Shungu DC, Millar WS, et al. Leukoencephalopathy and raised brain lactate from heroin vapor inhalation ("chasing the dragon"). *Neurology.* 1999;53:1765–1773.

21. Stern Y. MPTP-induced parkinsonism. *Prog Neurobiol.* 1990;34:107–114.

22. Przedborski S, Vila M. MPTP: a review of its mechanisms of neurotoxicity. *Clin Neurosci Res.* 2002;1:407–410.

23. Ng SKC, Brust JCM, Hauser WA, et al. Illicit drug use and the risk of new onset seizures: contrasting effects of heroin, marijuana, and cocaine. *Am J Epidemiol.* 1990;40:47–57.

24. Hershey LA. Meperidine and central neurotoxicity. *Ann Intern Med.* 1983;98:548–549.

25. Choucair AK, Ziter FA. Pentazocine abuse masquerading as familial myopathy. *Neurology.* 1984;34:524–527.

26. Finnegan LP. The effects of narcotics and alcohol on pregnancy and the newborn. *Ann NY Acad Sci.* 1981;362:136–157.

27. Peterson DR. SIDS in infants of drug-dependent mothers. *J Pediatr.* 1980;96:784–785.

28. Malanga CJ, Kosofsky BE. Mechanisms of action of drugs of abuse on the developing fetal brain. *Clin Perinatol.* 1999;26:17–37.

29. Nassaogne MC, Gressens P, Evrard P, et al. In contrast to cocaine, prenatal exposure to methadone does not produce detectable alterations in the developing mouse brain. *Brain Res Dev Brain Res.* 1998;110:61–67.

30. Steingart RA, Abu-Roumi M, Newman ME, et al. Neurobehavioral damage to cholinergic systems caused by prenatal exposure to heroin or phenobarbital: cellular mechanisms and the reversal of deficits by neural grafts. *Brain Res Dev Brain Res.* 2000;122:125–133.

31. Wilson GS, Desmond MM, Verniaud WM. Early development of infants of heroin-addicted mothers. *Am J Dis Child.* 1973;126:457–462.

32. Maynard EC. Maternal abuse of cocaine and heroin. *Am J Dis Child.* 1990;144:520–521.

33. Eyler FD, Behnke M, Conlon M, et al. Birth outcomes from a prospective, matched study of prenatal crack/cocaine use: II. Interactive and dose effects on neurobehavioral assessment. *Pediatrics.* 1998;101:237–241.

34. Lester BM, Lagasse L, Seifer R, et al. The Maternal Lifestyle Study (MLS): effects of prenatal cocaine or opiate exposure on auditory brain response at one month. *J Pediatr.* 2003;142:279–285.

35. Lakoski JM, Cunningham KA. Cocaine interaction with central monoaminergic systems: electrophysiological approaches. *Trends Pharmacol Sci.* 1988;9:177–180.

36. Gawin FH. Cocaine addiction: psychology and neurophysiology. *Science.* 1991;251:1580–1586.

37. Bartzokis G, Beckson M, Wirshing DA, et al. Choreoathetoid movements in cocaine dependence. *Biol Psychiatry.* 1999;45:1630–1635.

38. Brower KJ, Blow FC, Beresford TP. Forms of cocaine and psychiatric symptoms. *Lancet.* 1988;1:50.

39. Goldfrank LR, Hoffman RS. The cardiovascular effects of cocaine. *Ann Emerg Med.* 1991;20:165–175.

40. Campbell BG. Cocaine abuse with hyperthermia, seizures and fatal complications. *Med J Aust.* 1988;149:387–389.

41. Hollander JE, Hoffman RS. Cocaine. In: Goldfrank LR, Flomenbaum NE, Lewin NA, et al., eds. *Goldfrank's Toxicologic Emergencies.* 6th ed, Stamford, Conn: Appleton & Lange; 1998:1071–1089.

42. Randall T. Cocaine, alcohol mix in body to form even longer-lasting, more lethal drug. *JAMA.* 1992;267:1043–1044.

43. Uslaner J, Kalechstein A, Richter T, et al. Association of depressive symptoms during abstinence with the subjective high produced by cocaine. *Am J Psychiatry.* 1999;156:1444–1446.

44. Bozarth MA, Wise RA. Toxicity associated with long-term intravenous heroin and cocaine self-administration in the rat. *JAMA.* 1985;254:81–83.

45. Karch SB, Billingham ME. The pathology and etiology of cocaine-induced heart disease. *Arch Pathol Lab Med.* 1988;112:225–230.

46. Petty GW, Brust JCM, Tatemichi TK, et al. Embolic stroke after smoking "crack" cocaine. *Stroke.* 1990;21:1632–1635.

47. Levine SR, Brust JCM, Futrell N, et al. Cerebrovascular complications of the use of the "crack" form of alkaloidal cocaine. *N Engl J Med.* 1990;323:699–704.

48. Merkel PA, Koroshetz WJ, Irizarry MC, et al. Cocaine-associated cerebral vasculitis. *Semin Arthritis Rheum.* 1995;25: 172–183.

49. Kaufman MJ, Levin JM, Ross MH, et al. Cocaine-induced cerebral vasoconstriction detected in humans with magnetic resonance angiography. *JAMA*. 1998;279:376–380.

50. Powers RH, Madden JA. Vasoconstrictive effects of cocaine, metabolites and structural analogs on cat cerebral arteries. *FASEB*. 1990;4:A1095.

51. Wilpert-Lampen U, Seliger C, Zilker T, et al. Cocaine increases the endothelial release of immunoreactive endothelin and its concentration in human plasma and urine: reversal by coincubation with α-receptor antagonists. *Circulation*. 1998;98:385–390.

52. Nolte KB, Brass LM, Fletterick CF. Intracranial hemorrhage associated with cocaine abuse: a prospective autopsy study. *Neurology*. 1996;46:1291–1296.

53. Winberg S, Blaho K, Logan B, et al. Multiple cocaine-induced seizures and corresponding cocaine and metabolite concentrations. *Am J Emerg Med*. 1998;16:529–533.

54. Miller KA, Witkin JM, Ungared JT, et al. Pharmacological and behavioral characterization of cocaine-kindled seizures in mice. *Psychopharmacology*. 2000;148:78–82.

55. Choy-Kwong M, Lipton RB. Seizures in hospitalized cocaine users. *Neurology*. 1989;39:425–427.

56. Schwartz RH, Luxenberg MG, Hoffman NG. "Crack" use by American middle-class adolescent polydrug abusers. *J Pediatr*. 1991;118:150–155.

57. Weiner WJ, Rabinstein A, Levin B, et al. Cocaine-induced persistent dyskinesias. *Neurology*. 2001;56:964–965.

58. Richards JR. Rhabdomyolysis and drugs of abuse. *J Emerg Med*. 2000;19:51–56.

59. Davidson C, Gow AJ, Lee TH, et al. Methamphetamine neurotoxicity: necrotic and apoptotic mechanisms and relevance to human abuse and treatment. *Brain Res Rev*. 2001;36:1–22.

60. Seiden LS, Kleven MS. Lack of toxic effects of cocaine on dopamine or serotonin neurons in the rat brain. *NIDA Res Monogr*. 1988;88:276–289.

61. Smelson DA, Roy A, Santana S, et al. Neuropsychological deficits in withdrawn cocaine-dependent males. *Am J Drug Alcohol Abuse*. 1999;25:377–381.

62. Bolla KI, Rothman R, Cadet JL. Dose-related neurobehavioral effects of chronic cocaine use. *J Neuropsychiatry Clin Neurosci*. 1999;11:361–369.

63. Hoff AL, Riordan H, Morris L, et al. Effects of crack cocaine on neurocognitive function. *Psychiatry Res*. 1996;60:167–176.

64. Van Gorp WG, Wilkins JN, Hinkin CH, et al. Declarative and procedural memory functioning in abstinent cocaine abusers. *Arch Gen Psychiatry*. 1999;56:85–89.

65. Bolla KI, Funderburk FR, Cadet JL. Differential effects of cocaine and cocaine plus alcohol on neurocognitive performance. *Neurology*. 2000;54:2285–2292.

66. McLellan AT, Woody GE, O'Brien CP. Development of psychiatric disorders in drug abusers. *N Engl J Med*. 1979;301:1310–1313.

67. Langendorf FG, Tupper DE, Rottenberg DA, et al. Does chronic cocaine exposure cause brain atrophy? A qualitative MRI study. *Neurology*. 2000;54 (Suppl 3):A442–A443.

68. Bartzokis G, Beckson M, Lu PH, et al. Age-related brain volume reductions in amphetamine and cocaine addicts and normal controls: implications for addiction research. *Psychiatry Res*. 2000;98:93–102.

69. Bartzokis G, Beckson M, Hance DB, et al. Magnetic resonance imaging evidence of "silent" cerebrovascular toxicity in cocaine dependence. *Biol Psychiatry*. 1999;45:1203–1211.

70. Volkow ND, Hitzemann R, Wang G-J, et al. Long-term frontal metabolic changes in cocaine abusers. *Synapse*. 1992;11:184–190.

71. Tumeh SS, Nagel JS, English RJ, et al. Cerebral abnormalities in cocaine abusers: demonstration by SPECT perfusion brain scintigraphy. *Radiology*. 1990;176:821–824.

72. Holman BL, Carvalho PA, Mendelson J, et al. Brain perfusion is abnormal in cocaine-dependent polydrug users: a study using technetium-99m–HMPAO and ASPECT. *J Nucl Med*. 1991;32:1206–1210.

73. Li S-J, Wang Y, Pankiewicz J, et al. Neurochemical adaptation to cocaine abuse: reduction of *N*-acetyl aspartate in thalamus of human cocaine abusers. *Biol Psychiatry*. 1999;45:1481–1487.

74. Kosten TR. Pharmacotherapy of cerebral ischemia in cocaine dependence. *Drug Alcohol Dep*. 1998;49:133–144.

75. Storen EC, Wijdicks EFM, Crum BA, et al. Moyamoya-like vasculopathy from cocaine dependency. *Am J Neuroradiol*. 2000;21:1008–1010.

76. Ryan L, Ehrlich S, Finnegan L. Cocaine abuse in pregnancy: effects on the fetus and newborn. *Neurotoxicol Teratol*. 1987;9:295–299.

77. Bandstra ES, Morrow CE, Anthony JC, et al. Intrauterine growth of full-term infants: impact of prenatal cocaine exposure. *Pediatrics*. 2001;108:1309–1319.

78. Eyler FD, Behnke M, Conlon M, et al. Birth outcomes from a prospective, matched study of prenatal crack/cocaine use: I. Interactive and dose effects on health and growth. *Pediatrics*. 1998;101:229–237.

79. Eyler FD, Behnke M, Conlon M, et al. Birth outcomes from a prospective, matched study of prenatal crack/cocaine use: II. Interactive and dose effects on neurobehavioral assessment. *Pediatrics*. 1998;101:237–241.

80. Scher MS, Richardson GA, Day NL. Effects of prenatal cocaine/crack and other drug exposure on electroencephalographic sleep studies at birth and one year. *Pediatrics*. 2000;105:39–48.

81. Hoyme HE, Jones KL, Dixon SD, et al. Prenatal cocaine exposure and fetal vascular disruption. *Pediatrics*. 1990;85:743–747.

82. Chiriboga CA, Vibbert M, Malouf R, et al. Neurological correlates of fetal cocaine exposures: transient hypertonia of infancy and early childhood. *Pediatrics*. 1995;96:1070–1077.

83. Dempsey DA, Hajnal BL, Partridge JC, et al. Tone abnormalities are associated with maternal cigarette smoking during pregnancy in in utero cocaine-exposed infants. *Pediatrics*. 2000;106:79–85.

84. Frank DA, Augustyn M, Knight WG, et al. Growth, development, and behavior in early childhood following prenatal cocaine exposure: a systematic review. *JAMA*. 2001;285:1613–1625.

85. Hurt H, Malmed E, Betancourt L, et al. Children with in utero cocaine exposure do not differ from control subjects on intelligence testing. *Arch Pediatr Adolesc Med*. 1997;151:1237–1241.

86. Richardson GA, Coroy ML, Day NL. Prenatal cocaine exposure: effects on the development of school-age children. *Neurotoxicol Teratol*. 1996;18:627–634.

87. Wasserman GA, Kline JK, Bateman DA, et al. Prenatal cocaine exposure and school-age intelligence. *Drug Alcohol Dep*. 1998;50:203–210.

88. Warner TD, Behnke M, Eyler FD, et al. Diffusion tensor imaging of frontal white matter and executive functioning in cocaine-exposed children. *Pediatrics*. 2006;118:2014–2024.

89. Wilkins AS, Genova LM, Posten W, et al. Transplacental cocaine exposure: I. A rodent model. *Neurotoxicol Teratol*. 1998;20:215–226.

90. Hecht GS, Spear NE, Spear LP. Alterations in the reinforcing efficacy of cocaine in adult rats following prenatal exposure to cocaine. *Behav Neurosci*. 1998;112:410–418.

91. Church MW, Crossland WJ, Holmes PA, et al. Effects of prenatal cocaine on hearing, vision, growth, and behavior. *Ann NY Acad Sci*. 1998;846:12–28.

92. Mactutus CF. Prenatal intravenous cocaine adversely affects attentional processing in preweanling rats. *Neurotoxicol Teratol*. 1999;21:539–550.

93. Snyder-Keller A, Sam C, Keller RW. Enhanced susceptibility to cocaine and pentylenetetrazol-induced seizures in prenatally cocaine-treated rats. *Neurotoxicol Teratol.* 2000;22:231–236.

94. Iso A, Nakahara K, Barr GA, et al. Long-term intravenous perinatal cocaine exposure on the mortality of rat offspring. *Neurotoxicol Teratol.* 2000;22:165–173.

95. Baraban SL, Wenzel HJ, Castro PA, et al. Hippocampal dysplasia in rats exposed to cocaine in utero. *Brain Res Dev Brain Res.* 1999;117:213–217.

96. Murphy A, Ghazi I, Kokabi A, et al. Prenatal cocaine produces signs of neurodegeneration in the lateral habenula. *Brain Res.* 1999;851:175–182.

97. Morgan MA, Silavin SL, Randolf M, et al. Effect of intravenous cocaine on uterine blood flow in the gravid baboon. *Am J Obstet Gynecol.* 1991;164:1021–1027.

98. Iverson L. Cannabis and the brain. *Brain.* 2003;126:1252–1270.

99. Wilson RI, Nicoll RA. Endocannabinoid signaling in the brain. *Science.* 2002;296:678–682.

100. Otten EJ. Marijuana. In: Goldfrank LR, Flomenbaum NE, Lewin NA, et al., eds. *Goldfrank's Toxicologic Emergencies.* 6th ed. Stamford, Conn: Appleton & Lange; 1998:1121–1126.

101. Pope HG, Gruber AJ, Yurgelun-Todd D. The residual neuropsychological effects of cannabis: the current status of research. *Drug Alcohol Dep.* 1995;38:25–34.

102. Fletcher JM, Page JB, Francis DJ, et al. Cognitive correlates of long-term cannabis use in Costa Rican men. *Arch Gen Psychiatry.* 1996;53:1051–1057.

103. Lyketsos CG, Garrett E, Liang K-Y, et al. Cannabis use and cognitive decline in persons under 65 years of age. *Am J Epidemiol.* 1999;149:794–800.

104. Pope HG, Yurgelun-Todd D. The residual cognitive effects of heavy marijuana use in college students. *JAMA.* 1996;275:521–527.

105. Pope HG, Gruber AJ, Hudson JL, et al. Neuropsychological performance in long-term cannabis users. *Arch Gen Psychiatry.* 2001;275:909–915.

106. Solowij N, Stephens RS, Hoffman RA, et al. Cognitive functioning of long-term heavy cannabis users seeking treatment. *JAMA.* 2002;287:1123–1131.

107. Ehrenreich H, Rinn T, Kunert JH, et al. Specific attentional dysfunction in adults following early start of cannabis use. *Psychopharmacology.* 1999;142:205–301.

108. Bolla KI, Brown K, Eldreth D, et al. Dose-related neurocognitive effects of marijuana use. *Neurology.* 2002;59:1337–1343.

109. Koppel BS. Heavy marijuana use: the price of getting high. *Neurology.* 2002;59:1295.

110. Presberger G, Robinson JK. Spatial signal detection in rats is differentially disrupted by δ-9-tetrahydrocannabinol, scopolamine, and MK-801. *Behav Brain Res.* 1999;99:27–34.

111. Lawston J, Borella A, Robinson JK, et al. Changes in hippocampal morphology following chronic treatment with the synthetic cannabinoid WIN55, 212-2. *Brain Res.* 2000;877:407–410.

112. Varvel SA, Hamm RJ, Martin BR, et al. Differential effects of Δ-9-THC on spatial reference and working memory in mice. *Psychopharmacology.* 2001;157:147–150.

113. Johns A. Psychiatric effects of cannabis. *Br J Psychiatry.* 2001;178:116–122.

114. Bovasso GB. Cannabis abuse as a risk factor for depressive symptoms. *Am J Psychiatry.* 2001;158:2033–2037.

115. Brook DW, Brook JS, Zhang C, et al. Drug use and the risk of major depressive disorder, alcohol dependence, and substance use disorders. *Arch Gen Psychiatry.* 2002;59:1039–1044.

116. Patton GC, Caffey C, Carlin JB, et al. Cannabis use and mental health in young people: cohort study. *BMJ.* 2002;325:1195–1198.

117. Verdoux H, Gindre C, Sorbara F, et al. Effects of cannabis and psychosis vulnerability in daily life: an experience sampling test study. *Psychol Med.* 2003;33:23–32.

118. Fergusson DM, Harwood LJ, Swain-Campbell NR. Cannabis dependence and psychotic symptoms in young people. *Psychol Med.* 2003;33:15–21.

119. Roy JM, Tennant CC. Cannabis and mental health: more evidence establishes clear link between use of cannabis and mental illness. *BMJ.* 2002;325:1183–1184.

120. Degenhardt L, Hall W. Cannabis and psychosis. *Curr Psychiatry Rep.* 2002;4:191–196.

121. Zuckerman B, Frank DA, Hingson R, et al. Effects of marijuana and cocaine use on fetal growth. *N Engl J Med.* 1989;320:762–768.

122. Frank DA, Bauchner H, Parker S, et al. Neonatal body proportionality and body composition after in utero exposure to cocaine and marijuana. *J Pediatr.* 1990;117:622–626.

123. Fried PA, Makin JE. Neonatal behavioral correlates of prenatal exposure to marijuana, cigarettes, and alcohol in a low-risk population. *Neurotoxicol Teratol.* 1987;9:1–7.

124. Fried PA, Watkinson B. 36- and 48-month neurobehavioral follow-up of children prenatally exposed to marijuana, cigarettes, and alcohol. *J Dev Behav Pediatr.* 1990;11:49–58.

125. Fried PA, Smith AM. A literature review of the consequences of prenatal marijuana exposure: an emerging theme of a deficiency in aspects of executive function. *Neurotoxicol Teratol.* 2001;23:1–11.

126. Rodriquez-de-Fonseca F, Cabeira M, Fernandez-Ruiz JJ, et al. Effects of pre- and perinatal exposure to hashish extracts on the ontogeny of brain dopaminergic neurons. *Neuroscience.* 1991;43:713–723.

127. Hutchings DE, Brake SC, Banks AN, et al. Prenatal δ-9-tetrahydrocannabinol in the rat: effects on auditory startle in adulthood. *Neurotoxicol Teratol.* 1991;13:413–416.

128. Steinpreis RE. The behavioral and neurochemical effects of phencyclidine in humans and animals: some implications for modeling psychosis. *Behav Brain Res.* 1996;74:45–55.

129. Jansen KLR. A review of the nonmedical use of ketamine: use, users, and consequences. *J Psychoactive Drugs.* 2000;32:419–433.

130. McCarron MM, Schultze BW, Thompson GA, et al. Acute phencyclidine intoxication: incidence of clinical findings in 1000 cases. *Ann Emerg Med.* 1981;10:237–242.

131. McCarron MM, Schultze BW, Thompson GA, et al. Acute phencyclidine intoxication: clinical patterns, complications, and treatment. *Ann Emerg Med.* 1981;10:290–297.

132. Gorelick DA, Wilkins JN, Wong C. Outpatient treatment of PCP abusers. *Am J Drug Alcohol Abuse.* 1989;15:367–374.

133. Javitt DC, Zukin SR. Recent advances in the phencyclidine model of schizophrenia. *Am J Psychiatry.* 1991;148:1301–1308.

134. Svensson TH. Dysfunctional brain dopamine systems induced by psychotomimetic NMDA-receptor antagonists and the effects of antipsychotic drugs. *Brain Res Brain Rev.* 2000;31:320–329.

135. Ellison G. The N-methyl-D-aspartate antagonists phencyclidine, ketamine, and dizocilpine as both behavioral and anatomical models of the dementias. *Brain Res Brain Rev.* 1995;20:250–267.

136. Allen HL, Iversen LL. Phencyclidine, dizocilpine, and cerebrocortical neurons. *Science.* 1990;247:221.

137. Golden NL, Sokol RJ, Rubin IL. Angel dust: possible effects on the fetus. *Pediatrics.* 1980;65:18–20.

138. Wachsman L, Schuetz S, Chan LS, et al. What happens to babies exposed to phencyclidine (PCP) in utero? *Am J Drug Alcohol Abuse.* 1989;15:31–39.

139. Tabor BL, Smith-Wallace T, Yonekura ML. Perinatal outcome associated with PCP versus cocaine use. *Am J Drug Alcohol Abuse.* 1990;16:337–348.

140. Golden NL, Kuhnert BR, Sokol RJ, et al. Neonatal manifestations of maternal phencyclidine exposure. *J Perinat Med*. 1987;15:185–191.

141. Howard J, Kropenske V, Tyler R. The long-term effects on neurodevelopment in infants exposed prenatally to PCP. *NIDA Res Monogr*. 1986;64:237–251.

142. Chasnoff IJ, Burns KA, Burns WJ, et al. Prenatal drug exposure: effects on neonatal and infant growth and development. *Neurobehav Toxicol Teratol*. 1986;8:357–362.

143. Deutsch SI, Mastropaolo J, Rosse RB. Neurodevelopmental consequences of early exposure to phencyclidine and related drugs. *Clin Neuropharmacol*. 1998;21:320–332.

144. Abdel-Rahman MS, Ismail EE. Teratogenic effect of ketamine and cocaine in CF-1 mice. *Teratology*. 2000;61:291–296.

145. Giesch PJ, Strickland LV, Sanders-Bush E. Lysergic acid diethylamide–induced Fos expression in rat brain: role of serotonin-2A receptors. *Neuroscience*. 2002;114:707–713.

146. Isbell H. Comparison of the reactions produced by psilocybin and LSD-25 in man. *Psychopharmacologia*. 1959;1:29–38.

147. Ungerleider JT, Fisher DD, Fuller M, et al. The "bad trip": the etiology of the adverse LSD reaction. *Am J Psychiatry*. 1968;124:1483–1490.

148. Blaho K, Merigan K, Winberg S, et al. Clinical pharmacology of lysergic acid diethylamide: case reports and review of the treatment of intoxication. *Am J Therapeut*. 1997;4:211–221.

149. Abraham HD. Visual phenomenology of the LSD flashback. *Arch Gen Psychiatry*. 1983;40:884–889.

150. Abraham HD, Aldridge AM. Adverse consequences of lysergic acid diethylamide. *Addiction*. 1993;88:1327–1334.

151. Li J H, Lin L F. Genetic toxicology of abused drugs: a brief review. *Mutagenesis*. 1998;13:557–565.

152. Eller JL, Morton JM. Bizarre deformities in offspring of user of lysergic acid diethylamide. *N Engl J Med*. 1970;283:295.

153. Chan CC, Fishman M, Egbert PR. Multiple ocular anomalies associated with maternal LSD ingestion. *Arch Opthalmol*. 1978;96:282–284.

154. Alexander GJ, Miles B, Gold GM, et al. LSD: ingestion early in pregnancy produces abnormalities in offspring in rats. *Science*. 1967;157:459–460.

155. Henretig F. Inhalant abuse in children and adolescents. *Pediatr Ann*. 1996;25:47–52.

156. Brouette T, Anton R. Clinical review of inhalants. *Am J Addict*. 2001;10:79–94.

157. Bowen SE, Daniel J, Balster RL. Deaths associated with inhalant abuse in Virginia from 1987 to 1996. *Drug Alcohol Dep*. 1999;53:239–245.

158. Fornazzari L, Wilkinson D, Kapor B, et al. Cerebellar, cortical and functional impairment in toluene abusers. *Acta Neurol Scand*. 1983;67:319–329.

159. Kornfield M, Moser AB, Moser HW, et al. Solvent vapor abuse leukoencephalopathy: comparisons to adrenoleukodystrophy. *J Neuropathol Exp Neurol*. 1994;53:389–398.

160. Hormes JT, Filley CM, Rosenberg NL. Neurologic sequelae of chronic vapor abuse. *Neurology*. 1986;36:698–702.

161. Korobkin R, Asbury AK, Sumner AJ, et al. Glue-sniffing neuropathy. *Arch Neurol*. 1975;32:158–162.

162. Schaumburg H, Spencer P. Degeneration in central and peripheral nervous systems produced by pure n-hexane: an experimental study. *Brain*. 1976;99:183–192.

163. Iwata K, O'Keefe GB, Karanas A. Neurologic problems associated with chronic nitrous oxide abuse in a non-healthcare worker. *Am J Med Sci*. 2001;322:173–174.

164. Heyer EJ, Simpson DM, Bodis-Wollner I, et al. Nitrous oxide: clinical and electrophysiologic investigation of neurologic complications. *Neurology*. 1986;36:1618–1622.

165. Madarai B, Kapadia YK, Kerins M, et al. Methylene blue: a treatment for severe methaemoglobinaemia secondary to misuse of amyl nitrite. *Emerg Med J*. 2002;19:2700–2710.

166. Cairney S, Maruff P, Burns C, et al. The neurobehavioral consequences of petrol (gasoline) sniffing. *Neurosci Biobehav Rev*. 2002;26:81–89.

167. Valpey R, Sumi S, Copass MK, et al. Acute and chronic progressive encephalopathy due to gasoline sniffing. *Neurology*. 1978;28:507–510.

168. Mitchell ABS, Parsons-Smith BG. Trichloroethylene neuropathy. *BMJ*. 1969;1:422–423.

169. Weintraub E, Gandhi D, Robinson C. Medical complications due to mothball abuse. *South Med J*. 2000;93:427–429.

170. Jones HE, Balster RL. Neurobehavioral consequences of intermittent prenatal exposure to high concentrations of toluene. *Neurotoxicol Teratol*. 1997;19:305–313.

171. McMartin KI, Liau M, Kopecky E, et al. Pregnancy outcome following maternal organic solvent exposure: a meta-analysis of epidemiological studies. *Am J Ind Med*. 1998;34:288–292.

172. Khattak S, K-Moghtader G, McMartin K, et al. Pregnancy outcome following gestational exposure to organic solvents: a prospective controlled study. *JAMA*. 1999;281:1106–1109.

173. Woods JH, Katz JL, Winger G. Abuse liability of benzodiazepines. *Pharmacol Rev*. 1987;39:251–413.

174. Twyman RE, Rogers CJ, MacDonald RL. Differential regulation of γ-aminobutyric acid receptor channels by diazepam and phenobarbital. *Ann Neurol*. 1989;25:213–220.

175. Greenblatt DJ, Allen MD, Noel BJ, et al. Acute overdosage with benzodiazepine derivatives. *Clin Pharmacol Ther*. 1977;21:497–514.

176. Fialip J, Aumaitre O, Eschalier A, et al. Benzodiazepine withdrawal seizures: analysis of 48 case reports. *Clin Neuropharmacol*. 1987;10:538–544.

177. Hoeken PCS. Adverse effects of methaqualone. *CMAJ*. 1975;112:685–688.

178. Hansen AR, Kennedy KA, Ambre JJ, et al. Glutethimide poisoning. *N Engl J Med*. 1975;292:250–252.

179. Bender FH, Cooper JV, Dreyfus R. Fatalities associated with an acute overdose of glutethimide (Doriden) and codeine. *Vet Hum Toxicol*. 1988;30:332–333.

180. Nover R. Persistent neuropathy following chronic use of glutethimide. *Clin Pharmacol Ther*. 1967;8:283–285.

181. Marks P. Methaqualone and peripheral neuropathy. *Practitioner*. 1974;212:721–722.

182. Teehan BP, Maher JF, Carey JJH, et al. Acute ethchlorvynol (Placidyl) intoxication. *Ann Intern Med*. 1970;72:875–882.

183. Li J, Stokes SA, Woeckener A. A tale of novel intoxication: a review of the effects of γ-hydroxybutyric acid with recommendations for management. *Ann Emerg Med*. 1998;31:729–736.

184. Zvosec D, Smith SW, McCutcheon JR, et al. Adverse events, including death, associated with the use of 1,4-butanediol. *N Engl J Med*. 2001;344:87–94.

185. Ricaurte GA, McCann VD. Recognition and management of complications of new recreational drug use. *Lancet*. 2005;365:2137–2145.

186. Snead OC, Gibson KM. γ-Hydroxybutyric acid. *N Engl J Med*. 2005;352:2721–2732.

187. Allgulander C, Borg S, Vikander B. A 4–6 year follow-up of 50 patients with primary dependence on sedative and hypnotic drugs. *Am J Psychiatry*. 1984;141:1580–1582.

188. Rummans TA, Davis LJ, Morse RM, et al. Learning and memory impairments in older, detoxified, benzodiazepine-dependent patients. *Mayo Clin Proc*. 1993;68:731–737.

189. Tata PR, Rollins J, Collins M, et al. Lack of cognitive recovery following withdrawal from long-term benzodiazepine use. *Psychol Med*. 1994;24:203–213.

190. McAndrews MP, Weiss RT, Sandor P. Cognitive effects of long-term benzodiazepine use in older adults. *Hum Psychopharmacol Clin Exp.* 2003;18:51–57.

191. Vining EP, Mellitis ED, Dorsen MM, et al. Psychologic and behavioral effects of antiepileptic drugs in children: a double-blind comparison between phenobarbital and valproic acid. *Pediatrics.* 1987;80:165–174.

192. Reinish JM, Sanders SA, Mortensen EL, et al. In utero exposure to phenobarbital and intelligence deficits in adult men. *JAMA.* 1995;274;1518–1525.

193. Diaz J, Schain RJ, Bailey BG. Phenobarbital-induced brain growth retardation in artificially reared rat pups. *Biol Neonate.* 1977;32:77–82.

194. Reinisch JM, Sanders SA. Early barbiturate exposure: the brain, sexually dimorphic behavior, and learning. *Neurosci Biobehav Rev.* 1982;6:311–319.

195. Laegreid L, Olegard R, Wahlstrom J, et al. Abnormalities in children exposed to benzodiazepines in utero. *Lancet.* 1987;1:108–109.

CHAPTER 29

The Neurotoxicity of Ethanol and Related Alcohols

John C.M. Brust

INTRODUCTION

The terms *alcoholic* and *problem drinker* encompass those who are physically dependent on ethanol (i.e., they develop physical withdrawal symptoms and signs when they stop drinking), those who are addicted to ethanol (i.e., with or without physical dependence, craving for ethanol becomes a daily preoccupation), and those who, although abstinent most of the time, get into trouble when they drink. In the United States, it is estimated that 7% of all adults and 19% of adolescents are problem drinkers and that ethanol-related deaths exceed 100,000 per year, accounting for 5% of all mortality.[1,2] By various mechanisms, ethanol inflicts widespread tissue damage, especially on the central and peripheral nervous systems. Some of these mechanisms represent different forms of neurotoxicity.

ACUTE INTOXICATION

Ethanol is a central nervous system (CNS) depressant, indirectly affecting many neurotransmitter systems, including inhibition of excitatory glutamate receptors and facilitation of inhibitory γ-aminobutyric acid (GABA) receptors.[3] Early symptoms of euphoria and hyperactivity reflect disinhibition; as blood ethanol concentrations (BECs) rise, impaired judgment and ataxic gait progress to coma, respiratory depression, and death. Drinkers differ in their degrees of tolerance, which is related less to increased metabolism than to adaptive changes in the brain.[4] BEC by itself does not, therefore, predict the degree of intoxication. A naïve drinker might become comatose and apneic at 500 mg/dL, whereas someone physically dependent on ethanol might be fully alert at the same level. Ethanol metabolism follows zero-order kinetics, and BEC falls 10 to 25 mg/dL per hour.[5] For most adults, consuming 50 g of absolute ethanol produces a mildly intoxicating BEC of 100 mg/dL, which takes 6 hours to fall to zero, during which time ingestion of only 8 g of additional ethanol maintain the BEC at 100 mg/dL.

The treatment of someone stuporous or comatose from ethanol intoxication includes respiratory support in an intensive case unit.[6] No available pharmacological agent accelerates ethanol metabolism, and analeptic drugs such as amphetamine have no useful role. Obstreperous or violent patients require close observation; sedatives should be avoided. Ethanol intoxication can coexist with and mask subdural hematoma, meningitis, hepatic encephalopathy, and hypoglycemia. Other drugs, including sedatives, cocaine, opioids, and marijuana, are often taken with ethanol, sometimes in suicide attempts, and the acute effects of such combinations can be synergistic.

DEPENDENCE AND WITHDRAWAL

In contrast to other agents, such as opioids, cocaine, or tobacco, psychic dependence (craving, addiction) develops in only a minority of those who drink ethanol. As with other drugs, the pathophysiology of ethanol addiction is not well understood, but it clearly involves the so-called reward circuit, a complex limbic circuitry that includes dopaminergic projections from the ventral tegmental area of the midbrain to the nucleus accumbens and the prefrontal cortex. Addictive liability has considerable hereditary predisposition, albeit polygenetic rather than mendelian.[7] Physical dependence, on the other hand, is the result of neurotoxic effects on other parts of the CNS and is reflected in characteristic symptoms and signs when ethanol is abruptly withdrawn after prolonged heavy drinking.

Early withdrawal symptoms, usually within 48 hours of abstinence, include tremulousness, perceptual disturbances, and seizures.[8] Tremor, which is promptly relieved by ethanol, can be so coarse as to interfere with eating or even standing, and it is often accompanied by insomnia, easy startling, facial and conjunctival flushing, sweating, anorexia, nausea, tachypnea, tachycardia, and systolic hypertension. Except for inattentiveness and inability to remember events during a binge, mentation is usually intact. If drinking cannot continue, tremor can persist for weeks or longer.

Perceptual disturbances include illusions and hallucinations that are visual, auditory, tactile, olfactory, or a combination (alcoholic hallucinosis).[9] There may be paranoid auditory accusations or imagery of animals, insects, or people. Hallucinations tend to last minutes at a time over several days and can occur during active drinking or after more than a week of abstinence. Insight as to their unreality varies, but the sensorium is clear (i.e., this is not delirium tremens).

The term alcohol-related seizures refers to seizures that occur without preexisting epilepsy or a precipitant such as head injury or CNS infection. As a feature of early withdrawal, they are most often generalized tonic–clonic and occur singly or in a brief cluster; less than 10% progress to status epilepticus. Focal features, when present, do not consistently correlate with evidence of structural brain pathology.[10] In a case–control study of new-onset seizures, it was found that risk conferred by ethanol is dose related beginning at only 50 g of absolute ethanol daily.[11] The minimal duration of drinking sufficient to cause seizures is uncertain. As with hallucinosis, seizures can occur during active drinking or after many days of abstinence, suggesting more than one pathophysiological mechanism.[11] Excitotoxicity might play a major role. During prolonged intoxication, glutamate inhibition would lead to receptor up-regulation, with a hyperglutamatergic state during withdrawal. Repeated bouts of withdrawal might then cause permanent excitotoxic neuronal damage, lowering the threshold for seizures independent of abrupt abstinence.

Ethanol can precipitate seizures in known epileptics, but the amount required is disputed. Seizures in alcoholics can also be the result of underlying neuropathology such as meningitis, so even during early withdrawal a seizure workup should be done, including brain imaging and consideration of a spinal tap.

Transient parkinsonism and transient chorea have each occurred during ethanol withdrawal.[12]

In contrast to tremor, hallucinosis, and seizures, delirium tremens typically begins 48 to 72 hours after the last drink. Defining features include tremor, delirium (severe inattentiveness often accompanied by agitation, hallucinations, or fluctuating levels of alertness), and autonomic overactivity, with fever, tachycardia, hypertension, and profuse sweating.[13] Seizures during delirium tremens are unusual and mandate search for another cause. Symptoms typically begin and end abruptly and last from hours to a few days. Severe fluid loss and electrolyte imbalance are often present, and mortality from delirium tremens is reportedly as high as 15%, usually from other diseases such as pneumonia or cirrhosis but sometimes as the result of cardiac arrhythmia or unexplained shock.

Treatment of ethanol withdrawal depends on symptoms and severity.[13] Prevention or reduction of early symptoms can be accomplished with a sedative cross-tolerant with ethanol, usually a benzodiazepine such as lorazepam; in patients with abnormal liver function, a shorter-acting agent might be preferred. Neuroleptic drugs should be avoided; they are not cross-tolerant with ethanol, and they lower seizure threshold. Ethanol as a recognized tissue toxin is also a poor choice. Status epilepticus is treated in standard fashion. Delirium tremens calls for more aggressive treatment in an intensive care unit. Parenteral benzodiazepine administration is titrated to a dosage that produces sustained sedation, and careful attention is given to fluid and electrolyte imbalance, autonomic instability, hyperthermia, and possible coexisting illness such as hypoglycemia, pancreatitis, or sepsis. Heavy drinkers hospitalized for any reason should receive thiamine and multivitamins. An unavoidable complication of treating ethanol withdrawal with large doses of sedatives may be the precipitation of hepatic encephalopathy.

DISORDERS OF NUTRITIONAL DEFICIENCY: DOES DIRECT ETHANOL NEUROTOXICITY PLAY A ROLE?

Alcoholics are often deficient in thiamine, nicotinic acid, other B vitamins, and folate. They are therefore at risk for neurological diseases associated with malnutrition, including Wernicke-Korsakoff syndrome, cerebellar degeneration, amblyopia, polyneuropathy, and pellagra. There is no doubt, from both animal studies and reports of nutritional deprivation in nondrinkers, that avitaminosis can cause these disorders, but increasingly evidence shows that ethanol neurotoxicity either increases the risk of their development or modulates their clinical features.

Wernicke and Korsakoff syndromes share the same pathology, but they are clinically distinct.[14] Acute Wernicke syndrome consists of the triad of (1) abnormal mentation (inattentiveness, abulia, lethargy, impaired memory progressing without treatment to coma), (2) abnormal eye movements (most often nystagmus and abducens or horizontal gaze palsy, progressing to complete external ophthalmoplegia), and (3) truncal ataxia. There may be autonomic instability, with tachycardia and postural hypotension. The full symptomatic triad is not always present; autopsies describe Wernicke neuropathology (characteristic histological abnormalities within the medial thalamus and hypothalamus and the mesencephalic periaqueductal gray matter) in patients dying in coma in whom the diagnosis was unsuspected.[15]

Treatment of Wernicke syndrome with thiamine produces rapid clinical improvement, but if it is delayed the multidomain mental abnormalities may evolve into Korsakoff syndrome, a relatively selective and persistent amnestic disorder affecting both anterograde and retrograde memory.[16] There may also be residual nystagmus and gait unsteadiness. How often the Korsakoff amnestic disorder occurs without preceding Wernicke syndrome is uncertain and confounded by recognition that ethanol neurotoxicity alone can cause dementia.

Cerebellar cortical degeneration, with neuronal loss especially affecting the superior vermis, can affect nutritionally deficient alcoholics without Wernicke-Korsakoff syndrome.[17] Symptoms evolve over weeks or months and are less likely than the ataxia of Wernicke syndrome to improve with abstinence and vitamin replenishment.

Alcoholic amblyopia is a visual impairment that progresses over days or weeks, with centrocecal scotomas and temporal pallor of the optic discs.[18] Total blindness does not occur, and improvement, although often incomplete, follows vitamin replacement and abstinence.

Alcoholic polyneuropathy is present in most patients with Wernicke-Korsakoff syndrome, but more often it occurs alone.[19] Sensory symptoms usually precede weakness, including paresthesias and burning or lancinating pain in the feet. Impaired vibratory sensation and loss of ankle tendon reflexes are early signs; proprioception is usually preserved until later in the course. In some patients, weakness evolves so rapidly as to suggest Guillain-Barré syndrome.[20] Autonomic neuropathy occurs, although less often than with diabetic polyneuropathy.[21]

Are these disorders more likely to occur in nutritionally deficient heavy drinkers than in nutritionally deficient nondrinkers? The answer is unclear. In developing countries, thiamine deficiency is more likely to produce beriberi with cardiac failure and polyneuropathy than Wernicke-Korsakoff syndrome, and Wernicke syndrome in nondrinkers is far less likely to progress to Korsakoff amnesia than Wernicke syndrome in alcoholics.[22] (On the other hand, several of Korsakoff's original patients had not been heavy drinkers.[16]) Like episodic ethanol withdrawal, thiamine deficiency causes excessive glutamate release with the potential for excitotoxicity, and N-methyl-d-aspartate (NMDA) receptor blockers prevent Wernicke-Korsakoff pathology in thiamine-deficient animals.[23]

Cerebellar degeneration can occur with severe nutritional deprivation in nondrinkers.[24] On the other hand, animal studies demonstrate neurotoxic effects of ethanol on cerebellar granule and Purkinje cells, with neuronal damage blocked by NMDA receptor antagonists.[25,26]

A study in humans found that alcoholic polyneuropathy appears to be of two types.[27] Neuropathy in nonalcoholic patients with thiamine deficiency was motor dominant and acutely progressive, impaired both superficial and deep sensation, and caused predominantly large-fiber axonal loss. Neuropathy in alcoholics without thiamine deficiency was sensory dominant, slowly progressive, and painful with impaired superficial sensation, and it caused predominantly small-fiber axonal loss. Thiamine-deficient alcoholics had a mixture of the two forms.

Patients with optic atrophy have reportedly improved with nutritional supplement even though they continued drinking, but it is nonetheless possible that direct toxicity from ethanol (and from compounds in tobacco smoke) is contributory.

ETHANOL AS A DIRECT NEUROTOXIN

Alcoholic Dementia

Clinicians have long suspected that ethanol causes lasting cognitive impairment in the absence of nutritional deficiency, cerebral trauma, hepatic failure, or other indirect forms of brain injury. Many alcoholics demonstrate gradually progressive impairment affecting not only memory but other cognitive domains as well and without evidence of prior Wernicke syndrome, nutritional deficiency, or other apparent cause. Computerized axial tomography scanning reveals cerebral ventricular and sulcal enlargement unexplained by the pathological anatomy of Wernicke-Korsakoff syndrome, and the apparent brain shrinkage reportedly improves with abstinence.[28]

Animal studies using pair-fed controls confirm that ethanol is neurotoxic; in exposed animals, impaired memory and learning correlate with neuropathological change. Reported abnormalities include loss of hippocampal CA1 and CA3 pyramidal neurons, mossy fiber-CA3 synapses, and dentate granule cells; loss of cholinergic neurons in the basal forebrain; pathological changes in neurons of cerebral cortex, hypothalamus, and brainstem; and impaired pruning of redundant cortical synapses during early development.[29–34] Damage is dose related and especially likely with a binge pattern of drinking that produces high BECs.[30,35] In some studies, hippocampal cell loss began during chronic ethanol exposure and continued after withdrawal.[36] In other studies, hippocampal cell loss began only after ethanol administration was stopped.[36]

It is obviously more difficult to exclude nutritional deficiency in heavy drinkers with cognitive impairment, but evidence does support the existence of brain shrinkage and neuronal loss in "uncomplicated alcoholics."[37] Loss of cerebral white matter is at least partly reversible, although it is less clear that cognitive improvement follows morphological improvement. White matter loss, reflected in abnormal magnetic resonance imaging signals including diffusion-weighed images, is not the result of water loss but involves many structural elements.[38] Magnetic resonance spectroscopy identified cerebral white matter phospholipid damage in the absence of white matter volume loss.[39] Neuronal loss has been described most consistently in the superior frontal association cortex, hypothalamus, and cerebellum and less consistently in the hippocampus, amygdala, and locus ceruleus. Basal ganglia and nucleus basalis appear to be unaffected.[37] Magnetic resonance spectroscopy using the neuronal or axonal marker N-acetyl aspartate confirmed the special vulnerability of the frontal lobes in alcoholics,[40] and correlative studies of cognitive function have described abnormalities in planning, organization, problem solving, and abstracting, as well as disinhibition, perseveration, and lack of insight.[41,42] Cognitive impairment that precedes obvious morphological change is plausibly explained by early abnormalities of dendrites, receptors, and neurotransmitters.[37]

As with Wernicke-Korsakoff syndrome and other nutritionally related complications of alcoholism, glutamate excitotoxicity and oxidative stress might be the pathophysiological mechanism of alcoholic dementia.[43–45]

It is thus possible that some (or maybe most) cases of alcoholic dementia represent additive (or synergistic) effects of both thiamine deficiency and ethanol toxicity.

If ethanol is neurotoxic, is there a safe-dose threshold? A review of 19 published studies addressing this issue concluded that people drinking 5 or 6 "standard drinks" per day over extended periods demonstrated "cognitive inefficiencies," that 7 to 9 drinks per day resulted in "mild cognitive deficits," and that 10 or more drinks per day caused cognitive deficits of a degree encountered in frank alcoholics.[46] Some studies found that heavy ethanol consumption (average 418 g of ethanol per week) was a risk factor for reduced frontal lobe volume, whereas light consumption (88 g/week) and moderate consumption (181 g/week) were not.[47] Several studies, moreover, found that light to moderate ethanol intake *reduced* the risk of dementia compared to abstention and heavy drinking.[48–53] Considerable epidemiological evidence thus supports the view that ethanol's effects on cognition follow a "J-shaped curve," with light to moderate doses reducing the risk of dementia and heavy doses increasing the risk. A similar J-shaped curve reflects ethanol's effects on coronary artery disease, all causes of death, and ischemic stroke, but in older light-to-moderate drinkers, ethanol appears to protect against both vascular dementia and Alzheimer dementia.[53] The mechanism of protection is unclear. Some investigators found benefit most evident in wine drinkers, consistent with a protective effect of antioxidants in wine, especially red wine.[50] Ethanol itself also has antioxidant properties. Some investigators found that protection was greatest for subjects carrying the apolipoprotein E e4 allele and speculated that ethanol might block oxidation of the apolipoprotein, thereby preventing it from binding to β-amyloid.[51]

Not all studies have found a relationship between ethanol intake and risk of dementia. Moreover, a review of published studies demonstrating a protective effect of ethanol against death from all causes concluded that such studies were confounded by combining among the abstainers never drinkers and former drinkers (who might have given up ethanol for reasons of ill health).[54] Whether such confounding invalidates the protective effects of light-to-moderate ethanol consumption on cognition remains to be seen.

Fetal Alcohol Syndrome

Offspring of alcoholic mothers are at risk for fetal alcohol syndrome (FAS), the most prominent features of which are abnormal cognition and behavior, microcephaly, prenatal and postnatal growth reduction, and characteristic facies that includes short palpebral fissures, short upturned nose, hypoplastic philtrum, thin lips, hypoplastic maxilla, retrognathia in infancy, and macrognathia or prognathia in adolescence.[55] A minority of patients have additional anomalies involving eyes, mouth, ears, skeleton, heart, skin, muscles, or genitalia. In prospective controlled studies, FAS occurred independently of maternal malnutrition, tobacco, other drugs, and age.[56] Binge drinking at a critical period is more important than chronic exposure, and early gestation is the most vulnerable period, although subtle behavioral abnormalities in some subjects suggests that later exposure also confers risk.[55] Children of alcoholic mothers are often mentally retarded or intellectually borderline without other features of FAS. Older children are often hyperactive and clumsy with hypertonia or hypotonia. A 30-year follow-up of FAS children revealed facial dysmorphism, persistent growth failure, pronounced microcephaly, frequent mental retardation, and invariably, abnormal behavior.[57] Neuropathological abnormalities include microcephaly and anomalies of the cerebellum, corpus callosum, basal ganglia, and frontal and parietal cortex.[58–60]

Animal studies confirm that ethanol is a CNS teratogen. Carefully controlled animal models, including chickens, rodents, dogs, pigs, and primates, describe impaired learning and neurological, ocular, cardiac, and skeletal anomalies.[61–63] Monkeys subjected in utero to a binge pattern of ethanol consumption display nervous system and craniofacial abnormalities similar to human FAS.[64] In mice, a single exposure to ethanol at the equivalent of week 3 of human pregnancy developed typical features of FAS.[65] Exposed rodents display neuronal reduction in the hippocampus, as well as decreased myelinogenesis and decreased synthesis of DNA, RNA, and protein.[66,67]

The mechanism of ethanol's teratogenicity is unknown, and an extensive literature has addressed the possible contributions of vasospasm and CNS ischemia,[68] altered glutamate binding and apoptotic neurodegeneration,[69,70] inhibition of acetylcholine muscarinic receptors,[71] inhibition of a cell adhesion molecule necessary for neuronal migration,[72] retinoic acid toxicity,[73] nerve growth factor inhibition,[74] and deleterious effects of the ethanol metabolite acetaldehyde.[75]

A threshold of safety for fetal ethanol exposure has not been established. FAS may affect 1% of children whose mothers drink 1 oz of ethanol per day early in pregnancy and 30% of the offspring of heavy drinkers.[76] In some studies, ingestion as low as 0.1 oz daily carried risk for subtle neurological and behavioral effects.[77–79] It thus appears that there is no safe dose for what is probably the leading teratogenic cause of mental retardation in the Western world.

DISORDERS WITH UNCERTAIN TOXICITY

Alcoholic Myopathy

Three types of alcoholic myopathy exist along a spectrum.[80,81] Subclinical myopathy consists of elevated creatine kinase, sometimes with intermittent cramps or weakness. With chronic myopathy, there is progressive proximal weakness. Acute rhabdomyolysis with sudden severe weakness, muscle pain, myoglobinuria, and renal shutdown is sometimes superimposed on chronic myopathy. Symptoms often appear during a binge, and ethanol toxicity rather than nutritional deficiency is considered the likely cause. Nonalcoholic volunteers consuming large amounts of ethanol with adequate diets developed intracellular edema, lipid and glycogen accumulation, and abnormal mitochondria and sarcoplasmic reticulum.[82] Both ethanol and acetaldehyde produce reversible alterations of muscle sodium–potassium adenosine triphosphatase, fatty acid oxidation, protein synthesis, and calcium binding to troponin.[83] Whether chronic or acute, alcoholic myopathy improves with abstinence.[80]

Marchiafava-Bignami Disease

A rare disorder, Marchiafava-Bignami disease is defined by characteristic lesions in the corpus callosum and a variable clinical spectrum.[84] Early symptoms are typically mental, including mania, depression, paranoia, and dementia. There may ensue seizures, fluctuating hemiparesis, aphasia, abnormal movements, ataxia, and progression to coma and death over a few months. Some patients have a chronic course over years or improve either partially or completely.[85] Lesions consisting of demyelination in the medial zone of the corpus callosum and sometimes involving the cerebral white matter, basal ganglia, and middle cerebellar peduncle can be detected with magnetic resonance imaging.[86] The cause of Marchiafava-Bignami disease is unknown. It occurs almost exclusively in alcoholics, and neurotoxicity is suspected, but the nature of the toxicity is unclear.

Hepatic Encephalopathy

Alcoholic liver disease is mainly the result of direct or indirect toxicity, not nutritional deficiency, with oxidative stress playing a major role.[87,88] Hepatic failure results in encephalopathy with altered behavior, psychosis, or delirium progressing to coma; accompanying signs include tremor, asterixis, extensor posturing, and sometimes hemiparesis or other focal signs.[89,90] Seizures or myoclonus should prompt a search for other causes. The responsible encephalopathic toxins are not well-defined; candidates include ammonia, glutamine, short-chain fatty acids, mercaptans, tryptophan, quinolinic acid, false neurotransmitters such as octopamine, and exogenous or endogenous benzodiazepine agonists acting at GABA receptors.[7,91] Favoring the latter is the observation that encephalopathic symptoms can be briefly reversed by the benzodiazepine antagonist flumazanil.[92]

Stroke

As with coronary artery disease, light to moderate ethanol consumption reduces the risk of ischemic stroke, whereas heavy consumption increases the risk.[93,94] The result is a J-shaped curve resembling that which describes ethanol's effects on cognition. The risk of hemorrhagic stroke is increased at any level of consumption. Several mechanisms probably contribute to the association between drinking and stroke. Ethanol acutely and chronically raises blood pressure.[95] It lowers blood levels of low-density lipoproteins and raises levels of high-density lipoproteins.[96] It decreases fibrinolytic activity, raises levels of factor VIII, increases platelet reactivity, decreases erythrocyte aggregation, and elevates C reactive protein.[97–101] Ethanol has both vasodilatory and vasoconstrictive effects on cerebral blood vessels.[102] Folate deficiency in alcoholics results in hyperhomocysteinemia.[103]

ETHANOL SUBSTITUTES

Methanol

Methanol (methyl alcohol, wood alcohol) is present in industrial solvents, carburetor fluid, antifreeze, canned fuels, and other products. Contamination of bootleg spirits has led to epidemics of methanol poisoning.[104,105] Compared to ethanol, methanol produces less prominent inebriation; patients often display visual impairment, abdominal pain, and metabolic acidosis with a clear sensorium. Methanol is metabolized by alcohol dehydrogenase (ADH) to formaldehyde and formic acid. Formic acid, by inhibiting mitochondrial cytochrome oxidase, is toxic to neurons, including retinal ganglion cells. Visual loss often begins 12 or more hours after ingestion and progresses to complete blindness, with unreactive pupils and optic disc hyperemia. There may ensue delirium, seizures, coma, respiratory depression, bradycardia, and death. Treatment includes cardiac and respiratory support and intravenous ethanol, which competes with methanol for ADH, thereby slowing methanol's metabolism to toxic products. 4-Methylpyrazole (fomepizole), which inhibits ADH, can also slow metha-

nol metabolism.[106] Folate is given because it hastens metabolism of formic acid to carbon dioxide. Hemodialysis is recommended for patients who are symptomatic or have significant metabolic acidosis, a blood methanol concentration higher than 25 mg/dL, or renal compromise. Following treatment there may or may not be recovery of vision, and survivors may display abnormal movements such as parkinsonism or dystonia.[107] Autopsies show putaminal necrosis and widespread neuronal damage in cerebral cortex, cerebellum, brainstem, and spinal cord.[108]

Ethylene Glycol

Present in antifreeze and brake fluids, ethylene glycol is deliberately drunk as an ethanol substitute, and several thousand cases of ethylene glycol poisoning are reported yearly in the United States.[104] Within a few hours, inebriation is followed by nausea, vomiting, ataxia, nystagmus, ophthalmoparesis, myoclonus, seizures, delirium, hallucinations, and stupor or coma. Like methanol, ethylene glycol is metabolized by ADH. Metabolic acidosis is caused by glycolic acid metabolites, including oxylate, which chelates calcium, causing tetany and cardiac symptoms 24 to 72 hours after ingestion. Calcium oxylate crystals are often identified in urine, and their precipitation can cause renal failure several days later.[109] Common among survivors are cranial neuropathies, especially facial palsy, probably the result of oxylate crystal deposition.[110] As with methanol, treatment of ethylene glycol poisoning includes slowing of ADH action by giving competitive ethanol or the inhibitory agent 4-methylpyrazole. Other measures include forced diuresis, treatment of acidosis, and in severely affected patients, hemodialysis.[109]

Isopropanol

Present in rubbing alcohol, household cements, glass cleaners, and windshield deicers, isopropanol (isopropyl alcohol) is also deliberately ingested. Metabolized by ADH to acetone, isopropanol causes ketosis without lactic acidosis.[111] Vomiting and abdominal pain are prominent early symptoms. Ataxia and altered mental status may appear after several hours and in severe cases progress to coma with miosis, absent tendon reflexes, and hypothermia. Renal tubular necrosis, hemolytic anemia, myopathy, and cardiac failure can ensue. Treatment is supportive and includes continuous gastric lavage. (Isopropanol is secreted into the stomach.) Because the principal toxin is ethylene glycol itself, there is no need to slow the action of ADH. Hemodialysis is used for hypotensive or comatose patients.

REFERENCES

1. Doyle R. Deaths caused by alcohol. *Sci Am.* 1996;274:30–31.
2. Hanson GR, Li T-K. Public health implications of excessive alcohol consumption. *JAMA.* 2003;289:1031–1032.
3. Davis KM, Wu J-Y. Role of glutamatergic and GABAergic systems in alcoholism. *J Biomed Sci.* 2001;8:7–19.
4. Tabakoff B, Cornell N, Hoffman PL. Alcohol tolerance. *Ann Emerg Med.* 1986;15:1005–1012.
5. Holford NHG. Clinical pharmacokinetics of ethanol. *Clin Pharmacokinet.* 1987;13:273–292.
6. Koch-Weser J, Sellers EM, Kalent HL. Alcohol intoxication and withdrawal. *N Engl J Med.* 1976;294:757–762.
7. Brust JCM. *Neurological Aspects of Substance Abuse.* 2nd ed. Boston: Butterworth-Heinemann; 2004:19–42.
8. Fox A, Kay J, Taylor A. The course of alcohol withdrawal in a general hospital. *QJM.* 1997;90:253–261.
9. McMicken DB. Alcohol withdrawal syndromes. *Emerg Med Clin North Am.* 1990;8:805–819.
10. Hauser WA, Ng SKC, Brust JCM. Alcohol, seizures, and epilepsy. *Epilepsia.* 1988;29 (Suppl 2):S66–S78.
11. Ng SKC, Hauser WA, Brust JCM, et al. Alcohol consumption and withdrawal in new-onset seizures. *N Engl J Med.* 1988;319:666–673.
12. Neiman J, Lang AE, Fornazarri L, et al. Movement disorders in alcoholism: a review. *Neurology.* 1990;40:741–746.
13. Kosten TR, O'Connor PG. Management of drug and alcohol withdrawal. *N Engl J Med.* 2003;348:1786–1795.
14. Victor M, Adams RD, Collins GH. *The Wernicke-Korsakoff Syndrome.* 2nd ed. Philadelphia: FA Davis; 1989.
15. Caine D, Halliday GM, Kril JJ, et al. Operational criteria for the classification of chronic alcoholics: identification of Wernicke's encephalopathy. *J Neurol Neurosurg Psychiatry.* 1997;62:51–60.
16. Kopelman MD. The Korsakoff syndrome. *Br J Psychiatry.* 1995;166:154–173.
17. Victor M, Adams RD, Mancall EL. A restricted form of cerebellar cortical degeneration occurring in alcoholic patients. *Arch Neurol.* 1959;71:579–688.
18. Shimozono M, Townsend JC, Ilsen PD, et al. Acute vision loss resulting from complications of ethanol abuse. *J Am Optomet Assoc.* 1998;69:293–303.
19. Behse F, Buchthal F. Alcoholic neuropathy: clinical, electrophysiological, and biopsy findings. *Ann Neurol.* 1977;2:95–110.
20. Wöhrle JC, Spengos K, Steinke W, et al. Alcohol-related acute axonal polyneuropathy: a differential diagnosis of Guillian-Barré syndrome. *Arch Neurol.* 1998;55:1329–1334.
21. Novak DJ, Victor M. The vagus and sympathetic nerves in alcoholic polyneuropathy. *Arch Neurol.* 1974;30:273–284.
22. Homewood J, Bond NW. Thiamine deficiency and Korsakoff's syndrome: failure to find memory impairments following nonalcoholic Wernicke's encephalopathy. *Alcohol.* 1999;19:75–84.
23. Robinson JK, Mair RG. MK-801 prevents brain lesions and delayed-nonmatching-to-sample deficits produced by pyrithiamine-induced encephalopathy in rats. *Behav Neurosci.* 1992;106:623–633.
24. Mancall EL, McEntee WJ. Alterations of the cerebellar cortex-nutritional encephalopathy. *Neurology.* 1965;15:303–313.
25. Dlugos CA, Pentney RJ. Morphometric evidence that the total number of synapses on Purkinje neurons of old F344 rats is reduced after long-term ethanol treatment and restores to control levels after recovery. *Alcohol.* 1997;32:161–172.
26. Pantazis NJ, Dohrman DP, Thomas JD, et al. NMDA prevents alcohol-induced neuronal cell death of cerebellar granule cells in culture. *Alcohol Clin Exp Res.* 1995;19:846–853.
27. Koike H, Iljima M, Sugiura M, et al. Alcoholic neuropathy is clinicopathologically distinct from thiamine deficiency neuropathy. *Ann Neurol.* 2003;54:19–29.
28. Harper CJ, Kril J, Daly J. Are we drinking our neurons away? *BMJ.* 1987;294:534–536.
29. Bengoechea O, Gonzalo LM. Effects of alcoholization in the rat hippocampus. *Neurosci Lett.* 1991;123:112–114.
30. Collins MA, Corso TD, Neafsey EJ. Neuronal degeneration in rat cerebrocortical and olfactory regions during subchronic "binge" intoxication with ethanol: possible explanation for olfactory deficits in alcoholics. *Alcohol Clin Exp Res.* 1996;20:284–292.
31. Lundqvist C, Alling C, Knoth R, et al. Intermittent ethanol exposure of adult rats. Hippocampal cell loss after one month of treatment. *Alcohol.* 1995;30:737–748.
32. Ferrer I, Galofre E, Fabriques I, et al. Effects of chronic ethanol consumption beginning at adolescence: increased numbers of dendritic spines on cortical pyramidal cells in adulthood. *Acta Neuropathol.* 1989;78:528–532.
33. File SE, Mabbutt PS. Long-lasting effects on habituation and passive avoidance performance of a period of chronic ethanol administration in the rat. *Behav Brain Res.* 1990;36:171–178.
34. Arendt T, Henning D, Gray JA, et al. Loss of neurons in the rat basal forebrain cholinergic projection system after prolonged intake of ethanol. *Brain Res Bull.* 1988;21:563–569.
35. Benthius DJ, West JR. Ethanol-induced neuronal loss in the developing rats: increased brain damage with binge exposure. *Alcohol Clin Exp Res.* 1990;14:107–118.
36. Cadete-Leite A, Tavares MA, Paula-Barbosa MM. Alcohol withdrawal does not impede hippocampal granule cell progressive loss in chronic alcohol-fed rats. *Neurosci Lett.* 1988;86:45–50.
37. Harper C. The neurobiology of alcohol-specific brain damage, or does alcohol damage the brain? *J Neuropathol Exp Neurol.* 1998;57:101–110.
38. Kril JJ, Halliday GM. Brain shrinkage in alcoholics: a decade on and what have we learned? *Prog Neurobiol.* 1999;58:381–387.
39. Estilaei MR, Matson GB, Payne GS, et al. Effects of chronic alcohol consumption on the broad phospholipid signal in human brain: an in vivo 31P MRS study. *Alcohol Clin Exp Res.* 2001;25:89–97.
40. Schweinsburg BC, Taylor MJ, Alhassoon OM, et al. Clinical pathology in brain white matter of recently detoxified alcoholics: a 1H magnetic resonance spectroscopy investigation of alcohol-associated frontal lobe injury. *Alcohol Clin Exp Res.* 2001;25:924–934.
41. Brun A, Anderson J. Frontal dysfunction and frontal cortical synapse loss in alcoholism: the main cause of alcohol dementia? *Dement Geriatr Cogn Disord.* 2001;12:289–294.
42. Monnot M, Nixon S, Lovallo W, et al. Altered emotional perception in alcoholics: deficits in affective prosody comprehension. *Alcohol Clin Exp Res.* 2001;25:362–369.
43. Tsai G, Coyle JT. The role of glutamatergic neurotransmission in the pathophysiology of alcoholism. *Annu Rev Med.* 1998;49:173–184.
44. Chandler LJ, Newsom H, Sumners C, Crews F. Chronic ethanol exposure potentiates NMDA excitotoxicity in cerebral cortical neurons. *J Neurochem.* 1993;60:1578–1581.
45. Gotz ME, Janetzky B, Pohli S, et al. Chronic alcohol consumption and cerebral indices of oxidative stress: is there a link? *Alcohol Clin Exp Res.* 2001;25:717–725.
46. Parsons OA, Nixon SJ. Cognitive functioning in sober social drinkers: a review of the research since 1986. *J Stud Alcohol.* 1998;59:180–190.
47. Kubota M, Nakazaki S, Hirai S, et al. Alcohol consumption and frontal lobe shrinkage: study of 1432 non-alcoholic subjects. *J Neurol Neurosurg Psychiatry.* 2001;71:104–106.

48. Launer LJ, Feskens EJ, Kalmijn S, et al. Smoking, drinking, and thinking: the Zutphen Elderly Study. *Am J Epidemiol.* 1996;143:219–227.

49. Galanis DJ, Joseph C, Masaki KH, et al. A longitudinal study of drinking and cognitive performance in elderly Japanese American men: the Honolulu-Asia Aging Study. *Am J Public Health.* 2000;90:1254–1259.

50. Lemeshow S, Letenneur L, Dartigues JF, et al. Illustration of analysis taking into account complex survey considerations: the association between wine consumption and dementia in the PAQUID study. *Am J Epidemiol.* 1998;148:298–306.

51. Ruitenberg A, van Swieten JC, Witteman JCM, et al. Alcohol consumption and the risk of dementia: the Rotterdam Study. *Lancet.* 2002;359:281–286.

52. Truelson T, Thudium D, Gronbaek M. Amount and type of alcohol and risk of dementia: the Copenhagen City Heart Study. *Neurology.* 2002;59:1313–1319.

53. Mukamal KJ, Kuller LH, Fitzpatrick AL, et al. Prospective study of alcohol consumption and risk of dementia in older adults. *JAMA.* 2003;289:1405–1413.

54. Filmore KM, Kerr WC, Stockwell T, et al. Moderate alcohol use and reduced mortality risk: systematic error in prospective studies. *Addict Res Theory.* 2006;14:101–132.

55. Allebeck P, Olsen J. Alcohol and fetal damage. *Alcohol Clin Exp Res.* 1998;22 (Suppl 7):229S–322S.

56. Mattson SN, Riley EP, Gramling L, et al. Neuropsychological comparison of alcohol-exposed children with or without physical features of fetal alcohol syndrome. *Neuropsychology.* 1998;12:146–153.

57. Lemoine P, Lemoine P. Avenir des enfants de meres alcooliques (etude de 105 cas retrouves a l'age adult) et quelques constatations d'interet prophylactique. *Ann Pediatr.* 1992;29:226–235.

58. Roebuck TM, Mattson SN, Riley EP. A review of the neuroanatomical findings in children with fetal alcohol syndrome or prenatal exposure to alcohol. *Alcohol Clin Exp Res.* 1998;22:339–344.

59. Sowell ER, Mattson SN, Thompson PM, et al. Mapping callosal morphology and cognitive correlates: effects of heavy prenatal alcohol exposure. *Neurology.* 2001;57:235–244.

60. Archibald SL, Fennema-Notestine C, Riley EP, et al. A quantitative MRI study of subjects exposed to alcohol prenatally. *Dev Med Child Neurol.* 2001;43:148–154.

61. Chernoff GF. The fetal alcohol syndrome in mice: maternal variables. *Teratology.* 1980;22:71–75.

62. Ellis FW, Pick JR. An animal model of the fetal alcohol syndrome in beagles. *Alcoholism Clin Exp Res.* 1980;4:123–134.

63. Dexter JD, Tumbleson ME, Decker JD, et al. Fetal alcohol syndrome in Sinclair (S-1) miniature swine. *Alcoholism Clin Exp Res.* 1980;4:146–151.

64. Clarren SK, Bowden DM. Fetal alcohol syndrome: a new primate model for binge drinking and its relevance to human ethanol teratogenesis. *J Pediatr.* 1982;101:819–824.

65. Sulik KK, Lauder JM, Dehart DB. Brain malformations in prenatal mice following acute maternal ethanol administration. *Int J Dev Neurosci.* 1984;2:203–213.

66. Berman RF, Hannigan JH. Effects of prenatal alcohol exposure on the hippocampus: spatial behavior, electrophysiology, and neuroanatomy. *Hippocampus.* 2000;10:94–110.

67. Guerri C, Renau-Piqueras J. Alcohol, astroglia, and brain development. *Mol Neurobiol.* 1997;15:65–81.

68. Mukherjee AB, Hodgen GD. Maternal ethanol exposure induces transient impairment of umbilical circulation and fetal hypoxia in monkeys. *Science.* 1982;218:700–702.

69. Kumari M, Tucku MK. Ethanol and regulation of the NMDA receptor subunits in fetal cortical neurons. *J Neurochem.* 1998;70:1467–1473.

70. Ikonomidou C, Bittigau P, Ishimaru MJ, et al. Ethanol-induced apoptotic neurodegeneration and fetal alcohol syndrome. *Science.* 2000;287:1056–1060.

71. Costa LG, Guizzetti M. Muscarinic cholinergic receptor signal transduction as a potential target for the developmental neurotoxicity of ethanol. *Biochem Pharmacol.* 1999;57:721–726.

72. Ramanathan R, Wilkenmeyer MF, Mittal B, et al. Alcohol inhibits cell–cell adhesion mediated by human L1. *J Cell Biol.* 1996;133:381–390.

73. Zachman RD, Grummer MA. The interaction of ethanol and vitamin A as a potential mechanism for the pathogenesis of fetal alcohol syndrome. *Alcohol Clin Exp Res.* 1998;22:1544–1556.

74. Dow KE, Riopelle RI. Ethanol neurotoxicity: effects on neurite formation and neurotrophic factor production in vitro. *Science.* 1985;228:591–593.

75. O'Shea KS, Kaufman MH. The teratogenic effect of acetaldehyde: implications of the study of the fetal alcohol syndrome. *J Anat.* 1979;128:65–76.

76. Alpert J, Zuckerman B. High blood alcohol levels in women. *N Engl J Med.* 1990;323:60–66.

77. Streissguth AP, Barr HM, Martin DC. Maternal alcohol use and neonatal habituation assessed with the Brazelton Scale. *Child Dev.* 1983;54:1109–1118.

78. Ernhart CH, Wolf AW, Linn PL, et al. Alcohol-related birth defects: syndromal anomalies, intrauterine growth retardation, and neonatal behavioral assessment. *Alcohol Clin Exp Res.* 1985;9:447–453.

79. Mills JL, Graubard BI, Harley EE, et al. Maternal alcohol consumption and birth weight: how much drinking during pregnancy is safe? *JAMA.* 1984;252:1875–1879.

80. Estruch R, Sacanella E, Fernandez-Sola J, et al. Natural history of alcoholic myopathy: a 5 year study. *Alcohol Clin Exp Res.* 1998;22:2023–2028.

81. Fernandez-Sola J, Grav Junyent JM, Urbana-Marquez A. Alcoholic myopathies. *Curr Opin Neurol.* 1996;9:400–405.

82. Rubin E, Katz AM, Lieber CS, et al. Muscle damage produced by chronic alcohol consumption. *Am J Pathol.* 1976;83:499–515.

83. Psuzkin S, Rubin E. Adenosine diphosphate effect on contractility of human actomyosin: inhibition by ethanol and acetaldehyde. *Science.* 1975;188:1319–1320.

84. Kohler CG, Ances BM, Coleman AR, et al. Marchiafava-Bignami disease: literature review and case report. *Neuropsychiatry Neuropsychol Behav Neurol.* 2000;13:67–76.

85. Helenius J, Tatlisumak T, Soinne L, et al. Marchiafava-Bignami disease: two cases with favorable outcome. *Eur J Neurol.* 2001;8:269–272.

86. Yamashita K, Kobayashi S, Yamaguchi S, et al. Reversible corpus callosum lesions in a patient with Marchiafava-Bignami disease: serial changes on MRI. *Eur Neurol.* 1997;37:192–193.

87. Lieber CS. Hepatic, metabolic, and nutritional disorders of alcoholism: from pathogenesis to therapy. *Crit Rev Clin Lab Sci.* 2000;37:551–584.

88. Hagymasi K, Blazovics A, Lengyel G, et al. Oxidative damage in alcoholic liver disease. *Eur J Gastroenterol Hepatol.* 2001;13:49–53.

89. Gammal SH, Jones EA. Hepatic encephalopathy. *Med Clin North Am.* 1989;73:793–813.

90. Cadranel J-F, Lebiez E, Di Martino V, et al. Focal neurological signs in hepatic encephalopathy in cirrhotic patients: an underestimated entity? *Am J Gastroenterol.* 2001;92:515–518.

91. Jones EA, Schafer DF. Hepatic encephalopathy: a neurochemical disorder. *Prog Liver Dis.* 1986;8:525–540.

92. Barbaro G, DiLorenzo G, Soldini M, et al. Flumazenil for hepatic encephalopathy Grade III and IV in patients with cirrhosis: an Italian multicenter double-blind, placebo-controlled, cross-over study. *Hepatology.* 1998;28:374–378.

93. Sacco RL, Elkind M, Baden-Albala B, et al. The protective effect of moderate alcohol consumption on ischemic stroke. *JAMA.* 1999;281:53–60.

94. Reynolds K, Lewis LB, Nolen JDL, et al. Alcohol consumption and risk of stroke: a meta-analysis. *JAMA.* 2003;289:579–588.

95. Cushman WC. Alcohol consumption and hypertension. *J Clin Hypertens.* 2001;3:166–170.

96. van Tol A, Hendriks HD. Moderate alcohol consumption: effects on lipids and cardiovascular disease risk. *Curr Opin Lipid.* 2001;12:19–23.

97. Lacoste L, Hung J, Lam JY. Acute and delayed antithrombotic effects of alcohol in humans. *Am J Cardiol.* 2001;87:82–85.

98. Brust JCM. Stroke and substance abuse. In: Mohr JP, Choi DW, Grotta JC, Weir B, Wolf PA, eds. *Stroke: Pathophysiology, Diagnosis and Management.* New York: Churchill Livingstone; 2004:725–746.

99. Imhof A, Froehlich M, Brenner H, et al. Effect of ethanol consumption on systemic markers of inflammation. *Lancet.* 2001;357:763–767.

100. Crews FT, Steck JC, Chandler LJ, et al. Ethanol, stroke, brain damage, and excitotoxicity. *Pharmacol Biochem Behav.* 1998;59:981–991.

101. Hillbom M, Numminen H. Alcohol and stroke: pathophysiologic mechanisms. *Neuroepidemiology.* 1998;17:281–287.

102. Mayhan WG. Responses of cerebral arterioles during chronic ethanol exposure. *Am J Physiol.* 1992;262:H787–H791.

103. Cravo ML, Camilo ME. Hyperhomocysteinemia in chronic alcoholism. Relations to folic acid and vitamins B_6 and B_{12} status. *Nutrition.* 2000;16:296–302.

104. Burkhart KK, Kulig KW. The other alcohols. *Emerg Med Clin North Am.* 1990;8:913–928.

105. Swartz RD, Millman RP, Billi JE, et al. Epidemic methanol poisoning: clinical and biochemical analysis of a recent episode. *Medicine.* 1981;60:373–386.

106. Brent J, McMartin K, Phillips S, et al. Fomepizole for the treatment of methanol poisoning. *N Engl J Med.* 2001;344:424–429.

107. LeWitt PA, Martin SD. Dystonia and hypokinesis with putaminal necrosis after methanol intoxication. *Clin Neuropharmacol.* 1988;11:161–167.

108. McLean DR, Jacobs H, Mielke BW. Methanol poisoning: a clinical and pathological study. *Ann Neurol.* 1980;8:161–167.

109. Piagnerelli M, Lejeune P, Vanhaeverbeek M. Diagnosis and treatment of an unusual cause of metabolic acidosis: ethylene glycol poisoning. *Acta Clin Belg.* 1999;54:351–356.

110. Lewis LD, Smith BW, Mamourian AC. Delayed sequelae after acute overdoses or poisonings: cranial neuropathy related to ethylene glycol ingestion. *Clin Pharmacol Ther.* 1997;61:692–699.

111. Rich J, Scheife RT, Katz N, Caplan LR. Isopropyl alcohol intoxication. *Arch Neurol.* 1990;47:322–324.

CHAPTER 30

Neurotoxic Effects of Pharmaceutical Agents I: Anti-infectives

Melody Ryan

INTRODUCTION

The anti-infectives are a vast category of medications encompassing agents from aminoglycosides to antiretroviral agents. To effectively treat bacterial, fungal, and viral infections, many mechanisms of action have been employed, from agents that affect the bacterial cell wall to those that affect the viral organism's ability to replicate. As expected with such a variety of medications with a plethora of mechanisms of action, numerous neurotoxicities are associated with these medications. Well-recognized and significant neurotoxicities are discussed in this chapter by category of anti-infective.

AMINOGLYCOSIDES

Aminoglycosides are recognized to have multiple toxicities. Of those that affect the nervous system, ototoxicity and myasthenia gravis exacerbations are the most common. These agents have been in use for many years and continue to be a mainstay of treatment for gram-negative infections.

Ototoxicity

Ototoxicity is a well-known adverse effect of aminoglycoside administration. Less appreciated is vestibular toxicity that may be more common than hearing loss.[1] The prevalence of ototoxicity with hearing loss is usually reported as 3% to 25%, but when high-frequency audiograms are used for detection, hearing loss may be seen in up to 62% of patients treated with aminoglycosides.[2] Changes in hearing have been detected within days of aminoglycoside administration; however, aminoglycosides can remain in the cochlea for up to 11 months after administration; this retention is thought to be responsible for late-onset hearing loss.[2]

When horizontal canal vestibulo-ocular reflex testing was done on a series of 28 patients receiving aminoglycosides, 39% were found to have vestibular ototoxicity.[3] Decreases in response were first detected an average of 35 days after administration, with maximum decreases seen at 99 days. Recovery of normal responses took 4 to

10 months.[3] Vestibular toxicity has been reported after intravenous administration of all available aminoglycosides, after eardrops, and after inhaled tobramycin.[4,5]

Much interest has focused on identifying risk factors for ototoxicity development; however, the only consistently associated risk factor is a longer course of aminoglycoside treatment.[4] Many studies have also associated renal dysfunction with ototoxicity, but other studies have found no relationship.[6] Animal studies found higher inner ear gentamicin concentrations in animals without kidneys.[6] Associations with age, total aminoglycoside dose, and aminoglycoside serum concentrations have been inconsistent. Hearing loss is more common in people inheriting a particular mitochondrial DNA mutation (m.1555A>G). This mutation can predispose individuals to deafness in the absence of aminoglycoside therapy; however, this spontaneous hearing loss only occurs in 40% of individuals with this mutation. With aminoglycoside exposure, the deafness rate increases to 96% for individuals who carry this mutation. The prevalence of this mutation is low (0.0025% to 0.42%) and its variability may depend on the population studied.[7]

Ototoxicity appears to be due to both type I hair cell loss[6,8] and spiral ganglion cell loss.[8] The aminoglycoside may form reactive oxygen species that trigger apoptosis or necrotic cell death.[9] However, the precise mechanism of otoxicity is unknown.

Common symptoms include tinnitus, vertigo, disequilibrium, and nausea in those suffering from vestibular toxicity.[3] In one series of 35 patients with ototoxicity from gentamicin, all patients complained of imbalance, disequilibrium, and oscillopsia (sense of objects jumping). Only three patients had changes in hearing and five patients had vertigo.[6] If recovery occurs, it may be slow and incomplete.[1]

Some research has focused on use of antioxidants to prevent ototoxicity when aminoglycosides are administered. High-dose aspirin (1 g three times daily) reduced the incidence of hearing loss from 13% in the untreated group to 3% in the treated group; however, vestibular symptoms did not seem to be affected.[9] Likewise, hearing loss was prevented by N-acetylcysteine in hemodialysis patients taking gentamicin (25% treated versus 60% untreated, $p = 0.027$), but the number of patients reporting tinnitus and vertigo was not different between the groups.[2]

Myasthenic Syndrome

Aminoglycosides are thought to impair neuromuscular transmission by impairing the release of acetylcholine from the presynaptic terminal.[10,11] Thus, it is possible that they can induce myasthenic symptoms in patients without myasthenia gravis. However, most reports are of preexisting myasthenia gravis worsening after aminoglycoside treatment.[10]

β-LACTAMS

The β-lactams encompass the penicillins, the cephalosporins, and the carbapenams. The most commonly recognized neurotoxicity of this group of medications is seizure induction. Less commonly seen are myoclonus, encephalopathy, tremor, and myasthenia gravis exacerbations.

Seizures

Virtually all β-lactam antibiotics have been reported to cause seizures, including penicillins, cephalosporins, and carbapenams. There may be some differences among the various agents in incidence of seizures, but any difference is difficult to quantify. The incidence of seizures with imipenem is approximately 3%.[12] The β-lactams appear to have common risk factors for seizures, foremost of which is renal impairment leading to increased serum concentrations of the antibiotic.[13–15] Other risk factors include high β-lactam dose, history of seizures, underlying brain pathology, and conditions favoring increased cerebral penetration of the antibiotic (sepsis or central nervous system infection).[13–15] It does appear possible to anticipate patients at risk and adjust doses of the β-lactam to prevent seizures in some cases. In a case series of 75 critically ill patients who received imipenem at doses no higher than 2 g/day and dose adjusted for renal dysfunction, no increase in seizures was seen after imipenem initiation.[12]

β-Lactams are thought to cause seizures through competitive antagonism of brain γ-aminobutyric acid (GABA) at the GABA$_A$ receptor.[14] In the case of carbapenems (imipenem and meropenem), the degree of their antagonism correlates with the presence of a basic side chain on the second carbon atom of the carbapenem. The basic nature enhances the binding to the GABA$_A$ receptor.[16] Imipenem's side chain is more basic than meropenem's; this fact may be responsible for the high incidence of seizures in patients treated with imipenem.[16]

When electroencephalograms (EEGs) have been performed, they sometimes reveal epileptiform activity.[17] In addition, nonconvulsive status epilepticus has often been overlooked in patients with deteriorating mental status or altered levels of consciousness.[14,17–19] Symptoms generally abate after discontinuation of the β-lactam, but high-flux hemodialysis has been used to rapidly reduce concentrations of dialyzable medications.[20]

Another possible cause of seizures with meropenem lies in an interaction with valproic acid. Meropenem appears to enhance glucuronidation of valproic acid to cause a rapid decline in serum valproic acid concentrations. In patients treated with valproic acid before initiation of meropenem, serum concentrations of valproic acid decreased from a mean of 64.3 μg/mL before meropenem to a mean of 22.5 μg/mL (66% decrease) following the addition of meropenem. The decrease occurred within 24 hours of beginning meropenem. In 11 of the 20 patients who had EEG recordings, electroclinical deterioration was seen when meropenem was added; four of these patients had worsening or new-onset seizure activity.[21] It is, therefore, important to anticipate this drug–drug interaction that may precipitate seizures.

Myoclonus

Isolated case reports associate myoclonus with cephalosporin and imipenem administration.[22–25] One of these cases occurred after intraperitoneal administration in a patient with chronic renal failure and continuous ambulatory peritoneal dialysis.[25] EEG recordings are not available for these cases; thus, myoclonic seizure activity cannot be ruled out.

Encephalopathy

Mental confusion is a prominent symptom of β-lactam toxicity.[17] While some cases of confusion have been determined to be nonconvulsive status epilepticus, several reports suggestive of metabolic–toxic encephalopathies associated with cefepime administration are found in the literature.[17,26,27] EEGs typically have shown loss of background activity, increased slow rhythms in the θ- and δ-range, and triphasic waves.[17,27,28] Some cases have been fatal[27]; however, it is difficult to conclusively determine that the cefepime neurotoxicity caused mortality because these patients were already critically ill. Through their bactericidal activity, cephalosporins may cause endotoxin release that stimulates tumor necrosis factor-α. Tumor necrosis factor-α may be the mediator for toxic encephalopathy.[28]

Other Neurotoxicities

A flapping tremor was seen in two patients with renal dysfunction given imipenem. The tremor was thought to be distinct from seizure activity in these patients, although EEGs were not performed.[29] Worsening myasthenia gravis has been reported following ampicillin[30] and imipenem[10] treatment. The mechanisms of these neurotoxicities are unknown.

ERYTHROMYCINS

Various erythromycins including erythromycin,[31] clarithromycin,[32] azithromycin,[33] and telithromycin[34] have been associated with worsening myasthenia gravis. The mechanism by which they exert this effect is unknown.

QUINOLONES

Quinolones are commonly used antibiotics for many infections ranging from minor to serious illnesses. Neurotoxicities that can occur with this class of medications include seizures, myasthenic symptoms, rhabdomyolysis, paresthesias, peripheral neuropathy, optic neuropathy, myoclonus, tremor, and Tourette-like symptoms.

Seizures

Seizures have been reported with all quinolones.[35] Most seizures either have not been well described or have been generalized tonic–clonic in nature; however, there is one case report of a 63-year-old man given ciprofloxacin who developed myoclonus associated with cortical EEG activity on the second day of treatment.[36] While most reports of seizures with quinolones have followed oral or intravenous dosing, there is one case report associated with eardrop use. In this case, the patient had bilateral tympanostomy tubes for treatment of recurrent otitis media, which may have facilitated systemic absorption of the medication.[37] Cases have generally responded to medication cessation and treatment with benzodiazepines.

The mechanism by which quinolones cause seizures is not definitively known but may be due to competitive antagonism of the $GABA_A$ or $GABA_B$ receptors or to excitatory glutamate receptor occupation.[35] Affinity for the GABA receptor is not equal among the quinolones. Trovafloxacin (discontinued in the United States due to hepatotoxicity) has the highest affinity, followed by enoxacin, moxifloxacin, ciprofloxacin, ofloxacin, and gatifloxacin or levofloxacin. Trovafloxacin also has the highest incidence of seizures associated with its use.[38]

Neuromuscular Disorders

Myasthenic symptoms have been associated with levofloxacin, ciprofloxacin, ofloxacin, and norfloxacin. In several cases, the quinolone likely unmasked myasthenia gravis or worsened existing cases.[39] In a laboratory-based study, quinolones progressively decreased the amplitude of the miniature endplate potentials as drug concentrations were increased.[40] This finding may explain the exacerbation of myasthenia gravis with quinolone use.

The World Health Organization Collaborating Center for International Drug Monitoring received reports of 27 cases of rhabdomyolysis associated with levofloxacin; 4 were fatal.[41] Ofloxacin has also been associated with rhabdomyolysis.[42]

The Swedish Adverse Drug Reactions Advisory Committee received 30 reports of paresthesias, 19 reports of numbness, and 10 reports of pain while patients were taking norfloxacin, ciprofloxacin, or temafloxacin. Within

2 weeks of medication discontinuation, 71% of cases resolved.[43]

Individuals made self-reports to a Web site of 45 cases of symptoms compatible with a diagnosis of peripheral neuropathy; these were then verified by an investigator. Levofloxacin was implicated in 33 cases, ciprofloxacin in 11 cases, ofloxacin in 6 cases, lomefloxacin in 1 case, and trovafloxacin in 1 case. One-third of cases experienced symptoms within 24 hours. Both sensory and motor abnormalities were reported by 47% of subjects, 44% reported sensory abnormalities only, and 9% reported only motor abnormalities. Symptoms lasted for more than a month in 91% of cases.[44]

Optic Neuropathy

Two cases of optic neuropathy have been associated with ciprofloxacin use. In one case, the patient had been taking the medication for approximately 6 years. Improvement in visual acuity was seen soon after stopping the ciprofloxacin and continued to improve over 4 years. The patient's visual field testing also improved; however, color vision did not improve.[45] The other case had taken high doses of ciprofloxacin. Upon discontinuation, vision also improved.[46]

Movement Disorders

There is one case report of a patient who developed truncal myoclonic jerks during treatment with ciprofloxacin. These decreased but did not resolve until 1 year after therapy completion.[47]

Transient soft palate tremor was observed 3 days after inadvertent high-dose (2000 mg/day) ciprofloxacin treatment in one patient. Symptoms resolved 2 days after stopping ciprofloxacin.[48]

There is one case report of a Tourette-like syndrome consisting of spitting, profuse swearing, echolalia, echopraxia, automatisms, hypersalivation, and amnesia with ofloxacin. These symptoms resolved with therapy cessation.[49]

TRIMETHOPRIM–SULFAMETHOXAZOLE

Several movement disorders have been reported in patients taking trimethoprim–sulfamethoxazole. In addition, rhabdomyolysis has been reported with this medication.

Movement Disorders

Tremor, myoclonus, chorea, or a combination of these have been reported in nine patients treated with trimethoprim–sulfamethoxazole, most of whom had acquired immune deficiency syndrome (AIDS) or other immunocompromising conditions.[50] However, some patients have been immunocompetent.[51] In fact, the risk of developing neurotoxicity related to trimethoprim–sulfamethoxazole treatment may be related more to the higher doses used for *Pneumocystis* infections (trimethoprim–sulfamethoxazole at 20 and 100 mg/kg/day, respectively) than to the immunological status of the patient.[52] When 12 healthy subjects were given high-dose trimethoprim–sulfamethoxazole, all of them developed some central nervous system toxicity. These symptoms included headache, nervousness, fine tremors, lightheadedness, insomnia, and drowsiness.[52] Other reports of the tremor describe a high-frequency, action, or postural tremor.[50,51]

One possible cause of tremor is the mechanism of action for trimethoprim. It inhibits dihydrofolate reductase, leading to a deficit of tetrahydrobiopterin. Tetrahydrobiopterin is a cofactor for neurotransmitter production; thus, fewer neurotransmitters, particularly dopamine, are produced. The reduction in dopamine could lead to the movement disorders that have been described.[50] On withdrawal of the medicine, the conditions have generally abated over 2 to 5 days.[50] For patients in whom trimethoprim–sulfamethoxazole must be continued, it is possible that folic acid supplementation could counteract the movement disorder. However, there are no reports of its use in this situation.[50]

Rhabdomyolysis

Nine cases of rhabdomyolysis have been reported with trimethoprim–sulfamethoxazole. The mechanism by which this medication could cause this toxicity is unknown. Typically cases resolve when the agent is discontinued.[53,54]

METRONIDAZOLE

Metronidazole is another medication that has long been available. Several neurotoxicities have been associated with its use over this time. These include neuropathy, optic neuropathy, encephalopathy, and seizures.

Neuropathy

Neuropathy is the most commonly recognized neurotoxicity of metronidazole. Sensory and motor neuropathies are most common, but autonomic neuropathy has also been reported.[55] Neuropathies usually manifest after long-term treatment; however, one case in which the patient had only been treated for 2 or 3 days has been reported.[55–57] A sural nerve biopsy in one case found

341

axonal degeneration.[58] Often recovery is slow, taking months, and may be incomplete.[55,57,59]

Optic Neuropathy

Eight cases of optic neuropathy have been reported with metronidazole. The length of medication treatment before optic neuropathy development is quite broad (7 to 365 days). Daily metronidazole doses have ranged from 750 to 1200 mg in these cases. All patients had vision improvement when metronidazole was stopped, with six patients recovering normal vision.[60,61]

Encephalopathy

Symptoms including dysarthria, weakness, and ataxia have been grouped into an entity called metronidazole-induced encephalopathy (MIE).[62] In a series of seven patients, the average length of metronidazole treatment before development of symptoms was 25.4 days.[63] MIE is associated with bilateral, symmetrical hyperintense lesions on imaging. Combining imaging data from all available cases ($n = 20$), the lesion distribution is cerebellar dentate nuclei for 85%, midbrain for 55%, corpus callosum for 50%, pons for 35%, medulla for 30%, subcortical white matter of the hemisphere for 25%, and basal ganglia for 20%.[63] Diffusion-weighted imaging suggests symptoms are due to interstitial edema seen in these lesions.[62] This etiology is supported by the rapid resolution of symptoms following metronidazole discontinuation (mean 6.7 days).[63]

Seizures

Metronidazole has been rarely associated with seizures but generally only in large doses, after long courses of therapy, and in cases of severe renal dysfunction.[64,65] Metronidazole is metabolized to 1-(2-hydroxyethyl)-2-hydroxymethyl-5-nitroimidazole and 2-methyl-5-nitroimidazole-l-acetic acid. Serum concentrations of both of these metabolites increase in severe renal dysfunction.[66] A pharmacokinetic study conducted in 29 patients with varying degrees of renal function determined that significant accumulation is likely only if the patients' estimated creatinine clearances are less than 10 mL/min.[66]

LINEZOLID

Linezolid is a recently introduced addition to the antibiotic armamentarium. However, several neurotoxicities have been associated with its use. These include neuropathy, optic neuropathy, seizures, and leukoencephalopathy.

In addition, because it is a monoamine oxidase inhibitor, serotonin syndrome is a concern with this medication.

Neuropathy

There are 16 reported cases of linezolid-associated neuropathy; 6 of these had concomitant optic neuropathy.[67] Linezolid has been approved by the U.S. Food and Drug Administration for treatment for up to 28 days, but most patients who developed neuropathy had prolonged courses of therapy, with a median duration of 4 months (range 10 days to 6 months).[67] Following medication discontinuation, most patients showed some improvement, but complete recovery was not seen in any case.[67]

The bactericidal action of linezolid is to bind to 23S ribosomal RNA and inhibit bacterial protein synthesis. It has been hypothesized that linezolid may bind to mitochondrial 16S ribosomal RNA, which is important to human cells.[67] Most cases have reported a sensory-motor axonal neuropathy or sensory axonal neuropathy.[67] A skin biopsy in one patient demonstrated a small-fiber neuropathy with cutaneous nerve degeneration.[68]

Optic Neuropathy

Likely because the optic nerve is highly dependent on mitochondrial function, it is also affected by linezolid.[67] Twelve reported cases of optic neuropathy exist, six of which occurred in conjunction with peripheral neuropathy.[67] The median duration of linezolid therapy before development of optic neuropathy was 10 months (range 1 to 48 months).[67] Most patients had some visual field deficit with variable retinal findings.[67] In contrast to neuropathy, visual improvement or complete recovery was seen in all cases.[67]

Serotonin Syndrome

Linezolid is a reversible, nonselective monoamine oxidase inhibitor.[69] Thus, patients are at some risk for developing serotonin syndrome when they receive other serotonergic medications or when they consume large quantities of tyramine-containing foods. The risk of serotonin syndrome, however, may be small; in one retrospective study, only 2.8% of patients either who were receiving concomitant serotonin-specific reuptake inhibitors (SSRIs) or who had received SSRIs and linezolid within 2 weeks of each other developed serotonin syndrome.[70] In addition, in a study in which subjects were administered two 20-mg doses of dextromethorphan, no serotonin syndrome effects were seen.[69] However, the total dextromethorphan dose of 40 mg in this study was less than the maximum adult daily dose of 120 mg. To date, all reports of serotonin syndrome result from coadministration of linezolid with SSRIs or venlafaxine.[67] This finding is unsurprising because these agents are more commonly prescribed than other agents that may precipitate serotonin syndrome. Serotonin syndrome symptoms began a median of 4 days after linezolid was initiated. Resolution occurred within 1 to 9 days of medication cessation.[67] Symptoms of serotonin syndrome include the following clusters of clinical features: tremor and hyperreflexia; spontaneous clonus; muscle rigidity, body temperature above 38°C, and either ocular clonus or inducible clonus; ocular clonus and either agitation or diaphoresis; or inducible clonus and either agitation or diaphoresis.[71] Because of the seriousness of serotonin syndrome, the recommendation is to avoid concomitant use of medications that also increase serotonin (Table 1). Due to the long half-lives of the SSRIs, a 2-week washout period is recommended before beginning linezolid (5 weeks for fluoxetine).[67] However, because of the urgency of treating infection, it is not always possible to observe such a long washout period. Quantities of tyramine consumed should be less than 100 mg per meal; for many foods, even those rich in tyramines, this quantity is above the usually consumed amounts (Table 2).[69]

Other Neurotoxicities

Seizures have been reported in 2.8% of pediatric (birth to 11 years) patients taking linezolid for indications other than skin and soft tissue infection in the product information.[69] However, no case reports of seizures without other neurological findings are found in the literature.

There is one report of posterior reversible leukoencephalopathy syndrome presenting with seizures, disorientation, visual disturbance, and headache following linezolid treatment. The magnetic resonance imaging showed multifocal, mainly posterior, white and gray matter hyperintensivities on fluid-attenuated inversion recovery sequences and vasogenic edema on diffusion-weighted images. The patient recovered fully over 3 months when linezolid was stopped.[72]

AMPHOTERICIN B

Several adult and pediatric cases of leukoencephalopathy associated with parkinsonian features have been reported with amphotericin B. In most cases, these symptoms have occurred in individuals with high cumulative doses of the medication[73]; however, there are two cases with lower doses (less than 5 g total).[74] Most cases have been with the non-lipid-based formulation of amphotericin B, but one case involved lipid-based amphotericin B.[75] Symptoms associated with these cases include bradykinesia, akinesia, cogwheel rigidity, masklike facies, coarse resting tremor, mutism, and

Table 1: Selected Medications that May Precipitate Serotonin Syndrome[69]

Medication Classes	Individual Medications
Amphetamines	Bromocriptine
Ergotamines	Bupropion
Monoamine oxidase inhibitors	Buspirone
Selective norepinephrine reuptake inhibitors	Cocaine
Serotonin-specific reuptake inhibitors	Codeine
Triptans	Dextromethorphan
	Fentanyl
	Levodopa
	Lithium
	Pentazocine
	Phenylpropanolamine
	Pseudoephedrine
	Reserpine
	Tramadol
	Trazodone

Table 2: Tyramine Content of Selected Foods[69]

Food	Tyramine Content
Aged cheeses	0–15 mg/oz
Fermented or air-dried meats	0.1–8 mg/oz
Red wine	0–6 mg per 8 oz
Sauerkraut	8 mg per 8 oz
Soy sauce	5 mg/teaspoon
Tap beers	4 mg per 12 oz

hyperreflexia. Imaging and autopsy studies have found evidence of leukoencephalopathy.[73,74,76,77] In one case, carbidopa or levodopa was initiated, but no significant improvement was observed.[75]

It is difficult to establish the culpability of amphotericin B in most of these cases because of the immunosuppression of the underlying diseases, as well as other potentially causative therapies. However, in all of them, the temporal association with amphotericin B was strong. Cranial or total body irradiation may play a role in increasing permeability of the blood–brain barrier and thus the neurotoxicity of this medicine.[75]

NUCLEOSIDE REVERSE TRANSCRIPTASE INHIBITORS

Some nucleoside reverse transcriptase inhibitors (NRTIs), such as zalcitabine, didanosine, stavudine, and lamivudine, have been associated with peripheral neuropathy,[78] while others, such as zidovudine and abacavir, have not.[79] Overall, it appears that 15% to 30% of patients receiving didanosine, stavudine, or zalcitabine develop a peripheral neuropathy.[80] However, zalcitabine appears to be more neurotoxic than didanosine or stavudine,[78] with approximately 25% of zalcitabine-treated patients developing neuropathy after more than 9 months of therapy.[81] A retrospective database analysis found an incidence of 6.8 cases per 100 person-years for didanosine and 9.8 cases per 100 person-years for stavudine, with a dramatic increase to 17.5 cases per 100 person-years when didanosine and stavudine were used together. The relative risk of developing peripheral neuropathy was not different between stavudine and didanosine, but adding them together increased the risk 3.50 times that of didanosine alone ($p = 0.002$) and 2.23 times that of stavudine alone ($p = 0.04$).[80] Therefore, the combination of didanosine and stavudine is usually avoided.

Development of NRTI-associated neuropathy shows a clear relationship to dose of medication.[80] Other risk factors include low CD4 cell count, high viral load, older age, past history of peripheral neuropathy, and nutritional deficiencies.[80] In one trial, risk of peripheral neuropathy peaked around day 90 of treatment, suggesting that length of therapy is unlikely to be a risk factor for neuropathy.[82]

The mechanism by which NRTIs affect the peripheral nerves is likely associated with the mitochondrial toxicity they induce. NRTIs affect DNA polymerase-γ. This polymerase is required for mitochondrial DNA replication. If mitochondrial DNA replication is slowed, insufficient energy is generated for cellular function.[81] The peripheral nerves are heavy users of mitochondria and are, thus, severely affected. Indeed, the effects of NRTIs on the peripheral nerves mirror their effects on mitochondrial polymerase-γ, with zalcitabine having the most effect, followed by stavudine and lamivudine. The relatively nontoxic zidovudine and abacavir have the least mitochondrial effect.[81]

NRTIs usually induce a sensory axonal neuropathy.[78] However, human immunodeficiency virus (HIV) infection can also cause peripheral neuropathy; it is important to be able to distinguish between the two types. Clinically, NRTI-associated neuropathy may be more abrupt in onset and more painful than HIV-associated neuropathy.[78] A potential laboratory test to discern the etiology is measurement of venous lactate. In one small study, venous lactate concentrations were measured after at least 10 minutes of rest. The blood samples were collected without tourniquet or fist clenching. Patients with stavudine and neuropathy had higher mean lactate concentrations (3.16 ± 0.81 mmol/L) than those with neuropathy associated with HIV (1.8 ± 0.67 mmol/L) or those with stavudine therapy but without neuropathy (1.68 ± 0.4 mmol/L).[83] While this test has not become standard clinical practice, it may be helpful in situations in which medication continuation is essential.

Symptoms of NRTI-induced peripheral neuropathy are usually reversible after discontinuation of the NRTI.[80] In one study, patients had significant improvement 19 weeks after stopping zalcitabine.[84] Paradoxically, neuropathy pain may initially increase after cessation of therapy; this increased discomfort may last weeks to months.[79] In most cases, the implicated medication is changed to a less neurotoxic alternative. However, there are situations in which the patient requires the causative medication. Acetyl-L-carnitine at 1500 mg twice daily was used in one small, open-label study of 21 patients with NRTI-associated neuropathy. Pain improved in 15 patients. Acetyl-L-carnitine is an antioxidant; it also improves neuronal metabolic capacity and increases response to nerve growth factor.[85] One of these mechanisms could be responsible for the pain improvement in seen in this small study.

MEDICATIONS FOR TUBERCULOSIS

Of the medications used to treat tuberculosis, isoniazid and ethambutol are most often associated with neurotoxicities. Isoniazid has been linked to neuropathy and seizures. Ethambutol contributes to an optic neuropathy.

Isoniazid

Neuropathy

The most common neurotoxicity of isoniazid is peripheral neuropathy. The incidence of neuropathy is clearly dose related, with up to 20% of patients who receive 6 mg/kg/day of isoniazid without pyridoxine developing neuropathy.[86] Risks may be increased in patients previously prone to neuropathy, such as those with diabetes, alcoholism, or HIV.[86] Because tubercular infections are more common among immunosuppressed individuals, including those with HIV, a retrospective study was conducted to determine the incidence of peripheral neuropathy among patients taking both isoniazid and stavudine. There was a dramatic increase with the combination, resulting in neuropathy in 55% of individuals versus 11% of those taking stavudine alone.[87] Supplemental pyridoxine doses of 6 to 50 mg/day during isoniazid therapy are recommended for patients predisposed to neuropathy development.[86] Paradoxically, doses of pyridoxine above 50 mg/day may be associated with peripheral neuropathy.[88]

The elimination of isoniazid is through N-acetylation; N-acetylation speed is controlled through a polymorphic gene. The prevalence of the slow acetylator phenotype is 50% among American and European Caucasians and African-Americans and 10% among Japanese.[89] Those slow acetylators have an increased risk of developing neuropathy with isoniazid therapy.[89]

Seizures

Acute overdoses of isoniazid, particularly in doses above 30 mg/kg, may cause seizures.[90] Isoniazid inhibits the activity of pyridoxine phosphokinase and thus depletes pyridoxal-5'-phosphate. GABA concentrations depend on pyridoxal-5'-phosphate and quickly diminish, resulting in seizures.[90]

Benzodiazepines and barbiturates may be useful for treatment because of their action on the GABA receptor, but other antiepileptics are not helpful. Pyridoxine may be administered to restore GABA concentrations.[90] If the amount of the isoniazid overdose is known, pyridoxine should be administered at a dose equal to the ingestion of isoniazid by intravenous push at 1 g/minute. If the amount ingested is unknown, a less precise method of administering 5 g of pyridoxine every 5 to 10 minutes until seizures stop can be used.[90]

Ethambutol

Optic Neuropathy

An optic neuropathy is well known during ethambutol therapy. Its onset is typically 1.5 to 12 months after starting ethambutol.[91] The optic neuropathy is dose related, developing in 44% of patients given 60 to 100 mg/kg/day; 5% to 6% of patients given 25 mg/kg/day, and 1% or less of patients given 15 mg/kg/day.[91]

Symptoms include decreased visual acuity, visual fields defects, and blue–yellow color changes.[91] Vision often returns to normal when ethambutol is discontinued, but there are reports in which no visual improvement was noted.[91]

CONCLUSION

Many neurotoxicities arising from various anti-infectives have been discussed in this chapter. However, this discussion is by no means exhaustive. Case reports of neurotoxicities continue to surface daily. In addition, new medications, both within existing categories of anti-infectives and with new mechanisms of action, are continually being developed. There is difficulty in establishing causality in many of these cases, mainly because of the possibility of nervous system infection or fevers as additionally potentially causative factors. As has been demonstrated in the preceding material, not all agents within a therapeutic class of anti-infectives have the same risks for neurotoxicities. The clinician must, therefore, be vigilant and report new occurrences of neurotoxicity with these medications through the U.S. Food and Drug Administration's MedWatch reporting system, as well as through publication of case reports and case series.

REFERENCES

1. Seemungal BM, Bronstein AM. Aminoglycoside ototoxicity: vestibular function is also vulnerable. *BMJ.* 2007;335:952.
2. Feldman L, Efrati S, Eviatar E, et al. Gentamicin-induced ototoxicity in hemodialysis patients is ameliorated by N-acetylcysteine. *Kidney Int.* 2007;72:359–363.
3. Black FO, Gianna-Poulin C, Pesznecker SC. Recovery from vestibular ototoxicity. *Otol Neurotol.* 2001;22:662–671.
4. Moore RD, Smith CR, Lietman PS. Risk factors for the development of auditory toxicity in patients receiving aminoglycosides. *J Infect Dis.* 1984;149:23–30.
5. Edson RS, Brey RH, McDonald TJ, et al. Vestibular toxicity due to inhaled tobramycin in a patient with renal insufficiency. *Mayo Clin Proc.* 2004;79:1185–1191.
6. Ishiyama G, Ishiyama A, Kerber K, Baloh RW. Gentamicin ototoxicity: clinical features and the effect on the human vestibule-ocular reflex. *Acta Otolaryngol.* 2006;126:1057–1061.
7. Bitner-Glindzicz M, Rahman S. Ototoxicity caused by aminoglycosides is severe and permanent in genetically susceptible people. *BMJ.* 2007;335:784–785.
8. Hinojosa R, Nelson EG, Lerner SA, et al. Aminoglycoside ototoxicity: a human temporal bone study. *Laryngoscope.* 2001;111:1797–1805.
9. Chen Y, Huang WG, Zha DJ, et al. Aspirin attenuates gentamicin ototoxicity: from the laboratory to the clinic. *Hear Res.* 2007;226:178–182.
10. O'Riordan J, Javed M, Doherty C, Hutchinson M. Worsening of myasthenia gravis on treatment with imipenem/cilastatin. *J Neurol Neurosurg Psychiatry.* 1994;57:383.
11. Liu C, Hu F. Investigation on the mechanism of exacerbation of myasthenia gravis by aminoglycoside antibiotics in mouse model. *J Huazhong Univ Sci Technolog Med Sci.* 2005;25:294–296.
12. Koppel BS, Hauser WA, Politis C, et al. Seizures in the critically ill: the role of imipenem. *Epilepsia.* 2001;42:1590–1593.
13. Barrons RW, Murray KM, Richey RM. Populations at risk for penicillin-induced seizures. *Ann Pharmacother.* 1992;26:26–29.

14. Lam S, Gomolin IH. Cefepime neurotoxicity: case report, pharmacokinetic considerations, and literature review. *Pharmacother.* 2006;26:1169–1174.

15. Pestotnik SL, Classen DC, Evans RS, et al. Prospective surveillance of imipenem/cilastatin use and associated seizures using a hospital information system. *Ann Pharmacother.* 1993;27:497–501.

16. Norrby SR. Neurotoxicity of carbapenem antibiotics: consequences for their use in bacterial meningitis. *J Antimicrob Chemother.* 2000;45:5–7.

17. Chow KM, Szeto CC, Hui AC, et al. Retrospective review of neurotoxicity induced by cefepime and ceftazidime. *Pharmacother.* 2003;23:369–373.

18. Abanades S, Nolla J, Rodriguez-Campello A, et al. Reversible coma secondary to cefepime neurotoxicity. *Ann Pharmacother.* 2004;38:606–608.

19. Maganti R, Jolin D, Rishi D, Biswas A. Nonconvulsive status epilepticus due to cefepime in a patient with normal renal function. *Epilepsy Behav.* 2006;8:312–314.

20. Lin CS, Cheng CJ, Chou CH, Lin SH. Piperacillin/tazobactam-induced seizure rapidly reversed by high flux hemodialysis in a patient on peritoneal dialysis. *Am J Med Sci.* 2007;333:181–184.

21. Spriet I, Goyens J, Meersseman W, et al. Interaction between valproate and meropenem: a retrospective study. *Ann Pharmacother.* 2007;41:1130–1136.

22. Uchihara T, Tsukagoshi H. Myoclonic activity associated with cefmetazole, with a review of neurotoxicity of cephalosporins. *Clin Neurol Neurosurg.* 1988;90:369–371.

23. Chan S, Turner MR, Young L, Gregory R. Cephalosporin-induced myoclonus. *Neurology.* 2006;66:E20.

24. Frucht S, Eidelberg D. Imipenem-induced myoclonus. *Mov Disord.* 1997;12:621–622.

25. Rivera M, Crespo M, Teruel JL, et al. Neurotoxicity due to imipenem/cilastatin in patients on continuous ambulatory peritoneal dialysis. *Nephrol Dial Transplant.* 1999;14:258–259.

26. De Silva DA, Pan ABS. Cefepime-induced encephalopathy with triphasic waves in three Asian patients. *Ann Acad Med.* 2007;36:450–451.

27. Sonck J, Laureys G, Verbeelen. The neurotoxicity and safety of treatment with cefepime in patients with renal failure. *Nephrol Dial Transplant.* 2008;23:966–970.

28. Capparelli FJ, Diaz MF, Hlavnika A, et al. Cefepime- and cefixime-induced encephalopathy in a patient with normal renal function. *Neurology.* 2005;65:1840.

29. Campise M. Neurological complication during imipenem/cilastatin therapy in uraemic patients. *Nephrol Dial Transplant.* 1998;13:1895–1896.

30. Argov Z, Brenner T, Abramsky O. Ampicillin may aggravate clinical and experimental myasthenia gravis. *Arch Neurol.* 1986;43:255–256.

31. Absher JR, Bale JF Jr. Aggravation of myasthenia gravis by erythromycin. *J Pediatr.* 1991;119:155–156.

32. Pijpers E, van Rijswijk RE, Takx-Kohlen B, Schrey G. A clarithromycin-induced myasthenic syndrome. *Clin Infect Dis.* 1996;22:175–176.

33. Cadisch R, Streit E, Hartmann K. Exacerbation of pseudoparalytic myasthenia gravis following azithromycin (Zithromax). *Schweiz Med Wochenschr.* 1996;126:308–310.

34. Perrot X, Bernard N, Vial C, et al. Myasthenia gravis exacerbation or unmasking associated with telithromycin treatment. *Neurology.* 2006;67:2256–2258.

35. Kushner JM, Peckman HJ, Snyder CR. Seizures associated with fluoroquinolones. *Ann Pharmacother.* 2001;35:1194–1198.

36. Striano P, Zara F, Coppola A, et al. Epileptic myoclonus as ciprofloxacin-associated adverse effect. *Mov Disord.* 2007;22:1675–1676.

37. Orr CF, Rowe DB. Eardrop attacks: seizures triggered by ciprofloxacin eardrops. *Med J Aust.* 2003;178:343.

38. Quigley CA, Lederman JR. Possible gatifloxacin-induced seizure. *Ann Pharmacother.* 2004;38:235–237.

39. Gunduz A, Turedi S, Kalkan A, Nuhoglu I. Levofloxacin induced myasthenia crisis. *Emerg Med J.* 2006;23;662.

40. Sieb JP. Fluoroquinolone antibiotics block neuromuscular transmission. *Neurology.* 1998;50:804–807.

41. Korzets A, Gafter U, Dicker D, et al. Levofloxacin and rhabdomyolysis in a renal transplant patient. *Nephrol Dial Transplant.* 2006;21:3304–3305.

42. Hsiao SH, Chang CM, Tsao CJ, et al. Acute rhabdomyolysis associated with ofloxacin/levofloxacin therapy. *Ann Pharmacother.* 2005;39:146–149.

43. Hedenmalm K, Spigset O. Peripheral sensory disturbances related to treatment with fluoroquinolones. *J Antimicrob Chemother.* 1996;37:831–837.

44. Cohen JS. Peripheral neuropathy associated with fluoroquinolones. *Ann Pharmacother.* 2001;35:1540–1547.

45. Samarakoon N, Harrisberg J, Ell J. Ciprofloxacin-induced toxic optic neuropathy. *Clin Experiment Ophthalmol.* 2007;35:102–104.

46. Vrabec TR, Sergott RC, Jaeger EA, et al. Reversible visual loss in a patient receiving high-dose ciprofloxacin hydrochloride (Cipro). *Opthalmology.* 1990;97:707–710.

47. Post B, Koelman JHTM, Tijssen MAJ. Propriospinal myoclonus after treatment with ciprofloxacin. *Mov Disord.* 2004;19:595–597.

48. Cheung YF, Wong WW, Tang KW, et al. Ciprofloxacin-induced palatal tremor. *Mov Disord.* 2007;22:1038–1043.

49. Thomas RJ, Reagan DR. Association of a Tourette-like syndrome with ofloxacin. *Ann Pharmacother.* 1996;30:138–141.

50. Bua J, Marchetti F, Barbi E, et al. Tremors and chorea induced by trimethoprim–sulfamethoxazole in a child with *Pneumocystis* pneumonia. *Pediatr Infect Dis J.* 2005;24:934–935.

51. Patterson RG, Couchenour RL. Trimethoprim–sulfamethoxazole-induced tremor in an immunocompetent patient. *Pharmacotherapy.* 1999;19:1456–1458.

52. Stevens RC, Laizure SC, Williams CL, Stein DS. Pharmacokinetics and adverse effects of 20-mg/kg/day trimethoprim and 100-mg/kg/day sulfamethoxazole in healthy adult subjects. *Antimicrob Agents Chemother.* 1991;35:1884–1890.

53. Singer SJ, Racoosin JA, Viraraghavan R. Rhabdomyolysis in human immunodeficiency virus–positive patients taking trimethoprim–sulfamethoxazole. *Clin Infect Dis.* 1998;26:233–234.

54. Walker S, Norwood J, Thornton C, Schaberg D. Trimethoprim–sulfamethoxazole associated rhabdomyolysis in a patient with AIDS: case report and review of the literature. *Am J Med Sci.* 2006;331:339–341.

55. Hobson-Webb LD, Roach ES, Donofrio PD. Metronidazole: newly recognized cause of autonomic neuropathy. *J Child Neurol.* 2006;21:429–431.

56. Coxon A, Pallis CA. Metronidazole neuropathy. *J Neurol Neurosurg Psychiatry.* 1976;39:403–405.

57. Bradley WG, Karlsson IJ, Rassol CG. Metronidazole neuropathy. *BMJ.* 1977;2:610–611.

58. Takeuchi H, Yamada A, Touge T, et al. Metronidazole neuropathy: a case report. *Jpn J Psychiatry Neurol.* 1988;42:291–295.

59. Gupta BS, Baldwa S, Verma S, et al. Metronidazole induced neuropathy. *Neurol India.* 2000;48:192–193.

60. McGrath NM, Kent-Smith B, Sharp DM. Reversible optic neuropathy due to metronidazole. *Clin Experiment Ophthamol.* 2007;35:585–586.

61. Putnam D, Fraunfelder FT, Dreis M. Metronidazole and optic neuritis. *Am J Ophthalmol.* 1991;112:737.

62. Heaney CJ, Capeau NG, Lindell EP. MR imaging and diffusion-weighted imaging changes in metronidazole (Flagyl)–induced cerebellar toxicity. *Am J Neuroradiol.* 2003;24:1615–1617.

63. Kim E, Na DG, Kim EY, et al. MR imaging of metronidazole-induced encephalopathy: lesion distribution

and diffusion-weighted imaging findings. *Am J Neuroradiol.* 2007;28:1652–1658.

64. Beloosesky Y, Grosman B, Marmelstein V, Grinblat J. Convulsions induced by metronidazole treatment for *clostridium difficile*–associated disease in chronic renal failure. *Am J Med Sci.* 2000;319:338–339.

65. Herreman G, Krainik F, Betous F, et al. Convulsive seizures and polyneuritis in a patient with lupus treated with metronidazole. *Ann Med Interne.* 1981;132:398–403.

66. Houghton GW, Dennis MJ, Gabriel R. Pharmacokinetics of metronidazole in patients with varying degrees of renal failure. *Br J Clin Pharmacol.* 1985;19:203–209.

67. Narita M, Tsuji BT, Yu VL. Linezolid-associated peripheral and optic neuropathy, lactic acidosis, and serotonin syndrome. *Pharmacother.* 2007;27:1189–1197.

68. Chao CC, Sun HY, Chang YC, Hsieh ST. Painful neuropathy with skin denervation after prolonged use of linezolid. *J Neurol Neurosurg Psychiatry.* 2008;79:97–99.

69. Pfizer. Zyvox Prescribing Information. New York: Pfizer; March 2007.

70. Taylor JJ, Wilson JW, Estes LL. Linezolid and serotonergic drug interactions: a retrospective study. *Clin Infect Dis.* 2006;43:180–187.

71. Boyer EW, Shannon M. The serotonin syndrome. *N Engl J Med.* 2005;352:1112–1120.

72. Nagel S, Kohrmann M, Huttner HB, et al. Linezolid-induced posterior reversible leukoencephalopathy syndrome. *Arch Neurol.* 2007;64:746–748.

73. Ellis WG, Sobel RA, Nielsen SL. Leukoencephalopathy in patients treated with amphotericin B methyl ester. *J Infect Dis.* 1982;146:125–137.

74. Walker RW, Rosenblum MK. Amphotericin B–associated leukoencephalopathy. *Neurology.* 1992;42:2005–2010.

75. Manley TJ, Chusid MJ, Rand SD, et al. Reversible parkinsonism in a child after bone marrow transplantation and lipid-based amphotericin B therapy. *Pediatr Infect Dis J.* 1998;17:433–434.

76. Mott SH, Packer RJ, Vezina LG, et al. Encephalopathy with parkinsonian features in children following bone marrow transplantations and high-dose amphotericin B. *Ann Neurol.* 1995;37:810–814.

77. Devinsky O, Lemann W, Evans AC, et al. Akinetic mutism in a bone marrow transplant recipient following total-body irradiation and amphotericin B chemoprophylaxis: a positron emission tomographic and neuropathologic study. *Arch Neurol.* 1987;44:414–417.

78. Peltier AC, Russell JW. Advances in understanding drug-induced neuropathies. *Drug Saf.* 2006;29:23–30.

79. Moyle GJ, Sadler M. Peripheral neuropathy with nucleoside antiretrovirals: risk factors, incidence, and management. *Drug Saf.* 1998;19:481–494.

80. Moore RD, Wong WE, Keruly JC, McArthur JC. Incidence of neuropathy in HIV-infected patients on monotherapy versus those on combination therapy with didanosine, stavudine and hydroxyurea. *AIDS.* 2000;14:273–278.

81. White AJ. Mitochondrial toxicity and HIV therapy. *Sex Transm Inf.* 2001;77:158–173.

82. Arenas-Pinto A, Bhaskaran K, Dunn D, Weller IV. The risk of developing peripheral neuropathy induced by nucleoside reverse transcriptase inhibitors decreases over time: evidence from the Delta trial. *Antivir Ther.* 2008;13:289–295.

83. Brew BJ, Tisch S, Law M. Lactate concentrations distinguish between nucleoside neuropathy and HIV neuropathy. *AIDS.* 2003;17:1094–1096.

84. Berger AR, Arezzo JC, Schaumburg HH, et al. 2′, 3′ -dideoxycytidine (ddC) toxic neuropathy: a study of 52 patients. *Neurology.* 1993;43:358–362.

85. Hart AM, Wilson ADH, Montovani C, et al. Acetyl L carnitine: a pathogenesis based treatment for HIV-associated antiretroviral toxic neuropathy. *AIDS.* 2004;18:1549–1560.

86. West-ward Pharmaceutical. Isoniazid Product Information. Eatontown, NJ: West-ward Pharmaceutical; 2001.

87. Breen RAM, Lipman MCI, Johnson MA. Increased incidence of peripheral neuropathy with co-administration of stavudine and isoniazid in HIV-infected individuals. *AIDS.* 2000;14:615.

88. Nisar M, Watkin SW, Bucknall RC, Agnew RAL. Exacerbation of isoniazid induced peripheral neuropathy by pyridoxine. *Thorax.* 1990;45:419–420.

89. Relling MV. Polymorphic drug metabolism. *Clin Pharm.* 1989;8:852–863.

90. Morrow LE, Wear RE, Schuller D, Malesker M. Acute isoniazid toxicity and the need for adequate pyridoxine supplies. *Pharmacotherapy.* 2006;26:1529–1532.

91. Melamud A, Kosmorsky GS, Lee MS. Ocular ethambutol toxicity. *Mayo Clin Proc.* 2003;78:1409–1411.

CHAPTER 31

Neurotoxic Effects of Pharmaceutical Agents II: Psychiatric Agents

Melody Ryan and Kara A. Kennedy

INTRODUCTION

Psychiatric disorders, including depression, psychosis, and bipolar disorder, are common and gaining more acceptance in the United States. The most commonly used classes of medications for these disorders are antidepressants, antipsychotics, and lithium. Unfortunately, these medications are associated with significant neurotoxicities.

ANTIDEPRESSANTS

In the period between 1999 and 2002, 8% of the adult population in the United States reported using an antidepressant. The rate of use was quite different between females (10.6%) and males (5.2%).[1] The classes of antidepressants available include monoamine oxidase inhibitors (MAOIs), tricyclic antidepressants (TCAs), serotonin-specific reuptake inhibitors (SSRIs), and newer compounds designed to increase serotonin, norepinephrine, dopamine, or a combination of these (Table 1). Some neurotoxicities such as antidepressant discontinuation syndrome, serotonin syndrome, and poisoning are common to all antidepressants. Other neurological adverse effects are specific to certain medications.

An adverse effect surveillance system in psychiatric hospitals in Germany, Austria, and Switzerland studied severe adverse effects of antidepressants in 122,562 patients.[2] Neurological adverse effects occurred in approximately 0.11% of patients receiving TCAs alone, in about 0.06% of patients receiving SSRIs alone, and in about 0.04% of those receiving only mirtazapine, mianserin, venlafaxine, nefazodone, or reboxetine. The type of neurological effects differed among antidepressant classes: for TCAs, delirium and seizures were most common; for SSRIs, serotonin syndrome was most common; and for the other medications, delirium and seizures were most common.[2]

Depression is particularly common in patients with epilepsy, with a 20% to 55% prevalence rate and a suicide risk of three to five times that of the worldwide population.[3] Therefore, patients with epilepsy often require antidepressant treatment. However, most antidepressants have been reported to induce seizures. The risk is different for each class of medications and is discussed in more detail later.

Antidepressant Discontinuation Syndrome

Antidepressant discontinuation syndrome, sometimes called SSRI discontinuation syndrome, may occur in up to 30% of patients who abruptly discontinue antidepressants. It is more common in patients treated with antidepressants with shorter half-lives (see Table 1). In one

Table 1: Classes of Commonly Used Antidepressants and Their Half-lives

Monoamine Oxidase Inhibitors		Tricyclic Antidepressants		Serotonin-specific Reuptake Inhibitors		Serotonin and Norepinephrine Reuptake Inhibitors		Norepinephrine and Dopamine Reuptake Inhibitor		Noradrenergic and Specific Serotoninergic Antidepressant		Serotonin 2 Receptor Antagonists	
Agent	$t_{(1/2)}$ (h)	Agent	$t_{(1/2)}$ (h)	Agent	$t_{(1/2)}$ (h)	Agent	$t_{(1/2)}$ (h)	Agent	$t_{(1/2)}$ (h)	Agent	$t_{(1/2)}$ (h)	Agent	$t_{(1/2)}$ (h)
Phenelzine	11	Amitriptyline	9–27	Citalopram	24–48	Duloxetine	12	Bupropion	21	Mirtazapine	20–40	Nefazodone	1.5–18
Rasagaline*	1.3–3	Amoxapine	11–16	Escitalopram	27–32	Venlafaxine	3–7					Trazodone	7–8
Selegiline*	10	Clomipramine	20–30	Fluoxetine	24–72								
Tranylcypromine	1.5–3	Desipramine	7–60	Fluvoxamine	15								
		Doxepin	6–8	Paroxetine	21								
		Imipramine	6–18	Sertraline	26								
		Maprotiline†	51										
		Nortriptyline	28–31										
		Protriptyline	54–92										
		Trimipramine	16–40										

*Selective for monoamine oxidase B at standard doses for parkinsonism.
†Tetracyclic compound with similar properties to tricyclic antidepressant.

observational study of 171 patients supervised during antidepressant withdrawal, symptoms occurred in 30.8% of those withdrawing from clomipramine and 17.2% of patients stopping fluvoxamine or paroxetine and compared to only 1.5% of patients ceasing sertraline or fluoxetine, with their longer half-lives.[4]

Symptoms can begin as early as one day after discontinuation and resolve over a period of 3 weeks.[5] Symptoms vary among patients but may include dizziness, myalgias, tremor, myoclonus, lightheadedness, anxiety, agitation, irritability, lethargy, headache, vivid dreams, paresthesias, impaired short-term memory, gait instability, insomnia, nausea, fatigue, shortness of breath, diaphoresis, and chills.[5,6] Because symptoms may be so variable and are often confused with reemergence of the underlying psychiatric condition for which the antidepressant was prescribed, some attempts at more standard criteria for the definition of antidepressant discontinuation syndrome have been made recently.[7,8] A scale, the Discontinuation–Emergent Signs and Symptoms Scale, has been developed to assess patients for antidepressant discontinuation syndrome.[9] However, its use is generally limited to clinical trials.

Serotonin Syndrome

Serotonin syndrome is a risk with all classes of antidepressants. Some authors debate whether some cases dubbed neuroleptic malignant syndrome in case reports are actually serotonin syndrome.[10,11] Other authors have suggested that both syndromes reflect a disruption of the balance between serotonin and dopamine in the central nervous system.[12]

Symptoms of serotonin syndrome are wide ranging, and criteria have been suggested by Sternbach.[13] Other causes must be ruled out, and no antipsychotics may have been started or increased before symptom onset. At least three of the following features should be present: agitation, mental status changes, myoclonus, hyperreflexia, diaphoresis, shivering, tremor, diarrhea, incoordination, and fever.[13] The symptoms present in almost all cases of serotonin syndrome are fever, neuromuscular rigidity or hyperreflexia, and mental status changes.[14]

The combination of medications that increase synaptic serotonin concentrations is often to blame for serotonin syndrome. Some lesser-known medications that increase serotonin include dextromethorphan, meperidine, cocaine, selegiline, rasagaline, 3,4-methylenedioxymethamphetamine (the illicit drug Ecstasy), amphetamines, linezolid, and lithium. In addition, the triptan and ergotamine medications that may be taken only as needed for vascular headaches may increase serotonin.[14] Of the medications more commonly known to induce serotonin syndrome, MAOIs are probably the best known. MAOIs and SSRIs should not be used concomitantly and require a 2-week washout period—except for fluoxetine, which requires a 5-week washout due to its longer half-life. The selective MAO_B inhibitors, selegiline and rasagaline, are often used with caution in Parkinson's disease patients taking SSRIs. Of note, these agents lose their selectivity for MAO_B at higher doses and should be treated as nonselective in those cases. Particularly, the transdermal formulation of selegiline for depression should be considered a nonselective MAOI.

Serotonin syndrome symptoms usually begin within 24 hours of medication additions or increases but may be much sooner.[14] Symptoms usually resolve within 24 hours of medication cessation. Generally, discontinuation of the offending agent or agents and supportive care are the only therapies used for serotonin syndrome. However, in some cases, it may be necessary to administer a serotonin antagonist such as methysergide or cyproheptadine.[14]

Poisoning

Unfortunately, intentional toxic ingestions of antidepressants are common. In one series from Turkey, 350 patients who had ingested antidepressants were assessed. TCAs were the most common class of agents ingested (58.4%), followed by SSRIs (22.5%). Neurological symptoms were common in this population, with altered mental status in 35.7% (4.4% presenting in coma), seizures in 2.2%, and tremor in 0.5% of patients. Endotracheal intubation was 26 times more common in patients who experienced a seizure.[15]

Some patient characteristics have been identified to increase the risk of seizures in antidepressant overdoses. These include history of seizure, multisystem illnesses, cancer with brain metastases, electrolyte or endocrine imbalance, head injury, neurological abnormalities, and older age. In addition, patients who are undergoing substance withdrawal or who are taking other medications that may lower the seizure threshold or that increase the serum concentrations of antidepressants may be at increased risk for seizures during antidepressant overdose.[16]

Tricyclic Antidepressants

TCAs commonly cause anticholinergic adverse effects, as well as sedation from their effects on the muscarinic and histamine H_1-receptors (see Chapter 34). They are also implicated in seizures.[5] The mechanism by which TCAs cause seizures is not precisely known. However, animal studies suggest that the H_1-receptor blockade is more likely than increased serotonergic or muscarinic mechanisms to be the etiology.[17]

In the setting of therapeutic use, the risk of seizures with TCAs is low, between 0.4% and 2%.[16] However, clomipramine may have a higher risk than other TCAs. At doses less than 250 mg/day, the incidence was 0.5%;

at doses greater than 250 mg/day, the rate was 1.66%. When given to patients with obsessive compulsive disorder, the rate was 3%.[16]

In overdose situations, seizures appear to be more commonly seen. A Californian 2003 retrospective review of 386 poisoning cases resulting in seizures found 7.7% of these cases were associated with TCAs.[18] A similar study from this database in 1993 found TCAs accounted for 24.6% of cases. This decrease in number of poisonings due to TCAs is likely indicative of changing prescribing patterns.[18] In another retrospective review of 1561 patients admitted to a hospital in Turkey, 1.6% had seizures. Of those patients who experienced seizures, TCAs were the most common agent ingested ($n = 11$; 42%). Status epilepticus was present in 6 patients, and mechanical ventilation was necessary in 12 patients.[19] Supportive measures are usually needed with significant overdoses. Activated charcoal is usually advocated to prevent further absorption.[5]

Serotonin-specific Reuptake Inhibitors

Seizures and movement disorders are the two most common neurotoxicities reported with SSRIs. Rhabdomyolysis has been reported in only three subjects enrolled in an exercise trial. However, these were the only patients enrolled in the study taking SSRIs.[20]

Seizures

Generally, the risk of seizures with SSRIs is low (0.1%) and uniform across agents in this class.[16] In a comparison of data from Phase II and III clinical trials of antidepressants from 1985 to 2004, seizures were seen with small numbers of patients taking SSRIs: citalopram (0.3%), fluoxetine (0.2%), and paroxetine (0.07%). Escitalopram and sertraline were not associated with any seizures in this comparison. In this analysis, except for immediate-release bupropion, antidepressants were not statistically associated with seizures.[21] However, because these trials were highly controlled studies leading to U.S. Food and Drug Administration approval, most excluded patients with seizure histories.

To more carefully examine the risk of increased seizures in patients with epilepsy, four small trials have been conducted. A small, open-label study of 39 patients with epilepsy who started on citalopram did not find a seizure worsening; in fact, these patients saw an improvement in seizure frequency.[22] A second small, uncontrolled study of 17 patients with epilepsy initiated fluoxetine. All patients showed an improvement in seizures, and 6 of them had cessation of seizures.[23] Conversely, a prospective study of 100 adults with epilepsy who were started on sertraline found an increase in seizures in 6 patients.[24] One small, retrospective study of 36 children with epilepsy examined the risk of seizures with SSRI initiation.

Only 2 patients had worsening of seizures after starting SSRI treatment.[3]

Movement Disorders

A review of the literature by Gerber and Lynd revealed 127 reports of movement disorders associated with SSRI use.[25] The frequency of each disorder was as follows: akathisia, 24%; parkinsonism, 20%; dystonia, 15%; dyskinesia, 9%; bruxism, 8%; and tardive dyskinesia, 5%.[25] Tremor, myoclonus, restless legs syndrome, and tics have also been reported.[26–30]

A series of 21 patients who developed tremor while taking fluoxetine was reported. All patients developed a postural tremor. Onset was a mean of 54.3 days after treatment began. Tremor resolved in 10 patients at a mean of 35.5 days. The other 11 patients continued to have a tremor for more than 449 days.[27] Paroxetine has also been associated with tremor in 2 patients.[28]

In some studies, onset of, or worsening of, restless legs syndrome appears to be associated with SSRI use.[31–33] However, in other studies, SSRIs either have no effect on[34] or improve symptoms.[33] In one large, cross-sectional study, SSRI use was associated with developing restless legs syndrome (odds ratio 3.11, 95% confidence interval 1.66 to 5.79).[31] In one study of 66 patients treated with SSRIs for depression, 43 of whom had restless legs syndrome, 30 reported an improvement in restless legs symptoms; however, two patients who were previously free of restless legs syndrome developed it with SSRI initiation.[33]

Poisoning

The Toxic Exposure Surveillance System of the American Association of Poison Control Centers reported 48,204 ingestions of SSRIs in 2004. Main symptoms include central nervous system depression, seizures, cardiac electrical abnormalities, tremor, and serotonin syndrome.[5,35] Most symptoms occur within 4 hours of ingestion.[35]

SSRIs are considerably safer than TCAs in overdose situations. The fatal toxicity index (number of deaths per million prescriptions) is 2.02 to 13.4 for SSRIs compared to 19.1 to 34.14 for TCAs.[36,37] Seizures respond well to benzodiazepines.[5]

Other Antidepressants

Other antidepressants have been associated with neurotoxicity. Bupropion has been most associated with seizures, but a few movement disorders have also been reported. The serotonin and norepinephrine reuptake inhibitors, duloxetine and venlafaxine, have been only rarely associated with seizures outside of overdose situations. Mirtazapine has been implicated in movement disorders and rhabdomyolysis. Of the serotonin 2 receptor antagonists, trazodone and nefazodone, only nefazodone has been associated with rhabdomyolysis when used with simvastatin.

Bupropion

Soon after the introduction of bupropion, case reports of seizures began to emerge. Several case series and retrospective studies followed, establishing the link between immediate-release bupropion and seizures. A series of 279 patients admitted to the emergency department with new-onset seizures was reviewed. Of these, 1.4% were attributed to bupropion.[38] Higher doses (more than 450 mg/day) of immediate-release bupropion were associated with double the amount of seizures compared to lower doses.[40] Women were also more likely to have bupropion-related seizures than men.[40] Patients with bulimia may be predisposed to developing seizures when treated with bupropion, with an incidence of 15%.[41] Although no mechanism is known for this increased risk, bupropion should not be used in patients with bulimia.

Due to this increased risk of seizures, bupropion was reformulated as a sustained-release product to prevent higher peak concentrations that were thought to be associated with seizures in the immediate-release form.[16] In one study, the incidence of seizures in the immediate-release formulation was 0.4% while it was approximately 0.1% for the sustained-release formulation.[16] In a comparison of data from Phase II and III clinical trials of antidepressants from 1985 to 2004, bupropion immediate release ranked highest in number of seizures (0.6%). In comparison, bupropion sustained release ranked fifth (0.1%).[21] However, case reports of seizures, including status epilepticus, following extended-release bupropion administration and overdose exist.[42-44]

In seizures occurring in overdose situations, bupropion is well represented. A 2003 retrospective review of 386 poisoning cases resulting in seizures in California found 23% of cases were associated with bupropion.[18]

Movement disorders with bupropion are uncommon. Three case reports associate parkinsonism with bupropion use.[45,46] An additional two cases report dyskinesia in patients taking bupropion.[47,48]

Serotonin and Norepinephrine Reuptake Inhibitors

In clinical trials, duloxetine and venlafaxine had a low incidence of seizures (0.2% and 0.3%, respectively). No seizures occurred in these trials with extended-release venlafaxine.[16] However, 5.9% of seizures from a 2003 retrospective review of 386 poisoning cases were associated with venlafaxine.[18]

A separate review of 184 patients who overdosed on venlafaxine revealed 8.9% of patients experienced a seizure. Patients with seizures had higher creatine kinase serum concentrations than those who did not have seizures (mean concentration 317 U/L versus 91 U/L, respectively; $p < 0.001$). However, the creatine kinase serum concentration was increased with the increase in the amount of venlafaxine ingested in patients who did not have seizures. In the group that did not experience seizures, 43 patients (25.7%) had a creatine kinase serum concentration greater than 150 U/L and 6 patients (3.6%) had a creatine kinase serum concentration greater than 1000 U/L. Some elevations were not seen until after 12 hours following the ingestion.[49] This review suggests that creatine kinase concentrations may increase in venlafaxine overdose independently of seizures. Presumably, rhabdomyolysis may also be seen clinically, although it was not discussed in this report.

Mirtazapine

Movement disorders including akathisia, dystonia, and tremor have been seen in patients receiving mirtazapine.[50-52] In the two reported akathisia patients, mirtazapine was continued, with concomitant clonazepam in one case and with a reduced dose of mirtazapine in the other case.[50]

Three cases of rhabdomyolysis have been reported with mirtazapine. One case occurred after therapeutic doses[53] and the other two after overdose.[52,54]

Serotonin 2 Receptor Antagonists

Rhabdomyolysis has also been reported in patients treated with nefazodone in conjunction with simvastatin. Nefazodone is an inhibitor of the cytochrome P450 enzyme CYP3A4, which metabolizes simvastatin. This combination of medications increases simvastatin serum concentrations about 20 times.[55-58] Of the statin drugs, only fluvastatin is significantly metabolized by an enzyme other than CYP3A4; it is metabolized by CYP2C9, making it the preferred statin in a patient treated with nefazadone.[58]

ANTIPSYCHOTICS

Antipsychotic agents are commonly categorized into conventional, or "typical," antipsychotics and second-generation, or "atypical," antipsychotics (Table 2). This classification is based on the medications' mechanisms of action and adverse effect profiles. The conventional antipsychotics are notorious for their risk of drug-induced movement disorders, or extrapyramidal symptoms (EPSs). The newer agents are much less likely to cause EPSs[59]; however, there are differences in the rate of occurrence of EPSs among the agents in this class.[60] The typical agents can be divided into high-potency and low-potency medications (see Table 2). High-potency agents have more EPSs, while low-potency agents cause more sedative, hypotensive, and autonomic effects.

With regard to neurotoxicity, EPSs are the most common, troublesome, and notable drug effects. However,

Table 2:   Classification of Antipsychotics

Typical			Atypical
High Potency	**Medium Potency**	**Low Potency**	
Fluphenazine	Mesoridazine	Chlorpromazine	Aripiprazole
Haloperidol	Perphenazine	Thioridazine	Clozapine
Loxapine			Olanzapine
Molindone			Quetiapine
Pemozide			Risperidone
Thiothixene			Ziprasidone
Trifluoperazine			

neuroleptic malignant syndrome and ischemic stroke are serious neurological effects that may occur with this class of medications. The usual EPSs are acute dystonia, akathisia, parkinsonism, and tardive dyskinesia.[61] EPSs can be categorized into two groups separated by time of symptom onset. The first group includes acute dystonia, akathisia, and parkinsonism. These toxicities manifest with initial drug administration or early in drug treatment. The second group, tardive dyskinesias or dystonias, presents only after long-term use of antipsychotic medications.

Acute Dystonias

Acute dystonias are characterized by dystonic movements of the tongue, face, neck, limbs, extraocular muscles, or back. The patient's facial grimacing, torticollis, or oculogyric crisis may be misinterpreted as a hysterical reaction or seizure. The rates of dystonia range from 2.3% to 90% across all patients treated with antipsychotics.[62] Haloperidol and other high-potency medications are reported to cause dystonias in 30% to 40% of patients.[62] Men are more commonly affected than women.[62] Patients treated with these medications are at greatest risk of these effects in the first 1 to 5 days of treatment.

Patients affected with acute dystonias respond to parenteral anticholinergic agents, such as benztropine or diphenhydramine. These medications or other anticholinergics should be continued by oral administration for days to weeks after the initial symptoms. If continued antipsychotic therapy is necessary, the anticholinergic may be continued as an oral medication.

Akathisia

Akathisia is manifested by an inability to remain in a seated posture secondary to motor restlessness and a sensation of muscle quivering. Patients have an overwhelming need to be constant motion. Because of this internal sensation, patients may pace and appear agitated or psychotic. These behaviors may lead to further use of the precipitating drug; therefore, the proper diagnosis of this toxic manifestation is critical. Patients are often noncompliant with their antipsychotics if they experience significant akathisia while taking it, increasing the need for accurate identification of this toxicity.[62]

Onset of symptoms is typically within the first 14 days of antipsychotic use.[62] Akathisia is more common with high-potency antipsychotics, where rates can be as low as 8% or as high as 76%.[62] For treatment, anticholinergics can be used but are often only partially effective; therefore, dose reduction or drug substitution is often required. Patients may also respond to antianxiety agents, such as benzodiazepines or propranolol.[63]

Parkinsonism

A parkinsonian syndrome induced by antipsychotics is often distinguishable from idiopathic Parkinson's disease only by the patient's history and careful medication review. Patients will have a generalized slowing of volitional movement (bradykinesia) with masked facies and reduction in arm movements. Most notable is patients' stereotypical resting tremor with easily appreciated rigidity on examination. Onset of symptoms is typically within the first week of treatment initiation, but symptoms may evolve slowly over days to weeks.[62] As with other EPSs, it is more common with high-potency medications.

Treatment for parkinsonism typically includes anticholinergics or amantadine. Direct dopamine agonists or levodopa may exacerbate patients' underlying psychiatric illness.[62] Discontinuation of the antipsychotic may improve or resolve symptoms; however, symptoms have been reported in 11% of affected patients 1 year after discontinuation.[62]

Tardive Dyskinesia

Tardive dyskinesia clinically presents as stereotypical, repetitive, involuntary, ticlike choreiform movements of the face, eyelids, mouth, tongue, extremities, or trunk. Patients may also have slower athetosis or twisting movements, sustained dystonic postures, or akathisia. As the name tardive implies, this is a dyskinesia that occurs late, after months or years of neuroleptic use.

Patients taking typical antipsychotics are commonly affected, with a median occurrence rate of 24%. Tardive dyskinesia has been reported more commonly in women in some studies; however, this association is inconsistent.[64,65] Elderly patients are more commonly affected.[62] In one study, the rate of tardive dyskinesia was six times higher in patients over 55 years of age compared to younger patients.[66] Higher rates are reported in African American and lower rates in Asian populations.[62] The mechanism by which tardive dyskinesia occurs is not clearly defined. It is proposed that with antipsychotic-induced dopamine blockade a compensatory increase occurs in dopamine neurotransmission in the basal ganglia due to an up-regulation and increased sensitivity of dopamine receptors.

Discontinuation of the offending agent is often not practicable, as this patient population has required maintenance with antipsychotic medications for a long period. Even with discontinuation of the causative agent, patients' symptoms only gradually improve over several months, if ever. A younger age at onset has a more favorable prognosis, if the antipsychotic can be discontinued.[62] Dyskinesias may be diminished by changing to an atypical antipsychotic. Many other agents to improve dyskinesias have been attempted, but little success has been observed.[62] In conclusion, prevention or early detection of this neurological syndrome is critical, as treatment is not very effective.

Neuroleptic Malignant Syndrome

Neuroleptic malignant syndrome is a rare, but life-threatening, disorder characterized by fever, muscular rigidity, altered mental status, and autonomic dysfunction.[62] Creatine kinase may be elevated due to the muscle rigidity and may lead to rhabdomyolysis. Onset of symptoms is likely to occur within weeks of drug administration and can persist for days after stopping the neuroleptic. Overall incidence of neuroleptic malignant syndrome is about 0.2% of those treated with neuroleptics. The mortality is between 4% to 30%[67] but can be significantly decreased with early recognition, close monitoring, and aggressive treatment.

Treatment consists primarily of early recognition, discontinuation of triggering drugs, management of fluid balance, temperature reduction, and monitoring for complications.[68] Antipyretics and cooling blankets can help in temperature reduction. Aggressive intravenous hydration with normal saline should be used to correct dehydration and prevent acute renal failure secondary to rhabdomyolysis. Closely monitor kidney function, electrolytes, creatine kinase, and white blood cell count. In serious cases in which pharmacological treatment is necessary, dopamine agonists and dantrolene, a direct-acting muscle relaxant, may be used. If patients' symptoms are recognized early, dopamine agonist administration may prevent further progression of this potentially lethal syndrome. Dantrolene is also successful in treatment of symptoms and can be given parenterally. A review by Pelonero et al. concluded that most neuroleptic malignant syndrome patients have resolution of symptoms within 2 to 14 days without any notable sequelae.[68] In those who do have sequelae, these are not typically attributed to neuroleptic malignant syndrome itself but rather extreme hyperthermia, hypoxia, or other complications of the syndrome.

Ischemic Stroke

Antipsychotics have been associated with a statistically significant increased risk of stroke in patients with dementia in meta-analyses. This effect was originally reported with atypical agents.[69,70] However, typical agents also appear to increase stroke risk.[71–73]

LITHIUM

Despite other therapeutic options for bipolar disorder, lithium continues to be used often and neurological manifestations of toxicity are common. The therapeutic range for serum concentrations is narrow (0.6 to 1.2 mEq/L). The amount of lithium in cerebrospinal fluid or in the cerebral tissues may be quite different from the amount in the serum.[74] In addition, the elimination of lithium is closely correlated with renal function and averages about 20% of the glomerular filtration rate. Thus, dehydration, low-salt diets, diuretics, and nonsteroidal antiinflammatory medications have all been shown to decrease lithium elimination and lead to potential toxicity.[75] All of these factors lead to difficulty in maintaining patients at therapeutic serum concentrations without causing toxicity. Patients may exhibit symptoms of acute toxicity from overdoses, chronic ingestion, or from changes in elimination of lithium. Patients may also experience a persistent state dubbed syndrome of irreversible lithium-effectuated neurotoxicity (SILENT) following acute symptoms. In addition, a myasthenia gravis–like condition has been described with lithium use.

Acute Toxicity

Symptoms can range from mild (tremor, nausea, diarrhea, blurred vision, vertigo, confusion, ataxia, fatigue, apathy, and hyperreflexia) to severe (seizures, coma, cardiac dysrhythmia, and renal failure), and may cause death.[76] The encephalopathic picture includes altered mental status, dysarthria, ataxia, and nystagmus.[77] Postural and action tremors are the most common neurotoxic symptoms, and they may occur at serum concentrations in the higher therapeutic range. Choreoathetosis, tardive dystonia, and peripheral axonal neuropathy that improved after lithium cessation have been rarely observed.[78–80] In one report, a patient developed neuroleptic malignant syndrome with fever, tachypnea, muscle rigidity, rhabdomyolysis, acute renal insufficiency, mental confusion, and obtundation 10 days after an acute lithium overdose when his serum lithium concentration was 0.5 mEq/L.[74]

Treatment of Acute Toxicity

Treatment following acute lithium toxicity is aimed at decreasing serum lithium concentrations. In the case of overdose, gastric lavage or induced emesis may remove any undissolved medications; however, activated charcoal does not bind lithium and is not thought to be helpful in this situation. In patients with serious symptoms or lithium serum concentrations greater than 4 mEq/L, hemodialysis is recommended.[76] Peritoneal dialysis has also been effective.[81] It should be recognized that after ingestion of sustained-release formulations the peak serum concentrations may be delayed for 2 to 12 hours.[75,76] Following hemodialysis, rebound redistribution into the serum occurs. Thus, a 6- to 8-hour postdialysis serum concentration should be obtained, and further dialysis sessions may be necessary.[75] Elevated serum concentrations as late as 33 to 40 hours have been reported.[76]

Myasthenic Syndrome

A disorder of the neuromuscular junction has been reported after lithium administration at therapeutic serum concentrations. In six reported cases, four remitted after lithium cessation.[82–85] In two cases, symptoms of myasthenia gravis continued after stopping lithium and lithium apparently worsened subclinical cases of myasthenia gravis.[83,86] Patients with this syndrome experience weakness and fatigability, and when repetitive stimulation has been conducted, decremental response has been demonstrated. The mechanism by which lithium may cause myasthenic symptoms is unknown but may involve decreased acetylcholine synthesis or decreased numbers of acetylcholine receptors.[86,87]

Syndrome of Irreversible Lithium-Effectuated Neurotoxicity

Several cases and two case series of long-lasting cerebellar toxicity have been reported following acute toxicity.[77,88] Symptoms may include ataxic scanning articulation, truncal ataxia, broad-based ataxic gait, coarse finger-to-nose and heel-to-shin movements, dysdiadochokinesia, tremor, and dementia. The degree of serum lithium concentration elevation did not appear to be correlated with development of SILENT, and some patients developed problems with concentrations within the therapeutic range. Common conditions to these patients were somatic illness, dehydration, fever, renal dysfunction, and diuretic use; however, none of these apparently predisposing factors were present in all cases.[77,88]

Patients with SILENT commonly have cerebellar atrophy. Pathological findings may include extensive demyelination in peripheral nerves, loss of Purkinje cells with sparing of the surrounding basket cells, or gliosis of the cerebellar cortex. Elevated core body temperatures may contribute to loss of Purkinje cells, because this is also a common finding in neuroleptic malignant syndrome.[88,89]

The cerebellar toxicity of SILENT may be irreversible. Improvement is often seen in the first 6 to 12 months but only rarely after that. No evidence shows that hemodialysis for acute intoxication prevents permanent neurotoxicity.[89]

CONCLUSION

With the common use of psychiatric medications, particularly antidepressants, in the U.S. population, the neurotoxicities associated with these agents are more often encountered. The practitioner should be aware of the neurological issues surrounding antidepressants, antipsychotics, and lithium. With appropriate caution, some of these adverse effects may be preventable or detected early.

REFERENCES

1. National Center for Health Statistics. Health, United States, 2007: Chartbook on Trends in the Health of Americans. Hyattsville, Md: Department of Health and Human Services; 2007:88.

2. Degner D, Grohmann R, Kropp S, et al. Severe adverse drug reactions of antidepressants: results of the German multicenter drug surveillance program AMSP. *Pharmacopsychiatry*. 2004;37 (Suppl 1):S39–S45.

3. Thome-Souza MS, Kuczynski E, Valente KD. Sertraline and fluoxetine: safe treatments for children and adolescents with epilepsy and depression. *Epilepsy Behav*. 2007;10:417–425.

4. Coupland NJ, Bell CJ, Potokar JP. Serotonin reuptake inhibitor withdrawal. *J Clin Psychopharmacol*. 1996;16:356–362.

5. Sarko J. Antidepressants, old and new: a review of their adverse effects and toxicity in overdose. *Pharamcol Adv Emerg Med*. 2000;18:637–654.

6. Shelton RC. The nature of the discontinuation syndrome associated with antidepressant drugs. *J Clin Psychiatry*. 2006;67 (Suppl 4):3–7.

7. Black DW, Shea C, Dursun S, et al. Selective serotonin reuptake inhibitor discontinuation syndrome: proposed diagnostic criteria. *J Psychiatry Neurosci*. 2000;25:255–261.

8. Schatzberg AF, Haddad P, Kaplan EM, et al. Serotonin reuptake inhibitor discontinuation syndrome: a hypothetical definition. Discontinuation Consensus Panel. *J Clin Psychiatry*. 1997;58 (Suppl 7):5–10.

9. Rosenbaum JF, Fava M, Hoog SL, et al. Selective serotonin reuptake inhibitor discontinuation syndrome: a randomized clinical trial. *Biol Psychiatry*. 1998;44:77–87.

10. Isbister GK, Buckley NA. Clomipramine and neuroleptic malignant syndrome: literature on adverse reactions to psychotropic drugs continues to confuse. *BMJ*. 2005;330:790–791.

11. Haddow AM, Harris D, Wilson M, Logie H. Clomipramine-induced neuroleptic malignant syndrome and pyrexia of unknown origin. *BMJ*. 2004;329:1333–1335.

12. Ames D. Ecstasy, the serotonin syndrome, and neuroleptic malignant syndrome: a possible link? *JAMA*. 1993;269:869.

13. Sternbach H. The serotonin syndrome. *Am J Psychiatry*. 1991;148:705–713.

14. Lane R, Baldwin D. Selective serotonin reuptake inhibitor–induced serotonin syndrome: review. *J Clin Psychopharmacol*. 1997;17:208–221.

15. Unverir P, Atilla R, Karcioglu O, et al. A retrospective analysis of antidepressant poisonings in the emergency department: 11-year experience. *Hum Exper Toxicol*. 2006;25:605–612.

16. Montgomery SA. Antidepressants and seizures: emphasis on newer agents and clinical implications. *Int J Clin Pract*. 2005;59:1435–1440.

17. Ago J, Ishikawa T, Matsumoto N, et al. Mechanism of imipramine-induced seizures in amygdale-kindled rats. *Epilepsy Res*. 2006;72:1–9.

18. Thundiyil JG, Kearney TE, Olson KR. Evolving epidemiology of drug-induced seizures reported to a poison control center system. *J Med Toxicol*. 2007;3:15–19.

19. Citak A, Soysal DD, Ucsel R, et al. Seizures associated with poisoning in children: tricyclic antidepressant intoxication. *Pediatr Intern* 2006;48:582–585.

20. Labotz M, Wolff TK, Nakasone KT, et al. Selective serotonin reuptake inhibitors and rhabdomyolysis after eccentric exercise. *Med Sci Sports Exerc*. 2006;38:1539–1542.

21. Alper K, Schwartz KA, Kolts RL, Khan A. Seizure incidence in psychopharmacological clinical trials: an analysis of Food and Drug Administration (FDA) summary basis of approval reports. *Biol Psychiatry*. 2007;62:345–354.

22. Specchio LM, Iudice A, Specchio N, et al. Citalopram as treatment of depression in patients with epilepsy. *Clin Neuropharmacol*. 2004;27:133–136.

23. Favale E, Rubino V, Mainardi P, et al. Anticonvulsant effect of fluoxetine in humans. *Neurology*. 1995;45:1926–1927.

24. Kanner AM, Kozak AM, Frey M. The use of sertraline in patients with epilepsy: is it safe? *Epilepsy Behav*. 2000;1:100–105.

25. Gerber PE, Lynd LD. Selective serotonin reuptake inhibitor–induced movement disorders. *Ann Pharmacother*. 1998;32:692–698.

26. Ghika-Schmid F, Ghika J, Vuadens P, et al. Acute reversible myoclonic encephalopathy associated with fluoxetine therapy. *Mov Disord*. 1997;12:622–623.

27. Serrano-Duenas M. Fluoxetine-induced tremor: clinical features in 21 patients. *Parkinsonism Relat Disord*. 2002;8:325–327.

28. Lai H, Tolat R. Paroxetine-related tremor: while this SSRI can significantly improve mood, its adverse effect warrants second look. *Geriatrics*. 2005;60:18–20.

29. Altindag A, Yanik M, Asoglu M. The emergence of tics during escitalopram and sertraline treatment. *Int Clin Psychopharmacol*. 2005;20:177–178.

30. Ghanizadeh A. Sertraline and tic: case report. *Pharmacopsychiatry*. 2007;40:289–290.

31. Ohayon MM, Roth T. Prevalence of restless legs syndrome and periodic limb movement disorder in the general population. *J Psychosom Res*. 2002;534:547–554.

32. Leutgeb U, Martus P. Regular intake of non-opioid analgesics is associated with an increased risk of restless legs syndrome in patients maintained on antidepressants. *Eur J Med Res*. 2002;7:368–378.

33. Dimmitt SB, Riley GJ. Selective serotonin reuptake inhibitors can reduce restless legs symptoms. *Arch Intern Med*. 2000;160:712.

34. Brown LK, Dedrick DL, Doggett JW, Guido PS. Antidepressant medication use and restless legs syndrome in patients presenting with insomnia. *Sleep Med*. 2005;6:443–450.

35. Nelson LS, Erdman AR, Booze LL, et al. Selective serotonin reuptake inhibitor poisoning: an evidence-based consensus guideline for out-of-hospital management. *Clin Toxicol*. 2007;45:315–332.

36. Buckley NA, McManus PR. Can the fatal toxicity of antidepressant reactions be predicted with pharmacological and toxicological data? *Drug Saf*. 1998;18:369–381.

37. Henry JA, Alexander CA, Sener EK. Relative mortality from overdose of antidepressants. *BMJ*. 1995;310:221–224.

38. Pesola GR, Avasarala J. Bupropion seizure proportion among new-onset generalized seizures and drug-related seizures presenting to an emergency department. *J Emerg Med*. 2002;22:235–239.

39. Shepherd G. Adverse effects associated with extra doses of bupropion. *Pharmacotherapy*. 2005;25:1378–1382.

40. Davidson J. Seizures and bupropion: a review. *J Clin Psychiatry*. 1989;50:256–261.

41. Horne RL, Fergusson JM, Pope HG, et al. Treatment of bulimia with bupropion: a multicenter controlled trial. *J Clin Psychiatry*. 1988;49:262–266.

42. Rissmiller DJ, Campo T. Extended-release bupropion-induced grand mal seizures. *J Am Osteopath Assoc*. 2007;107:441–442.

43. Rosoff DM. Another case of extended-release bupropion-induced seizure. *J Am Osteopath Assoc*. 2008;108:189–190.

44. Morazin F, Lumbroso A, Harry P, et al. Cardiogenic shock and status epilepticus after massive bupropion overdose. *Clin Toxicol*. 2007;45:794–797.

45. Grandas F, Lopez-Manzaneres L. Bupropion-induced parkinsonism. *Mov Disord*. 2007;22:1830–1831.

46. Szuba MP, Leuchter AF. Falling backward in two elderly patients taking bupropion. *J Clin Psychiatry*. 1992;53:157–159.

47. Kohen I. Mirtazapine in bupropion-induced dyskinesias: a case report. *Mov Disord*. 2006;21:584–585.

48. Gardos G. Reversible dyskinesia during bupropion therapy. *J Clin Psychiatry*. 1997;58:218.

49. Wilson AD, Howell C, Waring WS. Venlafaxine ingestion is associated with rhabdomyolysis in adults: a case series. *J Toxicol Sci.* 2007;32:97–101.

50. Girishchandra BG, Johnson L, Cresp RM, Orr KGD. Mirtazapine-induced akathisia. *Med J Aust.* 2002;176:242.

51. Lu R, Hurley AD, Gourley M. Dystonia induced by mirtazapine. *J Clin Psychiatry.* 2002;63:452–453.

52. Kuliwaba A. Non-lethal mirtazapine overdose with rhabdomyolysis. *Aust NZ J Psychiatry.* 2005;39:312–313.

53. Khandata AB, Nurnberger JI, Shekhar A. Possible mirtazapine-induced rhabdomyolysis. *Ann Pharmacother.* 2004;38:1321.

54. Retz W, Maier S, Maris F, Rosler M. Non-fatal mirtazapine overdose. *Int Clin Psychopharmacol.* 1998;13:277–279.

55. Thompson M, Samuels S. Rhabdomyolysis with simvastatin and nefazodone. *Am J Psychiatry.* 2002;159:1607.

56. Skrabal MZ, Stading JA, Monaghan MS. Rhabdomyolysis associated with simvastatin–nefazodone therapy. *South Med J.* 2003;96:1034–1035.

57. Jacobsen RH, Wang P, Glueck CJ. Myositis and rhabdomyolysis associated with concurrent use of simvastatin and nefazodone. *JAMA.* 1997;277:296–297.

58. Karnik NS, Maldonado JR. Antidepressant and statin interactions: a review and case report of simvastatin and nefazodone-induced rhabdomyolysis and transaminitis. *Psychosomatica.* 2005;46:565–568.

59. Leucht S, Wahlbeck K, Hamann J. New generation antipsychotics versus low-potency conventional antipsychotics: a systematic review and meta-analysis. *Lancet.* 2003;361:1581–1589.

60. Gao K, Kemp DE, Ganocy SJ, et al. Antipsychotic-induced extrapyramidal side effects in bipolar disorder and schizophrenia: a systematic review. *J Clin Psychopharmacol.* 2008;28:203–209.

61. Haddad PM, Dursun SM. Neurological complications of psychiatric drugs: clinical features and management. *Hum Psychopharmacol Clin Exp.* 2008;23:15–26.

62. Sachdev PS. Neuroleptic-induced movement disorders: an overview. *Psychiatr Clin North Am.* 2005;28:255–274.

63. Lipinski JF Jr, Zubenko GS, Cohen BM, Barreira PJ. Propranolol in the treatment of neuroleptic-induced akathisia. *Am J Psychiatry.* 1984;141:412–415.

64. Yassa R, Jeste DV. Gender differences in tardive dyskinesia: a critical review of the literature. *Schizophr Bull.* 1992;18(4):701–715.

65. van Os J, Walsh E, van Horn E, et al. Tardive dyskinesia in psychosis: are women really more at risk? *Acta Psychiatr Scand.* 1999;99:288–293.

66. Saltz BL, Woener MG, Kane JM, et al. A prospective study of tardive dyskinesia incidence in the elderly. *JAMA.* 1991;66:2402–2406.

67. Andreassen MD, Pedersen S. Malignant neuroleptic syndrome: a review of epidemiology, risk factors, diagnosis, differential diagnosis and pathogenesis of MNS. *Ugeskr Laeger.* 2000;162:1366–1370.

68. Pelonero AL, Levenson JL, Pandurangi AK. Neuroleptic malignant syndrome: a review. *Psychiatr Serv.* 1998;49:1163–1172.

69. Schneider LS, Dagerman KS, Insel P. Risk of death with atypical antipsychotic drug treatment for dementia: meta-analysis of randomized placebo-controlled trials. *JAMA.* 2005;294:1934–1943.

70. Schneider LS, Dagerman K, Insel PS. Efficacy and adverse effects of atypical antipsychotics for dementia: meta-analysis of randomized placebo-controlled trials. *Am J Geriatr Psychiatry.* 2006;14:191–210.

71. Gill SS, Rochon PA, Hermann N, et al. Atypical antipsychotic drugs and risk of ischaemic stroke: population-based retrospective cohort study. *BMJ.* 2005;330:445–448.

72. Hermann N, Mamdani M, Lanctot KLK. Atypical antipsychotics and risk of cerebrovascular accidents. *Am J Psychiatry.* 2004;151:1113–1115.

73. Wang PS, Schneeweisee S, Avorn J, et al. Risk of death in elderly users of conventional vs. atypical antipsychotic medications. *N Engl J Med.* 2005;353:2335–2341.

74. Gill J, Singh H, Nugent K. Acute lithium intoxication and neuroleptic malignant syndrome. *Pharmacotherapy.* 2003;23:811–815.

75. Carson SW. Lithium. In: Evans WE, Schentag JJ, Jusko WJ, eds. *Applied Pharmacokinetics: Principles of Therapeutic Drug Monitoring.* 3rd ed. Vancouver, BC: Applied Therapeutics; 1992:34-1–34-36.

76. Borras-Blasco J, Sirvent AE, Navarro-Riz A, et al. Unrecognized delayed toxic lithium peak concentration in an acute poisoning with sustained release lithium product. *South Med J.* 2007;100:321–323.

77. Schou M. Long-lasting neurological sequelae after lithium intoxication. *Acta Psychiatr Scand.* 1984;70:594–602.

78. Chakrabarti S, Chand PK. Lithium-induced tardive dystonia. *Neurol India.* 2002;50:473–475.

79. Stemper B, Thurauf N, Neundorfer B, Heckmann JG. Choreoathetosis related to lithium intoxication. *Eur J Neurol.* 2003;10:743–744.

80. Johnston SRD, Burn DJ, Brooks DJ. Peripheral neuropathy associated with lithium toxicity. *J Neurol Neurosurg Psychiatry.* 1991;54:1019–1020.

81. El-Mallakh RS. Treatment of acute lithium toxicity. *Vet Hum Toxicol.* 1984;26:31–35.

82. Granacher RP. Neuromuscular problems associated with lithium. *Am J Psychiatry.* 1977;134:702.

83. Lipton ID. Myasthenia gravis unmasked by lithium carbonate. *J Clin Psychopharmacol.* 1987;7:57.

84. Neil JF, Himmelhoch JM, Licata SM. Emergence of myasthenia gravis during treatment with lithium carbonate. *Arch Gen Psychiatry.* 1976;33:1090–1092.

85. Ronziere T, Auzou P, Ozsancak C, et al. Syndrome myasthenique induit par le lithium. *Press Med.* 2000;29:1043–1044.

86. Alevizos B, Gatzonis S, Anagnostara C. Myasthenia gravis disclosed by lithium carbonate. *J Neuropsychiatry Clin Neurosci.* 2006;18:427–429.

87. Dilsaver SC. Lithium down-regulates nicotinic receptors in skeletal muscle: cause of lithium-associated myasthenic syndrome? *J Clin Psychopharmacol.* 1987;7:369–370.

88. Adityanjee, Munshi KR, Thampy A. The syndrome of irreversible lithium-effectuated neurotoxicity. *Clin Neuropharmacol.* 2005;28:38–49.

89. Niethammer M, Ford B. Permanent lithium-induced cerebellar toxicity: three cases and review of the literature. *Mov Disord.* 2007;22:570–573.

357

Neurotoxic Effects of Pharmaceutical Agents III: Neurological Agents

Kara A. Kennedy and Melody Ryan

INTRODUCTION

Pharmaceutical agents targeting the nervous system have the potential for many neurotoxic adverse effects. For these medications to exert their therapeutic effects, they must penetrate the blood–brain barrier to enter the central nervous system (CNS). The characteristics that allow drug penetration, and thus efficacy, also may produce adverse effects. This chapter describes the adverse neurological effects most commonly reported with use of common neurological medications. The two most common neurological drug classes with adverse CNS effects are anti-Parkinson's agents and antiepileptic medications. When prescribing these or any neurological drugs, the clinician must consider the potential for adverse effects. Awareness of these drugs' characteristics and potential toxic effects is crucial to making the optimal initial drug choice and maintaining appropriate vigilance throughout drug therapy. This chapter also provides insight into the management of these adverse effects.

ANTIEPILEPTIC MEDICATIONS

Because of their action on the CNS, antiepileptics have many associated neurological adverse and toxic effects. Note the distinction between neurological adverse effects, which may occur at therapeutic drug concentrations, and neurotoxic effects, which occur with drug overdose. The pharmacokinetics of these antiepileptic drugs are quite relevant in regards to neurotoxicity. The serum concentrations of these medications, particularly the older antiepileptics, are greatly affected by the individual drug properties, such as protein binding, metabolism, and drug elimination (Table 1). The relevance of these effects is described in some detail in the first subsection.

The symptoms, signs, and treatment of medication overdoses are discussed in this chapter. Benzodiazepines are the only antiepileptic medications with a specific antidote in cases of toxicity or overdose. The universal treatment for most toxicity cases is impediment of absorption, enhancement of elimination, and supportive care. The degree of aggressive treatment is tailored to the individual's symptoms and the individual drug's potential toxicities.

Keep in mind the risk of seizures with antiepileptic medication withdrawal. This risk should be considered with discontinuation of antiepileptic medications or with treatment of toxicity when serum drug concentrations lower rapidly or antagonism of the drug occurs. A slow taper or alternative drug substitution is typically recommended.

Phenytoin and Fosphenytoin

Phenytoin exerts its antiepileptic effects by prolonging the inactivation of voltage-dependent sodium channels in neuronal cell membranes.[4] Inactivation of these

Table 1: Pharmacokinetic Properties of Antiepileptic Medications[1-3]

	Therapeutic Range (μg/mL)	Elimination Half-Life (h)	Protein Binding	Elimination	CYP Enzymes
Carbamazepine	4–12	5–26 (highly variable)	75%	Hepatic	3A4 2C8 1A2 2C9
Ethosuximide	40–100	30–60	<10%	Hepatic	3A4
Gabapentin	2–20	5–7	None	Renal	—
Lamotrigine	1–15	29	55%	Hepatic	—
Levetiracetam	—	6–8 (longer in the elderly or renally impaired)	None	Renal	—
Oxcarbazepine	10–35	8–10 (active metabolite: MHD)	38% (active metabolite: MHD)	Hydroxylation, conjugation, then renal excretion	—
Pregabalin	—	6	None	Renal	—
Phenobarbital	15–40	75–120 (longer in children)	45–60%	Hepatic	2C9 2C19 CYP2EI
Phenytoin	10–20	7–24 (mean 20, dependent on serum drug level)	85–95%	Hepatic	2C9 (90%) 2C19
Tiagabine	0.001–0.234	5–9	96%	Hepatic	3A4
Topiramate	9–12	19–25	13–17%	Renal	—
Valproic acid	50–100	12–15 (adults) 14–17 (elderly) 30–60 (neonates)	85–95%	Hepatic	2C9 2C19
Zonisamide	20–30	46–69	30–60%	Hepatic ($^{2}/_{3}$), renal ($^{1}/_{3}$)	3A4

CYP, cytochrome P450; MHD, 10-monohydroxy.

channels hinders partly depolarized axons' abilities to rapidly transmit action potentials, as is needed for epileptic discharges.[5]

Phenytoin follows nonlinear, or zero order, elimination kinetics and has a narrow therapeutic index[6]; therefore, toxicity can occur with only small adjustments in drug dosage. Complicating matters further, 90% of phenytoin is bound to plasma proteins, primarily albumin (see Table 1).[7] Only the free, or nonprotein bound, drug is active. The bound drug cannot cross the blood–brain barrier, while the free drug passively crosses between plasma and cerebrospinal fluid[8]; therefore, cerebrospinal fluid phenytoin concentrations strongly correlate with free serum drug concentrations.[7] Subtle disturbances in protein-binding cause dramatic changes in the free phenytoin serum concentration, and, in turn, the active cerebrospinal fluid drug concentrations.[7] The percentage of bound drug, which ranges from 70% to 95%, is influenced by several factors, including serum albumin concentrations (nutritional status), comorbidities that affect

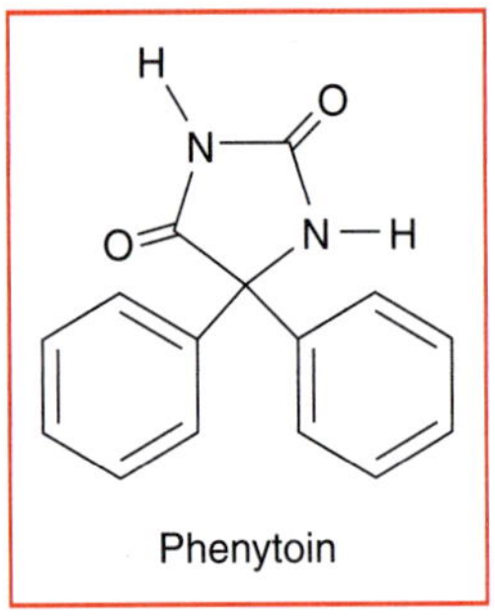

Figure 32-1. Chemical structure: phenytoin.

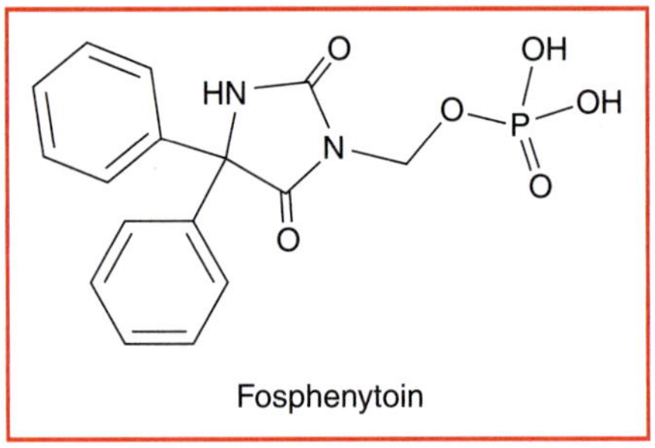

Figure 32-2. Chemical structure: fosphenytoin.

protein binding (such as uremia, renal, or hepatic disease), and use of additional medications that are highly bound to albumin.[6] Increased concentrations of free drug are also seen in neonates.[7] If a patient has evidence of toxicity while in the typically accepted therapeutic range, obtaining a free serum phenytoin concentration may be helpful.[6]

Most of the phenytoin is eliminated through hepatic metabolism by cytochrome P450 enzymes, specifically CYP2C9 and to a lesser extent CYP2C19. These enzymes are saturable, meaning that other drugs, using the same enzyme pathway, compete for metabolism. The net result can be prevention of phenytoin's metabolism, thus increasing phenytoin serum concentrations. Phenytoin metabolism is also notoriously affected by P450 enzyme inducers or inhibitors.

Due to phenytoin's poor water solubility, fosphenytoin, a water-soluble prodrug, was developed to avoid the adverse effects associated with intravenous phenytoin and its vehicles. Fosphenytoin is rapidly (8 to 15 minutes) converted into phenytoin in the liver and red blood cells.[7] Since fosphenytoin is rapidly converted to phenytoin, the signs of neurotoxicity are the same as those seen with phenytoin.[9]

A good correlation is observed between the total phenytoin concentration in plasma and the clinical effect. While the typically accepted therapeutic range of phenytoin is 10 to 20 μg/mL, therapy often must be individualized. Serum concentrations that produce toxicity vary among individuals as well; however, in general, signs and symptoms of toxicity tend to develop above plasma drug concentrations of 20 to 25 μg/mL. At this point, patients begin to manifest evidence of vestibulocerebellar disturbance.[6] Nystagmus is typically the first toxic manifestation of phenytoin. At plasma drug concentrations above 30 μg/mL, gait ataxia and diplopia are observed. At concentrations of 40 μg/mL and higher, patients become drowsy and may develop nausea and vomiting.[10] With higher concentrations, coma is possible. Occasionally, toxic concentrations of phenytoin may cause dyskinetic and dystonic involuntary

movements.[11,12] Ophthalmoplegia and impairment of color vision have been reported.[13] Lastly, paradoxical seizures have been reported at serum phenytoin concentrations greater than 30 μg/mL.[14] This effect was first reported by Levy and Fenichel in 1965.[15] Since that time, there have been infrequent case reports of paradoxical phenytoin-induced seizures associated with toxicity in the literature. Chua et al. reported three cases in which patients had serum phenytoin concentrations of 43.5, 46.5, and 38.3 μg/mL.[16] In general, this phenomenon is rare. Osorio et al. reported a review of 96 cases of phenytoin toxicity.[17] Only seven patients had seizures with supratherapeutic drug concentrations, and only two patients (2.1%) had a highly probable causal relationship between toxicity and seizure. The serum concentrations for these two patients were 93.2 and 69.7 μg/mL. In conclusion, paradoxical seizures associated with phenytoin toxicity are rare but can occur at high phenytoin concentrations.[17]

In addition, some adverse effects that appear are unrelated to dose or concentration of phenytoin. Electrophysiological evidence of peripheral neuropathy can occur many patients receiving phenytoin, but this phenomenon usually is not clinically significant.[18] Cerebellar atrophy has been reported with chronic phenytoin use.[19] Cognitive and psychological effects have also been reported. Aldenkamp et al. report impaired speed of information processing with phenytoin use.[20] Depression has been reported with phenytoin use, but the incidence is relatively low—around 1% of those treated.[21]

Phenobarbital and Primidone

Phenobarbital inhibits seizures by potentiation of synaptic inhibition through the γ-aminobutyric acid subtype A (GABA$_A$) receptor. Phenobarbital is metabolized hepatically via CYP2C9, with minor metabolism by CYP2C19 and CYP2EI.[7] The half-life of phenobarbital ranges from 75 to 120 hours after a single dose of the drug (see Table 1).[22] This long half-life makes phenobarbital users particularly vulnerable to toxic drug effects.

Phenobarbital's most common adverse effect is sedation. Almost all patients experience this effect upon initial drug use, but a tolerance develops with time. Patients tend to tolerate the drug better if they are started on a conservative initial dose with a gradual dosage increase.[23] Sedation, nystagmus, and ataxia are typically manifested at serum concentrations greater than 30 μg/mL during chronic therapy; however, during initiation or dose adjustment, these signs and symptoms of toxicity may be noted at lower serum concentrations.[7] As the serum drug concentration increases, the patient develops increased sleepiness, dysarthria, and incoordination. Higher concentrations can lead to stupor and coma. Serum drug concentrations greater than 70 μg/mL almost universally cause coma, regardless of previous experience with the medication. Death is likely to result from concentrations higher than 80 μg/mL.[24]

Children and the elderly may experience a paradoxical stimulant effect with use of phenobarbital. In one study, almost of half (n = 109) the children developed hyperactivity if treated daily with phenobarbital.[25] The mechanism for this paradoxical effect is not well defined but may be related to phenobarbital's effect on sleep organization.[26] Cognitive impairment and depression may also occur with use of phenobarbital in children.[27]

Treatment of toxic serum concentrations involves supportive therapy and enhancement of phenobarbital elimination from the body. Enhanced elimination is best accomplished through urine alkalinization and forced diuresis. Activated charcoal increases intestinal elimination of the drug.[28]

Primidone, a congener of phenobarbital, is similar to phenobarbital in its antiepileptic effects. The antiepileptic effects of primidone are secondary to primidone itself and its two active metabolites, phenobarbital and phenylethylmalonamide. Both metabolites accumulate with chronic primidone use.[7]

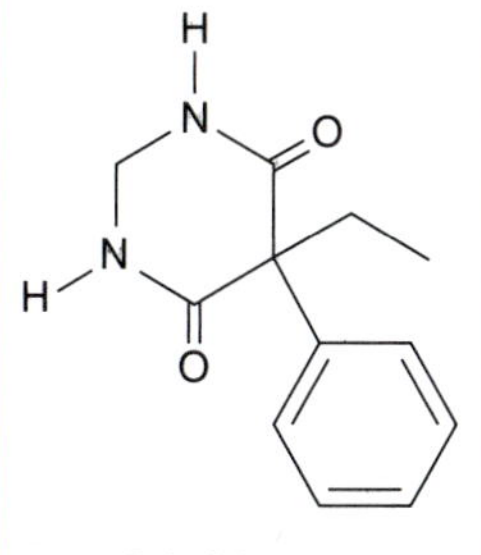

The dose required to cause adverse neurological effects is not clearly defined, as the effects are caused by both the parent drug and the active metabolites. Adverse effects are shared between phenobarbital, as discussed earlier, and primidone.

Unique to primidone, however, some patients report an acute toxicity rapidly after initial exposure, regardless of the dose. Patients may quickly develop significant drowsiness, dizziness, ataxia, nausea, and emesis directly after drug administration.[24] Some patients also report an acute sense of intoxication following dosing.[7] Rarely, an acute psychosis has been reported with primidone use.[28]

Overdose of primidone causes symptoms of CNS depression that correlate more closely with serum and cerebrospinal fluid primidone concentrations, rather than with phenobarbital or phenylethylmalonamide concentrations. Treatment includes supportive care and gastric lavage.[24]

Carbamazepine

Carbamazepine has a chemical structure closely related to the tricyclic antidepressants (Figure 32-4), but its antiepileptic effects are similar to phenytoin. It slows of the rate of recovery of voltage-activated sodium channels from inactivation.[7] Inactivation of voltage- and frequency-dependent sodium channels impairs the axons' ability to rapidly transmit action potentials, as is needed for epileptic discharges.[5] Most of the carbamazepine is converted to 10,11-carbamazepine epoxide, an active metabolite responsible for many of carbamazepine's toxic effects.[29] The accepted therapeutic concentration for seizure prevention is between 6 and 12 μg/mL.[30] Toxicity usually becomes apparent above 9 μg/mL (see Table 1).[7]

Half of patients taking carbamazepine report adverse effects, but only 5% to 10% discontinue the drug.[31] CNS effects are common with initiation of the drug but are usually mild and transient.[30] Drowsiness, vertigo, and incoordination are all common (incidence greater than 20%) symptoms with therapeutic drug doses. Diplopia, sedation, and nystagmus may also occur but are somewhat less common (reported rate of 10% to 20%). Tremor, cognitive disturbance, and headache are rarely

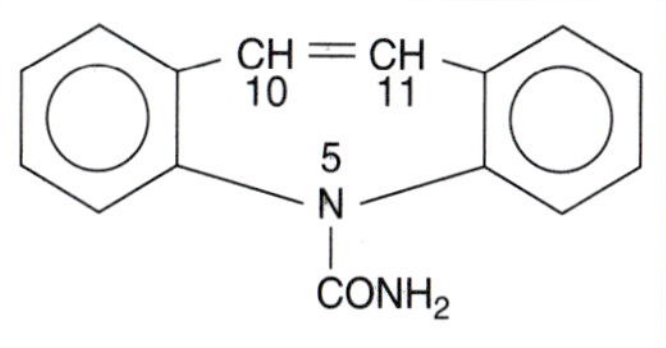

Figure 32-3. Chemical structure: primidone.

Figure 32-4. Chemical structure: carbamazepine.

reported (1% to 9%).[32] Dystonia and choreoathetosis have been reported with supratherapeutic serum drug concentrations.[33]

Acute intoxication may lead to increased seizure frequency, hyperirritability, respiratory depression, stupor, and coma.[7] The adverse effects of 30 children with carbamazepine overdose were documented as follows: lethargy (93%), ataxia (50%), coma (27%), seizures (20%), need for intubation (20%), nystagmus (13%), and minor arrhythmias (10%).[32] The smallest reported lethal ingestion in adults is 60 g. There are reports of a 6-year-old child who survived a 10-g ingestion and a 3-year-old child who survived a 5-g ingestion.[32] Weaver et al. described stages of neurotoxicity categorized by serum carbamazepine concentrations. At concentrations of 11 to 15 μg/mL, drowsiness and ataxia are evident. At concentrations between 15 and 25 μg/mL, patients experience combativeness, hallucinations, and choreiform movements. At concentrations above 25 μg/mL, patients develop seizures and coma.[34] A similar correlation was reported in 2008 by Brahmi et al., with a direct relationship between carbamazepine concentrations and Glasgow Coma Scale scores.[35] Two cases of status epilepticus after massive carbamazepine overdose have been reported.[36] Coma has been attributed, at least partly, to sodium channel suppression of neurotransmission,[35,37] whereas seizures are thought to be largely related to powerful anticholinergic effects of the drug.[38] Other concomitant anticholinergic signs reported in massive overdose include agitation, hyperreflexia, and bilateral mydriasis.[35]

Supportive care and treatment of hemodynamic instability are critical in the treatment of overdose. In addition to supportive care, carbamazepine overdose is treated by prevention of further drug absorption, as well as enhancement of drug elimination.[39] Gastric lavage and treatment with activated charcoal prevent further drug absorption.[40] Charcoal hemoperfusion and high-efficiency hemodialysis used in combination or alone are effective in significantly reducing drug concentrations.[39]

Due to the incidence of seizures with carbamazepine overdose, continuous electroencephalogram (EEG) monitoring may afford some benefit in acute treatment and in regards to prognosis.[32] Seizures should be treated with benzodiazepines and phenytoin or fosphenytoin.[32]

Oxcarbazepine

Oxcarbazepine, a keto analogue of carbamazepine, is rapidly metabolized to an active metabolite, a 10-monohydroxy derivative. Oxcarbazepine was developed to mimic the efficacy of carbamazepine while minimizing the side effects of the original drug.[41] The

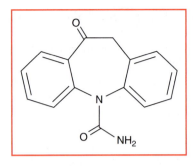

Figure 32-5. Chemical structure: oxcarbazepine.

mechanism of action is similar to carbamazepine, but unlike carbamazepine, oxcarbazepine is not metabolized to an epoxide metabolite (which is responsible for many of carbamazepine's toxic effects).[29]

The most common adverse CNS effects include headache (37%), somnolence (22%), and dizziness (20%).[42] These are mild to moderate in severity. Ataxia and diplopia have been reported but have a very low incidence (2.0% and 0.5%, respectively).[43] Six failed suicide attempts by oxcarbazepine overdose were reported by the manufacturer.[42] The symptoms in these cases of overt toxicity were reportedly magnification of the gastrointestinal and CNS adverse effects seen at therapeutic doses of the drug.[42] Few published reports show acute toxicity with oxcarbazepine. A case report by van Opstal et al. documented an overdosage of more than 100 tablets of oxcarbazepine; this patient experienced no life-threatening situations and fully recovered.[29] Again, the low incidence of adverse effects is attributed to the absence of the epoxide metabolite in oxcarbazepine metabolism.

Ethosuximide

Ethosuximide lowers the threshold calcium currents (T currents) in thalamic neurons. These currents, in turn, affect the oscillatory activity of thalamocortical neurons, which are generators of the 3-Hz spike-and-wave rhythms of patients with absence epilepsy. The drug is metabolized by CYP3A4 enzymes in the liver

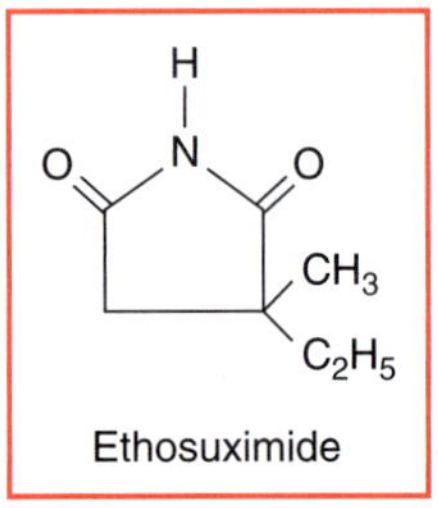

Ethosuximide

Figure 32-6. Chemical structure: ethosuximide.

and is renally excreted (see Table 1).[44] Ethosuximide's most common side effects are gastrointestinal and neurological. Drowsiness (average incidence 7%) can occur at the initiation of therapy but is easily alleviated with dose reduction. Other infrequent (less than 6% incidence) CNS-related effects include lethargy, fatigue, dizziness, ataxia, hiccoughs, headaches, and behavioral changes.[45] Headaches occur with approximately 14% of children using ethosuximide. This effect does not appear to be dose dependent and does not resolve with decreasing the dosage.[44]

Psychiatric problems, ranging from anxiety and depression to visual and auditory hallucinations, have been reported. Young adults or patients with a history of psychiatric illness are at highest risk for these adverse effects. It has been proposed that these psychiatric effects are secondary to "forced normalization" that may occur with seizure control.[44] Forced normalization is the concept that an antagonism exists between seizures and abnormal behavior. With seizure remission and normalization of electroencephalographic activity (as may occur with antiepileptic treatment), there is an increase in these patients' dysfunctional or psychotic behavior. This phenomenon was first reported by Landolt in 1953,[45a] but its existence remains controversial.[46] There has been debate about the existence of ethosuximide-induced seizures, but most studies have found no evidence for such claims.[47] With long-term ethosuximide therapy, parkinsonism has been reported.[48]

Acute overdoses of ethosuximide may present with nausea, vomiting, and CNS depression. Symptoms may progress to stupor and coma. Treatment includes supportive care, impediment of further drug absorption, and enhancement of drug elimination.[47]

Valproic Acid

Valproic acid is available in the form of valproate sodium and divalproex sodium, both of which are rapidly converted to valproic acid once administered. Valproic acid's mechanism of action appears to be related to an indirect increase in regional brain GABA levels, an inhibitory neurotransmitter.[49] It also inhibits T-type calcium channels.[50]

When valproic acid serum concentrations are within therapeutic range, CNS effects, such as somnolence and

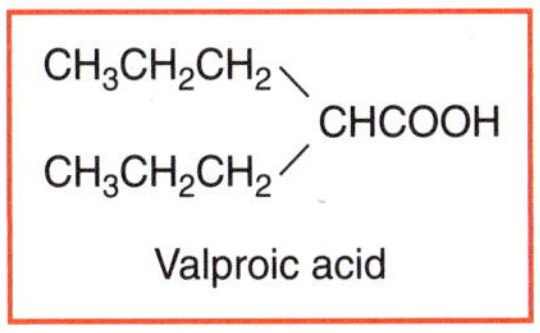

Figure 32-7. Chemical structure: valproic acid.

dizziness, occur in up to 25% of patients but are most often mild in severity and resolve with dose reduction.[51] Movement disorders, such as tremor or parkinsonism, can occur with valproic acid use. Chronic treatment with valproic acid causes symptomatic tremor in about 10% of patients.[52] The tremor may be alleviated by dosage decrease, discontinuation of the medication, or use of a symptomatic agent, such as propranolol or amantadine.[52] Parkinsonism is reported to occur in approximately 5% of patients on valproic acid.[53,54] The odds of having parkinsonism are five times higher with valproic acid than with other antiepileptic drugs.[53] The symptoms are quickly resolved by discontinuation of the medication.[53]

Rare case reports document reversible dementia and cerebral pseudoatrophy with the use of valproic acid. Papazian et al. reported two cases of children who developed severe cognitive and behavioral deterioration analogous to a neurodegenerative process with corresponding cortical and cerebellar atrophy on neuroimaging. These symptoms and the neuroimaging findings resolved after discontinuation of valproic acid.[55]

Reports exist of valproic acid–induced stupor, which are not dose related. In one study of seven patients with valproic acid–related stuporous episodes, the patients' EEG recordings revealed spike-and-wave discharges or continuous sharp theta- and delta-waves. All patients' symptoms resolved within 24 to 72 hours after discontinuation of the drug.[56] The mechanism behind these changes is not well defined.

This presentation is distinct from hyperammonemic encephalopathy. Hyperammonemic encephalopathy typically occurs during the first weeks of therapy, is manifested by excess drowsiness and lethargy, and can be directly linked to elevated ammonia levels. Ammonia concentrations should be checked in patients on valproic acid therapy who develop alterations in mental status or cognitive function.[51] Discontinuation of the drug reverses this disorder.

In frank valproic acid overdose, CNS depression may occur with progression to coma and respiratory depression. Cerebral edema and increased intracranial pressure have been reported.[57]

Management of acute valproic acid ingestion requires supportive care and close attention to the airway.[49] Gastric lavage and activated charcoal are helpful if administered early. L-carnitine supplementation decreases ammonia levels, but its exact role in valproic acid toxicity is still being defined. Intravenous L-carnitine supplementation is clearly indicated for valproic acid–induced hepatotoxicity, overdose, and other acute metabolic crises associated with carnitine deficiency.[58] A recent toxicology article by Chan et al. reports two cases of acute valproic acid poisoning with CNS depression and raised ammonia level without hepatotoxicity. For either valproic acid overdose with hyperammonemia or valproic acid–induced hyperammonemic encephalopathy and hepatotoxicity, the authors recommend administration of intravenous L-carnitine at a dose of 50 mg/kg every 8 hours for the initial 24 hours with further individual assessment.[59]

Benzodiazepines

Benzodiazepines increase $GABA_A$ receptor activity. This activity increases the frequency of channel-opening events, which increases chloride ion conductance, leads to inhibition of the action potential, and thus decreases the likelihood of seizures.[7] Benzodiazepines can be used as preventive antiepileptics or in emergent treatment of status epilepticus. Common side effects include weakness, headache, blurred vision, and vertigo. Drowsiness, lightheadedness, slowed reaction time, motor incoordination, impaired cognitive and motor function, confusion, and anterograde amnesia are well-documented effects of benzodiazepines. Benzodiazepine behavioral side effects occurred in 15% of people prescribed benzodiazepines for epilepsy in one study. The four most reported behavioral side effects were aggression, irritability, hyperactivity, and agitation.[60] Euphoria, hallucinations, and hypomanic behavior have also been reported.[7] In a so-called disinhibition reaction, patients may exhibit bizarre uninhibited behavior. Paranoia, depression, and suicidal ideation have also been reported but are rare effects and appear to be dose related.[7]

Lastly, reports point to a paradoxical proconvulsant effect with use of benzodiazepines,[61–63] but it is a rare occurrence. Lennox-Gastaut patients are particularly vulnerable to this rare paradoxical effect. It has been proposed that the benzodiazepine decrease following a peak concentration may induce a rapid EEG rhythm that is characteristic of tonic seizures.[61]

In an overdose situation, benzodiazepines have a dose-dependent ventilatory depressant effect. They also can cause a modest decrease in arterial blood pressure with a resultant increase in heart rate (due to a decrease of systemic vascular resistance). High doses of benzodiazepines can lead to severe respiratory or cardiovascular depression. However, benzodiazepine ingestions are rarely fatal unless the benzodiazepines are taken concurrently with another drug, such as ethanol.[7] Flumazenil is useful in reversing benzodiazepine-induced sedation, as well as diagnosing or treating benzodiazepine overdose.[64] However, with this rapid reversal of benzodiazepines in patients with epilepsy, seizures should be anticipated.

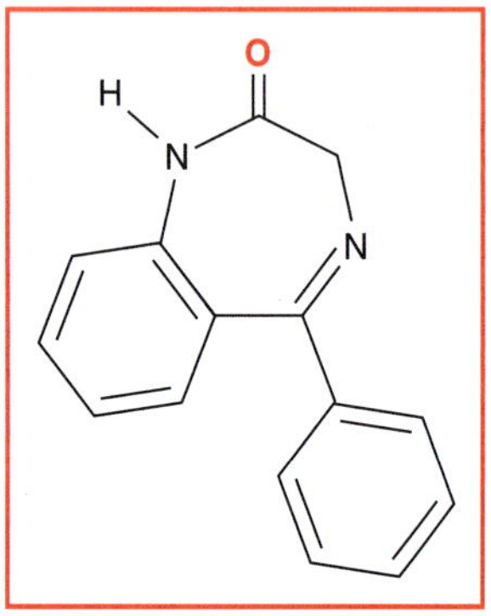

Gabapentin and Pregabalin

Structurally, gabapentin is a GABA molecule covalently bound to a lipophilic cyclohexane ring. It was designed to act centrally as a GABA agonist, but its exact mechanism of action is unknown.[7]

Overall, gabapentin is well tolerated. The most common adverse effects include somnolence, dizziness, ataxia, and fatigue. By combining the safety data from multiple placebo-controlled trials ($n = 1160$), Chadwick reported somnolence in 24.4%, dizziness in 20.3%, ataxia in 17.4%, fatigue in 14.7%, nystagmus in 15%, tremor in 15%, and diplopia in 10.7% of patients.[65] Asconapé et al. reported a 12.5% incidence of gabapentin-associated myoclonus in their chart review of 104 patients.[66] Rare cases of choreoathetosis have been reported.[67,68] Behavioral changes, such as irritability and aggression, have also been reported. These effects tend to occur in children with attention-deficit/hyperactivity disorder or developmental delay.[69] Adverse effects are typically observed within the first 1 to 2 weeks of treatment but resolve with acclimation to the drug.

Klein-Schwartz et al. reported 20 cases of gabapentin overdose, with doses ranging from 50 mg to 35 g. One-half of the cases involved children and adolescents. Of the patients, 9 developed symptoms of drowsiness, dizziness, nausea or vomiting, tachycardia, and hypotension early after ingestion. Most patients had resolution of symptoms within 10 hours. In addition, 7 cases were managed at home, with 4 patients asymptomatic. None of the patients required hospital admission.[70]

Figure 32-8. Core chemical structure: benzodiazepines.

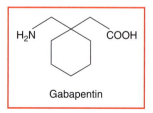

Figure 32-9. Chemical structure: gabapentin.

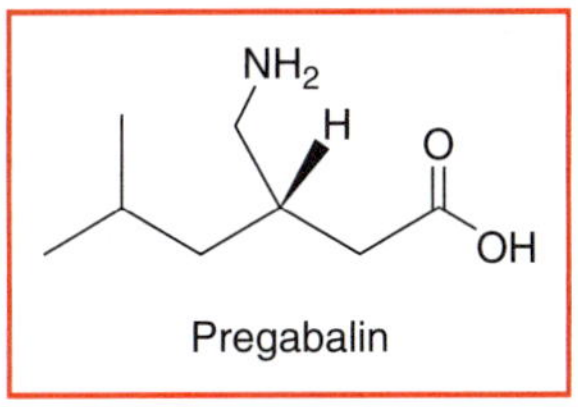

Figure 32-10. Chemical structure: pregabalin.

Pregabalin is a GABA analogue similar in structure to gabapentin (Figure 32-10). Although the exact mechanism of action is unknown, pregabalin's mechanism of action is thought to be similar to that of gabapentin.[71]

With pregabalin use, Kugler et al. reported dizziness (29%), somnolence (21%), and ataxia (13%),[72] all at incidences similar to those reported with gabapentin. Huppertz et al. reported pregabalin-induced myoclonus at a rate comparable to that seen with gabapentin.[73] The drug manufacturer reported an accidental overdose of 8 g of pregabalin with no notable clinical consequences.[74] Spiller et al. report a case of pregabalin overdose with an estimated ingestion of 1.5 g. The 59-year-old patient developed mild transient somnolence but no other adverse effects or sequelae.[75]

Lamotrigine

Lamotrigine is a phenyltriazine derivative. The mechanism of action is largely attributed to the drug's ability to delay the recovery from inactivation of recombinant sodium channels,[76] but its complete mechanism of action is not fully understood. The most common adverse neurological effects with lamotrigine use are dizziness (50%), ataxia (24%), blurred vision (23%), diplopia (33%), and somnolence (14%).[77]

Overdose with lamotrigine has been reported. Various single-case reports describe nystagmus,[78] choreiform dyskinesia,[79] stupor,[80] or drug-induced status epilepticus.[81] The largest aggregate of cases reported are from Lofton and Klein-Schwartz, who collected data reported

to the American Association of Poison Control Centers Toxic Exposure Surveillance System on single-substance exposures to lamotrigine from 2000 to 2001. Of 493 cases, most patients (52.1%) exposed to lamotrigine in overdose experienced no toxic clinical effects. The most common clinical effects reported in overdose were drowsiness or lethargy (20.9%), vomiting (11%), nausea (5.1%), ataxia (4.9%), dizziness or vertigo (4.5%), and tachycardia (4.3%). Major clinical effects included coma ($n = 6$), seizures ($n = 8$), and respiratory depression ($n = 3$). No deaths were reported.[82] Overdose has been reported in the pediatric population at a dose as low as 500 mg, or 25 mg/kg. This dose caused ataxia, drowsiness, acute confusion, emesis, and seizure exacerbation.[83]

Treatment of lamotrigine toxicity should begin with gastric lavage or activated charcoal to decrease drug absorption. Lamotrigine-induced seizures should be treated with benzodiazepines. Sodium bicarbonate can be administered to normalize serum pH. No data report on the value of hemodialysis or hemoperfusion in treatment of lamotrigine toxicity.[84]

Levetiracetam

Levetiracetam, a pyrrolidine, has an unknown mechanism of action.[7] Levetiracetam is well tolerated; the main adverse neurological effects are fatigue, impaired coordination, and behavioral disturbances. These adverse events were typically mild to moderate in severity and were reported most often within the initial 4 weeks of therapy.[85] According to the three major clinical trials done in 2000 to assess the safety and efficacy of levetiracetam, 14.7% of patients reported fatigue, 13% reported behavioral instability, and 3.4% reported impaired coordination.[86-88] These symptoms were dose dependent. Dizziness was also reported at the higher doses of leviteracetam.[88] Asthenia and headache were reported but did not show a clear dose–effect relationship.

Barrueto et al. reported the first intentional levetiracetam overdose, in which a 38-year-old reportedly

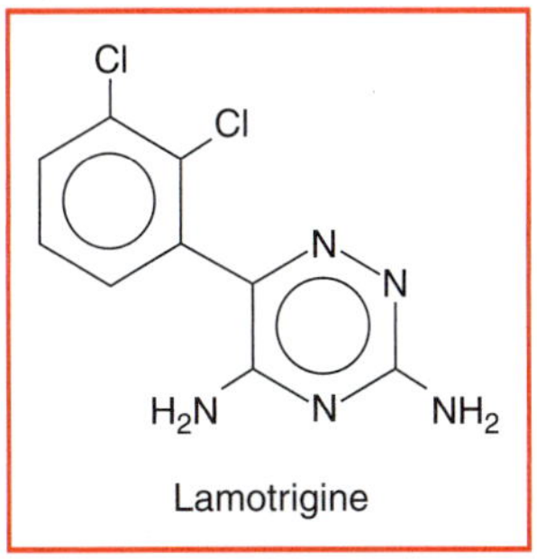

Figure 32-11. Chemical structure: lamotrigine.

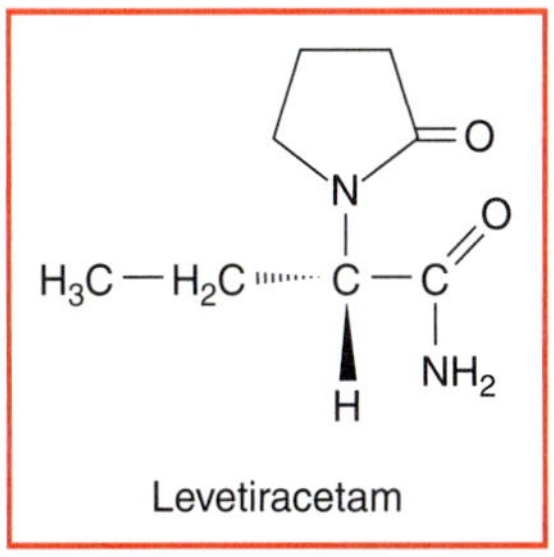

Figure 32-12. Chemical structure: levetiracetam.

ingested 30 g of levetiracetam.[89] The patient's serum drug concentration was 400 μg/mL 6 hours after ingestion. The patient presented with sedation and respiratory depression, which required intubation. The next day, the patient's respiratory depression and sedation resolved, allowing extubation. Even at serum drug concentrations 10- to 40-fold higher than therapeutic concentrations, first-order pharmacokinetics was appreciated.[89] A case report found two children who suffered from accidental overdose of 4 and 10 times their recommended dosage yet had no reported side effects.[90] Treatment of levetiracetam overdose consists of decreasing drug absorption by use of activated charcoal, followed by supportive care.[84]

Tiagabine

Tiagabine is a derivative of nipecotic acid. Tiagabine exerts antiepileptic effects by blocking GABA uptake into neurons and glia. GABA uptake inhibition sustains the level of endogenously released GABA at the synapse,[91] thus preventing synchronous neuronal firing and seizures. The main adverse effects include dizziness (27%), asthenia (20%), nervousness (10%), and tremor (9%).[92] These effects typically occur soon after drug administration and are mild to moderate in severity.[7]

Spiller et al. reported the cumulative results of 57 single-drug tiagabine overdoses.[93] Neurotoxicity included lethargy, seizures, status epilepticus, coma, confusion, agitation, tremors, dizziness, dystonias or abnormal posturing, and hallucinations. Other symptoms included respiratory depression, tachycardia, hypertension, and hypotension. The mean dose for development of seizures was 224 mg and for coma and respiratory depression was 270 mg. The lowest dose of tiagabine to cause multiple seizures and coma was 96 mg.[93] Symptoms tend to be rapid in onset and have a rapid resolution (within 12 to 24 hours). Activated charcoal and supportive care are recommended for treatment of tiagabine overdose.[84]

Topiramate

Topiramate is a sulfamate-substituted monosaccharide. It has multiple mechanisms of action. It reduces voltage-gated sodium currents in cerebellar granule cells and may act on the inactivated state of the channel in a manner similar to that of phenytoin. In addition, topiramate enhances GABA and limits activation of glutamate receptors.[7] Generally, topiramate is well tolerated. The adverse CNS effects are typically mild to moderate in nature. Adverse CNS effects can be divided into three categories: (1) cognitive-related dysfunction, (2) psychiatric or behavioral effects, and (3) somnolence or fatigue. In the monotherapy epilepsy controlled trial, 15% to 24% of patients experienced one or more cognitive-related adverse event. Specifically, difficulty with concentration and attention occurred at an incidence of 7% to 8%. Memory impairment is seen in 5% to 10% of patients. Psychomotor slowing, or slowing of all movements that require higher-order executive planning, programming, and execution, can be appreciated in 3% to 5% of patients. Kockelmann et al. reported a significant improvement in frontal lobe function-associated measures such as verbal fluency and working memory upon discontinuation of topiramate.[94] Depression was reported in 7% to 9% of patients, anxiety in 4% to 6%, and mood problems in 2% to 5%. Somnolence occurred in 9% to 15% of patients at respective doses of 50 to 400 mg daily. These events typically occurred during the titration phase of the drug.[95] Paresthesias (13% to 20%) may also occur and are likely related to carbonic anhydrase inhibition. This effect is also dose related and responds to dosage decrease.[96] Adverse effects are less prevalent if the initial dosing is titrated slowly and the lowest effective dose is used.[97]

Lofton and Klein-Schwartz examined the outcome of 567 patients reported to the American Association of Poison Control Centers for toxic topiramate exposure.[98] Of the patients, 62.1% experienced no toxicity. The most common clinical effects reported were drowsiness or lethargy (15.5%), dizziness or vertigo (4.9%), agitation (4.9%), confusion (3.9%), nausea (2.6%), and vomiting (2.5%). Patients treated with gastrointestinal decontamination experienced less serious outcomes than those

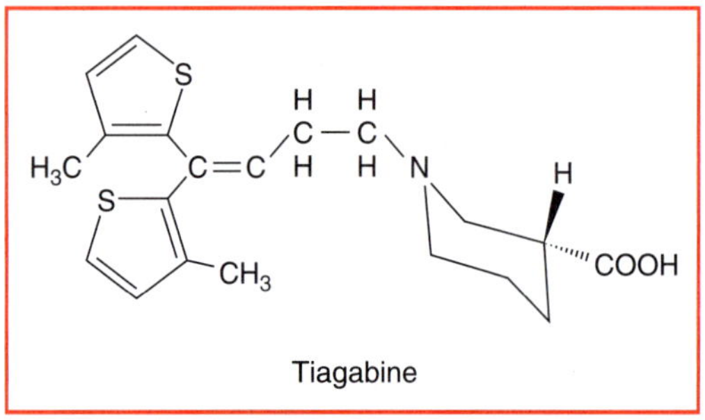

Figure 32-13. Chemical structure: tiagabine.

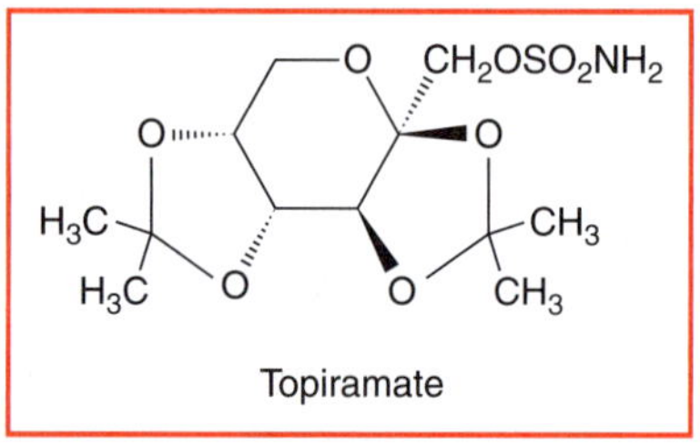

Figure 32-14. Chemical structure: topiramate.

without decontamination.[98] Hemodialysis is recommended in cases with severe neurological effects. Hemodialysis is particularly beneficial in patients with an underlying metabolic acidosis.[84]

Zonisamide

Zonisamide is a sulfonamide derivative.[7] It appears to work through inhibition of T-type calcium currents, prolongation of voltage-gated sodium channels inactivation, and possibly inhibition of glutamate release.[99] In general, zonisamide is well tolerated.[7] The most common neurological adverse effects are fatigue (3.3 to 22.5%), ataxia (3.3 to 11.3%), headache (5 to 15.9%), somnolence (5.2 to 18.3%), confusion (5.6 to 10.6%), dizziness (6.9 to 16.9%), nervousness (8.8 to 9.9%), and abnormal thinking (9.7 to 11.3%).[99] Psychomotor slowing and difficulty with concentration were reported during the first month of treatment at doses above 300 mg/day. Speech and language problems were more commonly seen after 6 to 10 weeks of treatment and at doses above 300 mg/day. These effects were typically mild to moderate in severity.[100]

Limited information exists on the effects of zonisamide dosages greater than 800 mg/day. The drug manufacturer reports three suicide attempts of patients who ingested an unknown amount of the zonisamide. All three patients were hospitalized with CNS symptoms. In one case, the patient's plasma drug concentration was 100.1 μg/mL 31 hours after drug ingestion. The patient was comatose with cardiovascular depression. The patient recovered to alertness 5 days after presentation.[100] Only one case report has occurred of acute zonisamide overdose associated with death. The patient intentionally ingested 4.8 g of zonisamide in a suicide attempt. This case is complicated by ingestion of multiple substances, so the death cannot be clearly attributed to zonisamide.[101]

Antiepileptic agents are powerful tools in the treatment of epilepsy. As with all medications, their use has advantages and disadvantages. The risks and benefits of drug use must be considered when choosing the appropriate antiepileptic agent, and therapy often requires individualization. Providers must be aware of the various adverse effects associated with each prescribed drug.

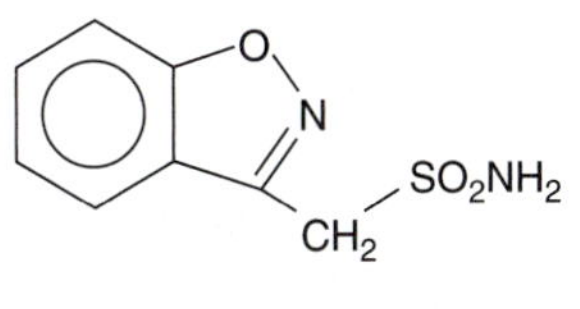

Figure 32-15. Chemical structure: zonisamide.

Box 32-1 FDA Warning

Recently, the U.S. Food and Drug Administration (FDA) issued a class warning regarding suicidal ideation for the antiepileptic medications.[102] An FDA analysis determined that patients receiving 1 of 11 antiepileptic medications* had twice the risk (0.43%) of suicidal ideation or behavior compared to those receiving placebo (0.22%). This effect was observed as early as week 1 of treatment through week 24. This effect was consistently noted among all 11 antiepileptic drugs analyzed. The FDA will likely extend the warning for risk of suicidality as a classwide effect. With this noted increased risk of suicidality, health-care providers must be hypervigilant to signs and symptoms of suicidality upon initiation and during treatment with antiepileptics.

*Carbamazepine, felbamate, gabapentin, lamotrigine, levetiracetam, oxcarbazepine, pregabalin, tiagabine, topiramate, valproate, zonisamide.

Recognition and early treatment of adverse neurological effects have a great impact on patient outcome and quality of life (Box 1).

ANTI-PARKINSON'S AGENTS

Anti-Parkinson's agents are commonly prescribed and effective in the treatment of some symptoms of Parkinson's disease. This varied group of medications exerts its effects by increasing dopaminergic activity. This neurotherapeutic effect, unfortunately, precipitates adverse neurological effects. This section discusses those undesired adverse effects and the best approach to resolution of these symptoms.

The medications commonly used to treat Parkinson's disease include levodopa, dopamine-receptor agonists, catechol-O-methyltransferase inhibitors, monoamine oxidase type B inhibitors, anticholinergics, and amantadine (Table 2). With the exception of the anticholinergics, all these agents modulate Parkinson's disease symptoms by either a direct or an indirect effect on dopamine or its metabolism, with the net result of increasing dopamine effects. Anticholinergics work by blocking muscarinic receptors within the striatum. These medications are discussed in greater depth in Chapter 33.

The D_1 and D_2 dopaminergic receptors are abundant in the striatum and are the predominant receptors involved in the treatment of Parkinson's disease.[7] Levodopa may cause confusion, hallucinations, delusions, agitation, and psychosis, particularly in older patients. Other medications, including dopamine agonists, catechol-O-methyltransferase inhibitors, and amantadine, may also cause confusion and hallucinations.

Table 2: Drugs Used in Treatment of Parkinson's Disease

ANTICHOLINERGICS

Benztropine

Trihexyphenidyl

MAO$_B$ INHIBITORS

Rasagiline

Selegiline

DOPAMINE PRECURSOR

Levodopa

DOPAMINE AGONISTS

Apomorphine

Bromocriptine

Pramipexole

Ropinirole

COMT INHIBITORS

Entacapone

Tolcapone

MISCELLANEOUS

Amantadine

MAO$_B$, monoamine oxidase type B; COMT, catechol-O-methyltransferase.

Dopamine agonists may cause a disinhibition syndrome, with behavior notable for compulsive buying, excessive gambling, or hypersexuality.[103] Grosset et al. report that 8% of patients taking dopamine agonists had pathological gambling.[104] Voon et al. reported a prevalence of disinhibition syndrome of 0.7% in levodopa treatment alone compared to 13.5% with dopamine agonist use.[105] The mechanism of this behavior is not well defined but is likely complicated by use of a dopamine agonist in a vulnerable host. It has been proposed that this behavior may be attributable to disproportionate stimulation of dopamine D$_3$ receptors, which are located predominately in the limbic system.[106] Higher doses of dopamine agonists generally increase the risk of disinhibited behavior.[103,104] Mamikonyan et al.

report that a significant decrease in drug dosage or drug discontinuation significantly reduces or resolves symptoms of disinhibition, even if offset by an increase in levodopa treatment.[107]

Long-term use of levodopa may lead to motor fluctuations, dyskinesias, and dystonias. Olanow et al.[107a] reported that these complications occur in more than half of the patients after 5 to 10 years of treatment. Many attribute the fluctuations in motor symptoms to the natural disease course. With progressive degeneration of dopaminergic neurons, the buffering capacity of plasma levodopa levels decreases. Because of levodopa's short half-life (90 minutes), the patient cannot tolerate this quick rise and fall of plasma levodopa concentrations and, thus, manifests motor fluctuations.[108] Because of the potential for worsening motor fluctuations with levodopa treatment, clinicians have debated when levodopa therapy should be started. To address the controversy surrounding the potential neurotoxic effects of levodopa use, the ELLDOPA study compared early Parkinson's disease patients treated with carbidopa-levodopa (at one of three doses) versus those treated with placebo. The groups were treated for 40 weeks with the medication or placebo, followed by withdrawal of treatment for 2 weeks to assess for motor fluctuation with drug withdrawal. At 42 weeks, all subjects treated with levodopa showed less evidence of Parkinson's symptoms when compared to placebo. The decrease in parkinsonism was directly proportional to the dose of levodopa, suggesting that levodopa may actually have neuroprotective properties.[109,110]

Several drug classes are used in the treatment of Parkinson's disease. All of these medications modulate dopamine to exert their beneficial effect. Correspondingly, the primary adverse neurological effects, namely, psychobehavioral effects and movement disorders, are attributed primarily to the drugs' dopaminergic effects. The balance of dopaminergic replacement with avoidance of excessive stimulation is the goal of treatment.

CONCLUSION

As expected, nervous system–altering drugs can cause numerous unwanted neurological effects. These medications must penetrate the blood–brain barrier to exert their desired effects. This, in turn, makes the patient vulnerable to various adverse CNS effects. Anti-Parkinson's drugs and antiepileptics are the most common neurological drugs to cause neurotoxicity. These effects are typically dose related, but some may occur regardless of drug dosage and serum concentrations. With drug overdose, associated risk arises of serious neurological consequences. Awareness of these drugs' potential adverse effects can guide the provider in patient care in regards to both making the appropriate initial drug choice, while considering the patient's characteristics and vulnerabilities, and increasing recognition of symptoms once the patient presents with drug-induced neurological disease.

REFERENCES

1. Shorvon S, Perucca E, Fish D, Dodson E, eds. *The Treatment of Epilepsy*. 2nd ed. Maiden, Ma: Blackwell Science; 2004.
2. Walker MC, Patsalos PN. Clinical pharmacokinetics of new antiepileptic drugs. *Pharmacol Ther*. 1995;67:351–384.
3. Anderson GD. A mechanistic approach to antiepileptic drug interactions. *Ann Pharmacother*. 1998;32:554–563.
4. Macdonald RL. Cellular actions of antiepileptic drugs. In: Eadie MJ, Vajda FJE, eds. *Antiepileptic Drugs: Pharmacology and Therapeutics*. Berlin: Springer; 1999:123–150.
5. Eadie MJ. Phenytoin. In: Shorvon S, Perucca E, Fish D, Dodson E, eds. *The Treatment of Epilepsy*. Maiden, Ma: Blackwell Science; 2004:475–488.
6. Morita D, Glauser T. Phenytoin and fosphenytoin. In: Wyllie E, Gupta A, Lachhwani DK, eds. *The Treatment of Epilepsy: Principles and Practice*. 4th ed. Philadelphia: Lippincott Williams & Wilkins; 2005:785–803.
7. Brunton LL, Lazo JS, Parker KL, eds. *Goodman & Gilman's: The Pharmacological Basis of Therapeutics*. 11th ed. New York: McGraw-Hill; 2006.
8. Woodbury D. Pharmacology of anticonvulsant drugs in CSF. In: Woods J, ed. *Neurobiology of Cerebrospinal Fluid*. vol 2. New York: Plenum Press; 1983:615–628.
9. Ramsay RE, DeToledo J. Intravenous administration of fosphenytoin: options for the management of seizures. *Neurology*. 1996;46(6 Suppl 1):S17–S19.
10. Kutt H, Winters W, Kokenge R, McDowell F. Diphenylhydantoin metabolism, blood levels, and toxicity. *Arch Neurol*. 1964;11:642–648.
11. McLellan DL, Swash M. Choreo-athetosis and encephalopathy induced by phenytoin. *BMJ*. 1974;2:204–205.
12. Montenegro MA, Scotoni AE, Cendes F. Dyskinesia induced by phenytoin. *Arq Neuropsiquiatr*. 1999;57:356–360.
13. Bayer AU, Thiel HJ, Zrenner E, et al. Color vision tests for early detection of antiepileptic drug toxicity. *Neurology*. 1997;48:1394–1397.
14. Stilman N, Madeu JC. Incidence of seizures with phenytoin toxicity. *Neurology*. 1985;35:1769–1772.
15. Levy LL, Fenichel GM. Diphenylhydantoin activated seizures. *Neurology*. 1965;15:716–722.
16. Chua HC, Venketasubramanian N, Tan CB, Tjia H. Paradoxical seizures in phenytoin toxicity. *Singapore Med J*. 1999;40:276–277.
17. Osorio I, Burnstine TH, Remler B, et al. Phenytoin-induced seizures: a paradoxical effect at toxic concentrations in epileptic patients. *Epilepsia*. 1989;30:230–234.
18. Mochizuki Y, Suyehiro Y, Tanizawa A, et al. Peripheral neuropathy in children on long-term phenytoin therapy. *Brain Dev*. 1981;3:375–383.
19. Lee SK, Mori S, Kim DJ, et al. Diffusion tensor MRI and fiber tractography of cerebellar atrophy in phenytoin users. *Epilepsia*. 2003;44:1536–1540.
20. Aldenkamp AP, Alpherts WC, Diepman L, et al. Cognitive side-effects of phenytoin compared with carbamazepine in patients with localization-related epilepsy. *Epilepsy Res*. 1994;19:37–43.
21. Mula M, Sander JW. Negative effects of antiepileptic drugs on mood in patients with epilepsy. *Drug Saf*. 2007;30:555–567.
22. Dodson WE, Rust RS. Phenobarbital: mechanisms of action. In: Levy RH, Mattson RH, Meldrum BS, eds. *Antiepileptic Drugs*. 4th ed. New York: Raven Press; 1995:371–375.
23. Feely M, O'Callaghan N. Phenobarbitone in previously untreated epilepsy. *J Neurol Neurosurg Psychiatr*. 1980;43:365–368.
24. Michelucci R, Tassinar CA. Phenobarbital, primidone, and other barbiturates. In: Wyllie E, Gupta A, Lachhwani DK, eds. *The Treatment of Epilepsy: Principles and Practice*. 4th ed. Philadelphia: Lippincott Williams & Wilkins; 2005:461–474.
25. Wolf SM, Forsythe A. Psychology, pharmacotherapy and new diagnostic approaches. In: Meinardi H, Rowan AJ, eds. *Advances in Epileptology*. Amsterdam: Swets & Zeitlinger; 1977:124–127.
26. Geladze TSH. Hyperactive behavior in children as a complication of antiepileptic treatment. *Zh Nevropatol Psikhiatr Im S S Korsakova*. 1987;87:1791–1796.
27. Cramer JA, Mattson RH. Phenobarbital: toxicity. In: Levy RH, Mattson RH, Meldrum BS, eds. *Antiepileptic Drugs*. 4th ed. New York: Raven Press; 1995:409–419.
28. Berg JM, Berlinger WG, Goldberg MJ, et al. Acceleration of the body clearance of phenobarbital by oral activated charcoal. *N Engl J Med*. 1982;307:642–644.
29. van Opstal JM, Janknegt R, Cilissen J, et al. Severe overdosage with the antiepileptic drug oxcarbazepine. *Br J Clin Pharmacol*. 2004;58:329–331.
30. Guerreiro CA, Guerreiro MM. Carbamazepine and oxcarbazepine. In: Wyllie E, Gupta A, Lachhwani DK, eds. *The Treatment of Epilepsy: Principles and Practice*. 4th ed. Philadelphia: Lippincott Williams & Wilkins; 2005:761–774.
31. Pellock JM. Carbamazepine side effects in children and adults. *Epilepsia*. 1987;28 (Suppl 3):S64–S70.
32. Sillanpaa M. Carbamazepine. In: Shorvon S, Perucca E, Fish D, Dodson E, eds. *The Treatment of Epilepsy*. 2nd ed. Maiden, Ma: Blackwell Science; 2004:352–353.
33. Jacome D. Carbamazepine-induced dystonia. *JAMA*. 1979;241:2263.
34. Weaver DF, Camfield P, Fraser A. Massive carbamazepine overdose: clinical and pharmacologic observations in five episodes. *Neurology*. 1988;38:755–759.
35. Brahmi N, Kouraichi N, Abderrazek H, et al. Clinical experience with carbamazepine overdose: relationship between serum concentration and neurological severity. *J Clin Psychopharmacol*. 2008;28:241–243.
36. Spiller HA, Carlisle RD. Status epilepticus after massive carbamazepine overdose. *J Toxicol Clin Toxicol*. 2002;40:81–90.
37. Van Calker D, Steber R, Klotz KN, Greil W. Carbamazepine distinguishes between adenosine receptors that mediate different second messenger responses. *Eur J Pharmacol*. 1991;206:285–290.
38. Schmidt S, Schmitz BM. Signs and symptoms of carbamazepine overdose. *J Neurol*. 1995;242:169–173.
39. Pilapil M, Petersen J. Efficacy of hemodialysis and charcoal hemoperfusion in carbamazepine overdose. *Clin Toxicol*. 2008;46:342–343.
40. Anon. Position statement and practice guidelines in the use of multi-dose activated charcoal in the treatment of acute poisoning. *J Toxicol Clin Toxicol*. 1999;36:731–751.
41. Tecoma ES. Oxcarbazepine. *Epilepsia*. 1999;40 (Suppl 5):S37–S46.
42. Novartis Pharmaceuticals. Trileptal (Oxcarbazepine) Package Insert. East Hanover, NJ: Novartis Pharmaceuticals; 2000.
43. Glauser TA, Nigro M, Sachdeo R, et al. Adjunctive therapy with oxcarbazepine in children with partial seizures. *Neurology*. 2000;54:2237–2244.

44. Sabers A, Dam M. Ethosuximide and other succinimides. In: Shorvon S, Perucca E, Fish D, Dodson E, eds. *The Treatment of Epilepsy.* 2nd ed. Maiden, Ma: Blackwell Science; 2004:414–420.

45. Browne T. Ethosuximide (Zarontin) and other succinimides. In: Browne T, Feldman R, eds. *Epilepsy, Diagnosis and Management.* Boston: Little, Brown; 1983:215–224.

45a. Landolt. Some clinical EEG correlations in epileptic psychoses (twilight states). *EEG Clin Neurophysiol.* 1953;5:121.

46. Krishnamoorthy ES, Trimble MR, Sander JW, Kanner AM. Forced normalization at the interface between epilepsy and psychiatry. *Epilepsy Behav.* 2002;3:303–308.

47. Glauser TA. Ethosuximide. In: Wyllie E, Gupta A, Lachhwani DK, eds. *The Treatment of Epilepsy: Principles and Practice.* 4th ed. Philadelphia: Lippincott Williams & Wilkins; 2005:817–827.

48. Goldensohn ES, Hardie J, Borea ED. Ethosuximide in the treatment of epilepsy. *JAMA.* 1962;180:840–842.

49. Sztainkrycer MD, Huang EE, Bond GR. Acute zonisamide overdose: a death revisited. *Vet Hum Toxicol.* 2003;45:154–156.

50. Coulter DA, Huguenard JR, Prince DA. Characterization of ethosuximide reduction of low-threshold calcium current in thalamic neurons. *Ann Neurol.* 1989;25:582–593.

51. Arroyo S. Valproate. In: Shorvon S, Perucca E, Fish D, Dodson E, eds. *The Treatment of Epilepsy.* 2nd ed. Maiden, Ma: Blackwell Science; 2004:528–539.

52. Karas BJ, Wilder BJ, Hammond EJ, Bauman AW. Treatment of valproate tremors. *Neurology.* 1983;33:1380–1382.

53. Zadikoff C, Munhoz RP, Asante AN, et al. Movement disorders in patients taking anticonvulsants. *J Neurol Neurosurg Psychiatry.* 2007;78:147–151.

54. Jamora D, Lim SH, Pan A, et al. Valproate-induced parkinsonism in epilepsy patients. *Mov Disord.* 2007;22:130–133.

55. Papazian O, Cañizales E, Alfonso I, et al. Reversible dementia and apparent brain atrophy during valproate therapy. *Ann Neurol.* 1995;38:687–691.

56. Marescaux C, Warter JM, Micheletti G, et al. Stuporous episodes during treatment with sodium valproate: report of seven cases. *Epilepsia.* 1982;23:297–305.

57. Marklund N, Enblad P, Ronne-Engström E. Neurointensive care management of raised intracranial pressure caused by severe valproic acid intoxication. *Neurocrit Care.* 2007;7:160–164.

58. De Vivo DC, Bohan TP, Coulter DL, et al. L-carnitine supplementation in childhood epilepsy: current perspectives. *Epilepsia.* 1998;39:1216–1225.

59. Chan YC, Tse ML, Lau FL. Two cases of valproic acid poisoning treated with L-carnitine. *Hum Exp Toxicol.* 2007; 26:967–969.

60. Kalachnik JE, Hanzel TE, Sevenich R, Harder SR. Benzodiazepine behavioral side effects: review and implications for individuals with mental retardation. *Am J Mental Retard.* 2002;107:376–410.

61. DiMario FJ Jr, Clancy RR. Paradoxical precipitation of tonic seizures by lorazepam in a child with atypical absence seizures. *Pediatr Neurol.* 1988;4:249–251.

62. Amand G, Evrard P. Le lorazepam injectable dans les etats de mal epileptique. *Rev EEG Neurophysiol Clin.* 1976;6:532–533.

63. Waltregny A, Dargent J. Preliminary study of parenteral lorazepam in status epilepticus. *Acta Neurol Belg.* 1975;75:219–229.

64. Olkkola KT, Ahonen J. Midazolam and other benzodiazepines. *Handb Exp Pharmacol.* 2008;182:335–360.

65. Chadwick D. Gabapentin. *Lancet.* 1994;343:89–91.

66. Asconapé J, Diedrich A, DellaBadia J. Myoclonus associated with the use of gabapentin. *Epilepsia.* 2000;41:479–481.

67. Buetefisch CM, Gutierrez A, Gutmann L. Choreoathetotic movements: a possible side effect of gabapentin. *Neurology.* 1996;46:851–852.

68. Chudnow RS, Dewey RB Jr, Lawson CR. Choreoathetosis as a side effect of gabapentin therapy in severely neurologically impaired patients. *Arch Neurol.* 1997;54:910–912.

69. Lee DO, Steingard RJ, Cesena M, et al. Behavioral side effects of gabapentin in children. *Epilepsia.* 1996;37:87–90.

70. Klein-Schwartz W, Shepherd JG, Gorman S, Dahl B. Characterization of gabapentin overdose using a poison center case series. *J Toxicol Clin Toxicol.* 2003;41:11–15.

71. McLean MJ, Gidal BE. Gabapentin and pregabalin. In: Wyllie E, Gupta A, Lachhwani DK, eds. *The Treatment of Epilepsy: Principles and Practice.* 4th ed. Philadelphia: Lippincott Williams & Wilkins; 2005:855–868.

72. Kugler AR, Robbins JL, Strand JC, et al. Pregabalin overview: a novel CNS-active compound with anticonvulsant activity [paper]. 56th Annual Meeting of American Epilepsy Society, Dec 11, 2002, Seattle, Washington.

73. Huppertz HJ, Feuerstein TJ, Schulze-Bonhage A. Myoclonus in epilepsy patients with anticonvulsive add-on therapy with pregabalin. *Epilepsia.* 2001;42:790–792.

74. Pfizer Pharmaceuticals. Lyrica (Pregabalin) Prescribing Information. Revised. New York: Pfizer Pharmaceuticals; 2007.

75. Spiller HA, Bratcher R, Griffith JR. Pregabalin overdose with benign outcome. *Clin Toxicol.* 200830:1–2.

76. Xie X, Lancaster B, Peakman T, Garthwaite J. Interaction of the antiepileptic drug lamotrigine with recombinant rat brain type IIA Na+ channels and with native Na+ channels in rat hippocampal neurones. *Pflugers Arch.* 1995;430:437–446.

77. Matsuo F, Gay P, Madsen J, et al. Lamotrigine high-dose tolerability and safety in patients with epilepsy: a double-blind, placebo-controlled, eleven-week study. *Epilepsia.* 1996;37: 857–862.

78. O'Donnell J, Bateman DN. Lamotrigine overdose in an adult. *J Toxicol Clin Toxicol.* 2000;38:659–660.

79. Miller MA, Levsky ME. Choreiform dyskinesia following isolated lamotrigine overdose. *J Child Neurol.* 2008;23:243.

80. Sbei M, Campellone JV. Stupor from lamotrigine toxicity. *Epilepsia.* 2001;42:1082–1083.

81. Hasan M, Lerman-Sagie T, Lev D, Watemberg N. Recurrent absence status epilepticus (spike-and-wave stupor) associated with lamotrigine therapy. *J Child Neurol.* 2006;21:807–809.

82. Lofton AL, Klein-Schwartz W. Evaluation of lamotrigine toxicity reported to poison centers. *Ann Pharmacother.* 2004; 38:1811–1815.

83. Daana M, Nevo Y, Tenenbaum A, et al. Lamotrigine overdose in a child. *J Child Neurol.* 2007;22:642–644.

84. Doyon S. Overdose of Newer Anticonvulsants. ToxAlert. Baltimore: Maryland Poison Center; 2006:22.

85. Harden C. Safety profile of levetiracetam. *Epilepsia.* 2001;42 (Suppl 4):36–39.

86. Cereghino JJ, Biton V, Abou-Khalil B, et al. Levetiracetam for partial seizures: results of a double-blind, randomized clinical trial. *Neurology.* 2000;55:236–242.

87. Shorvon SD, Löwenthal A, Janz D, et al. Multicenter double-blind, randomized, placebo-controlled trial of levetiracetam as add-on therapy in patients with refractory partial seizures. *Epilepsia.* 2000;41:1179–1186.

88. Ben-Menachem E, Falter U. Efficacy and tolerability of levetiracetam 3000 mg/d in patients with refractory partial seizures: a multicenter, double-blind, responder-selected study evaluating monotherapy. *Epilepsia.* 2000;41:1276–1283.

89. Barrueto F Jr, Williams K, Howland MA, et al. A case of levetiracetam (Keppra) poisoning with clinical and toxicokinetic data. *J Toxicol Clin Toxicol.* 2002;40:881–884.

90. Awaad Y. Accidental overdosage of levetiracetam in two children caused no side effects. *Epilepsy Behav.* 2007;11:247.

91. Suzdak PD, Jansen JA. A review of the preclinical pharmacology of tiagabine: a potent and selective anticonvulsant GABA uptake inhibitor. *Epilepsia*. 1995;36:612–626.

92. Leppik IE, Gram L, Deaton R. Safety of tiagabine: summary of 53 trials. *Epilepsy Res*. 1999;33:235–246.

93. Spiller HA, Winter ML, Ryan M, et al. Retrospective evaluation of tiagabine overdose. *Clin Toxicol*. 2005;43:855–859.

94. Kockelmann E, Elger CE, Helmstaedter C. Significant improvement in frontal lobe associated neuropsychological functions after withdrawal of topiramate in epilepsy patients. *Epilepsy Res*. 2003;54:171–178.

95. Ortho-McNeil Neurologics. Topamax Prescribing Information. Revised. Titusville, NJ: Ortho-McNeil Neurologics, division of Ortho-McNeil-Janssen Pharmaceuticals; 2008.

96. Cross JH. Topiramate. In: Shorvon S, Perucca E, Fish D, Dodson E, eds. *The Treatment of Epilepsy*. 2nd ed. Maiden, Ma: Blackwell Science; 2004:515–527.

97. Privitera MD. Topiramate: a new antiepileptic drug. *Ann Pharmacother*. 1997;31:1164–1173.

98. Lofton AL, Klein-Schwartz W. Evaluation of toxicity of topiramate exposures reported to poison centers. *Hum Exp Toxicol*. 2005;24:591–595.

99. Welty TE. Zonisamide. In: Wyllie E, Gupta A, Lachhwani DK, eds. *The Treatment of Epilepsy: Principles and Practice*. 4th ed. Philadelphia: Lippincott Williams & Wilkins; 2005:891–899.

100. Eisai. Zonegran (Zonisamide) Prescribing Information. Woodcliff Lake, NJ: Eisai; 2007.

101. Sztajnkrycer MD. Valproic acid toxicity: overview and management. *J Toxicol Clin Toxicol*. 2002;40:789–801.

102. U.S. Food and Drug Administration, Center for Drug Evaluation and Research. Suicidality and Antiepileptic Drugs. Available at: http://www.fda.gov/cder/drug/infopage/antiepileptics/default.htm. Accessed August 14, 2008.

103. Weintraub D, Siderowf AD, Potenza MN, et al. Association of dopamine agonist use with impulse control disorders in Parkinson disease. *Arch Neurol*. 2006;63:969–973.

104. Grosset KA, Macphee G, Pai G, et al. Problematic gambling on dopamine agonists: not such a rarity. *Mov Disord*. 2006;21:2006–2008.

105. Voon V, Hassan K, Zurowski M, et al. Prevalence of repetitive and reward-seeking behaviors in Parkinson disease. *Neurology*. 2006;67:1254–1257.

106. Dodd ML, Klos KJ, Bower JH, et al. Pathological gambling caused by drugs used to treat Parkinson disease. *Arch Neurol*. 2005;62:1377–1381.

107. Mamikonyan E, Siderowf AD, Duda JE, et al. Long-term follow-up of impulse control disorders in Parkinson's disease. *Mov Disord*. 2008;23:75–80.

107a. Olanow CW, Watts RL, Koller WC. An algorithm (decision tree) for the management of Parkinson's disease (2001): treatment guidelines. *Neurology*. 2001;56(11 Suppl 5): S1–S88.

108. Fahn S, Parkinson Study Group. Does levodopa slow or hasten the rate of progression of Parkinson's disease? *J Neurol*. 2005; 252 (Suppl 4):IV37–IV42.

109. Fahn OD, Shoulson I, Kleburtz K, et al. Levodopa and the progression of Parkinson's disease. *N Engl J Med*. 2004;351: 2498–2508.

110. Fahn S. A new look at levodopa based on the ELLDOPA study. *J Neural Transm Suppl*. 2006;70:419–426.

CHAPTER 33

Neurotoxic Effects of Pharmaceutical Agents IV: Cancer Chemotherapeutic Agents

Arthur D. Forman, Christina A. Meyers, and Victor A. Levin

INTRODUCTION

While chemotherapy is a primary treatment in the management of cancer, its acute and/or persistent adverse effects on the functioning of the human nervous system can, at times, have profound effects on patient quality of life. These potential adverse effects include seizures; severe ataxia; acute encephalopathy characterized by confusion, sleep disturbance, and agitation that may resolve after treatment; and quadriplegia. Less severe problems are more common, including chronic cognitive dysfunction and peripheral neuropathy that less often impair patient function permanently and more often cause disturbing paresthesia, ataxia, pain, autonomic dysfunction, or a combination of these. Table 1 lists many neurotoxic effects of commonly used anticancer agents.

Any consideration of cancer therapy's toxicity on the nervous system must take into account the impact of the disease itself on the nervous system. Cancer, through the host's response to the illness, has widespread non-metastatic effects on both the central and the peripheral nervous systems, which makes study of neurotoxicity challenging. Evidence of peripheral neuropathy can be found in more than half of patients with lung cancer before initiation of any therapy, if looked for carefully.[1,2]

Similarly, central nervous system effects are widespread, particularly cognitive impairment resulting from vascular effects and/or inflammatory mediator activation or local cytokine release. Beyond these indirect effects, neoplasms can, of course, metastasize to the nervous system, which must be considered in any suspected instance of neurotoxicity.

Unfortunately, the mechanisms by which cytoreductive therapies work are often intertwined with their side effects, challenging the rational management of nervous system toxicity related to anticancer treatment. Preexisting neurological disease, which may have been subclinical, may also have a significant impact on neurological toxicity. Moreover, neurotoxicity from cancer therapy presents a greater risk for neonates and elderly patients than for other age groups.

PERIPHERAL NEUROTOXICITY

Neuropathy is the most commonly encountered paraneoplastic disorder, and its prevalence makes study of peripheral neurotoxicity difficult. Peripheral neuropathy is the most common neurotoxic effect of systemic therapy, as peripheral nerves are far more vulnerable than

Table 1:   Common Neurotoxic Anticancer Therapies

Drug or Drug Class	Use	Toxic Effect	Severity	Onset	Recovery	Therapy
Vinca alkaloids	Lymphomas, leukemias, solid tumors	Neuropathy, cranial neuropathy	Moderate to severe	Acute to subacute	Usually complete	Symptomatic management, possibly sulfur antioxidant compounds
Taxanes	Breast and other solid tumors	Neuropathy	Moderate	Acute to subacute	Usually complete	Symptomatic management, possibly sulfur antioxidant compounds
Platinum compounds	Solid tumors including gynecological, gastrointestinal, and lung	Neuropathy	Moderate to severe	Subacute to chronic	At least 20% do not recover	Symptomatic management, possibly sulfur antioxidant compounds
Bortezomib	Multiple myeloma, lymphoma	Neuropathy	Moderate	Subacute	Usually complete	Symptomatic management, possibly sulfur antioxidant compounds
Thalidomide	Multiple myeloma, central nervous system tumors	Neuropathy, sedation	Moderate, limited	Acute	Usually complete	Symptomatic management, possibly sulfur antioxidant compounds
Methotrexate	Leukemia, lymphoma, solid tumors	Neuropathy (rare), optic neuropathy (infrequent), myelopathy (rare), encephalopathy, leukoencephalopathy	Moderate to severe	Subacute to chronic	Usually incomplete	Folinic acid
Cytosine arabinoside	Leukemia, lymphoma	Neuropathy (infrequent), myelopathy (intrathecal), cerebellopathy, encephalopathy	Moderate to severe	Acute to subacute	Good for neuropathy, fair for encephalopathy, poor for cerebellopathy	Possibly antioxidants
Ifosfamide	Solid tumors, broad activity	Seizures, encephalopathy	Severe	Acute to subacute	Usually complete	Supportive care, anticonvulsants, methylene blue
Busulfan	Transplant conditioning	Seizures	Moderate	Acute	Complete	Anticonvulsants
Asparaginase	Acute lymphocytic leukemia	Seizures, cortical vein thrombosis	Moderate to severe	Acute to subacute	Often complete	Anticonvulsants, supportive care
Hormonal manipulations	Breast, prostate, and gynecological cancers	Sleep disturbance, hot flashes, cognitive impairment	Mild to moderate	Subacute to chronic	Good	Antidepressants, supportive care

central neurons. Peripheral nerves have a blood–nerve capillary barrier that is less robust at protecting from extraneous substances than the blood–brain barrier of the central nervous system. The sensory neurons' cell bodies lay outside the protection of the central nervous system's blood–brain barrier, which is why sensory symptoms predominate in many neurotoxic neuropathies. Furthermore, peripheral nerves have by far the largest surface area of any cell, which places them at great vulnerability to toxins. Oxidative stress is another consequence of peripheral nerves' enormous surface area. The nerves' external membrane is particularly susceptible, being composed largely of lipids. Peripheral nerves are richly endowed with antioxidant systems, chiefly in the form of the superoxide dismutases, of which there are multiple forms in nerve tissues. Oxidative stress is increased in cancer and its therapy, adding to the peripheral nerves' vulnerability to toxins.

Unlike central nervous system neurons, peripheral nerves have the capacity to regenerate. Peripheral nerves therefore can heal completely from toxic insults, provided that the cell body, which is centrally located, is intact. Recovery from various insults may take months to years depending on variables such as age, concurrent metabolic disturbances such as diabetes, or exposure to other toxins such as alcohol or other chemotherapy. While a nerve is recovering, ironically, patients may experience more symptoms such as paresthesias or cramping because immature nerve sprouts are irritable.

General Treatment Measures

Symptomatic management is important for patients with treatment-related peripheral neuropathy because the neuropathic symptoms often dominate and have a significant impact on quality of life. Table 2[3] lists some of these treatments. Painful dysesthesias are treated with gabapentin or pregabalin; the latter may have a more rapid onset of benefit. Amitriptyline in doses lower than those used to treat depression can ease neuropathic pain but adds to the risk of orthostatic hypotension and dysautonomia. The more complex antidepressant duloxetine may help, particularly if there is accompanying depression. While neuropathic pain is relatively resistant to narcotics, many patients benefit from their use. Occasional patients benefit from the use of capsaicin cream applied to the painful extremities. Cramps are treated effectively with quinine sulfate, usually about one-third to one-half the dose found in available capsules. Patients with serum hypomagnesia, hypocalcemia, or both should be given supplements because these deficiencies may contribute to cramping and other neuropathic symptoms. Dietary

Table 2:	Treatments for Neuropathic Pain	
Class	**Example**	**Typical Dose**
Tricyclic drugs	Amitriptyline	10–75 mg at bedtime
	Nortriptyline	25–75 mg at bedtime
	Imipramine	25–75 mg at bedtime
Anticonvulsants	Gabapentin	300–1200 mg tid
	Carbamazepine	200–400 mg tid
	Pregabalin	100 mg tid
5-Hydroxytryptamine, norepinephrine uptake inhibitors	Duloxetine	30–60 mg daily
Narcotics	Oxycodone	5 to 10 mg 3 hourly prn
	Hydromorphone	2 to 4 mg 2 hourly prn
TRPV1 receptors	Capsaicin cream	0.025–0.075% applied tid–qid
Membrane stabilizers	Quinine sulfate	100–150 mg at night

TRPV1, transient receptor potential cation channel, subfamily V, member 1.
Modified from American Diabetes Association. Standards of medical care in diabetes: 2007. *Diabetes Care.* 2007;30 (Suppl 1):S4–S41.

measures to provide adequate sources of thiamine and antioxidants may help speed recovery.

Vinca Alkaloids

The vinca alkaloids, mitotic spindle poisons derived from the periwinkle plant, include vincristine, vinblastine, vinorelbine, and vindesine. The mitotic spindle has close homology with the axonal transport mechanism of peripheral nerve, which becomes damaged by these poisons through the same mechanisms that give this drug class activity against malignancies. Patients often experience toxic effects acutely in the form of cramps or paresthesia that may arise even as the drug is being given.[4] More often they develop numbness and tingling paresthesia ("walking on clouds or pillows") toward the end of their therapy. As with most toxic axonal neuropathies, the parts of the body most distant from the center are affected earliest and most severely. Numbness in feet and toes is the predominant symptom in what is called a length-dependent or dying back neuropathy. Fingers and hands may be affected as well.[5,6] Painful paresthesia is not uncommon and may arise well after the drug has been administered. The vinca alkaloids often affect autonomic fibers and may cause cranial neuropathies which can recover rapidly following cessation of therapy.[7] Recovery from vinca-induced neuropathy is usually excellent, although it may be protracted and depends on the patient having no further insults to peripheral nerves.

Taxanes and Other Mitotic Spindle Poisons

The taxanes, which include paclitaxel and docetaxel, are also plant-derived spindle poisons, although they work through a different mechanism than the vinca alkaloids, causing spasm of the spindle rather than paralysis. The clinical pattern of neuropathy is similar to that seen with the vinca alkaloids, although the neurotoxic effects of the taxanes seem to plateau in many patients.[8] Paclitaxel is administered with cremophor, which may increase its neurotoxicity; overall, paclitaxel has greater neurotoxicity than docetaxel[9] but less hematological toxicity. Albumin-bound paclitaxel preparations may provide more rapid recovery from neurotoxic effects,[10] in addition to avoiding allergic responses to the castor oil–derived cremophor solvent. Some newer noncremophor paclitaxel preparations may be more neurotoxic, but this may reflect better delivery of the drug.[11,12] Ixabepilone, a epothilone analogue, is a recently approved mitotic spindle toxin that has activity in breast cancer refractory to the taxanes. Early reports suggest that ixabepilone is less neurotoxic than the other mitotic spindle toxins.[13]

Heavy Metals

Cisplatin, carboplatin, oxaliplatin, and arsenicals are heavy-metal chemotherapy agents used to treat a range of malignancies. The heavy metals all cause axonal neuropathy in which sensory symptoms predominate. The platinum compounds are the most problematic of peripheral neurotoxins because of their activity in many tumors and the neuronal cell body damage that they cause. Arsenicals have restricted use only in some leukemias and have other toxic effects that limit their use. The onset of symptoms is not as rapid as for the mitotic spindle poisons, but the effects are cumulative. Unlike most other oncological peripheral neurotoxins, the heavy metals appear to cause irreversible injury to the cell body, and some patients do not recover following cessation of their chemotherapy. As the sensory neuron cell body is relatively less protected in the dorsal root ganglion, the heavy metals, like the mitotic spindle poisons, tend to produce sensory symptoms both first and most severely.

Unfortunately, platinum accumulates in dorsal root ganglion neurons and is poorly cleared with time.[14] Both small and large nerve fibers are affected to a varying degree in individual patients, producing symptoms ranging from pain, autonomic dysfunction,[15] and distal paresthesia to ataxia. Patients may develop Lhermitte's sign, perhaps due to the profound effects platinum may have on proprioceptive fibers[16] and consequent effects on dorsal columns within the spinal cord. This sign is an electrical shocklike sensation that travels up and down the spine. Lhermitte's sign is associated with dorsal column injury, due to secondary myelin loss following severe injury to proprioception fibers. Platinum compounds also affect hearing to a greater extent than other chemotherapeutic peripheral neurotoxins.[17] Ototoxicity may be a greater risk for patients with darkly pigmented irises.[18]

The mechanisms by which the heavy metals cause neuronal injury are still inadequately understood but likely relate to the heavy metal poisoning the superoxide dismutases, the main protective system against oxidation in nerves. This mechanism has been best demonstrated for lead intoxication in the central nervous system. A direct apoptotic response of dorsal root ganglion neurons that correlates with DNA adduct formation has been demonstrated[19]; unfortunately, DNA adduct formation is also a mechanism by which platinum exerts its benefits in tumor reduction.

Uniquely among the heavy-metal chemotherapy drugs, oxaliplatin has been reported to cause a hyperexcitability syndrome consisting of eyelid twitching, severe limb tremors, slurred speech, and teeth chattering associated with increased tone on neurological examination. Infusion of magnesium and calcium with pregabalin has been reported to help reverse this remarkable state.[20] Hypomagnesemia increases the risk of developing neuropathy, and as the platinum compounds can cause magnesium wasting, this must be closely monitored and carefully corrected.[21] Magnesium infusions have been used to counter the peripheral neurotoxic effects of the platinum compounds, but they also may diminish their efficacy.

Peripheral neurotoxicity limits dose intensification of the platinum drugs. Given these drugs' activity in a host of tumor types, efforts to find neuroprotective therapies have focused on platinum chemotherapies. The most widely used strategy centers on using sulfur-containing antioxidants such as amifostine, glutathione (or its precursor acetylcysteine), and α-lipoic acid. Both amifostine and glutathione must be administered parenterally, as oral absorption is poor. Both have been reported in controlled series to lessen the neurotoxicity of platinum chemotherapy. Acetylcysteine, commercially available as a mucolytic, supplies the sulfur-containing amino acid cysteine component of the naturally occurring tripeptide glutathione. α-Lipoic acid is a naturally occurring, sulfur-containing nutritional supplement that is highly soluble in lipids and water. Clinical trials of these compounds hold promise both for neuroprotection and for augmenting recovery from neurotoxic effects.[22–24]

Other proposed treatments for platinum neuropathy have included recombinant nerve growth factor,[25] erythropoietin,[26] and neuroprotective peptides such as adrenocorticotropic hormone analogues. These have shown promise in laboratory trials but have yet to prove useful clinically.[27]

Thalidomide

Thalidomide gained notoriety shortly after its introduction for producing severe fetal deformities, doubtless related to its suppression of blood vessel formation during development. More than 75% of patients treated with thalidomide develop a peripheral neuropathy, but fortunately this evolves gradually and may plateau.[28] Thalidomide is used to treat multiple myeloma, a disease often associated with peripheral neuropathy, which is independent of treatment and arises from multiple mechanisms. The peripheral neurotoxic mechanism may relate to the drug's effects on the microcirculation of nerves,[29] although other mechanisms may be responsible as well. A recently developed analogue, lenalidomide, may have less neurotoxic effects while maintaining efficacy.

Bortezomib

The proteasome inhibitor bortezomib is being used increasingly to treat multiple myeloma and mantle cell lymphomas. It causes a sensory neuropathy in a high percentage of patients, which has been reported to develop rapidly in some. It is often used to treat multiple myeloma, which itself causes neuropathy. Ironically, multiple myeloma is also treated with thalidomide, another peripheral neurotoxin. Lenalidomide has been reported to improve neuropathic symptoms in patients with bortezomib-induced neuropathy.[30] Bortezomib has also been reported to cause rhabdomyolysis.

Cytosine Arabinoside, Methotrexate, and 5-Fluorouracil

The antimetabolites cytosine arabinoside (cytarabine), methotrexate, and 5-fluorouracil have been reported to cause neuropathy, but clinically this is an uncommon occurrence and is usually mild. At high doses, cytosine arabinoside has been reported to cause a rapidly progressive demyelinating neuropathy with features similar to acute demyelinating polyradiculoneuropathy (Guillain-Barré syndrome).[31,32] A severe axonal neuropathy has been described with methotrexate, even when administered at low doses.[33,34] Optic neuropathy and anosmia in

association with encephalopathy have been reported in patients receiving high-dose intravenous cytosine arabinoside therapy.[35]

Corticosteroids

With long-term use, corticosteroids produce a myopathy that typically affects proximal appendicular and axial muscles. The earliest change on biopsy is simplification of mitochondrial cristae seen on electron microscopy. The myopathy may be associated with minor changes on electrophysiological testing, and muscle enzyme levels are not increased when tested. Acetylcysteine and carnitine have been reported to speed recovery, which is the rule once the corticosteroid therapy is stopped.

CENTRAL NEUROTOXICITY

The neurobehavioral effects of most cancer therapy agents tend to be nonspecific and diffuse, except for those that have a mechanism of action that affects focal brain regions[36] or biological response modifiers that are known to regulate particular proinflammatory cytokines, neurotransmitters, and neuroendocrine hormones.[37] Other potential mechanisms for these effects include direct neurotoxic effects leading to cortical atrophy or demyelination and microvascular changes.[38]

Regrettably, among patients treated for cancer today, the term "chemo-brain" is being used with increasing frequency to describe perceived cognitive declines resulting from chemotherapy. While these symptoms may resolve once treatment is completed, the changes appear to be persistent for a subset of patients. Unfortunately, there are no reliable methods for identifying or predicting which patients might be at risk for these symptoms. Memory loss, decreased information-processing speed, reduced attention, anxiety, depression, and fatigue are common changes reported during and after chemotherapy,[39] and it has been estimated that as many as one-third of patients undergoing systemic chemotherapy evince declines in cognitive function that interfere with their quality of life.[40]

Estimates of the prevalence of chemotherapy-related cognitive decline in breast cancer survivors are as high as 75%.[41–46] These changes are often subtle but occur in several domains. In a recently published prospective, randomized, longitudinal trial, Wefel et al. found an association between cognitive dysfunction and chemotherapy in a subgroup of women with nonmetastatic breast carcinoma.[47] Patients received a baseline assessment before initiation of chemotherapy with 5-fluorouracil, doxorubicin, and cyclophosphamide, approximately 3 weeks following the completion of chemotherapy, and again at

1 year after treatment. Within-subject analyses revealed that 61% of patients evinced a decline in cognitive function between the baseline assessment and the assessment just after the cessation of chemotherapy. Cognitive decline occurred most often in domains of attention, learning and memory, and processing speed. One year after chemotherapy, only 45% had improved back to baseline, while 45% did not recover and 10% had a mixed pattern of improvement and stabilization of cognitive performance.

Certain chemotherapeutic agents are known to be especially toxic to the central nervous system. For example, CI-980, an agent structurally and functionally similar to colchicine, causes a significant decline in learning and memory by selectively blocking choline acetyltransferase in the hippocampus and basal forebrain, areas of the brain involved in memory consolidation.[36] In patients with acute leukemia, central nervous system complications of high-dose cytarabine include cerebellar dysfunction, seizures, optic neuropathy, leukoencephalopathy, and cognitive changes including confusion, disorientation, and memory loss.[18,49] The mechanism of cytarabine neurotoxicity is unknown; however, the agent readily crosses the blood–brain barrier and in high doses may damage Purkinje cells in the cerebellum.[49,50] Other models suggest that cytarabine-induced neuronal apoptosis is mediated by oxidative stress.[51] Patients treated with 5-fluorouracil may develop a cerebellar syndrome characterized by dysarthria, ataxia, dizziness, and nystagmus that generally resolves within a few weeks of discontinuing treatment.[52] Changes in emotional functioning and cognition have been reported in patients with androgen-independent prostate cancer treated with the angiogenesis inhibitor TNP-470.[53] In that study, the dose-limiting toxic effect (reversible on cessation of therapy) was neuropsychiatric in nature and was attributed to frontal subcortical system dysfunction.

Biological Response Modifiers

Biological response modifiers such as interferon or the interleukins, like many chemotherapy agents, have been associated with development of cognitive dysfunction. Some biological response modifiers may also cause psychiatric symptoms such as depression or hallucinations that may require additional treatment. The side effect profile for interferon-α is an important consideration because neurotoxicity may prohibit patients from gaining maximum benefit from treatment.[37] Approximately 11% of patients treated with interferon elect to discontinue treatment because of adverse effects to the central nervous system.[54] Negative effects are seen immediately after initiation of treatment, as many patients experience flulike symptoms (e.g., fever, chills, and body aches). In most cases, these symptoms are transient and are responsive to treatment with a nonsteroidal antiinflammatory

agent.[55] In normal, healthy controls, a single dose of 1.5 million international units has been shown to decrease reaction time 6 and 10 hours after injection.[56] Most cancer patients who receive interferon receive higher doses than this for longer periods. Fatigue tends to be the most serious side effect, often persisting for the duration of treatment, and is the symptom reported most often across trials. It is estimated that between 70% and 100% of patients undergoing interferon treatment experience fatigue and that 10% to 40% require dose reduction.[57] Psychiatric symptoms, usually increased depression, are reported in 15% to 50% of patients receiving interferon treatment,[58–60] although the clinical picture may vary to include mania.

Both astrocytes and, to a lesser extent, neurons are richly endowed with receptors for these inflammatory mediators, so this toxic effect is hard to avoid with their use. Symptomatic therapy with antidepressants or psychostimulants has helped some patients.

Corticosteroids and Other Immune Modulators

Even when given over a limited period for treatment of an acute condition, corticosteroids often cause insomnia and may cause frank psychosis and mood disorders after only a few weeks.[61] Steroid receptors are widely distributed throughout the central nervous system, particularly the limbic system, which almost certainly is responsible for these toxic effects. Withdrawal of the steroid helps with this toxicity, usually within days. Often antidepressants and neuroleptics are needed to control these symptoms. The sleep disturbance and possibly the psychiatric toxic effects can be minimized by administering the corticosteroids on a schedule that mimics their normal diurnal pulse rhythm.[62]

The powerful immunosuppressants tacrolimus (FK-506) and cyclosporine inhibit calcineurin, a phosphatase enzyme that acts on calmodulin. This system is important both in immune function and in the central nervous system, particularly the endothelial cells, oligodendroglia, and neurons.[63] The toxic effects of these agents may develop subacutely or even rapidly, sometimes manifested as seizures and encephalopathy. Alterations noted on flair sequences of magnetic resonance images are often most prominent in the parieto-occipital white matter and are consistent with development of vasogenic edema,[64] which may be an important mechanism of toxicity. Low serum cholesterol levels predispose to this toxic effect.[65] Withdrawal of the drug usually results in improvement within 72 hours.

Methotrexate

Acute methotrexate neurotoxicity often manifests as seizures, confusion, and generalized cognitive deficits and is similar in presentation to the late-delayed effects of radiotherapy in their more chronic form.[66] Methotrexate-related cognitive declines have been reported on measures of intellectual and memory function.[67,68] Animal models point to disruption of learning and memory function via preferential effects on the CA4 area of the hippocampus.[69] High-dose methotrexate given intravenously can cause a leukoencephalopathy that may have imperceptible effects or progress subacutely to severe cognitive impairment and a spastic quadriparesis or even quadriplegia.[70]

Treatment of methotrexate encephalopathy includes high-dose folinic acid, which acts to rescue tissues from the effects of methotrexate on folate metabolism.[71] Methotrexate causes more injury when given intravenously according to a high-dose protocol then when given intrathecally at low dose, which is usually well tolerated unless administered close to irradiation. A relationship between tumor burden and methotrexate toxicity is likely, particularly in leukemia in which a cerebral tumor lysis syndrome may contribute to the pathogenesis of injury. Methotrexate toxicity seems greater when patients have central nervous system involvement by leukemia and may be exacerbated by tumor lysis. Methotrexate also has direct toxic effects on astrocytes in experimental models,[72] which likely contributes to the encephalopathy and is probably responsible for the occasional episodes of acute cerebral edema reported following methotrexate therapy.[72-74] Aminophylline has been reported to reverse methotrexate-induced neurotoxicity in some children.[75]

Less often, methotrexate has been implicated in myelopathy, although this happens mainly with lymphomas and leukemias, disorders that have been associated with occult myelopathy even in patients not given methotrexate. Intrathecal administration of methotrexate has rarely been associated with myelopathy.[76] Administered intrathecally, methotrexate penetrates throughout the spinal cord, with highest concentrations in the substania gelatinosa and the peripheral white matter, areas most affected by the myelopathy.[77] Fibrosing arachnoiditis has been found on pathological study of cases of myelopathy, in some cases following intrathecal therapy.

Cytosine Arabinoside

Cytosine arabinoside can cause a pancerebellar syndrome due to profound loss of Purkinje cells.[78] This dramatic toxic effect clinically mimics the cerebellopathy rarely seen as an effect of treatment with phenytoin and is one of the few causes of an acquired adult onset pancerebellar syndrome. The often-acute clinical presentation includes ataxia, dysarthria, and nystagmus and often is associated with delirium. While the mechanism of this syndrome is not completely understood, experimental models have shown that cytarabine causes apoptosis of cerebellar granule neurons which project to Purkinje cells.[79] The risk of this toxic effect increases with age[80] and cumulative dose.[81] The incidence of this toxic effect has been reported to vary with the manufacturer's preparation of cytosine arabinoside[82] and is increased by combination therapy, particularly with methotrexate. Once Purkinje cell death has occurred, it is unlikely that therapy will help, but some suggest that therapy with antioxidants helps in early cases, and flushing the cerebrospinal fluid proved beneficial in at least one instance.[83]

Thalidomide

Thalidomide was originally developed as a hypnotic and is quite sedating. Because of this, it is usually given at night, but many patients find it sedating during the day following treatments. The sedation quickly lessens once the drug is discontinued. The analogue lenalidomide is less sedating.

Ifosfamide

The cyclophosphamide analogue ifosfamide causes a generalized encephalopathy characterized by confusion, stupor, seizures, and coma. The incidence of ifosfamide neurotoxicity may be as high as 30%, and it is thought to be dose dependent. Symptoms are typically reversible and include confusion, seizures, hallucinations, weakness, and cranial nerve dysfunction.[52] Both convulsive seizures and nonconvulsive status have been described.[84] Fortunately, of the many patients treated with ifosfamide who develop central nervous system toxicity, a large number recover within 72 to 96 hours after the drug is discontinued. Intermediate metabolites of the drug are believed to be responsible for the encephalopathy, and methylene blue infusions have proved helpful in both treating and preventing the ifosfamide-induced encephalopathy.[85]

Busulfan

Seizures are sufficiently frequent when the alkylating agent busulfan is given that anticonvulsant therapy should be administered prophylatically.[86] Encephalopathy or other central nervous system toxic effects have not been seen; with anticonvulsant therapy, this drug can be given safely.

Asparaginase

Asparaginase, used almost exclusively in the management of acute lymphocytic lymphoma, can cause cortical vein thrombosis, which can lead to venous obstruction and infarction. Seizures and alterations of mental status are common when this occurs. Although these patients are usually desperately ill, recovery is often surprisingly complete. This drug is often combined with methotrexate or cytosine arabinoside and may contribute to their toxicity.

Intra-arterial Chemotherapy

Cisplatin, a broad-spectrum agent used in the treatment of testicular, urological, ovarian, head, neck, brain, and lung cancers, has been associated with problems in perception, memory, executive function, and attention,[87] but the precise mechanisms of these effects remain unclear. Such effects may relate to complex interactions between the host response to therapy, both metabolic and immunological, and the central nervous system. Since intra-arterial administration for the treatment of brain tumors can lead to subacute brain necrosis, this route of administration has been limited.

Hormonal Therapy

Hormonal ablation is a mainstay of treatment for breast and prostate cancers and is used in some gynecological malignancies. Patients undergoing antiestrogen therapy have noted hot flashes, mood disturbances, and cognitive impairment, as well as headaches. Receptors for the sex hormones are found throughout the brain, so it should come as no surprise that manipulations of these may produce complex effects on cognitive and emotional function. Hormonal ablation has been studied more in women than in men; it seems to affect verbal memory and processing speed,[88] although the effect is less pronounced in men. The role of the underlying malignancy is difficult to separate from that of the hormonal manipulation in these patients.

CONCLUSION

Treatment-related neurotoxicity is not universal among cancer patients. Some individuals are able to tolerate treatment with little physical discomfort and no obvious neurocognitive impairments, while others develop significant toxic effects that seriously compromise their quality of life and prevent them from resuming their usual social and occupational roles. Any adverse effects of cancer treatment must always be considered, however, in the light of potential therapeutic benefits. The nature of cancer-related neurocognitive and neurobehavioral dysfunction has yet to be fully characterized. Increased inclusion of neuropsychological evaluations in clinical research will further our understanding of the nature, severity, and mechanisms underlying neurocognitive

dysfunction in the patient with cancer. Multidisciplinary investigations are essential.

Advances in neuropsychology, cognitive neuroscience, genomics, proteonomics, molecular epidemiology, functional neuroimaging, neuroimmunology, and traditional oncological disciplines will ultimately contribute to understanding the relationships among disease, treatment, and host factors in the manifestation of altered neurocognitive and neurobehavioral function. These multidisciplinary investigations will identify which agents are most neurotoxic in the context of different treatment regimens, the course of the neurocognitive and neurobehavioral dysfunction, the cognitive and neurobehavioral domains most affected, the mechanisms for these effects, the host risk factors that contribute to the expression of these neurotoxic effects, and which neuroprotective or rehabilitative therapies are most efficacious in preventing or treating these adverse symptoms. Strategies for prevention are limited because the mechanisms that produce the toxic effects are often fundamental to the agent's efficacy in treating malignancy. Study of symptomatic relief measures needs to include both efficacy and effects on tumor activity.

Acknowledgments

The authors wish to thank Kay Hyde for assistance with manuscript preparation and Kathryn Hale for editorial assistance.

REFERENCES

1. Teravainen H, Larsen A. Some features of the neuromuscular complications of pulmonary carcinoma. *Ann Neurol.* 1977;2: 495–502.
2. Paul T, Katiyar BC, Misra S, Pant GC. Carcinomatous neuromuscular syndromes: a clinical and quantitative electrophysiological study. *Brain.* 1978;101(1):53–63.
3. American Diabetes Association. Standards of medical care in diabetes: 2007. *Diabetes Care.* 2007;30 (Suppl 1):S4–S41.
4. Haim N, Barron SA, Robinson E. Muscle cramps associated with vincristine therapy. *Acta Oncol.* 1991;30(6):707–711.
5. Legha SS. Vincristine neurotoxicity: pathophysiology and management. *Med Toxicol.* 1986;1(6):421–427.
6. Bradley WG, Lassman LP, Pearce GW, Walton JN. The neuromyopathy of vincristine in man: clinical, electrophysiological and pathological studies. *J Neurol Sci.* 1970;10(2):107–131.
7. Annino DJ Jr, MacArthur CJ, Friedman EM. Vincristine-induced recurrent laryngeal nerve paralysis. *Laryngoscope.* 1992;102(11):1260–1262.
8. Cavaletti G, Bogliun G, Marzorati L, et al. Peripheral neurotoxicity of taxol in patients previously treated with cisplatin. *Cancer.* 1995;75(5):1141–1150.
9. Katsumata N. Docetaxel: an alternative taxane in ovarian cancer. *Br J Cancer.* 2003;89 (Suppl 3):S9–S15.

10. Gradishar WJ. Albumin-bound paclitaxel: a next-generation taxane. *Expert Opin Pharmacother.* 2006;7(8):1041–1053.

11. Veronese ML, Flaherty K, Kramer A, et al. Phase I study of the novel taxane CT-2103 in patients with advanced solid tumors. *Cancer Chemother Pharmacol.* 2005;55(5):497–501.

12. Kim TY, Kim DW, Chung JY, et al. Phase I and pharmacokinetic study of Genexol-PM, a cremophor-free, polymeric micelle-formulated paclitaxel, in patients with advanced malignancies. *Clin Cancer Res.* 2004;10(11):3708–3716.

13. Perez EA, Lerzo G, Pivot X, et al. Efficacy and safety of ixabepilone (BMS-247550) in a phase II study of patients with advanced breast cancer resistant to an anthracycline, a taxane, and capecitabine. *J Clin Oncol.* 2007;25(23):3407–3414.

14. Gregg RW, Molepo JM, Monpetit VJ, et al. Cisplatin neurotoxicity: the relationship between dosage, time, and platinum concentration in neurologic tissues, and morphologic evidence of toxicity. *J Clin Oncol.* 1992;10(5):795–803.

15. Rosenfeld CS, Broder LE. Cisplatin-induced autonomic neuropathy. *Cancer Treat Rep.* 1984;68(4):659–660.

16. Inbar M, Merimsky O, Wigler N, Chaitchik S. Cisplatin-related Lhermitte's sign. *Anticancer Drugs.* 1992;3(4):375–377.

17. Waters GS, Ahmad M, Katsarkas A, Stanimir G, McKay J. Ototoxicity due to *cis*-diamminedichloroplatinum in the treatment of ovarian cancer: influence of dosage and schedule of administration. *Ear Hear.* 1991;12(2):91–102.

18. Barr Hamilton RM, Matheson LM, Keay DG. Ototoxicity of *cis*-platinum and its relationship to eye colour. *J Laryngol Otol.* 1991;105:7–11.

19. Ta LE, Espeset L, Podratz J, Windebank AJ. Neurotoxicity of oxaliplatin and cisplatin for dorsal root ganglion neurons correlates with platinum–DNA binding. *Neurotoxicology.* 2006;27(6):992–1002.

20. Saif MW, Hashmi S. Successful amelioration of oxaliplatin-induced hyperexcitability syndrome with the antiepileptic pregabalin in a patient with pancreatic cancer. *Cancer Chemother Pharmacol.* 2008;61(3):349–354.

21. Ashraf M, Scotchel PL, Krall JM, Flink EB. *cis*-Platinum-induced hypomagnesemia and peripheral neuropathy. *Gynecol Oncol.* 1983;16(3):309–318.

22. Pirovano C, Balzarini A, Bohm S, Oriana S, Spatti GB, Zunino F. Peripheral neurotoxicity following high-dose cisplatin with glutathione: clinical and neurophysiological assessment. *Tumori.* 1992;78(4):253–257.

23. Pisano C, Pratesi G, Laccabue D, et al. Paclitaxel and cisplatin-induced neurotoxicity: a protective role of acetyl-L-carnitine. *Clin Cancer Res.* 2003;9(15):5756–5767.

24. Treskes M, van der Vijgh WJ. WR2721 as a modulator of cisplatin- and carboplatin-induced side effects in comparison with other chemoprotective agents: a molecular approach. *Cancer Chemother Pharmacol.* 1993;33(2):93–106.

25. Apfel SC, Arezzo JC, Lipson L, Kessler JA. Nerve growth factor prevents experimental cisplatin neuropathy. *Ann Neurol.* 1992;31(1):76–80.

26. Bianchi R, Brines M, Lauria G, et al. Protective effect of erythropoietin and its carbamylated derivative in experimental cisplatin peripheral neurotoxicity. *Clin Cancer Res.* 2006;12(8):2607–2612.

27. Windebank AJ, Smith AG, Russell JW. The effect of nerve growth factor, ciliary neurotrophic factor, and ACTH analogs on cisplatin neurotoxicity in vitro. *Neurology.* 1994;44(3 Pt 1):488–494.

28. Plasmati R, Pastorelli F, Cavo M, et al. Neuropathy in multiple myeloma treated with thalidomide: a prospective study. *Neurology.* 2007;69(6):573–581.

29. Kirchmair R, Tietz AB, Panagiotou E, et al. Therapeutic angiogenesis inhibits or rescues chemotherapy-induced peripheral neuropathy: taxol- and thalidomide-induced injury of vasa nervorum is ameliorated by VEGF. *Mol Ther.* 2007;15(1):69–75.

30. Badros A, Goloubeva O, Dalal JS, et al. Neurotoxicity of bortezomib therapy in multiple myeloma: a single-center experience and review of the literature. *Cancer.* 2007;110(5):1042–1049.

31. Borgeat A, De Muralt B, Stalder M. Peripheral neuropathy associated with high-dose Ara-C therapy. *Cancer.* 1986;58(4):852–854.

32. Rodriguez V, Kuehnle I, Heslop HE, Khan S, Krance RA. Guillain-Barré syndrome after allogeneic hematopoietic stem cell transplantation. *Bone Marrow Transplant.* 2002;29(6):515–517.

33. Balachandran C, McCluskey PJ, Champion GD, Halmagyi GM. Methotrexate-induced optic neuropathy. *Clin Exp Ophthalmol.* 2002;30(6):440–441.

34. Clare G, Colley S, Kennett R, Elston JS. Reversible optic neuropathy associated with low-dose methotrexate therapy. *J Neuroophthalmol.* 2005;25(2):109–112.

35. Hoffman DL, Howard JR Jr, Sarma R, Riggs JE. Encephalopathy, myelopathy, optic neuropathy, and anosmia associated with intravenous cytosine arabinoside. *Clin Neuropharmacol.* 1993;16(3):258–262.

36. Meyers CA, Kudelka AP, Conrad CA, Gelke CK, Grove W, Pazdur R. Neurotoxicity of CI-980, a novel mitotic inhibitor. *Clin Cancer Res.* 1997;3(3):419–422.

37. Valentine AD, Meyers CA, Kling MA, Richelson E, Hauser P. Mood and cognitive side effects of interferon-α therapy. *Semin Oncol.* 1998;25(1 Suppl 1):39–47.

38. Saykin AJ, Ahles TA, McDonald BC. Mechanisms of chemotherapy-induced cognitive disorders: neuropsychological, pathophysiological, and neuroimaging perspectives. *Semin Clin Neuropsychiatry.* 2003;8(4):201–216.

39. Meyers CA, Abbruzzese JL. Cognitive functioning in cancer patients: effect of previous treatment. *Neurology.* 1992;42(2):434–436.

40. Ferguson RJ, Ahles TA. Low neuropsychologic performance among adult cancer survivors treated with chemotherapy. *Curr Neurol Neurosci Rep.* 2003;3(3):215–222.

41. Ahles TA, Saykin AJ, Furstenberg CT, et al. Neuropsychologic impact of standard-dose systemic chemotherapy in long-term survivors of breast cancer and lymphoma. *J Clin Oncol.* 2002;20(2):485–493.

42. Brezden CB, Phillips KA, Abdolell M, Bunston T, Tannock IF. Cognitive function in breast cancer patients receiving adjuvant chemotherapy. *J Clin Oncol.* 2000;18(14):2695–2701.

43. Schagen SB, van Dam FS, Muller MJ, Boogerd W, Lindeboom J, Bruning PF. Cognitive deficits after postoperative adjuvant chemotherapy for breast carcinoma. *Cancer.* 1999;85(3):640–650.

44. Tchen N, Juffs HG, Downie FP, et al. Cognitive function, fatigue, and menopausal symptoms in women receiving adjuvant chemotherapy for breast cancer. *J Clin Oncol.* 2003;21(22):4175–4183.

45. van Dam FS, Schagen SB, Muller MJ, et al. Impairment of cognitive function in women receiving adjuvant treatment for high-risk breast cancer: high-dose versus standard-dose chemotherapy. *J Natl Cancer Inst.* 1998;90(3):210–218.

46. Wieneke MH, Dienst ER. Neuropsychological assessment of cognitive functioning following chemotherapy for breast cancer. *Psychooncology.* 1995;4:61–66.

47. Wefel JS, Lenzi R, Theriault RL, Davis RN, Meyers CA. The cognitive sequelae of standard-dose adjuvant chemotherapy in women with breast carcinoma: results of a prospective, randomized, longitudinal trial. *Cancer.* 2004;100(11):2292–2299.

48. Hwang TL, Yung WK, Estey EH, Fields WS. Central nervous system toxicity with high-dose Ara-C. *Neurology.* 1985;35(10):1475–1479.

49. Schwartz J, Alster Y, Ben-Tal O, Lowenstein A. Visual loss following high-dose cytosine arabinoside (ARA-C). *Eur J Haematol.* 2000;64(3):208–209.

50. Salinsky MC, Levine RL, Aubuchon JP, Schutta HS. Acute cerebellar dysfunction with high-dose ARA-C therapy. *Cancer.* 1983; 51(3):426–429.

51. Geller HM, Cheng KY, Goldsmith NK, et al. Oxidative stress mediates neuronal DNA damage and apoptosis in response to cytosine arabinoside. *J Neurochem.* 2001;78(2):265–275.

52. Lipp HP. Neurotoxicity (including sensory toxicity) induced by cytostatics. In: Lipp HP, ed. *Anticancer Drug Toxicity Prevention, Management, and Clinical Pharmacokinetics.* New York: Marcel Dekker; 1999:431–454.

53. Logothetis CJ, Wu KK, Finn LD, et al. Phase I trial of the angiogenesis inhibitor TNP-470 for progressive androgen-independent prostate cancer. *Clin Cancer Res.* 2001;7(5):1198–1203.

54. Spiegel RJ. α-Interferons: a clinical overview. *Urology.* 1989; 34(4 Suppl):75–79; discussion, 87–96.

55. Meyers CA, Valentine AD. Neurological and psychiatric effects of immunological therapy. *CNS Drugs.* 1995;3:56–68.

56. Smith A, Tyrrell D, Coyle K, Higgins P. Effects of interferon-α on performance in man: a preliminary report. *Psychopharmacology (Berl).* 1988;96(3):414–416.

57. Malik UR, Makower DF, Wadler S. Interferon-mediated fatigue. *Cancer.* 2001;92(6 Suppl):1664–1668.

58. Valentine AD, Meyers CA. Neurobehavioral effects of interferon therapy. *Curr Psychiatry Rep.* 2005;7(5):391–395.

59. Dieperink E, Willenbring M, Ho SB. Neuropsychiatric symptoms associated with hepatitis C and interferon-α: a review. *Am J Psychiatry.* 2000;157(6):867–876.

60. Meyers CA, Scheibel RS, Forman AD. Persistent neurotoxicity of systemically administered interferon-α. *Neurology.* 1991;41(5): 672–676.

61. Patten SB, Neutel CI. Corticosteroid-induced adverse psychiatric effects: incidence, diagnosis and management. *Drug Saf.* 2000; 22(2):111–122.

62. Weissman DE, Janjan NA, Erickson B, et al. Twice-daily tapering dexamethasone treatment during cranial radiation for newly diagnosed brain metastases. *J Neurooncol.* 1991;11(3):235–239.

63. McDonald JW, Goldberg MP, Gwag BJ, Chi SI, Choi DW. Cyclosporine induces neuronal apoptosis and selective oligodendrocyte death in cortical cultures. *Ann Neurol.* 1996;40(5):750–758.

64. Ahn KJ, Lee JW, Hahn ST, et al. Diffusion-weighted MRI and ADC mapping in FK506 neurotoxicity. *Br J Radiol.* 2003; 76(912):916–919.

65. de Groen PC. Cyclosporine, low-density lipoprotein, and cholesterol. *Mayo Clin Proc.* 1988;63(10):1012–1021.

66. Taphoorn MJ, Klein M. Cognitive deficits in adult patients with brain tumours. *Lancet Neurol.* 2004;3(3):159–168.

67. Ochs J, Mulhern R, Fairclough D, et al. Comparison of neuropsychologic functioning and clinical indicators of neurotoxicity in long-term survivors of childhood leukemia given cranial radiation or parenteral methotrexate: a prospective study. *J Clin Oncol.* 1991;9(1):145–151.

68. Mulhern RK, Wasserman AL, Fairclough D, Ochs J. Memory function in disease-free survivors of childhood acute lymphocytic leukemia given CNS prophylaxis with or without 1,800 cGy cranial irradiation. *J Clin Oncol.* 1988;6(2):315–320.

69. Madhyastha S, Somayaji SN, Rao MS, Nalini K, Bairy KL. Hippocampal brain amines in methotrexate-induced learning and memory deficit. *Can J Physiol Pharmacol.* 2002;80(11): 1076–1084.

70. Abelson HT. Methotrexate and central nervous system toxicity. *Cancer Treat Rep.* 1978;62(12):1999–2001.

71. Cohen IJ, Stark B, Kaplinsky C, et al. Methotrexate-induced leukoencephalopathy is treatable with high-dose folinic acid: a case report and analysis of the literature. *Pediatr Hematol Oncol.* 1990;7(1):79–87.

72. Gregorios JB, Gregorios AB, Mora J, Marcillo A, Fojaco RM, Green B. Morphologic alterations in rat brain following systemic and intraventricular methotrexate injection: light and electron microscopic studies. *J Neuropathol Exp Neurol.* 1989;48(1):33–47.

73. Enevoldson TP. Acute cerebral oedema induced by methotrexate. *BMJ.* 1989;299(6697):516.

74. Hughes PJ, Lane RJ. Acute cerebral oedema induced by methotrexate. *BMJ.* 1989;298(6683):1315.

75. Bernini JC, Fort DW, Griener JC, Kane BJ, Chappell WB, Kamen BA. Aminophylline for methotrexate-induced neurotoxicity. *Lancet.* 1995;345(8949):544–547.

76. Bay A, Oner AF, Etlik O, Yilmaz C, Caksen H. Myelopathy due to intrathecal chemotherapy: report of six cases. *J Pediatr Hematol Oncol.* 2005;27(5):270–272.

77. Burch PA, Grossman SA, Reinhard CS. Spinal cord penetration of intrathecally administered cytarabine and methotrexate: a quantitative autoradiographic study. *J Natl Cancer Inst.* 1988; 80(15):1211–1216.

78. Winkelman MD, Hines JD. Cerebellar degeneration caused by high-dose cytosine arabinoside: a clinicopathological study. *Ann Neurol.* 1983;14(5):520–527.

79. Courtney MJ, Coffey ET. The mechanism of Ara-C-indiced apoptosis of differentiating cerebellar granule neurons. *Eur J Neurosci.* 1999;11(3):1073–1084.

80. Gottlieb D, Bradstock K, Koutts J, Robertson T, Lee C, Castaldi P. The neurotoxicity of high-dose cytosine arabinoside is age-related. *Cancer.* 1987;60(7):1439–1441.

81. Graves T, Hooks MA. Drug-induced toxicities associated with high-dose cytosine arabinoside infusions. *Pharmacotherapy.* 1989;9(1):23–28.

82. Jolson HM, Bosco L, Bufton MG, et al. Clustering of adverse drug events: analysis of risk factors for cerebellar toxicity with high-dose cytarabine. *J Natl Cancer Inst.* 1992;84(7):500–505.

83. Pellier I, Leboucher B, Rachieru P, Ifrah N, Rialland X. Flushing out of cerebrospinal fluid as a therapy for acute cerebellar dysfunction caused by high dose of cytosine arabinoside: a case report. *J Pediatr Hematol Oncol.* 2006;28(12):837–839.

84. Kilickap S, Cakar M, Onal IK, et al. Nonconvulsive status epilepticus due to ifosfamide. *Ann Pharmacother.* 2006;40(2):332–335.

85. Pelgrims J, De Vos F, Van den Brande J, Schrijvers D, Prove A, Vermorken JB. Methylene blue in the treatment and prevention of ifosfamide-induced encephalopathy: report of 12 cases and a review of the literature. *Br J Cancer.* 2000;82(2):291–294.

86. Vassal G, Deroussent A, Hartmann O, et al. Dose-dependent neurotoxicity of high-dose busulfan in children: a clinical and pharmacological study. *Cancer Res.* 1990;50(19):6203–6207.

87. Troy L, McFarland K, Littman-Power S, et al. Cisplatin-based therapy: a neurological and neuropsychological review. *Psychooncology.* 2000;9(1):29–39.

88. Shilling V, Jenkins V, Fallowfield L, Howell T. The effects of hormone therapy on cognition in breast cancer. *J Steroid Biochem Mol Biol.* 2003;86(3–5):405–412.

CHAPTER 34

Neurotoxic Effects of Pharmaceutical Agents V: Miscellaneous Agents

Melody Ryan and Kara A. Kennedy

INTRODUCTION

Many commonly used medications have adverse neurotoxic effects. This chapter reviews those effects not discussed elsewhere in this text. The chapter is necessarily wide ranging, encompassing cardiovascular medications, cholesterol-lowering medications, respiratory medications, corticosteroids, anticholinergics, antihistamines, metoclopramide, and analgesics. The neurotoxic effects of these medications are also comprehensive from parkinsonism to tinnitus.

CARDIOVASCULAR MEDICATIONS

Digoxin, amiodarone, and lidocaine are among the most commonly used antiarrhythmic medications. Each of these agents is associated with neurotoxicity syndromes. Digoxin has been linked with delirium or encephalopathy. Amiodarone has a host of neurotoxicities associated with its use, including peripheral neuropathy, optic neuropathy, and movement disorders. Lidocaine has been associated with transient neurological symptoms (TNSs)

following local administration and with seizures when high systemic concentrations are achieved. Antihypertensives are remarkably free of significant, persistent neurological adverse effects. However, reports of exacerbation of myasthenia gravis exist for β-adrenergic blockers and calcium channel blockers.

Antiarrhythmics

Digoxin

One set of symptoms associated with digoxin toxicity has been termed *delirium* or *encephalopathy*. Symptoms of anxiety, depression, delirium, and hallucinations were reported by 4% of patients in double-blind, placebo-controlled trials of digoxin.[1] Other reports suggest that fatigue, tearfulness, emotional lability, paranoia, psychomotor retardation, and cognitive problems are also common with digoxin toxicity. Several reports note the absence of depressed mood, even though other symptoms of depression are common.[2,3] The generally accepted therapeutic range for digoxin is 0.8 to 2 ng/mL,[1] but note that these symptoms have been reported in patients with serum concentrations as low as 0.6 ng/mL, particularly in elderly patients with a preexisting neurological insult (e.g., stroke or meningioma).[4–6]

Withdrawal or reduction of the digoxin resolves these problems as the serum concentration decreases. Generally, improvement is seen within 3 days, with complete resolution within 1 week. Other symptoms of digoxin toxicity, such as cardiac abnormalities, nausea, or anorexia, may be present. In particular, mood or cognitive changes, in conjunction with gastrointestinal symptoms, in a patient taking digoxin should be a signal to the clinician to consider digoxin toxicity as a potential cause. In most cases, immediate removal of digoxin activity is not necessary. However, if life-threatening digoxin intoxication is present (e.g., ventricular fibrillation), digoxin immune antigen-binding fragments may be used.[7]

Amiodarone

Neurotoxicity occurs often with amiodarone and, in some cases, appears to be dose dependent. Peripheral and optic neuropathies have been reported, although the link between amiodarone and optic neuropathy has been the object of debate. Tremor is also commonly reported; however, parkinsonism has only been seen occasionally. Amiodarone is used to prevent several types of arrhythmias, including life-threatening ventricular fibrillation. The decision to stop treatment with amiodarone because of adverse effects must be made in consultation with the patient and the patient's cardiologist, carefully weighing the advantages and disadvantages of continued therapy.

Peripheral Neuropathy

In two studies, approximately 6% of patients taking amiodarone developed peripheral neuropathy.[8,9] However, in another observational prospective study, only 2% of patients reported peripheral neuropathy (0.65 incidence for 100 person-years).[10] The cause of peripheral neuropathy is unknown. A rat study in which amiodarone was injected directly into nerves found acute motor axon degeneration, which regenerated slowly.[11] In humans, peripheral neuropathy may resolve slowly, but the patient may have residual symptoms.[12]

Optic Neuropathy

The link between amiodarone and optic neuropathy has been discussed often in the literature. One study estimated the incidence at 1.76% over 5 years in amiodarone-treated subjects compared to 0.3% in age-matched controls.[13] However, these cases were not matched for other diseases, including hypertension and diabetes, that may also influence the development of optic neuropathy. Therefore, the findings could be incidental. One of the authors of this study has even suggested recently that the association could have occurred by chance.[14] A study of 1835 patients, 793 of whom received amiodarone, was prospectively constructed to examine the question of amiodarone-associated optic neuritis. No patient developed optic neuritis during the course of treatment. Following exact binomial 95% confidence interval calculations, the authors concluded that it is possible that in a similar population a maximum of 0.13% would develop optic neuritis.[15]

Findings seen in optic neuropathy that developed in amiodarone-treated patients include a spectrum of problems, among them optic disc swelling and hemorrhages, visual difficulties without disc changes, and unilateral or bilateral optic neuropathy. If bilateral, optic neuropathy has affected both eyes either simultaneously or sequentially.[16] A case series of 55 patients with amiodarone-associated optic neuropathy found median time to onset was 4 months after starting amiodarone. Onset was insidious in 43% of patients and acute in 28%. Visual acuity problems ranged from mild to severe, with 18% having legal blindness (20/200 or worse). Visual field loss was seen in 91% of patients, and 40% had color vision loss. Visual field loss was usually permanent. Most patients (85%) had optic disc edema, but 15% had retrobulbar optic neuropathy. Disc edema resolved over a median 3 months, even if amiodarone was continued.[17]

Regular ophthalmic examination, including funduscopy and slip-lamp examinations, has been recommended during amiodarone therapy.[12] However, patients may have optic disc edema that is asymptomatic.[16] In one small series, four patients taking amiodarone who developed asymptomatic optic disc edema did not progress to optic neuropathy.[18] This finding and the need for continued antiarrhythmic therapy in many patients raises the question of how to respond when a patient develops asymptomatic optic disc edema; no prudent answer has been suggested. At this time, the clinician should treat each case individually.

Movement Disorders

Tremor and ataxia are commonly seen during amiodarone treatment, with estimates ranging from 1% to 35%.[10,19] The tremor is usually a bilateral 6- to 10-Hz action tremor of the upper extremities.[20] These adverse effects are clearly dose related and often respond to a decrease in dose and resolve with medication cessation.[19] One case report found an amiodarone-associated ataxia responsive to acetazolamide 250 mg twice daily while amiodarone was continued.[21]

Parkinsonism, with varying degrees of symptoms, has been described in several case reports.[20,22,23] In one case, symptoms began 2 years after starting amiodarone,[22] but the others had more rapid onset. In one case, a dose-related parkinsonian resting tremor in one leg was seen.[20] In another, the sole symptom was akinesia.[23] All of these effects have been reversible when amiodarone was discontinued.

Lidocaine

Lidocaine is commonly used locally for anesthesia and systemically for ventricular arrhythmias. Adverse neurological effects of spinal anesthesia are TNSs, occurring in a significant proportion of patients undergoing regional anesthesia. Systemic lidocaine use is associated with seizures.

Transient Neurological Symptoms after Spinal Anesthesia

TNSs usually involve bilateral pain or dysesthesia in the back and buttocks following spinal anesthesia. The pain radiates to the legs in approximately half the patients affected by TNSs. Onset is within 24 hours of the spinal anesthesia, and duration is between 6 and 96 hours.[24,25] The neurological examination is normal, and no muscular weakness is detected.[24] In studies of TNSs, none of 1437 patients sustained any permanent neurological damage following development of symptoms.[26]

The etiology of TNSs is unknown, but many causes, including direct local anesthetic neurotoxicity, pooling of local anesthetics within the subarachnoid space, and irritation of the dorsal root ganglion by the anesthetic, have been postulated.[24] TNSs are significantly more common with lidocaine than other local anesthetics, with a relative risk of 4.47 (95% confidence interval = 2.17 to 9.20).[26] Other risk factors appear to be the use of vasoconstrictors such as epinephrine in association with lidocaine, diabetes, and the use of the lithotomy position.[24,25] In particular, positioning of the patient has a dramatic effect on the development of TNSs. The lithotomy position is associated with a 37% incidence of TNSs, compared to only a 4% to 8% incidence for patients in the supine position.[24] The concentration and baricity (ratio of density of anesthetic solution to density of cerebrospinal fluid) do not appear to affect the risk of TNS development.[25,27]

TNSs have been effectively treated with administration of nonsteroidal antiinflammatory drugs such as ibuprofen and with warm heat. Opioids are moderately effective, and muscle relaxants such as cyclobenzaprine may be beneficial if muscle spasms are present.[24]

Seizures

Lidocaine has well-defined, dose-related neurotoxicities. The therapeutic range for lidocaine is 2 to 6 µg/mL when used for arrhythmias.[28] Fasciculations and tinnitus usually occur at serum concentrations of 6 to 8 µg/mL, while seizures and obtundation are usually seen at concentrations above 8 µg/mL.[28] In one study, seizures were seen when serum lidocaine concentrations were above 22 µg/mL. These concentrations were obtained following infusions of very high doses (11.2 and 16.5 mg/kg) of lidocaine.[29] Of note, systemic concentrations leading to seizures can be obtained after local application of lidocaine, although these isolated cases usually involve a medication error, resulting in overapplication. Subcutaneous administration, bladder instillation, and dermatological application have all been implicated in cases of generalized seizures.[30,31]

At low serum concentrations (0.5 to 4 µg/mL), lidocaine has an anticonvulsive effect.[30] Lidocaine is being used to treat status epilepticus, particularly in countries like Japan, where neither lorazepam nor fosphenytoin is available.[32] Neonates and children are usually treated with 2 mg/kg as a bolus over 20 minutes, followed with a 2 to 6 mg/kg/hr infusion.[33] Two retrospective studies found effectiveness for status epilepticus in 56.7%[32] and 93%[33] as a second-line treatment. No serum lidocaine concentrations were available in either of these studies.

Antihypertensives

While lightheadedness and fatigue are common adverse effects of many antihypertensives, they are likely related to the blood pressure–lowering effects of these agents and are predictable. Other neurotoxic effects are uncommon; however, myasthenia gravis has been reported with both β-adrenergic blockers and calcium channel blockers.

Class warnings for β-adrenergic blockers and calcium channel blockers exist for worsening myasthenia gravis based on several case reports.[34] While the mechanism for calcium channel blocker worsening of myasthenia gravis is unknown, β-adrenergic blockers are thought to either inhibit acetylcholine release or block acetylcholine receptor sites.[34] Two studies by the same investigators that administered propranolol and verapamil intravenously to patients moderately affected by myasthenia gravis did not find any significant decrease in muscle strength or fatigability. The authors concluded that emergency use of these agents should not be withheld for patients with myasthenia gravis.[35,36] The second study also examined 2 weeks of oral administration with verapamil and propranolol. Similarly, no significant decrease in muscle strength or fatigability was seen.[36]

CHOLESTEROL-LOWERING MEDICATIONS

Three of the categories of cholesterol-lowering medications—statins, fibric acid derivatives, and ezetimibe—have been reported to cause neurotoxicity. The 3-hydroxy-3-methylglutaryl–coenzyme A (HMG-CoA) reductase inhibitors, more commonly called *statins*, are the most commonly prescribed cholesterol-lowering medications. Approximately 25 million patients worldwide and 12 million patients in the United States have been treated with statins.[37] Statins have been implicated in various muscular conditions, including myalgia, rhabdomyolysis, and myasthenic syndromes, as well as peripheral neuropathy. Fibric acid derivatives and ezetimibe have been reported to cause myopathies.

Statins

Myopathy

For clarity, a clinical advisory panel composed of members from the American College of Cardiology, American Heart Association, and National Heart, Lung, and Blood Institute has defined the various myopathies associated with statin therapy in the following way: *myopathy* is any disease of muscles, *myalgia* is muscle ache or weakness without creatine kinase (CK) elevation, *myositis* consists of muscle symptoms with increased CK levels, and *rhabdomyolysis* consists of muscle symptoms with marked CK elevation (typically more than 10 times the upper limit of normal [ULN]) and with creatinine elevation (brown urine and urinary myoglobin).[38]

The incidence of muscular disorders with statins has been somewhat exaggerated by the press. With the exception of cerivastatin, which was voluntarily withdrawn by the manufacturer in 2001 due to rhabdomyolysis, the rate of muscular problems is about the same among statins.[39] Myalgias are the most common disorder, occurring in 0.3% to 33% of patients prescribed a statin. Myopathy occurs at an incidence of 5 to 11 per 100,000 patient-years, and rhabdomyolysis has an incidence range of 1.6 to 3.4 per 100,000 patient-years.[39,40] These rates show a fairly rare occurrence of serious muscular problems with statins. This can be contrasted with the rate of fatal rhabdomyolysis with cerivastatin of 1.9 deaths per 1 million prescriptions, 10 to 50 times higher than for other statins.[38] A large, epidemiological study with a strict definition of rhabdomyolysis of hospitalization and CK greater than 10 times the ULN calculated a composite incidence rate for therapy with atorvastatin, pravastatin, or simvastatin monotherapy of 0.44 per 10,000 person-years.[41] However, the outcome of rhabdomyolysis can be quite severe, with approximately 10% of cases being fatal.[42]

Several factors that increase the risk of myopathies have been identified. These include intrinsic patient factors, lifestyle factors, and medication factors. Patient factors are advanced age, low body mass index, Asian race, underlying myopathy, hypothyroidism, biliary-tract obstruction, and renal or hepatic dysfunction.[37,39] Genetic testing in patients who developed myopathies while on statins found that 10% had an underlying, subclinical metabolic myopathy or were carriers for a metabolic myopathy.[43] Lifestyle-related factors include sporadic heavy exercise, heavy alcohol consumption, and crack cocaine use.[39] Medication-related factors include the dose of the statin, as well as drug–drug interactions that may increase statin serum concentrations, such as

inhibition of metabolism. Myopathy occurrence has been shown to correlate with statin dosage but not with low-density lipoprotein reduction.[39]

The cause of statin-associated muscular problems is unknown; however, it is well recognized that increased serum concentrations of statins increase the risk of myopathies. Atorvastatin, lovastatin, and simvastatin are all metabolized by CYP3A4.[37] Several commonly prescribed medications, including clarithromycin, ketoconazole, itraconazole, miconazole, nafazodone, and nicardipine, as well as grapefruit juice, inhibit this enzyme and increase concentrations of these medicines. Statins also undergo glucuronidation with uridine diphosphate glucuronosyl transferases 1A1 and 1A3. The fibric acid derivative, gemfibrozil completes with statins for these enzymes and thus increases the serum concentrations of statins when administered concomitantly.[39]

Pathologies that have been proposed to explain the effect of statins on muscles include an aberration in coenzyme Q10, a statin-induced immune problem, or increased apoptosis.[37,39] A reduction in coenzyme Q10 concentrations is seen in some patients taking statins; however, it is not well correlated with development of myopathies.[39,44] HMG-CoA reductase is responsible for production of isoprenoids. These lipids control myofiber apoptosis, and a depletion of them could trigger increased muscle cell destruction.[39] Finally, a proposed theory is that a threshold level of cholesterol is needed to for muscle cell membranes and that statins reduce cholesterol levels excessively. However, myopathies are not found in people with inherited disorders that result in low cholesterol, nor are myopathies correlated with the amount low-density lipoprotein reduction.[39]

Myopathy symptoms seen with statin-induced myopathies are not different from other causes of myopathy. Myalgias, weakness, fatigue, low back and proximal muscle pain, and generalized aching are the most common complaints.[39] However, if rhabdomyolysis develops, renal failure and death may occur. Mean time to onset of any muscle symptoms after statin initiation is 1 month[45]; however, in patients who develop rhabdomyolysis, the mean time is 6.3 months after therapy is started.[46] Resolution of muscle complaints usually takes about 2 months following statin discontinuation.[42]

Investigation of muscle complaints in patients taking statins has been addressed by the National Lipid Association Statin Safety Assessment Task Force (Figure 34-1).[40] At this time, routine CK measurements for patients on statins without symptoms are not recommended. For those patients who may be at risk for development of myopathies (e.g., elderly patients and those with liver disease), a baseline CK may be considered.[40] Treatment for rhabdomyolysis may require hospitalization with intravenous hydration and urine alkalinization to prevent myoglobin precipitation in the renal tubules.[39]

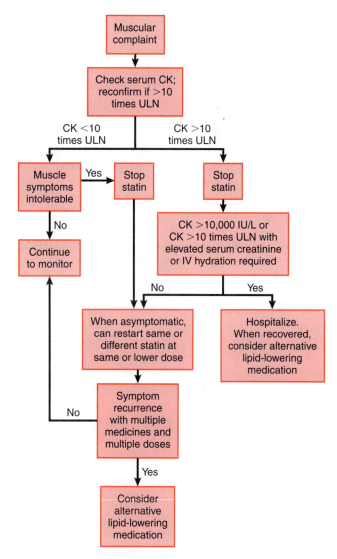

Figure 34-1. Assessment of muscular complaints in patients taking statins. (Adapted from McKenney JM, Davidson MH, Jacobson TA, Guyton JR. Final conclusions and recommendations of the National Lipid Association Statin Safety Assessment Task Force. *Am J Cardiol.* 2006;97[Suppl]:89C–94C.)

There has been some interest in administering coenzyme Q10 supplements to patients to prevent myopathies with statins. If the proposed pathology of reduced coenzyme Q10 concentrations plays a part in development of myopathy, it would be expected that supplementation might prevent myopathy. However, the two studies that have been conducted came to conflicting conclusions. One study was a double-blind, placebo-controlled trial that enrolled 44 patients who previously experienced myalgia with a statin. Subjects were randomized to receive coenzyme Q10 at 200 mg/day or placebo in conjunction with simvastatin. No difference was seen between the groups in the ability to tolerate

the simvastatin.[47] The second study randomized 32 patients who experienced muscle pain while taking statins to either coenzyme Q10 at 100 mg/day or vitamin E at 400 IU/day. Patients in the coenzyme Q10 group had decreased pain severity and interference with their daily activities, while those in the vitamin E group experienced no change.[48] Larger studies are necessary before recommending coenzyme Q10 to patients to prevent myopathies with statins.

Myasthenic Syndrome

Myasthenia gravis–type symptoms of weakness and fatigability have been reported after treatment with statins. Six cases have been reported. Two cases had positive single-fiber electromyographs, two cases had positive repetitive stimulation electromyographs, and two cases did not receive electromyographs. Four of these patients had positive acetylcholine receptor antibodies. All patients developed symptoms within 1 to 2 weeks of statin initiation. Some patients experienced recovery when the statin was discontinued, but others improved without full recovery. Two patients had recurrence of symptoms when rechallenged with another statin.[49]

The mechanism by which this myasthenic syndrome developed is unknown. The myotoxic nature of the statins could be unmasking subclinical myasthenia gravis. Alternatively, the statin might induce formation of antibodies to the neuromuscular junction.[49]

Peripheral Neuropathy

Several types of peripheral neuropathy have developed in patients taking statins. Again, decreases in serum concentrations of coenzyme Q10 in some patients given statins has been hypothesized as a mechanism for development of neuropathy. It has been further proposed that decreased coenzyme Q10 induces apoptosis of the myotubes, inhibits guanosine triphosphate signaling–related binding proteins, and inhibits the formation of selenoproteins.[44]

Development of statin-related neuropathy appears to be uncommon, but patients taking statins have been shown to have an increased risk of peripheral neuropathy in two retrospective, case–control studies. The odds ratio appears to be between 1.22 and 14.2.[50,51] Most cases that have been reported develop a sensorimotor axonal neuropathy that resolves after stopping treatment.[44] However, persistent small-fiber neuropathy and acute onset polyneuropathy have also been described.[44] The acute onset polyneuropathy has occurred within 24 hours after starting a statin but more usually has been within 1 to 2 years of initiation. Recovery may occur as soon as 2 weeks, but full recovery may take 9 months and some patients continue to have residual effects.[52–54] In one case, intravenous immune globulin was administered, but recovery was incomplete and took 12 weeks.[52]

Fibric Acid Derivatives

The two fibric acid derivatives that are available in the United States are gemfibrozil and fenofibrate. Myopathy can be seen with both of these agents, but it is more common with gemfibrozil (15.7 per 1 million prescriptions versus 8.8 per 1 million prescriptions). Likewise, gemfibrozil-associated rhabdomyolysis occurs more often than that associated with fenofibrate.[55] For the fibric acid derivatives as a class, the summary point estimate of incidence of myopathy was 2.82 per 10,000 person-years.[41] However, there is a marked difference between these agents when they are combined with statins. Because gemfibrozil inhibits the glucuronidation of statins, its use results in higher statin plasma concentrations.[56] Therefore, the risk of rhabdomyolysis when gemfibrozil is combined with a statin is 10 to 15 times the risk of a fenofibrate–statin combination.[39]

Ezetimibe

Ezetimibe, a recent introduction in lipid management, decreases cholesterol absorption from the small intestine. Three case reports exist of elevated CK in patients using ezetimibe as monotherapy.[57,58] Two of the patients were asymptomatic,[58] and one developed myopathy.[57] All of them had developed myalgia and/or CK elevations during treatment with other cholesterol-lowering mediations. One patient was determined to have impaired fatty acid oxidation.[57] Reports of muscle-related adverse effects, with CK increases less than 3 times the ULN, were reported in 24% of ezetimibe-treated patients in one study of patients who had previously experienced muscle-related adverse effects to statins.[59]

Overall, myopathies have been strongly related to statins, with some relationship to fibric acid derivatives and ezetimibe. In addition, peripheral neuropathy is emerging as a previously unknown adverse effect of statins. Patients experiencing these symptoms may be treated with lower doses or different agents. For patients who experience muscular problems with multiple classes of lipid-lowering medications, bile acid resins such as cholestyramine may be tolerated.[37]

RESPIRATORY MEDICINES

Several medication classes employed for respiratory disorders cause some degree of neurotoxicity. Theophylline and β-adrenergic agonists have been associated with tremor. Theophylline also is implicated in seizures, particularly in overdoses. Leukotriene antagonists are a relatively new class of medications, but an emerging literature is linking them to a peripheral neuropathy associated with Churg-Strauss syndrome.

Theophylline

Theophylline is not used as often for respiratory disorders in the United States as it once was, largely due to the advent of inhaled therapies. However, it still has significant worldwide use and merits careful attention because of its narrow therapeutic range (5 to 20 μg/mL) and its significant toxicities.

Seizures

Most seizures that have been reported in patients taking theophylline are generalized and many are self-limiting. However, status epilepticus has been seen in several case series, and one case of infantile spasms has been reported in a 6-month-old infant.[60] In two reports of case series of theophylline toxicity, 8.1% to 38% of patients experienced seizures.[61,62] In the largest series, including 356 patients over a 10-year period, the mean serum theophylline concentration was 60 μg/mL and 10.7% of patients had serum concentrations of more than 100 μg/mL. Seven patients in this series experienced status epilepticus.[62] Another case series of 41 patients, who were admitted for other conditions but who developed status epilepticus during hospitalization, found a high prevalence (27%) of theophylline treatment. Only one of these patients had a supratherapeutic serum concentration.[63]

It is difficult to identify risk factors for theophylline-associated seizures because many patients have seizures without other signs of toxicity and with serum concentrations below 20 μg/mL. One study compared 10 children who had experienced seizures during theophylline treatment to 27 children who had not experienced seizures in an attempt to discover risk factors for seizures. Children who experienced seizures were more likely to be younger than 1 year, but no other risk factors emerged. Total serum theophylline concentrations were available for only three children, and they were all below 10 μg/mL. No estimations of unbound serum concentrations were available for these children.[64] However, protein binding of theophylline in the serum is lower in neonates and could lead to an increase in unbound fraction of the medication that is available to cross the blood–brain barrier.[65] A second case series of 54 children with theophylline-associated seizures found the mean serum concentration at the time of seizure within the therapeutic range (10.79 ± 4.66 μg/mL). No correlation was seen between serum concentrations and duration of seizures.[66]

Several mechanisms by which theophylline may cause seizures have been proposed: it may decrease the seizure threshold, it may inhibit the binding of adenosine to its receptor and/or inhibit the production of adenosine, or it may decrease the production of γ-aminobutyric acid (GABA) or directly inhibits the GABA receptor.[66] Under normal circumstances, adenosine suppresses the release of excitatory amino acids; therefore, if adenosine is decreased, more excitatory amino acids could be released, which might cause a seizure. Theophylline is also known to antagonize the actions of benzodiazepines, possibly at the GABA receptor. In this case, the inhibitory effect of GABA might be ameliorated.[66]

Treatment of theophylline-associated seizures has proved difficult. One study compared theophylline-associated seizures to non-theophylline-associated seizures. Only 45.5% of theophylline-associated cases were successfully treated with diazepam compared to 68% of non-theophylline-associated cases. Phenytoin was used as a second-line therapy in eight cases and was efficacious in only three. A higher percentage also required barbiturates and endotracheal intubation compared to patients with non-theophylline-associated seizures.[66] Phenytoin is usually considered much less effective in the treatment of theophylline-associated seizures; thus, benzodiazepines and barbiturates are recommended.[67]

Movement Disorders

A course muscle tremor of myoclonus is often seen in patients with theophylline intoxication. In one case series, 40% were thus affected. The mean serum theophylline concentration in the whole series was 60 μg/mL.[62] Tremor usually resolves as serum concentrations decrease or after the theophylline is discontinued. Acute facial and limb dyskinesias have been reported after bolus dosing of theophylline in three children. Movements subsided over a period of days after theophylline discontinuation.[68,69]

Treatment of Theophylline Intoxication

In the situation of acute overdoses of theophylline, administration of activated charcoal is effective in removal of medication.[67] However, large amounts of theophylline often induce vomiting, and hemodialysis or extracorporeal removal with charcoal hemoperfusion may be necessary. Peritoneal dialysis is ineffective for theophylline removal.[67]

The need for anticonvulsants should be anticipated. Prophylactic phenobarbital therapy has been recommended in some cases with high serum theophylline concentrations (>100 μg/mL) or when the patient is thought to be at higher risk for seizures.[67] The risk of respiratory depression when using the combination of a benzodiazepine and barbiturate should be considered, particularly in patients who likely have some underlying respiratory disorder.

β-Adrenergic Agonists

Tremor is a common occurrence with the β-adrenergic agonists, even at therapeutic doses (Table 1). There are differences among the agents and the dosage forms. Systemic dosing, such as intravenous or oral, is associated with the highest reported prevalence of tremor, while inhaled formations have substantially lower prevalence. Usually, the tremor is transient and is often benign.

A mechanism has been proposed to account for tremor associated with β-adrenergic agonist use. When the agonist stimulates the β_2-adrenergic receptors on the extracellular membrane of the skeletal muscle, the sodium/potassium/ATPase pump activates. Potassium is driven intracellularly, causing a drop in serum potassium. The onset of hypokalemia corresponds to onset of tremor in animal studies when intravenous salbuterol was administered.[79] However, this may be an incidental finding in that stimulation of the β_2-adrenergic receptors may cause both hypokalemia

Table 1:   Tremor Reported with Selected β-Adrenergic Agonists

Medication	Dosage Form	Percentage of Patients with Tremor
Albuterol	Solution for nebulization Inhaler Extended-release tablets	20%[70] 7%[71] 24.2%[72]
Arformoterol	Solution for nebulization	<2%[73]
Formoterol	Inhaler	1.9%[74]
Levalbuterol	Solution for nebulization	6.8%[75]
Metaproterenol	Solution for nebulization Inhaler Tablets	2.5%/16.6%*[76] 1–4%[76] 16.9%[76]
Pirbuterol	Inhaler	6%[77]
Terbutaline	Intravenous	7.8%/38%†[78]

*2.5% in adults; 16.6% in children.
†7.8% with a 0.25-mg dose; 38% with a 0.5-mg dose.

and tremor without a causative relationship between the two.

Leukotriene Antagonists

The leukotriene antagonists, montelukast and zafirlukast, have been associated with Churg-Strauss syndrome. This syndrome is a disseminated small-vessel granulomatous vasculitis that is associated with some neurological manifestations, along with the more common symptoms of fever, weight loss, hypereosinophilia, asthma, allergic rhinitis, eosinophilic pneumonia and gastroenteritis, cardiomyopathy, and purpuric rash.[80] The American College of Rheumatology diagnostic criteria for Churg-Strauss syndrome require four or more of the following signs and symptoms: asthma, eosinophilia of more than 10% on white blood cell differential, mononeuropathy or polyneuropathy, nonfixed pulmonary infiltrate on chest x-ray, paranasal sinus abnormality, and biopsy containing a blood vessel with extravascular eosinophils.[81] The neurological symptom of peripheral neuropathy is usually a late symptom that occurs because of ischemic nerve injury caused by systemic vasculitis.

Churg-Strauss syndrome has often been reported following dose reduction or discontinuation of corticosteroids. In this so-called form frusta, it appears that the corticosteroids have suppressed the Churg-Strauss syndrome symptoms, which are only revealed when the steroid dose is lowered.[82] Indeed, this appears to be the case for some reports with the leukotriene antagonists.[80,83] However, two cases of Churg-Strauss syndrome after zafirlukast[84] and two after montelukast[85,86] initiation have been reported in which no systemic steroids were being used. Some patients' symptoms improve after the leukotriene antagonist has been discontinued, even without immunosuppressant therapy. However, most continue to have neurological deficits.

CORTICOSTEROIDS

Corticosteroids are commonly used in neurological, immunological, and respiratory disorders. Muscle wasting and myopathy are well-recognized adverse effects of corticosteroids. However, the myopathy can be particularly problematic when it involves the respiratory muscles in patients with preexisting respiratory disease. Psychosis is also a well-recognized adverse effect of corticosteroids and is covered in Chapter 33. However, dementia associated with corticosteroid use is less common and often overlooked.

Myopathy

Myopathies may occur in 7% to 64% of patients treated with corticosteroids.[87,88] Most research has centered on the myopathies associated with the chronic administration of corticosteroids,[88] but patients given these medications acutely may also be affected.[89] One retrospective study of patients given corticosteroids for acute asthma exacerbations for which they were mechanically ventilated found myopathy in 10.4% of patients. This rate increased to 30% for patients who received both corticosteroids and neuromuscular blocking agents.[89] There are also case reports of myopathy following high-dose inhaled steroids that likely achieved pharmacologically active systemic concentrations.[90] No relationship between dose or duration of steroid therapy and development of myopathy has been detected.[88] The more potent, fluorinated steroids (dexamethasone, triamcinolone) are more likely to cause myopathy, but cases with nonfluorinated steroids have also been observed.[88]

The specific mechanism by which corticosteroids induce myopathy is unclear. Muscle biopsies often are nonspecific. It is thought that corticosteroids inhibit protein synthesis, mainly in type II muscle fibers, and reduce the expression of insulin-like growth factor-1, which may increase apoptosis of muscle cells.[88,91]

Patients usually present with proximal weakness, atrophy, and myalgia.[88] One study found decreased survival in eight patients with chronic obstructive pulmonary disease and corticosteroid-associated myopathy compared to age, sex, and degree of airflow obstruction-matched patients with chronic obstructive pulmonary disease ($p < 0.025$).[92] Treatment usually consists of discontinuation of the corticosteroid, taking care to provide a gradual decrease for patients who have been on long-term therapy. Resolution may take weeks to months.[88]

Dementia

Dementia associated with corticosteroid administration is not common; most information on this effect has been via case reports.[93–95] However, there is one estimate from a closed health system in which 6 out of 1500 patients who were given corticosteroids (0.4%) developed dementia.[95] Risk factors for development of dementia with corticosteroids are unknown. Doses of prednisone have been as low as 30 mg/day but as high as 300 mg/day. Most doses of prednisone have been higher than 60 mg/day. Three of 11 patients reported to have steroid-associated dementia in case reports also had steroid-associated psychosis, but the others did not.[93,95]

It is thought that corticosteroids mainly affect the hippocampus to produce symptoms of dementia. Animal studies show dendritic atrophy in hippocampal CA3 neurons and hippocampal pyramidal cell loss when cells are exposed to elevated corticosteroid concentrations. Some of these histological changes in animals have been reversible upon corticosteroid discontinuation.[96]

The cases reported in the literature have shown deficits of functioning, as well as on neuropsychological tests such as verbal and performance intelligence quotient, memory tests, and associative fluency.[95] All patients have improved following corticosteroid cessation, but some deficits ranging from mild to moderate have continued.[93–95,97] No reports of dementia-specific treatments such as cholinesterase inhibitors exist.

ANTICHOLINERGICS

Because anticholinergics are commonly used medications, anticholinergic toxicity is relatively prevalent. In 2006, 6296 unintentional and 382 intentional anticholinergic ingestions were reported to the American Association of Poison Control Centers.[98] In addition to the commonly used anticholinergic compounds (Table 2), there are more than 500 additional compounds with anticholinergic properties. These agents include many commonly used medications, such as antihistamines, low-potency antipsychotics, tricyclic antidepressants, sedative hypnotics, and narcotics.[99] The anticholinergic properties of some atypical antipsychotics are often overlooked. Clozapine binds to the central nervous system (CNS) muscarinic receptors; olanzapine is also a potent muscarinic receptor antagonist.[100]

Both the young and the elderly are particularly susceptible to anticholinergic effects. Toxicity from diphenoxylate–atropine in the pediatric population has been reported numerous times. Transdermal scopolamine, which is commonly used for motion sickness, has been reported to cause blurred vision and even hallucinations and psychosis in both children and elderly people.[101,102] Children have suffered from systemic anticholinergic toxicity with the use of conjunctivally administered ophthalmic drops.[99] The elderly often take multiple medications that have anticholinergic properties, contributing to the likelihood of experiencing neurotoxicity from these medicines.[103]

The neurological effects of anticholinergics are dose dependent. At low doses, patients may have blurred vision from impaired accommodation. At moderate doses,

Table 2:	Selected Anticholinergic Medications	
Agent	**Description**	**Indication**
Atropine	Naturally occurring tertiary amine antimuscarinic	Inhibition of secretions during surgery, diagnosis of sinus node dysfunction, cardiopulmonary resuscitation
Benztropine	Antimuscarinic	Parkinson's disease
Clidinium	Synthetic quaternary ammonium antimuscarinic	Gastrointestinal disorders
Dicyclomine	Synthetic tertiary amine antimuscarinic	Gastrointestinal disorders
Glycopyrrolate	Synthetic quaternary ammonium antimuscarinic	Inhibition of secretions during surgery
Hyoscyamide	Naturally occurring tertiary amine antimuscarinic	Gastrointestinal disorders
Ipratropium	Synthetic quaternary ammonium antimuscarinic	Respiratory disorders
Oxybutynin	Synthetic tertiary amine antimuscarinic	Overactive bladder
Scopolamine	Naturally occurring tertiary amine antimuscarinic	Motion sickness, inhibition of secretions during surgery
Tiotropium	Synthetic quaternary ammonium antimuscarinic	Respiratory disorders
Tolterodine	Synthetic tertiary amine antimuscarinic	Overactive bladder
Trihexyphenidyl	Antimuscarinic	Parkinson's disease

patients become mildly agitated and have difficulty with speaking and swallowing. At high doses, pupils are intensely mydriatic and nonreactive, vision is significantly blurred, ataxia may become prominent, and mental status can be significantly altered. Patients may also experience restlessness, excitement, hallucinations, delirium, and seizures.

Acute intoxication leads to symptoms within minutes to hours after ingestion. Symptoms may also result from an accumulation of medication, or its metabolites, after long-term use. Anticholinergic syndrome is classically described as the following constellation of symptoms: "red as a beet, dry as a bone, hot as a hare, blind as a bat, mad as a hatter, full as a flask."[104] Each of these colorful descriptions refers to a manifestation of cholinergic blockade: The sweat glands are innervated by muscarinic receptors. With the absence of appropriate heat dissipation via sweat loss, the patient compensates with cutaneous vasodilatation, which is referred to as *atropine flush* or "red as a beet." Muscarinic antagonism leads to anhidrosis, or the symptom of "dry as a bone." In the same manner, the patient develops anhydrotic hyperthermia, or is "hot as a hare." Both pupillary constriction and accommodation with near vision are controlled by muscarinic input. Antagonism at these receptor sites produces nonreactive mydriasis and impaired accommodation, or blurry vision—described as "blind as a bat." Muscarinic receptor blockade within the CNS may precipitate anxiety, agitation, confusion, disorientation, visual hallucinations, bizarre behavior, delirium, psychosis, coma, and seizures. This presentation is described as "mad as a hatter." Lastly, the patient's detrusor muscle and urethral sphincter are controlled by muscarinic receptors. Muscarinic blockade leads to urinary retention, otherwise described as "full as a flask."

Treatment of acute anticholinergic overdose may be necessary. If the medication was orally ingested, efforts to limit intestinal absorption should be made with charcoal or gastric lavage. In patients with severe symptoms, physostigmine can be given to reverse the anticholinergic effects. If seizures occur, benzodiazepines are often effective. Benzodiazepines may also be used to treat agitation or drug-induced psychosis because antipsychotic use is relatively contraindicated due to antipsychotics' potential additive anticholinergic effects.

ANTIHISTAMINES

The chemical histamine is found throughout the body and is involved in the allergic response, is a regulator of gastric acid secretion, and is a modulator of neurotransmitter release in the central and peripheral nervous systems. There are three histamine receptor classes, designated H_1, H_2, and H_3; medications have been developed to specifically

Table 3:   Classification of Selected Antihistamines

H_1 RECEPTOR ANTAGONISTS
Nonselective (First Generation)
Azatadine
Brompheniramine
Carbinoxamine
Chlorpheniramine
Clemastine
Cyproheptadine
Dexchlorpheniramine
Diphenhydramine
Hydroxyzine
Phenindamine
Pheniramine
Pyrilamine
Triprolidine
Peripherally Selective (Second Generation)
Azelastine
Certirizine
Desloratadine
Fexofenadine
Loratadine
H_2 RECEPTOR ANTAGONISTS
Cimetidine
Famotodine
Nizatidine
Ranitidine

antagonize each of these receptors (Table 3). The first H_1-receptor antagonists helped treat allergy symptoms but caused significant sedation; thus, the second-generation or "nonsedating" H_1-receptor antagonists were developed. H_2-receptor antagonists were developed to block gastric acid production. H_3-receptor antagonists are not used therapeutically.

H_1-Receptor Antagonists

The H_1-receptor antagonists reversibly and competitively inhibit the H_1-receptor sites. This group of antihistamines has a significant effect on the CNS. H_1 receptors are found throughout the CNS. Curiously, endogenous plasma concentrations of histamine are quite low, but there are relatively large amounts of histamine in cerebrospinal fluid.[105] It is theorized that histamine is a neurotransmitter within the CNS. Likely because of the ubiquity of histamine, the first-generation H_1 blockers have the dual characteristics of both a CNS stimulant and a CNS depressant. The effect depends on the dosage, specific H_1 antagonist, and recipient response. Agitation, restless, and anxiety may occur at standard antihistamine doses. Euphoria, insomnia, and tremors are also potential adverse neurological effects. Extreme CNS excitation, such as convulsions, is a manifestation of H_1-receptor antagonist neurotoxicity. In an analysis of the San Francisco Bay Area Poison Control Center's database, diphenhydramine accounted for 7% of 233 seizure reports associated with overdose.[106] CNS depression, such as somnolence or slowed cognitive response, is a typical adverse effect of the first-generation H_1 antagonists, even at therapeutic doses.[105] Diphenhydramine is notorious for this side effect and is opportunistically used for the treatment of insomnia. Retrospective and prospective case studies of diphenhydramine poisonings show a dose–response relationship for neurotoxicities.[107] Somnolence was a prominent symptom at ingestions ranging from 0.3 to 2.5 g. Agitation, confusion, and hallucinations were also seen with lower and midrange ingestions (0.5 to 4 g). The more severe symptoms of delirium, psychosis, seizures, and coma were only seen at ingestions greater than 1 g. At ingestions above 1.5 g, seizures were seen in 19%, delirium was seen in 13%, and coma was seen in 9% of patients in the retrospective study. In the prospective analysis, ingestions above 1.5 g resulted in seizures in 22%, delirium in 11%, and coma in 11% of patients.

Additional adverse effects of dizziness, tinnitus, incoordination, diplopia, and fatigue may occur. These may largely be attributable to the anticholinergic activity of many first-generation H_1 antagonists. Chlorpheniramine, cyproheptadine, doxylamine, hydroxyzine, diphenhydramine, meclizine, and promethazine have potent muscarinic antagonist properties, leading to many of the adverse CNS effects of these medications at therapeutic, but especially at supratherapeutic, doses. See the Anticholinergics section for a more detailed description of the adverse neurological effects attributed to muscarinic receptor blockade.

The second-generation H_1-receptor antagonists are lipophobic and therefore do not readily cross the blood–brain barrier. Thus, second-generation H_1-receptor antagonists do not typically cause CNS effects.[108–110] The nonsedating H_1 blockers have an affinity to occupy CNS H_1 receptors that ranges from 0% with fexofenadine to 30% with cetirizine.[111]

There are case reports of rhabdomyolysis associated with overdoses of first-generation H_1-receptor antagonists.[112] Thus far, rhabdomyolysis has not been associated with second-generation H_1-receptor antagonists.[113]

H_2-Receptor Antagonists

A review of CNS toxicity reported in the literature or to the U.S. Food and Drug Administration from 1977 to 1989 revealed 1374 cases; 64% were associated with cimetidine, 29% with ranitidine, 5% with famotidine, and 2% with nizatidine.[114] Symptoms associated with H_2-receptor antagonists include confusion or disorientation (45%); agitation, hostility, or delirium (22%); hallucinations (18%); obtundation or somnolence (7%); mental status changes (5%); and psychosis or paranoia (3%). Symptoms usually occurred within 2 weeks of starting therapy, and all resolved within 1 week of discontinuation of the H_2-receptor antagonist.

Other case reports reveal additional neurotoxicities of H_2-receptor antagonists. Five cases of optic neuropathy have been associated with cimetidine administration.[115] Dystonic reactions have also been observed after cimetidine and ranitidine administration.[116,117]

METOCLOPRAMIDE

Metoclopramide is widely used as an antiemetic and prokinetic agent. Its action comes from antagonizing dopamine (D_1 and D_2) receptors centrally in the chemoreceptor trigger zone and peripherally in myenteric neurons.[118] Because of this blockade, several movement disorders have been associated with metoclopramide use, particularly extrapyramidal effects. Chorea has also been reported.[119] Neurotoxicities may be acute in onset, as in dystonia, or may develop over a longer period, as in parkinsonism. They may also be life threatening, as in neuroleptic malignant syndrome. As illustrated in the epidemiological studies that follow, metoclopramide is often overlooked as a potentially causative agent for extrapyramidal effects.

An epidemiological review of extrapyramidal reactions associated with metoclopramide use was performed. All reports made between 1964 and 1982 to the Adverse Reactions Register of the Committee on the Safety of Medicine of the United Kingdom were examined. For the review, 479 reports were collected; 455 were dystonic or dyskinetic reactions, 20 were parkinsonism, and 4 were tardive dyskinesia. When compared to the number of prescriptions in the United Kingdom, the incidence of extrapyramidal reactions appears to be between 0.001% and 0.005% each year.[120]

A case series of 16 patients with metoclopramide-associated movement disorders found tardive dyskinesia in 10 patients, parkinsonism in 5 patients, tardive dystonia in 1 patient, and akathisia in 1 patient. While most patients were elderly at the onset (mean age 63 years), the range spanned adulthood (24 to 85 years). Women were more commonly affected (3:1). Therapy with metoclopramide continued for an average of 6 months after the onset of symptoms before recognition of neurotoxicity.[121]

A case–control study of 53 patients treated with metoclopramide and 51 controls found a relative risk of 4.0 (95% confidence interval = 1.5 to 10.5) for drug-induced parkinsonism and a nonsignificant relative risk of 1.67 (95% confidence interval = 0.93 to 2.97) for tardive dyskinesia among those exposed to metoclopramide.[122]

In a large database review, acute dystonic–dyskinetic reactions were more common in women (70%) and usually occurred 24 to 72 hours after treatment initiation.[120] Metoclopramide is metabolized by cytochrome P450 enzyme 2D6. Patients may possess polymorphisms for the gene that codes for this enzyme, causing them to metabolize substrates of this enzyme faster or slower than the general population. In two patients with acute dystonic reactions to metoclopramide, genetic testing revealed that both patients were slow metabolizers.[123] Three cases of laryngeal dystonia leading to acute upper airway obstruction have been reported following doses of metoclopramide.[124,125] If the dystonia is recognized and related to metoclopramide, intravenous diphenhydramine may be administered with good results.[126]

A form of tardive dyskinesia can develop in patients given metoclopramide. As the descriptor tardive suggests, it usually develops more slowly. In a retrospective review of 434 patients with tardive dyskinesia, the causative agent appeared to be metoclopramide in 39.4%. In this study, the incidence of metoclopramide-associated tardive dyskinesia appeared to be rising compared to other agents (i.e., typical antipsychotics); it was implicated in 24% of cases from 1988 to 1993 and in 34.5% of cases between 2000 and 2006.[118]

In the literature, 18 cases of neuroleptic malignant syndrome have been reported following metoclopramide administration; 4 have been lethal.[119] Renal dysfunction, seen in 5 cases, may predispose patients to developing neuroleptic malignant syndrome.[128]

In contrast to the acute dystonias and dyskinesias, parkinsonism may take longer to develop. In a large database review, seven patients developed symptoms within 3 days, six developed symptoms between 3 and 28 days, and seven developed symptoms more than 28 days after treatment initiation. Two of these patients took metoclopramide for more than 5 years before exhibiting symptoms of parkinsonism. In this review, parkinsonism occurred more often in women (75%).[120]

The features of metoclopramide-associated parkinsonism are clinically indistinguishable from those of idiopathic Parkinson's disease.[129] In one case series, 24 patients were identified as having drug-induced parkinsonism (29% treated with metoclopramide). Most of these patients had been diagnosed with Parkinson's disease and were being treated for that disorder. The mean time to diagnosis of drug-induced parkinsonism was 1.8 years, and none of these patients received a diagnosis of drug-induced parkinsonism before evaluation by a movement disorder clinic, although many had been examined by other neurologists.[129] This underrecognition of metoclopramide as a causative agent for drug-induced parkinsonism highlights the need for a careful pharmacotherapy review for patients presenting with this movement disorder. After withdrawal of metoclopramide, recovery is often complete but may take several months.[120]

When metoclopramide is associated with akathisia, it usually occurs acutely in the context of parenteral administration. A prospective study was used to determine whether metoclopramide infusion rate affected the development of metoclopramide-associated akathisia. In the study, 300 subjects were randomized to receive either 10 mg of metoclopramide as an intravenous bolus over 2 minutes or 10 mg of metoclopramide in 100 mL of normal saline as a 15-minute intravenous infusion. The group treated with bolus metoclopramide was 5.27 times more likely to experience akathisia than the infusion group (24.7% versus 5.8%). All patients who developed akathisia did so within an hour of the dose of metoclopramide.[130]

A prospective study designed to determine the preferred agent for treating metoclopramide-induced akathisia randomized 56 patients. Subjects were given either 2 mg of intravenous midazolam or 20 mg of intravenous diphenhydramine. Both medications equally relieved the symptoms of akathisia; however, with midazolam subjects reported significant relief within the first 5 minutes, while relief provided by diphenhydramine took more than 15 minutes.[131]

ANALGESICS

Among agents classified as analgesics—aspirin, acetaminophen, nonsteroidal antiinflammatory agents, and opioids—only aspirin and opioids have significant neurotoxicity. Aspirin overdose can be associated with various neurological symptoms. The association of Reye's syndrome with aspirin use is controversial. Opioids have been associated with seizures and movement disorders. The synthetic opioid tramadol has also been implicated in serotonin syndrome.

Aspirin

Reye's Syndrome

Reye's syndrome usually begins with a flulike, upper respiratory, or gastrointestinal viral illness. In the United States, Reye's syndrome is most often linked to influenza or varicella infection.[132] After a few days, profuse vomiting begins and an abrupt clinical deterioration follows. Encephalopathy with delirium, stupor, or lethargy may follow.[132,133] Mortality occurs in 25% to 50% of cases, with the remainder of patients usually recovering without sequelae.[133]

Aspirin was associated with Reye's syndrome in the 1980s with large epidemiological studies.[134–137] In 1982, the U.S. Food and Drug Administration required a warning label regarding the possible association of aspirin with Reye's syndrome.[138] The number of Reye's syndrome cases in the United States has declined from a high of approximately 550 cases from 1979 to 1980 to the present number of less than 10 per year.[138]

Some scientists believe that aspirin is a necessary cofactor in viral illnesses that results in Reye's syndrome in susceptible individuals.[132] Other authors have argued that aspirin was simply present in many cases of Reye's syndrome but that it was not causative, that numerous patients with inborn errors of metabolism were misdiagnosed as Reye's syndrome, and that the original epidemiological studies were biased and methodologically flawed.[133] A study meant to control for biases and correct methodological problems from previous studies was undertaken in the late 1980s. It too found an association between Reye's syndrome and aspirin administration, with 88% of cases compared to 17% of controls receiving aspirin during the initial febrile illness.[139]

Criteria were developed in the 1980s by Hall et al. and Gauthier et al. to more specifically define Reye's syndrome so that it can be distinguished from metabolic disorders that might clinically mimic Reye's syndrome.[134,140] The criteria developed by Hall et al. are straightforward and include clearly defined prodrome, vomiting, elevated liver enzymes, elevated plasma ammonia, cerebrospinal fluid white blood cell count of 8×10^9 per liter or fewer, and

fatty liver on histology. Investigation of alternative diagnoses is required, and the presence of atypical features makes Reye's syndrome less likely.[134]

With these criteria in mind, several reanalyses of case series reported as Reye's syndrome have been undertaken.[132,138] A reanalysis with the Hall criteria of 49 Australian patients originally diagnosed with Reye's syndrome in the 1980s revealed that 13 of these cases were unlikely to be Reye's syndrome. In addition, upon reanalysis, 9 patients were considered to have probable Reye's syndrome and 27 were thought to have possible Reye's syndrome. Also upon reanalysis, 15 patients were diagnosed with inborn errors of metabolism.[138] Another reanalysis of 632 cases of Reye's syndrome reported between 1981 and 2001 found 164 cases with a disorder other than Reye's syndrome, 81 of which were inherited metabolic disorders.[132]

The evidence for a causal role of aspirin in Reye's syndrome is still disputed. At this time, it is usual clinical practice in the United States to not give aspirin to children under 16 years of age for febrile or viral illnesses.

Intoxication

U.S. poison control centers received 40,405 reports of aspirin poisonings in 2004. Of these, 44% involved children younger than 6 years.[141] Neurological symptoms reported following exposure include tinnitus, lethargy, confusion, and seizures.[141] Onset of symptoms may occur between 1 and 24 hours following aspirin ingestion.[141]

Few reports exist in the literature regarding neurological manifestations of aspirin and other salicylate intoxication. In mild to moderate intoxication, patients may have tinnitus and lethargy; however, in severe intoxications, encephalopathy, coma, seizures, and cerebral edema may be seen.[142] Cerebral dysfunction may include symptoms ranging from confusion to coma.[143] Histopathological reports following aspirin intoxication are rare, but autopsy results from a 34-year-old woman who had ingested 15 g over 3 days showed centrum semiovale and deep cerebellar white matter myelin damage with preservation of axons. White matter edema was pronounced.[143]

Clinical Correlate

A 38-year-old man with a history of schizophrenia presented to a community hospital with respiratory distress, altered mental status, hearing loss, and headache. He rapidly worsened, requiring intubation. Computerized tomography scan of the head revealed generalized cerebral edema. Antibiotics were empirically given for meningoencephalitis. He was emergently transferred to my university medical center. Initial physical examination findings there included hypotension, tachypnea, tachycardia, temperature of 100.8°F, obtundation, intact brainstem reflexes, symmetrical withdrawal to pain, and diffuse upper motor neuron signs. General laboratory studies revealed mild, acute renal failure secondary to dehydration, hyperchloremia, and metabolic acidosis with respiratory compensation. Imaging studies are in Figure 34-2A and B. The patient's family offered that the patient, whom they described as "compulsive," had taken two bottles of aspirin over the previous 2 days for headache. Salicylate serum concentration was 46.5 mg/dL (>25 mg/dL is toxic). With hemodialysis, the patient's renal function returned to normal and his salicylate concentration declined; he was asymptomatic at discharge 1 week later.

Opioids

Movement Disorders

Movement disorders seen with opioids can include muscular rigidity and myoclonus. Choreiform movements appear to be associated only with methadone.

Muscular Rigidity

Muscular rigidity is rare, but when seen it usually occurs during induction of anesthesia in nonparalyzed patients or during emergence from anesthesia.[144] These symptoms have been reported up to 5 hours after cessation of anesthesia.[144] The opioid is thought to cause glottic closure, and in unventilated patients, this may precipitate ventilatory difficulties.[144] The area of the brain thought to be involved with this toxicity is the locus ceruleus.[144] If the patient is only undergoing spinal anesthesia when the muscular rigidity occurs, it can be resolved with administration of general anesthesia.[145] Administration of a neuromuscular blocker or naloxone can also treat this effect.[144]

Myoclonus

Myoclonus has been reported following treatment with diamorphine, fentanyl, hydromorphone, meperidine, methadone, morphine, and sufentanil.[146] Myoclonus is usually seen in conjunction with hyperalgesia. Hyperalgesia does not appear to be an opioid tolerance but rather an increase in pain sensitivity that occurs rapidly.[147] The incidence range for myoclonus is quite broad, from 2.7% to 87%.[148] The risk of developing myoclonus is correlated with presence of spinal cord cancer lesions, renal failure, and dehydration.[148] The development of myoclonus may also be associated with the concomitant use of dopamine receptor antagonists,

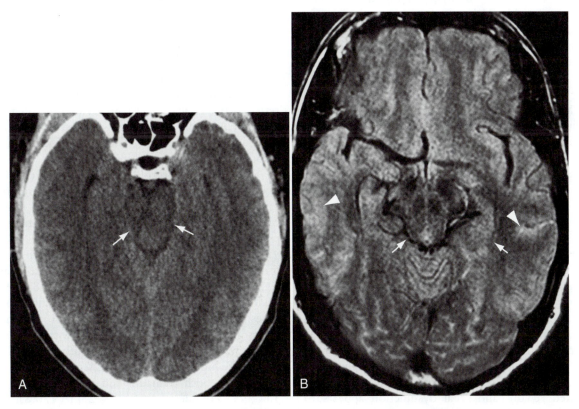

Figure 34-2. *(A)* Axial noncontrast computerized tomograph (at time of presentation) at level of midbrain demonstrating generalized cerebral edema and effacement of the perimesencephalic cisterns *(arrows)*. *(B)* Fluid-attenuated inversion recovery axial image (48 hours after presentation) at level of the midbrain. Note patchy regions of cortical hyperintensity *(arrowheads)*. Quadrigeminal cistern is effaced *(small arrows)*.

including antipsychotics and antiemetics.[149] A retrospective study of 191 patients with cancer pain revealed that 80 patients (42%) required switching to an alternative opioid. Of those switches, 11% occurred because of myoclonus.[150]

Although the exact mechanism by which opioids cause myoclonus is unknown, theories include activation of the δ-opioid receptors or inhibition of the glycine or N-methyl-d-aspartate receptors by morphine or metabolites of morphine.[146,151] Particular attention has focused on the morphine-3-glucuronide (M3G) metabolite. Rats have developed myoclonus after administration of high-dose morphine and M3G.[152] Renal failure may cause accumulation of M3G and may explain the association between myoclonus and renal dysfunction.[148] The hyperalgesia may also be due to analgesic effects of M3G.[153]

Reports on the effect of naloxone, a opioid antagonist, on myoclonus are mixed.[147,149] However, the need for rapid reversal is rare. In some cases in which myoclonus is mild and patients have good pain control, the opioids are continued. Other management options include reduction of opioid dose (if pain is adequately controlled), change of opioids, or administration of benzodiazepines, baclofen, or dantroline.[146,151] There are reports of two cases of morphine-induced myoclonus that resolved within 24 hours of starting gabapentin.[151] Intravenous clonidine has also been used for the management of methadone-induced myoclonus in a 96-day-old infant.[153]

Other Movement Disorders

There are several case reports of choreiform movements following use of methadone for cancer-related pain,[154] reflex sympathetic dystrophy,[155] and substance abuse treatment.[156,157] In all of these cases, other opioids did not cause recurrence of this movement disorder and symptoms resolved within approximately 1 week after cessation of methadone.

Seizures

Seizures have been reported with most commonly used opioids, including fentanyl, alfentanil, sulfentanil, pentazocine, morphine, codeine, and oxycodone.[158] However, meperidine is the opioid analgesic most commonly associated with seizures. It is metabolized to an active form, normeperidine. It is thought that the normeperidine is responsible for the neurotoxicity associated with meperidine, including hallucinations, tremor, myoclonus, and seizures.[159] Normeperidine is eliminated renally, and renal dysfunction appears to increase the risk of seizures.[159] In patients with normal renal function, seizures are uncommon unless meperidine doses exceed 600 mg/day.[159,160]

Tramadol

Tramadol is a synthetic analgesic that binds to the μ-opioid receptors, increases serotonin release, and weakly inhibits norepinephrine and serotonin reuptake.[161] It is metabolized by the cytochrome P450 enzymes 2D6 and 3A4. Thus, inhibitors of these enzymes such as quinidine, fluoxetine, paroxetine, amitriptyline, ketoconazole, and erythromycin may increase the serum concentrations and the risk for adverse effects of tramadol.[162] The use of multiple medications that lower the seizure threshold, increase serotonin, or both should be undertaken cautiously, if at all, with tramadol.[163]

Several case reports associate serotonin syndrome with the concomitant use of tramadol and serotonin-specific reuptake inhibitors,[164,165] tricyclic antidepressants,[166] mirtazapine,[167,168] and venlafaxine.[168] There are also rare reports of patients taking only tramadol who have developed serotonin syndrome.[169] In one case, elevated cerebrospinal fluid serotonin concentrations were seen in conjunction with symptoms of serotonin syndrome.[170]

Seizures are also a concern in patients taking tramadol. Several epidemiological studies have been performed to help discern the incidence of seizures and risk factors associated with seizures in patients taking tramadol.[161,171,172] A case–control study with a large U.S. database found the hazard of a seizure diagnosis was higher for patients who received more tramadol prescriptions: 2.2 for those with 1 prescription compared to 6.1 for those with more than 10 prescriptions.[172] However, this study found a low incidence (>1%) of seizures in patients with no other seizure risk factors.[172] In contrast, a retrospective review of 97 patients seen in a first seizure clinic in Australia found eight patients with tramadol-associated seizures (8.2%). These events occurred within 1 to 365 days of tramadol initiation.[171]

A nested case–control study using the General Practice Research Database from the United Kingdom determined the incidence of new-onset seizures in patients receiving a prescription for tramadol. Patients with preexisting epilepsy or brain tumor were excluded. Thus, 11,383 subjects were identified with tramadol prescriptions, 59 of whom had a seizure diagnosis (0.52%). Further analysis revealed that 48% of those having a seizure had a predisposing condition for seizures (e.g., head trauma, stroke, or degenerative disease). The odds ratio for seizures with tramadol exposure was not higher than that for other opioids in this study. The highest odds ratio was seen for those patients exposed to both tramadol and other opioids (OR = 30.6; 95% confidence interval = 2.0 to 470.8). Among those patients also exposed to antidepressants, use of tricyclic antidepressants and serotonin-specific reuptake inhibitors increased the odds of seizures in a statistically significant fashion (OR = 4.1 and 7.9, respectively).[161] At this time, it appears that the risk of seizures with tramadol in patients without epilepsy or other risk factors for seizures is low.

CONCLUSION

The number of medications that can cause neurotoxicity is vast, and their effects are myriad. However, the common theme among these agents is that their neurotoxicities are often unrecognized for long periods, even by specialists. This ongoing issue underscores the importance of a thorough review of pharmacotherapy whenever an unexplained neurological symptom emerges in a patient.

REFERENCES

1. GlaxoSmithKline. Lanoxin Product Information. Research Triangle Park, NC: GlaxoSmithKline; 2006.
2. Wamboldt FS, Jefferson JW, Wamboldt MZ. Digitalis intoxication misdiagnosed as depression by primary care physicians. *Am J Psychiatry.* 1986;143:219–221.
3. Shear MK, Sacks MH. Digitalis delirium: report of two cases. *Am Psychiatric Assoc.* 1978;135:109–110.
4. El-Mallakh RS, Hedges S, Casey D. Digoxin encephalopathy presenting as mood disturbance. *J Clin Psychopharm.* 1995; 15:82–83.
5. Eisendrath SJ, Sweeney MA. Toxic neuropsychiatric effects of digoxin at therapeutic serum concentrations. *Am J Psychiatry.* 1987;144:506–507.
6. Eisenman DP, McKegney FP. Delirium at therapeutic serum concentrations of digoxin and quinidine. *Psychosomatics.* 1994; 35:91–93.
7. GlaxoSmithKline. Digibind Product Information. Research Triangle Park, NC: GlaxoSmithKline; 2003.
8. Harris L, McKenna WJ, Rowland E, et al. Side effects of long-term amiodarone therapy. *Circulation.* 1983;67:45–51.
9. Waxman HL, Groh WC, Marchlinski FE, et al. Amiodarone for control of sustained ventricular tachyarrhythmia: clinical and electrophysiologic effects in 51 patients. *Am J Cardiol.* 1982; 50:1066–1074.
10. Bongard V, Marc D, Philippe V, et al. Incidence rate of adverse drug reactions during long-term follow-up of patients newly treated with amiodarone. *Am J Ther.* 2006;13:315–319.
11. Santoro L, Barbieri F, Nucciotti R, et al. Amiodarone-induced experimental acute neuropathy in rats. *Muscle Nerve.* 1992; 15:788–795.
12. Wyeth Pharmaceuticals. Cordarone Product Information. Philadelphia: Wyeth Pharmaceuticals; 2004.
13. Feiner LA, Younge BR, Kazmier FJ, et al. Optic neuropathy and amiodarone therapy. *Mayo Clin Proc.* 1987;62:702–717.
14. Younge BR. Amiodarone and ischemic optic neuropathy. *J Neuroophthalmol.* 2007;27:85–86.
15. Mindel JS, Anderson J, Johnson G, et al. Absence of bilateral vision loss from amiodarone: a randomized trial. *Am Heart J.* 2007;153:837–842.
16. Murphy MA, Murphy JF. Amiodarone and optic neuropathy: the heart of the matter. *J Neuroophthalmol.* 2005;25:232–236.
17. Johnson LN, Krohel GB, Thomas ER. The clinical spectrum of amiodarone-associated optic neuropathy. *J Natl Med Assoc.* 2004; 96:1477–1491.
18. Almog Y, Goldstein M. Visual outcome in eyes with asymptomatic optic disc edema. *J Neuroophthalmol.* 2003;23:204–207.
19. Morady F, Sauve MJ, Malone P, et al. Long-term efficacy and toxicity of high-dose amiodarone therapy for ventricular tachycardia or ventricular fibrillation. *Am J Cardiol.* 1983;52:975–979.
20. Werner EG, Olanow CW. Parkinsonism and amiodarone therapy. *Ann Neurol.* 1989;25:630–632.
21. Onofrj M, Thomas A. Acetazolamide-responsive periodic ataxia induced by amiodarone. *Mov Disord.* 1999;14:379–381.
22. Dotti MT, Federico A. Amiodarone-induced parkinsonism: a case report and pathogentic discussion. *Mov Disord.* 1995;10:233–234.
23. Malaterre HR, Renou C, Kallee K, Gauthier A. Akinesia and amiodarone therapy. *Int J Cardiol.* 1997;59:107–108.
24. Pollock JE. Neurotoxicity of intrathecal local anaesthetics and transient neurological symptoms. *Best Pract Res Clin Anaesth.* 2003;17:471–484.
25. Faccenda KA, Finucane BT. Complications of regional anaesthesia: incidence and prevention. *Drug Saf.* 2001;45:413–442.
26. Zaric D, Christiansen C, Pace NL, Punjasawadwong Y. Transient neurologic symptoms (TNS) following spinal anaesthesia with lidocaine versus other local anaesthetics. *Cochrane Database Syst Rev.* 2005;(4):CD003006.
27. Bersani G, Raitano A, Stobbia G, Girotti R. Baricity in spinal anaesthesia: pharmaceutical aspects. *Eur J Hosp Pharm.* 1999;5:83–87.
28. Pieper JA, Johnson KE. Lidocaine. In: Evans WE, Schentag JJ, Jusko WJ, eds. *Applied Pharmacokinetics: Principles of Therapeutic Drug Monitoring.* 3rd ed. Vancouver, BC: Applied Therapeutics; 1992:21-1–21.37.
29. Wikinski JA, Usubiaga JE, Morales RL, et al. Mechanism of convulsions elicited by local anesthetic agents: I. Local anesthetic depression of electrically induced seizures in man. *Anesth Analg.* 1970;49:504–510.
30. Rincon E, Baker RL, Iglesias AJ, Duarte AM. CNS toxicity after topical application of EMLA cream on a toddler with molluscum contagiosum. *Pediatr Emerg Care.* 2000;16:252–254.
31. Clapp CR, Poss WB, Cilento BG. Lidocaine toxicity secondary to postoperative bladder instillation in a pediatric patient. *Urology.* 1999;53:1228.
32. Hattori H, Yamano T, Hayashi K, et al. Effectiveness of lidocaine infusion for status epilepticus in childhood: a retrospective multi-institutional study in Japan. *Brain Dev.* 2008;30:504–512.
33. Shany E, Benzaquen O, Watemberg N. Comparison of continuous drip of midazolam or lidocaine in the treatment of intractable neonatal seizures. *J Child Neurol.* 2007;22:255–259.
34. Micromedex. Drug-Induced Myasthenia Gravis: Drug Consults. Greenwood Village, CO: Thomson Healthcare; 2008.
35. Jonkers I, Swerup C, Pirskanen R, et al. Acute effects of intravenous injection of β-adrenoreceptor and calcium channel antagonists and agonists in myasthenia gravis. *Muscle Nerve.* 1996;19:959–965.
36. Matell G, Bjelak S, Jonkers I, et al. Calcium channel and β-receptor antagonists and agonists in MG. *Ann NY Acad Sci.* 1998;13:785–788.
37. Baker SK, Samjoo IA. A neuromuscular approach to statin-related myotoxicity. *Can J Neurol Sci.* 2008;35:8–21.
38. Pasternak RC, Smith SC, Bairey-Merz CN, et al. ACC/AHA/NHLBI advisory on the use and safety of statins. *J Am Coll Cardiol.* 2002;40:568–573.
39. Harper CR, Jacobson TA. The broad spectrum of statin myopathy: from myalgia to rhabdomyolysis. *Curr Opin Lipidol.* 2007;18:401–408.

40. McKenney JM, Davidson MH, Jacobson TA, Guyton JR. Final conclusions and recommendations of the national lipid association statin safety assessment task force. *Am J Cardiol.* 2006;97(Suppl):89C–94C.

41. Graham DJ, Staffa JA, Shatin D, et al. Incidence of hospitalized rhabdomyolysis in patients treated with lipid-lowering drugs. *J Am Med Assoc.* 2004;292:2585–2590.

42. Ahn SC. Neuromuscular complications of statins. *Phys Med Rehabil Clin North Am.* 2008;19:47–59.

43. Vladutiu GD, Simmons Z, Isackson PJ, et al. Genetic risk factors associated with lipid-lowering drug-induced myopathies. *Muscle Nerve.* 2006;34:153–162.

44. Peltier AC, Russell JW. Advances in understanding drug-induced neuropathies. *Drug Saf.* 2006;29:23–30.

45. Bruckert E, Hayem G, Dejager S, et al. Mild to moderate muscular symptoms with high-dosage statin therapy in hyperlipidemic patients: the PRIMO study. *Cardiovasc Drugs Ther.* 2005;19:403–414.

46. Hansen KE, Hildebrand JP, Ferguson EE, et la. Outcomes in 45 patients with statin induced myopathy. *Arch Intern Med.* 2005;165:2671–2676.

47. Young JM, Florkowski CM, Molyneux SL, et al. Effect of coenzyme Q10 supplementation on simvastatin-induced myalgia. *Am J Cardiol.* 2007;100:1400–1403.

48. Caso G, Kelly P, McNurlan MA, Lawson WE. Effect of coenzyme Q10 on myopathic symptoms in patients treated with statins. *Am J Cardiol.* 2007;99:1409–1412.

49. Purvin V, Kawasaki A, Smith KH, Kesler A. Statin-associated myasthenia gravis: report of 4 cases and review of the literature. *Medicine.* 2006;85:82–85.

50. Corrao G, Zambon A, Bertu L, et al. Lipid lowering drugs prescription and the risk of peripheral neuropathy: an exploratory case–control study using automated databases. *J Epidemiol Community Health.* 2004;58:1047–1051.

51. Gaist D, Jeppesen U, Andersen M, et al. Statins and risk of polyneuropathy: a case–control study. *Neurology.* 2002;58:1333–1337.

52. Rajabally YA, Varakantam V, Abbott RJ. Disorder resembling Guillain-Barré syndrome on initiation of statin therapy. *Muscle Nerve.* 2004;30:663–666.

53. Phan T, McLeod JG, Pollard JD, et al. Peripheral neuropathy associated with simvastatin. *J Neurol Neurosurg Psychiatry.* 1995;58:625–628.

54. Jacobs MB. HMB-CoA reductase inhibitor therapy and peripheral neuropathy. *Ann Intern Med.* 1994;120:970.

55. Davidson MH, Armani A, McKenney JM, Jacobson TA. Safety considerations with fibrate therapy. *Am J Cardiol.* 2007;99(Suppl):3C–18C.

56. Jones PH, Davidson MH. Reporting rate of rhabdomyolysis with fenofibrate + statin versus gemfibrozil + any statin. *Am J Cardiol.* 2005;95:120–122.

57. Havranek JM, Wolfsen AR, Warnke GA, Phillips PS. Monotherapy with ezetimibe causing myopathy. *Am J Med.* 2006;119:285–286.

58. Meas T, Cimadevilla C, Timsit J, et al. Elevation of CKP induced by ezetimibe in monotherapy: report on two cases. *Diabetes Metab.* 2006;32:364–366.

59. Stein EA, Ballantyne CM, Windler E, et al. Efficacy and tolerability of fluvastatin XL 80 mg alone, ezetimibe alone, and the combination of fluvastatin XL 80 mg with ezetimibe in patients with a history of muscle-related side effects with other statins. *Am J Cardiol.* 2008;101;490–496.

60. Shields MD, Hicks EM, Macgregor DF, Richey S. Infantile spasms associated with theophylline toxicity. *Acta Paediatr.* 1995;84:215–217.

61. Henderson A, Wright DM, Pond SM. Management of theophylline overdose patients in the intensive care unit. *Anaesth Intensive Care.* 1992;20:56–62.

62. Shannon M. Life-threatening events after theophylline overdose: a 10-year prospective analysis. *Arch Intern Med.* 1999;159:989–994.

63. Delanty N, French JA, Labar DR, et al. Status epilepticus arising de novo in hospitalized patients: an analysis of 41 patients. *Seizure.* 2001;10:116–119.

64. Miura T, Kimura K. Theophylline-induced convulsion in children with epilepsy. *Pediatrics.* 2000;105:920.

65. Edwards DJ, Zarowitz BJ, Slaughter RL. Theophylline. In: Evans WE, Schentag JJ, Jusko WJ, eds. *Applied Pharmacokinetics: Principles of Therapeutic Drug Monitoring.* 3rd ed. Vancouver, BC: Applied Therapeutics; 1992:13-1–13-38.

66. Yoshikawa H. First-line therapy for theophylline-associated seizures. *Acta Neurol Scand.* 2007;115(Suppl 186):57–61.

67. Purdue Pharmaceutical Products. Uniphyl Product Information. Stamford, Conn: Purdue Pharmaceutical Products; 2004.

68. Deleted in proof.

69. Deleted in proof.

70. Astra USA. Albuterol Sulfate Solution for Inhalation Product Information. Westborough, Mass: Astra USA; 1998.

71. Schering. Proventil HFA Inhalation Aerosol Product Information. Kenilworth, NJ: Schering; 1999.

72. DAVA Pharmaceuticals. Vospire ER Product Information. Fort Lee, NJ: DAVA Pharmaceuticals; 2006.

73. Sepracor. Brovana Product Information. Marlborough, Mass: Sepracor; 2006.

74. Schering. Foradil Product Information. Kenilworth, NJ: Schering; 2006.

75. Sepracor. Xopenex Inhalation Solution Product Information. Marlborough, Mass: Sepracor; 2007.

76. Boehringer Ingelheim. Alupent Product Information. Ridgefield, CT: Boehringer Ingelheim; 1998.

77. 3M Pharmaceuticals. Maxair Product Information. Northridge, Calif: 3M Pharmaceuticals; 2003.

78. SICOR Pharmaceuticals. Terbutaline Sulfate Injection Product Information. Irvine, Calif: SICOR Pharmaceuticals; 2004.

79. Tesfamariam B, Waldron T, Seymour AA. Quantitation of tremor in response to β-adrenergic receptor stimulation in primates: Relationship with hypokalemia. *J Pharmacol Toxicol Methods.* 1998;40:201–205.

80. Boccagni C, Tesser F, Mittino D, et al. Churg-Strauss syndrome associated with the leukotriene antagonist montelukast. *Neurol Sci.* 2004;25:21–22.

81. Masi AT, Hunder GG, Lie JT, et al. The American College of Rheumatology 1990 criteria for the classification of Churg-Strauss syndrome (allergic granulomatosis and angiitis). *Arthritis Rheum.* 1990;33:1094–1100.

82. Lilly CM, Churg A, Lazarovich M, et al. Asthma therapies and Churg-Strauss syndrome. *J Allergy Clin Immunol.* 2002;109:S1–S20.

83. Michael AB, Murphy D. Montelukast-associated Churg-Strauss syndrome. *Age Aging.* 2003;32:551–552.

84. Green RL, Vayonis AG. Churg-Strauss syndrome after zafirlukast in two patients not receiving systemic steroid treatment. *Lancet.* 1999;353:725–726.

85. Oberndorfer S, Beate U, Sabine U, et al. Churg-Strauss syndrome during treatment of bronchial asthma with a leucotriene receptor antagonist presenting with polyneuropathy. *Neurologia.* 2004;19:135–138.

86. Villena V, Hidalgo R, Sotelo MT, Martin-Escribano P. Montelukast and Churg-Strauss syndrome. *Eur Respir J.* 2000;15:626.

87. Batchelor TT, Taylor LP, Thaler HT, et al. Steroid myopathy in cancer patients. *Neurology.* 1997;46:1234–1238.

88. Owczarek J, Jasinska M, Orszulak-Michalak D. Drug-induced myopathies: an overview of the possible mechanism. *Pharmacol Rep.* 2005;57:23–34.

89. Behbehani NA, Al-Mane F, D'yachkova Y, et al. Myopathy following mechanical ventilation for acute severe asthma: the role of muscle relaxants and corticosteroids. *Chest.* 1999;115:1627–1631.

90. DeSwert LF, Wouters C, de Zegher F. Myopathy in children receiving high-dose inhaled fluticasone. *N Engl J Med.* 2004; 350:1157–1159.

91. Lee MC, Wee GR, Kim JH. Apoptosis of skeletal muscle on steroid-induced myopathy in rats. *J Nutr.* 2005;135: 1806S–1808S.

92. Decramer M, de Bock V, Dom R. Functional and histologic picture of steroid-induced myopathy in chronic obstructive pulmonary diseases. *Am J Respir Crit Care Med.* 2996;153: 1958–1964.

93. Sacks O, Shulman M. Steroid dementia: an overlooked diagnosis? *Neurology.* 2005;64:707–709.

94. Wolkowitz OM, Lupien SJ, Bigler E, et al. The "steroid dementia syndrome": an unrecognized complication of glucocorticoid treatment. *Ann NY Acad Sci.* 2004;1032:191–194.

95. Varney NR, Alexander B, MacIndoe JH. Reversible steroid dementia in patients without steroid psychosis. *Am J Psychiatry.* 1984;141:369–372.

96. Sapolsky RM. Glucocorticoids, stress and exacerbation of excitotoxic neuron death. *Semin Neurosci.* 1994;6:323–331.

97. Sacks O, Shulman M. Steroid dementia: a follow-up. *Neurology.* 2007;68:622.

98. Bronstein AC, Spyker DA, Cantilena LR Jr, et al. 2006 annual report of the American Association of Poison Control Centers' National Poison Data System (NPDS). *Clin Toxicol.* 2007;45:815–917.

99. Brown JH, Taylor P. Muscarinic receptor agonists and antagonists. In: Brunton LL, Lazo JS, Parker K, eds. *Goodman and Gillman's The Pharmacological Basis of Therapeutics.* 11th ed. New York: McGraw-Hill Medical; 2006:183–200.

100. Richelson E. Receptor pharmacology of neuroleptics: relation to clinical effects. *J Clin Psychiatry.* 1999;60(Suppl 10):5–14.

101. Wilkinson JA. Side effects of transdermal scopolamine. *J Emerg Med.* 1987;5:389–392.

102. Ziskind AA. Transdermal scopolamine-induced psychosis. *Postgrad Med.* 1988;84:73–76.

103. Feinberg M. The problems of anticholinergic adverse effects in older patients. *Drugs Aging.* 1993;3:335–348.

104. Anticholinergic Poisoning Rapid Overview. UpToDate 2008. Accessed July 14, 2008.

105. Skidgel RA, Erdos EG: Histamine, bradykinin, and their antagonists. In: Brunton LL, Lazo JS, Parker K, eds. *Goodman and Gillman's The Pharmacological Basis of Therapeutics.* 11th ed. New York: McGraw-Hill Medical; 2006:629–653.

106. Olson KR, Kearney TE, Dyer JE, et al. Seizures associated with poisoning and drug overdose. *Am J Emerg Med.* 1993; 11:565–568.

107. Radovanovic D, Meier PJ, Guirguis M, et al. Dose-dependent toxicity of diphenhydramine overdose. *Hum Exp Toxicol.* 2000;19:489–495.

108. Chishty M, Reichel A, Siva J, et al. Affinity for the P-glycoprotein efflux pump at the blood–brain barrier may explain the lack of CNS side-effects of modern antihistamines. *J Drug Target.* 2001;9:223–228.

109. Chen C, Hanson E, Watson JW, Lee JS. P-glycoprotein limits the brain penetration of nonsedating but not sedating H$_1$ antagonists. *Drug Metab Dispos.* 2003;31:312–318.

110. Timmerman H. Factors involved in the absence of sedative effects by the second-generation antihistamines. *Allergy.* 2000;55(Suppl 60):5–10.

111. Tashiro M, Mochizuki H, Iwabuchi K, et al. Roles of histamine in regulation of arousal and cognition: functional neuroimaging of histamine H$_1$ receptors in human brain. *Life Sci.* 2002;72:409–414.

112. Khosla U, Ruel KS, Hunt DP. Antihistamine-induced rhabdomyolysis. *South Med J.* 2003;96:1023–1026.

113. Adesanya H. Lack of association between fexofenadine and rhabdomyolysis. *Am J Health Syst Pharm.* 2004;61:724–725.

114. Cantu TG, Korek JS. Central nervous system reactions to histamine-2 receptor blockers. *Ann Intern Med.* 1991;114: 1027–1034.

115. Sa'adah MA, Al Salem M, Ali AS, et al. Cimetidine-associated optic neuropathy. *Eur Neurol.* 1999;42:23–26.

116. Peiris RS, Peckler BF. Cimetidine-induced dystonic reaction. *J Emerg Med.* 2001;21:27–29.

117. Davis BJ, Aul EA, Granner MA, Rodnitzky RL. Ranitidine-induced cranial dystonia. *Clin Neuropharmacol.* 1994;17: 489–491.

118. Kenney C, Hunter C, Davidson A, Jankovic J. Metoclopramide: an increasingly recognized cause of tardive dyskinesia. *J Clin Pharmacol.* 2008;48:379–384.

119. Dubow JS, Leikin J, Rezak M. Acute chorea associated with metoclopramide use. *Am J Ther.* 2006;13:543–544.

120. Bateman DN, Rawlins MD, Simpson JM. Extrapyramidal reactions with metoclopramide. *BMJ.* 1985;291:930–932.

121. Deleted in proof.

122. Ganzini L, Casey DE, Hoffman WF, Mccall AL. The prevalence of metoclopramide-induced tardive dyskinesia and acute extrapyramidal movement disorders. *Arch Intern Med.* 1993;153:1469–1475.

123. van der Padt A, van Schaik RHN, Sonneveld P. Acute dystonic reaction to metoclopramide in patients carrying homozygous cytochrome P450 2D6 genetic polymorphisms. *Netherlands J Med.* 2006;64:160–162.

124. Newton-John H. Acute upper airway obstruction due to supraglottic dystonia induced by a neuroleptic. *Br Med J.* 1988;297: 964–965.

125. Tait PA. Supraglottic dystonic reaction to metoclopramide in a child. *Med J Aust.* 2001;174:607–608.

126. Yis U, Ozdemir D, Dumna M, Unal N. Metoclopramide induced dystonia in children: two case reports. *Eur J Emerg Med.* 2005;12:117–119.

127. Deleted in proof.

128. Fujita Y, Yasukawa T, Mihira M, et al. Metoclopramide in a patient with renal failure may be an increased risk of neuroleptic malignant syndrome. *Intensive Care Med.* 1996;22:717.

129. Esper CD, Factor SA. Failure of recognition of drug-induced parkinsonism in the elderly. *Mov Disord.* 2008;23:401–404.

130. Parlak I, Atilla R, Cicek M, et al. Rate of metoclopramide infusion affects the severity and incidence of akathisia. *Emerg Med J.* 2005;22:6231–624.

131. Parlak I, Erdur B, Parlak M, et al. Midazolam vs. diphenhydramine for the treatment of metoclopramide-induced akathisia: a randomized controlled trial. *Acad Emerg Med.* 2007;14: 715–721.

132. Glasgow JFT. Reye's syndrome: the case for a causal link with aspirin. *Drug Saf.* 2006;29:1111–1121.

133. Orlowski JP, Hanhan UA, Fiallos MR. Is aspirin a cause of Reye's syndrome? A case against. *Drug Saf.* 2002;25: 225–231.

134. Hall SM, Plaster PA, Glasgow JFT, et al. Preadmission antipyretics in Reye's syndrome. *Arch Dis Child.* 1988;63: 857–866.

135. Halprin TJ, Holtzhauer FJ, Campbell MS, et al. Reye's syndrome and medication use. *J Am Med Assoc.* 1982;248:687–691.

136. Hurwitz ES, Barrett MJ, Bregman D, et al. Public health service study of Reye's syndrome and medications: report of the main study. *J Am Med Assoc.* 1987;257:1905–1911.

137. Waldman RJ, Hall WN, McGee H, et al. Aspirin as a risk factor in Reye's syndrome. *J Am Med Assoc.* 1982;247:3089–3094.

138. Orlowski JP. Whatever happened to Reye's syndrome? Did it ever really exist? *Crit Care Med.* 1999;27:1582–1587.

139. Forsyth BW, Horwitz RI, Acampora D, et al. New epidemiologic evidence confirming that bias does not explain the aspirin–Reye's syndrome association. *J Am Med Assoc.* 1989;261:2517–2524.

140. Gauthier M, Guay J, Lacroix J, et al. Reye's syndrome: a reappraisal of diagnosis in 49 presumptive cases. *Am J Dis Child.* 1989;143:1181–1185.

141. Chyka PA, Erdman AR, Christianson G, et al. Salicylate poisoning: an evidence-based consensus guidelines for out-of-hospital management. *Clin Toxicol.* 2007;45:95–131.

142. Thomson Healthcare. Salicylates. POISINDEX® System [Internet database]. Greenwood Village, Colo: Thomson Healthcare. Updated periodically.

143. Rauschka H, Aboul-Enein F, Bauer J, et al. Acute cerebral white matter damage in lethal salicylate intoxication. *Neurotoxicology.* 2007;28:33–37.

144. Roy S, Fortier LP. Fentanyl-induced rigidity during emergence from general anesthesia potentiated by venlafexine. *Can J Anesth.* 2003;50:32–35.

145. Kitagawa N, Oda M, Totoki T. Meperidine-induced muscular rigidity during spinal anesthesia? *Anesth Analg.* 2006;103: 490–491.

146. Sarhill N, Davis MP, Walsh D, Nouneh C. Methadone-induced myoclonus in advanced cancer. *Am J Hospice Pall Care.* 2001; 18:51–53.

147. Ferris DJ. Controlling myoclonus after high-dosage morphine infusions. *Am J Health Syst Pharm.* 1999;56:1009–1010.

148. Mercadante S. Pathophysiology and treatment of opioid-related myoclonus in cancer patients. *Pain.* 1998;74:5–9.

149. Lauterbach EC. Hiccup and apparent myoclonus after hydrocodone: review of the opiate-related hiccup and myoclonus literature. *Clin Neuropharmacol.* 1999;22:87–92.

150. de Stoutz ND, Bruera E, Suarez-Almazor M. Opioid rotation for toxicity reduction in terminal cancer patients. *J Pain Symptom Manage.* 1995;10:378–384.

151. Mercadante S, Villari P, Fulfaro F. Gabapentin for opioid-related myoclonus in cancer patients. *Support Care Cancer.* 2001;9:205–206.

152. Yaksh TL, Harty GJ, Onofrio BM. High doses of spinal morphine produce a nonopiate receptor–mediated hyperesthesia: clinical and theoretic implications. *Anesthesiology.* 2986;64:590–597.

153. McClain BC, Probst LA, Pinter E, Hartmannsgruber M. Intravenous clonidine use in a neonate experiencing opioid-induced myoclonus. *Anesthesiology.* 2001;95:549–550.

154. Lussier D, Cruciani RA. Choreiform movements after a single dose of methadone. *J Pain Symptom Manage.* 2003;26:688–691.

155. Clark JD, Elliott J. A case of a methadone-induced movement disorder. *Clin J Pain.* 2001;17:375–377.

156. Bonnet U, Banger M, Wolstein J, Gastpar M. Choreoathetoid movements associated with rapid adjustment to methadone. *Pharmacopsychiatry.* 1998;31:143–145.

157. Wasserman S, Yahr MD. Choreic movements induced by the use of methadone. *Arch Neurol.* 1980;37:727–728.

158. Klein M, Rudich Z, Gurevich B, et al. Controlled-release oxycodone-induced seizures. *Clin Ther.* 2005;27:1815–1818.

159. Seifert CF, Kennedy S. Meperidine is alive and well in the new millennium: evaluation of meperidine usage patterns and frequency of adverse drug reactions. *Pharmacotherapy.* 2004;24: 776–783.

160. Marinella M. Meperidine-induced generalized seizures with normal renal function. *South Med J.* 1997;90:556–558.

161. Gasse C, Derby L, Vasilakis-Scaramozza C, Jick H. Incidence of first-time idiopathic seizures in users of tramadol. *Pharmacotherapy.* 2000;20:629–634.

162. Ortho-McNeil. Ultram ER Product Information. Raritan, NJ: Ortho-McNeil; 2007.

163. Ripple MG, Pestaner JP, Levine BS, Smialek JE. Lethal combination of tramadol and multiple drugs affecting serotonin. *Am J Forensic Med Pathol.* 2000;21:370–374.

164. John AP, Koloth R. Severe serotonin toxicity and manic switch induced by combined use of tramadol and paroxetine. *Aust NZ J Psychiatry.* 2007;41:192–193.

165. Kesavan S, Sobala GM. Serotonin syndrome with fluoxetine plus tramadol. *J R Soc Med.* 1999;92:474–475.

166. Kitson R, Carr B. Tramadol and severe serotonin syndrome. *Anaesthesia.* 2005;60:934–935.

167. Duggal HS, Fetchko J. Serotonin syndrome and atypical antipsychotics. *Am J Psychiatry.* 2002;159:672–673.

168. Houlihan DJ. Serotonin syndrome resulting from coadministration of tramadol, venlafaxine, and mirtazapine. *Ann Pharmacother.* 2004;38:411–413.

169. Garrett PM. Tramadol overdose and serotonin syndrome manifesting as acute right heart dysfunction. *Anaesth Intensive Care.* 2004;32:575–577.

170. Mittino D, Mula M, Monaco F. Serotonin syndrome associated with tramadol-sertraline coadministration. *Clin Neuropharmacol.* 2004;27:150–151.

171. Labate A, Newton MR, Vernon GM, Berkovic SF. Tramadol and new-onset seizures. *Med J Aust.* 2005;183:42–43.

172. Gardner JS, Blough D, Drinkard CR, et al. Tramadol and seizures: a surveillance study in a managed care population. *Pharmacotherapy.* 2000;20:1223–1431.

CHAPTER 35 ••••

Organic Solvents

Jordan A. Firestone and Sidney M. Gospe, Jr.

INTRODUCTION

Solvents constitute a diverse group of chemical substances that are ubiquitous in our modern, industrialized societies. Exposures to these volatile organic compounds commonly occur in the workplace and in the residential environment. Solvent intoxication is well described, producing both acute and chronic neuropsychiatric syndromes, involving multiple elements of the central and peripheral nervous systems, and occurring through both direct and indirect mechanisms, including multisystem organ dysfunction. Solvent intoxication may present as a transient dysphoria or constitute a life-threatening emergency with complex neuropsychiatric consequences.

An array of organic solvents has been in common use since the industrial revolution. Solvents can be characterized by their physical properties, such as volatility and lipid solubility, which can be predicted by chemical structure–function relationships. These properties determine their toxicokinetic profiles, bioavailability, tissue distribution, biotransformation, and excretion, thus predicting risk and hazard to the nervous system and other end organs. Relatively few solvents have been rigorously tested for neurotoxic effects; however, a few examples have been well documented through animal and human research. In this chapter, we illustrate important principles of solvent neurotoxicity using a few prototypical examples and provide some practical suggestions regarding recognition and management of common clinical scenarios.

It is beyond the scope of this chapter to provide a detailed review of the variety of systemic health effects that may occur following solvent intoxication, although some of these endpoints, such as carcinogenesis, closely inform risk assessment. For more information, refer to source regulatory documents published by the National Institute of Occupational Safety and Health and the U.S. Environmental Protection Association (EPA), topical reviews by the International Agency for Research on Cancer and the Agency for Toxic Substances and Disease Registry, or standard textbooks of general toxicology and neurotoxicology.[1,2]

Brief History

Solvents have been used in various forms since antiquity. The value of organic solvents lies in their defining ability to remain chemically stable while dissolving various useful substances, such as fats, waxes, and resins. Their ease of combustion has always been a mixed blessing. Alchemists experimenting with coal tar pitch were the first to purify and characterize various solvent constituents. It should be noted that their use of crude isolates remains somewhat the norm today, with many products constituting enriched mixtures of several chemically related compounds (e.g., Stoddard solvent and gasoline) and patterns of population exposures involving a complex assortment of solvents, including not only the undesirable residues of industrial contamination from a previous era (e.g., trichloroethylene in groundwater) but also as an oft-sought complement to our daily lives (e.g., ethanol in a wine glass).

Innumerable practical applications for solvents were developed during 19th-century industrialization, and with these came reports of solvent neurotoxicity, such as the neuroepidemiological studies of workers in the mid-1800s in whom a range of neurological deficits were traced to carbon disulfide exposures from vulcanization of rubber.[3,4] The distillation of coal tar, and subsequently petroleum, led to the large-scale production of novel organic compounds, several of which have been used for medicinal purposes as inhalational anesthetics and many others which have been used in myriad industrial applications.

During the early part of the 20th century, extensive research characterized a variety of solvent exposures and a range of corresponding health effects, defining the toxicology of organic solvents and related occupational health and industrial hygiene issues. During the 1970s, the number of publications in both scientific and lay literature increased following concerns, on the one hand, about the subclinical effects demonstrated through technical advances in biological monitoring[5] and, on the other hand, about the recognition of the neuropsychosocial effects of voluntary self-exposure to extremely high levels of toluene and other volatile substances.[6,7] Following the 1980 Superfund legislation, many stakeholders became interested in defining action levels for various contaminants. Trichloroethylene (TCE) became a priority contaminant, as there was already an extensive literature regarding its uses in medicine and industry. Contemporary issues involve quantitative risk assessments for populations with low-level environmental exposures to solvents. While these have been generally reassuring, the uncertainty of many implicit assumptions attracts ongoing debate.

Common Exposure Pathways

The prevalence of substantial solvent exposure in the industrial setting should not be underestimated. Estimates from the National Occupational Hazard Survey indicate that nearly 10 million Americans are potentially exposed to organic solvents at work.[8] Worldwide production of these chemicals is substantial; for example, in 2003 worldwide production of xylenes was 18.28 million

metric tons, toluene was 9.46 million metric tons, and solvent mixtures such as white spirit and other naphthas were 6.12 million and 206.64 million metric tons, respectively.[9]

Common solvent-containing products available for both industrial and residential use include adhesives and fixatives, paints, lacquers, thinners, strippers, and degreasers; alcohols, fuels, and antifreeze; agricultural products; foodstuffs; cosmetics; and pharmaceuticals. Some compounds, including refrigerant and propellant gases such as Freon, pesticides such as DDT, and polychlorinated biphenyls have been phased out of production due to environmental concerns such as ozone depletion, disruption of natural ecosystems, and persistent bioaccumulation. Most routine exposures occur in occupational settings, with activities such as painting, construction, and furniture finishing; metal degreasing and finishing; mechanical and refrigeration systems maintenance; rubber, plastic, textile and leather production; and dry cleaning. Solvent exposures from these activities occur primarily through two routes, inhalation and cutaneous contact, both of which can be significant. Ingestion also occurs, typically from unintentional or accidental exposures.

INDUSTRIAL HYGIENE CONSIDERATIONS

Absolute risk assessment is often difficult, because exposure monitoring is not routinely performed in a standardized fashion. Fortunately, with improved exposure assessment and effective industrial hygiene controls, it is possible to limit exposures by addressing the two primary routes of exposure: inhalation and cutaneous contact.

With solvents, the two primary routes of exposure, inhalation and cutaneous contact, are also the two primary targets for interventions that can reduce exposures. In applying the hierarchy of controls, the preferred "materials substitution" has characterized the field for decades so that changing exposure patterns continually pose potential new hazards. Engineering controls with process isolation and local exhaust ventilation are essential to effective prevention. Solvent vapors are typically heavier than air and tend to sink toward the floor, which predicts that downdraft ventilation would be optimal. As always, adequate makeup air is essential.

It is important to select personal protective equipment that is rated to withstand contact with the particular solvent to be used. Skin protection requires selection of coverings that are resistant to the solvent in use, recognizing that gloves may need to be changed periodically because they may only withstand a few minutes of direct solvent contact and even vapor exposures may compromise glove integrity. Solvents typically have favorable warning properties that provide a large margin of safety for inhalation exposure, with the odor threshold much lower than the neurotoxicity threshold. In most situations, a half-face negative pressure respirator with charcoal-based organic vapor cartridge is adequate to prevent substantial neurotoxicity from inhalation. However, in certain situations this would be inappropriate, such as for substances that are odorless (carbon monoxide), that have an unfavorable odor–toxicity threshold ratio (methylene chloride), or that produce particularly rapid sensory fatigue, habituation, or paralysis (carbon disulfide, toluene).[10] In situations in which the atmosphere may be immediately hazardous to life, or in which work is done in a confined space with limited natural ventilation, the indicated method of respiratory protection is a supplied airline hood or self-contained breathing apparatus.

Consultation with a certified industrial hygienist can provide invaluable guidance in devising effective preventive interventions. All of these measures must be supported by appropriate administrative controls that enforce compliance with standard policies promoting worker safety and health.

TOXICOKINETIC CONSIDERATIONS

Common organic solvents (Figure 35-1) are classified as aliphatic hydrocarbons, cyclic hydrocarbons, aromatic hydrocarbons, halogenated hydrocarbons, ketones, amines, esters, alcohols, aldehydes, and ethers. Their properties are readily found in standard organic chemistry texts and in the *CRC Handbook of Chemistry and Physics*.[11]

Bioavailability of solvents is determined by their physical properties, notably their volatility, which predicts inhalation exposure, and lipid–water partition coefficient, which predicts transcutaneous uptake.[12] The kinetics of these pathways predicts the health effects of a given solvent. For example, the sharp onset and brief duration of action of toluene makes it more likely to be abused than acetone, which has a much slower onset with less powerful effect.

The development of halogenated hydrocarbons helped reduce the combustion hazard while providing a series of solvents with a range of useful properties.[13] This group of agents includes chlorinated aliphatic hydrocarbons such as methyl chloride, methylene chloride, 1,1,1-trichloroethane, and TCE; chlorinated aromatic hydrocarbons such as polychlorinated biphenyls and DDT; and chlorofluorocarbons such as Freon and other refrigerants and propellants. However, the new chemistry brought new challenges. One notable phenomenon is the tendency of chlorinated aliphatic hydrocarbons to "crack" when heated so that solvents such as carbon tetrachloride can produce poison gases (hydrogen chloride and phosgene) that are directly and acutely harmful to cardiorespiratory function.[14] Other concerns relate to the biological stability of polychlorinated compounds, which results in biopersistence and concentration in ecological systems.

Solvent toxicodynamics can be largely explained on the basis of general class effects. The prevailing model holds that solvents exert their effects largely through nonspecific physicochemical effects that modulate membrane fluidity and perturb the hydrophobic force regulating macromolecular interactions. Solvents inflict much of their damage through lipid peroxidation, leading to mitochondrial dysfunction, failure of electron transport and energy production, and collapse of membrane integrity.[15–17] As essential energy-dependent housekeeping functions begin to fail, axonal transport is disturbed, and there is evidence for solvent-related damage to neurofilament structures resulting in a length-dependent, dying-back axonopathy. The mixed central–peripheral axonopathy that results can account for neuropathic deficits involving multiple structures.

Solvent effects on shared biotransformation pathways can explain many interactions observed with mixed exposures. The effects of many solvents on the liver involve the P450 microsomal ethanol oxidizing system (MEOS), including CYP2E1.[18,19] These are exemplified by the interactions between ethanol and toluene.[20–22] Acute doses of ethanol compete with toluene for biotransformation, thereby delaying excretion and potentiating the effects of each. Conversely, regular use of ethanol induces CYP2E1 activity, thereby speeding excretion and attenuating the effects of both compounds. Genetic differences with variable patterns of expression of the MEOS may help explain the observed interindividual variation in solvent effects and may account partly for the phenomena of tolerance, dependence, and withdrawal.

Interactions

It is not always possible to delineate a clinical neurotoxic syndrome that is specific to a particular solvent. Rather, it is necessary to consider a differential diagnosis that addresses the interactions of multiple contributing factors. First, the major pathophysiological effects of solvents could be considered class effects, since many solvents share essential physical–chemical properties. Second, exposure to multiple solvents is the norm because many commercial products contain a mixture

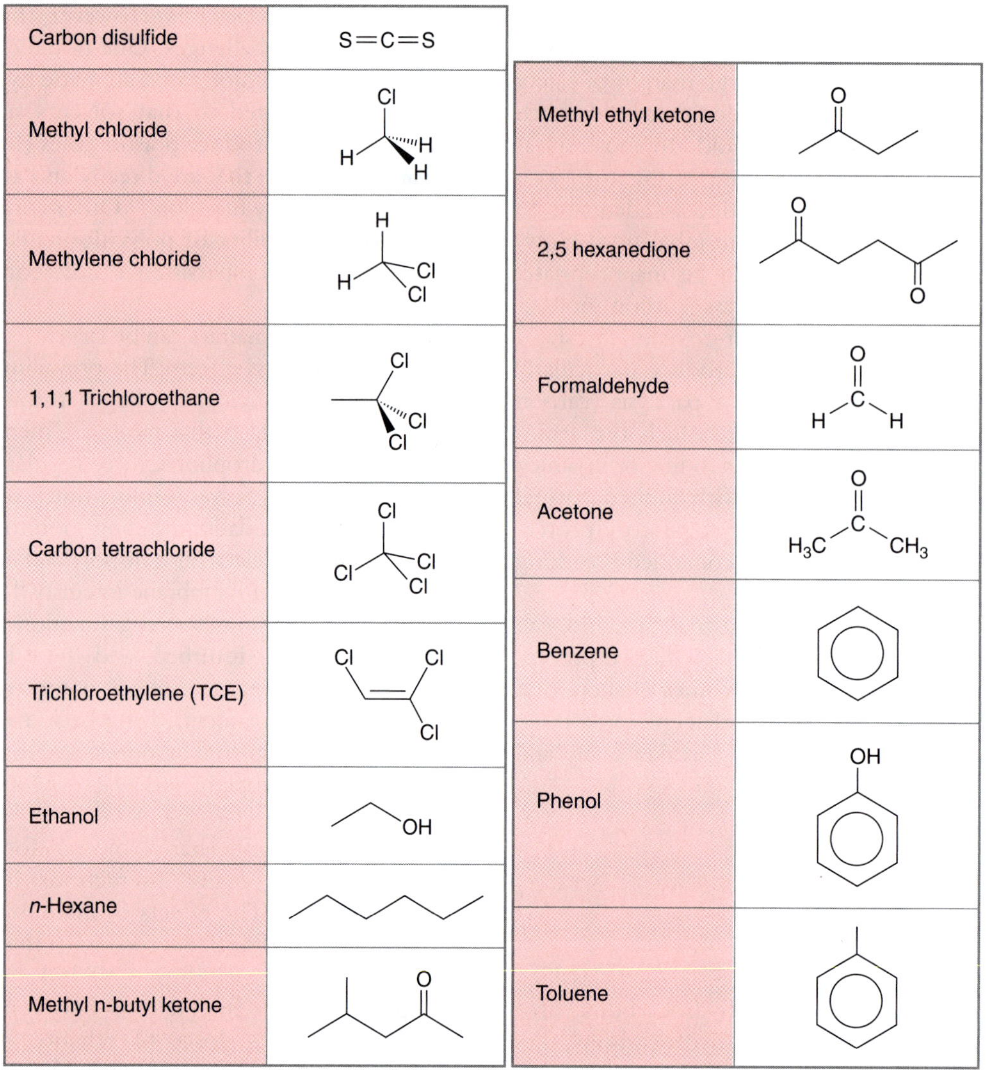

Carbon disulfide	S=C=S	Methyl ethyl ketone	
Methyl chloride		2,5 hexanedione	
Methylene chloride		Formaldehyde	
1,1,1 Trichloroethane		Acetone	H₃C—C(=O)—CH₃
Carbon tetrachloride		Benzene	
Trichloroethylene (TCE)		Phenol	
Ethanol	OH		
n-Hexane		Toluene	
Methyl n-butyl ketone			

Figure 35-1. Chemical structures of some common organic solvents.

of solvents and workers and hobbyists use multiple solvent-containing products. Third, the potential adverse health effects of the solutes contained within these products, such as dye pigments, resins, and heavy metals, must be taken into account. Fourth, preexisting comorbid conditions and genetic factors can modulate individual susceptibility to solvent neurotoxicity. Fifth, the competitive metabolic interactions between mixed exposures can modulate the toxicokinetics of biotransformation processes, as illustrated earlier with mixed exposures involving toluene and various patterns of alcohol use. Clearly, it is important to consider alcohol and drug use history, evidence of past toxin exposure, history of head injury, and evidence of diabetes or other metabolic conditions when evaluating the etiology of a given case of neuropathy or encephalopathy.

CLINICAL CONSIDERATIONS

Clinical Syndromes

At least three specific criteria must be demonstrated to confirm that a particular solvent is neurotoxic in humans.[23] First, the solvent or solvent mixture needs to produce a consistent pattern of clinical neurological dysfunction. Second, a similar disorder should be induced in experimental animals under equivalent exposure conditions. Third, pathological findings need to be correlated with the neurobehavioral deficits that have been described. Although this level of evidence does not exist for all compounds, the neurotoxic effects of several organic solvents have been well studied, and in certain circumstances specific mechanisms of neurotoxicity have been demonstrated. Specific chemicals discussed here are not intended as a comprehensive list but rather as prototypical examples that illustrate common principles.

The various presentations of solvent neurotoxicity should be familiar to most neurologists who have evaluated the various central and peripheral syndromes that accompany acute or chronic alcohol intoxication—after all, ethanol is a solvent. These can include the gamut of encephalopathy with cognitive decline and peripheral neuropathy with sensorimotor deficits. Recognizing solvent exposures and intervening to prevent permanent adverse health effects requires the astute clinician to maintain a high index of suspicion when alerted by the right historical context.

The most common presentation is an acute central nervous system delirium, with mixed cortical and subcortical features. Dysphoria accompanies these rapid changes in neuronal function, producing elation and euphoria in some, cephalgia and malaise in others. Some volatile solvents have a high abuse potential due to the rapid onset of peak effect, with rapid return back to steady state. With continued, high-level exposure, the acute encephalopathy can progress to "narcotic" suppression of respiratory centers with hypopnea and hypoxia, a mixed respiratory and metabolic acidosis, concomitant circulatory collapse, and tissue ischemia. One of the most severe consequences is acute cardiac arrhythmia attributed to adrenergic sensitization. If the victim is fortunate enough to survive the initial acute intoxication, subacute evolution of multiorgan system damage may produce multiple metabolic disturbances with associated secondary neurological dysfunction. Neurological syndromes related to these various metabolic, hepatotoxic, nephrotoxic, circulatory, and carcinogenic effects are no doubt familiar to many and may be reviewed in standard medical texts.

In cases of recurrent, moderate exposure, central manifestations commonly begin with insidious personality changes. Irritability and erratic behavior presage cognitive decline, in which even subtle, subcortical attentional deficits can limit mental agility and short-term memory. Insidious onset of autonomic and sensorimotor peripheral nerve dysfunction is seen most commonly in the context of chronic exposures. Episodic dyspnea may be another indication of exposure to irritant solvent vapors, and cross-shift spirometry may demonstrate reversible bronchoconstriction. The irritant properties of solvents may also trigger mucosal or dermal symptoms, which can be managed with improved industrial hygiene controls, guided by formal worksite evaluation with representative air-quality testing.

Clinical assessment should involve a comprehensive history to characterize exposures and a detailed neurological examination to characterize the diagnostic syndrome. Ancillary testing should address common, treatable causes, assessing metabolic systems with complete blood count, blood chemistry with electrolytes, renal and hepatic function tests, thyroid status, vitamin B_{12}, thiamine, and folate. In the setting of recent exposure, an increased osmolar gap may prompt more specific toxicological testing guided by the exposure history. To optimize the utility of laboratory analysis, it is important to consider timing relative to most recent exposure. Although contemporary techniques that couple chromatography and mass spectrometry can provide precise identification and quantification of particular chemical agents,[24] a detailed occupational and environmental exposure history remains essential to guide efficient use of laboratory testing.

Toxic Encephalopathy

Much of the initial work on organic solvent toxicity originated in Scandinavia, where a neurobehavioral syndrome in painters leading to early retirement was first described.[25] Interestingly, there is a spectrum of response to solvent intoxication, with similar exposures perceived either as euphoria, with pleasurable symptoms of narcosis, sedation, and giddiness, or as dysphoria, with aversive symptoms of mucosal irritation, headache, and disorientation. The former are experienced by solvent abusers, while the latter are experienced by those with chemical intolerance. This interindividual variation likely reflects variable neuropsychiatric responses to the phenomena of tolerance and habituation, as well as genetic variation in kinetics of biotransformation pathways or in dynamics of neurotransmitter systems.

The diffuse neuropathological effects of acute solvent intoxication reflect neurophysiological abnormalities involving multiple central brain regions. With increasingly intense or prolonged exposures, the severity of acute impairment may increase along the spectrum of delirium. Progressive alteration in consciousness may lead to stupor, anesthesia, and coma, with severe neurological depression producing secondary hypopnea complicated by asphyxia with hypoxia, cardiac sensitization to sympathetic tone, dysrhythmia, and possible death.

Recurrent solvent exposures, either in the occupational setting or as a consequence of intentional self-exposure (inhalant abuse), may initially produce transient symptoms of mild encephalopathy that may disappear when the individual is away from work or during periods of abstinence. This intermittent pattern of symptoms can be a tip-off to an association with an unrecognized chemical exposure. Another clue in some workers is a solvent withdrawal syndrome, with headaches and lassitude occurring on the first day away from work. These symptoms may be ameliorated with recreational (or medicinal) alcohol use, a confounder that potentially obscures the occupational connection. Eventually, neurobehavioral abnormalities may become persistent, evolving into a progressive encephalopathy if a pattern of regular exposure is maintained.

Chronic high-level exposure may lead to global cognitive impairment, including deficits in memory, attention, energy, and personality. These chronic neurobehavioral effects of solvents are a well-described form of dementia.[26–29] The extent of exposure required to achieve this degree of impairment is uncertain, as exposure levels are seldom monitored and hygienic measures may be inconsistently applied. However, it appears that the severest cases typically only occur following repeated exposures intense enough to produce transient acute encephalopathy.

In response to increasing concern about solvent neurotoxicity, two international meetings were conducted in 1985 to define the spectrum of encephalopathic signs and symptoms found in solvent-exposed workers. Although the specific descriptions differ slightly, each group yielded comparable consensus classification schemes that parallel the severity of the condition.[30,31]

Type 1: Organic Affective Syndrome

Organic affective syndrome has minimal severity; it consists of symptoms only, characterized by fatigue, memory difficulties, poor concentration, loss of motivation, irritability, and mild mood disturbance. These symptoms are reversible with the elimination of exposure, and neuropsychological testing does not reveal abnormalities.

Type 2A: Mild Chronic Toxic Encephalopathy

This type of mild chronic toxic encephalopathy is characterized by persistent personality or mood change. These patients have an obvious sustained change in personality and affect. Fatigue, reduced impulse control, loss of initiative, depression, and aggression may be noted. Psychometric assessments are usually normal. It is not certain whether or not these behavioral symptoms are reversible.

Type 2B: Mild Chronic Toxic Encephalopathy

Mild chronic toxic encephalopathy type 2B has the mood disturbance seen in 2A, along with concomitant impairment in intellectual function. Those affected have difficulty concentrating, impaired memory, and reduced learning capacity. Minor neurological signs may be present, and neuropsychiatric testing demonstrates cognitive impairment. With cessation of solvent exposure, the syndrome may persist or improve, but symptom progression does not occur.

Type 3: Severe Chronic Toxic Encephalopathy

Severe chronic toxic encephalopathy has pronounced severity, with global deterioration in intellectual and memory function. These patients often meet the criteria for dementia described in the *Diagnostic and Statistical Manual,* fourth edition, along with abnormal neurological signs and neuroradiological findings. Neuropsychological testing demonstrates severe deficits. This condition is rarely seen without a history of intense exposures producing repeated acute intoxications, notably in solvent abusers. It can be progressive as long as exposures continue. Once exposures have terminated, a period of "coasting" may occur before progression ceases. Severe symptoms are essentially irreversible.

PROTOTYPICAL SOLVENT NEUROTOXINS

Toluene Neurotoxicity

Toluene (methylbenzene) is one of the best-studied aromatic solvents commonly found in both industrial and residential environments.[32] Toluene-containing products include paints, lacquers, glues, and cleaning agents. Consequently, this substance may be encountered by a large variety of workers, including printers, machinists, assemblers, shoemakers, and floor layers. Workers are not the only individuals at risk of exposure; individuals involved in home improvement projects may use toluene-containing products, and toluene has been found along with other solvents in residences adjacent to commercial facilities.[33]

As with all solvents, toluene's bioavailability is predicted by its lipid solubility. It is readily absorbed by the respiratory tract, and inhalation is the most common route of exposure. Transcutaneous absorption also occurs, although less readily than for other aromatic solvents such as phenol, a difference that can be explained on the basis of their relative lipid–water solubility ratios. Toluene can also be readily absorbed through the gastrointestinal tract, and rare cases of oral ingestion should be handled as a medical emergency.[34]

Once absorbed, toluene is rapidly distributed in lipid-rich structures throughout the body, notably the brain and adipose tissue. In the brain, toluene is preferentially distributed to lipid-rich regions, primarily the white matter. This has been demonstrated in animal studies, as well as from analysis of human brain tissue obtained at autopsy following chronic toluene abuse.[35,36] Well-described neuroradiological findings in toluene-based inhalant abusers also correlate with a white matter distribution.[26]

Toluene is a well-recognized substance of abuse, as predicted by its sharp pharmacokinetic profile, and much of our knowledge of toluene's clinical neurotoxicity comes from case reports of inhalant abusers.[6,7,37] Euphoria is the effect desired by inhalant abusers, who expose themselves to high levels of toluene, often by inhaling vapors from a rag soaked in the solvent or from a paper bag into which paint or another solvent-based aerosol product has been sprayed. Slang terms for this form of substance abuse include "huffing" and "bagging." There is a higher prevalence in some communities among young teenage children, who preferentially select glues, spray paints, shoe polishes, or other commercial products that contain toluene as the principle solvent.

Experimental studies of toluene provide an excellent example of toxicological dose–response. Subjects exposed to toluene vapors at increasing concentrations have demonstrated a gradation of clinical effects paralleling exposure intensity.[38–40] Low-level exposure at 100 ppm resulted in eye irritation, with some subjects reporting headache, dizziness, and a sense of intoxication. At 200 ppm, euphoria was reported and reaction time was reduced. At levels between 400 and 800 ppm, increasing degrees of inebriation resulted. Traumatic falls and other accidents may occur with moderate levels of acute intoxication, and with deeper levels of intoxication consequences such as asphyxiation and hypothermia may become life threatening. These latter effects are most concerning for solvent abusers, who often expose themselves to very high levels of 4,000 to 12,000 ppm, taking repetitive deep breaths over several minutes.[41,42]

With increasing recognition of the neurotoxic hazards of toluene and other solvents, occupational exposure limits have become more restrictive over time. The American Conference of Governmental Industrial Hygienists reduced the threshold limit value for toluene from 200 ppm in the 1940s to 100 ppm in the 1970s and then to its current level of 50 ppm in 1992.[43] Fortunately, there have been fewer instances of excessive occupational exposure over time, and fatal toluene intoxication has rarely been reported in the occupational setting.[44] Nonetheless, the total morbidity from toluene intoxication is difficult to assess because effects on concentration, reaction time, and executive functions may increase risk of accidental injury.

While many clinical reports of chronically exposed workers have been published, the question of whether neurotoxic effects can be attributed to chronic occupational toluene exposure has been controversial. Most of these individuals were exposed not only to toluene but also to many other solvents, and distinguishing between the residual effects of prior episodes of acute, high-level intoxication and the insidious effects of chronic, low-level exposures is not always possible. It is also important to remember that causality cannot be inferred from case reports that lack a comparison group.

Epidemiological studies of worker groups exposed to toluene have yielded inconsistent results, largely reflecting variable methodology. Various occupational groups have been studied, including workers in rotogravure printing, painting, and textile production. Clinical assessments often rely on different techniques for neuropsychiatric, electrophysiological, radiological, and pathological testing. These differences make it difficult to draw direct comparisons between studies.

Perhaps the biggest challenge in epidemiological studies is the uncertainty in estimating wide-ranging historic exposures. In one occupational study, chronic exposure to toluene at levels in the 200- to 300-ppm range was not associated with differences in clinical neurological, electrophysiological, or neuropsychological tests.[45] In another study, psychiatric interviews indicated significantly increased prevalence of mild chronic encephalopathy, comparable to types 1 and 2A, with toluene exposures that had been previously documented above 1000 ppm, although they were within acceptable standards at the time of the investigation.[46] Using duration of employment as a surrogate measure of cumulative exposure, another study demonstrated exposure-related variance in memory and simple reaction time.[47] The gold standard of prospectively monitoring vapor concentrations in workers' breathing zones has rarely been done.

While uncertainty remains regarding the possibility of chronic effects of occupational toluene exposure, a substantial literature has been published describing persistent neurobehavioral deficits in inhalant abusers who have been self-exposed to toluene-containing products (and in some circumstances to pure toluene) at high levels for many years.[7,26,48] These individuals develop a toxic leukoencephalopathy manifesting primarily as a subcortical dementia, the severity of which correlates with the extent of white matter involvement seen on neuroradiological studies.[49] Affected individuals demonstrate a combination of apathy, inattention, visual–spatial deficits, disturbed working memory, and impaired executive function in the setting of preserved language. Thus, they share similarities with cognitive findings in patients with other disorders of white matter, including multiple sclerosis, Binswanger's disease, and cerebral autosomal dominant arteriopathy with subcortical infarcts and leukoencephalopathy (CADASIL).[26,27] The point in the evolution of this disorder at which the condition becomes irreversible is unpredictable; there have been reports of solvent abusers who develop a remission following a period of abstinence.[50] Cerebellar, brainstem, and long-tract signs may be present,[48,49] and although classic length-dependent peripheral neuropathy is not a common feature, optic and auditory neuropathy with visual decline and sensorineural hearing loss have been reported.[51]

Ototoxic effects of toluene have been studied both in humans and in experimental animals. Several studies have provided evidence of an interaction between toluene exposure and noise, leading to functional auditory deficits.[52] Occupational exposures to toluene and noise produce a greater relative risk of hearing loss than that experienced from exposure to noise alone.[53,54]

Animal studies have provided evidence for a synergistic interaction between toluene and noise, with tissue analysis showing noise-induced injury to stereocilia and toluene-induced injury to outer hair cells.[55,56] These findings support the idea that brainstem auditory evoked responses may be a sensitive tool to screen workers or inhalant abusers for early signs of toluene-related neurotoxicity.[29]

The structural effects of toluene neurotoxicity can be demonstrated using magnetic resonance imaging (MRI). Findings in patients with toluene-abuse leukoencephalopathy may include diffuse atrophy, increased white matter T_2-signal in the periventricular regions, and poor gray–white matter differentiation (Figure 35-2).[29] Hypointensity of the thalami and basal ganglia have also been reported on T_2-weighted images using a more powerful, 1.5-T magnetic field.[57] In a series of 14 patients with toluene-abuse leukoencephalopathy, neuropsychological deficits were first noted in a subject after 2 years of solvent abuse, whereas white matter abnormalities on conventional MRI were first noted in a subject who had been abusing toluene for 14 years.[27] It is possible that diffusion tensor imaging or magnetic resonance spectroscopy will be sensitive to subtle abnormalities developing after shorter intervals of exposure.[26,58]

White matter abnormalities have also been described in the setting of occupational exposure to toluene and other solvents. A cohort of workers exposed to various solvents including toluene from 5 to 28 years reported several nonspecific neurobehavioral symptoms, such as memory loss, dizziness, headache, and fatigue. Subtle white matter changes with hypointensity of the thalami and basal ganglia were seen on 1.5-T field-strength MRI, whereas the MRI abnormalities were not seen in unexposed, symptom-free controls.[58] The authors did not correlate the abnormalities detected by MRI with type of solvent, length of exposure, or pattern of neurobehavioral symptoms.

A limited amount of neuropathological material from toluene-abusing patients has been examined. In a patient who had abused toluene-containing paint for many years, autopsy revealed thinning of the corpus callosum, with microscopic pallor of the cerebral and cerebellar white matter and relative sparing of the subcortical U-fibers. Axonal and neuronal loss was not noted in this case (Figure 35-3). While this patient did not have imaging performed, the neuropathological findings correlated with the abnormal features on MRI of other toluene-abusing patients.[28] In two other cases, similar white matter pathology was noted, with less evidence of axonal loss compared to the degree of myelin reduction.[59] Of particular interest in these two cases was electron microscopic evidence of periodic acid-Schiff-positive granules containing clusters of trilaminar inclusions. These abnormalities, as well as biochemical evidence for increased levels of very long chain fatty acids, were similar to changes seen in patients with adrenoleukodystrophy. However, in the toluene abusers there was less evidence of inflammation, no lipid-containing macrophages, and only patchy, incomplete loss of myelin. The clinical deficits in these patients with toluene abuse, taken together with the neuroradiological and neuropathological findings, indicate that toluene has significant neurotoxic effects on white matter and that myelin damage may be a primary consequence of toluene intoxication.[28]

In the setting of inhalant abuse, toluene has also been demonstrated to have teratogenic effects. An animal model of toluene embryopathy has been developed. Pups from dams exposed to toluene during pregnancy have demonstrated intrauterine growth retardation, along with a reduced brain volume, cellularity, and myelination.[60,61] This model has demonstrated delayed and reduced neurogenesis, along with abnormal neuronal migration, which could serve as the basis of the neurodevelopmental abnormalities noted in affected children of toluene-abusing mothers.[62] A constellation of dysmorphic features and neurodevelopmental deficits have been described as fetal solvent syndrome or toluene embryopathy.[63-67] These infants have intrauterine growth retardation, microcephaly, and micrognathia and other facial anomalies, and over time they demonstrate variable degrees of developmental delay, hyperactivity, and cerebellar deficits. This pattern in many ways resembles the well-described fetal alcohol syndrome. Concerns about this syndrome have prompted attention to limit occupational exposures to women of childbearing age, even

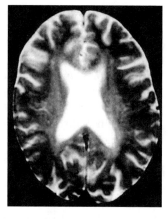

Figure 35-2. Toluene leukoencephalopathy as demonstrated by brain magnetic resonance imaging. Axial T_2-weighted image demonstrating severe, diffuse cerebral white matter hyperintensity and marked ventricular enlargement. (Filley CM, Halliday W, Kleinschmidt-DeMasters BK. The effects of toluene on the central nervous system. *J Neuropathol Exp Neurol.* 2004;63:1–12).

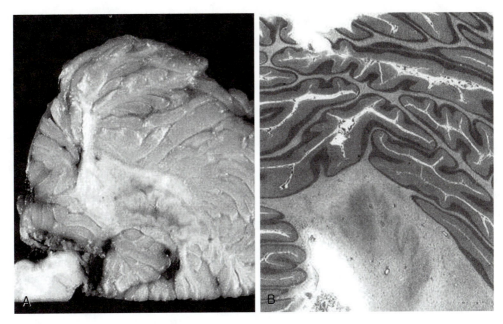

Figure 35-3 Autopsy case of toluene leukoencephalopathy. *(A)* Discoloration of the white matter of the cerebellar hemisphere. *(B)* Low-power view of the cerebellum stained with Luxol fast blue–periodic acid-Schiff shows the severe, near-total myelin loss, except for relative preservation in the fleece and hilum of the dentate nucleus. (Filley CM, Halliday W, Kleinschmidt-DeMasters BK. The effects of toluene on the central nervous system. *J Neuropathol Exp Neurol.* 2004;63:1–12).

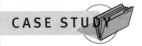

CASE STUDY

A 36-year-old man accompanied by his wife is brought by ambulance to the emergency department for evaluation of altered mental status, left arm swelling, and rib bruising. Approximately 30 minutes before arrival, the man had been stripping paint from a bathroom and his wife heard a crashing noise from that part of the home. She went to investigate and discovered her husband lying on the bathroom floor with his left arm draped over the bathtub. His body was limp and he did not respond to her questions. A strong chemical smell was present within the small bathroom, which was poorly ventilated. Examination in the emergency department noted bruising and swelling of the left forearm and contusions over the left side of the chest. The man was awake and complaining of dizziness and nausea with slurred speech; he could not describe the nature of his injury. His neurological examination was significant for nystagmus on horizontal gaze, and there was no evidence of lateralized motor or sensory deficit. A cranial computerized tomography scan was unremarkable, and radiographs demonstrated a left ulnar fracture. Over the course of 2 hours, the man's mental status returned to normal. At the request of the emergency department physician, his wife retrieved the label from the paint stripper container, which indicated that the product contained a mixture of methanol, toluene, acetone, and Stoddard solvent.

though this condition has not been reported in children of women with occupational exposures.

Trichloroethylene Neurotoxicity

TCE provides a prototypical example of a solvent that can produce a combined system disorder affecting the nervous system at multiple locations.[68] The neurotoxic effects of such solvents produce a combination of symptoms referable to both the central and the peripheral nervous systems, with neurons in the brain, spinal cord, and peripheral nerves affected by similar pathophysiology. As with other halogenated hydrocarbons, inhalation of TCE at low to moderate levels may produce a self-limited toxic encephalopathy, characterized by nausea, headache, lightheadedness, and cognitive dysfunction.[7] Intense acute exposures to TCE can produce specific clinical effects such as cranial neuropathies and cardiac arrhythmias. Although persistent neurobehavioral deficits from chronic occupational exposure to TCE are not well established,[7,23] a recent study suggests that exposed workers may be at an increased risk of developing Parkinson's disease or parkinsonism.[68a]

TCE saw heavy industrial use during the early and middle decades of the 20th century, particularly as a vapor degreaser for metal parts before finish steps in the manufacturing process. In the 1940s, TCE saw use as a general anesthetic agent and was a popular agent due to its nonflammability. Through the mid-1970s, it was used in the food-processing industry to extract oils and fats from vegetables. TCE has also been used in dry cleaning, paint removal, adhesives, and typewriter correction fluid, providing many opportunities for exposures in occupational and residential settings, as well as inhalant abuse. Since the 1980s, in the United States TCE has been eliminated as a component of these products due to concerns of possible carcinogenicity.[69] The National Toxicology Program has determined that TCE is "reasonably anticipated to be a human carcinogen,"[68] and the International Agency for Research on Cancer has determined that TCE is "probably carcinogenic to humans"[68]. TCE has been used by the U.S. EPA as a priority contaminant in the context of risk assessment for Superfund site remediation because it is so commonly found and because there is an extensive scientific and clinical database regarding TCE.

TCE may spontaneously degrade, producing several toxic substances, including hydrogen chloride, phosgene, and dichloroacetylene. In a remarkable example of medical investigation, it was recognized that patients receiving TCE general anesthesia were at the greatest risk of developing trigeminal and other cranial neuropathies when the soda lime used as an absorbent in anesthesia circuits would react with TCE to accelerate the production of dichloroacetylene.[7,23,70,71] Once this relationship was established and anesthesia circuits were modified, TCE-related anesthetic toxicity was no longer a clinical problem. Of course, this did not eliminate the risk of toxic cranial neuropathy due to occupational exposures to impure mixtures or following heat-induced "cracking" and degradation of TCE to dichloroacetylene.

The first reports of a reversible toxic trigeminal neuropathy secondary to industrial TCE exposure appeared in 1915, and shortly thereafter TCE inhalation was prescribed as a treatment for trigeminal neuralgia.[72] Reports of a similar reversible trigeminal neuropathy appeared relatively soon after its clinical introduction as an anesthetic.[73–75] Affected patients noted circumoral numbness or paresthesias that eventually spread to involve a bilateral sensory loss in the distribution of the trigeminal nerve. Case studies of some patients indicate more extensive involvement of cranial nerves, with trigeminal involvement producing facial numbness and masseter weakness, optic nerve involvement producing visual disturbance, and facial nerve involvement producing facial weakness.[76]

In experimental animals, dichloroacetylene has been demonstrated to morphologically disrupt both sensory and motor nuclei of the trigeminal nerve and motor nuclei of the facial and oculomotor nerves.[77] Similar pathology was noted at autopsy in a worker exposed to TCE and its decomposition products; the worker developed subacute progression of brainstem dysfunction, with loss of gag and dysphagia necessitating placement of a tracheostomy. Postmortem examination nearly 2 months later demonstrated lesions affecting multiple structures bilaterally in the dorsal brainstem and reticular formation, trigeminal nerve nuclei and tracts, and nucleus and tractus solitarius.[78] The range of variability is illustrated by another case, in which a worker exposed to TCE developed a transverse myelopathy of the cervicothoracic junction, with motor, sensory, and sphincteric symptoms, as well as optic neuropathy, despite no apparent trigeminal involvement.[79]

A recent study of 30 workers who were chronically exposed to TCE for between 8 and 33 years suggests that long-term occupational exposure to this agent may lead to striatonigral toxicity.[68a] These individuals were employed in a factory where the solvent was used as a metal degreaser. The employees whose workstations were proximate to vats of TCE and who were exposed by both the respiratory and dermal routes developed Parkinson's disease, while workers whose duties were conducted at more distant sites, but who still had chronic respiratory exposure, had some features of parkinsonism. While this was not a formal epidemiologic study, and some of the workers may have been co-exposed to other potential neurotoxic substances, the authors conclude that there is a strong link between TCE exposure and clinical striatonigral dysfunction. To strengthen their conclusion, the authors also studied the effects of oral TCE exposure on rats and demonstrated both loss of dopaminergic neurons within the substantia nigra with a concomitant loss of striatonigral fibers and dysfunction mitochondrial complex I activity. As such, the neurotoxicity of TCE may share a similar mechanism with 1-methyl-4-phenyl-1,2,3,6-tetrahydropyridine (MPTP). TCE inhalation has also been associated with sudden death due to cardiac dysrhythmia in a clinical syndrome of sudden sniffing death first described in inhalant abusers.[80] These affected individuals had abused various commercial products containing halogenated hydrocarbons or occasionally other solvents such as toluene. Subsequently, sudden death was reported in inhalant abusers exposed to typewriter correction fluid containing TCE and 1,1,1-trichloroethane.[81] In many instances, these individuals were noted to collapse after running or being startled, suggesting that TCE sensitizes the heart to circulating catecholamines, thereby increasing the risk of ventricular dysrhythmia.[82,83] To discourage the abuse of typewriter correction fluid, mustard oil was added to the product in the early 1980s.[81] Shortly thereafter, TCE was removed from these products; most correction fluids are now water based.

n-Hexane Neurotoxicity

n-Hexane neurotoxicity provides one of the best-characterized models of toxin-induced neuropathy.[84] It manifests clinically as a mixed sensorimotor, length-dependent, dying-back, axonal polyneuropathy that is identified by a stocking-glove sensory disturbance and distal weakness. The condition has long been recognized as an occupational neuropathy.[85,86] Electrodiagnostic testing may reveal conduction block as an early feature of the disease.[87] Loss of myelinated fibers is evident on sural nerve biopsy.[88,89] Prognosis in mild to moderate cases is optimistic for gradual recovery, but in severe cases symptoms may not fully resolve, although they may stabilize once exposure is ended.

Human exposures to n-Hexane are ubiquitous in modern industrialized societies. It is a natural constituent of crude oil, and in its pure form, n-hexane is a colorless, highly flammable liquid. It has been used as a means to extract essential oils. In common commercial applications it is found as a component of mixed solvents used in various cleaning agents and degreasers or in adhesives in printing, textile, and shoemaking industries.

The molecular pathophysiology of hexane has been extensively studied.[4] The pathology of hexane neuropathy involves axonal swelling with accumulation of neurofilaments, cross-linking of cytoskeletal proteins, and associated dysfunctional axonal transport.[88,90,91] Evidence from a rodent model demonstrates that the molecular mechanisms producing these pathological changes are common to a family of solvent compounds that interact with lysine residues in various cellular proteins.[89]

The effects of n-hexane have been traced to 2,5-hexanedione, the γ-diketone metabolite.[85,92,93] The enzymatic pathways involved in hexane metabolism can be potentiated by concomitant exposures to other solvents, notably methyl ethyl ketone (MEK) and methyl n-butyl ketone (MBK). Interestingly, MBK is also metabolized to 2,5-hexanedione,[94] encouraging the impression that MEK is a less hazardous substitute. While this may be true, it turns out that MEK coexposure potentiates the effects of n-hexane exposure, producing more severe damage than hexane alone.[95,96] This again illustrates the complexity of risk assessment in the setting of mixed solvent exposures.

Mixed Solvent Neurotoxicity

Perhaps the most common context in which solvent neurotoxicity occurs is in the setting of mixed solvent exposures. Workers commonly encounter multiple materials in the course of their occupational duties, and many products are formulated as mixtures. Common examples are white spirit and Stoddard solvent.[97] These products are also known by many common names, including mineral spirit, mineral turpentine, naphtha safety solvent, and dry-cleaning safety solvent. These solvent mixtures, obtained from refined crude petroleum, contain a combination of aliphatic, alicyclic, and aromatic organic compounds and are commonly used as degreasers, spot removers, dry-cleaning fluids, or paint and lacquer thinners.

Mixtures are the norm—a fundamental challenge in exposure assessment and risk characterization. It is difficult to extrapolate results from experiments done in a laboratory setting using purified substances to the sort of complex real-world exposures in which people encounter various materials over time. Only rarely is it possible to quantify exposures at a level of detail that supports quantitative risk assessment at the individual level. Instead, it is necessary to apply general principles of preventive medicine and industrial hygiene while maintaining a strong precautionary approach.

PUBLIC HEALTH CONSIDERATIONS

Over the past 2 centuries, since Delpech first described carbon disulfide intoxication in workers and subsequently studied the effects of exposures on experimental animals,[98] many reports have been published regarding central and peripheral neurotoxicity, as well as systemic toxicity of these various chemicals. Although it is fair to say that great strides have been made in protecting workers in developed countries from hazardous occupational exposures, and that solvent levels routinely encountered have fallen substantially through the past 100 years, it is still true that protective measures are not consistently implemented. This is especially true of small to medium employers, of those who may be independently engaged in cottage industries, and of hobby enthusiasts who are unlikely to have had formal training in hazard reduction. Individuals and small-business owners working outside a regulated work environment are often ill-prepared to ensure their employees have a "safe and healthful working environment," as required by the U.S. Occupational Safety and Health Administration (OSHA) general duty clause. Consulting someone learned in the occupational health ramifications of solvent exposures may be necessary to effectively advocate for worksite improvements. Specific guidance regarding the legal requirements and public health regulations in a given jurisdiction is available from a regional office of OSHA or the EPA or from a state department of public health.

Despite the progress that has been made on many fronts, workers and their communities remain particularly vulnerable in countries where occupational and environmental public health regulations are underdeveloped or ineffective. These problems are aggravated during periods of extreme economic growth, like the growth that occurred in 19th-century Europe and that characterized China at the early part of the 21st century. Today, workers are still vulnerable to neurotoxicity from carbon disulfide, which continues to be used in rayon production operations overseas. Even here in the United States, solvents remain an underappreciated hazard, as illustrated by a report of hexane exposures in auto mechanics.[99]

The molecular and cellular pathophysiology of solvent neurotoxicity is increasingly well-described. Solvents have been demonstrated to have substantial neurotoxic effects to both the central and the peripheral nervous systems. In the setting of inhalant abuse, exposures can produce severe, irreversible, toxic leuko-encephalopathy, clinically characterized as a white matter dementia. In the setting of chronic occupational exposures, there are well-characterized syndromes of neuropathy and encephalopathy. Nonetheless, substantial gaps remain in our knowledge of the precise mechanism underlying the adverse health effects of solvent exposures. Well-designed epidemiological studies of subjects and matched control workers using clinical neurological assessments, standardized neuropsychometric testing, and advanced imaging modalities are needed to better elucidate the mechanisms of neurotoxicity of organic solvents.

REFERENCES

1. Klaasen CD, ed. *Casarett & Doull's Toxicology: The Basic Science of Poisons.* 6th ed. New York: McGraw-Hill; 2001.
2. Spencer PS, Schaumburg HH, Ludolph AC, eds. *Experimental and Clinical Neurotoxicology.* 2nd ed. New York: Oxford University Press; 2000.
3. Beauchamp RO Jr, Bus JS, Popp JA, et al. A critical review of the literature on carbon disulfide toxicity. *Crit Rev Toxicol.* 1983;11:169–278.
4. Graham DG, Amarnath V, Valentine WM, et al. Pathogenetic studies of hexane and carbon disulfide neurotoxicity. *Crit Rev Toxicol.* 1995;25:91–112.
5. Angerer J. Biological monitoring of workers exposed to organic solvents: past and present. *Scand J Work Environ Health.* 1985;11(Suppl 1):45–52.
6. Comstock EG, Comstock BS. Medical evaluation of inhalant abusers. *NIDA Res Monogr.* 1977;15:54–80.
7. Sharp CW, Rosenberg NL. Inhalants. In: Lowinson JH, Ruiz P, Millman RB, et al., eds. *Substance Abuse: A Comprehensive Textbook.* 4th ed. Philadelphia: Lippincott Williams & Wilkins; 2005:336–366.
8. National Institute for Occupational Safety and Health. Organic Solvent Neurotoxicity. Cincinnati, Ohio: NIOSH; 1987.
9. United Nations Department of Economic and Social Affairs. 2003 Industrial Commodity Statistics Yearbook: Productions Statistics (1994–2003). New York: UN, 2006.
10. Andersen I, Lundqvist GR, Molhave L, et al. Human response to controlled levels of toluene in six-hour exposures. *Scand J Work Environ Health.* 1983;9:405–418.
11. Lide DR, ed. *CRC Handbook of Chemistry and Physics.* 88th ed. Boca Raton, Fla: CRC Press; 2007.
12. Sato A, Nakajima T. A structure–activity relationship of some chlorinated hydrocarbons. *Arch Environ Health.* 1979;34:69–75.
13. Armstrong SR, Green LC. Chlorinated hydrocarbon solvents. *Clin Occup Environ Med.* 2004;4:481–496, vi.
14. Nieuwenhuizen MS, Groeneveld FR. Formation of phosgene during welding activities in an atmosphere containing chlorinated hydrocarbons. *AIHAJ.* 2000;61:539–543.
15. Goldstein DB. The effects of drugs on membrane fluidity. *Annu Rev Pharmacol Toxicol.* 1984;24:43–64.
16. Revilla AS, Pestana CR, Pardo-Andreu GL, et al. Potential toxicity of toluene and xylene evoked by mitochondrial uncoupling. *Toxicol In Vitro.* 2007;21:782–788.
17. Sajbidor J. Effect of some environmental factors on the content and composition of microbial membrane lipids. *Crit Rev Biotechnol.* 1997;17:87–103.
18. Hewitt NJ, Lecluyse EL, Ferguson SS. Induction of hepatic cytochrome P450 enzymes: methods, mechanisms, recommendations, and in vitro–in vivo correlations. *Xenobiotica.* 2007;37:1196–1224.
19. Tanaka E, Terada M, Misawa S. Cytochrome P450 2E1: its clinical and toxicological role. *J Clin Pharm Ther.* 2000;25:165–175.
20. Imbriani M, Ghittori S. Effects of ethanol on toluene metabolism in man. *G Ital Med Lav Ergon.* 1997;19:177–181.
21. Pryor GT, Howd RA, Uyeno ET, et al. Interactions between toluene and alcohol. *Pharmacol Biochem Behav.* 1985;23:401–410.
22. Wallen M, Naslund PH, Nordqvist MB. The effects of ethanol on the kinetics of toluene in man. *Toxicol Appl Pharmacol.* 1984;76:414–419.
23. Spencer PS, Schaumburg HH. Organic solvent neurotoxicity: facts and research needs. *Scand J Work Environ Health.* 1985;11(Suppl 1):53–60.
24. Imbriani M, Ghittori S. Gases and organic solvents in urine as biomarkers of occupational exposure: a review. *Int Arch Occup Environ Health.* 2005;78:1–19.
25. Gregersen P, Mikkelsen S, Klausen H, et al. Chronic cerebral syndrome in painters: dementia due to inhalation or is it of cryptogenic origin? *Ugeskr Laeger.* 1978;140:1638–1644.
26. Filley CM, Halliday W, Kleinschmidt-DeMasters BK. The effects of toluene on the central nervous system. *J Neuropathol Exp Neurol.* 2004;63:1–12.
27. Filley CM, Heaton RK, Rosenberg NL. White matter dementia in chronic toluene abuse. *Neurology.* 1990;40:532–534.
28. Rosenberg NL, Kleinschmidt-DeMasters BK, Davis KA, et al. Toluene abuse causes diffuse central nervous system white matter changes. *Ann Neurol.* 1988;23:611–614.
29. Rosenberg NL, Spitz MC, Filley CM, et al. Central nervous system effects of chronic toluene abuse: clinical, brainstem evoked response and magnetic resonance imaging studies. *Neurotoxicol Teratol.* 1988;10:489–495.
30. Cranmer JM, Golberg L. Human aspects of solvent neurobehavioral effects: report on the workshop session on clinical and epidemiological topics. *Neurotoxicology.* 1986;7:43–56.
31. World Health Organization and Nordic Council Of Ministers. Chronic effects of organic solvents on the central nervous system and diagnostic criteria: Report on a Joint WHO/Nordic Council of Ministers Working Group, Copenhagen, 10-14 June 1985. Copenhagen: World Health Organization, Regional Office for Europe; Oslo: Nordic Council of Ministers, 1985.

32. Agency for Toxic Substances and Disease Registry. Toxicological Profile for Toluene. Atlanta, Ga: U.S. Department of Health and Human Services, Public Health Service; 2000.

33. Verhoeff AP, Suk J, van Wijnen JH. Residential indoor air contamination by screen printing plants. *Int Arch Occup Environ Health*. 1988;60:201–209.

34. Ameno K, Fuke C, Ameno S, et al. A fatal case of oral ingestion of toluene. *Forensic Sci Int*. 1989;41:255–260.

35. Ameno K, Kiriu T, Fuke C, et al. Regional brain distribution of toluene in rats and in a human autopsy. *Arch Toxicol*. 1992;66:153–156.

36. Gospe SM Jr, Calaban MJ. Central nervous system distribution of inhaled toluene. *Fund Appl Toxicol*. 1988;11:540–545.

37. Carroll E. Notes on the epidemiology of inhalants. *NIDA Res Monogr*. 1977;15:14–27.

38. von Oettingen WF, Neal PA, Donahue DD. The toxicity and potential dangers of toluene. *JAMA*. 1942;118:579–584.

39. Carpenter CP, Shaffer CB, Weil CS, et al. Studies on the inhalation of 1:3-butadiene, with a comparison of its narcotic effect with benzol, toluol, and styrene, and a note on the elimination of styrene by the human. *J Ind Hyg Toxicol*. 1944;26:69–78.

40. Ogata M, Tomokuni K, Takatsuka Y. Urinary excretion of hippuric acid and m- or p-methylhippuric acid in the urine of persons exposed to vapours of toluene and m- or p-xylene as a test of exposure. *Br J Ind Med*. 1970;27:43–50.

41. Bruckner JV, Peterson RG. Evaluation of toluene and acetone inhalant abuse: I. Pharmacology and pharmacodynamics. *Toxicol Appl Pharmacol*. 1981;61:27–38.

42. Bruckner JV, Peterson RG. Evaluation of toluene and acetone inhalant abuse: II. Model development and toxicology. *Toxicol Appl Pharmacol*. 1981;61:302–312.

43. American Conference of Governmental Industrial Hygienists. Documentation of the Threshold Limit Values and Biological Exposure Indices. 7th ed. Cincinnati, Ohio: ACGIH; 2001.

44. Takeichi S, Yamada T, Shikata I. Acute toluene poisoning during painting. *Forensic Sci Int*. 1986;32:109–115.

45. Cherry N, Hutchins H, Pace T, et al. Neurobehavioural effects of repeated occupational exposure to toluene and paint solvents. *Br J Ind Med*. 1985;42:291–300.

46. Larsen F, Leira HL. Organic brain syndrome and long-term exposure to toluene: a clinical, psychiatric study of vocationally active printing workers. *J Occup Med*. 1988;30:875–878.

47. Iregren A. Effects on psychological test performance of workers exposed to a single solvent (toluene): a comparison with effects of exposure to a mixture of organic solvents. *Neurobehav Toxicol Teratol*. 1982;4:695–701.

48. Hormes JT, Filley CM, Rosenberg NL. Neurologic sequelae of chronic solvent vapor abuse. *Neurology*. 1986;36:698–702.

49. Rosenberg NL, Grigsby J, Dreisbach J, et al. Neuropsychologic impairment and MRI abnormalities associated with chronic solvent abuse. *J Toxicol Clin Toxicol*. 2002;40:21–34.

50. Wiedmann KD, Power KG, Wilson JT, et al. Recovery from chronic solvent abuse. *J Neurol Neurosurg Psychiatry*. 1987;50:1712–1713.

51. Ehyai A, Freemon FR. Progressive optic neuropathy and sensorineural hearing loss due to chronic glue sniffing. *J Neurol Neurosurg Psychiatry*. 1983;46:349–351.

52. Sliwinska-Kowalska M, Prasher D, Rodrigues CA, et al. Ototoxicity of organic solvents: from scientific evidence to health policy. *Int J Occup Med Environ Health*. 2007;20:215–222.

53. Morata TC, Dunn DE, Kretschmer LW, et al. Effects of occupational exposure to organic solvents and noise on hearing. *Scand J Work Environ Health*. 1993;19:245–254.

54. Chang SJ, Chen CJ, Lien CH, et al. Hearing loss in workers exposed to toluene and noise. *Environ Health Perspect*. 2006;114:1283–1286.

55. Brandt-Lassen R, Lund SP, Jepsen GB. Rats exposed to toluene and noise may develop loss of auditory sensitivity due to synergistic interaction. *Noise Health*. 2000;3:33–44.

56. Lataye R, Campo P. Combined effects of a simultaneous exposure to noise and toluene on hearing function. *Neurotoxicol Teratol*. 1997;19:373–382.

57. Unger E, Alexander A, Fritz T, et al. Toluene abuse: physical basis for hypointensity of the basal ganglia on T_2-weighted MR images. *Radiology*. 1994;193:473–476.

58. Thuomas KA, Moller C, Odkvist LM, et al. MR imaging in solvent-induced chronic toxic encephalopathy. *Acta Radiol*. 1996;37:177–179.

59. Kornfeld M, Moser AB, Moser HW, et al. Solvent vapor abuse leukoencephalopathy: comparison to adrenoleukodystrophy. *J Neuropathol Exp Neurol*. 1994;53:389–398.

60. Gospe SM Jr, Zhou SS, Saeed DB, et al. Development of a rat model of toluene-abuse embryopathy. *Pediatr Res*. 1996;40:82–87.

61. Gospe SM Jr, Zhou SS. Toluene abuse embryopathy: longitudinal neurodevelopmental effects of prenatal exposure to toluene in rats. *Reprod Toxicol*. 1998;12:119–126.

62. Gospe SM Jr, Zhou SS. Prenatal exposure to toluene results in abnormal neurogenesis and migration in rat somatosensory cortex. *Pediatr Res*. 2000;47:362–368.

63. Toutant C, Lippmann S. Fetal solvents syndrome. *Lancet*. 1979,1:1356.

64. Hersh JH, Podruch PE, Rogers G, et al. Toluene embryopathy. *J Pediatr*. 1985;106:922–927.

65. Hersh JH. Toluene embryopathy: two new cases. *J Med Genet*. 1989;26:333–337.

66. Arnold GL, Kirby RS, Langendoerfer S, et al. Toluene embryopathy: clinical delineation and developmental follow-up. *Pediatrics*. 1994;93:216–220.

67. Pearson MA, Hoyme HE, Seaver LH, et al. Toluene embryopathy: delineation of the phenotype and comparison with fetal alcohol syndrome. *Pediatrics*. 1994;93:211–215.

68. Agency for Toxic Substances and Disease Registry. Toxicological Profile for Trichloroethylene (TCE): Atlanta: U.S. Department of Health and Human Services, Public Health Service; 1997.

68a. Gash DM, Rutland K, Hudson, ML, et al. Trichloroethylene: Parkinsonism and complex 1 mitochondrial neurotoxicity. *Ann Neurol*. 2008;63:184–192.

69. Ong CN, Koh D, Foo SC, et al. Volatile organic solvents in correction fluids: identification and potential hazards. *Bull Environ Contam Toxicol*. 1993;50:787–793.

70. Anders MW. Formation and toxicity of anesthetic degradation products. *Annu Rev Pharmacol Toxicol*. 2005;45:147–176.

71. Greim H, Wolff T, Hofler M, et al. Formation of dichloroacetylene from trichloroethylene in the presence of alkaline material: possible cause of intoxication after abundant use of chloroethylene-containing solvents. *Arch Toxicol*. 1984;56:74–77.

72. Glaser MA. Treatment of trigeminal neuralgia with trichloroethylene. *JAMA*. 1931;96:916–920.

73. Hewer CL. Trichloroethylene as a general analgesic and anaesthetic. *Proc R Soc Med*. 1942;35:463–468.

74. Hewer CL. Further observations on trichloroethylene. *Proc R Soc Med*. 1943;36:463–465.

75. Enderby GEH. The use and abuse of trichloroethylene. *BMJ*. 1944;2:300–302.

76. Feldman RG. Trichloroethylene. In: Vinken PJ, Gruyn GW, eds. *Handbook of Clinical Neurology: I. Intoxications of the Nervous System*. vol 36. Amsterdam: North-Holland Publishing; 1979:457–464.

77. Reichert D, Ewald D, Henschler D. Generation and inhalation toxicity of dichloroacetylene. *Food Cosmet Toxicol*. 1975;13:511–515.

78. Buxton PH, Hayward M. Polyneuritis cranialis associated with industrial trichloroethylene poisoning. *J Neurol Neurosurg Psychiatry.* 1967;30:511–518.

79. Sagawa K, Nishitani H, Kawai H, et al. Transverse lesion of spinal cord after accidental exposure to trichloroethylene. *Int Arch Arbeitsmed.* 1973;31:257–264.

80. Bass M. Sudden sniffing death. *JAMA.* 1970;212:2075–2079.

81. King GS, Smialek JE, Troutman WG. Sudden death in adolescents resulting from the inhalation of typewriter correction fluid. *JAMA.* 1985;253:1604–1606.

82. White JF, Carlson GP. Epinephrine-induced cardiac arrhythmias in rabbits exposed to trichloroethylene: potentiation by ethanol. *Toxicol Appl Pharmacol.* 1981;60:466–471.

83. White JF, Carlson GP. Epinephrine-induced cardiac arrhythmias in rabbits exposed to trichloroethylene: role of trichloroethylene metabolites. *Toxicol Appl Pharmacol.* 1981;60:458–465.

84. Agency for Toxic Substances and Disease Registry. Toxicological Profile for n-Hexane. Atlanta: U.S. Department of Health and Human Services, Public Health Service; 1999.

85. Governa M, Calisti R, Coppa G, et al. Urinary excretion of 2,5-hexanedione and peripheral polyneuropathies workers exposed to hexane. *J Toxicol Environ Health.* 1987;20:219–228.

86. Rizzuto N, De Grandis D, Di Trapani G, et al. n-Hexane polyneuropathy: an occupational disease of shoemakers. *Eur Neurol.* 1980;19:308–315.

87. Pastore C, Izura V, Marhuenda D, et al. Partial conduction blocks in n-hexane neuropathy. *Muscle Nerve.* 2002;26:132–135.

88. Puri V, Chaudhry N, Tatke M. n-Hexane neuropathy in screen printers. *Electromyogr Clin Neurophysiol.* 2007;47:145–152.

89. Tshala-Katumbay DD, Palmer VS, Kayton RJ, et al. A new murine model of giant proximal axonopathy. *Acta Neuropathol.* 2005;109:405–410.

90. DeCaprio AP. Molecular mechanisms of diketone neurotoxicity. *Chem Biol Interact.* 1985;54:257–270.

91. Tahti H, Engelke M, Vaalavirta L. Mechanisms and models of neurotoxicity of n-hexane and related solvents. *Arch Toxicol.* 1997;19(Suppl):337–345.

92. Couri D, Milks M. Toxicity and metabolism of the neurotoxic hexacarbons n-hexane, 2-hexanone, and 2,5-hexanedione. *Annu Rev Pharmacol Toxicol.* 1982;22:145–166.

93. Couri D, Milks MM. Hexacarbon neuropathy: tracking a toxin. *Neurotoxicology.* 1985;6:65–71.

94. Bos PM, de Mik G, Bragt PC. Critical review of the toxicity of methyl n-butyl ketone: risk from occupational exposure. *Am J Ind Med.* 1991;20:175–194.

95. Noraberg J, Arlien-Soborg P. Neurotoxic interactions of industrially used ketones. *Neurotoxicology.* 2000;21:409–418.

96. Yu RC, Hattis D, Landaw EM, et al. Toxicokinetic interaction of 2,5-hexanedione and methyl ethyl ketone. *Arch Toxicol.* 2002;75:643–652.

97. Agency for Toxic Substances and Disease Registry. Toxicological Profile for Stoddard Solvent. Atlanta: U.S. Department of Health and Human Services, Public Health Service, 1995.

98. O'Flynn RR, Waldron HA. Delpech and the origins of occupational psychiatry. *Br J Ind Med.* 1990;47:189–198.

99. Centers for Disease Control and Prevention. n-Hexane-related peripheral neuropathy among automotive technicians: California, 1999–2000. *MMWR.* 2001;50:1011–1013.

Other Organic Chemicals

Sidney M. Gospe, Jr.

INTRODUCTION

While workers, as well as homeowners and hobbyists, may be at risk of exposure to and neurotoxicity from volatile organic substances that are primarily used for their solvent properties (see Chapter 35), exposure to certain other neurotoxic organic chemicals is a potential hazard for individuals involved with the synthesis and fabrication of plastics and with synthetic rubbers and textiles. In each of these industries, raw materials are derived from petroleum distillates, which are then polymerized in various ways to form a specific resin. Depending on the industry in question, the resin may then be reacted with additional chemicals or mixed with certain additives to form secondary or tertiary substances, which are in turn fabricated into a final product such as plastic pipes or synthetic fabrics. As with organic solvents, the raw materials used in these industries are volatile. Workers may therefore be exposed to these substances not only by cutaneous contact but also via the respiratory route. Some volatile monomeric substances used in these industries, such as ethylene, propylene, and vinyl chloride, have asphyxiant and anesthetic properties that upon inhalation may lead to an acute encephalopathy. Many raw materials, resins, and secondary products have caustic, irritant, or allergic properties that may result in respiratory, mucous membrane, and dermal toxicity, and others may have hepatotoxic, nephrotoxic, or carcinogenic properties. While clinical neurotoxicity is relatively uncommon for workers involved in the manufacturing of plastics and other "synthetics," when this does occur, affected individuals may demonstrate various central and peripheral nervous system effects. This chapter briefly summarizes the neurotoxic effects of several chemicals that pose risks to workers involved in their synthesis and manufacturing and in some cases to users of the end product.

VINYL CHLORIDE

Vinyl chloride is used primarily in the manufacturing of polyvinyl chloride (PVC) resin, a common plastic used in the fabrication of pipes, packaging materials, and insulation. The worldwide production of PVC is extensive, estimated at 59 billion pounds in 2002.[1] At room temperature, vinyl chloride is a flammable, colorless gas that has anesthetic properties. As inhalation exposure levels rise, exposed volunteers report an increasing degree of nonspecific encephalopathic symptoms, including dizziness, ataxia, irritability, and headache.[2–5] Peripheral neuropathy with both sensory and motor manifestations has been described in some exposed workers. A mild distal axonopathy manifested by weakness, reduced reflexes,

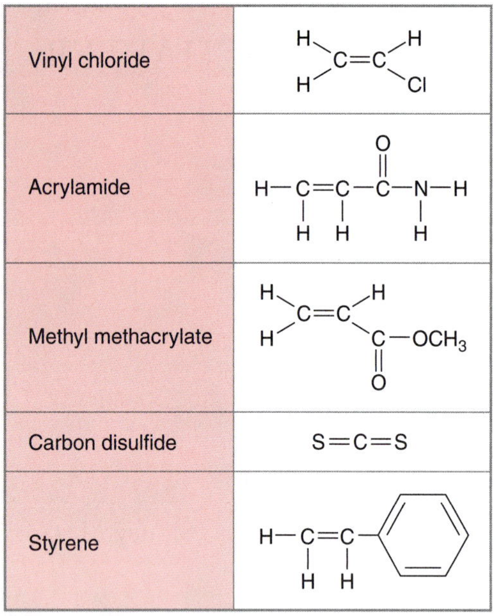

Vinyl chloride	
Acrylamide	
Methyl methacrylate	
Carbon disulfide	$S=C=S$
Styrene	

Figure 36-1. Chemical structures.

and paresthesia, along with denervation on electromyography, has been described in affected individuals.[2–6] Rheumatological symptoms including Raynaud's phenomenon and scleroderma have been reported,[7] as well as a case of polymyositis associated with Jo-1 antibodies.[8] As such, it is not certain whether the peripheral neuropathy is due to a specific neurotoxic effect of vinyl chloride or is a secondary effect of vascular compromise. In 1974, the recognition of the risk of hepatic angiosarcoma in workers exposed to vinyl chloride led to a reduction in time-weighted average (TWA) workplace exposure levels from 500 ppm to 1 ppm, which concomitantly led to a reduced risk of vinyl chloride-induced encephalopathy among exposed workers.[1,9] While primary malignancies of other organs including the brain have been reported, the relationship between brain tumors and vinyl chloride exposure is not well established.[9,10]

ACRYLICS

Acrylics represent a class of plastics composed of polymers manufactured from several monomeric acrylic esters, including ethyl acrylate, methyl acrylate, acrylamide, and methylmethacrylate; the latter two having well-established peripheral nervous system toxicity. Workers are exposed to acrylamide through the use of grouts containing the chemical, as well as in the manufacturing of polyacrylamide resins. While acrylamide monomer is neurotoxic, the polyacrylamide resins are considered to be nontoxic; however, a small amount of the toxic

monomer may be present within the resin and products fabricated from polyacrylamide resin.[11,12] These products are used in industrial settings including water treatment plants, in ore-processing facilities, and in research laboratories that perform chromatography and electrophoresis. In the 1981 to 1983 National Occupational Exposure Survey, it was estimated that greater than 10,000 U.S. workers were exposed to acrylamide monomer while between 100,000 to 200,000 laboratory workers were exposed to polyacrylamide gels.[13,14] Workers are exposed to acrylamide primarily by the dermal route; gastrointestinal and inhalation exposure may also occur.

While acrylamide has dermal irritant properties and at high doses may result in encephalopathy, this substance is best recognized as a peripheral neurotoxin. As such, exposure results in a central–peripheral distal axonopathy, with foci of axonal swelling and accumulations of neurofilaments and other degenerative changes (i.e., dying-back process) felt to be due to an abnormality of axonal transport.[15–17] More recent research suggests that the site of acrylamide neurotoxicity may be at multiple nerve terminals within both the central and the peripheral nervous systems and that retrograde axonal loss is a secondary phenomenon; cerebellar Purkinje cell injury was also noted.[18]

Clinically, workers intoxicated by acrylamide monomer suffer from dermatitis, along with distal numbness and paresthesia, reduced tendon reflexes, and loss of vibration sensation and proprioception. Excess sweating of the hands and feet is a common finding, and signs of more significant autonomic dysfunction such as orthostasis may develop. In workers with more significant intoxication, nonspecific encephalopathic symptoms including ataxia may develop.[11,12,19] Hemoglobin adducts of acrylamide in blood represent an indicator of exposure, and a clinical dose–response association can be demonstrated between symptoms of peripheral nervous system toxicity and levels of these hemoglobin adducts.[20] Electrodiagnostic studies demonstrated reduced to absent sensory nerve action potentials, while motor nerve conduction velocities were normal or slightly reduced. Sural nerve biopsy of affected individuals has noted loss of large-diameter myelinated axons, as well as signs of nerve fiber regeneration.[21] Clinical recovery varies depending on the degree of intoxication, with severely exposed individuals developing chronic ataxia, weakness, and sensory loss.

Comparable to acrylamide monomer, methylmethacrylate monomer has been associated with peripheral neurotoxicity. Examples of peripheral neuropathy[22,23] and abnormal olfaction (hyposmia and parosmia)[24] have been reported in dental technicians exposed to methylmethacrylate monomer and resins while fabricating orthodontic appliances and dental prostheses. In one affected worker, sural nerve biopsy demonstrated a reduction in both large myelinated fibers and unmyelinated axons, similar to changes described in acrylamide intoxication.[22]

CARBON DISULFIDE

Since its introduction into industry in the mid-1800s for the vulcanization of rubber, carbon disulfide has had numerous commercial uses, including serving as a key component in the production of viscous rayon and cellophane and as a solvent in adhesives and cleaners. Since carbon disulfide is a volatile substance, workers are exposed to this chemical primarily via inhalation.[25] The neurotoxicity of carbon disulfide was recognized shortly after its first uses in the rubber industry,[26] and numerous reports of clinical central and peripheral nervous system toxicity have been published.[25,27] Similar to other organic solvents (see Chapter 35), depending on exposure conditions, carbon disulfide intoxication may result in both acute and chronic toxic encephalopathy. Nonspecific signs and symptoms of central nervous system dysfunction including nausea, dizziness, headache, delirium, extrapyramidal and cerebellar signs, as well as frank psychiatric disturbances such as mania and psychosis, have been reported. Chronic motor and neuropsychological deficits, together with cerebral atrophy on computed tomography, have been demonstrated in some workers with a history of chronic exposures.[28,29] Similar features of cortical atrophy, along with lesions within the subcortical white matter and basal ganglia (Figure 36-2), have been demonstrated on magnetic resonance imaging in rayon factory workers with encephalopathic symptoms,[30] while subcortical lacunae were noted in a retrospective clinical study.[31] The pathophysiology of these imaging findings has not been established; however, concomitant computed tomography angiography and perfusion studies suggest that these changes may be secondary to a cerebral microangiopathy rather than to central demyelination.[30]

The threshold limit value (TLV) for carbon disulfide is 10 ppm on a TWA for an 8-hour workday.[32] The risk of developing chronic neuropsychiatric symptoms is greater in workers with higher levels of carbon disulfide exposure, such as those who work in spinning rooms where viscous rayon fibers were made (mean TWA 19.2 ppm), as opposed to those workers who worked in areas where secondary production steps occur and where carbon disulfide levels are lower (mean TWA 4.2 ppm).[33] In a cross-sectional study of workers exposed to carbon disulfide in a viscous rayon factory where exposures fluctuated up to 65.7 ppm but were generally less than the TLV of 10 ppm (mean 4.02 ppm), there was no increase in either subjective neurological symptoms or abnormalities on

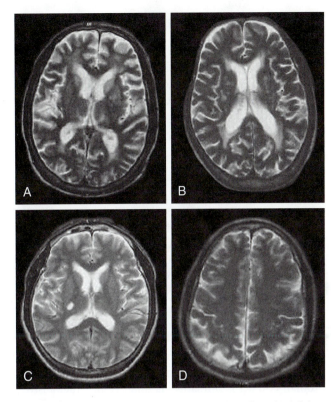

Figure 36-2. T$_2$-weighted magnetic resonance imaging of the brain in four patients with carbon disulfide intoxication. Two patients (*A* and *B*) had multiple high signal intensity lesions in the subcortical white matter and basal ganglia; a third patient (*C*) was found to have a right basal ganglia hyperintensity lesion; and the fourth patient (*D*) demonstrated evidence of mild cortical atrophy. (Chuang, W-L, Huang, C-C, Chen, C-J, et al. Carbon disulfide encephalopathy: cerebral microangiopathy. *Neurotoxicology.* 2007;28:387–393.)

neurological and neuropsychological examination of exposed workers compared with unexposed matched control workers from the same factory.[34]

The peripheral nervous system is another site of carbon disulfide toxicity. Chronically exposed workers may demonstrate a subclinical neuropathy characterized by distal motor hypoexcitability or slowing of both sensory and motor conduction velocities,[35,36] but such changes may not be present when exposure levels are generally below the TLV.[37] In cases of overt clinical toxicity, workers may develop distal numbness, sensory loss, and weakness, together with reduced tendon reflexes.[38] A distal axonopathy characterized by neurofilamentous axonal swellings primarily affecting long, large myelinated fibers has been noted in experimental animals.[39–41] Covalent cross-linking of neurofilament proteins has been demonstrated to underlie the axonal swellings. A similar cross-linking of both the red blood cell membrane protein spectrin and the α-chain of hemoglobin has been produced by carbon disulfide exposure, and these changes correlate with the alterations noted in the axonal swellings. These observations suggest that these biochemical changes in spectrin and hemoglobin may serve as biomarkers in workers at risk for carbon disulfide exposure.[42] This form of employee screening may be preferable to electrodiagnostic studies.

STYRENE

Styrene monomer is used extensively in both the plastics and the synthetic rubber industries. Applications of styrene include polystyrene plastic packaging materials for foods and numerous commercial products; expanded polystyrene foam, which is a ubiquitous material used for insulated shipping containers, disposable coffee cups, and many other purposes; and the production of resins such as styrene–butadiene polymer used for synthetic rubber and unsaturated polyester resin (fiberglass). As is the case with the other chemicals discussed in this chapter, styrene is volatile and a mucous membrane irritant. Human contact is primarily via inhalation, while gastrointestinal and skin exposures also lead to absorption of the chemical.[43] Presently, the TLV for styrene is 20 ppm on a TWA for an 8-hour workday.[32]

There is limited epidemiological evidence for carcinogenic and hepatotoxic effects of styrene. Clinical studies of volunteers and workers exposed to styrene have demonstrated toxicity to both the central and the peripheral nervous systems; however, the number of studies of styrene clinical neurotoxicity is small when compared to those of other organic chemicals. Acute exposure to styrene via inhalation at 376 ppm for 25 minutes resulted in nausea, a sense of inebriation, and headache, along with abnormal performance on the Romberg test.[44] Similar exposure conditions resulted in an insignificant reduction in reaction time with no change in manual dexterity or perceptual speed.[45] In a study of workers in a plant that manufactured fiberglass and reinforced plastics, workers who were exposed to 22 ppm of styrene had no specific acute or chronic symptoms related to their exposure, but when compared to unexposed control workers, they did have significant alterations in the continuous performance test and vibration threshold, suggesting an adverse effect of styrene on both central and peripheral nervous system function, respectively.[46] In contrast, a study of normal volunteers exposed to various styrene exposure scenarios that adhered to local industrial standards failed to demonstrate either symptoms of altered mood and neurological function or abnormal performance on neuropsychological testing.[47]

Chronic exposure to styrene has been noted to result in alterations in neurobehavioral and neurophysiological measurements. For example, in a study of employees involved in fiberglass boat construction that compared former workers exposed to higher styrene concentrations, current workers exposed to lower styrene concentrations, and matched control unexposed workers, the duration of exposure and the interaction between exposure duration and exposure concentration were noted to be the best predictors of impaired visuomotor and perceptual speed performances. This study suggested that less than 10 years of exposure to 37 ppm of styrene may lead to chronic neurotoxic effects.[48] Abnormal electroencephalogram (EEGs), including localized slow activity, diffuse θ-activity, and bilateral spike and wave discharges were noted in 24% of 96 workers chronically exposed to styrene in plants producing reinforced plastic products, with abnormal EEGs being present in more than one-third of workers who had high-level exposures. Those with low-level styrene exposures had the same frequency of abnormal EEGs as were found in a normal population. Electrodiagnostic studies were performed on 40 of the subjects who noted the most neurobehavioral symptoms, but there was no evidence of motor or sensory nerve conduction slowing.[49,50] A neurophysiology study of styrene workers exposed to 22 ppm demonstrated abnormal conduction of myelinated sensory fibers, as well as reduced variability of the R–R interval of the electrocardiogram, indicative of autonomic dysfunction; motor conduction velocity and short-latency somatosensory evoked potentials were not affected by styrene exposure.[51] Similarly, mild sensory nerve conduction slowing was recorded in 23% of fiberglass workers exposed to less than 50 ppm of styrene and in 71% of workers exposed to more than 100 ppm of styrene. Sensory nerve conduction slowing was not present in five workers exposed to more than 100 ppm of styrene who had been on the job for less than 4 weeks, suggesting that duration of exposure was also a factor in the development of peripheral neurotoxicity. Central nervous system effects were evaluated by assessing reaction time. This measurement was slower in workers with high styrene exposure burdens but did not specifically depend on the overall length of exposure.[52] Decreased color discrimination due to styrene exposure has been documented in several studies, and assessment of alterations in color vision may be a sensitive indicator of styrene toxicity. Significant differences in the color confusion index and other assessments of color discrimination have been reported in workers exposed to styrene at levels spanning the range of the current TLV of 20 ppm.[43] In particular, one study estimated that impaired color vision could be detected at exposure levels of 4 ppm, with a 95% upper confidence interval of 26 ppm.[53]

Workers involved in the synthesis of resins and the fabrication of various products that contain plastics and "synthetics," as well as some users of the final products, are at risk of exposure to neurotoxic organic compounds. At present, we have only a partial understanding of the basic toxicological mechanisms that underlie the effects of these substances on the nervous system. In many circumstances, the epidemiology of occupational exposures and the clinical toxicity of these chemicals have been studied on a limited basis. Additional research is clearly needed in each of these fundamental areas.

REFERENCES

1. Agency for Toxic Substances and Disease Registry. Toxicological Profile for Vinyl Chloride. Atlanta: U.S. Department of Health and Human Services, Public Health Service; 2006.

2. Langauer-Lewowicka H, Kurzbauer H, Byczkowska Z, Wocka-Marek T. Vinyl chloride disease: neurological disturbances. *Int Arch Occup Environ Health*. 1983;52:151–157.

3. Lilis R, Anderson H, Nicholson WJ, Daum S, Fischbein AS, Selikoff IJ. Prevalence of disease among vinyl chloride and polyvinyl chloride workers. *Ann NY Acad Sci*. 1975;246:22–41.

4. Spirtas R, McMichael AJ, Gamble J, Van Ert M. The association of vinyl chloride exposures with morbidity symptoms. *Am Ind Hyg Assoc J*. 1975;36:779–789.

5. Suciu I, Prodan L, Ilea E, Paduraru A, Pascu L. Clinical manifestations in vinyl chloride poisoning. *Ann NY Acad Sci*. 1975;246:53–69.

6. Perticoni GF, Abbritti G, Cantisani TA, Bondi L, Mauro L. Polyneuropathy in workers with long exposure to vinyl chloride: electrophysiological study. *Electromyogr Clin Neurophysiol*. 1986;26:41–47.

7. Kahn MF, Bourgeois P, Aeschlimann A, de Truchis P. Mixed connective tissue disease after exposure to polyvinyl chloride. *J Rheumatol*. 1989;16:533–535.

8. Serratrice J, Granel B, Pache X, et al. A case of polymyositis with anti-histidyl-t-RNA synthetase (Jo-1) antibody syndrome following extensive vinyl chloride exposure. *Clin Rheumatol*. 2001;20:379–382.

9. Sass JB, Castleman B, Wallinga D. Vinyl chloride: a case study of data suppression and misrepresentation. *Environ Health Perspect*. 2005;113:809–812.

10. Mundt KA, Dell LD, Austin RP, Luippold RS, Noess R, Bigelow C. Historical cohort study of 10,109 men in the North American vinyl chloride industry, 1942–72: update of cancer mortality to 31 December 1995. *Occup Environ Med*. 2000;57:774–781.

11. National Institute for Occupational Safety and Health. NIOH and NIOSH Basis for an Occupational Health Standard. Acrylamide: A Review of the Literature. Atlanta: U.S. Department of Health and Human Services, Centers for Disease Control, Public Health Service; 1991.

12. Smith EA, Oehme FW. Acrylamide and polyacrylamide: a review of production, use, environmental fate and neurotoxicity. *Rev Environ Health*. 1991;9:215–228.

13. Environmental Protection Agency. Preliminary Assessment of Health Risks from Exposure to Acrylamide. Washington, DC: U.S. Environmental Protection Agency, Office of Toxic Substances; 1988.

14. National Institute for Occupational Safety and Health. National Occupational Exposure Survey. Available at: http://www.cdc.gov/noes/. Accessed May 24, 2008.

15. Gold BG, Griffin JW, Price DL. Slow axonal transport in acrylamide neuropathy: different abnormalities produced by single-dose and continuous administration. *J Neurosci*. 1985;5:1755–1768.

16. Miller MS, Spencer PS. Single doses of acrylamide reduce retrograde transport velocity. *J Neurochem*. 1984;43:1401–1408.

17. Schaumburg HH, Arezzo JC, Spencer PS. Delayed onset of distal axonal neuropathy in primates after prolonged low-level administration of a neurotoxin. *Ann Neurol*. 1989;26:576–579.

18. LoPachin RM, Balaban CD, Ross JF. Acrylamide axonopathy revisited. *Toxicol Appl Pharmacol*. 2003;188:135–153.

19. Spencer PS, Schaumburg HH. A review of acrylamide neurotoxicity: I. Properties, uses and human exposure. *Can J Neurol Sci*. 1974;1:143–150.

20. Hagmar L, Tornqvist M, Nordander C, et al. Health effects of occupational exposure to acrylamide using hemoglobin adducts as biomarkers of internal dose. *Scand J Work Environ Health*. 2001;27:219–226.

21. Fullerton PM. Electrophysiological and histological observations on peripheral nerves in acrylamide poisoning in man. *J Neurol Neurosurg Psychiatry*. 1969;32:186–192.

22. Donaghy M, Rushworth G, Jacobs JM. Generalized peripheral neuropathy in a dental technician exposed to methyl methacrylate monomer. *Neurology*. 1991;41:1112–1116.

23. Sadoh DR, Sharief MK, Howard RS. Occupational exposure to methyl methacrylate monomer induces generalised neuropathy in a dental technician. *Br Dent J*. 1999;186:380–381.

24. Braun D, Wagner W, Zenner HP, Schmahl FW. Disabling disturbance of olfaction in a dental technician following exposure to methyl methacrylate. *Int Arch Occup Environ Health*. 2002;75 Suppl:S73–S74.

25. Agency for Toxic Substances and Disease Registry. Toxicological Profile for Carbon Disulfide. Atlanta: U.S. Department of Health and Human Services, Public Health Service; 1996.

26. O'Flynn RR, Waldron HA. Delpech and the origins of occupational psychiatry. *Br J Ind Med*. 1990;47:189–198.

27. Beauchamp RO Jr, Bus JS, Popp JA, Boreiko CJ, Goldberg L. A critical review of the literature on carbon disulfide toxicity. *Crit Rev Toxicol*. 1983;11:169–278.

28. Aaserud O, Gjerstad L, Nakstad P, et al. Neurological examination, computerized tomography, cerebral blood flow and neuropsychological examination in workers with long-term exposure to carbon disulfide. *Toxicology*. 1988;49:277–282.

29. Peters HA, Levine RL, Matthews CG, Chapman LJ. Extrapyramidal and other neurologic manifestations associated with carbon disulfide fumigant exposure. *Arch Neurol*. 1988;45:537–540.

30. Chuang WL, Huang CC, Chen CJ, Hsieh YC, Kuo HC, Shih TS. Carbon disulfide encephalopathy: cerebral microangiopathy. *Neurotoxicology*. 2007;28:387–393.

31. Cho SK, Kim RH, Yim SH, Tak SW, Lee YK, Son MA. Long-term neuropsychological effects and MRI findings in patients with CS2 poisoning. *Acta Neurol Scand*. 2002;106:269–275.

32. American Conference of Governmental Industrial Hygienists. Documentation of the Threshold Limit Values and Biological Exposure Indices. 7th ed. Cincinnati, Ohio: ACGIH; 2001.

33. Krstev S, Perunicic B, Farkic B, Banicevic R. Neuropsychiatric effects in workers with occupational exposure to carbon disulfide. *J Occup Health*. 2003;45:81–87.

34. Reinhardt F, Drexler H, Bickel A, et al. Neurotoxicity of long-term low-level exposure to carbon disulphide: results of questionnaire, clinical neurological examination and neuropsychological testing. *Int Arch Occup Environ Health*. 1997;69:332–338.

35. Johnson BL, Boyd J, Burg JR, Lee ST, Xintaras C, Albright BE. Effects on the peripheral nervous system of workers' exposure to carbon disulfide. *Neurotoxicology*. 1983;4:53–65.

36. Vasilescu C, Florescu A. Clinical and electrophysiological studies of carbon disulphide polyneuropathy. *J Neurol*. 1980;224:59–70.

37. Reinhardt F, Drexler H, Bickel A, et al. Electrophysiological investigation of central, peripheral and autonomic nerve function

in workers with long-term low-level exposure to carbon disulphide in the viscose industry. *Int Arch Occup Environ Health*. 1997;70:249–256.

38. Chu CC, Huang CC, Chen RS, Shih TS. Polyneuropathy induced by carbon disulphide in viscose rayon workers. *Occup Environ Med*. 1995;52:404–407.

39. Jirmanova I, Lukas E. Ultrastructure of carbon disulphide neuropathy. *Acta Neuropathol*. 1984;63:255–263.

40. Juntunen J, Linnoila I, Haltia M. Histochemical and electron microscopic observations on the myoneural junctions of rats with carbon disulfide induced polyneuropathy. *Scand J Work Environ Health*. 1977;3:36–42.

41. Sills RC, Harry GJ, Morgan DL, Valentine WM, Graham DG. Carbon disulfide neurotoxicity in rats: V. Morphology of axonal swelling in the muscular branch of the posterior tibial nerve and spinal cord. *Neurotoxicology*. 1998;19:117–127.

42. Valentine WM, Amarnath V, Amarnath K, et al. Covalent modification of hemoglobin by carbon disulfide: III. A potential biomarker of effect. *Neurotoxicology*. 1998;19:99–107.

43. Agency for Toxic Substances and Disease Registry. Draft Toxicological Profile for Styrene. Atlanta: U.S. Department of Health and Human Services, Public Health Service; 2007.

44. Stewart RD, Dodd HC, Baretta ED, Schaffer AW. Human exposure to styrene vapor. *Arch Environ Health*. 1968;16:656–662.

45. Gamberale F, Hultengren M. Exposure to styrene: II. Psychological functions. *Work Environ Health*. 1974;11:86–93.

46. Tsai SY, Chen JD. Neurobehavioral effects of occupational exposure to low-level styrene. *Neurotoxicol Teratol*. 1996;18:463–469.

47. Ska B, Vyskocil A, Tardif R, et al. Effects of peak concentrations on the neurotoxicity of styrene in volunteers. *Hum Exp Toxicol*. 2003;22:407–415.

48. Viaene MK, Pauwels W, Veulemans H, Roels HA, Masschelein R. Neurobehavioural changes and persistence of complaints in workers exposed to styrene in a polyester boat building plant: influence of exposure characteristics and microsomal epoxide hydrolase phenotype. *Occup Environ Med*. 2001;58:103–112.

49. Harkonen H. Relationship of symptoms to occupational styrene exposure and to the findings of electroencephalographic and psychological examinations. *Int Arch Occup Environ Health*. 1977;40:231–239.

50. Seppalainen AM, Harkonen H. Neurophysiological findings among workers occupationally exposed to styrene. *Scand J Work Environ Health*. 1976;2:140–146.

51. Murata K, Araki S, Yokoyama K. Assessment of the peripheral, central, and autonomic nervous system function in styrene workers. *Am J Ind Med*. 1991;20:775–784.

52. Cherry N, Gautrin D. Neurotoxic effects of styrene: further evidence. *Br J Ind Med*. 1990;47:29–37.

53. Campagna D, Gobba F, Mergler D, et al. Color vision loss among styrene-exposed workers neurotoxicological threshold assessment. *Neurotoxicology*. 1996;17:367–373.

CHAPTER 37 ····

Botulinum Neurotoxin

Peter J. Osterbauer

INTRODUCTION

Botulinum neurotoxin (BoNT) is hailed as the deadliest neurotoxin known to man.[1–3] Initially identified in 1895 by Emile van Ermengem,[4] BoNT is produced by *Clostridium botulinum*, a gram-negative, anaerobic, rod-shaped bacteria, which forms spores that are highly resistant to destruction by heat, surviving for up to 2 hours at temperatures of 100°C.[1,5] Spores can be found worldwide in soil, in freshwater and saltwater sediments, and in the intestinal tracts of various animals.[1,5] The toxin itself is best produced in anaerobic, alkalinic environments with low concentrations of salt and sugar.[1,5] There are seven subtypes (A to G) (Table 1), with types A, B, and E being the most common causes of human botulism.[1,2,5] Although the spores are highly resistant to heat, the toxin is rendered harmless when exposed to a temperature of at least 85°C for 5 minutes.[1]

The syndrome known as *botulism*, which is addressed later in more detail, was first described by Justinus Kerner in the 19th century.[6] It is most often acquired by ingesting the preformed toxin in undercooked foods, which have been prepared in a manner favoring proliferation of spores and subsequent production of the neurotoxin.[1] Clinical BoNT intoxication, however, can be introduced by various routes, including inhalation, proliferation in the gut by *C. botulinum* with subsequent toxin production, contamination of open wounds, or even iatrogenically,[1,7] and its high potential for lethality makes it a prime agent for bioterrorism.[4] The toxin does not penetrate intact skin, nor is it transmissible from person to person.[1] Despite its serious potential for toxicity, BoNT is also being used at low therapeutic doses successfully in various clinical applications.

PATHOPHYSIOLOGY AND MECHANISM OF ACTION

Although antigenically distinct, each of the seven subtypes is similar in structure and function. BoNT is a 150-kDa molecule consisting of a 100-kDa heavy chain and a 50-kDa light chain, linked together by a disulfide bond.[1,2,4] The heavy chain is responsible for binding to the plasma membrane of presynaptic motor neurons, and it facilitates internalization via receptor-mediated endocytosis.[1,4] The light chain is a zinc-dependent endopeptidase, which is responsible for the actual toxicity upon the neuron.[1,4] Once inside the cell, the disulfide bond is broken, allowing the light chain to irreversibly bind to soluble N-ethylmaleimide-sensitive fusion attachment receptor (SNARE) proteins, subsequently cleaving peptide

Table 1: Botulinum Neurotoxin Subtype Characteristics

BoNT SUBTYPE	TARGET PROTEIN	PREDOMINANT GEOGRAPHIC LOCATION	MISCELLANEOUS
A	SNAP-25	Rocky Mountains, Western US	Most Potent
B	Synaptobrevin	Allegheny Range, Eastern US	Requires Intracellular Tubules for Action
C	Syntaxin & SNAP-25	Mainly Seen in Animals	Poorly Absorbed from Intestine
D	Synaptobrevin	Mainly Seen in Animals	Poorly Absorbed from Intestine
E	SNAP-25	Baltic Sea, Alaska, Great Lakes States	Associated with Ingestion of Contaminated Fish
F	Synaptobrevin	Not Specified	Produced by *C. baratii*
G	Synaptobrevin	Not Specified	Rarely Implicated in Botulism Cases

bonds.[1,8] This prevents fusion of acetylcholine vesicles with the presynaptic cell membrane, ultimately resulting in failure of nerve impulse transmission (Figure 37-1; see color plate).[1,2,4] Fusion of vesicles containing norepinephrine, glutamate, substance P, and calcitonin gene–related peptide is also prevented, which may be partly responsible for some of the toxin's clinical effects. The toxic effect of BoNT absolutely depends on the cleavage of the disulfide bond, allowing the light chain to fulfill its purpose.[4,9] Although there is no definitive evidence to date, it is not believed that BoNT enters the central nervous system.[4]

CLINICAL PRESENTATION OF BOTULISM

Clinical symptoms generally occur within 24 to 72 hours of exposure; however, it has been reported that symptoms can manifest as early as 2 hours or as late as 5 days after presumed exposure.[1,5] The usual presentation is one of symmetrical cranial nerve palsies, followed by a progressive, descending paralysis.[1,5,7] Sensation and cognition are spared.[1] Anticholinergic symptoms can also occur.[1,5,10] A classical diagnostic pentad of dry mouth, nausea or vomiting, dysphagia, diplopia, and fixed dilated pupils has been suggested; however, a case of foodborne botulism sparing the extraocular muscles has been described, calling into question the validity of this classical pentad.[10]

Infantile botulism, often acquired from consuming tainted honey, has also been well described. This should be suspected in any child younger than 1 year who presents with feeding problems (poor sucking and swallowing), change in pitch or volume of crying, poor head control (caused by weakness of neck musculature), ptosis, and descending paralysis.[1,5] Other symptoms, such as constipation and lethargy, may be overlooked, given their general nature. It has been postulated that infantile botulism may be one cause of the sudden infant death syndrome (SIDS).[5]

Differential Diagnosis

A differential diagnosis of botulism would include myasthenia gravis, Lambert-Eaton syndrome, Guillain-Barré syndrome (GBS) and its variants, tick paralysis, stroke, diphtheria, or exposure to other toxins, such as organophosphates or other nerve agents, carbon monoxide, or neuromuscular junction blockers.[11] Although it is usually possible to differentiate botulism from other potential etiologies, it must be remembered that the syndrome can progress quickly, so time is of the essence. If a strong clinical suspicion for botulism exists, treatment should not be delayed.

A standard edrophonium (Tensilon) test can help differentiate botulism from myasthenia gravis; however, a weak positive response to this test can sometimes be seen with botulism.[11] Repetitive stimulation and single-fiber electromyography studies may also be helpful but might not be available in a timely manner or, in some cases, at all.

Traditional GBS presents as an ascending paralysis, in contrast to the descending paralysis classically seen in botulism; however, variants of GBS, such as the

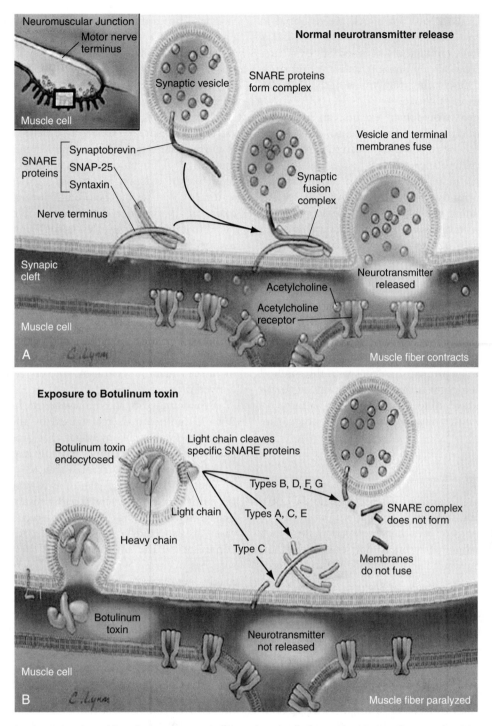

Figure 37-1. Mechanism of action of botulinum neurotoxin (see color plate). (Horowitz BZ. Botulinum toxin. *Crit Care Clin.* 2005;21:825–839.)

Miller-Fischer type, can present with descending paralysis instead. The GBSs usually present with sensory findings, which are absent in botulism. Also, the classic albuminocytological dissociation seen in GBS would be absent in botulism. Care must be taken with cerebrospinal fluid results, however, since the albuminocytological dissociation may not be seen early in the course of GBS. It should also be noted that botulism can produce a slight increase in cerebrospinal fluid protein.[11]

Like GBS, tick paralysis typically presents in an ascending pattern and is often accompanied by sensory complaints.[11] History of potential tick exposure and a careful examination to look for a tick are essential in ruling this out.

Stroke syndromes can typically be ruled out by a careful history, neurological examination, and imaging studies. Symmetrical, descending paralysis would also be an unusual presentation of stroke.

Absence of fever would help exclude an infectious etiology, such as diphtheria. Exposure to other toxic agents can normally be ruled out by a careful history and laboratory tests (where appropriate).

Unfortunately, a rapid test to assess for botulism does not yet exist. Currently, the most sensitive and specific means for confirming the presence of intoxication with BoNT is the mouse bioassay.[1,5,12] This method involves collecting potentially infected bodily substances from the patient, such as blood, stool, vomitus, or wound swabs, as well as the potentially contaminated food source if available. Portions of these substances are then injected into mice, half of which have been previously inoculated with antitoxin specific for BoNT and half of which are unprotected. Botulism is confirmed if the unprotected mice subsequently die while exhibiting signs of BoNT intoxication.[1,5,12] The primary drawback with this method from a clinical standpoint is that it can be difficult to coordinate and can take up to 4 days to yield a positive result.[1,12] Other potential means of confirming botulism are being developed.[1,12,13]

Treatment

The first step in addressing a suspected case of botulism, after ensuring stability of the patient, would be to notify the state and/or local health department, which sets in motion a chain of events to help ensure containment of the toxic source and availability of the appropriate antitoxin.[1,14]

With regard to direct patient care, top priority is given to managing the standard "ABCs" of airway, breathing, and circulation. Given the potential for rapid symptomatic decline, careful and frequent attention must be paid to the patient's neurological and respiratory function, and means of mechanical ventilation should be close at hand in the event that intubation is required.[1,14]

If the route of exposure is known, other specific measures can be taken to try to prevent further spread of the toxin. Activated charcoal, cathartics, or enemas can be considered in cases of foodborne intoxication.[1,11] Potentially infected wounds should be thoroughly cleaned to remove any *C. botulinum* spores that may be present.[1] Treatment with agents with potential inhibitory effects at the neuromuscular junction, such as aminoglycosides, clindamycin, and polymyxin B, and agents containing magnesium should be avoided.[1,11] Since botulism is not contagious, specific isolation precautions are not necessary,[1] although standard precautions should be observed, as with any patient.

The only known definitive treatment for botulism at this time is administration of a botulism antitoxin,[14] of which there are presently two types available to the public. A trivalent, equine-derived antitoxin, effective against BoNT types A, B, and E, is the standard treatment in most cases of botulism.[1,2,14] One vial of antitoxin is diluted 1:10 in normal saline and delivered intravenously over 30 to 60 minutes.[1,14] A limitation of this antitoxin is the possibility of an allergic reaction, given that it is derived from horse serum.[1,14] Skin testing before administration of the antitoxin can be considered[14]; however, it must be remembered that time is of the essence, so this may not be feasible in every situation. In any event, the treating providers must be prepared to handle an anaphylactic event.

A human-derived antitoxin, effective against BoNT types A and B (baby-BIG), is available from the California State Health Department for treatment of patients in whom the equine-derived antitoxin is contraindicated or who experience an adverse reaction to the trivalent antitoxin.[1,2,14] Baby-BIG is also recommended for the treatment of infantile botulism, rather than the equine-derived product.[14]

A third antitoxin, an equine-derived, heptavalent (types A to G) antitoxin, is maintained by the U.S. Army.[1,14] This, however, is an investigational product and would likely only be released under extreme circumstances, such as in the event of a bioterrorist attack.[1]

There is also some question as to when to administer the antitoxin or whether to administer it at all. Some believe that it should be administered empirically in all cases of suspected botulism,[14] while others recommend administering the antitoxin only if the suspected exposure has occurred within the past 72 hours.[1] Unfortunately, an distinct therapeutic window has yet to be established.[2] All things being considered, I tend to favor empirical treatment, regardless of time of exposure.

(See Chapter 55 for additional information about botulinum toxin.)

Prognosis

As previously explained, the effect of BoNT on presynaptic neurons is irreversible, once the toxin binds to the SNARE proteins. Recovery of nerve transmission takes place by axonal rearborization, which can take months.[4,11,15] Therefore, many factors may affect overall prognosis, such as the elapsed time between exposure and treatment, the need for mechanical ventilation, and of course the premorbid baseline health status of the individual patient. With appropriate treatment, mortality is estimated to be 10% or less.[5,16]

Little is known with regard to the long-term effects of botulism. One study suggests that botulism survivors may continue to experience persistent health, functional, and psychosocial problems for several years after recovery.[17] Factors thought to predict poorer overall health after recovery from botulism include need for mechanical ventilation, older age, and region of residence.[17]

Prevention

Active immunization against BoNT is available as a pentavalent (types A to E) vaccine through the Centers for Disease Control and Prevention (CDC), requiring three initial doses, plus an annual booster.[1] Multiple other means of prevention are also being explored. A mucosal vaccine against types A, B, and E looks to be promising but is still in development.[18,19]

IATROGENIC BOTULISM

Currently, there are reportedly more than 100 clinical uses for BoNT.[3] Beside the well-known cosmetic uses, headaches, blepharospasm, strabismus, cervical dystonia, and hyperhidrosis are just a few of the conditions being successfully treated with BoNT.[3,20,21] Many other potential uses are constantly being explored, even in the realm of cancer treatment.[22]

With the use of BoNT for clinical purposes comes the possibility of human error. Clinical botulism has been known to occur with therapeutic use, even when proper dosing guidelines have been followed.[1,23] This is rare, however, and is believed to be caused by BoNT unintentionally entering the bloodstream.[1] Regardless of the route of intoxication, treatment would not differ from that described earlier.

There is one further caveat with regard to clinical use of BoNT. Anesthesiologists often employ a train-of-four (TOF) technique using a peripheral nerve stimulator to assess the level of induced paralysis during surgery. Facial muscles, such as the orbicularis oculi muscles, are often among those tested with this procedure. Patients who have been treated with BoNT injections into facial musculature may produce inaccurate TOF readings when obtained from affected facial musculature; therefore, information about BoNT injections should be obtained during the preanesthesia history, and obtaining baseline TOF readings should be strongly considered.[24]

PUBLIC HEALTH CONCERNS

The most common cause of botulism in the United States is foodborne illness associated with home-canned foods and Native Alaskan meals.[1] BoNT as a potential weapon of biological warfare has also been well documented.[1,14,25,26] From a public health standpoint, the most important consideration is early recognition of a potential breakout so that appropriate measures to treat the afflicted and prevent further spread can be taken in a timely fashion. As previously stated, the state or local health department, the CDC, or all of these should be notified at the first indication of a potential breakout.

CONCLUSION

Botulinum toxin, one of the deadliest toxins known, is a prime example of a double-edged sword. In the right hands, it can be used to treat potentially disabling medical conditions. In the wrong hands, it could be used as a veritable weapon of mass destruction. Most often, intoxication with BoNT is the result of careless or inexperienced hands involved in food preparation. Regardless of the means of exposure, the clinical signs and symptoms, diagnosis, and treatment are essentially the same. Early recognition and treatment are the primary keys to preventing death and long-term consequences.

CASE STUDY

A 42-year-old man presents with nausea and vomiting, which began several hours after a family reunion picnic 2 days ago. Initially, he assumed that he had eaten too much, so he was not overly concerned. However, as time progressed, he began to notice double vision and difficulty swallowing. When his wife observed that he was having difficulty with his speech, she rushed him to the local emergency department, afraid that he may have had a stroke.

Initial history did not reveal any significant risk factors for cerebral ischemia. He was previously healthy, exercised regularly, and was not taking any prescribed medications. He denied any associated pain symptoms but did comment that bright lights seemed to bother him more than usual. Further history revealed that during the picnic he was the only one who received a serving of a three-bean salad before the bowl was accidentally knocked over. As far as they were aware, no one else from the picnic became ill.

The patient was afebrile, with normal vital signs. Positive findings on physical examination included mild, bilateral ptosis; slightly abnormal extraocular movements; a diminished gag reflex;

Continued

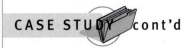

CASE STUDY cont'd

and dilated, poorly reactive pupils. There was also some subtle weakness of the proximal muscles of the upper extremities, but sensation was intact, and deep tendon reflexes, although somewhat sluggish, were essentially normal. Dysarthria was apparent, but mentation was fully intact, and there was no evidence of aphasia.

Complete blood count, electrolytes, and liver, kidney, and thyroid function tests were all normal. Drug and alcohol screens were negative. Electrocardiogram revealed a normal sinus rhythm, and a noncontrast computerized tomography scan of the head showed no evidence of mass or ischemia. A lumbar puncture was performed to look for evidence of a possible acute demyelinating syndrome, but cerebrospinal fluid studies were normal. Edrophonium was not available to help rule out a myasthenic syndrome.

Given the overall clinical picture, the emergency department physician suspected foodborne botulism and notified the state health department. Arrangements were subsequently made to obtain the trivalent, equine-derived antitoxin. In the meantime, the patient was admitted to the hospital's intensive care unit for close monitoring of neurological and pulmonary function. The antitoxin arrived and was administered within hours, and although the upper extremity weakness progressed to some extent, the patient's respiratory status remained intact and intubation was not required. Although it took several weeks, the patient eventually made a full recovery, with no relapse in symptoms.

REFERENCES

1. Villar RG, Elliott SP, Davenport KM. Botulism: the many faces of botulinum toxin and its potential for bioterrorism. *Infect Dis Clin North Am.* 2006;20:313–327.
2. Ravichandran E, Gong Y, Al Saleem FH, et al. An initial assessment of the systemic pharmacokinetics of botulinum toxin. *J Pharmacol Exp Ther.* 2006;318(3):1343–1351.
3. Lang AM. Considerations for the use of botulinum toxin in pain management. *Lippincotts Case Manag.* 2006;11(5):279–282.
4. Mahajan ST, Brubaker L. Botulinum toxin: from life-threatening disease to novel medical therapy. *Am J Obstet Gynecol.* 2007;196:7–15.
5. Plorde JJ. Clostridia, gram-negative anaerobes, and anaerobic cocci. In: Ryan KJ, Champoux JJ, Drew WL, et al., eds. *Sherris Medical Microbiology: An Introduction to Infectious Diseases.* 3rd ed. Stamford, Conn: Appleton & Lange; 1994:302–303.
6. Aoki, KR. Botulinum toxin: a successful therapeutic protein. *Curr Med Chem.* 2004;11(23):3085 [abstract].
7. Brook I. Botulism: the challenge of diagnosis and treatment. *Rev Neurol Dis.* 2006;3(4):182–189.
8. Lim EC, Seet RC. Botulinum toxin, quo vadis? *Med Hypotheses.* 2007;69(4):718–723.
9. Fischer A, Montal M. Crucial role of the disulfide bridge between botulinum neurotoxin light and heavy chains in protease translocation across membranes. *J Biol Chem.* 2007;282(40):29604–29611.
10. Gdynia HJ, Huber R, Kastrup A, et al. Atypical botulism sparing palsy of extraocular muscles. *Eur J Med Res.* 2007;12(7):300–301.
11. Arnon SS, Schechter R, Inglesby TV, et al. Botulinum toxin as a biological weapon: medical and public health management. *JAMA.* 2001;285:1059–1070.
12. Cai S, Singh BR, Sharma S. Botulism diagnostics: from clinical symptoms to in vitro assays. *Crit Rev Microbiol.* 2007;33(2):109–125.
13. Wang J, Gao S, Zhang Q, et al. Avian eyelid assay: a new diagnostic method for detecting botulinum neurotoxin serotypes A, B, and E. *Toxicon.* 2007;49(7):1019–1025.
14. Lawrence DT, Kirk MA. Chemical terrorism attacks: update on antidotes. *Emerg Med Clin North Am.* 2007;25:582–584.
15. Martin CO, Adams HP. Neurological aspects of biological and chemical terrorism: a review for neurologists. *Arch Neurol.* 2003;60:21–25.
16. Taillac PP, Kim J. CBRNE: Botulism, 6/6/2006. Available at: http://www.emedicine.com/emerg/topic64.htm. Accessed January 4, 2008.
17. Gottlieb SL, Kretsinger K, Tarkhashvili N, et al. Long-term outcomes of 217 botulism cases in the Republic of Georgia. *Clin Infect Dis.* 2007;45(2):174–180.
18. Fujihashi K, Staats HF, Kozaki S, et al. Mucosal vaccine development for botulinum intoxication. *Expert Rev Vaccines.* 2007;6(1):35–45.
19. Ravichandran E, Al-Saleem FH, Ancharski DM, et al. Trivalent vaccine against botulinum toxin serotypes A, B, and E that can be administered by the mucosal route. *Infect Immune.* 2007;75(6):3043–3054.
20. Evers F. Status on the use of botulinum toxin for headache disorders. *Curr Opin Neurol.* 2006;19(3):310–315.
21. Jancovic J, Hunter C, Dolimbek BZ, et al. Clinico-immunologic aspects of botulism toxin type B treatment of cervical dystonia. *Neurology.* 2006;67(12):2233–2235.
22. Ansiaux R, Gallez B. Use of botulinum toxins in cancer therapy. *Expert Opin Investig Drugs.* 2007;16(2):209–218.
23. Rossi RP, Strax TE, Di Rocco A. Severe dysphagia after botulinum toxin B injection to the lower limbs and lumbar paraspinal muscles. *Am J Phys Med Rehabil.* 2006;85(12):1011–1013.
24. Miller L, Neustein S. Neuromuscular blockade monitoring complicated by the unknown preoperative cosmetic use of botulinum toxin. *Anesthesiology.* 2006;105(4):862.
25. Greenfield RA, Brown BR, Hutchins JB, et al. Microbiological, biological, and chemical weapons of warfare and terrorism. *Am J Med Sci.* 2002;323:326–340.
26. Patocka J, Splino M, Merka V. Botulism and bioterrorism: how serious is this problem? *Acta Medica (Hradec Kralove).* 2005;48(1):23–28.

CHAPTER 38

Tetanus Toxin

D. Brandon Burtis and Michael R. Dobbs

Definition: Tetanus is defined by the acute onset of hypertonia or by painful muscular contractions (usually of the muscles of the jaw and neck) and generalized muscle spasms without other apparent medical cause. This definition, published in 1997, is approved by the Council of State and Territorial Epidemiologists.[1]

INTRODUCTION

Tetanus is an acute illness characterized by uncontrolled, severe contraction of voluntary skeletal muscles, generalized tonic activity, or both that may, in severe cases, lead to respiratory failure and death.[2–5] The organism responsible is *Clostridium tetani*—an obligate anaerobic gram-positive rod with terminal round endospores.[6] This heat-sensitive bacterium is found as spores worldwide in soil and gut flora of animals, including horses, sheep, cattle, dogs, cats, rats, guinea pigs, and chickens. The endospores produced by *C. tetani* are highly resistant to extreme environmental conditions, allowing for survival for up to 40 years. They can survive most antiseptics and autoclaving at 249.8°F (121°C) for 10 to 15 minutes.[7] Endospores are a complex, multilayer encapsulated form of the organism consisting of polysaccharides, dipiclonic acid, and high calcium content.[8] The organism itself is heat sensitive and requires anaerobic conditions such as found in superficial skin wounds to thrive.

EPIDEMIOLOGY

Because of effective vaccination programs, tetanus is rare in developed countries such as the United States. However, it remains a serious problem worldwide (Table 1).[9]

Since the routine introduction of a childhood immunization and national surveillance system began in 1947, the incidence of tetanus in the United States has greatly decreased from 560 cases (approximately 0.4 cases per 100,000 population) reported per year to a total of 20 cases (0.01 cases per 100,000) reported in 2003.[7,10,11] The death-to-case ratio also decreased from 30 to approximately 10%.[7] It is believed that the increased rural to urban migration with a consequent decrease in exposure to tetanus spores may also have contributed to declines in mortality, especially during the first half of the 20th century.[12]

From 1980 to 2000, 70% of U.S. cases reported were among people 40 years and older. From 1980 to 1990,

Table 1:	2006 Global Tetanus Figures
14,529 reported cases	
290,000 estimated deaths (2000–2003)	
79% estimated DTP3 coverage	
World Health Organization data.	

21% were among people 40 years and younger. The age distribution shift during 1991 to 1995 was attributed to both a reduction in cases reported for the elderly and an increase in cases reported among the young. People 40 years and younger accounted for 28% of reported cases from 1991 to 1995 and then 42% of reported cases from 1996 to 2000.[7] Injection-drug users in California accounted for most of this increase during this period.[13–15] Heroin users, in particular, diluted this drug with quinine, which may actually support the growth of *C. tetani*.[7,12] Almost all cases of tetanus reported either have been never vaccinated or have completed the primary series but have not had a booster in the previous 10 years.[12]

The number of neonatal cases reported in the United States has been only 2 since 1989.[12] Neither of the infants' mothers were immunized. However, the number of neonatal cases worldwide range from 300,000 to 500,000 deaths per year.[16–18] This accounts for nearly 50% of the 1 million cases. Infant deaths in developing countries reached nearly 560,000 in 1993.[7] In 1999 and 2000, the number of neonatal deaths attributed to tetanus decreased dramatically to roughly 215,000 and 200,000, respectively.[12,19]

From 1998 to 2000, acute injuries or wound injuries preceded tetanus in the United States in 94 (73%) of the 129 cases. Among the most common wound types were puncture wounds (50%), lacerations (33%), and abrasions (9%).[7] The most common puncture wound involved stepping on a "rusty" nail. Other puncture wounds involved barbed wire, splinters, animal or insect bites, self-piercings, and self-performed tattoos. The environment in which acute injuries occurred were indoors or at home (45%); in the yard, in a garden, or on a farm (31%); and at other outdoor locations (23%).[7]

TRANSMISSION

Transmission typically occurs by implantation of contaminated soil into penetrating wounds.[20,21] There is no person-to-person transmission. Interestingly, 10% to 20% of reported cases demonstrate no evidence of injury or wound during both history and physical examination.[22] The organism is also found as a natural inhabitant of the skin of individuals who show no sign or symptoms of tetanus.[3] The incidence is higher in hot, damp climates with soil rich in organic matter, especially manure-treated soil. The spore is commonly found in the intestines of nonhuman and agricultural animals.[7,8,12]

PATHOPHYSIOLOGY

The etiology of tetanus was discovered in 1884, but records from 5th century BC contain probable clinical descriptions of tetanus. It was not until 1889 that Kitasato isolated the organism from a human case. He injected this unknown organism to produce tetany in an animal. He later postulated the possibility of neutralizing the exotoxin by antibodies.[8]

The natural barrier of the human skin provides protection from *C. tetani*.[21,23] Once this pathogen gains entry beyond the protective skin layer, *C. tetani* produces two exotoxins.[7] The first exotoxin is called tetanolysin. Its activity is uncertain. The second exotoxin, called tetanospasmin, is responsible for the muscular contractions called tetanus, also known as "lockjaw." All strains of *C. tetani* appear to produce the same toxin.[8]

Tetanospasmin, a 150-kDa peptide, prevents the release of inhibitory neurotransmitters at the central nervous system, leading to disinhibition of end-organ tissues and uncontrolled skeletal muscle contractions. This exotoxin released by *C. tetani* consists of a two-chain molecule bound by a disulfide bond.[24] The heavy or β-chain (100 kDa) binds to disialogangliosides, GT1β and GD1β, found on the membranes at the neuromuscular junction.[24] It allows entry before being transported retrograde by the peripheral nerves to enter the central nervous system. The toxin can also spread hematogenously or lymphatically from the site of injury. The gene for tetanospasmin is encoded within a plasmid.

The second chain of tetanospasmin, the light or α-chain (50 kDa), is a zinc metalloendopeptidase that provides the pathogenic inhibitory property of tetanospasmin.[24] It acts by cleaving synaptobrevin (a vesicle-associated membrane protein) at a single point. Synaptobrevin is necessary for the exocytosis of intracellular vesicles containing neurotransmitters.[24] This mutated chain prevents the release of glycine and γ-aminobutyric acid (GABA),[8] leading to the disinhibition and unregulated control of agonistic and antagonistic skeletal muscles by excitatory neurotransmitters at the spinal synapses. The rapid frequency of firing at the neuromuscular junction increases above the threshold to achieve "tetanus"—a sustained maximal contraction of the motor unit. Tetanospasmin is also postulated to act at the level of the autonomic nervous system, leading to associated dysautonomia with severe cases characterized by labile hypertension, arrhythmias, and hyperpyrexia.[25] Accordingly, if the patient survives beyond the acute phase of tetanus, autonomic dysfunction becomes a major cause of death.[26,27] Cardiac arrhythmias and myocardial infarction are not uncommon.[26] Case reports suggest that elevated levels of serum catecholamines are present during autonomic instability.[28–31] There may be disinhibition at the presynaptic level of the interomediolateral cell column and adrenal medulla or vagal nerve.[25] This disinhibition leads to the alternating imbalance between sympathetic storm and parasympathetic activity. Fortunately, the heart cannot be tetanized because the longer refractory period of cardiac muscle compared to skeletal muscle protects it from this neurotoxin.[8,24]

DIAGNOSIS AND MANIFESTATIONS

The diagnosis of tetanus is made clinically.[32,33] There are no diagnostic or predictive laboratory findings. The examiner must have a high index of suspicion to make the correct diagnosis and mitigate further complications as much as possible. The importance of accurate diagnosis is made apparent by the high mortality rate without appropriate treatment. Mortality is reported to be higher than 50% and appears to depend on the severity and treatment. Even with excellent intensive care, mortality remains as high as 20%.[22]

The onset and severity of disease is variable and depends on the degree of prior immunization, the amount of toxin introduced to a tetanus-prone wound, and the age or overall general health of the individual.[34] Incubation ranges from 3 days to 3 weeks (average 8 days) after the wound depending on the initial site of entry of the organism. Neonatal onset can begin between 4 and 14 days (average 7 days) after delivery. The distance of the wound from the central nervous system helps determine the length of the incubation period. Furthermore, a shorter incubation period increases the mortality rate.[7] The symptoms typically begin as its original name "lockjaw." Lockjaw, or trismus, manifests as severe muscular stiffness of the muscles of the lower face and jaw, including the masseters (Figure 38-1). Muscle spasms then normally descend to involve the muscles of the neck; the chest, abdomen, and back; and eventually the extremities.

Familiar clinical signs include the following:

- Lockjaw or trismus
- Laryngospasm—diaphragmatic spasms leading to transient periods of hypoxia
- Dysphagia due to severe muscle spasms upon swallowing[35]

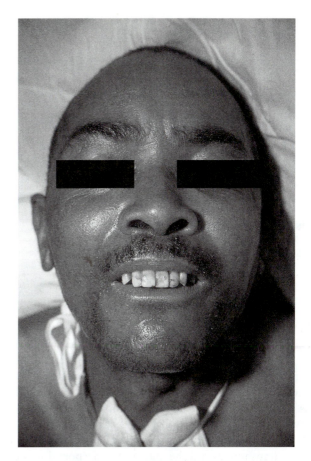

Figure 38-1. Lockjaw, or trismus, may result in a sneering appearance called risus sardonicus. (From the Centers for Disease Control and Prevention's Public Health Image Library, ID No 2857.)

- Diffuse hyperreflexia as the afferent input stimulates the contraction of skeletal muscle
- Risus sardonicus or a sneering appearance
- Opisthotonus, sometime resembling decorticate posturing
- Tonic contractions of agonist–antagonist skeletal muscles mimicking convulsions

These may be accompanied by sympathetic activity such as the following:

- Hypertension
- Tachycardia or arrhythmia
- Diaphoresis
- Pyrexia
- Urinary and bowel incontinence

Several types of tetanus are described in the literature.[36,37] The generalized form makes up nearly 80% of all cases. This typically begins with trismus, followed by dysphagia and neck stiffness.[38] The pattern continues

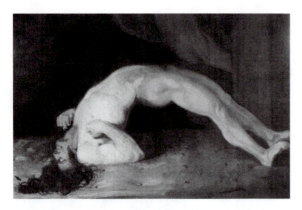

Figure 38-2. *Tetanus.* Painting by Sir Charles Bell, 1809, shows characteristic opisthotonic spasms seen in severe disease.

in a descending fashion to involve all skeletal muscles (Figure 38-2), along with other autonomic symptoms. Generalized tetanus involves frequent, severe muscle tonic spasms lasting several minutes and peaking on average 17 days after inoculation. These spasms continue for as long as 3 to 4 weeks, while complete recovery takes several months.[7] This is probably because of the time it takes to synthesize new presynaptic vesicles containing neurotransmitters and the antegrade transport down the distal axon to the synaptic bouton.[39]

Neonatal tetanus is a form of generalized tetanus and a leading cause of infant mortality worldwide (Figure 38-3). It is often associated with the use of nonsterile instruments when cutting the umbilical cord. The unhealed stump provides an easy entry site for *C. tetani*. The tetanic newborn would not have acquired passive immunity from the mother who never received primary immunization.

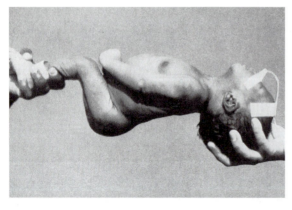

Figure 38-3. Neonatal tetanus with opisthotonos. (From the Centers for Disease Control and Prevention's Public Health Image Library, ID No 6374.)

Cephalic tetanus, often associated with otitis media or head trauma,[40–42] is another manifestation of the disease. In these cases, bacteria can often be isolated from the middle ear.[7,8,20] Cephalic tetanus most often presents as trismus, often preceded by other cranial nerve impairments.[43] Flaccid paralysis of the cranial nerves may occur for nerves 7, 6, 3, 4, and 12.[43] Cephalic tetanus has a mortality rate of 15% to 30% if it progresses to the generalized form.[43]

Local tetanus, the last type, has an incidence of 13% with a rare mortality of less than 1%.[7] The spasms begin locally surrounding the injury and resolve without sequelae. However, bear in mind that a localized muscle spasm could represent the initial onset of a generalized form rather than local tetanus.[25] Local tetanus can also progress to a mild generalized form and continue for weeks before finally subsiding. This is often found in patients with incomplete or partial immunity.[7,44,45]

Some consideration should include the following disorders or diseases. Trismus can be caused by an infection of the peritonsillar area and an odontogenic abscess or as a dystonic reaction from certain medications,[25] including dopaminergic agonist. Focal muscles may be affected by myopathies or neuropathies. However, the muscles are typically weak on examination rather than the expected rigidity of tetanus. Also, sensory changes may be found with the neuropathies.[25] Strychnine poisoning has been known to lead to tetanus-like activity. Strychnine acts by inhibiting the release of glycine similar to tetanospasmin but has no effect on GABA release.[25] Hypocalcemia can also resemble tetanus, but a routine total serum or ion calcium level helps rule this out.[25] Cephalic tetanus may resemble Bell's palsy, central nervous system tumor, or stroke if trismus is initially absent.[25] However, progression to trismus leads to the correct diagnosis.

Spatula Test

The spatula test has been reported in literature as a reliable although perhaps dangerous way of demonstrating tetanus.[46] In this bedside test, a sterile soft-tipped instrument is introduced into the posterior pharynx. The normal reaction of a noninfected individual includes the gag reflex with expelling of the instrument. However, in tetanus, the muscles spasms of the posterior pharynx manifest, as well as trismus. The *American Journal of Tropical Medicine and Hygiene* in 1995 reported a sensitivity of 94% and a specificity of nearly 100%.[46]

Diagnostic Studies

The diagnosis of tetanus is most often established by clinical manifestations alone and by exclusion of other etiologies. Laboratory studies may help rule out other possibilities in the differential diagnosis. Routine studies including complete blood count and basic metabolic panel are typically normal. White blood cell count can rarely be elevated during acute infections from wounds, but the amount of neurotoxin is so small that the body usually does not mount any significant immune reaction. Muscle enzymes are expected to become elevated during the progression of the disease. Normal calcium levels rule out hypocalcemia. Strychnine levels may be checked if strychnine poisoning is reasonably suspected. Lumbar puncture may demonstrate an elevated opening pressure, particularly during tonic contractions. However, the cerebrospinal fluid is often diagnostically unremarkable. Bone fractures may be found on plain films but may not show rupturing of muscle or tendons. Directed magnetic resonance imaging may disclose muscle or tendon damage and can be performed as clinically indicated.

Laboratory Identification

Presence of tetanus toxin can be demonstrated in a two-mouse model. The suspect material or pus is injected at the root of the tails of two mice. One of these mice has been previously protected with antitoxin. The other mouse will contract disease if the neurotoxin is present.[8]

Testing is commonly performed by enzyme-linked immunoabsorbent assay. The presence of tetanus toxoid antibodies helps support the examiner's clinical suspicion of exposure immediately or over a period of 1 to 3 months afterward. Any result of at least 0.16 IU/mL is indicative of an antibody response. Patients with titers of 0.01 IU/mL to as high as 1.0 IU/mL have been observed in mild cases of tetanus. An absence of serum antibody following vaccination or exposure may indicate an immune deficiency, including from congenital, acquired, or iatrogenic sources. (See also Chapter 17.)

MANAGEMENT

Toxin Neutralization

Proper management involving neutralizing tetanospasmin, removing the source of the toxin, and providing supportive care for muscle spasms, respiration, and autonomic instability greatly improves survival of individuals with either clinically suspected or actual disease.[47,48] Tetanospasmin is one of the most potent toxins known to man based purely on weight. The estimated lethal dose equals only 2.5 ng/kg.[7] Human tetanus immunoglobulin (TIG) is still an important part of treatment today for the prevention of tetanus. No consensus exists on the dose of intramuscular TIG; the dose recommended varies from 500 to 6000 IU. Typically, a dose of 3000 to 5000 IU for adults and children is injected around the site of injury if identified.[7] However, a retrospective study performed by Blake et al. found that a lower dose of 500 IU was as effective as larger dosages but also required fewer injections and less adverse reactions including reflex spasms.[49] The half-life of human TIG is 25 days, which adds greater benefit.[25] This immunoglobulin binds to any unbound neurotoxin before entering the nervous system or blood or lymphatic vessels and has no effect once the neurotoxin has gained entry into the neuron. In case TIG is not available, equine TIG or intravenous immunoglobulin may be used as a substitute to remove any unbound toxin.[7,25] Also, human TIG is considered safe during pregnancy.[25]

Intrathecal TIG had initially gained little support.[50–58] Theoretically, intrathecal TIG could potentially bind to tetanospamin during its transfer from the postsynaptic terminal to the presynaptic bouton. Unfortunately, either poorly designed and too few studies have shown little to either support or refute this treatment. One randomized, blinded study performed by Vikal et al. showed no benefit to intrathecal immunoglobulin.[59,60] Furthermore, a meta-analysis by Abrutyn and Berlin also concluded that there is insufficient evidence to support TIG.[56] Formal studies are needed at this time to settle this question and to better define the risk of this procedure.

Wound Care and Antibiotics

Debridement of the identified wound is extremely important to limit the severity of this disease. Debridement includes the removal of foreign material and necrotic tissue to prevent any suitable condition for this anaerobe to survive.[8,20] Antimicrobial treatment with metronidazole is used to decrease the number of spore-forming bacteria in the wound.[61] Penicillin has long been used as the antibiotic for *C. tetani*. However, reports indicate that penicillin theoretically could increase the risk of muscle spasm due to its GABA antagonist activity.[41,43,62] Therefore, metronidazole for a course of 10 days has replaced this as the antibiotic of choice due to its penetration through vascular compromised abscess and wounds.[3,39,61] Other antibiotics include clindamycin and erythromycin for its anaerobic coverage.[62]

Supportive Care

One of several major complications includes respiratory failure. Great care must be taken while attempting to intubate for fear of causing involuntary laryngospasm and potential hypoxic injury. Endotracheal intubation allows airway protection and adequate oxygen supplementation. However, a tracheostomy would be preferable for mechanical ventilation during the 3- to 4-week course of the disease to prevent continued laryngospasm leading to hypoxia or patient discomfort.

Muscle relaxants and sedatives are the mainstay of symptomatic treatment of tetanus. Benzodiazepines are the drug of choice, sometimes requiring extremely large dosages, typically infused intravenously. Case reports recommend as much as 3400 mg of diazepam and 1440 mg of midazolam over a 24-hour period.[63–74] In extreme cases, or if benzodiazepines fail, generalized tonic activity may respond to curare-like agents including vecuronium, with a long half-life and less cardiovascular side effects,[75–77] or succinylcholine if rapid initial muscle paralysis is needed. Other potential agents include dantrolene,[78,79] which acts at the sarcoplasmic reticulum; intrathecal baclofen,[80–82] a GABA agonist; or topically applied mephenesine,[83] a centrally acting muscle relaxant.

Treatment of autonomic dysfunction proves challenging as α- and β-blockade result in potential reflex worsening of symptoms such as tachycardia and hypertension, respectively, or an increased risk of sudden death.[25,27,84] Intravenous labetalol has been commonly recommended due to its combination of β- and α-antagonist activity. Other agents include intravenous magnesium,[85–88] which blunts catecholamine release; clonidine,[86,89] an α-antagonist; and nifedipine, a calcium channel blocker. Morphine and fentanyl also act centrally by decreasing the sympathetic outflow with subsequent control of hypertension and tachycardia,[27,30] along with additional sedation. However, fentanyl may be the better choice, as morphine suppresses myocardial function and can induce histamine release. Finally, epidural anesthesia can successfully control autonomic instability by blocking the preganglionic sympathetic neurons.[25,31,90]

Other supportive care[91,92] includes proper nutrition, with a recommended caloric intake of 3500 to 4000 calories with more than 150 g of protein via a percutaneously placed gastrostomy tube due to the increased metabolic demand from constant muscular contractions. Strict bed rest with a nonstimulating environment is also ideal for these patients. Minor stimuli including light or noise can induce muscle spasms.[25]

Complications

Complications are common during tetanus and must be managed emergently and preventively to decrease the morbidity or mortality rate. These include the following:

- Airway obstruction from laryngospasms
- Respiratory arrest secondary to respiratory muscle spasms
- Heart failure or arrhythmia
- Anoxic brain injury
- Spine and/or long-bone fractures
- Muscle or ligament tears

Prolonged hospitalization also leads to severe complications and must be met with protective caution:

- Aspiration pneumonia, a common late complication found in 50% to 70% of autopsy cases[7]
- Nosocomial infection secondary to indwelling catheters, decubitus ulcers, and hospital-acquired pneumonia
- Stress peptic ulcers
- Deep venous thrombosis or pulmonary embolus
- Generalized decompensation

PREVENTION

In 1889, Kitasato reported the possibility of neutralizing tetanus with antibodies. In 1897, Nocard demonstrated the protective effects by passively transferring antitoxin. U.S. soldiers and U.S. armed services of World War I in 1918 were passively immunized as a treatment and prophylaxis. Desombey developed the tetanus toxoid in 1924 for active immunization. This later became widely used by the armed services during World War II.[7]

The tetanus toxoid is the inactivated form of the virulent exotoxin produced by *C. tetani*. The exotoxin becomes inactivated when processed with formaldehyde. This toxoid is combined with another inactivated toxin produced by diphtheria to form the "DT" vaccine used today. It is believed that the killed component of *Bordetella pertussis* acts as an adjunct for conferring immunity to diphtheria, tetanus, and pertussis (DTaP) versus DT alone.[93–95] Currently, two toxoids are available: the absorbed (aluminum salt precipitated) and the fluid toxoid. The toxoid is standardized for potency in animal tests in the United States according to Food and Drug Administration regulations. Although the rate of seroconversion is roughly equal, the absorbed toxoid is preferred because the antitoxin response reaches higher titers and seems to be longer lasting than that following the fluid toxoid.[7]

Tetanus toxoid is available as a single antigen preparation.[96] It is also combined for pediatric (DT, DTaP) and adult (Td, TdaP) preparations. A single antigen preparation for either tetanus or diphtheria is not recommended because both vaccines require similar scheduling and booster requirements for proper immunization.[93] The pediatric formulation (DT) contains a similar amount of tetanus toxoid compared to adult formulation (Td) but also contain three to four times more diphtheria toxoid. In 2005, two tetanus toxoid, reduced diphtheria and acellular pertussis (TdaP), vaccine brands were licensed for use by the U.S. Food and Drug Administration. Boostrix is approved for ages 10 to 18 years; Adacel is approved for ages 11 to 64 years. A multiple antigenic preparation became available in recent years, called

Pediarix, combining vaccines for DTaP, inactivated poliovirus, and hepatitis B.[20]

Vaccination became routine in the United States beginning in 1947.[7,93,97] The schedule depends on the patients' age and previous history of a single vaccine dose. The schedule for the primary series for ages 6 weeks to 7 years recommends five doses of pediatric formulation (DT/DTaP) at 2, 4, 6, 15, to 18 months and 4 to 6 years. The first three doses should be separated by at least 4 weeks. The fourth dose should not proceed less than 6 months or should be administered before 12 months of age. The fifth dose may not be necessary if the fourth dose was administered after the child's fourth birthday. However, if the child is 12 months or older when the first dose was provided, then a total of three doses is currently recommended. The third dose, again, should not be administered less than 6 to 12 months following the second dose. Children younger than 7 years still need the pediatric formula, whereas patients 7 years or older require an adult formula even if the primary series has not been completed. If the primary series had not been completed before 7 years of age, the Advisory Committee on Immunization Practices recommends that at least one (but not all) adult TDaP be administered in place of Td. It is preferable to administer as the first dose. Interruption and/or delay of the recommended schedule should not reduce the response to the vaccine when finally completed. There is also no need to restart the series, regardless of the time elapsed between doses. The tetanus disease does not confer immunity due to the very small amount of toxin required to produce illness.[7]

Children 7 years and older, adolescents, and adults to 64 years of age require a three-dose series of vaccination.[98–102] The preferred schedule begins with TdaP followed by two doses of Td, each separated by at least 4 to 8 weeks. TdaP may be substituted for any one of the three-dose series.[103,104] At least two doses can provide some protection against disease, but one dose shows little protection.[20]

After completion of the primary series, the minimal protective level of 0.001 IU/mL nears 100% efficacy.[7] Since this level naturally decreases over time, a routine booster every 10 years is recommended to maintain adequate antitoxin titer levels. Some patients may receive protection for life, but most do not. A small percentage of the population requires a booster before the recommended 10 years as their antibody titers decrease below the minimum protective level. The first booster may be given at age 11 to 12 if more than 5 years have lapsed since the last dose. The Advisory Committee on Immunization Practices recommends that this dose be administered as TDaP.[7] If a dose is given for wound management, the next dose is not needed until the recommended 10-year booster. More frequent boosters have resulted in an increased incidence and severity of local adverse reactions.[7] During wound management, a booster of Td or TdaP is recommended for unclean or minor wounds if the last dose was administered more than 5 years prior.[93]

CONCLUSION

Tetanus is the only vaccine-preventable disease that is infectious but not contagious. Tetanus disease does not confer immunity due to the very small amount of toxin required to produce illness. Herd immunity also does not play a role in protecting individuals against tetanus. These endospores by *C. tetani* are found in the soil worldwide, which potentiates a global problem. Proper management includes neurotoxin neutralization, wound debridement, antibiotics, muscle relaxants, and intensive supportive care. Mortality remains high. Vaccination is effective in preventing disease transmission.

REFERENCES

1. Centers for Disease Control and Prevention. Case definitions for infectious conditions under public health surveillance. *MMWR Recomm Rep.* 1997;46;1–55.
2. National Institutes of Health. Tetanus. Available at: http://www.nlm.nih.gov/medlineplus/ency/article/000615.htm. Accessed May 23, 2008.
3. Sanford JP. Tetanus: forgotten but not gone. *N Engl J Med.* 1995;332(12):812–813.
4. Weber LE, Greenhouse AH. Update of tetanus. *Semin Neurol.* 1983;3:88–93.
5. Alfery DD, Rauscher LA. Tetanus: a review. *Crit Care Med.* 1979;7:176–180.
6. Smith JW, MacIver AG. Growth and toxin production of *Tetanus bacilli* in vivo. *J Med Microbiol.* 1974;7(4):497–504.
7. Centers for Disease Control and Prevention. Epidemiology and Prevention of Vaccine Preventable Diseases, 10th edition-revised 2008. http://www.cdc.gov/vaccines/pubs/pinkbook/downloads/table-of-contents-508.pdf. Accessed May 23, 2008.
8. Mims C, Playfair J, Roitt I, Wakelin D, Williams R. *Medical Microbiology.* 2nd ed. London: Mosby; 1998:310, 448, 520.
9. Armitage P, Clifford R. Prognosis in tetanus: use of data from therapeutic trial. *J Infect Dis.* 1978;138:1–8.
10. Centers for Disease Control and Prevention. Tetanus surveillance: United States, 1991–1994. *MMWR.* 1997;46:15–25.
11. Gergen PJ, McQuinllan GM, Kiely M, et al. A population-based serologic survey of immunity to tetanus in the United States. *N Engl J Med.* 1995;332:761–813.
12. Nagachinta T, Cortese MM, Roper MH, Pascual FB, Murphy T. Tetanus. In: *VPD Surveillance Manual.* 3rd ed. Available at: http://www.cdc.gov/vaccines/pubs/surv-manual/downloads/chpt13_tetanus.pdf. Accessed May 23, 2008.
13. Centers for Disease Control and Prevention. Tetanus among injecting-drug users: California, 1997. *MMWR.* 1998;47(8):149–151.
14. Beeching NJ, Crowcroft NS. Tetanus in injecting drug users. *BMJ.* 2005;330:208–209.

15. Levinson A, Marska RL, Shein MK. Tetanus in heroin addicts. *JAMA*. 1955;157:658–660.

16. Centers for Disease Control and Prevention. Progress toward the global elimination of neonatal tetanus, 1988–1993. *MMWR*. 1994;43:885–894.

17. Dietz V, Galazka A, Loon F, et al. Factors affecting the immunogenicity and potency of tetanus toxoid: implications for the elimination of neonatal and non-neonatal tetanus as public health problems. *Bull WHO*. 1997;75:81–93.

18. World Health Organization. Expanded Program on Immunization: Immunization Policy. Document WHO/EPI/GEN/95.03. Geneva: WHO; 1996.

19. World Health Organization. State of the World's Vaccines and Immunization. Publication WHO/GPV/96.04. Geneva: WHO; 1996.

20. Centers for Disease Control and Prevention. Prevention of Specific Infectious Diseases. Available at: http://wwwn.cdc.gov/travel/yellowBookCh4-Tetanus.aspx. Accessed May 23, 2008.

21. Searl SS. Minor trauma, disastrous results. *Surv Ophthalmol*. 1987;31:337.

22. Pascual FB, McGinley EL, Zanardi LR, Cortese MM, Murphy TV. Tetanus surveillance: United States, 1998–2000. *MMWR Surveill Summ*. 2003;52(SS-3):1–8.

23. Schwartz E, Rodeisperger E. Skin and soft tissue infections. In: Schillinger D, Harwood-Nuss A, eds. *Infections in Emergency Medicine*. vol. 2. New York: Churchill Livingstone; 1990:63–113.

24. Cook TM, Protheroe RT, Handel JM. Tetanus: a review of the literature. *Br J Anaesth*. 2001;87:477–487.

25. Hsu, SS, Groleau, G. Tetanus in the emergency department: A current review. *J Emerg Med*. 2001;20;4:357–365.

26. Trujillo MH, Castillo A, Espana J, et al. Impact of intensive care management of the prognosis of tetanus. *Chest*. 1987;92:63–65.

27. Wright DK, Lalloo UG, Nayiager S, et al. Autonomic nervous system dysfunction in severe tetanus: current perspectives. *Crit Care Med*. 1989;17:371–375.

28. Domenighetti GM, Savary G, Stricker H. Hyperadrenergic syndrome in severe tetanus: extreme rise in catecholamines responsive to labetolol. *BMJ*. 1984;288:1483–1484.

29. Kerr JH, Corbert JL, Pryst-Roberts C, et al. Involvement of the sympathetic nervous system in tetanus. *Lancet*. 1968;2:236–241.

30. Moughabghab AV, Prevost G, Scolovsky C. Fentanyl therapy controls autonomic hyperactivity in tetanus. *Br J Clin Pract*. 1996;50:477–478.

31. Southorn PA, Blaise GA. Treatment of tetanus-induced autonomic nervous system dysfunction with continuous epidural blockade. *Crit Care Med*. 1986;14:251–252.

32. Veronesi R, Focaccia R. The clinical picture. In: Veronesi R, ed. *Tetanus: Important New Concepts*. Amsterdam: Excerpta Medica; 1981:183–206.

33. Bleck TP. Tetanus: dealing with the continuing clinical challenge. *J Crit Illn*. 1987;41:41–52.

34. Crone NE, Reeder AT. Severe tetanus in immunized patients with high anti-tetanus titers. *Neurology*. 1992;42:761–764.

35. Hetzler DC, Hilsinger RL. The otolaryngologist and tetanus. *Otolaryngol Head Neck Surg*. 1986;95:511.

36. Phillips LA. A classification of tetanus. *Lancet*. 1967;1(7501):1216–1217.

37. Husada T, Rampengan TH, Harjanto IG, Arif IG, Munir M. Neonatal tetanus: evaluation of treatment and a proposal for classification of severity. *Paediatr Indones*. 1976;16:345–354.

38. Stoll BJ. Tetanus. *Pediatr Clin North Am*. 1979;26:415–431.

39. Bleck TP, Brauner JS. Tetanus. In: Scheld WM, Whitely RJ, Durack DT, eds. *Infections of the Central Nervous System*. 2nd ed. Philadelphia: Lippincott-Raven; 1997:629–653.

40. Edlich RF, Silloway KA, Haines PC, et al. Tetanus. *Compreh Ther*. 1986;12:12–21.

41. Weinstein L. Tetanus. *N Engl J Med*. 1973;289:1293–1296.

42. DeMoraes-Pinto MI, Oruambo RS, Igbagiri FP, et al. Neonatal tetanus despite immunization and protective antitoxin antibody [letter]. *J Inf Dis*. 1995;171:1076–1077.

43. Jagoda A, Riggio S, Burgieres T. Cephalic tetanus: a case report and review of the literature. *Am J Emerg Med*. 1988;6:128–130.

44. Passen EL, Anderson BR. Clinical tetanus despite a "protective" level of toxin-neutralizing antibody. *JAMA*. 1986;255:1171–1173.

45. Spenny JG, Lamb RN, Cobbs CG. Recurrent tetanus. *South Med J*. 1971;64:859.

46. Apte NM, Karnard DR. Short report: the spatula test—a simple bedside test to diagnose tetanus. *Am J Trop Med Hyg*. 1995;53:386–387.

47. Sun KO, Chan YW, Cheung RTF, So PC, Yu YL, Li PCK. Management of tetanus: a review of 18 cases. *J R Soc Med*. 1994;87:135–137.

48. Stubbe M, Mortelmans L, Desruelles D, et al. Improving tetanus prophylaxis in the emergency department: a prospective, double-blind cost-effectiveness study. *Emerg Med J*. 2007;24:648–653.

49. Blake PA, Feldman RA, Buchanan TM, et al. Serologic therapy of tetanus in the United States, 1965–1971. *JAMA*. 1976;235:42–44.

50. Miranda-Filho Dde B, Ximenes RA, Barone AA, Vaz VL, Vieira AG, Albuquerque VM. Randomised controlled trial of tetanus treatment with antitetanus immunoglobulin by the intrathecal or intramuscular route. *BMJ*. 2004;328(7440):615.

51. Sanders RKM, Martyn B, Joseph R, Peacock ML. Intrathecal antitetanus serum (horse) in the treatment of tetanus. *Lancet*. 1977;1:974–977.

52. Gupta PS, Goyal S, Kapoor R, Batra VK, Jain BK. Intrathecal human tetanus immunoglobulin in early tetanus. *Lancet*. 1980;2:439–440.

53. Keswani NK, Singh AK, Upadhyana KD. Intrathecal tetanus anti-toxin in moderate and severe tetanus. *J Indian Med Assoc*. 1980;75:67–69.

54. Ildirim I. Intrathecal treatment of tetanus with antitetanus serum and prednisolone mixture. International Conference on Tetanus, São Paulo. *PAHO Scient Public*. 1972;253:119–126.

55. Thomas PP, Crowell EB, Mathew M. Intrathecal anti-tetanus serum (ATS) and parenteral betamethasone in treatment of tetanus. *Trans R Soc Trop Med Hyg*. 1982;76:620–623.

56. Abrutyn E, Berlin JA. Intrathecal therapy in tetanus, a meta-analysis. *JAMA*. 1991;266:2262–2267.

57. Miranda-Filho D de B, et al. Randomised control trial of tetanus treatment with antitetanus immunoglobulin by the intrathecal or intramuscular route. *BMJ* 2004;28:615–617.

58. Agarwal M, Thomas K, Peter JV, Jeyaseelan L, Cherian AM. A randomised double-blind sham controlled study of intrathecal human anti-tetanus immunoglobulin in the management of tetanus. *Natl Med J India*. 1998;11:209–212.

59. Vakil BJ, Mehta AJ, Tulpule TH. Recurrent tetanus. *Postgrad Med J*. 1964;40:601–603.

60. Vakil BJ, Armitage P, Clifford RE, et al. Therapeutic trial of intracisternal human tetanus immunoglobulin in clinical tetanus. *Trans R Soc Trop Med Hyg*. 1979;73:579–583.

61. Ahmadsyah I, Salim A. Treatment of tetanus: an open study to compare the efficacy of procaine penicillin and metronidazole. *BMJ Clin Res Ed*. 1985;291(6496):648–650.

62. Centers for Disease Control and Prevention. Diphtheria, tetanus, and pertussis: recommendations for vaccine use and other preventive measures. Recommendations of the Immunization Practices Advisory Committee (ACIP). *MMWR*. 1991;40:1–28.

63. Weinberg WA. Control of the neuromuscular and convulsive manifestations of severe systemic tetanus: case report with a new drug Valium (diazepam). *Clin Pediatr.* 1964; 71:226–228.

64. Femi-Pearse D. Experience with diazepam in tetanus. *BMJ.* 1966;2:862–865.

65. Hendrickse RG, Sherman PM. Tetanus in childhood: report of a therapeutic trial of diazepam. *BMJ.* 1966;2:860–862.

66. Grewal RS, Sharma BK. Valium in the treatment of tetanus. *Indian Pract.* 1969;22:643.

67. Vassa NT, Doshi HV, Yajnik VH, Shah SS, Joshi KR, Patel SH. Comparative clinical trial of diazepam with other conventional drugs in tetanus. *Postgrad Med J.* 1974;50:755–758.

68. Joseph A, Pulimood BM. Use diazepam in tetanus: a comparative study. *Indian J Med Res.* 1978;68:489–491.

69. Gupta SM, Takkar VP, Verma AK. A retrospective study of tetanus neonatorum and comparative assessment of diazepam in its treatment. *Indian J Pediatr.* 1979;16:343–347.

70. Billimoria RB, Chhabra RB, Satoskar RB. Evaluation of diazepam alone and in combination with chlorpromazine or propranolol in the therapy of tetanus. *J Postgrad Med.* 1981;27:80–85.

71. Keswan NK, Singh AK, Singh DR. Continuous intravenous therapy in severe tetanus. *J Indian Med Assoc.* 1983;81:64–65.

72. Sugitha N, Suwendra P, Suraatmaja SA. High dosage diazepam as single antispasmodic agent in the treatment of neonatal tetanus. *Paediatr Indones.* 1983;23:163–172.

73. Okuonghae HO, Airede AI. Neonatal tetanus: incidence and improved outcome with diazepam. *Dev Med Child Neurol.* 1992;34:448–453.

74. Okoromah CAN, Lesi FEA. Diazepam for treating tetanus (Cochrane Review). In: *The Cochrane Library.* Issue 1. Chichester, UK: John Wiley & Sons; 2004.

75. Udwadia FE, Lall A, Udwadia ZF, Sekhar M, Vora A. Tetanus and its complications: intensive care and management experience in 150 Indian patients. *Epidemiol Infect.* 1987;99:675–684.

76. Edmondson RS, Flowers MW. Intensive care in tetanus: management, complications and mortality in 100 cases. *BMJ.* 1979;1:1401–1404.

77. Harding-Goldson HE, Hanna WJ. Tetanus: a recurring intensive care problem. *J Trop Med Hyg.* 1995;98:179–184.

78. Bernal OR, Bender MA, Lacy ME. Efficacy of dantrolene sodium in management of tetanus in children. *J R Soc Med.* 1986;79:277–281.

79. Farquhar I, Hutchinson A, Curran J. Dantrolene in severe tetanus. *Intensive Care Med.* 1988;14:249–256.

80. Brock H, Moosbauer W, Gabriel C. Treatment of severe tetanus by continuous intrathecal infusion of baclofen [letter]. *J Neurol Neurosurg Psych.* 1995;59:193–194.

81. Pellanda A, Caldiroli D, Vaghi GM, et al. Treatment of severe tetanus by intrathecal infusion of baclofen [letter]. *Intensive Care Med.* 1993;19:59.

82. Mulle H, Borner U, Zierski I, et al. Intrathecal baclofen in tetanus [letter]. *Lancet.* 1986;1:317–318.

83. Smitz S, Conen AI, Sadoz B. Mephenesine in tetanus [letter]. *J Am Geriatr Soc.* 1995;43:836–837.

84. King WW, Cave DR. Use of esmolol to control autonomic instability of tetanus. *Am J Med.* 1991;4:425–428.

85. Lipman J, James MFM, Erskine J, Plit ML, Eidelman J, Esser JD. Autonomic dysfunction in severe tetanus: magnesium sulfate as an adjunct to deep sedation. *Crit Care Med.* 1987;15:987–988.

86. Sutton DN, Tremlett MR, Woodcock TE, et al. Management of autonomic dysfunction in severe tetanus: the use of magnesium sulfate and clonidine. *Intensive Care Med.* 1990;16:75–80.

87. James MFM, Manson EDM. The use of magnesium sulfate infusion in the management of severe tetanus. *Intensive Care Med.* 1995;11:5–12.

88. Attygalle D, Rodrigo N. Magnesium sulphate for the control of spasms in severe tetanus: can we avoid sedation and artificial ventilation? *Anaesthesia.* 1997;52:956–962.

89. Brown JL, Sinding H, Mathias CJ. Autonomic disturbance in severe tetanus: failure of parental clonidine to control blood pressure. *J Infect.* 1994;29:67–71.

90. Quintero MLM, Ansuategui M, Mederos DL, et al. Epidural anesthesia for sympathetic overactivity in severe tetanus [letter]. *Crit Care Med.* 1987;15:801.

91. Chandy ST, Peter JV, John L, et al. Betamethasone in tetanus patients: an evaluation of its effect on the mortality and morbidity. *J Assoc Physicians India.* 1992;40:373–376.

92. Paydas S, Akogly TF, Akkiz H, et al. Mortality-lowering effect of systemic corticosteroid therapy in severe tetanus. *Clin Ther.* 1988;10:276–280.

93. Centers for Disease Control and Prevention. Diphtheria, tetanus, and pertussis: recommendations for vaccine use and other preventive measures. Recommendations of the Immunization Practices Advisory Committee (ACIP). *MMWR Recomm Rep.* 1991;40(RR-10):1–28.

94. Orenstein WA, Weisfeld JS, Halsey NA. Diphtheria and tetanus toxoids and pertussis vaccine, combined. In: *Recent Advances in Immunization: A Bibliographic Review.* Scientific Pub No 451. Washington, DC: Pan American Health Organisation, 1983:30–51.

95. Edsall G, Altman JS, Gaspar AJ. Combined tetanus–diphtheria immunization of adults: use of small doses of diphtheria toxoid. *Am J Public Health.* 1954;44:1537–1545.

96. Thwaites CL, Farrar JJ. Preventing and treating tetanus: the challenge continues in the face of neglect and lack of research. *BMJ.* 2003;326:117–118.

97. Allen T, Audet D. Tetanus prophylaxis: protocols require further change and simplification [editorial]. *J Emerg Med.* 1993;11:757–758.

98. Stegr MM, Maczek C, Berger P, et al. Vaccination against tetanus in elderly: do recommended strategies give sufficient protection? *Lancet.* 1996;348:762.

99. Karalliedde L, Cumberland N, Alexander C. Unfinished business: adult immunization against tetanus. *World Health Forum.* 1995;16:374–376.

100. Scher KS, Balders A, Wheeler WE, et al. Inadequate tetanus protection among the elderly. *South Med J.* 1985;78:153.

101. Alagappan K, Rennie W, Kwiatkowski T, et al. Seroprevalence of tetanus antibodies among adults older than 65 years. *Ann Emerg Med.* 1996;28:18–21.

102. Balestra DJ, Littenberg B. Should adult tetanus immunization be given as a single vaccination at age 65? A cost-effectiveness analysis. *J Gen Int Med.* 1993;8:405–412.

103. Centers for Disease Control and Prevention. Preventing tetanus, diphtheria, and pertussis among adolescents: use of tetanus toxoid, reduced diphtheria toxoid and acellular pertussis vaccines. Recommendations of the Advisory Committee on Immunization Practices (ACIP). *MMWR Recomm Rep.* 2006;55(RR-3):1–34.

104. Centers for Disease Control and Prevention. Preventing tetanus, diphtheria, and pertussis among adults: use of tetanus toxoid, reduced diphtheria toxoid and acellular pertussis vaccines. Recommendations of the Advisory Committee on Immunization Practices (ACIP). *MMWR Recomm Rep.* 2006;55 (RR-17);1–33.

CHAPTER 39

Diphtheria

Delia Bethell, Jeremy Farrar, and Tran Tinh Hien

INTRODUCTION

Diphtheria is an acute and potentially highly lethal infection of the upper respiratory tract caused by toxigenic strains of *Corynebacterium diphtheriae*. Today diphtheria is extremely rare in the developed world, yet it remains a threat in countries with poor vaccine coverage. During the 1990s, a huge epidemic occurred in parts of the former Soviet Union, with smaller outbreaks reported in several other countries. With increasing migration of people around the world, clinicians working in developed countries may encounter diphtheria in people moving from countries where the disease remains a problem.[1]

HISTORICAL PERSPECTIVE

Since ancient times, diphtheria has been one of the most feared childhood diseases, characterized by devastating outbreaks. Before the introduction of antitoxin in the 1890s, mortality in some epidemics exceeded 50%. During the World War II, more than 1 million cases were reported, including 50,000 deaths. In 2007, there were still an estimated 5000 deaths from diphtheria, of which 4000 were in children under 5 years of age.

PATHOGENESIS

C. diphtheriae are slender, pleomorphic, gram-positive rods or clubs. There are four biotypes: *gravis, intermedius, belfanti,* and *mitis,* any of which can cause diphtheria if the biotype is exotoxin producing. Early manifestations of diphtheria, including pseudomembrane formation, result from an inflammatory reaction to the multiplying toxigenic *C. diphtheriae*. The pseudomembrane is adherent to underlying tissues and bleeds when pulled away (Figure 39-1).[2]

    C. diphtheriae does not usually pass beyond the pseudomembrane site; it is the toxin that is responsible for the later complications of diphtheria. Diphtheria toxin is a 535-residue, 62-kDa exotoxin. It consists of two factors: spreading factor B attaches to the cell membrane, allowing lethal factor A to enter the cell. Factor A catalyses the nicotinamide adenine dinucleotide-positive-dependent adenosine diphosphate ribosylation of eukaryotic elongation

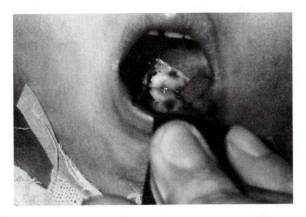

Figure 39-1. Membrane of diphtheria.

factor 2, preventing protein synthesis. The toxin inhibits protein synthesis in mammalian cells. It is an incredibly potent toxin; a single molecule of factor A is sufficient to kill a mammalian cell. Locally, the toxin causes tissue necrosis and, when absorbed into the bloodstream, systemic complications.

The toxin exerts its main clinically important changes on the myocardium, peripheral nerves, and kidneys. Common cardiac changes include fatty degeneration of cardiac muscle (myocarditis) and infiltration of the interstitium with leucocytes, which may involve the conduction fibers, leading to conduction problems. Although the heart can recover completely from these effects, severe fibrosis and scarring may lead to cardiac failure and death in late convalescence. Mural endocarditis may cause embolism, leading to cerebral infarction and hemiplegia. Endocarditis is extremely rare. Neuritic changes may be seen in the nerves to the heart during the late paralytic stage of the disease. Diphtheria toxin also causes demyelination and degeneration of both sensory and motor nerves by inhibition of myelin synthesis by the Schwann cells. It affects the nerves to the eye, palate, pharynx, larynx, heart, and limb muscles. It is unclear whether the toxin crosses the blood–brain barrier to cause central lesions.

EPIDEMIOLOGY

Man is the only known reservoir for *C. diphtheriae*. In most cases, transmission to susceptible individuals results in transient pharyngeal carriage rather than disease. Spread is via respiratory droplets or direct contact with skin lesions. Cutaneous diphtheria is more contagious than respiratory diphtheria, and chronic skin infections are the main reservoir in environments of poverty and overcrowding. Patients may become carriers of the infection and continue to harbor the organism for weeks or months.

Diphtheria remains a significant health problem in countries with poor vaccine coverage. In these settings, children generally meet *C. diphtheriae* early, sometimes becoming a carrier, and young children may suffer severe or fatal attacks of diphtheria. Recent serological studies in several countries indicate that up to 50% of adults are susceptible to diphtheria, with a significant trend of decreasing immunity with increasing age. This potential risk assumes particular significance given changing demographics and global migration patterns.[3]

Immunity to systemic disease depends on the presence of immunoglobulin G antitoxin antibodies. Type-specific protection against carriage and mild forms of local disease is induced by antibodies to the variable K-antigens of the bacterial cell wall. Infection does not always confer protective immunity, and outbreaks of mild disease have been reported even in highly vaccinated populations. In endemic countries, protective immunity is boosted naturally through circulating strains of toxigenic *C. diphtheriae*.

Diphtheria is a devastating but preventable disease. A large gap in the immunity of adults poses an outbreak risk but is probably not sufficient to sustain a large diphtheria epidemic. However, an immunity gap in adults coupled with the presence of large numbers of susceptible children and adolescents creates the potential for an extensive epidemic. In countries of the former Soviet Union, economic hardship, large urban migration, and low vaccination coverage probably all contributed to the outbreak of the 1990s.[4,5]

CLINICAL FEATURES

Early Features

Diphtheria has an incubation period of 2 to 5 days and presents acutely in a variety of forms, classified according to the location of the pseudomembrane.

Anterior Nasal

Anterior nasal diphtheria is usually unilateral and relatively mild unless it coexists with other forms. The nasal discharge is initially watery and then purulent and blood stained. The nostril may be sore or crusted, and a thin pseudomembrane can sometimes be seen within the nostril itself.

Tonsillar (Faucial)

Tonsillar is the commonest form of diphtheria. Malaise, sore throat, and moderate fever develop gradually. At the onset of symptoms, only a small, yellow–gray spot of pseudomembrane may be present on one or both tonsils, easily mistaken for other types of tonsillitis. The surrounding areas are dull and inflamed. Over the next few days, the pseudomembrane enlarges and may extend to cover the uvula, soft palate, oropharynx, nasopharynx, or larynx. There is tender cervical lymphadenopathy, nausea, vomiting, and painful dysphagia.

Tracheolaryngeal

Some 85% of tracheolaryngeal presentations are secondary to faucial diphtheria, but occasionally there may be no pharyngeal pseudomembrane. Initial symptoms include fever, hoarseness, and a nonproductive cough. Over the next day or two, as the pseudomembrane and associated edema spread, the patient can become increasingly dyspneic, with severe chest recession, cyanosis, and eventual asphyxiation unless the obstruction is relieved. Tracheostomy brings instant relief if the obstruction is confined to the larynx and upper trachea. In a minority of cases, the pseudomembrane also involves the bronchi and bronchioles and tracheostomy has little effect.

Malignant

The malignant onset is rapid, with high fever, tachycardia, hypotension, and cyanosis. Pseudomembrane spreads from the tonsils to cover much of the nasopharynx. It has a thick edge, and as this advances the earlier parts become necrotic and foul smelling. There is gross cervical lymphadenopathy. Individual lymph nodes are difficult to feel because of surrounding edema; this is the characteristic "bull neck" of malignant diphtheria. The patient may bleed from the mouth, nose, or skin. Cardiac involvement with heart block occurs within a few days. Acute renal failure may ensue. Survival is unlikely.

Cutaneous

In contrast to respiratory forms, cutaneous diphtheria is usually chronic but mild. The morphological features of individual lesions can be extremely variable, as *C. diphtheriae* can colonize any preexisting skin lesion (such as impetigo, scabies, surgical wounds, or insect bites) without altering their picture. However, the ulcerative form is the most frequent and typical. Initially vesicular or pustular, filled with straw-colored fluid, it soon breaks down to leave a punched-out ulcer several millimeters to a few centimeters across. Common sites are the lower legs, feet, and hands. During the first 1 to 2 weeks, it is painful and may be covered with a dark pseudomembrane. After this separates, a hemorrhagic base is seen, sometimes with a serous or serosanguineous exudate. The surrounding tissue is edematous and pink or purple. Spontaneous healing to leave a depressed scar usually takes 2 to 3 months, sometimes much longer. Systemic complications, such as myocarditis, are rare. Occasionally, the affected limb becomes paralyzed.[6]

Other Sites

A mild conjunctivitis may accompany faucial diphtheria. Occasionally, a pseudomembrane forms in the lower conjunctiva and spreads over the cornea, causing considerable damage. Dysphagia may indicate that pseudomembrane has spread from the tonsils to the esophagus. Other parts of the gastrointestinal tract are not usually affected, but melena with colicky abdominal pain is described. Diphtheria may spread by fingers from the throat to vulva or penis, causing localized sores. *C. diphtheriae* occasionally invades the vagina and cervix, allowing the absorption of toxin. Endocarditis is rare.

Later Complications

Patients surviving acute diphtheria may develop one or more later complications. These result from delayed effects of the toxin following hematogenous spread. The risk and severity of complications correlates directly with the extent of the pseudomembrane and the delay in administration of antitoxin.

Neurological

Neurological complications usually appear 4 to 8 weeks after the onset of the disease, when the patient appears to be recovering, and occur in up to 20% of infected patients. The generalized neuropathy produces a rapidly ascending hypotonic paralysis and should be considered in the differential diagnosis of a patient presenting with a Guillain-Barré–like syndrome. A history of travel to a potentially endemic region is important. Palatal paralysis is relatively common and may be seen from the third week onward. The patient develops a nasal voice and regurgitates fluids through the nose. This usually resolves within a week or so. A little later, there may be blurred vision from paralysis of accommodation, and diphtheria can present with papillary dilatation due to damage to the ciliary nerves or a transient squint from external rectus paralysis. About the sixth or seventh week, more sinister paralyses may develop involving muscles to the pharynx, larynx, chest, and limbs. The nerves to the heart may be affected, causing tachycardia and dysrhythmias. In severe cases, patients may become profoundly hypotonic over a few hours and can die from respiratory arrest. However, if intensive-care facilities and skilled staff are available, complete recovery over the following weeks or months should ensue.

Cardiovascular

Approximately 10% of patients with diphtheria develop myocarditis, usually those with clinically severe infection. The frequency of cardiac involvement is much greater when the antitoxin administration is delayed for more than 48 hours after the onset of symptoms.

Cardiac toxicity usually appears after the first week of illness. Patients complain of upper abdominal pain and may vomit. They become lethargic and tired, but they usually remain fully conscious throughout. Examination reveals a rapid, thready pulse with hypotension. At this stage, profound shock may lead to death. In less severe cases, congestive cardiac failure may develop, with a displaced apex beat, gallop rhythm, and murmurs audible over all areas of the heart. Profound bradycardia may result from heart block.[7,8]

Electrocardiography is the best way to demonstrate cardiac involvement. The most common abnormalities are T wave inversion in one or more chest leads and prolonged QTc intervals. There may be right or left axis deviation, bundle-branch block, or heart block. Occasionally, atrial fibrillation or tachyarrhythmias are seen, and 24-hour electrocardiogram monitoring is helpful. Although most patients surviving myocarditis recover completely, the presence of left bundle-branch block at discharge is associated with poor long-term outcome.[9,10]

DIFFERENTIAL DIAGNOSIS

Clinical diagnosis is difficult where diphtheria is rare. The differential diagnosis includes infectious mononucleosis, streptococcal or viral tonsillitis, peritonsillar abscess, oral thrush, and leukemia and other blood dyscrasias. The bull neck of malignant diphtheria may be mistaken for mumps. In adults, secondary syphilis can sometimes cause a glairy (resembling egg white) exudate on the tonsils and may be accompanied by rash and laryngitis.

Clinical Investigation

Bacterial culture of *C. diphtheriae* is the mainstay of investigation. Material for culture should be obtained, preferably, from the edges of the mucosal lesions and inoculated onto appropriate selective media. The quality of the specimens from the swabs of the throat lesions is crucial to establishing a diagnosis. Suspected colonies may be tested for toxin production by gel precipitation (Elek test), guinea-pig inoculation, or enzyme immunoassay. Direct smears of infected areas of the throat are often used for diagnostic purposes but are only of value in experienced hands. More reliably, the diphtheria toxin gene may be detected directly in clinical specimens using polymerase chain reaction techniques.

Criteria for Diagnosis

In areas where diphtheria is relatively common and during outbreaks, the disease should be suspected in any patient with exudate in the throat. Treatment must not be delayed until the disease is confirmed, except in cases of suspected cutaneous diphtheria without associated respiratory symptoms.

TREATMENT

Antitoxin is the mainstay of treatment, but to be maximally effective it must be given before the toxin has reached tissues such as the heart and kidneys, preferably within 48 hours of the onset of symptoms. This means it must be given empirically before bacteriological confirmation. Dosage depends on the site of primary infection, the extent of pseudomembrane, and the delay between onset of symptoms and antitoxin administration. Between 20,000 and 40,000 units are given for faucial diphtheria of less than 48-hour duration or for cutaneous infection, 40,000 to 80,000 units for faucial in excess of 48 hours or for laryngeal infection, and 80,000 to 100,000 units for malignant diphtheria. For doses higher than 40,000 units, a portion is given intramuscularly followed by the bulk of the dose intravenously after an interval of 30 minutes to 2 hours. Anaphylaxis can occur following antitoxin administration, and adrenaline (epinephrine) should always be available.

Antibiotics are given to eradicate the organism and prevent further toxin production. Benzylpenicillin at 150,000 to 250,000 U/kg/day (90 to 150 mg/kg/day) is given intravenously in four to six divided doses in children age 1 month to 12 years. In adults, the dose is 12 million to 20 million U/day (7.2 to 12 g/day) in four to six divided doses. Oral penicillin V is substituted when the patient is able to swallow. Erythromycin may be used for penicillin-sensitive individuals, but it may not be as effective in eradicating carriage. Antibiotic therapy should continue for 10 to 14 days.

Facilities for urgent tracheostomy should always be available in case of respiratory obstruction. Indications include increasingly labored breathing and agitation. This procedure is life saving in many cases. Most tracheostomies can be closed after just a few days. Steroids are of no benefit in preventing myocarditis or neuritis.

Patients with signs or symptoms of cardiac involvement need to be managed in intensive-care units. Oxygen should be given. Temporary cardiac pacing is useful in patients with heart block but is of doubtful value in cases of malignant diphtheria. An isoprenaline infusion may buy valuable time while the patient is transferred to a center with facilities for pacing. Digoxin has been used in congestive cardiac failure.

No specific treatment exists for neuritis. The severest cases need mechanical ventilation and intragastric or intravenous feeding. With skilled nursing care, full recovery can be expected. Patients recovering from clinical disease should complete active immunization during convalescence.

PREVENTION

Diphtheria toxoid is highly effective in conferring protection against clinical disease. Circulating antitoxin levels of less than 0.01 IU/mL are considered nonprotective, while levels of 0.01 IU/mL may confer some protection. Levels of 0.1 IU/mL or more are considered fully protective, and levels above 1.0 IU/mL are associated with long-term protective immunity. The potency of diphtheria vaccine is reduced in children age 7 years and older so that reactogenicity is minimized.

Where diphtheria is endemic, the primary course alone should be sufficient to prevent an epidemic of diphtheria, as natural mechanisms such as frequent skin infections caused by *C. diphtheriae* probably contribute to maintaining immunity. One or two DT or DTP booster doses may need to be added to the routine schedule in areas at increased risk of diphtheria. Adults in developing countries do not require routine immunization.

Aggressive action is needed in the event of a diphtheria outbreak. Groups at risk should be immunized, cases should be promptly diagnosed and managed, and close contacts should be identified so that the spread of infection can be halted. A single dose of DTP should be used for children under 3 years of age, with a single dose of DT used for children over 3 years and adults. Additional doses of vaccine are needed in nonimmunized individuals.

REFERENCES

1. World Health Organization. Diphtheria. Available at: http://www.who.int/topics/diphtheria/en. Accessed February 5, 2009.
2. Crowcroft NS, White JM, Efstratiou A, George R. Screening and toxigenic corynebacteria spread. *Emerg Infect Dis.* 2006;12(3):520–521.
3. Wren MW, Shetty N. Infections with *Corynebacterium diphtheriae*: six years' experience at an inner London teaching hospital. *Br J Biomed Sci.* 2005;62(1):1–4.
4. Rakhmanova G, Lumio G, Groundstroem KW, et al. Diphtheria outbreak in St. Petersburg: clinical characteristics of 1,860 adult patients. *Scand J Infect Dis.* 1996;28:37–40.
5. Mikhailovich VM, Melnikov VG, Mazurova IK, et al. Application of PCR for detection of toxigenic *Corynebacterium diphtheriae* strains isolated during the Russian diphtheria epidemic, 1990 through 1994. *J Clin Microbiol.* 1995;33(11):3061–3063.
6. Hofler W. Cutaneous diphtheria. *Int J Dermatol.* 1991;30:845–847.
7. Celik T, Selimov N, Vekilova A, et al. Prognostic significance of electrocardiographic abnormalities in diphtheritic myocarditis after hospital discharge: a long-term follow-up study. *Ann Noninvasive Electrocardiol.* 2006;11(1):28–33.
8. Bethell DB, Dung MN, Loan HT, et al. Prognostic value of electrocardiographic monitoring in severe diphtheria. *Clin Infect Dis.* 1995;20:1259–1265.
9. Dung NM, Kneen R, Kiem N, et al. Treatment of severe diphtheritic myocarditis by temporary insertion of a cardiac pacemaker. *Clin Infect Dis.* 2002;35(11):1425–1429.
10. Jayashree M, Shruthi N, Singi S. Predictors of outcome in patients with diphtheria receiving intensive care. *Indian J Pediatr.* 2006;43:155–160.

CHAPTER 40 ••••

Seafood Neurotoxins I: Shellfish Poisoning and the Nervous System

Pratap Chand

INTRODUCTION

Human shellfish poisoning can occur after eating clams, mussels, oysters, scallops, cockles, starfish, and crustaceans contaminated by toxins.[1] Herbivorous dinoflagellates are the primary transvectors that accumulate the toxins via feeding in their digestive organs and soft tissues, apparently without harm to themselves. Shellfish consume dinoflagellate organisms while feeding, and the poison is stored in their bodies.[2] This toxin has been found in these seafoods every month of the year, and butter clams have been known to store the toxin for up to 2 years. Shellfish poisoning is more common during red tides, when sea waters turn a reddish color because of the presence of large numbers of dinoflagellates (Figure 40-1; see color plate). These dinoflagellates produce at least 12 toxins, which are tetrahydropurines and are heat and acid stable. Saxitoxin was the first characterized and the best understood, and it produces paralysis.[3] Humans, birds, and fish can all be affected by paralytic shellfish poisoning toxins.[4] Shellfish contaminated by toxins do not have an abnormal taste, smell, or color; the toxins are water soluble and are not destroyed by acid, heating, or cooking.[5] Shellfish poisoning can produce four clinical syndromes—paralytic shellfish poisoning, neurotoxic shellfish poisoning, diarrheal shellfish poisoning, and amnesic shellfish poisoning (Table 1).

SHELLFISH TOXINS

The main toxins responsible for each of the shellfish syndromes are as follows[5]:

Paralytic shellfish poisoning—saxitoxin
Neurotoxic shellfish poisoning—brevetoxin
Diarrheal shellfish poisoning—okadaic acid
Amnesic shellfish poisoning—domoic acid

Paralytic Shellfish Poisoning

Gonyaulacoid dinoflagellates, the source of paralytic shellfish poisoning (PSP) marine toxins, develop algal blooms throughout the world (Figure 40-2; see color plate) for unknown reasons, although various factors have been studied, including change in weather, upwellings, temperature, turbulence, salinity, and transparency.[6] PSP is a significant problem on both the East and the West coasts of the United States[5] and is caused by several closely related species in the genus *Alexandrium* (Figure 40-3). On the East Coast, PSP is a serious and recurrent problem from Maine to Massachusetts and along the coasts of Connecticut, Long Island (New York), and New Jersey. On the West Coast, PSP is a recurrent annual problem along the coasts of northern California, Oregon,

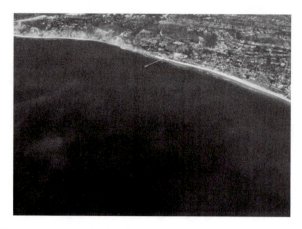

Figure 40-1. A red tide off the coast of La Jolla, California (see color plate). (Courtesy of Wikipedia.)

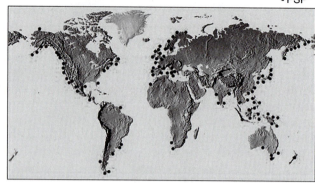

Figure 40-2. Worldwide prevalence of paralytic shellfish poisoning in 2006 (see color plate). (Courtesy of U.S. National Office for Harmful Algal Blooms/Woods Hole Oceanographic Institution.)

Washington, and Alaska. Florida red tides affect humans, wildlife, fishery resources, and the regional tourist-related economy. One of the highest concentrations of PSP in the world is reported to be in the shellfish in southeast Alaska.[7]

Toxins

There are at least 21 molecular forms of PSP-associated toxins. Collectively, these PSP toxins are termed *saxitoxins,* deriving the name from the butter clam, *Saxidomus giganteus,* from which the toxin was originally extracted and identified. In mice, the saxitoxin LD50 parentally is 3 to 10 μg/kg body weight and orally is 263 μg/kg body weight.[8] Humans are the most sensitive to saxitoxin; the

oral dose in humans for death is 1 to 4 mg (5000 to 20,000 mouse units) depending upon the general and physical condition of the patient. It is rapidly absorbed through the gastrointestinal tract and excreted in the urine.

The saxitoxins act by blocking sodium (Na+) ion movement through voltage-dependent Na+ channels in nerve and muscle cell membranes and have recently been found to also bind to calcium and potassium channels and neuronal nitric oxide synthase.[9] Conduction block occurs principally in motor neurons and muscle. Saxitoxin inhibits the temporary permeability of Na+ ions by binding tightly to a receptor site on the outside surface of the membrane close to the external orifice of the Na+ channel. The resulting widespread blockade

Table 1: Syndromes of Shellfish Poisoning				
Disease	**Toxin**	**Dinoflagellate**	**Symptoms or Signs**	**Treatment**
Paralytic shellfish poisoning	Saxitoxin	Alexandrium	Headache, nausea, dizziness, pain, vomiting, anuria, paralysis, respiratory failure	Supportive Symptomatic Ventilation
Neurotoxic shellfish paralysis	Brevetoxin	Gymnodinium	Vomiting, rectal burning, myalgia, paresthesias, ataxia reversal of hot–cold sensation, vertigo, tremor, dysphagia, weakness, mydriasis, decreased reflexes	Supportive Symptomatic
Diarrheal shellfish poisoning	Okadaic acid	Dinophysis	Diarrhea, nausea, vomiting	Supportive Symptomatic
Amnesic shellfish poisoning	Domoic acid	Pseudonitzschia	Vomiting, abdominal cramps, diarrhea severe headache, loss of short-term memory, seizures, myoclonus, coma, hemiparesis, ophthalmoplegia, motor and sensory motor neuronopathy	Supportive Symptomatic

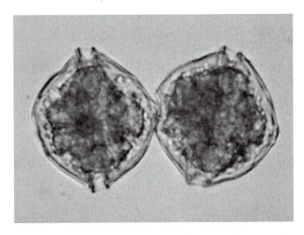

Figure 40-3. *Alexandrium fundyense.* (Courtesy of National Science Foundation.)

prevents impulse generation in peripheral nerves and skeletal muscles. Saxitoxin has a direct effect on skeletal muscle by blocking the muscle action potential without depolarizing cells; it abolishes peripheral nerve conduction but with no curare-like action at the neuromuscular junction.[9]

Clinical Features

PSP develops usually within minutes after eating a contaminated shellfish, most commonly a mussel, clam, or oyster. From 5 to 30 minutes after consumption, there is slight perioral tingling progressing to numbness, which spreads to face and neck in moderate cases. Muscle weakness causing difficulty swallowing or speaking may occur. Other symptoms include sense of throat constriction, headache, dizziness, nausea, vomiting, rapid pain, and anuria.[5] There is no loss of consciousness, and the reflexes are unaltered, except for perhaps pupillary size; sight may be temporarily lost. In severe cases within 2 to 12 hours there is complete paralysis, and death may occur from respiratory failure if the victims are not provided ventilatory support.[7] The symptoms may last for 6 to 12 hours, after which most victims start to recover gradually but may continue to feel weak for a week or more.[10] Some people have died after eating just one clam or mussel, others after eating many—each with a small amount of poison. The Guatemalan 1987 outbreak on the Pacific coast had a case fatality rate of 14%, which was even higher in young children (50%). It is possible that children may be more sensitive to PSP toxins than adults.[11] In addition, the access to emergency medical services in acute cases is crucial to the prognosis.

Nerve conduction studies in eight patients with PSP showed normal motor and sensory conduction velocities and amplitudes. The proximal conduction times, as assessed by F waves, showed delayed conduction and decreased frequency, which returned to normal in a few weeks.[12] The somatosensory evoked potentials confirmed normal peripheral and central sensory conduction. In another study, serial electrophysiological observations in a patient with acute bulbar and respiratory paralysis following ingestion of saxitoxin-contaminated clams showed prolonged distal motor and sensory latencies, slowed nerve conduction velocities, and moderately diminished amplitudes at the outset. All values returned to normal over 5 days.[13] These findings, the result of incomplete Na+ channel blockade, distinguish PSP from most other acute paralytic illnesses.

Diagnosis

The clinical scenario is the primary method of diagnosis initially. Recent shellfish ingestion, often but not always associated with a known red tide, and acute gastrointestinal illness with neurological symptoms forms the classic presentation. The differential diagnoses of an acute gastrointestinal illness with recent shellfish ingestion would be bacterial or viral gastroenteritis or recent organophosphate pesticide poisoning.

It is important to obtain samples of contaminated tissues and their source. Each PSP epidemic is associated with different mixtures of the PSP toxins; this complicates the laboratory analysis of contaminated tissues. The mouse bioassay (time to death) of food extract was the conventional diagnostic method, but it cannot distinguish between tetrodotoxin and other PSP toxins. A mouse unit is defined as the minimum amount needed to cause the death of an 18- to 22-g white mouse in 15 minutes.[14] Alternative methods include radioimmunoassay and indirect enzyme-linked immunoabsorbent assay (ELISA).[15] High-performance liquid chromatography (HPLC) analysis methods for all PSP toxins have been developed with good correlation with mouse bioassay in terms of quantification.[16] Human serum assays using HPLC have detected shellfish toxin but are not yet commercially available to clinicians.[17] Research in this area is ongoing, and reliable serum assays for several of these specific toxins would be useful for diagnosis.

Treatment

In general, care is primarily symptomatic and supportive. Supportive measures are the basis of treatment for PSP, especially maintenance of the airway and ventilatory support with artificial ventilation in severe cases. Without supportive treatment, up to 75% of severely affected people die within 12 hours.[18] It is important not to underestimate the seriousness of PSP. Once the symptoms begin to appear, the victim must be transported immediately to a medical care facility. Application of life support services at the medical care facility may be necessary to sustain the life of the victim. Nasogastric or orogastric lavage may be performed if the patient presents within

1 hour of ingestion, but this is often unnecessary. If gastric lavage is performed, the use of isotonic Na+ bicarbonate solution for lavage has been suggested because many shellfish toxins have reduced potency in an alkaline environment. Care must be taken concerning aspiration with the neurologically compromised patient. Gastrointestinal decontamination with activated charcoal is recommended for patients who present within 4 hours of ingestion. The greatest danger is respiratory paralysis. Close monitoring for at least 24 hours and aggressive airway management at any sign of respiratory compromise should prevent severe morbidity and mortality. Reduction of symptoms normally occurs within 9 hours, and complete recovery usually occurs within 24 hours. Lactic acidosis can be seen in experimental animals and possibly humans and can be treated by assisted ventilation, fluid therapy, and periodic monitoring of the blood pH. It is possible that the fluid therapy also assists in the renal excretion of toxin.[18] The prognosis for PSP is quite good, especially if the patient has passed the initial 12 hours of illness without needing breathing support. Most deaths occur during this period if breathing help is not available.

Neurotoxic Shellfish Poisoning

With the ingestion of contaminated shellfish, neurotoxic shellfish poisoning (NSP) presents as a milder syndrome of gastroenteritis with neurological symptoms compared with PSP. The classic causative organism, *Gymnodinium breve*, is a dinoflagellate restricted to the Gulf of Mexico and the Caribbean, although similar species occur throughout the world.[19] As *G. breve* cells die and break up, they release powerful neurotoxins, known collectively as *brevetoxins*.[5] NSP is found especially during red tides in the late summer and autumn months almost every year off the west coast of Florida with massive fish and bird kills. Walker was the first to record NSP in 1880 on the west coast of Florida. The associated red tides are often characterized by patches of discolored water, dead or dying fish, and respiratory irritants in the air. Since then, NSP has been reported from the Gulf of Mexico, the east coast of Florida, and the North Carolina coast.[20]

Toxin

Brevetoxins, the cause of NSP, are made by the dinoflagellate *Ptychodiscus brevis* and consist of two types of lipid-soluble toxins: hemolytic and neurotoxins.[21] The major brevetoxin produced is PbTx-2, followed by lesser amounts of PbTx-1 and PbTx-3. Fish, birds, and mammals are all susceptible to the brevetoxins. The mouse LD50 is 0.20 mg/kg body weight (range 0.15 to 0.27) intraperitoneally. In human cases of NSP, the brevetoxin concentrations present in contaminated clams have been reported to be 30 to 18 µg (range 78 to 120 µg/mg).

Brevetoxins are polycyclic ethers that bind to and stimulate Na+ flux through voltage-gated Na+ channels in nerve and muscle. These toxins are depolarizing substances that open voltage-gated Na+ ion channels in cell walls, leading to uncontrolled Na+ influx into the cell.[4] This alters the membrane properties of excitable cell types in ways that enhance the inward flow of Na+ ions into the cell; this current can be blocked by external application of tetrodotoxin.[18] Like the other marine toxins, the brevetoxins are tasteless, odorless, and heat and acid stable. These toxins cannot be easily detected nor removed by food preparation procedures.[5] Brevetoxin can be assayed by using a mouse bioassay, ELISA, and antibody radioimmunoassay.

Clinical Features

The illness encountered with NSP is milder than that with PSP. Symptom onset ranges from 15 minutes to 18 hours after ingestion, and the duration of toxicity ranges from 1 to 72 hours (usually <24 h) after ingestion.[22] Presenting symptoms include gastroenteritis; rectal burning; paresthesias of the face, trunk, and limbs; myalgias; ataxia; and reversal of hot–cold sensations. Other less common features include vertigo, tremor, dysphagia, motor weakness, bradycardia, decreased reflexes, and mydriasis.[23] Symptoms may last from several hours to a few days.

Treatment

Treatment of NSP is mostly symptomatic, with attention to fluid and electrolyte imbalance; the neurological symptoms are self-limiting, and patients recover spontaneously; respiratory compromise is not encountered as in PSP.[5]

Diarrheal Shellfish Poisoning

Diarrheal shellfish poisoning (DSP) is a gastrointestinal illness without neurological manifestations reported worldwide caused by the consumption of contaminated shellfish.[24] The causative organisms are the marine dinoflagellates *Dinophysis* and *Procentrum*, although there is an uneven distribution among species and location of toxin production. These dinoflagellates are widely distributed but do not always form red tides.

Toxin

The associated toxins produced by the *Dinophysis* dinoflagellates are okadaic acid and its derivatives. At least nine toxins are produced by these dinoflagellates that bind to intestinal epithelial cells and increase their permeability; these have collectively been called *pectenotoxins*.[25] *D. fortii* at levels of 200 cell/L in mussels and scallops becomes toxic for humans; the minimal amount of DSP toxins required to induce disease in humans was 12 mouse units. Pectenotoxin 1 causes liver damage in mice under similar circumstances. Okadaic acid is lipophilic. It is a potent inhibitor of protein phosphorylase phosphatase 1 and 2A in the cytosol of the mammalian cells that dephosphorylate serine and threonine.[26] It probably causes diarrhea by stimulating the phosphorylation that controls Na+ secretion by intestinal cells. Okadaic acid also acts through the variations of cellular concentration of the calcium ion second messenger. It strongly increases the L-type inward calcium current in isolated guinea pig cardiac myocytes.

Clinical Features

DSP is a self-limited diarrheal disease without known chronic sequelae. Gastroenteritis develops shortly after ingestion and generally lasts 1 to 2 days. There is no evidence of neurotoxicity, and no fatal cases have ever been reported. Diarrhea was the most commonly reported symptom, closely followed by nausea and vomiting, with onset 30 minutes to 12 hours from ingestion.[27] Complete clinical recovery is seen even in severe cases within 3 days.

Diagnosis

A mouse bioassay using an intraperitoneal injection of toxin extracts with a 24-hour waiting period is used in Japan and shellfish with DSP toxin levels greater than 50 mouse units per kilogram are banned; similar surveillance systems have been established in the European countries.[24] An HPLC method for detection of DSP toxins is available and is used in Sweden for monitoring purposes.[28]

Treatment

Treatment is symptomatic and supportive with regards to short-term diarrhea and accompanying fluid and electrolyte losses. In general, hospitalization is not necessary; fluid and electrolytes can usually be replaced orally. Other diarrheal illnesses associated with shellfish consumption, such as bacterial or viral contamination, should be ruled out.[24,27] Okadaic acid undergoes enterohepatic recycling that could be interrupted by charcoal administration.

Amnesic Shellfish Poisoning

Amnesic shellfish poisoning (ASP) is caused by the consumption of shellfish contaminated with the neurotoxin domoic acid produced by diatoms in the genus *Pseudonitzschia* (see Figure 40-3). It may cause permanent short-term memory loss in victims, hence the name. It was first reported from Canada in 1987 and involved 150 reported cases, 19 hospitalizations, and four deaths after consumption of contaminated mussels. Later it was identified as a continuing problem in the Washington state and Oregon. After an initial gastroenteritis with neurological symptoms, some people with ASP develop apparent permanent neurological deficits.[5]

Domoic acid production has been confirmed for three species of *Pseudonitzschia* on the West Coast of the United States—*P. australis, P. multiseries,* and *P. pungens.* Domoic acid poisoning first became a noticeable problem in 1991, when pelicans and cormorants in Monterey Bay (California) died or suffered from unusual neurological symptoms similar to ASP. That same year, domoic acid was identified in razor clams and Dungeness crabs on the Oregon and Washington coasts. Since 1991, *Pseudonitzschia* species and domoic acid have recurred in Monterey Bay, but with relatively low cell numbers and concentrations. Toxic *Pseudonitzschia* species are present in the Northeast and Gulf of Mexico, and low levels of domoic acid have been detected in shellfish on the East Coast, but not at levels that necessitate quarantine.

Toxin

Domoic acid is structurally similar to the excitatory neurotransmitter glutamate.[29] Domoic acid binds to and stimulates the kainic acid glutamate receptor in the central nervous system, which allows Na+ influx and a small amount of potassium efflux with resulting neuronal depolarization. Lesions in the human brain, with necrosis of the glutamate-rich hippocampus and amygdala in autopsied cases, have been reported in the ASP cases and are similar to those seen in rats after kainic acid intravenous administration.[30] When rats are exposed experimentally to domoic acid and its analogues, they experience limbic seizures, memory and gait abnormalities, and degeneration of the hippocampus. In animals, domoic acid is 3 times more potent than kainic acid and 30 to 100 times more potent than glutamic acid. Novelli et al. demonstrated that domoic acid from mussels is more neurotoxic for cultured human neurons than is purified domoic acid.[31] This increase is believed to be due to domoic acid potentiation, even in subtoxic amounts, of the excitotoxic effect of glutamic and aspartic acids. Glutamic and aspartic acids are present in high concentrations in mussel tissue. This neurotoxic synergism may occur through a reduction in the voltage-dependent Mg2+ block at the *N*-methyl-d-aspartate (NMDA) receptor–associated channel, following activation of non-NMDA receptors by domoic acid. In humans, domoic acid appears to cause a nonprogressive acute neuronopathy involving anterior horn cells or a diffuse axonopathy predominantly affecting motor axons. The acute neuronal hyperexcitation syndrome presumably results from the stimulus of central and possibly peripheral neurons, followed by chronic loss of function in neural systems susceptible to excitotoxic degeneration (hippocampus and anterior horn cells of spinal cord).

Clinical Features

Gastroenteritis followed by headache and short-term memory loss is the typical scenario. In some cases, there followed confusion, hallucinations, loss of memory, and disorientation. Seizures, myoclonus, coma, hemiparesis, and ophthalmoplegia were noted in the most severe cases. The acute symptom frequencies were the following: vomiting (76%), abdominal cramps (50%), diarrhea (4%), severe headache (43%), and loss of short-term memory (25%). The mortality rate is 3%.[32] Permanent neurological sequelae, especially cognitive dysfunction, were most likely in people who developed neurological illness with 48 hours, in males, in older patients (>60 years), and in younger people with preexisting illnesses such as diabetes, chronic renal disease, and hypertension with a history of transient ischemic attacks. Teitelbaum et al. studied 14 patients with severe neurological disease. In neuropsychological testing performed several months after the acute episode, 12 patients had severe antegrade memory deficits with relative preservation of other cognitive functions and 11 had clinical and electromyographic evidence of pure motor or sensory motor neuronopathy or axonopathy.[30] Positron emission tomography results in 4 patients showed decreased glucose metabolism in the medial temporal lobes. The neuropathology for the 4 fatal cases revealed neuronal necrosis and loss, predominantly in the hippocampus and amygdala. All 14 patients with severe neurological disease reported confusion and disorientation within 1.5 to 48 hours after consumption. The maximal neurological deficits were seen 4 hours after ingestion in those least affected and 72 hours after ingestion in those most affected, with maximal improvement 24 hours to 12 weeks after ingestion. Acute coma was associated with the slowest recovery. Seizures ceased by 4 months but were frequent for up to 8 weeks.[30]

Diagnosis

The mouse assay, HPLC, mass spectrometry, and ELISA techniques have been developed for detection of domoic acid from contaminated shellfish.[33]

Treatment

Treatment of ASP is mainly supportive and symptomatic. Intensive care is required for those who have severe manifestations with unstable blood pressure, respiratory difficulties, and coma. Teitelbaum noted that seizures responded to intravenous diazepam and phenobarbital and were resistant to phenytoin in three patients.[30]

PREVENTION OF SHELLFISH POISONING

As with many marine toxin–induced diseases, the initial or index cases are often the tip of the iceberg. Any cases of PSP should be reported to the appropriate public health authorities for follow-up to ascertain other cases and to prevent further spread. A major problem is underreporting of PSP by people experiencing minor symptoms. In some instances, if victims had reported their PSP symptoms to a medical facility, more serious consequences could have been averted. Every effort should be made to obtain contaminated materials and their source. The most effective form of PSP prevention is to eliminate human contact with contaminated shellfish and other transvectors. Preventive measures include avoiding eating shellfish from an area with a high incidence of PSP. Purchasing shellfish from a seafood retailer or shellfish farm that sells only tested products is also a prudent measure.

Cooking the shellfish does not prevent this disease. Routine surveillance of shellfish beds for known toxins and closures of the beds by monitoring the amount of toxins using the mouse assay are common practice throughout the world.[34] In the United States, PSP levels in edible shellfish greater than 800 μg of PSP per kilogram by mouse assay means that commercial beds are closed until they are monitored below this level; this action level is more than 10 times lower than the lowest level associated with human outbreaks. In Canada, it is recommended that commercial shellfish operations should be closed if concentrations of domoic acid exceed 20 μg/g wet weight in shellfish. Furthermore, there is active monitoring of algal blooms with fish and bird kills.

Ozonation can remove low levels of toxins from soft-shell clams but not if the clams have retained toxin for long periods; some industrial canning processes may lead to a decrease in PSP concentration.[27,34] The feasibility and effectiveness of degrading saxitoxins through chlorination is being investigated. Biological controls to attack the red tide have been considered, such as using parasitic dinoflagellates like *Amoebophrya ceratii* that parasitizes various dinoflagellates responsible for PSP.[35] Shellfish management regulations include a biotoxin control plan that is implemented during red tides to reduce the risk to humans from consumption of toxic mollusks. While some illness related to shellfish consumption occasionally has occurred, in general the highly cautionary regulations have been quite effective in preventing NSP.

REFERENCES

1. Sobel J, Painter J. Illnesses caused by marine toxins. *Clin Infect Dis.* 2005;41:1290–1296.
2. Ciminiello P, Fattorusso E. Bivalve molluscs as vectors of marine biotoxins involved in seafood poisoning. *Prog Mol Subcell Biol.* 2006;43:53–82.
3. Van Dolah FM. Marine algal toxins: origins, health effects, and their increased occurrence. *Environ Health Perspect.* 2000;108 (Suppl 1):133–141.

4. Baden DG. Marine food-borne dinoflagellate toxins. *Int Rev Cytol*. 1983;82: 99–150.

5. Baden DG, Fleming LE, Bean JA. Marine toxins. In: deWolf FA, ed. *Handbook of Clinical Neurology: Intoxications of the Nervous System*. Part II. Natural Toxins and Drugs. Amsterdam: Elsevier; 1995:141–175.

6. Anderson D. Toxic algal blooms and red tides: a global perspective. In: Okaichi T, Anderson D, Nemoto T, eds. *Biology, Environmental Science and Toxicology*. New York: Elsevier; 1989.

7. Gessner BD, Middaugh JP. Paralytic shellfish poisoning in Alaska: a 20-year retrospective analysis. *Am J Epidemiol*. 1995;141:766–770.

8. Erker EF, Slaughter LJ, Bass EL, et al. Acute toxic effects in mice of an extract from the marine algae *Gonyaulax monilata*. *Toxicon*. 1985;23:761–767.

9. Llewellyn LE. Saxitoxin: a toxic marine natural product that targets a multitude of receptors. *Nat Prod Rep*. 2006;23:200–222.

10. Isbister GK, Kiernan MC. Neurotoxic marine poisoning. *Lancet Neurol*. 2005;4:219–228.

11. Rodrigue DC, Etzel RA, Hall S, et al. Lethal paralytic shellfish poisoning in Guatemala. *Am J Trop Med Hyg*. 1990;42:267–271.

12. de Carvalho M, Jacinto J, Ramos N, et al. Paralytic shellfish poisoning: clinical and electrophysiological observations. *J Neurol*. 1998;245:551–554.

13. Long RR, Sargent JC, Hammer K. Paralytic shellfish poisoning: a case report and serial electrophysiologic observations. *Neurology*. 1990;40:1310–1312.

14. Park DL, Adams WN, Graham SL, et al. Variability of mouse bioassay for determination of paralytic shellfish poisoning toxins. *J Assoc Off Anal Chem*. 1986;69:547–550.

15. Usleber E, Dietrich R, Burk C, et al. Immunoassay methods for paralytic shellfish poisoning toxins. *J AOAC Int*. 2001;84:1649–1656.

16. Hungerford JM. Committee on Natural Toxins and Food Allergens: marine and freshwater toxins. *J AOAC Int*. 2006;89:248–269.

17. Gessner BD, Bell P, Doucette GJ, et al: Hypertension and identification of toxin in human urine and serum following a cluster of mussel-associated paralytic shellfish poisoning outbreaks. *Toxicon*. 1997;35:711–722.

18. Brown CK, Shepherd SM. Marine trauma, envenomations, and intoxications. *Emerg Med Clin North Am*. 1992;10:385–408.

19. Fleming LE, Stinn J. Shellfish poisonings. *Travel Med*. 1999;3: 1–6.

20. Stommel EW, Watters MR. Marine neurotoxins: Ingestible toxins. *Curr Treat Options Neurol*. 2004;6:105–114.

21. Poli M, Mende TJ, Baden DG. Brevetoxins, unique activators of voltage-sensitive sodium channels bind to specific sites in rat brain synaptosomes. *Mol Pharmacol*. 1986;30:129–135.

22. Poli MA, Musser SM, Dickey RW, et al. Neurotoxic shellfish poisoning and brevetoxin metabolites: a case study from Florida. *Toxicon*. 2000;38:981–993.

23. Morris P, Campbell DS, Taylor TJ, et al. Clinical and epidemiological features of neurotoxic shellfish poisoning in North Carolina. *Am J Public Health*. 1991;81:471–473.

24. Aune T, Yndstad M. Diarrhetic shellfish poisoning. In: IR Falconer, ed. *Algal Toxins in Seafood and Drinking Water*. London: Academic Press; 1993:87–104.

25. Burgess V, Shaw G. Pectenotoxins: an issue for public health: a review of their comparative toxicology and metabolism. *Environ Int*. 2001;27:275–283.

26. Haystead TAJ, Sim ATR, Carling D, et al. Effects of the tumor promoter okadaic acid on intracellular protein phosphorylation and metabolism. *Nature*. 1989;337:78–81.

27. Halstead BW. *Poisonous and Venomous Marine Animals of the World*. 2nd ed, revised. Princeton, NJ: Darwin Press; 1988.

28. Lee JS, Murata M, Yasumoto T. Analytical methods for determination of diarrhetic shellfish toxins. In: Natori S, Hashimoto K, Ueno Y, eds. *Mycotoxins and Phycotoxins*. Amsterdam: Elsevier; 1989:327–334.

29. Chandrasekaran A, Ponnambalam G, Kaur C. Domoic acid–induced neurotoxicity in the hippocampus of adult rats. *Neurotox Res*. 2004;6:105–117.

30. Teitelbaum JS, Zatorre RJ, Carpenter S, et al. Neurologic sequelae of domoic acid intoxication due to the ingestion of contaminated mussels. *N Engl J Med*. 1990;322:1781–1787.

31. Novelli A, Kispert J, Fernandez-Sanchez T, et al. Domoic acid–containing toxic mussels produce neurotoxicity in neuronal cultures through a synergism between excitatory amino acids. *Brain Res*. 1992;577:41–48.

32. Jeffery B, Barlow T, Moizer K, et al. Amnesic shellfish poison. *Food Chem Toxicol*. 2004;42:545–557.

33. Lawrence JF, Charbonneau CF, Menard C, et al. Liquid chromatographic determination of domoic acid in shellfish products using the paralytic shellfish poison extraction procedure of the association of official analytical chemists. *Journal of Chromatogr*. 1989:462:349–356.

34. Silver MW. Protecting ourselves from shellfish poisoning. *Am Sci*. 2006;94:316–325.

35. Viviani R. Eutrophication, marine biotoxins, human health. *Sci Total Environ*. 1992;Suppl:631–662.

CHAPTER 41

Seafood Neurotoxins II: Other Ingestible Marine Biotoxins—Ciguatera, Tetrodotoxin, Cyanotoxins

Michael R. Watters

INTRODUCTION

The most common neurological syndrome resulting from ingested marine biotoxins is ciguatera (reef fish poisoning). A less common but perhaps more well-known syndrome occurs with tetrodotoxin (Figure 41-1) following ingestion of affected pufferfish (fugu). Both occur with saltwater fish and affect neuronal sodium channels to produce acute syndromes. Ciguatoxin (Figure 41-2) opens sodium channels, while tetrodotoxin blocks sodium channels. More ubiquitous are cyanobacteria, found in terrestrial, freshwater, and brackish environments. Cyanobacteria produce β-N-methylamino-L-alanine (BMAA) (Figure 41-3), a nonessential amino acid that mimics glutamate excitoxicity and is found in high concentrations in brain tissues of Guamanian patients with amyotrophic lateral sclerosis (ALS)–parkinsonism–dementia complex and North American patients with sporadic ALS and Alzheimer's disease. BMAA may play an important role in the genetic–environmental neuropathology of more insidiously evolving syndromes of neurodegeneration. It occurs in high concentration in the seeds and roots of cycad palms, in food made from cycad-based flour, and with consumption of fruit bats (flying foxes) or other animals feeding on cycad seeds. Toxic cyanobacterial blooms may occur in freshwater, municipal, and residential water supplies or in aquaculture, and represent an increasing environmental hazard in several parts of the world through ingesting contaminated seafood, drinking contaminated water, or recreationally using lakes and rivers containing high concentrations of toxic cyanobacteria (Figure 41-4).

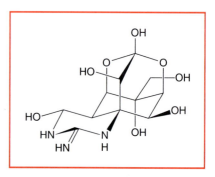

Figure 41-1. Tetrodotoxin.

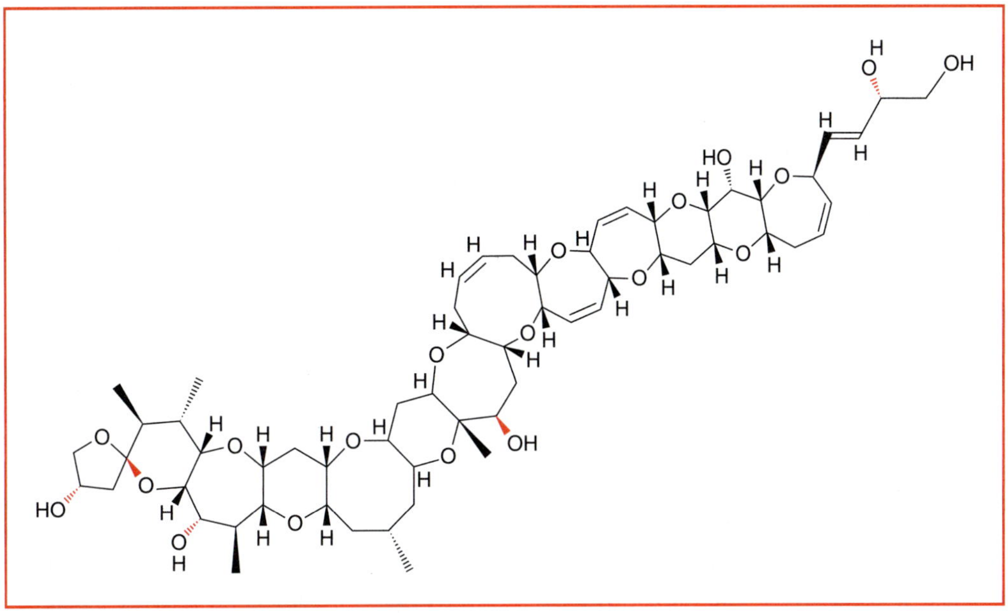

Figure 41-2. Chemical structure of the ciguatoxin CTX₁.

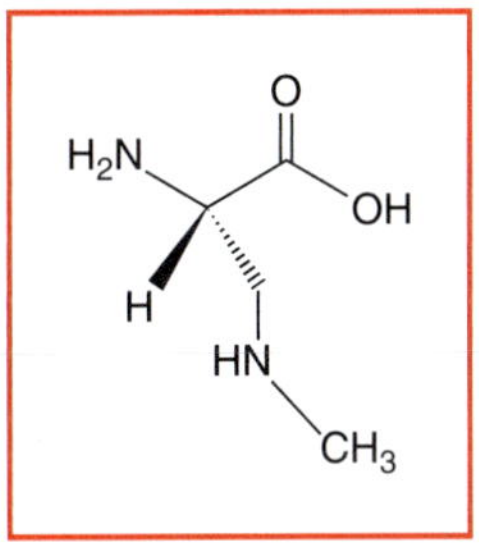

Figure 41-3. β-N-methylamino-L-alanine.

CIGUATERA: REEF FISH POISONING

Food poisoning producing gastrointestinal and sensorimotor symptoms beginning within 24 hours of ingestion of tropical reef fish or their predators is termed *ciguatera*.[1] Monoclonal antibody techniques have identified at least four separate neurotoxins that may be associated with the syndrome of ciguatera: ciguatoxin, maitotoxin, scaritoxin, and palytoxin. The vast majority of cases of ciguatera can be attributed to ciguatoxin. Each of these toxins is produced by microorganisms ingested by the small herbivorous reef fish and then passed along the food chain to omnivores and carnivores feeding along the coral reef. Affected fish may contain these microorganisms within their digestive glands, and the elaborated toxins tend to accumulate

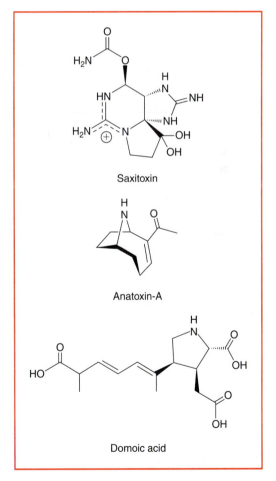

Saxitoxin

Anatoxin-A

Domoic acid

Figure 41-4. Examples of neurotoxins released from algal blooms.

within other visceral organs (particularly the liver), roe, and brain of the consuming fish. Clinical symptoms may vary, depending upon the predominant toxin. Ciguateric toxins are heat stable and unaffected by cooking, freezing, or salting of affected fish, which look, taste, and smell normal. These properties allow clinical cases to appear in unexpected locations far removed from the reef environment. Toxin-laden fishmeal prepared from affected reef fish may contaminate poultry, livestock, or farm-raised salmon fed such fishmeal.

Ciguatoxin

Ciguatoxin (CTX) is a lipophilic toxin elaborated by the dinoflagellate microorganism *Gamberdiscus toxicus,* a unicellular protozoan dinoflagellate capable of photosynthesis, which exists symbiotically with the macroalgae found along tropical reefs. CTX biosynthesis may be affected by multiple factors, including water temperature, runoff of fertilizers and phosphates, dredging, rainfall, salinity, nutrient exhaustion, and bioluminescence.[2] Symptoms result from CTX action on peripheral neuronal sodium channels, which binds to site 5 of the presynaptic sodium voltage-gated ion channels. These are clustered at the myelin clefts of the nodes of Ranvier.[3] Opening of the sodium voltage-gated ion channels induces spontaneous and repetitive action potentials in response to a single electrical stimulus, causing trains of repetitive endplate potentials that can trigger muscle action potentials, as well as resulting in time-dependent swelling of the nodes of Ranvier as water follows the influx of sodium in response to opening of the sodium channels, to impair salutatory nerve conduction.[4] Initial symptoms result from hyperactivity of autonomic neurons, causing nausea, emesis, and diarrhea. These symptoms typically appear within the initial 8 hours following ingestion of toxic fish, followed over the subsequent 10 to 18 hours by headache, myalgias, and loss of tendon reflexes.[5,6] By 24 hours, sensory symptoms predominant, manifested by perioral and limb paresthesias, dysesthesias, and pruritus. These sensory symptoms gradually evolve over the ensuing 2 to 5 days into paradoxical sensory disturbances, such as feeling heat as cold, and vice versa. Such paradoxical sensory perceptions are the clinical hallmark of CTX but may also occur with some shellfish toxins associated with red tides. Sensory symptoms may transiently recur with subsequent ingestion of foods containing low concentrations of CTX (e.g., chicken fed fishmeal from reef fish). Recurrent exposures to CTX may result in a persistent sensorimotor polyneuropathy. Prostration, fatigue, and weakness are present in approximately half of patients.[7] Fatigue may persist chronically as a syndrome of chronic fatigue. Titers of monoclonal antibody to CTX have been shown to be elevated in 96% of 115 patients carrying the diagnosis of chronic fatigue syndrome, compared to only 11% of 37 normal subjects, suggesting a possible link between subclinical ciguatera and chronic fatigue syndrome.[8]

Treatment of CTX-associated ciguatera includes attention to volume repletion from gastrointestinal loss and early use of mannitol. Mannitol has been shown in vitro to reverse the nodal swelling induced by CTX.[9] Prospective uncontrolled trials have demonstrated dramatic clinical improvement and shortening of the course compared to historic controls (class II evidence) when given to patients within the initial 10 hours (mean) after onset of symptoms.[10,11] The usual dose of mannitol is 1 gm/kg given intravenously as a 20% solution.[5] Delays in mannitol therapy beyond 18 hours (mean) after onset of symptoms were shown to result in no benefit compared with normal saline when studied in a prospective randomized controlled clinical trial of 50 patients.[12] However, there are anecdotal case reports of patients responding to mannitol after more than 24 hours of symptoms.[10] These data suggest that patients with acute ciguatera due principally to CTX are more likely to show benefit from mannitol if it is given as soon as possible once the clinical diagnosis has been established.[1]

Maitotoxin

The dinoflagellate *G. toxicus* not only elaborates lipophilic CTX but also is capable of producing an aqueous fraction, maitotoxin (MTX). Release of MTX may influence control of the size of the dinoflagellate colony.[13] MTX appears to activate voltage-dependent calcium channels, particularly within adrenergic nerve endings, to produce bradycardia and hypotension, which may respond to volume repletion.[1] Ciguatera associated with MTX appears only infrequently. In a series of 327 cases of ciguatera in Hawaii, bradycardia and hypotension were found in only 5% of patients.[7]

Scaritoxin

Ingestion of parrotfish (family Scaridae) may produce a syndrome of typical acute ciguatera. This is followed 5 to 10 days later by the tardive onset of a cerebellar syndrome, manifested by tremor and gait ataxia lasting for several weeks.[1] In a series of 327 cases of ciguatera in Hawaii, such cerebellar signs occurred in less than 10% of cases.[7] The presumptive toxin has been termed *scaritoxin.* Little is known about the physiology, source, or structure of this toxin.

Palytoxin

Palytoxin (PTX) was first discovered to be present in a soft Hawaiian coral (*Palythoa* species) in 1971.[14] PTX and its derivatives are elaborated by some sea anemones

(*Radianthus macrodactyylus*), dinoflagellates (genus *Ostreopsis*), red algae (*Chondria armata*), and marine worms (*Hermodice carunculata*) and may be found in mackerel, crabs, or seaweed harvested from affected areas.[15] High doses of PTX result in fatal cardiac arrhythmias and heart failure. This ciguateric syndrome is distinguishable by the presence of muscle spasms. The sustained muscle contractions occur partly because of impaired release of endothelial nitric oxide.[16] At very low concentration, PTX stimulates the activation of several mitogen-activated protein kinases and matrix metalloproteinases to promote carcinogenesis and formation of superoxide radicals.[15] No known treatment exists for PTX exposure, although animals given sublethal doses of PTX parenterally were partially protected against a subsequent lethal dose if given hydrocortisone before receiving PTX. Fortunately, fatal ciguatera associated with PTX is quite rare. In the largest ($n = 3,009$) published series of ciguatera cases, fatalities occurred in less than 0.1% of patients.[17]

TETRODOTOXIN

Tetrodotoxin (TTX) and anhydrotetrodotoxin (easily converted to TTX) are produced by marine bacteria of the Vibrionaceae family and selectively block the action potentials of voltage-gated sodium channels along nerves, skeletal and cardiac muscle membranes .[18] This occurs without change in the resting membrane potentials. TTX binds to site 1 of the sodium channel to block the influx of sodium.[3] TTX-sensitive sodium channels are found along all sensory neurons, muscle membranes, and some motor axons, where they are found in highest density at the myelin clefts and are responsible for the initiation of the axonal action potential.[2] TTX-resistant sodium channels are not opposed by potassium current and may not inactivate completely following sensory nerve action potentials, which may play an important role in nociceptor sensitization.[19] TTX-resistant channels allow some marine creatures to tolerate TTX, including the Australian blue-ringed and blue-spotted octopuses, pufferfish, Japanese ivory and trumpet shellfish, California newts, some flatworms, and the colored frogs of Central America.[1]

TTX is concentrated in the liver and roe of the pufferfish, in the visceral organs and skin of newts and colored frogs, and in the oral venom glands of the blue octopuses. Clinical intoxication occurs following ingestion of affected pufferfish or Japanese shellfish, an envenomating bite by the Australian blue octopuses, or contact with the skin of pufferfish or colored frogs. TTX is not found in all pufferfish of the same species nor found in those bred in captivity, although TTX may be transferred passively when captive puffers are fed livers from TTX-containing pufferfish.[1] In Japan, eating pufferfish (fugu) is considered a delicacy. Fugu is served only in licensed Japanese restaurants, with chefs specially trained in preparing the fleshy meat and avoiding contact with skin, visceral organs, or roe. However, enough TTX may be retained within the flesh to produce mild symptoms of toxicity and afford the thrill of flirting with death. More than 150 people per year are intoxicated by eating fugu in Japan, with about 20 annual deaths.[1] Eating pufferfish is prohibited in the United States.

Clinical symptoms of TTX poisoning usually begin within minutes of envenomation by blue octopus, contact with the skin of a colored frog or newt, or ingestion of fugu, although symptoms may be delayed by several hours.[5,20] Initial symptoms include euphoria and paresthesias around the lips and tongue and then more generalized paresthesias. These symptoms are usually followed by nausea, emesis, diarrhea, and increasing paralysis (limb and bulbar) with loss of brainstem and tendon reflexes.[7] Fatalities usually result from respiratory insufficiency with hypoxic encephalopathy, hypotension, and cardiac arrhythmias. Fatality rates range from 13% to 80%, with most fatal cases occurring within the initial half hour.[1] Treatment is supportive, particularly cardiovascular and ventilatory. TTX poisoning from fugu is easier to avoid than to treat.

CYANOTOXINS

Cyanobacteria are known to produce a diversity of cyanotoxins, with increasing toxic blooms in freshwater and brackish water environments.[21] The use of manures and fertilizers are conducive to the growth of cyanobacteria in freshwater fishponds and shrimp ponds, resulting in dominating cyanobacterial blooms for substantial periods of the growth cycles.[22] Carp and catfish cultures have a high risk of cyanobacteria blooms, while tilapia, milkfish, and shrimp farming carry a somewhat lower risk. With abundant sunshine, cyanobacteria may bloom then decompose to result in an increase in the ammonia content of the pond, with a concurrent decrease in dissolved oxygen content and a disturbance of pH, each of which potentially affecting survival of the aquaculture indirectly. The earliest reports of cyanobacterial lethality were published in the late 19th century, reporting on the death of sheep after drinking water from a lake in South Australia, with subsequent reports of animal fatalities among flamingos, dogs, cattle, and rhinoceros.[23] Extensive fish kills during planktonic cyanobacterial blooms have become a frequent occurrence in freshwater lakes in China in recent time.[24] Similar occurrences have been reported recently in Ireland, Germany, Brazil, Australia, the United States, and Turkey.[25] Human exposures may occur from ingestion of toxic fish, contaminated water supplies, cutaneous exposure from recreational activities amid toxic blooms or among aquaculture workers, or ingestion of dietary supplements made from cyanobacteria. Cyanobacterial neurotoxins include anatoxin (AN-α) and its analogs, as well as BMAA.

One AN-α analog is AN-α(s), with the *s* nomenclature indicating that salivation is stimulated because of AN-α(s) inhibition of acetylcholinesterase. AN-α(s) has been reported to be responsible for fatalities among ducks, swine, and dogs.[26] Humans have been affected by contaminated drinking water in Brazil and Australia, as well as 70 deaths in Brazil associated with use of contaminated hemodialysis solutions.[23]

BMAA is a potent neurotoxin produced by cyanobacteria of the genus *Nostoc,* which live symbiotically among the roots of cycad palm trees *(Cycas micronesica)* in Guam and elsewhere in the tropics.[27] BMAA accumulates in the seeds of the cycads, which may be consumed by flying fox bats and other animals that feed on the cycad seeds. Guamanians use the cycad seeds to make flour for tortillas and soups. Biomagnification of BMAA exposure occurs with ingestion of the bats, which are considered a delicacy by the indigenous Chomorros of Guam.[28] Monkeys fed high doses of BMAA develop features of human ALS and dementia, and BMAA induces selective loss of motor neurons in spinal cord cultures.[27] BMAA is incorporated into neuronal proteins, and accumulation may contribute to protein misfolding and altered protein functional expression. Motor and cognitive dysfunction occurs in rodents that have received subcutaneous BMAA or have been fed cycad-based diets.[29,30] BMAA has been found in high concentrations within the brains of ALS–parkinsonism–dementia complex patients in Guam and within the brains of North American patients with sporadic Alzheimer's disease or ALS.[27] BMAA is structurally similar to glutamate and promotes excitatory neurotoxicity by increasing intracellular calcium, with activation of AMPA–kainate receptor–dependent mechanisms of neuronal injury.[27] Cyanotoxins therefore represent an important public health issue, with the potential to produce acute fatal illness and to contribute to the subsequent insidious development of neurodegenerative disorders affecting motor and cognitive performance.

CONCLUSION

Neurotoxins that may be acquired through ingestion of various seafoods include the ciguateric toxins (CTX, MTX, scaritoxin, PTX), TTX, and cyanotoxins (ANs and BMAA). Other ingestible toxins include saxitoxins, brevetoxins, okadaic acid, and domoic acid (discussed in Chapter 40). Ciguatera has a distinct clinical syndrome of acute gastrointestinal dysautonomia, followed by sensory disturbances that include paradoxical perceptions to temperature, and may be attenuated by prompt treatment with intravenous mannitol. TTX is not treatable, can only be supported with mechanical ventilation until recovery occurs, and is more easily avoided than managed. Cyanotoxins are ubiquitous substances that may slowly accumulate within the central nervous system and contribute to neurodegeneration of motor and cognitive pathways.

REFERENCES

1. Watters MR. Tropical marine neurotoxins: venoms to drugs. *Sem Neurol.* 2005;25(3):278–289.
2. Watters MR. Neurologic marine biotoxins. *Continuum.* 2008;14(5):81–101.
3. Watters MR. Marine neurotoxins as a starting point to drugs. In: Botana LM, ed. *Seafood and Freshwater Toxins: Pharmacology, Physiology, and Detection.* 2nd ed. Boca Raton, Fla: Taylor & Francis/CRC Press; 2008:889–897.
4. Benoit E, Mattei C, Ouanounou G, et al. Ionic mechanisms involved in the nodal swelling of myelinated axons caused by marine toxins. *Cell Mol Biol Lett.* 2002;7(2):317–321.
5. Stommel EW, Watters MR. Marine neurotoxins: ingestible toxins. *Curr Treat Options Neurol.* 2004;6:105–114.
6. Pearn J. Neurology of ciguatera. *J Neurol Neurosurg Psychiatry.* 2001;70:4–8.
7. Watters MR. Organic neurotoxins in seafoods. *Clin Neurol Neurosurg.* 1995;97:119–124.
8. Hokama Y, Uto GA, Palafox NA, et al. Chronic phase lipids in sera of chronic fatigue syndrome (CFS), chronic ciguatera fish poisoning (CCFP), hepatitis B, and cancer with antigenic epitope resembling ciguatoxin, as assessed with MAb-CTX. *J Clin Lab Anal.* 2003;17:132–139.
9. Benoit E, Juzans P, Legrand AM, et al. Nodal swelling produced by ciguatoxin induces selective activation of sodium channels in myelinated nerve fibers. *Neuroscience.* 1996;71:1121–1131.
10. Palafox NA, Jain LG, Pinano AX, et al. Successful treatment of ciguatera fish poisoning with intravenous mannitol. *JAMA.* 1988;259:2740–2742.
11. Pearn J, Lewis R. Ciguatera and mannitol: experience with a new treatment regimen. *Med J Aust.* 1989;151:77–80.
12. Schnorf H, Taurarii M, Cundy T. Ciguatera fish poisoning: a double-blind randomized trial of mannitol therapy. *Neurology.* 2002;58:873–880.
13. MacKenzie L. Ecobiology of the brevetoxin, ciguatoxin, and cyclic imine producers. In: Botana LM, ed. *Seafood and Freshwater Toxins: Pharmacology, Physiology, and Detection.* 2nd ed. Boca Raton, Fla: Taylor & Francis/CRC Press; 2008:433–476.
14. Moore RE, Scheuer PJ. Palytoxin: a new marine toxin from a coelenterate. *Science.* 1971;172:495.
15. Munday R. Occurrence and toxicology of palytoxins. In: Botana LM, ed. *Seafood and Freshwater Toxins: Pharmacology, Physiology, and Detection.* 2nd ed. Boca Raton, Fla: Taylor & Francis/CRC Press; 2008:693–713.
16. Taylor RJ, Smith NC, Langford MJ, et al. Effect of palytoxin on endothelium-dependent and -independent relaxation in rat aortic rings. *J Appl Toxicol.* 1995;15:5–12.

17. Bagnis R, Kuberski T, Lamgier S. Clinical observations on 3,009 cases of ciguatera (fish poisoning) in the South Pacific. *Am J Trop Med Hyg.* 1979;28:1067–1073.

18. Narahashi T. Tetrodotoxin. In: Spencer PS, Schaumburg HH, eds. *Experimental and Clinical Neurotoxicology.* 2nd ed. Oxford, United Kingdom: Oxford University Press; 2000:1162–1164.

19. Reisner L. Biologic poisons for pain. *Curr Pain Headache Rep.* 2004;8:427–434.

20. Watters MR, Stommel EW. Marine toxins: envenomations and contact toxins. *Curr Treat Options Neurol.* 2004;6:115–123.

21. Codd GA, Azevedo SMFO, Bagchi SN, et al. Executive Summary. Cyanonet a Global Network for Cyanobacterial Bloom and Toxin Risk Management: Initial Situation Assessment and Recommendations. Paris: International Hydrological Programme, UNESCO; 2005:1.

22. Ito E. Toxicology of azaspiracid-1: acute and chronic poisoning, tumorigenicity, and chemical structure relationship to toxicity in a mouse model. In: Botana LM, ed. *Seafood and Freshwater Toxins: Pharmacology, Physiology, and Detection.* 2nd ed. Boca Raton, Fla: Taylor & Francis/CRC Press; 2008:775–784.

23. Welker M. Cyanobacterial hepatotoxins: chemistry, biosynthesis, and occurrence. In: Botana LM, ed. *Seafood and Freshwater Toxins: Pharmacology, Physiology, and Detection.* 2nd ed. Boca Raton, Fla: Taylor & Francis/CRC Press; 2008:825–843.

24. Kaya K. Asia: Eastern Asia, Cyanonet a Global Network for Cyanobacterial Bloom and Toxin Risk Management: Initial Situation Assessment and Recommendations. Paris: International Hydrological Programme, UNESCO; 2005:33.

25. Smith PT. Cyanobacterial toxins in aquaculture. In: Botana LM, ed. *Seafood and Freshwater Toxins: Pharmacology, Physiology, and Detection.* 2nd ed. Boca Raton, Fla: Taylor & Francis/CRC Press; 2008:787–806.

26. James KJ, Dauphard J, Crowley J, et al. Cyanobacterial neurotoxins, anatoxin-A and analogues: detection and analysis. In: Botana LM, ed. *Seafood and Freshwater Toxins: Pharmacology, Physiology, and Detection.* 2nd ed. Boca Raton, Fla: Taylor & Francis/CRC Press; 2008:809–822.

27. Mash DC. Cyanobacterial toxins in neurodegeneration. *Continuum.* 2008;14(5):138–149.

28. Wilson JM, Khabazian I, Wong MC, et al. Behavioral and neurological correlates of ALS–parkinsonism–dementia complex in adult mice fed washed cycad flour. *Neuromolecular Med.* 2002;1:207–221.

29. Banack SA, Cox PA. Biomagnification of cycad neurotoxins in flying foxes: implications for ALS–PDC in Guam. *Neurology.* 2003;61:387–389.

30. Dawson R, Marschall EG, Chan KC, et al. Neurochemical and neurobehavioral effects of neonatal administration of β-N-methylamino-L-alanine and 3,3′-iminodipropionitrile. *Neurotoxicol Teratol.* 1998;20:181–192.

Marine Envenomations

Pratap Chand

INTRODUCTION

The presence of poisonous biting and stinging marine creatures has been recorded historically from inscriptions from the tomb of the Egyptian Pharoah Ti (2700 BC) and later from the writings of Aristotle and Pliny. A considerable amount of literature has accumulated about jellyfish stings and the mortality and morbidity related to it from Australian and American researchers.[1] Other marine stinging organisms and the clinical manifestations from these have been documented in the literature. Many neurotoxins have been identified from marine stinging organisms, and their molecular mechanisms have been elucidated. Various neurological disorders associated with marine stings have been reported and range from myopathy, peripheral neuropathy, and autonomic dysfunction to seizures, coma, and death. This chapter reviews the neurological manifestations of marine stings, pathophysiological mechanisms, and methods of treatment.

JELLYFISH

The commonest cause of human marine stings reported worldwide is from jellyfish, which have more than 10,000 species, with more than 100 species that are toxic to humans. Jellyfish have four classes: Hydrozoa (Portuguese man-of-war), Scyphozoa (true jellyfish), Cubozoa (box jellyfish), and Anthozoa (sea anemones and corals).[1] Jellyfish have a single gastrovascular cavity opening, which is used for digestion and circulation, and a set of tentacles (Figure 42-1). The tentacles are covered with nematocysts, which are specialized stinging apparatus, and consist of a poison sac with an attached sharp hollow tube armed with barbs. Mechanical and chemical stimulation of the sensory hairs surrounding the pressurized nematocyte results in a calcium-mediated bioelectric signal that causes an opening of its lid, allowing the ejection of the nematocyst into the prey to express the venom.[2] Nematocysts are distributed on all parts of the tentacles of the jellyfish and may stick to ensnare or penetrate prey for both defense and

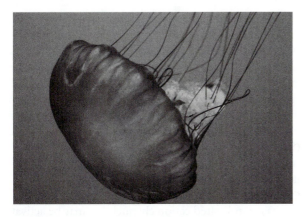

Figure 42-1. Sea nettle jellyfish, *Chrysaora quinquecirrha*. (Courtesy of Wikipedia.)

feeding. The nematocyst is capable of penetrating up to a depth of 0.9 mm, anchors the tentacles to the prey, and injects the toxins into the microvasculature of the dermal tissue, which is absorbed into the systemic circulation. Different types of venoms have been isolated from different species of jellyfish. The venoms may vary within the same animal and from one nematocyst to another. They contain various polypeptide toxins. The composition of the toxins include catecholamines, vasoactive amines (histamine, serotonin), kinins, collagenases, hyaluronidases, proteases, phospholipases, fibrinolysins, dermatotoxins, cardiotoxins, neurotoxins, nephrotoxins, myotoxins, and antigenic proteins.[3] The protein component of the toxin tends to be heat labile, tends to be nondialyzable, and is degradable by proteolytic agents. The toxins cause sodium and calcium ion transport abnormalities at the cellular level via the creation of nonselective pores in the cell membrane, disrupt cellular membranes, release inflammatory mediators, and act as direct toxins on the myocardium, nervous tissue, hepatic tissue, and kidneys.[4]

Clinical Features of Jellyfish Stings

In the United States, jellyfish stings occur most commonly during the summer along the coastal regions. About 1 to 2 million stings occur annually in the Chesapeake Bay area, and about 200,000 occur annually along the Florida coast.[5] Jellyfish stings occur worldwide in tropical oceans, especially between latitudes 30° south to 45° north, because of a high natural concentration of coelenterates.[6,7] Contact with toxic jellyfish causes a range of conditions, from cutaneous rashes to cardiovascular and respiratory collapse.[8,9] The effects of jellyfish stings are usually mild, except those caused by species in the South Pacific, such as the box jellyfish

or Portuguese man-of-war. A recent epidemiological study of 118 cases of jellyfish stings from the Texas Gulf Coast showed that 0.8% had no effect, 80.5% had minor effects, and 18.6% had moderate effects.[10] Box jellyfish venom has a median lethal dose of 40 µg/kg, which makes it the most potent marine toxin and has caused 72 deaths worldwide from neuromuscular and respiratory paralysis, drowning, and cardiovascular collapse.[7,11] The sting of the Portuguese man-of-war (Figure 42-2; see color plate) is more painful than that of a common jellyfish sting and has been responsible for two reported deaths. The toxins in the venom have been found to induce a calcium flux into cells by increasing membrane permeability.[12,13] Children are most susceptible to the effects of toxins because of their smaller body surface area and lower body weight as compared to the volume of toxins injected during envenomation. Older adults are more susceptible than younger adults because of their decreased physiological reserves and concurrent debilitation.

Mild envenomation may cause local skin contact reactions—burning pain, pruritus, soft tissue edema, angioedema, erythematous papules, and blisters in a whiplike pattern.[5] Ocular contact reactions include

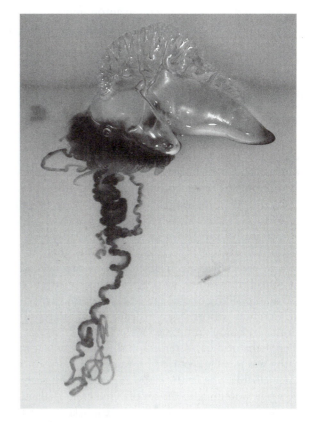

Figure 42-2. Portuguese man-of-war, *Physalia physalis* (see color plate). (Courtesy of Wikipedia.)

conjunctival hyperemia, corneal inflammation, iritis, secondary glaucoma, and mydriasis due to sphincter myotoxicity.[5,8] Moderate or severe envenomation is associated with systemic symptoms like headache, nausea, myalgia, headache, chills, or pallor following the initial localized reaction. Cardiovascular problems include arrhythmias, cardiac failure, peripheral and coronary vasospasm, and cardiovascular collapse or arrest. Respiratory complications include laryngeal edema, bronchospasm, pulmonary edema, acute respiratory distress syndrome, hypoxia, and respiratory failure.[9]

Neurological manifestations have included anxiety and agitation, seizures, signs of raised intracranial pressure, and coma.[14,15] Sánchez-Rodríguez et al. isolated a neurotoxin from the venom of the Caribbean box jellyfish, *Carybdea marsupialis*. A small fraction of the purified protein neurotoxin injected into crabs produced convulsions, paralysis, and death.[16] Autonomic dysfunction following jellyfish sting was first reported by Chand and Selliah from Penang in Malaysia when a Chinese fisherman developed reversible parasympathetic dysautonomia with abdominal distension and constipation due to adynamic ileus, retention of urine, absence of lacrimation, and failure of erection after a jellyfish sting.[17] Another report from Singapore by Ponampalam documented the occurrence of isolated paralytic ileus following a jellyfish sting on the forearm of a tourist in Sumatra in Indonesia.[18] The causes of these autonomic symptoms are unclear and are hypothesized to be due to alteration of sodium and calcium ion transport on autonomic nerve fibers. Other reports on autonomic symptoms attributable to the box jellyfish *Chironex fleckeri* in the Indo-Pacific region include vasospasm, cardiac irregularities, dysphonia, and ophthalmic abnormalities.[19-21] Coelenterate venoms can also target the myocardium, Purkinje fiber, atrioventricular node, or aortic ring.[19] Prolonged urinary incontinence lasting 20 months and associated with biliary dyskinesia requiring surgical intervention was reported by Burnett and Burnett in a 16-year-old girl following an abdominal sting by jellyfish, identified later from pictures as *Chrysaora fuscescens*.[22] Cases of the Irukandji syndrome, caused by the jellyfish *Carukia barnesi*, have symptoms that mimic excessive catecholamine release, with severe headache, intense pallor, sweating, nausea, vomiting, prostration, a sense of impending doom, and severe systemic hypertension. Cerebral hemorrhage and death have been reported with the Irukandji syndrome.[11,23]

Peripheral nerve involvement in the form of ulnar neuropathy was initially reported by Laing and Harrison following jellyfish sting to the elbow region of a 21-year-old male while swimming in the sea off Phuket in Thailand.[24] Following recovery from systemic anaphylaxis, he had signs of an ulnar palsy, with reduced nerve conduction velocity across the elbow. Surgical exploration of the nerve revealed nerve edema but no compression. Recovery from the neuropathy occurred over a period of 4 months. Peel and Kandler reported the case of an 18-year-old female who sustained a jellyfish sting on her right wrist and subsequently developed complete radial, ulnar, and median nerve palsies distal to the site of the sting, which recovered fully over the next 10 months. The neuropathy was postulated to be due to a direct neurotoxic effect of the jellyfish venom.[25] Jellyfish and other cnidarian envenomations cause severe pain, and there is recent evidence that this pain is mediated through the effect of the venom on the transient receptor potential vanilloid subtype 1, a nonselective ligand-gated cation channel that may be activated by various exogenous and endogenous stimuli.[26] These receptors are found in the central and peripheral nervous systems and are involved in the transmission and modulation of pain, as well as the integration of diverse painful stimuli. There has also been research into myotoxins that explain some neurological manifestations of jellyfish stings. Two myotoxins, T_1 and T_2, with molecular weights of approximately 600,000 and 150,000, respectively, were isolated by Endean et al. from *C. fleckeri*. The toxins produced contractures of skeletal (diaphragm) musculature of the rat and of smooth (ileum and vas deferens) and atrial musculature of the guinea pig.[27] Ghosh et al., working on tentacle extracts from the jellyfish *Acromitus rabanchatu* from the Bay of Bengal, isolated a toxin (T-Ar) with a molecular weight of 182,000 Da that could induce a direct paralyzing effect on the muscle membrane.[28]

Clinical Management of Jellyfish Stings

Treatment usually consists of nematocyst deactivation, pain control, local wound care, symptomatic treatment, support of the vital organs in which function is affected, and use of antivenin for box jellyfish envenomation. Capture of the responsible jellyfish should not be necessary because the nematocysts imbedded in the patient can be preserved and sent for identification. Physicians should be aware that stings can occur through surgical gloves.[29] Initial treatments include removing the patient from water to prevent drowning, checking adequate airway ventilation and perfusion, and providing supportive care (e.g., central venous monitoring, fluids, inotropic support, and pressors for hypokinetic cardiac failure). Immobilization and sedation help prevent rapid absorption of venom resulting from muscle movement. A lymphatic–venous compression bandage proximally to the sting site to reduce venous and lymphatic flow of the venom (but not to stop arterial flow) is useful and should be removed only when the provider is ready to render systemic support and the antivenin has been initiated.[29]

Local skin treatment involves rinsing the wound with sterile normal saline to prevent nematocyte activation and immediate inactivation of nematocyte discharge by soaking the wound in 5% acetic acid for 15 to 30 minutes. After the inactivation, any visible tentacles should be carefully removed with forceps. Topical anesthetics and cold pack compresses at the sting site (after nematocyst removal) are useful for the severe pain following stings.[30] The use of freshwater, direct application of ice, and rubbing of the skin may trigger unfired nematocytes and are to be avoided. Hot compresses tend to increase systemic uptake of venom. Antihistamines and topical and systemic corticosteroids for severe local reactions, as well as to decrease the probability of serum sickness symptoms from the antivenin, are useful provided no secondary concurrent infection is present. Muscle relaxants (e.g., benzodiazepines or methocarbamol) can help severe local spasms. Narcotic analgesias are appropriate for severe local pain not responding to topical anesthetics. Tetanus shots are useful as a prophylactic measure, and systemic antibiotics should be administered if signs of secondary infection exist.[30]

Antivenin for box jellyfish envenomation is manufactured by the Commonwealth Serum Laboratories (CSL) of Melbourne, Australia. Unfortunately, the antivenin is ineffective if the toxin already has entered a cell. Anaphylaxis is rare but can be treated with airway support, oxygen, intravascular resuscitation, epinephrine, H_1 and H_2 blockers, steroids, and a β_2-agonist nebulizer. Catecholamine-excess hypertension as seen with the Irukandji syndrome is best treated with phentolamine. Ophthalmic treatments should include nonaqueous topical anesthetic drops followed by copious irrigation with isotonic normal saline. Ophthalmic steroids decrease the corneal inflammatory response. Beta-blockers and carbonic-anhydrase inhibitors are used for documented increased intraocular pressure resulting from the corneal jellyfish sting.[29]

Experimental treatments include monoclonal antibody against jellyfish toxin,[31] verapamil adjunct to antivenin for decreasing venom-induced cardiotoxicity,[32] and gadolinium for inhibiting nematocyte firing through blockade of the calcium-permeable mechanosensitive ion channels involved in nematocyte activation.[33]

BLUE-RINGED OCTOPUS

The blue-ringed octopus (*Hapalochlaena maculosa*), which is less than 5 inches in diameter, has blue rings on its body and luminous tentacles (Figure 42-3; see color plate). It is found in the Indo-Pacific Ocean area and is especially common to southern Australia.[34] It is not an aggressive animal, and when contact occurs, it

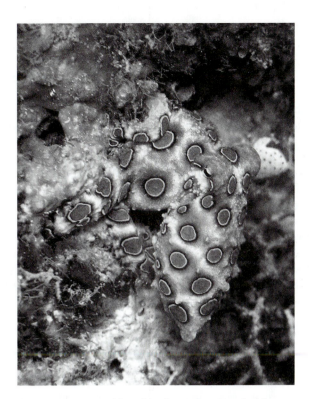

Figure 42-3. Greater blue-ringed octopus, *Hapalochlaena lunulata* (see color plate). (Courtesy of Wikipedia.)

is often accidental. The toxin in the venom from the salivary glands of the octopus initially named maculotoxin was later found to be tetrodotoxin, a neurotoxin that specifically inhibits sodium channel function, producing presynaptic somatic nerve blockade.[35] Other chemicals found in the venom include serotonin, hyaluronidase, tyramine, histamine, octopamine, taurine, acetylcholine, and dopamine. The toxin has been found to be distributed in all body parts, with high concentrations in the arms followed by the abdomen and cephalothorax of the octopus.[36]

Clinical Features of Octopus Stings

Tetrodotoxin blocks sodium channels and produces a dose-dependent flaccid voluntary paralysis with respiratory failure and autonomic nerve dysfunction and hypotension; the sting is often fatal. The stung victim may develop numbness, nausea, vomiting, changes in vision, difficulty in swallowing, and muscle paralysis requiring artificial ventilation until a hospital can be reached.[37] The symptoms vary in severity, with children being the most at risk because of their small body size. The victim might be saved if artificial respiration starts before marked cyanosis and hypotension develop.

Clinical Management of Octopus Stings

First aid treatment is pressure on the wound and rescue breathing. It is essential, if rescue breathing is required, that it be continued until the victim begins to breathe, which may be some hours. It is essential that immediate and full-time respiratory support be given—artificial respiration or rescue breathing even if the victim appears to be not responding.[38] Tetrodotoxin poisoning can result in the victim being fully aware of the surroundings but unable to breathe. Because of the paralysis that occurs, the victim has no way of signaling for help or indicating distress. Respiratory support until medical assistance arrives ensures that the victim will generally recover well. Hospital treatment involves respiratory assistance until the toxin is washed out of the body. Victims who live through the first 24 hours generally go on to make a complete recovery.[38]

CONE SHELLS

Cone shells are marine snails and are found in reef environments throughout the world. They prey upon other marine organisms, detecting the prey primarily with chemoreceptors and immobilizing them with unique venoms contained in a hollow, poison-filled barbed tooth.[39] The bright colors and patterns of cone snails are attractive to the eye, and people tend to pick up the live animals and are stung in this manner (Figure 42-4). Eighteen species of cone shell may sting humans, and there have been 30 recorded cases of human envenomation by cone shells with some fatal outcomes.[40]

The peptide toxins in the venom called conotoxins target an array of ion channels.[41] α-Conotoxins bind to and inhibit the acetylcholine receptors and cause flaccid paralysis of skeletal muscle, with respiratory paralysis and sometimes death. The neurotoxins of some species, such as *Conus geographus,* are selective for the muscle-type acetylcholine receptor, while the neurotoxins of other species are selective for the neuronal-type acetylcholine receptor. μ-Conotoxins close voltage-dependent sodium channels in muscles and within neurons, causing flaccid paralysis of skeletal muscle. Thus, μ-conotoxins block voltage-gated sodium channels in muscles. δ-Conotoxins produce skeletal muscle rigidity and paralysis, keeping voltage-gated sodium channels open. κ-Conotoxins block voltage-gated potassium channels. ω-Conotoxins block voltage-gated calcium channels and block conduction at the neuromuscular junctions of skeletal muscles, causing flaccid muscle paralysis.[41] Conantokins are peptides that target major excitatory *N*-methyl-d-aspartate glutamate receptors, which are ligand-gated calcium channels.[42] The conantokins have been synthesized and characterized in several animal models of human pathologies, including pain, convulsive disorders, stroke, and Parkinson's disease. The potential pharmacological selectivity of the conantokins, coupled with their efficacy in preclinical models of disease and favorable safety profiles, indicates that these peptides represent both novel probes for *N*-methyl-d-aspartate receptor function and an important class of compounds for continued investigation as human therapeutics.[42] The interest in conotoxins as therapeutic agents has resulted in a synthetic derivative of an ω-conotoxin MVIIA, which is now available as a new class of nonaddictive analgesic up to 1000 times more potent than morphine.[43]

Clinical Features of Cone Shell Stings

A sharp pain is usually felt at the site of the sting, and the site may develop a reaction or a bluish tinge. Minor envenomations cause pain, swelling, and localized numbness that often subside within hours of onset. One or more of the following symptoms might be reported upon presentation: swelling and pain in the involved body part; numbness, either localized to the extremity or more generalized; nausea, dysphagia, or vomiting; malaise, weakness, or paralysis; aphonia; areflexia; apnea; pruritus; or diplopia. Recovery after several hours of assisted respiration has also been documented. Serious envenomations are associated with a rapid progression of symptoms, including paralysis, respiratory arrest, cardiac failure, and death.[44] Fatalities have been documented, usually secondary to respiratory failure.[45]

Clinical Management of Cone Shell Stings

The initial treatment includes keeping the patient calm and inactive and maintenance of airway, ventilation, circulation, and intravenous lines for administration of fluids and medications. The toxins are heat labile, and immersion of the affected extremity in nonscalding hot

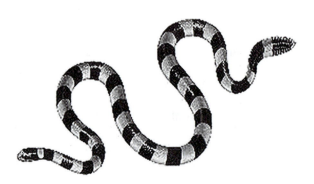

Figure 42-4. Sea snake, *Laticauda Colubrina*. (Courtesy of Wikipedia.)

water may inactivate the toxins and provide pain relief. Pressure bandages help inhibit venous and lymphatic drainage of the toxins from the affected extremity. Severe envenomation with respiratory paralysis requires intubation and ventilation. Intravenous analgesics might be required. Cardiac arrhythmias and coagulopathies may occur and need treatment. There is no antivenin at present, and care is entirely supportive in nature.[46] Mild envenomations should resolve in 6 to 8 hours. The patient might require oral analgesics for pain control. Oral antibiotics are indicated only in the presence of signs of infection at the envenomation site and are not indicated routinely. If the envenomation is not initially fatal, full recovery occurs within several weeks. Paresthesia is usually the last symptom to resolve.[46]

SEA SNAKES

Sea snakes, which comprise approximately 70 species, are the most abundant and widely dispersed group of poisonous reptiles in the world; most sea snake species are members of the family (Figure 42-5; see color plate). Hydrophiidae and are characterized by vertically flattened tails and nostrils with valvelike flaps. Sea snakes are found predominantly in tropical and subtropical waters in the western Pacific and Indian oceans, often in protected coastal waters and near river mouths.[46] The pelagic sea snake, *Pelamis platurus,* has a remarkably wide geographical range, which reaches the western coasts of North and South America from the Baja peninsula to Ecuador, along with the waters around Hawaii. In the United States, Hawaii is the

only state where sea snakes are found. Internationally, sea snake envenomations occur throughout the serpents' geographical ranges, but accurate data about the incidence of envenomation are not available. Victims most commonly are fishermen bitten while handling nets or after stepping on a snake. Generally, sea snakes are not aggressive and do not strike humans unless provoked.[46]

The venom apparatus of sea snakes is fairly rudimentary, consisting of two to four short, hollow maxillary fangs associated with a pair of venom glands. The venom ducts open near the tips of the fangs. Nearly 80% of sea snake bites fail to produce significant envenomation, and bites may be inconspicuous, painless, and free of edema. However, sea snake venom is extremely potent, and a complete envenomation by an adult sea snake may contain enough venom to kill adult people. The clinically relevant toxins in sea snake venom are neurotoxins and myotoxins. The primary neurotoxin causes peripheral paralysis by competitively binding to postsynaptic nicotinic acetylcholine receptors at the neuromuscular junction. Potent myotoxins account for the significant muscle necrosis, with consequent myoglobinemia and hyperkalemia that may occur following envenomation. Sea snakes are closely related to Australian elapids; some paraspecificity exists between sea snake antivenom and Australian elapid antivenom.[47]

Clinical Features of Sea Snake Envenomation

Symptoms are attributable to multiple organ systems, with neurological symptoms predominating. They may occur as early as 5 minutes or as late as 8 hours following the bite, but they usually occur within 2 hours.[46] Generalized muscle aches and pains and nonspecific weakness are usually the first symptoms, followed by symptoms of anxiety—nausea, vomiting, dizziness, dry throat, shallow breathing, dry throat, and rapid pulse. Muscle pain on movement and stiffness of neck, face, trunk, arm, and thigh may occur. Myoglobinuria may be evident 3 to 6 hours after the envenomation and can lead to secondary renal failure; hyperkalemia and deaths have been reported. Creatine kinase, serum glutamic oxaloacetic transaminase, and potassium levels rise in the serum with muscle necrosis, and leukocytosis higher than 20,000 cu/mm suggests significant envenomation.[46] True paralysis can occur within minutes to hours after the bite and is characterized by blurred vision, mydriasis, ptosis, ophthalmoplegia, drooling, dysphagia, dysarthria, respiratory distress, and finally apnea.[47] The clinical signs include muscle weakness, ascending paralysis, dysphagia, dysarthria, hypersalivation, trismus, ptosis, ophthalmoplegia, areflexia, and respiratory failure. Cardiac arrest may occur due to hyperkalemia.[46]

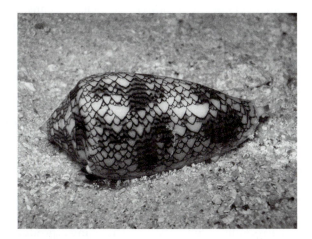

Figure 42-5. Cone shell, *Conus textile.* (see color plate). (Courtesy of Wikipedia.)

Clinical Management of Sea Snake Envenomation

Management consists of first aid application of compression bandages and immobilization of the limb until the patient has reached a medical facility. Attention to airway, breathing, circulation, intravenous access, cardiac monitoring, and continuous pulse oximetry are indicated. An electrocardiogram is useful to look for signs of hyperkalemia, including peaked T waves, a widened QRS complex, or ventricular arrhythmias. Supportive measures include endotracheal intubation and mechanical ventilation, as clinically indicated. Tetanus prophylaxis is important.

Indications for antivenom use are signs of envenomation and include shock, respiratory distress, generalized myalgias, trismus, moderate to severe pain with passive movement of extremities, myoglobinuria, elevated creatine kinase (>600 IU/L), altered level of consciousness, hyperkalemia, or leukocytosis.[47] The antivenom should be administered as soon as possible in these cases. The agent of choice is polyvalent sea snake antivenom against *Enhydrina schistosa* (CSL, Melbourne, Australia). Before antivenom administration, if time permits, skin testing to assess for allergy to horse serum is advised, but it is not mandatory if the patient is unstable. The results of skin testing are not completely reliable. If antivenom is not available, dialysis should be considered since sea snake neurotoxin is of low enough molecular weight to be dialyzable. Furthermore, dialysis can be lifesaving in cases of severe hyperkalemia. Aggressive hydration and diuresis can help promote renal myoglobin clearance. Urine alkalinization may be of some benefit in cases of myoglobinuria. Before the development of sea snake antivenom, the mortality rate associated with sea snake bites was approximately 10%. With timely administration of antivenom and aggressive supportive care, the mortality rate is currently much lower.[48]

STONEFISH

The stonefish is the most dangerous of known venomous fish and is found in the shallow tropical marine waters of the Pacific and Indian oceans, ranging from the Red Sea to the Queensland Great Barrier Reef. It has a mottled greenish to mostly brown color, which aids in its ability to camouflage itself among the rocks of many tropical reefs (Figure 42-6; see color plate). Its main habitat is on coral reefs, near and about rocks, or dormant in the mud or sand.[49,50] Its dorsal area is lined with spines that release the venom, which consists of a mixture of proteins, including the hemolytic stonustoxin, the neurotoxic trachynilysin, and the cardioactive cardioleputin and verrucotoxin.[51]

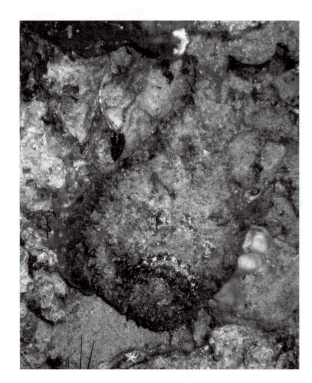

Figure 42-6. Stonefish (see color plate). (Courtesy of Wikipedia.)

The venom is protein based, is thermolabile, and can be partially denatured by the application of a hot compress to the injury site.

Clinical Features of Stonefish Stings

The venom of stonefish causes severe pain, with possible shock, paralysis, and tissue death depending on the depth of the penetration. Severe envenomation can be fatal to humans if not given medical attention within a couple of hours. Immediately after a sting from members of the *Synanceia* (stonefish) genus, excruciating and incapacitating localized pain occurs. This pain may spread to involve the entire limb and regional lymph nodes, peaking around 60 to 90 minutes and lasting up to 12 hours if untreated. Mild subsequent pain may persist for days to weeks.[50] Systemic symptoms of nausea, muscle weakness, and dyspnea may occur. Puncture wounds from the spines are often multiple and have a surrounding ring of bluish cyanotic tissue. Later, edema, erythema, and warmth may involve the entire limb, although it rarely results in tissue necrosis in the absence of secondary infection.[52] Vesicle formation, particularly of the hands, may be followed by rapid tissue sloughing, cellulitis, and surrounding hypesthesia. The stings produced by the spines can also induce respiratory weakness, damage to the cardiovascular system, convulsions, and paralysis, sometimes leading to death. Typically, surviving victims suffer localized nerve damage occasionally leading to atrophy of adjoining muscle tissues. The severity of envenomation depends on multiple factors, including the offending species, the number of stings, and the age and underlying health of the victim.[52]

Clinical Management of Stonefish Stings

Immediate first aid treatment requires immobilization of venom at the penetration site by firm constrictive bandaging or by managed tourniquet sited between wound and proximal flexure. Prehospital care should address recognition of the injury as a potential envenomation, gentle removal of visible spines, direct pressure to control bleeding, administration of analgesia, and transport for definitive medical evaluation. Recognition of serious systemic symptoms and prompt attention to airway, breathing, circulation, cardiopulmonary resuscitation, and treatment for anaphylaxis are lifesaving.[53] Hot water immersion is widely recommended as effective initial treatment for envenomations after removal of visible spines and sheath to inactivate the thermolabile components of the venom. The affected limb should be immersed in water no warmer than 114°F, or 45°C, with care not to inflict thermal burns. Emergency management of stonefish envenomations includes prompt analgesia, wound management, antivenom administration, and supportive treatment for significant envenomations.[54] Wound debridement and surgical removal of embedded spines are indicated when they are in proximity to joints, nerves, or vessels because retained spines continue to envenomate. Retained fragments also act as foreign bodies, causing inflammation and later granuloma formation and leading to delayed healing and secondary infection. Adjunctive regional or local anesthesia offers reliable, prompt, and prolonged analgesia, allowing simultaneous debridement of the wound. Parenteral analgesics and or sedatives may be needed for patients with wounds that are difficult to immerse or anesthetize or for people exhibiting significant anxiety reactions to the envenomation. Tetanus prophylaxis is indicated in all patients with insufficient immunization histories. Stonefish antivenom from Australia's CSL is recommended only for predilution intramuscular usage. In serious envenomations, a slow intravenous administration of antivenom diluted in 50 to 100 mL of isotonic sodium chloride solution and run through at least 20 minutes is preferable.[54] This is a hyperimmunized equine antisera, and there are risks of allergic reaction and serum sickness in the recipient. Skin testing and or pretreatment with subcutaneous epinephrine and an intramuscular antihistamine, adding an intramuscular corticosteroid for known hypersensitivity, should precede administration.[54]

CONCLUSION

Marine stings and envenomation pose significant hazards to unwary travelers and those who use the sea for sport, recreation, or their livelihood. Many are unwittingly stung on accidental contact with various marine stinging organisms. The toxins of these organisms contain many toxic proteins with effects on different organ systems, including the central, peripheral, and autonomic nervous systems. Specific neurotoxins have been identified from the venoms, and their molecular mechanisms have been elucidated. Various neurological clinical manifestations have been described after marine stings and include myopathy, peripheral neuropathy, autonomic dysfunction, seizures, coma, and death. Jellyfish, the blue-ringed octopus, cone shells, sea snakes, and stonefish are some marine organisms whose stings result in neurological symptoms and signs. Guidelines exist for general principles of management of marine stings and specific treatments of neurological and other organ system–related complications. Specific antivenins are commercially available for box jellyfish, sea snake, and stonefish envenomations and should be used when indicated. Prevention includes awareness of the habitats, appearances and dangers associated with marine stinging organisms, and avoidance of contact with them. An interesting result of research into the venoms of marine stinging organisms has been the recent finding of the therapeutic potential of derivatives from the toxins, and the first in this line has been the production of a potent analgesic from the conotoxin of the cone shell.

REFERENCES

1. Williamson JA, Fenner PJ, Burnett JW. *Venomous and Poisonous Marine Animals: A Medical and Biological Handbook.* Sydney, Australia: New South Wales Press; 1996.
2. Holstein T, Tardent P. An ultrahigh-speed analysis of exocytosis: nematocyst discharge. *Science.* 1984;223:830–833.
3. Hessinger HA. Nematocyst venoms and toxins. In: Hessinger DA, Lenhoff HM, eds. *Biology of Nematocysts.* San Diego, Calif: Academic Press; 1988:333–369.
4. Burnett JW, Bloom DA, Imafuku S, et al. Coelenterate venom research 1991–1995: clinical, chemical and immunological aspects. *Toxicon.* 1996;34:1377–1383.
5. Burnett JW. Human injuries following jellyfish stings. *Md Med J.* 1992;41:509–513.
6. Chand RP, Victor R. Marine stings in the Gulf of Oman. In: Williamson JA, Fenner PJ, Burnett JW. *Venomous and Poisonous Marine Animals: A Medical and Biological Handbook.* Sydney, Australia: New South Wales Press; 1996.
7. Fenner PJ, Williamson JA. Worldwide deaths and severe envenomation from jellyfish stings. *Med J Aust.* 1996;165:658–661.
8. Burnett JW. Clinical manifestations of jellyfish envenomation. *Hydrobiologia.* 1991;216/217:629–635.

9. Burnett JW, Calton GJ, Burnett HW. Jellyfish envenomation syndromes. *J Am Acad Dermatol.* 1986;14:100–106.

10. Forrester MB. Epidemiology of jellyfish stings reported to poison centers in Texas. *Hum Exp Toxicol.* 2006;25:183–186.

11. Fenner PJ, Hadok JC. Fatal envenomation by jellyfish causing Irukandji syndrome. *Med J Aust.* 2002;177:362–363.

12. Stein MR, Marraccini JV, Rothschild NE, Burnett JW. Fatal Portuguese man-o'-war *(Physalia physalis)* envenomation. *Ann Emerg Med.* 1989;18:312–315.

13. Edwards L, Hessinger DA. Portuguese man-of-war *(Physalia physalis)* venom induces calcium influx into cells by permeabilizing plasma membranes. *Toxicon.* 2000;38:1015–1028.

14. Tibballs J. Australian venomous jellyfish, envenomation syndromes, toxins and therapy. *Toxicon.* 2006;48:830–859.

15. Fenner PJ, Heazlewood RJ. Papilloedema and coma in a child: undescribed symptoms of the "Irukandji" syndrome. *Med J Aust.* 1997;167:650.

16. Sánchez-Rodríguez J, Torrens E, Segura-Puertas L. Partial purification and characterization of a novel neurotoxin and three cytolysins from box jellyfish *(Carybdea marsupialis)* nematocyst venom. *Arch Toxicol.* 2006;80:163–168.

17. Chand RP, Selliah K. Reversible parasympathetic dysautonomia following stinging attributed to the box jelly fish *(Chironex fleckeri)*. *Aust NZ J Med.* 1984;14:673–675.

18. Ponampalam R. An unusual case of paralytic ileus after jellyfish envenomation. *Emerg Med J.* 2002;19:357–358.

19. Burnett JW, Weinrich D, Williamson JA, Fenner PJ, Lutz LL, Bloom DA. Autonomic neurotoxicity of jellyfish and marine animal venoms. *Clin Auton Res.* 1998;8:125–130.

20. Burnett JW. Dysphonia: a new addition to jellyfish envenomation syndromes. *Wilderness Environ Med.* 2005;16:117–118.

21. Burnett HW, Burnett JW. Prolonged blurred vision following coelenterate envenomation. *Toxicon.* 1990;28:731–733.

22. Burnett JW. Prolonged urinary incontinence and biliary dyskinesia following abdominal contact with jellyfish tentacles. *Wilderness Environ Med.* 2006;17:180–186.

23. Little M, Pereira P, Mulcahy R, Cullen P, Carrette T, Seymour J. Severe cardiac failure associated with presumed jellyfish sting. Irukandji syndrome? *Anaesth Intensive Care.* 2003;31:642–647.

24. Laing JH, Harrison DH. Envenomation by the box jellyfish: an unusual cause of ulnar nerve palsy. *J R Soc Med.* 1991;84:115–116.

25. Peel N, Kandler R. Localized neuropathy following jellyfish sting. *Postgrad Med J.* 1990;66:953–954.

26. Cuypers E, Yanagihara A, Karlsson E, Tytgat J. Jellyfish and other cnidarian envenomations cause pain by affecting TRPV1 channels. *FEBS Lett.* 2006;580:5728–5732.

27. Endean R. Separation of two myotoxins from nematocysts of the box jellyfish *(Chironex fleckeri)*. *Toxicon.* 1987;25:483–492.

28. Ghosh TK, Gomes A, Chaudhuri AK. Isolation of a toxin from jellyfish *Acromitus rabanchatu* and its effect on skeletal muscle. *Toxicon.* 1993;31:873–880.

29. Watters MR, Stommel EW. Marine neurotoxins: envenomations and contact toxins. *Curr Treat Options Neurol.* 2004;6:115–123.

30. Nimorakiotakis B, Winkel KD. Marine envenomations: I. Jellyfish. *Aust Fam Physician.* 2003;32:969–974.

31. Collins SP, Comis A, Marshall M, Hartwick RF, Howden ME. Monoclonal antibodies neutralizing the haemolytic activity of box jellyfish *(Chironex fleckeri)* tentacle extracts. *Comp Biochem Physiol B.* 1993;106:67–70.

32. Bloom DA, Burnett JW, Hebel JR, Alderslade P. Effects of verapamil and CSL antivenom on *Chironex fleckeri* (box-jellyfish)–induced mortality. *Toxicon.* 1999;37:1621–1626.

33. Salleo A, La Spada G, Barbera R. Gadolinium is a powerful blocker of the activation of nematocytes of *Pelagia noctiluca*. *J Exp Biol.* 1994;187:201–206.

34. Williamson JA. The blue-ringed octopus. *Med J Aust.* 1984;140:308–309.

35. Sheumack DD, Howden ME, Spence I, Quinn RJ. Maculotoxin: a neurotoxin from the venom glands of the octopus *Hapalochlaena maculosa* identified as tetrodotoxin. *Science.* 1978;199:188–189.

36. Yotsu-Yamashita M, Mebs D, Flachsenberger W. Distribution of tetrodotoxin in the body of the blue-ringed octopus *(Hapalochlaena maculosa)*. *Toxicon.* 2007;49:410–412.

37. Williamson JA. The blue-ringed octopus bite and envenomation syndrome. *Clin Dermatol.* 1987;5:127–133.

38. Walker DG. Survival after severe envenomation by the blue-ringed octopus *(Hapalochlaena maculosa)*. *Med J Aust.* 1983;2:663–665.

39. Halstead BW. *Dangerous Marine Animals that Bite, Sting, Shock, and Are Non-Edible.* Centreville, Md: Cornell Maritime Press; 1980.

40. Nimorakiotakis B, Winkel KD. Marine envenomations: II. Other marine envenomations. *Aust Fam Physician.* 2003;32:975–979.

41. Terlau H, Olivera BM. Conus venoms: a rich source of novel ion channel-targeted peptides. *Physiol Rev.* 2004;84:41–68.

42. Layer RT, Wagstaff JD, White HS. Conantokins: peptide antagonists of NMDA receptors. *Curr Med Chem.* 2004;11:3073–3084.

43. Watters MR. Tropical marine neurotoxins: venoms to drugs. *Semin Neurol.* 2005;25:278–289.

44. Auerbach PS. Marine envenomations. *N Engl J Med.* 1991;325:486–493.

45. Rice RD, Halstead BW. Report of fatal cone shell sting by *Conus geographus* Linnaeus. *Toxicon.* 1968;5:223–224.

46. Brown CK, Shepherd SM: Marine trauma, envenomations and intoxications. *Emerg Med Clin North Am.* 1992;10:385–408.

47. Auerbach PS. Management of wilderness and environmental emergencies. In: ***, eds. *Wilderness Medicine.* 4th ed. St. Louis: Mosby; 2001:1492–1497.

48. Guenin DG, Auerbach PS. Trauma and envenomations from marine fauna. In: Tintinalli ***, et al., eds. *Emergency Medicine: A Comprehensive Study Guide.* 4th ed. ***: McGraw-Hill; 1996:868–873.

49. Cunningham P, Goetz P. *Pisces Guide to Venomous & Toxic Marine Life of the World.* Houston: Pisces Books; 1996:102–114.

50. Burnett JW. Aquatic adversaries: stonefish. *Cutis.* 1998;62:269–270.

51. Khoo HE. Bioactive proteins from stonefish venom. *Clin Exp Pharmacol Physiol.* 2002;29:802–806.

52. Perkins RA, Morgan SS. Poisoning, envenomation, and trauma from marine creatures. *Am Fam Physician.* 2004;69:885–890.

53. Lyon RM. Stonefish poisoning. *Wilderness Environ Med.* 2004;15:284–288.

54. Currie BJ. Marine antivenoms. *J Toxicol Clin Toxicol.* 2003;41:301–308.

CHAPTER 43

Neurotoxic Animal Poisons and Venoms

Terri L. Postma

INTRODUCTION

The world is filled with opportunities to encounter venomous and poisonous animals. Throughout history, these creatures permeate mythology and theological writings and have been used in zootherapy.[1] Medicinal uses have been recorded for many. Snakes, for example, are mentioned in both the Bible and the Talmud and represent modern medicine in the form of the caduceus. The scorpion was used by early Muslim physicians. The venom of the giant centipede is used as a poor man's cancer treatment in India. The toxin of the *Bufo* toad is found in love elixirs sold in China. The witches' coven in Shakespeare's *Macbeth* makes reference to the salamander as they mix their brew.

As is clear throughout this chapter, the epidemiology of envenomations is challenging. When regions attempt to keep statistics on envenomations and poisonings, they are often inaccurate. Many fatal encounters occur in remote areas of the world and go unreported. Often, the victim is unaware of an envenomation causing local or mild systemic reactions or the history of bite or sting is difficult to verify, particularly in the case of children. Therefore, world experts vary widely in their estimates. Consensus opinion estimates 50,000 fatalities annually from envenomations and a total number of cases exceeding 1 million.[2]

The toxins are produced for the survival of the species; that is, toxins are mainly used for obtaining sustenance, for defense of territory or against predators, and for increasing the chance of species survival. These toxins have developed in fascinating ways. The actions of toxins are complex and are the object of study around the world. Studies of these toxins have given us insights into coagulopathies, neurotransmitter release and neuromuscular junction physiology, and pathophysiology of pain. Many toxins are under investigation for their potential use in treating diseases such as pain syndromes and stroke. Others, such as some spider invertebrate-specific toxins, have the potential to be developed as insecticides. Although many components of venom produce clinically significant effects, this chapter focuses on neurotoxin function, clinical effect, and treatment. Similarly, although there is a vast and fascinating array of aquatic creatures that produce toxins of clinical significance and importance, discussion in this chapter is limited to encounters with land-dwelling creatures.

The basic principles of treatment are generally the same for all envenomations or poisonings. Recognition of envenomation and correct identification of the species is paramount to accurate treatment and prognosis.

Knowledge of appropriate first aid measures and immediate transportation of the victim to a full-care facility is also important. First aid measures as outlined by the World Health Organization (International Programme on Chemical Safety) include patient reassurance, immobilization of the wound, avoidance of injury from application of a tourniquet or excision of the wound, avoidance of aspirin for pain treatment, removal of restrictive jewelry and watches, and basic life support.[3]

Once transported to a hospital or clinic, a detailed history should be obtained, including species, amount of exposure (i.e., one or multiple injections, quantity of consumption), and time of envenomation or poisoning, which helps in determining prognosis. Onset, timing, and progression of symptoms should be documented. Specific symptoms may give clues as to the type of toxin encountered. Ptosis, for example, is a specific clue indicating a neurotoxic envenomation. Laboratory workup should include complete blood count, comprehensive metabolic panel, coagulation analysis including fibrinogen, and creatine kinase. Venom detection kits are available in some parts of the world, notably Australia for identification of snakebite, and provide timely and useful information.

Supportive care and symptomatic treatment are the mainstays for victims and may require a host of specialists: hematologists, nephrologists, cardiologists, plastic surgeons, neurologists, and intensive care specialists, to name a few. Because some toxin effects are delayed, no matter how clinically stable a patient appears when presenting to the emergency room, that patient should be given immediate attention and observed closely for signs and symptoms of cardiac and respiratory dysfunction, which can develop suddenly. When antivenom is available, consideration must be given to accuracy of species identification, severity of illness, and risks associated with treatment.

ARACHNIDS

Spiders

It is impossible to estimate the number of spider bites sustained by humans annually. Most are insignificant, causing only mild local pain, and go unreported. Several attempts have been made to report the epidemiology of spider bite. In 2006, the American Association of Poison Control Centers reported that 30% of more than 14,600 spider bites in the United States were identified as *Latrodectus* (black widow) or *Loxosceles* (brown recluse) spiders. Of those, 17.5% resulted in clinically moderate to severe reactions with no deaths recorded.[4] In Australia, a prospective trial revealed that 84% of severe envenomations over a 27-month period were perpetrated by *Latrodectus hasselti* (redback) spiders.[5] Over a 100-year period, 26 deaths were recorded in Australia, attributable to *Atrax* species.[6] In Chile, a 40-year retrospective analysis of approximately 1300 bites revealed only 45% could be attributed to spiders, the majority from *Loxosceles* species.[7] The Brazilian Health Ministry states that 4836 spider bites were reported over a 10-year period, revealing 38% attributable to *Phoneutria* species, and from 1990 to 1993, 42% of nearly 11,400 spider bites were attributable to or suspected to be perpetrated by *Phoneutria* species.[8,9]

With few exceptions, all spiders produce venom. Like snakes, most spider bites are considered "dry," or ineffective. Spider bites are made even more ineffective by the inability of their chelicerae (fangs) to penetrate through clothing and skin. Fortunately, therefore, less than 25 genera pose a medically significant threat to humans. A few families of spiders cause primarily neurotoxic effects in humans: Theridiidae, Hexathelidae, Ctenidae, and Actinopodidae. Within these families, three genera (*Atrax*, *Latrodectus*, and *Phoneutria*) are known to cause death in humans. Two others (*Hadronyche* and *Missulena*) may be responsible for causing severe symptoms and possible death.

Other families cause primarily necrotoxic effects: Agelenidae, Theraphosidae, and Sicariidae. Within them, envenomation from only one genus (*Loxosceles*) causes known death. Although several species of wolf spiders, hobo spiders, yellow sac spiders, and others have reportedly resulted in severe systemic symptoms or local necrosis, prospective trials have not clearly confirmed that they are a great threat and most appear to cause only local pain or mild systemic symptoms.[10,11] This chapter focuses on spiders responsible for producing clinically severe neurological symptoms. The most vulnerable to severe effects are children and the chronically ill or elderly.

Predominantly Neurotoxic Spider Envenomations

Family: Ctenidae
Genus: *Phoneutria*
Species: *P. nigriventer, P. keyserlingi, P. fera* (Brazilian wandering spider, Brazilian armed spider, banana spider)

Family: Theridiidae
Genus: *Achaearanea, Latrodectus, Steatoda*
Species: *L. mactans* (black widow spider), *L. hasselti* (redback spider), *L. tredecimguttatus* (malmignatte or European black widow spider), *L. indistinctus* (button spider), *Steatoda* species (false widow spiders)

Family: Hexathelidae
Genus: *Atrax, Hadronyche*
Species: *A. robustus* (Sydney funnel-web spider), *H. versuta* (Blue Mountains funnel-web spider), *H. formidabilis* and *cerberea* (northern and southern tree-dwelling funnel-web spider), *H. infensa* (Toowoomba funnel-web spider)

Family: Actinopodidae
Genus: *Missulena*
Species: *M. bradleyi* (eastern mouse spider)

Toxins A review article by Rash and Hodgson[12] divides neurotoxins by site of action:

1. Sodium channel slow inactivators—These toxins are isolated from *Atrax* and *Hadronyche* species(d-atracotoxin, robustoxin, versutoxin), and *P. nigriventer* (PhTx2). d-Atracotoxin inhibits tetrodotoxin-sensitive sodium channels; slows activation, causing prolonged action potential duration; and causes repetitive firing in autonomic and motor nerve fibers.[13] PhTx2 causes lacrimation, hind limb paralysis, priapism, convulsions, and death when injected into mice.[14] Venom from *M. bradleyi* facilitates neurotransmitter release in both smooth and skeletal muscle.[15]

2. Glutamate receptor toxins—Glutamate is an important neurotransmitter of the invertebrate neuromuscular system, as well as in the central nervous system (CNS) of mammals. PhTx4 was isolated from *P. nigriventer* and was demonstrated to inhibit glutamate uptake in the rat CNS.[16]

3. Calcium channel blockers—ω-Agatoxins and other fractions from *Agelenopsis* species have been shown to block frog neuromuscular transmission via their action on the L-type calcium channel.[17] They also block calcium channels in guinea pig cerebellar Purkinje cells.[18] Several fractions isolated from *P. nigriventer* block calcium channels and induce paralysis in mice.[14,19] HWTX-1, a peptide isolated from *Selenocosmia huwena* (Chinese bird spider), exhibits neuromuscular blocking activity in mice.[20]

4. Toxins stimulating neurotransmitter release—a-Latrotoxin (*Latrodectus* species) stimulates massive presynaptic transmitter release (acetylcholine, norepinephrine, glutamate, dopamine, γ-aminobutyric acid) throughout the nervous system by means of exocytosis via calcium dependent and independent mechanisms, resulting in vesicle depletion and paralysis.[21,22]

Several other neurotoxins have been identified that affect the mammalian nervous system via potassium or chloride receptor block, by postsynaptic acetylcholine (ACh) channel block, or by mechanisms not clearly understood. Still more neurotoxins have been identified that exhibit their effects primarily or exclusively on the invertebrate neuromuscular systems in various ways, leading to the suggestion that insect-specific compounds may be developed for use in agriculture.[23,24]

Clinical Presentation

Brazilian Wandering, Armed, or Banana Spider *Phoneutria* are impressive spiders reaching body sizes up to 3.5 centimeters and leg spans up to 15 centimeters. They are nocturnal, hunting at night, and hiding in dark places during the day. They do not make webs, thus the designation

---

Box 1 Wandering Spiders in the News

In March 2007, a woman from Snoqualmie, Washington, bought a box of bananas from a local store. Several days later, she found a quarter-sized egg sac in one bunch of bananas and a dead spider on the kitchen floor among her children's toys. A local expert identified the spider as a species of *Phoneutria*.

In April 2005, a chef in the United Kingdom was bitten by a giant spider while cleaning a freezer at work. Thinking his friends would never believe such a story, he took a picture of it with his cell phone. Soon after, his hand began to swell and he experienced tremors, hypertension, and lightheadedness. He reported feeling tightness in his chest and hypertension. Hospital staff sent the picture to experts who identified the spider as *P. nigriventer* and recommended appropriate antivenom and treatment.[25,26]

"wandering," and are known to turn up outside their South American territory via transport in banana shipments (Box 1). They are aggressive, and their name, *Phoneutria*, is Greek for "murderess." Their large chelicerae inflict painful stings, causing immediate sweating and local piloerection. Within 30 minutes, symptoms become systemic and include hyper- or hypotension, tachy- or bradycardia, diaphoresis, nausea, abdominal cramping, hypothermia, priapism, vertigo, convulsions, blurred vision, and rarely, death.[9,27]

Widow and False Widow Spider Spiders from the *Latrodectus* species are found worldwide. Some better known examples are the North American *L. mactans* (Figure 43-1), the Mediterranean *L. tredecimguttatus*, the African *L. indistinctus*, and the Australian *L. hasselti*.

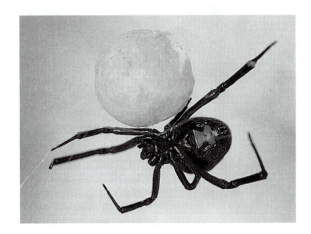

Figure 43-1. Example of a black widow (*Latrodectus mactans*) spider with egg sac. (Reprinted from Auerbach P. *Wilderness Medicine*. 5th ed. St. Louis: Mosby; 2007.)

Females are always more venomous than males. These spiders make webs in various places: in trees, on fences, under stones, and in cracks and crevices of buildings. Thus, they are suited for both urban and rural living and come into contact with humans often. Naturally timid, they prefer to run but will bite if trapped.

Latrodectism (Figure 43-2), describes the clinical syndrome following envenomation by widow spiders of the *Latrodectus* species. Victims experience generalized pain and muscle cramping within minutes to hours of the bite, and systemic effects may be delayed by as much as 12 hours. Muscle spasms spread from the bite site, and the patient may experience classic symptoms such as a rigid abdomen, priapism, or "facies latrodectismica" (contortion of face resembling tetanus, also associated with lacrimation, photophobia, and miosis).[28] Other symptoms include diaphoresis, nausea, vomiting, paresthesias, tremor, malaise, restlessness, insomnia, acute psychosis, delirium, hypertension, oliguria, and brady- or tachycardia, all of which usually resolve over 3 to 7 days.[2,28,29] Death by *Latrodectus* species has been well documented by various causes, including primary neurological dysfunction.[2]

Steatodism describes the clinical syndrome following envenomation by the false widow. It is similar to latrodectism, but symptoms are milder. Victims experience moderate to severe local pain, nausea, headache, fatigue, and malaise.[30]

Funnel-Web Spider

The large funnel-web spiders (body length 1.5 to 4.5 centimeters) are exclusively found in Australia, and all species of *Atrax* and *Hadronyche* are potentially dangerous to man. The best studied is *A. robustus*, which has a suspected envenoming rate of 10% to 25%.[31] Males have more potent venom than females and are therefore more responsible for severe envenoming.[6] Fast-onset clinical reactions range from minor or local and mild to severe and systemic, including autonomic effects (diaphoresis, salivation, lacrimation, piloerection, miosis, mydriasis), cardiovascular effects (hypertension, hypotension, tachycardia, bradycardia), neurological effects (pupil dilation, headache, oral paresthesia, muscle fasciculations, muscle spasms, confusion, cerebral edema), and pulmonary edema. Other systemic complaints include vomiting, abdominal pain, local pain, and metabolic acidosis.[6,11]

Mouse Spider

In a review of the literature, most mouse spider *(Missulena)* bites resulted in minor or moderate local effects, such as paresthesias, numbness, or pain. Rarely, patients reported mild systemic symptoms such as headache, nausea, or vomiting. One case of severe systemic effects was reported in a 19-month-old child, who then responded to funnel-web antivenom.[31a] The review concluded that, overall, mouse spider bites do not appear to be a major medical problem, causing only 2.5% severe envenoming compared to 10% to 25% for funnel-web spiders.[31]

Treatment

Brazilian Wandering, Armed, or Banana Spider

For *Phoneutria* species, wound cleansing, immobilization, antihistamines, opiates for pain, tetanus prophylaxis, and antivenom are available and useful.[29] In Brazil, local anesthetic nerve blocks have been performed to alleviate pain.[31b] Most victims recover within 24 to 48 hours with supportive care measures alone, but approximately 2.3% require antivenom, which is available for severe envenoming.[9]

Widow and False Widow Spider

Most victims of *Latrodectus* bites present with only mild or moderate symptoms and may warrant observation for 3 to 6 hours. Be aware, however, that rare cases have developed symptoms up to 24 hours following the bite. The definitive treatment for latrodectism is antivenom,[32] the

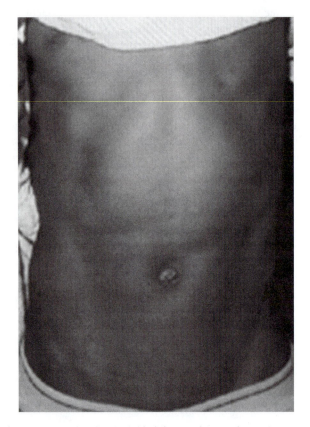

Figure 43-2. The classic rigid abdomen that results severe envenomation by *Latrodectus* species and is part of the clinical syndrome known as latrodectism. (Reprinted from Habif T. *Clinical Dermatology.* 4th ed. St. Louis: Mosby; 2004.)

results of which can be dramatic, reversing symptoms in as little as a few minutes. Widow antivenom has also shown excellent cross-reactivity within the Theridiidae family and has successfully treated severe envenomation by false widow bites.[30] Use of antivenom for widow bites carries a very low risk of adverse events, as demonstrated by Sutherland and Trinca,[32] who concluded that only 0.54% of 2062 patients receiving antivenom for widow bites developed anaphylaxis and that this was a result of giving undiluted antivenom IV instead of IM. Despite this minimal risk, most experts advocate administration in only severe cases.[11,27,33,34] Other treatment measures for pain control have included the use of neostigmine, opioid analgesics, calcium gluconate, or muscle relaxors, which may have limited efficacy and pose other risks to the patient.[21,35] Home remedies have included immersion in hot water and dancing, although some have proposed the bite of a spider was merely an excuse to dance in an era of prohibition (Box 2). Overall, prognosis is good, even in those presenting with systemic symptoms, with a death rate of only 5% to 8% in studies conducted before the availability of antivenom.[37]

Funnel-Web Spider   The Sutherland technique of pressure immobilization bandage, developed as first aid for snake bite, is recommended for initial treatment of funnel-web spider bite.[21,38] Antivenom has become an effective therapy for patients exhibiting systemic symptoms[21,39,40] and has been shown to shorten the course of symptoms and reduce hospital length of stay.[22] In a review by Isbister et al.,[6] 28 of 29 (97%) patients experienced a complete reversal of symptoms in response to the antivenom, while adverse events were recorded in only 3 of 75 patients. Laboratory studies can give an indication of systemic involvement and should include complete blood count, comprehensive metabolic panel, coagulation studies, creatine kinase, arterial blood gas, and urinary catecholamines. Other treatment is symptomatic and supportive as needed.

Box 2   Tarantism

Tarantism is a disorder characterized by frenzied dancing in an effort to cure the effects of spider bite or scorpion sting. It is thought to have originated in southern Italy as early as AD 1000 but reached epidemic proportions in the seventeenth century. The curative jig has since been named tarantella. Whether it developed as an attempt to dispel the toxic effects of *Latrodectus* or an effort to circumvent local restrictions on dancing is debated. Regardless, it remains an intriguing history that can be further explored by reading Russell's excellent review.[36]

Mouse Spider and Other Funnel Web Spiders   Treatment for *Missulena* and *Hadronyche* species is primarily supportive care. For rare cases of severe systemic symptoms, consider funnel-web antivenom, which has been successfully used.[10,24,28,41] Successful use of *A. robustus* antivenom for reversal of symptoms by other funnel-web species was also suggested by in vitro studies.[40]

Predominantly Necrotoxic Spiders with Some Neurotoxicity

Family: Sicariidae
Genus: *Loxosceles*
Species: *L. reclusa* (brown recluse spider), *L. laeta, L. gaucho, L. intermedia*

Toxin   Various spiders are blamed for unexplained necrotic lesions of the skin, but few have been proven.[11] There have been cases of misdiagnosis, and the clinician should consider other causes of necrotic lesions when the spider was not definitively identified.[11,42] The best described spiders of this group are *Loxosceles* species, which are found in the tropical and subtropical regions of the Western Hemisphere. *Loxosceles* species are shy but ubiquitous, being found in both rural and urban settings, and they thrive within human habitats. They are rarely the cause of serious human envenomations. In fact, not a single envenomation in more than 6 years was reported by one household in Kansas found to be infested with more than 2000 *L. reclusa*.[43] Sphingomyelinase D, isolated from the venom of *Loxosceles* species, is thought to be responsible for spreading necrosis.

Clinical Presentation   The brown recluse *(L. reclusa)* is shy, typically only biting when trapped. The bite is rarely felt, but evidence and reason for the bite are often discovered when the spider corpse is later found in the bedsheets or under clothing. Bites range from unremarkable to progressive local necrosis. Rarely, systemic symptoms can arise 2 to 3 days following the bite, and the syndrome is referred to as loxoscelism. Systemic symptoms can include nausea, vomiting, arthralgias, disseminated intravascular coagulation, vascular or renal damage, and convulsions.[27,44] Occasional deaths have been reported, notably in South America.[21]

Treatment   Antivenom is available, but efficacy reports are mixed and controlled studies are needed to better determine the role it plays.[45] It may only be useful in patients exhibiting severe necrosis and systemic effects and when given within 4 hours of the bite.[29] Treatment should include elevation and immobilization of limb without pressure, analgesics (not antiplatelets) for pain control, antihistamines, and tetanus prophylaxis.[27] Patients may require other supportive measures, such as blood transfusion or hemodialysis. Necrotic lesions should be monitored carefully for secondary infection, and IV antibiotics may be necessary. Studies have not supported the use of steroids, early surgical excision, dapsone, or hyperbaric oxygen.[11,46]

Scorpions

Family: Buthidae
Genus: *Androctonus, Buthotus (Hottentotta),Buthus, Centruroides, Leiurus, Mesobuthus, Parabuthus, Tityus*
Species: *A. australis* (yellow fat-tailed scorpion), *A. crassicauda, B. tamulus* (Indian red scorpion) *C. exilicauda* (or *C. sculpturatus*, Arizona bark scorpion), *C. suffusus* (Durango scorpion), other *Centruroides* species, *L. quinquestriatus* (deathstalker), *M. tamulus, P. granulatus, P. transvaalicus, T. trinitatus, T. serrulatus* (Brazilian yellow scorpion), other *Tityus* species

Family: Scorpionidae
Genus: *Hemiscorpius, Heterometrus, Pandinus*
Species: *H. swammerdami, H. bengalensis*

Commonly thought of as arid-region dwellers, scorpions are amazingly adaptable and are found in tropical and subtropical regions and even the Himalayas. A vast majority of neurotoxic species are found in the Buthidae family (Figure 43-3A and B;), although notable exceptions are found in the Scorpionidae family. Scorpions envenomate humans via accidental contact and pose mortality risk to the very young, infirm, or elderly. Stings are commonly reported in Central and South America, the southwestern United States, Africa, India, the Middle East, and Asia. Worldwide epidemiological data are unreliable since many stings and deaths occur in rural areas and go unreported; however, it is estimated that 5000 deaths due to scorpion stings occur yearly.[47]

Scorpions grasp with their claws and then sting by arching their tails over their heads. *Parabuthus* species is unique in its ability to spray aerosolized venom up to 2 feet. While every scorpion should be treated with caution, an interesting evolutionary development seems to have occurred and may be applied as a rule of thumb: the more slender the claw, the more deadly the sting.

Toxin

Like many toxins found in the wild, scorpion venom contains several substances, including histamine releasers, protease inhibitors, serotonin, phospholipase, and hyaluronidase.[48,49] Various neurotoxic substances have also been isolated from scorpion venom.

Most scorpion neurotoxins appear to affect the presynaptic voltage-gated sodium and potassium channels, as well as calcium-activated potassium channels of peripheral nerves and muscles.[50-53] The synergistic actions result in persistent depolarization and repetitive firing, with subsequent autonomic neurotransmitter (notably ACh and norepinephrine) release.[49] Interesting selective differences are seen in scorpion toxins for vertebrate versus invertebrate sodium channels, leading some to suggest that the study of scorpion venom may be used in the development of novel insecticides.[54,55]

Other compounds from Scorpionidae family venom have been isolated that appear to bind to postsynaptic muscarinic receptors, thus directly affecting the autonomic nervous system.[49]

Clinical Presentation

Most scorpion stings are limited to severe localized pain or paresthesias.[47] Systemic effects are less common, but when they occur, they can be lethal—typically appearing in less than 6 hours and resolving over days. Neurotoxins in scorpion venom can produce massive catecholamine release, particularly in children, creating an "autonomic storm" in

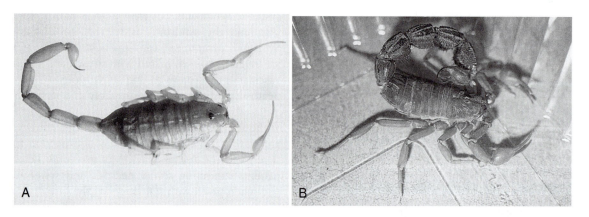

Figure 43-3. Examples of neurotoxic scorpions: Arizona bark scorpion (*Centruroides exilicauda; A*) and South African (*Parabuthus transvaalicus; B*). Note the fine pincers, which are typical for highly venomous species of scorpion. (Reprinted from Auerbach P. *Wilderness Medicine.* 5th ed. St. Louis: Mosby; 2007.)

which both the sympathetic and the parasympathetic nervous systems are overstimulated.[49,56] Sympathetic overstimulation causes tachycardia and cardiac dysfunction,[56] and hypertension is sometimes so severe that it results in encephalopathy.[64] This has been well described following stings from scorpions such as *M. tamulus, L. quinquestriatus,* and *A. australis.*[56,57] Parasympathetic overdrive results in salivation, bronchospasm, dysphagia, diaphoresis, hypotension, and severe pulmonary edema. Other systemic symptoms include thermoregulatory dysfunction, priapism, restlessness or agitation, roving eye movements, encephalopathy, photophobia, nystagmus, convulsions or severe trembling that can be mistaken for seizures, and coma.[57–59]

Treatment

As always, identification of the species of scorpion is extremely helpful in determining prognosis. The victim should undergo careful examination and observation for systemic symptoms. Localized pain can be treated with analgesics, but CNS-depressing medications should be avoided.[60,61] For severe systemic reactions, treatment can be difficult. Nearly every system can be affected, and the patient must be monitored for lethal arrhythmias, respiratory failure, and acid–base disturbances. Neurological manifestations, as an isolated effect or often as a result of cardiac or pulmonary dysfunction, are associated with poor outcomes.[57,62] In a retrospective study, Biswal et al.[63] found that children displaying systemic reactions from scorpion sting and who received antihistamines and steroids before arrival at the hospital had a worse outcome compared to those that did not. Similarly, Curry et al.[60] report that they have seen no benefit from these medications or good rationalization for their use based on the pathophysiology of scorpion venom action.

Gueron[56] recommends an "intensive supportive approach directed toward the overstimulated autonomic nervous system," i.e., control of blood pressure and pulmonary edema with agents such as hydralazine, dobutamine, prazosin, or nifedipine. Indeed, neurological symptoms often improve with this approach.[57,64] Prazosin therapy in particular is recommended based on its pharmacokinetic profile,[61] and those using prazosin therapy report significantly improved outcomes in children exhibiting systemic symptoms, especially if initiated early.[63,65,66]

Recommendations for antivenom use vary geographically. Controversy exists over its use not only because of the potential for anaphylaxis and serum sickness but also because of cost and efficacy. Delays in administration greater than 1 hour appear to hamper its effectiveness.[47] Once the toxin has triggered an autonomic storm, antivenom may be of limited use. Although in a shortcut review of the literature, Foex and Wallis[67,68] reported that IV antivenom appears to reduce serum venom concentrations, they also concluded that there was little evidence to suggest antivenom administration improves clinical outcome. However, one large prospective trial, which looked at the effect of a uniform antivenom treatment protocol of more than 2000 cases in Saudi Arabia, reported a lower incidence of systemic symptoms following IV antivenom administration, a significant overall reduction in mortality, and only mild secondary early reactions that could be medically managed.[61] Similarly, Curry et al.[60] reported that nearly all patients receiving IV antivenom therapy for severe *C. sculpturatus* envenomations had resolution of neurological symptoms within an hour and only mild side effects. Likewise, others in Mexico routinely treat scorpion sting victims with antivenom and report good results.[69] Most experts are in agreement that antivenom should be strongly considered when life-threatening systemic symptoms are present.[69]

As a penetrating wound, consideration should be given for tetanus vaccination in scorpion stings. Prognosis is generally good if the victim survives 24 to 48 hours without severe systemic complications from the sting.

Ticks

Family: Ixodid (hard), Argasid (soft)
Genus: *Amblyomma, Argas, Dermacentor, Haemaphysalis, Hyalomma, Ixodes, Ornithodoros, Rhipicentor, Rhipicephalus*
Species: *A. americanum* (Lone Star tick), *A. maculatum, D. andersoni* (Rocky Mountain wood tick), *D. variabilis* (American dog tick), *H. transiens, H. truncatum* (bontpoot tick), *I. scapularis* (black-legged tick or deer tick), *I. holocyclus* (Australian marsupial tick), *I. pacificus* (western black-legged tick), *I. cornuatus*

In addition to the number of well-known infectious diseases transmitted by various tick species that cause neurological deficits, more than 60 species of ticks produce toxins are capable of producing what is known as *tick paralysis*[70] (Figure 43-4A); however, only approximately 25 have been documented to do so.[71–74] The tick emits the toxin from its salivary glands, the largest organ in its body, during a blood meal, resulting in progressive ascending paralysis and death if not removed. Ticks with toxins have a worldwide distribution, and tick paralysis is not an uncommon problem for domestic and companion animals. Fortunately, tick paralysis in humans is relatively rare, although there have been occasional outbreaks.[73,75,76] Those at greatest risk seem to be small children and those exposed to areas with a high tick burden, with peak incidence in spring and summer. A general rule is the longer the attachment for feeding, the greater the likelihood of paralysis. Therefore, tick paralysis is reported most often as a result of gravid female attachment, although there are isolated reports in the literature of a male tick *(H. transiens)*, nongravid females, and ticks in

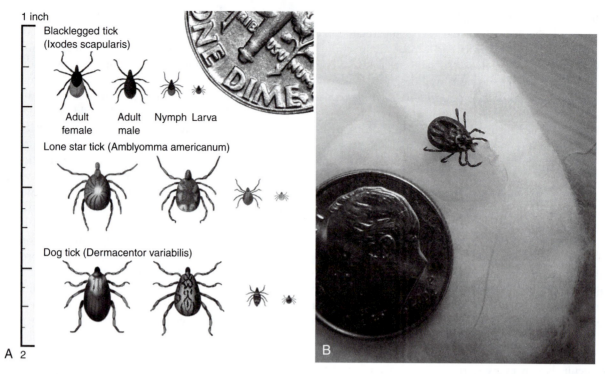

Figure 43-4. *A,* The size and stages of various tick species that are commonly known to cause tick paralysis. *B,* In addition to transmitting disease, the American dog tick *(Dermacentor variabilis)* can cause tick paralysis. This is an adult female removed from the author's dog. Note the intact mouth parts embedded in the dermis of the host. (*A,* Reprinted from Goldman L, Ausiello D. *Cecil Medicine.* 23rd ed. Philadelphia: Saunders; 2007; *B,* Courtesy of T. Postma.)

nymphal stages causing paralysis.[77] Most reported cases occur in North America and Australia, although isolated cases have been reported in South America, Eastern Europe, the Middle East, and Africa.[74,77] Before the 1950s, the reported mortality rate from tick bites in North America exceeded 10%, and Rose[78] suggested this was due to a lack of awareness by the medical community and late presentation to a medical doctor. Decreased mortality can be further attributed to modern intensive care.

Toxin

The toxin or toxins from ticks responsible for causing trouble in beast and human alike have not been fully identified to date. A toxin was partially purified from *I. holocyclus* by Kaire in 1966[79] and named holocyclotoxin. It is thought to be a polypeptide. Later studies suggest it acts on the presynaptic motor nerve terminals to inhibit ACh release, possibly by reducing calcium availability.[80] Injection of the toxoid has been shown to induce immunity in domestic animals.[81,82]

Clinical Presentation

Most cases of tick paralysis occur in the spring or summer months, when ticks are actively seeking hosts.[73,74] Clinically, tick paralysis can be easily mistaken for Guillain-Barré

syndrome or botulism (Box 3), which should be considered in the differential diagnosis.[72] Symptoms begin 2 to 7 days following tick bites depending on the species, beginning with an ascending, flaccid paralysis and gait instability that may progress quickly, leading to respiratory failure and death. Patients may also present with bulbar weakness and ophthalmoplegia, particularly in Australia. Facial nerve palsy has also been described.[84,85] Deep tendon reflexes are hypoactive or absent.[74,77,86] Patients typically do not exhibit changes suggestive of systemic infection, i.e., elevations in white blood cell count, temperature, or cerebrospinal fluid abnormalities. Neurophysiological studies in animals affected by the toxin of *Ixodes* species and humans paralyzed by *Dermacentor* species (see Figure 43-4B) demonstrate reduced nerve conduction and decreased muscle action potential amplitudes. However, defects in neuromuscular transmission have only been reported in *Ixodes* toxicity, suggesting that this may account for the difference in severity between the Australian and the North American species.[83]

Treatment

An antitoxin is the usual treatment for animals afflicted by tick paralysis, but it is not used in humans due to the high risk of anaphylactic reaction and serum sickness. Therefore, treatment primarily involves finding the tick

Box 3   Tick Paralysis

A 4-year-old boy was admitted to a Children's Hospital in Kentucky for progressive weakness. His weakness had begun 2 days before admission after having become generally irritable. He had no fever or recent illness. His parents report living in a rural community in a house backing up to a forest where the children routinely play. On physical examination, the child was irritable and noted to have external ophthalmoplegia. He had marked weakness of his lower extremities, more distally than proximally, and had diminished reflexes bilaterally. On examination of the scalp, an engorged female tick was removed from behind the right ear. The species was later identified by an expert as *D. andersoni*. The tick was carefully removed with forceps, making sure all mouth parts were extracted, and the child was examined for other ticks. He was monitored for cardiac, respiratory, and swallowing difficulties. Within 24 hours, the child began to recover motor function. Within 3 days following removal of the tick, the child had recovered the ability to walk and reflexes returned to normal.

and removing it (Figure 43-5) followed by supportive care measures. Once the tick is removed, symptoms begin to resolve within hours to days in North America, while in Australia, symptoms have been found to persist and patients can even deteriorate for up to 4 days after tick removal.[74] Complete recovery seems to occur much faster after removal of North American species compared to Australian species, where recovery can take up to several weeks.[72]

HYMENOPTERA

Hymenoptera are classified into two broad categories, social and solitary. In general, the venom of social insects is used for defense of the colony and typically produces only local or allergic reactions in predators, although some

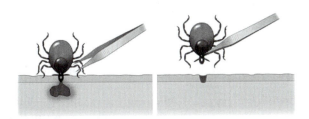

Figure 43-5.   The proper way to remove a tick. (Reprinted from Goldman L, Ausiello D. *Cecil Medicine*. 23rd ed. Philadelphia: Saunders; 2007.)

neurotoxic peptides such as apamin have been isolated from social species. The venom from solitary insects, however, tends to be much more potent, causing paralysis of prey for feeding and reproduction (Box 4). Although in dispute, some have suggested that the earliest recorded death by an insect sting was that of Pharoah Menes (2621 BC). Most fatalities from a single or few insect stings are due to immunoglobulin E (IgE)–mediated anaphylactic reactions. Systemic reactions can occur from multiple stings such as in defense of a nest. Half of all deaths occur within 30 minutes of the sting, and patients may be at risk

Box 4   Neurotoxic and Zombie Insects

Medically important families are mentioned in the main text; however, many insects use extremely effective neurotoxins regularly within their environment for survival of their species:

- Parasitoid wasps (Terebrantes) use neurotoxins to particular ghoulish advantage to paralyze prey as a food source for offspring. Wasps of the family Pompilidae (notably the tarantula hawk, *Hemipepsis* and *Pepsis* species), for example, paralyze spiders and then drag them to a prepared burrow, where an egg is deposited on the abdomen of the living spider. The spider becomes a fresh meal for the wasp larvae upon hatching. One of the most unique strategies is employed by *Ampulex compressa*, which turns a cockroach into a zombie slave. The wasp first injects a neurotoxin that transiently paralyzes the cockroach and then positions himself over the cockroach's head, where he neatly stings again, injecting a second neurotoxin directly into the CNS and causing the cockroach to engage in intense grooming behavior. After this, the cockroach is sluggish and responsive only to the wasp, which picks up an antennae and leads it "like a dog on a leash" to the place where it will in time become a suitable meal for the wasp's offspring.[87]
- Wasps from the *Hymenoepimecis* species attack and temporarily paralyze the orb spider (*Plesiometa argyra*) to lay an egg on the spider's abdomen. The spider regains normal function over the next 2 weeks while the larva hatches, makes a small hole in the spider abdomen, and begins to feed off the spider's hemolymph. Finally, the larva chemically induces the spider to weave a variant of its orb web into a special protective pupal cocoon. The larva then molts, kills, and eats the helpful host.[88]
- Soldier aphids of the genus *Tuberaphis* defend aphid colonies by injecting a venom that produces paralysis and death in moth larvae,[89] and many other insect orders, such as Neuroptera, Diptera, and Coleoptera, produce paralyzing and lethal neurotoxins for defense or providing a food source for young.[90]

up to 12 days later.[91] Treatment is mainly supportive. Venom immunotherapy regimens are highly effective and provide long-term protection against future systemic reactions in 97% of patients treated. The Joint Council of Allergy, Asthma, and Immunology published practice parameters in 2003 stating that "venom immunotherapy should be strongly considered in patients with a history of systemic reaction to a hymenoptera sting (especially if the reaction was associated with respiratory or cardiovascular symptoms) and patients with demonstrable evidence of specific IgE antibodies."[92] Occasionally, neurological sequelae have been documented, and those are the focus of this discussion.

Bees and Wasps

Family: Apidae
Genus: *Apis*
Species: *A. mellifera* (Africanized "killer" honeybee), *A. cerana* (Asian honeybee), *A. dorsata* (giant honeybee)

Family: Vespidae
Genus: *Dasymutilla* (velvet ant), *Dolichovespula* and *Vespula* (yellow jackets), *Polistes* (paper wasps), *Vespa* and *Provespa* (hornets)
Species: *D. maculate* (bald-faced hornet), *V. mandarainia* (Asian hornet)

Bees are found throughout the world except Antarctica and are social or solitary. Social bees, such as the honeybee, typically attack only to defend their territory or when the colony is threatened. They are most dangerous when attacking in a swarm. The Africanized "killer" bee is particularly aggressive when it comes to territory defense and chases threats farther than other species, reportedly even up to 2 miles. Jumping into a body of water to avoid being overtaken does not work with these insects, which have been known to patrol the area for up to an hour in search of their foe. It has been suggested that once a social bee stings its victim an alarm pheromone is released that signals the others in the colony to attack.[93,94]

Similarly, wasps are either social or solitary. Social wasps also aggressively defend their nests when disturbed or threatened. Solitary wasps normally use their sting to kill prey for food or to temporarily paralyze prey to permit egg laying in or on the host (see Box 4). Wasps lack barbs on their stingers and are therefore able to attack multiple times—unlike honeybees, which can only sting once before the barb embeds and detaches the apparatus from the insect.

Several interesting case reports can be found in the literature describing life-threatening neurological dysfunction from single wasp or bee stings. The 1964 Academy of Allergy survey of 2606 reactions determined that 2.8% were delayed by several days following the sting.[95] A study conducted in the United States revealed that of 100 fatal cases from hymenoptera stings 7% were associated with CNS involvement.[96]

Toxin

Bee and wasp venom contains a cocktail of substances, including mast-cell degranulation protein, hyaluronidase, acid phosphatase and lysophospholipase, histamine, dopamine, norepinephrine, and serotonin. Melittin facilitates ion diffusion across cell membranes, breaking down the resting potential and leading to the sensation of pain. Melittin also works with phospholipase to hemolyze red blood cells.[91,97] Apamin, a peptide, is the major neurotoxin in honeybees. It is permeable to the blood–brain barrier and thus has direct CNS effects. Peripherally, it selectively and potently affects the potassium permeability of cell membranes and causes convulsions when injected into rats.[98]

Several neurotoxins have been isolated from wasp venom, some of which are insect specific[99–102]:

1. Bradykinin-related peptides are presynaptic blockers of nicotinic acetylcholine (nACh) receptors in the insect CNS and may induce smooth muscle contraction in mammals.
2. Pompilidotoxins (*Anoplius samariensis* and *Batozonellus maculifrons*) block sodium channel inactivation in both vertebrates and invertebrates.
3. Philanthotoxins (*Philanthus triangulum*) block postsynaptic glutamate receptors and nACh receptors.
4. Microbracotoxin (*Microbracon* species) is a presynaptic neuromuscular signal blocker that causes irreversible flaccid paralysis in lepidopteran larvae.

Clinical Presentation

Honeybees sting only once before the stinger falls off, but wasps may sting multiple times. The most common lethal reaction to a single hymenopteran sting involves IgE-mediated anaphylaxis and resultant pulmonary edema, intravascular hemolysis, renal failure, and shock. Mass envenomations pose a greater threat for systemic reactions from increased venom load. Honeybee colonies typically reach up to 40,000 workers, which can inflict thousands of stings, and systemic toxic reactions are more likely to occur following envenomation by only 50 or more wasp stings.

Reported neurological symptoms include local paresthesias, headache, dizziness, nausea and vomiting, muscle aches, and rarely, cerebrovascular infarcts.[91,103,104] Others have reported bilateral ptosis and a clinical picture similar to myasthenia gravis following wasp sting. Repetitive stimulation showed decremental response, and in one case the patient was treated with an acetylcholinesterase inhibitor.[150,106] Typically, these symptoms are immediate and often in the context of IgE-mediated reactions. Interestingly, many reports are available describing pure neurological dysfunction that appears days to weeks following a single envenomation, leading to the suggestion that there may be a delayed immunological response or hypersensitivity reaction component to the illness.[107] Multiple reports are available describing acute demyelinating syndromes affecting both the CNS and the peripheral nervous system.[108] Clinically, patients may present with quickly progressive motor weakness and areflexia, paresthesias, encephalopathy, or vision changes associated with optic neuritis. When peripheral nerves are affected, nerve conduction studies reveal increased latencies and absent F waves. Antimyelin antibodies have been isolated.[109] Centrally, magnetic resonance imaging shows hyperintense T2 lesions in the subcortical white matter, and autopsy has documented white matter necrosis and demyelination in multiple areas of the brain, spinal cord, and optic nerves. Cerebrospinal fluid analysis in these patients has shown elevated protein without pleocytosis.[95,107,110,111]

Treatment

In the case of bee envenomation, remove the stinger as quickly as possible. It has been suggested that the stinger may continue to deliver venom for up to 1 minute after the sting, even if detached from the body of the insect. Admission for observation should be strongly considered for patients exhibiting any systemic symptoms. Anaphylactic reactions are managed with diphenhydramine, epinephrine, steroids, or a combination of these. Colloids and vasopressors may be required for treatment of shock. Supportive measures also include monitoring airway and cardiac function. Basic labs should be drawn assessing for renal, cardiac, and electrolyte dysfunction. Myoglobin, prothrombin time, and partial thromboplastin time should be drawn. Some patients may require respiratory support or hemodialysis. When patients present with acute demyelinating disease, some have been treated with IV steroids, IV immunoglobulin, or plasma exchange.

Overall, prognosis is good. With medical treatment, patients with more than 1000 bee stings have been known to survive.

Ants

Family: Formicidae
Genus: *Dinoponera, Paraponera, Solenopsis, Myrmecia*
Species: *P. clavata* (bullet ant), *S. invicta* (red fire ant), *S. richteri* (black fire ant), *Myrmecia species* (jack jumper, bull ant)

Hundreds of thousands of people are stung by ants each year. As with other hymenoptera, most deaths are a result of anaphylaxis.[112,113] Neurotoxins have been isolated from several ant species, notably, South and Central American fire ants and the South American bullet ant. The fire ant was imported to North America and other parts of the world through shipping routes in the early 1900s. It is aggressive and has become such a health risk in North America that authorities have introduced phorid flies, the ants' natural predator from South America, to combat the invasion.[114] As a result of the health risk, the fire ant has been more thoroughly studied and reported upon.

The Amazonian bullet ant (*P. clavata*) is carnivorous and large, growing up to 3 centimeters long. Fortunately, these ants are not particularly aggressive, but they vigorously defend their nest after emitting an eerie stridulant warning to the intruder.

Australian *Myrmecia* species (jack jumper and bull ants) are aggressive and have large mandibles. Although they can deliver a painful bite, no neurotoxin has been identified and deaths appear to occur from anaphylactic reactions alone.

Toxin

Isosolenopsin A, a piperidine alkaloid, has been isolated from the fire ant. It is the substance responsible for causing the burning sensation for which the ant is named. This toxin has potent cardiovascular depressant effects and produces seizures in rats.[115] Its mechanism of action has been suggested to affect neurotransmitter function by inhibition of neuronal nitric oxide synthase, which may cause neurotoxicity in humans after mass envenomations.[116]

Poneratoxin, a neurotoxic peptide isolated from bullet ants, affects the excitability of nerve and muscle fibers by its action on voltage-gated sodium channels.[117]

Ectatomin, a peptide isolated from *Ectatomma tuberculatum*, is a potent inhibitor of calcium currents in rat myosites[118] (Table 1).

Clinical Presentation

Fire ants sting in a line or semicircular pattern, inflicting multiple injections. At this site, the victim commonly develops a sterile pustule that necroses over the course of days. The pustules are pruritic and, if broken, put the patient at risk for severe infection. Anaphylactic shock is the most common severe reaction to single fire ant stings. Systemic reactions have been described after mass envenomations and may represent venom toxicity rather than anaphylaxis.[115] These reactions may include rhabdomyolysis, acute renal failure, nephrotic syndrome [118a,119] and neurological complications such as mental status changes, mononeuropathy, seizures, and stroke, typically in conjunction with anaphylaxis.[120–122]

The bullet ant (*P. clavata* and *Dinoponera* species) is so named for its powerful and potent sting. Intense excruciating pain, which reaches its peak after approximately

Table 1: Identified Ant Neurotoxins

Family/Genus	Common Name	Toxin	Mechanism	Clinical	Treatment
Formicidae/ *Paraponera*	Bullet ant	Poneratoxin	Action on voltage-gated sodium channels	Intense pain, paralysis, tremors	Antihistamines, epinephrine, supportive care
Formicidae/ *Solenopsis*	Red fire ant Black fire ant	Isosolenopsin A	Inhibition of neuronal nitric oxide synthase	Intense pain, cardiovascular depressant, seizures	Antihistamines, epinephrine, supportive care
Formicidae/ *Ectatomma*	No common name (*E. tuberculatum*)	Ectatomin	Inhibition of rat myosite calcium current	Possible inhibition of cardiac muscle contraction?	Not reported to be clinically relevant in humans

24 hours, follows the sting of a single worker ant. Systemic reactions may include diaphoresis, nausea, vomiting, tachycardia, lymphadenopathy, cardiac arrhythmias, local edema, and hematochezia.[123] Rare neurological complications include limb paralysis and paresthesia, trembling, and malaise[123–125] (Box 5).

In an extensive review of the literature, Klotz et al.[126] describe several other species associated with systemic clinical effects, most of which appear secondary to anaphylactic reactions, with some neurological manifestations such as lethargy, paresthesias, and dizziness.

Treatment

As with other hymenoptera, treatment for ant stings is mainly supportive. Medications typically used are antihistamines, epinephrine, and steroids for anaphylactic reactions. Those with systemic reactions, particularly following mass envenomations, should be monitored for neurological and cardiac dysfunction. It has been suggested that steroids and antihistamines may worsen the outcome for those with toxic systemic illness.[115,122,127]

BIRDS

Family: Pachycephalidae
Genus: *Pitohui*
Species: *P. dichrous* (hooded), *P. ferrugineus* (rusty), *P. kirhocephalus* (variable)

Family: Phasianidae
Genus: *Coturnix*
Species: *C. coturnix* (common quail)

Recently, scientific interest has turned to the study of neurotoxins in birds. Human poisoning thought to be a direct result of ingestion by certain birds has been known since ancient times. Accounts have been documented in several Muslim texts; by Pliny the Elder, Didymus of Alexandria, and Aristotle; and in the Bible[128–131] (Box 6). Folklore about inedible birds exists in Aztec culture[132] and among the natives of New Guinea, who call their local pitohuis *nanisani*, the word also used to describe the numbing sensation around the mouth resulting from contact with the toxin.[133]

Similar to poison dart frogs, birds appear to sequester toxins from their environment through their diet.[134,135] Depending on what and how much is consumed, the birds may become more or less poisonous. The European quail, for example, seems only to be toxic along its western migratory paths during its spring migration to the south.[128,130,131] It has also been suggested that people with certain genetic predispositions may be more susceptible than others since it has been noted not everyone sharing a meal becomes affected.[128,136,137]

Box 5   South American Native Initiation Rites

In South America, the Satere-Mawe, an Amazonian tribe, use *P. clavata* during rites of passage to manhood. For the test, ants are smoked out of their colonies. While they are stunned, they are secured by their midsections to a woven mat with stingers directed inward. Once the ants recover, the mat is applied to an abdomen, arm, or leg of a boy who withstands excruciating sting after sting for up to 30 minutes. The goal is to show no emotion. If the boy fails, he remains a boy in the eyes of the tribe. If he succeeds, he is eligible for marriage and leadership positions within the tribe. Following the rite, the new man is ill for a week and limbs may be paralyzed. He is put to bed while the rest of the tribe celebrates his achievement.[116–118]

Box 6   Putative Example of Coturnism from Ancient Times

4 The rabble with them began to crave other food, and again the Israelites started wailing and said, "If only we had meat to eat! 5 We remember the fish we ate in Egypt at no cost—also the cucumbers, melons, leeks, onions and garlic. 6 But now we have lost our appetite; we never see anything but this manna!"

***

18 Tell the people: "Consecrate yourselves in preparation for tomorrow, when you will eat meat. The LORD heard you when you wailed, 'If only we had meat to eat! We were better off in Egypt!' Now the LORD will give you meat, and you will eat it. 19 You will not eat it for just one day, or two days, or five, ten or twenty days, 20 but for a whole month—until it comes out of your nostrils and you loathe it—because you have rejected the LORD, who is among you, and have wailed before him, saying, "Why did we ever leave Egypt?"

***

31 Now a wind went out from the LORD and drove quail in from the sea. It brought them down all around the camp to about three feet above the ground, as far as a day's walk in any direction. 32 All that day and night and all the next day the people went out and gathered quail. No one gathered less than ten homers. Then they spread them out all around the camp. 33 But while the meat was still between their teeth and before it could be consumed, the anger of the LORD burned against the people, and he struck them with a severe plague. 34 Therefore the place was named Kibroth Hattaavah, because there they buried the people who had craved other food.

Numbers 11:4–34 (New International Version).

Interest was renewed with the identification of specific toxins from the New Guinea pitohuis by Dumbacher.[138] Overall, birds pose little threat to humans unless consumed or incidentally contacted.

Toxin

Toxicity in birds is believed to be a function of sequestration. To date, several toxins have been isolated from birds (Table 2). The best studied is from the *Pitohui*. Dumbacher isolated a steroid alkaloid toxin similar to batrachotoxin, the potent neurotoxin in poison dart frogs of the Dendrobatidae family, and named it homobatrachotoxin. The toxin binds to voltage-gated sodium channels, leading to depolarization of cell membranes at a site different from tetrodotoxin (TTX) and saxitoxin. The greatest concentration of the toxin is found in the feathers of the breast and epidermis. Dumbacher et al.[139] suggested the transfer of batrachotoxin-laden feathers to

nests may provide protection to eggs. They have also suggested that the presence of this toxin may provide adult birds protection from lice.[140] Similar toxins have since been identified in several related and unrelated species of bird also found in New Guinea.[139]

Aparicio et al.[134] performed studies on quail following an epidemic of quail poisoning on the Greek isle of Lesbos, which suggested that quail become toxic from the ingestion of *Galeopsis ladanum* seeds and identified several alkaloid toxins, including stachydrine.[134,141] Interesting historical reports exist of poisoning by ruffed grouse (partridge) in North America in the late 1800s. This bird was believed to become toxic through ingestion of mountain laurel (*Kalmia latifolia*) during hard winters. Mountain laurel is a recognized source of andromedotoxin.[141,142]

Clinical Presentation

Contact with pitohuis produces local irritation, numbness, tingling, and burning that can last for several hours. Ingestion is avoided by locals, but whether because of the unpleasant taste or a systemic effect caused by the toxin is unknown. Presumably, it would produce effects similar to that of batrachotoxin if ingested (see discussion under the Frogs and Toads section). Studies show it causes convulsions and death when injected into mice.[138]

Coturnism describes the clinical syndrome following ingestion of quail. Patients typically present within hours of consuming the bird with muscle pain, vomiting, lower limb paralysis, and acute rhabdomyolysis.[129,131]

Treatment

There is no known antidote for avian neurotoxins. Treatment is supportive. Patients suffering acute rhabdomyolysis from quail ingestion should be treated with forced hydration and urinary alkalinization. Some may require hemodialysis. Illness is typically self-limiting and resolves within 10 days. Although prognosis is good, deaths have been described.[129,143,144]

MAMMALS

Family: Ornithorhynchidae
Genus: *Ornithorhynchus*
Species: *O. anatinus* (duckbill platypus)

The egg-laying, venom-producing, duckbilled mammal, found in the rivers and streams of Australia, created quite a controversy when first introduced to the Western world years ago. It is one of few mammals known to produce venom, along with various shrews

Table 2: Known and Putative Avian Neurotoxins

	Toxin	Location	References
KNOWN			
Pitohuis (hooded, rusty, variable)	Batrachotoxins	New Guinea	Drumbacher 1992
Ifrita kowaldi (blue-capped)	Batrachotoxins	New Guinea	Drumbacher 2000
Plectropterus gambensis (spur-winged goose)	Cantharidin	North Benin	Carrel and Eisner 1974
UNDER INVESTIGATION			
Ergaticus ruber (red warbler)	Unidentified alkaloid	Mexico	Escalante and Daly 1994
Bonasa umbellus (ruffed grouse or partridge)	Andromedotoxin	North America	Wilson 1829, Comstock 1837, Bicknell 1960
Coturnix coturnix (European quail)	Stachydrine Unidentified alkaloids	Southern France, Greece, Algeria	Sergent 1942, Ouzonellis 1970, Grivetti 1980, Aparicio 1999, others
Phaps (common and brush bronzewing)	Monofluoroacetate	Australia	Gardner and Bennetts 1957, Main 1981
Conuropsis carolinensis (Carolina parakeet)	Unknown	North America	Wilson and Bonaparte 1800s, Audubon 1929

Dumbacher JP, Pruett-Jones S. Avian chemical defense. In: Nolan V Jr, Ketterson ED, eds. *Current Ornithology*. vol 13. New York: Plenum Press; 1996:137–174.

Weldon PJ, Rappole JH. A survey of birds odorous or unpalatable to humans: possible indications of chemical defense. *Journal of Chemical Ecology*. 1997;23:2609–2633.

(notably *Blarina brevicauda*) and the Caribbean solenodon, none of which are responsible for severe envenomations in humans (Box 7). The venom of the duck-billed platypus is made in crural glands and injected via spurs located behind hind leg of the male. It is thought to be used primarily to establish its territory during breeding season or in defense from predators.[148] The

platypus was hunted to near extinction for its fur but has been designated a protected species since 1905. Naturally shy, few human envenomations by this creature have been recorded.

Toxin

To date, the neurotoxin from the platypus has not been fully elucidated. Studies have suggested the venom forms slow-kinetic cation channels that modify membrane potentials,[149] contains a C-type natriuretic peptide and defensin-like peptides,[150–152] and may directly target putative nociceptors.[150]

Clinical Presentation

Following envenomation by the platypus, the victim experiences immediate excruciating pain that is long lasting and intense. Case reports suggest this particular pain may develop into a hyperalgesia lasting up to several months.[153,154] Marked edema, which occurs over several

---

Box 7   Other Clinically Insignificant Venomous Mammals

The Caribbean solenodon, Eurasian water shrew, and Northern short-tailed shrew delivers a venomous bite. Mice develop respiratory distress, paralysis, and convulsions when injected with the venom.[145,146]

The slow loris secretes a toxin from a gland near the elbow. Grooming transfers the toxin to its mouth, where a bite can result in painful swelling. Mothers spread the toxin onto their young for protection before leaving them to seek food.[147]

hours, can extend to involve the entire limb.[154,155] One patient experienced wasting of muscle mass in the affected limb and limitation of finger flexion months following envenomation.[154]

Treatment

No antivenom for platypus envenomation is available. Treatment, therefore, is aimed toward pain control and reducing associated edema. Treatments have included ice, elevation and immobilization of the affected limb, and liberal use of opiates and analgesics. Steroids have not proven to be effective. Tonkin and Negrine[155] also included antibiotics in their treatment regimen and reported worsening of symptoms when removed. In one report, the victim's severe pain did not respond to morphine but responded well to a regional nerve block of 0.5% bupivicaine.[154]

CENTIPEDES

Family: Scolopendromorpha
Genus: *Ethmostigmus, Scolopendra*
Species: *E. rubripes* (giant centipede), *S. gigantean* (giant centipede), *S. subspinipes* (Vietnamese centipede), *S. heros* (desert centipede)

While several large species of centipedes are found throughout the world, those within the *Scolopendra* genus are most often involved in human accidents requiring therapeutic intervention. The giant centipede *S. gigantean* is an impressive carnivorous arthropod that uses its venom effectively to subdue frogs, mice, bats, birds, and other small prey. In Brazil, a study from 1998 to 2000 reported that nearly 17% of all envenomations were attributable to centipede species.[156] Since these arthropods are becoming popular pets, the clinician may encounter an envenomation outside its usual territories.

Toxin

Centipede venom is a cocktail of several substances, including histamine, serotonin, cardiotoxin, and a quinoline alkaloid.[157–159] Research has suggested a possible muscarinic target.[160] The venoms of other centipedes are used in Chinese folk medicine to combat rheumatism, convulsions, tetanus, heart attacks, kidney stones, skin problems, and dementia.[158,161] It is also used in India as a last-resort cancer treatment, leading researchers to investigate potential antitumor properties of centipede venom. Bhagirath et al.[162] demonstrated that daily injections of the venom from *S. viridicornis* did inhibit the mean growth of tumors in mice.

Clinical Presentation

Adverse events can be seen following centipede envenomation or ingestion. They range from local symptoms, including pain, necrosis, and edema,[163,163a] to rare systemic symptoms, such as anaphylaxis, diaphoresis, chills, fever, paresthesias, rhabdomyolysis, hyperthermia, nausea, acute coronary ischemia, anxiety, and depression.[164–167] Acute renal failure, rhabdomyolysis, and multifocal neuropathies were reported after a Chinese man drank alcohol in which a centipede was soaked.[168] Rare reports of death from centipede bites are found in the literature.[168a,169]

Treatment

Treatment of centipede envenomation or ingestion is aimed at symptomatic relief, which occurs in 2 to 24 hours. Pain and pruritus may last several weeks. Recommendations include using hydrocortisone or analgesics.[170] Cepharanthine is commonly used in Japan.[164] Tetanus immunization is also recommended.[171] (Boxes 8 and 9.)

Box 8   Venomous Millipedes

Several species of millipede are reported to cause deleterious effects. Millipedes secrete a toxic substance when trapped, producing local mahogany skin discoloration, edema, blisters, burning, and paresthesias that can last up to several days. Some millipedes are capable of potentially serious injury to eyes by spraying their toxin up to 25 centimeters. The neurotoxin in the venom responsible for the development of pain and paresthesias has not been isolated. Symptoms are typically self-limiting and are treated with pain medication and steroids.[172–174]

Box 9   Venomous Caterpillars

Serious human injuries from caterpillar encounters are reported from many areas around the world, including North and South America, Europe, Australia, and China. Injuries range from urticarial dermatitis and asthma to renal failure and intracerebral hemorrhage from the venom of the *Lonomia* caterpillar. Neurological symptoms can include pain, headache, or hemorrhagic stroke. No neurotoxin has been identified from this group.[175,176]

REPTILES

Snakes

Family: Elapidae (subfamilies Elapinae, and sea snakes Hydrophiinae and Laticaudinae)

Genus: *Acanthophis, Aipysurus, Aspidelaps, Astrotia, Boulengerina, Bungarus, Dendroaspis, Elapsoidea, Enhydrina, Hemachatus, Homoroselaps, Hydrophis, Lapemis, Laticauda, Micropechis, Micrurus, Naja, Notechis, Ophiophagus, Oxyuranus, Pseudechis, Pseudonaja, Walterinnesia*

Species: *Acanthophis* species (death adder), *Bungarus* species (krait), *Dendroaspis* species (black/green mamba), *Hydrophis* species (sea snake), *Micrurus* species (coral snake), *Naja* species (cobra), *Notechis* species (tiger snake), *O. hannah* (king cobra), *O. microlepidotus* (Australian inland taipan), *W. aegyptia* (black desert cobra)

Snakes produce some of the most varied neurotoxins in the animal kingdom. With few exceptions, notably Antarctica, Ireland, and New Zealand, snakes populate nearly every land mass in the world. Approximately 200 of the 3000 species of snake are known to be lethal. Nearly 200 other species produce toxins but are not lethal to humans. Fatality estimates from snake bites range from 40,000 to 150,000 annually.[177,178] Reports from the World Health Organization and others suggest tens of thousands of deaths yearly in the Southeast Asia region alone and an additional yearly fatality rate of up to 15,000 in the Indian subcontinent,[179–181] which has higher concentrations of venomous snakes and less access to health care and antivenom.

Venomous snakes are found in nearly all taxonomic families. With few exceptions, the venom is delivered via hollowed curved fangs in order to immobilize or kill prey or to be used in self-defense. Most snake venom is a mixture of several compounds that function as neurotoxins, hemotoxins, cardiotoxins, nephrotoxins, necrotoxins, myotoxins, or cytotoxins. Toxin concentration per strike is variable, depending on such things as season, age, or species; in fact, even in the most venomous species, strikes can be ineffective or "dry." Clinical reaction to snake envenomation ranges from no symptoms from a dry bite to severe local necrosis to systemic effects such as respiratory failure, paralysis, or end-organ failure. Other victims develop long-lasting and life-threatening coagulopathies.

Treatment of the victim can be aided by definitive identification of snake species. Attempting to capture the snake is usually not recommended, as this may result in additional victims. First aid measures to be avoided include tourniquet, ice, electric shock, and cutting or suctioning the wound. Instead, first aid should include calming the victim, immobilizing the limb, and transportation of the victim to the nearest trauma facility where consultation with a regional toxicology expert is helpful in determining administration of antivenom. As of the time of writing, a comprehensive list of available species-specific and regional polyvalent antivenoms can be found at www.toxinfo.org/antivenoms/synopsis.html. Skin testing for horse serum sensitivity before administration of antivenom is controversial. It costs valuable time when systemic symptoms are already present, no improvement in outcome has been proven, and the only benefit may be medicolegal.[182] Wounds should be monitored for signs of secondary infection, and tetanus prophylaxis should be considered. Patients should be admitted for 24-hour observation even if symptoms are only initially minor or mild because some neurotoxins have late onset.

Four families contain snakes that produce neurotoxic venom: Elapidae (cobras, coral snakes, mambas, kraits, sea snakes), Viperidae (vipers, rattlesnakes, copperheads, cottonmouths, adders), Colubridae (mangrove snakes, vine snakes, boomslangs, tree snakes, twig snake), and Atractaspidae (stiletto snakes, mole vipers). Two families, Elapidae and Viperidae, account for most human fatalities associated with neurotoxic envenomations. The following discussion focuses on elapids (Figure 43-6; see color plate).

The Elapidae family contains some of the most neurotoxic creatures in the world. They are mainly found in tropical or subtropical regions, typically have a distinct hood that covers the head, have short fangs, and are active. Some elapids envenomate with quick, stabbing strikes similar to those of viperids, but in general they are slightly slower due to the proteroglyphic (fixed) construction of their fangs.

Toxin

Myriad toxins have been isolated from the species of the interesting Elapidae family. The majority block ACh transmission by competitively binding to the postsynaptic nicotinic and muscarinic ACh receptors or by presynaptic inhibition of ACh release, which prevents muscle contraction.[183,184] The better-known examples of neurotoxins that interrupt postsynaptic binding are krait α-bungarotoxin and naja cobrotoxin (Figure 43-7). Inhibition of ACh release is accomplished effectively by phospholipase A2 toxins such as krait β-bungarotoxin.[185] Phospholipase A2 neurotoxins are responsible for severe paralysis in bite victims. The opposite is true of other neurotoxins such as mamba dendrotoxin, which presynaptically facilitates ACh release. Likewise, fasciculin, isolated from *D. augusticeps* (mamba), appears to inhibit acetylcholinesterase, causing severe fasciculations lasting up to 7 hours in victims.[186] Other neurotoxins from this

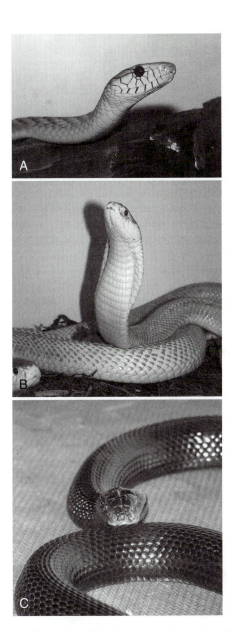

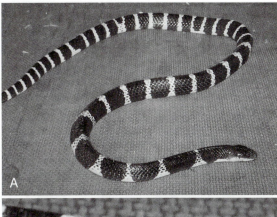

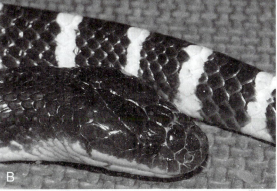

Figure 43-7. The banded krait *(Bungarus multicinctus)* produces paralyzing bungarotoxin and is responsible for many fatalities in some parts of the world. (Courtesy of Kentucky Reptile Zoo, T. Postma.)

Figure 43-6. Examples of highly neurotoxic species of snake: the Western green mamba *(Dendroaspis viridis; A)*; the monocled cobra *(Naja kaouthia, Suphan phase)* shown rearing and beginning to hood *(B)*; and the black desert cobra *(Walterinnesia aegyptia; C)*. (Courtesy of Kentucky Reptile Zoo, T. Postma.)

family act directly on smooth muscle to inhibit cardiac contractility.[187] Acanmyotoxin, isolated from the death adder, is a rare example of elapid myotoxin.

Clinical Presentation

Snake bite from elapids may be painful or painless. Sleeping victims may be unaware of bites from the krait, for example, which typically occur during the night. Symptoms usually manifest within minutes to hours; however, some symptoms from krait and coral snake envenomations may be delayed up to 10 hours.[188] Initial symptoms from elapid envenomation may include local swelling and necrosis (Figure 43-8), euphoria, headache, confusion, hypotension, and nausea. Cranial nerve paralysis often ensues, including ptosis (Figure 43-9), ophthalmoplegia, and dysphagia. Patients may experience severe peripheral paralysis and localized paresthesias. Initial paralysis may progress to respiratory failure and death or may be replaced by overexcitation, causing fasciculations, cramps, and muscle spasms. Although bleeding is not a major consideration following elapid envenomation, victims have been reported to develop significant coagulopathies[189,190] (Box 10).

Treatment

In general, the most effective first aid treatment for neurotoxic snake bite is pressure immobilization, followed by graded cautious release, a technique developed by Sutherland in Australia (Figure 43-10). Pressure immobilization has been shown to delay the systemic spread of toxin in monkeys,[191] and it has been adopted as a standard first aid measure in Australasia and Africa.[188] This technique can increase

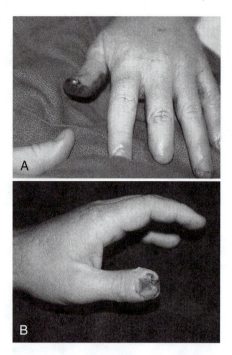

Figure 43-8. *A,* This photo was taken hours after envenomation by *Naja nivea. B,* One week later, the patient has developed osteomyelitis and the extent of the injury is better observed. (Courtesy of Kentucky Reptile Zoo, Keith Gad.)

Box 10   Kentucky Reptile Zoo

Jim Harrison, founder and director of the Kentucky Reptile Zoo in Slade, Kentucky, is one of few in the world who risk snake envenomation to obtain venom for research purposes and for antivenom production. Although every precaution is taken to avoid accidents, they have occurred. He reports one of the most severe envenomations he experienced was in 1997 by a cobra *(N. nivea).* Minutes after being caught by one fang on the tip of the thumb of his left hand, he experienced pain, weakness, and numbness of the left hand and double vision. He also experienced bradycardia, mental status changes, hypothermia, fasciculations, and respiratory failure requiring intubation. He received an initial 10 vials of SAVP polyvalent antivenom and then another 5 vials upon arrival at the University of Kentucky Medical Center. He recovered within 12 hours and was discharged the next day in good condition. He later developed and was treated for osteomyelitis in the affected thumb, which has never ceased causing him needle-like pain (Figure 43-8).

Jim and his wife, Kristen Wiley, have made significant contributions to the scientific and medical communities through their research and knowledge of venomous reptiles and continue their work today.

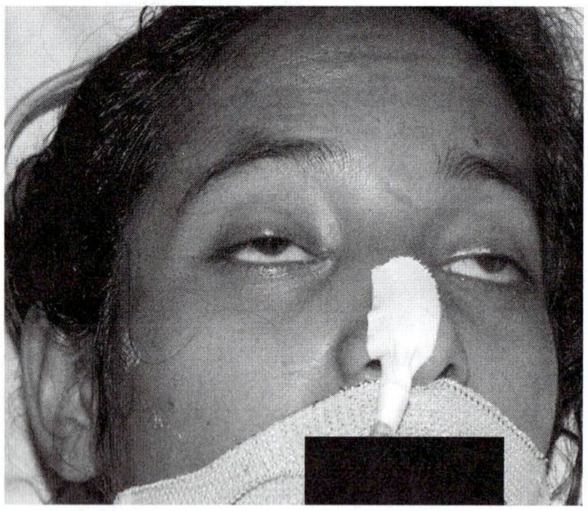

Figure 43-9. Ptosis is an important clinical finding and suggests systemic neurotoxicity. Any patient exhibiting ptosis must be monitored carefully for signs of cardiovascular and respiratory collapse. This patient was envenomated by a krait. (Reprinted from Auerbach P. *Wilderness Medicine.* 5th ed. St. Louis: Mosby; 2007.)

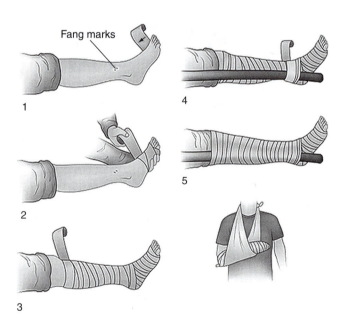

Figure 43-10. The Sutherland pressure-immobilization technique is employed to prevent the spread of neurotoxin via the lymphatic system following envenomation and is an important first aid technique. (Reprinted from Auerbach P. *Wilderness Medicine.* 5th ed. St. Louis: Mosby; 2007.)

local ischemia, so it is not recommended for nonneurotoxic snake bite such as in North America or other parts of the world, where most bites result mainly in local tissue necrosis. The patient should be admitted for observation and assessed for signs of coagulopathy or disseminated intravascular coagulation. If the species of snake is known, antivenom is available and can be used, although many are ineffective if not given immediately or if given in small quantities. This may be due to the irreversible binding of some toxins. If the species of snake is unknown, polyvalent antivenom is available; however, monovalent antivenom is always preferable because of lower risk of serum sickness and anaphylaxis. Therefore, polyvalent antivenom is reserved for those with life-threatening bites when the snake species cannot be definitively determined.[188] Neostigmine can be given but may only be initially effective or be effective to counter the effect of postsynaptic-blocking venoms.[192] Maintain vigilance for signs and symptoms of cardiotoxicity or neurotoxicity, which may develop without warning and lead to respiratory distress and need for mechanical ventilatory support. The site of the wound should be assessed for signs of infection and necrosis. Surgical consult may be required. Fasciotomies, however, should be performed only when compartmental pressures are documented to be greater than 30 mm Hg.[193]

Overall, the most important treatment for snake bite victims is vigilance, supportive care, and recruitment of a knowledgeable specialist. Because of the intricacies and potential life-threatening nature of snakebite, assistance from specialists knowledgeable in treating snakebite should be sought immediately to help direct region-specific care.

Lizards

Family: Helodermatidae
Genus: *Heloderma*
Species: *H. horridum* (Mexican beaded lizard), *H. suspectum* (Gila monster)

The Mexican beaded lizard (Figure 43-11) and the Gila monster (Figure 43-12) are both inhabitants of central and southwest North America. They have powerful jaws and razor-sharp teeth, which either slash or grip and chew the victim's flesh, releasing toxic venom from a paramandibular sack through grooves in the teeth. Typically nonaggressive, most helodermatid envenomations have involved handling lizards in captivity. Although the venom contains potent neurotoxins, few cases have been reported in the literature. Even fewer have resulted in death, none in the past 75 years.[194]

Monitor lizards from the family Veranidae are a group of carnivorous lizards found in Africa, India, Asia, and Australia. Although most researchers accept that the deleterious effects from the bites of these lizards is a result of deadly bacteria (*Pasteurella multocida*), a recently controversial suggestion has been made that

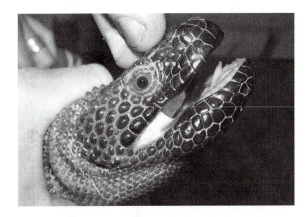

Figure 43-11. A Mexican beaded lizard demonstrating the beading for which it is named and its strong jaws. Multiple small but venomous teeth can be seen along the gum line. (Courtesy of Kentucky Reptile Zoo, T. Postma.)

the acute clinical signs and symptoms from its bite may be the result of weak venom.[195]

Toxin

Similar to elapid venom, helodermatid venom is comprised of a mix of protein and nonprotein substances, including such things as serotonin, bradykinin-releasing substance, phospholipase A2, and hyaluronidase.[194] Two substances, gilatoxin and helothermine, are neurotoxic. Gilatoxin is a component of both Gila monster and Mexican beaded lizard venom. It appears to be a presynaptic neurotoxin that produces hypothermia, lethargy, convulsions, restlessness, partial paralysis of hind limbs, and death in mice. It also appears to

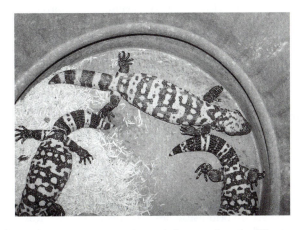

Figure 43-12. Nonaggressive and slow moving, the Gila monster is a well-known venomous reptile found in desert regions of the southwest United States. (Courtesy of Kentucky Reptile Zoo, T. Postma.)

contain a kallikrein-like substance that produces hypotension in mice.[196] Helothermine from *H. horridum* is also a kallikrein-like substance that produces hypothermia in mice, blocks calcium channels in rat cerebellar granule cells, and is thought to target the ryanodine receptor.[197–199]

Clinical Presentation

Theoretically, these lizards continue to inject toxin as long as they have contact with the victim, so clinical reactions may be more severe with prolonged attachment time. Most bites result in excruciating pain and localized swelling. Patients often report lightheadedness, diaphoresis, nausea and vomiting, hypotension, angioedema, and lymphangitis.[200] Anaphylaxis and myocardial infarction have been reported.[201] Pain has been described as radiating or burning with hyperesthesia.[194] Despite the neurotoxic action of helodermatid venom, few neurological symptoms are reported. One patient complained of lethargy and was noted to have moderate miosis.[202] Others noted fingertip paresthesias in the wounded extremity, radiating "burning" pain, severe localized myalgias, and headache.[202,203]

Treatment

Few fatal cases have been reported outside the Indo-Pacific region; however, one such case was reported in North America when a young man accepted a dare and swallowed five rough-skinned newts.[206] The first order of business in the treatment of helodermatid envenomations may be removal of the animal itself. Heloderms have been reported to remain engaged for up to 30 minutes. If the victim arrives with lizard still attached, experts recommend manually prying the jaw open with a stiff object.[200] Others have suggested administering hot water or flame to the jaw or submerging the lizard in cold water to subdue it.[194,204] Take care no one else comes into contact with the animal. Pain control, often difficult to manage, can be attempted with IV morphine, which may provide some relief. Although no significant coagulopathies have been reported from helodermatid bites, antiplatelet analgesics should be avoided. Place the extremity in a neutral position. One victim reported increased pain when the wounded arm was lowered,[194] and it seemed to be exacerbated by cold compresses in another.[203]

Basic labs should be obtained to assess for coagulopathies, in addition to complete blood count, blood chemistries, and electrocardiography, to monitor cardiorespiratory function. Vasopressors have been used for severe hypotension and anaphylaxis. Wounds are susceptible to secondary infection, and although cases report prophylactic antibiotic use, these are not routinely administered. Tetanus immunizations should be updated as needed. Most symptoms resolve within 6 to 12 hours, but overnight observation may be advisable for severe bites.[194]

Newts and Salamanders

Family: Salamandridae
Subfamily: Pleurodelinae
Genus: *Cynops, Notophthalmus, Taricha, Triturus*
Species: *C. pyrrhogaster* (Japanese newt), *N. viridescens* (red-spotted newt, eastern newt), *Taricha torosa* (California newt), *Taricha granulosa* (rough-skinned newt), *Taricha rivularis* (red-bellied newt)

Subfamily: Salamandrinae
Genus: *Salamandra*
Species: *S. maculosa, S. salamandra* (fire salamander)

Throughout medieval times, the salamander was considered a "pestilent beast most venomous (sic)" and as such was to be avoided. It was said to mortally poison all wells, fountains, and fruit trees in which it lived so that a man would die upon drinking or eating from them.[205] Today, salamanders have become popular as pets. Newts and salamanders are naturally found in North America, Europe, the Middle East, and Asia. Like some species of frogs, the more toxic species may be brightly colored. The California newt is rather plain colored on its dorsum but when threatened rises up to expose its brightly colored underside. If attacked, newts and salamanders secrete neurotoxins from their skin. Some salamanders also spray noxious substances in defense.

Toxin

Newt neurotoxin was isolated from its eggs and initially called tarichatoxin. Later it was also discovered to be secreted from skin and to be the same chemical compound as TTX found elsewhere in nature[207,208] (Box 11). Unlike puffer fish, however r, newts appear to produce TTX de novo; that is, even in captivity, newts continued to produce TTX.[208] Yotsu et al.[212] identified TTX in nine species of newt. They determined that toxin levels were highest in *T. granulosa* and *N. viridescens* followed by *Cynops* species. TTX binds to pores of voltage-gated presynaptic sodium channels blocking action potentials and unbinds slowly. Some predators, such as garter snakes, have adapted to the toxin,[213,214] and this observation supported the finding of the identification of two types of sodium receptors: TTX-r (resistant) and TTX-s (sensitive).[215]

Approximately nine steroidal alkaloids have been isolated from salamanders, recently reviewed by Daly et al.[216] Interestingly, the fire salamander is used in Slovenia to concoct "salamander brandy," a home alcohol that reportedly has hallucinogenic and aphrodisiac properties.[217]

Box 11   Tetrodotoxin Tidbits

- TTX was first isolated and named in 1909 by Japanese scientist Yoshizumi Tahara.
- TTX is most commonly associated with puffer fish but has also been isolated from various marine life, toads, and worms, in addition to newt species.
- Newts lay eggs protected by a gel-like membrane, which have been found to contain levels of TTX that correlate with maternal levels.[209]
- Unlike other organisms that lose toxicity in captivity, *Taricha granulosa* toxin levels increase in long-term captivity, suggesting that the toxin is produced by the newt rather than by a dietary source.[193]
- TTX was hypothesized by Davis[210] to be used in the making of Haitian zombies. In fact, TTX was isolated, albeit in very low doses,[211] from the so-called zombie drug Davis procured from voodoo witch doctors. He postulated that the belief of the victim, in conjunction with a toxic dose of the drug, may induce coma that is indistinguishable from death and may be subsequently reversed by an antidote containing atropine and scopolamine, resulting in a person who behaves as a zombie.

Table 3:   **Clinical Grading System for Tetrodotoxin Poisoning**

Grade 1	Perioral numbness and paresthesias, with or without gastrointestinal symptoms
Grade 2	Numbness of tongue, face, and other areas (distal); early motor paralysis and incoordination; slurred speech; normal reflexes
Grade 3	Generalized flaccid paralysis; respiratory failure; aphonia; fixed dilated pupils; patient still conscious
Grade 4	Severe respiratory failure with hypoxia; hypotension; bradycardia; cardiac arrhythmias; unconsciousness may occur

Isbister GK, Son J, Wang F, et al. Puffer fish poisoning: a potentially life-threatening condition. *Med J Aust.* 2002;177(11–12):650–653.

Clinical Presentation

Symptom onset from TTX exposure by newt ingestion is typically acute and includes a burning sensation and then numbness and tingling on the lips and tongue ingestion, followed by lightheadedness and paresthesias of face and extremities. The patient may experience headache, nausea, vomiting, diarrhea, and ataxia. In severe cases, the patient may experience a rapid ascending paralysis, increasing respiratory distress, mental status changes, convulsions, arrhythmias, and hypotension. Coma may ensue, and the patient may exhibit fixed, nonreactive pupils and loss of brainstem reflexes. Death can occur within 4 to 6 hours of ingestion[206,207,218,219] (Table 3).

Most exposures to the steroidal alkaloids of salamanders cause only a local skin irritation and a transient local anesthetic effect; however, ingestion in large amounts can cause restlessness, salivation, tachypnea, respiratory failure, hypertension, hallucinations, and convulsions.[220]

Treatment

Since there is no known antidote for TTX, treatment is largely supportive. Initial treatment involves administration of activated charcoal. Maintain a low threshold for mechanical airway support if respiratory failure ensues. Monitor cardiac function for arrhythmias, and treat hypotension as indicated with pressor agents. Symptoms may last several days. Prognosis is reportedly good if the patient survives the first 24 hours.[206,207,218,221] Few fatal cases have been reported outside the Indo-Pacific region; however, one such case was reported in North America when a young man accepted a dare and swallowed five rough-skinned newts.[206]

Wash hands after handling salamanders. Treatment is primarily supportive care.

Frogs and Toads

Family: Bufonidae
Genus: *Bufo*
Species: *B. alvarius* (Colorado river toad, Sonoran desert toad), *B. marinus* (Cane toad)

Family: Dentrobatidae
Genus: *Dendrobates, Phyllobates*
Species: *Dendrobates* species (poison dart frogs), *P. bicolor, P. terribilis*

Frogs and toads are found in tropical and subtropical regions. The most poisonous frogs (*Phyllobates* species) are found in Columbia (Figure 43-13). *B. alvarius* inhabit the southwestern United States, and *Bufo* species are depicted in the art of the Aztecs and Mayans as far back as 2000 BC. Because these creatures pose little threat to humans except when ingested or handled, information on epidemiology, clinical consequences, and treatment recommendations is limited.

Toxin

Bufo toads contain bufotenine (5-OH-DMT) and an alkaloid tryptamine (5-MeO-DMT), a potent hallucinogenic. Experts have concluded that psychotropic effects are most likely from contact with *B. alvarius*.[222] Bufotoxin is a toxic cardiac glycoside, which is dried and used as a preparation

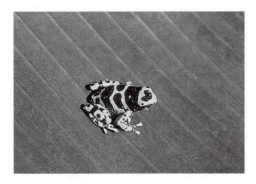

Figure 43-13. Poison dart frogs, such as the one pictured here, are beautiful but deadly creatures found in South America. (Reprinted from Auerbach P. *Wilderness Medicine.* 5th ed. St. Louis: Mosby; 2007.)

in Chinese medicine.[223] Trace amounts of morphine have also been detected from *B. marinus*.[224]

Dendrobates and *Phyllobates* species contain several alkaloids. Batrachotoxins are the principle toxins found in *Phyllobates* species, potent inhibitors of sodium channel deactivation causing persistent ACh release, and are used in Columbian Indian blowguns to poison darts for hunting.[225,226] Other alkaloids include pumiliotoxins and histrionicotoxins.[226]

Clinical Presentation

When *Bufo* species are ingested, toxicity ensues, including hemiparesis, muscle jerking and twitching, convulsions, altered mental status, slurred speech, headache, nausea, vomiting, severe dyspnea, and death.[227,228] Digoxin-like toxicity, cardiac arrhythmias, and heart block has been described in men ingesting homeopathic aphrodisiacs containing *Bufo* venom.[229–232] Auditory and visual hallucinations without toxicity are reported when *Bufo* venom is dried and smoked.[222]

Clinical consequences of encounters with injection of venom from *Phyllobates* or *Dendrobates* species include paralysis, ataxia, dyspnea, and convulsions. Reportedly, oral ingestion did not produce clinical consequences.[225,233]

Treatment

Treatment of *Bufo* toxicity is supportive. Steroids and phenobarbital were used in one case of *B. alvarius* toxicity.[227] For cardioglycoside toxicity, administration of digoxin-specific Fab fragments prevented death in young men poisoned by *Bufo* venom.[234]

No antidote is known for treatment of poison dart frog injection,[225] but studies have suggested that TTX prevents the clinical effects of batrachotoxin.[233]

CONCLUSION

In summary, neurotoxins developed and produced by creatures in the wild are used to attack the CNS and the peripheral nervous system of mammals and invertebrates through an amazing array of mechanisms. Envenomation of humans is usually accidental or in defense but this poses a significant threat to life in some parts of the world. Treatment of neurotoxic envenomations remains a challenge to the clinician. More investigation and research of these fascinating toxins is needed for a better understanding of the human nervous system and to reduce global mortality associated with envenomations.

Acknowledgments

Thanks to Jim Harrison and Kristen Wiley of the Kentucky Reptile Zoo for their generosity with suggestions and access to reptiles, resources, and medical records.

REFERENCES

1. Lev E. Traditional healing with animals (zootherapy): medieval to present-day Levantine practice. *J Ethnopharmacol.* 2003;85:107–118.
2. White J. Poisonous and venomous animals: the physician's view. In: Meier J, White J, eds. *Handbook of Clinical Toxicology of Animal Venoms and Poisons.* Boca Raton, Fla: CRC Press; 1995:9–26.
3. Henry JA, Wiseman H. *Management of Poisoning: A Handbook for Health Care Workers.* Geneva: World Health Organization, United Nations Environment Programme, International Labour Organization; 1997.
4. Bronstein AC, Spyker DA, Cantilena LR Jr, et al. 2006 Annual report of the American Association of Poison Control Centers' National Poison Data System (NPDS). *Clin Toxicol.* 2007;45:815–917.
5. Ibister GK, Gray MR. A prospective study of 750 definite spider bites with expert spider identification. *Q J Med.* 2002;95:723–731.
6. Isbister G, Gray MR, Balit CR, et al. Funnel web spider bite: a systematic review of recorded clinical cases. *Med J Aust.* 2005;182:407–411.
7. Schenone H. Diagnosis in 1348 patients which consulted for a probable spider bite or insect sting. *Bol Chil Parasitol.* 1996;51:20–27.
8. Lucas SM, Meier J. Biology and distribution of spiders of medical importance. In: Meier J, White J, eds. *Handbook of Clinical Toxicology of Animal Venoms and Poisons.* Boca Raton, Fla: CRC Press; 1995:239–258.
9. Bucaretchi F, de Deus Reinaldo DR, Hyslop S, et al. A clinico-epidemiological study of bites by spiders of the genus *Phoneutria. Rev Inst Med Trop Sao Paulo.* 2000;42:17–21.
10. Isbister GK, White J. Clinical consequences of spider bites: recent advances in our understanding. *Toxicon.* 2004;43:477–492.
11. Vetter RS, Isbister GK. Medical aspects of spider bites. *Annu Rev Entomol.* 2008;53:409–429.

12. Rash LD, Hodgson WC. Pharmacology and biochemistry of spider venoms. *Toxicon.* 2002;40:225–254.

13. Nicholson GM, Walsh R, Little MJ, et al. Characterization of the effects of robustoxin, the lethal neurotoxin from the Sydney funnel-web spider *Atrax robustus*, on sodium channel activation and inactivation. *Pflugers Arch-Eur J Physiol.* 1998;436:117–126.

14. Rezende L Jr, Cordeiro MN, Oliveira EB, et al. Isolation of neurotoxic peptides from the venom of the "armed" spider *Phoneutria nigriventer. Toxicon.* 1991;29:1225–1233.

15. Rash L, Birinyi-Strachan LC, Nicholson GM, et al. Neurotoxic activity of venom from the Australian eastern mouse spider (*M. badleyi*) involves modulation of sodium channel gating. *Br J Pharmacol.* 2000;130:1817–1824.

16. Mafra RA, Figueiredo SG, Diniz DR, et al. PhTx4, a new class of toxins from *Phoneutria nigriventer* spider venom, inhibits the glutamate uptake in rat brain synaptosomes. *Brain Res.* 1999;831:297–300.

17. Bindokas VP, Adams ME. ω-Aga-I: a presynaptic calcium channel antagonist from the venom of the funnel-web spider, *Agelenopsis aperta. J Neurobiol.* 1989;20:171–188.

18. Llinas R, Sgimori M, Lin JW, et al. Blocking and isolation of a calcium channel from neurons in mammals and cephalopods utilizing a toxin fraction (FTX) from funnel-web spider poison. *Proc Natl Acad Sci USA.* 1989;86:1689–1693.

19. Codeiro M, de Figueiredo SG, Valentim A, et al. Purification and amino acid sequences of six Tx3 type neurotoxins from the venom of the Brazilian "armed" spider *Phoneutria nigriventer* (Keys). *Toxicon.* 1993;31:35–42.

20. Liang S, Zhang D, Pan X, et al. Properties and amino acid sequence of huwentoxin-I, a neurotoxin purified from the venom of the Chinese bird spider *Selenocosmia huwena. Toxicon.* 1993;31:969–978.

21. White J, Cardoso JL, Fan HW. Clinical toxicology of spider bites. In: Meier J, White J, eds. *Handbook of Clinical Toxicology of Animal Venoms and Poisons.* Boca Raton, Fla: CRC Press; 1995:259–329.

22. Nicholson GM, Graudins A. Spiders of medical importance in the Asia-Pacific: atracotoxin, latrotoxin and related spider neurotoxins. *Clin Exp Pharmacol Physiol.* 2002;29:785–794.

23. Figueiredo SG, Garcia ME, Valentim A, et al. Purification and amino acid sequence of the insecticidal neurotoxin Tx4(6–1) from the venom of the "armed" spider *Phoneutria nigriventer* (Keys). *Toxicon.* 1995;33:83–93.

24. Nicholson GM, Graudins A, Wilson HI, et al. Arachnid toxinology in Australia: from clinical toxicology to potential applications. *Toxicon.* 2006;48:872–898.

25. Holcomb K. Stowaway Spider Spooks Snoqualmie Family. Available at: http://www.king5.com/topstories/stories/NW_030307WABbananaspiderSW.17855c0e.html. Accessed February 5, 2009.

26. DeBruxelles S. Bitten Chef Saved His Life by Snapping Lethal Spider. Available at: http://www.timesonline.co.uk/article/0,,2-1587022,00.html. Accessed February 5, 2009.

27. Gomez MV, Kalapothakis E, Guatimosim C, et al. *Phoneutria nigriventer* venom: A cocktail of toxins that affect ion channels. *Cell Mol Neurobiol.* 2002;22:579–588.

28. Maretic Z. Latrodectism: variations in clinical manifestations provoked by *Latrodectus* species of spiders. *Toxicon.* 1983;21:457–466.

29. Diaz JH. The global epidemiology, syndromic classification, management, and prevention of spider bites. *Am J Trop Med Hyg.* 2004;71:239–250.

30. Isbister GK, Gray MR. Effects of envenoming by comb-footed spiders of the genera *Steatoda* and *Achaearanea* (family Theridiidae: Araneae) in Australia. *J Toxicol Clin Toxicol.* 2003;41:809–819.

31. Isbister GK. Mouse spider bites (*Missulena* spp.) and their medical importance. A systematic review. *Med J Aust.* 2004;180:225–227.

31a. Rendle-Short H. Mouse spider envenomation [abstract]. Proceedings of the Australian and New Zealand intensive care society scientific meeting. Brisbane:The Society 1985:25.

31b. Fleury CT. Local anesthesia in stings of poisonous animals. *Rev Bras Anestesiol.* 1964;14:89–90.

32. Sutherland SK, Trinca JC. Survey of 2,144 cases of redback spider bites: Australia and New Zealand, 1963–1976. *Med J Aust.* 1978;2:620–623.

33. Clark RF. The safety and efficacy of antivenin *Latrodectus mactans. J Toxicol Clin Toxicol.* 2001;39:125–127.

34. Sutherland SK. Antivenom use in Australia: premedication, adverse reaction, and the use of venom detection kits. *Med J Aust.* 1993;157:734–739.

35. Key GF. A comparison of calcium gluconate and methocarbamol (Robaxin) in the treatment of latrodectism (black widow spider envenomation). *Am J Trop Med Hyg.* 1981;30:273–277.

36. Russell JF. Tarantism. *Med Hist.* 1979;23:404–425.

37. Bettini S. Epidemiology of latrodectism. *Toxicon.* 1964;104:93–102.

38. Sutherland S. New first-aid measures for envenomation: with special reference to bites by the Sydney funne-web spider (*Atrax robustus*). *Med J Aust.* 1980;1:378–379.

39. Sutherland SK. Antivenom to the venom of the male Sydney funnel-web spider *Atrax robustus:* preliminary report. *Med J Aust.* 1980;2:437–441.

40. Graudins A, Wilson D, Alewood PF, Broady KW, et al. Cross-reactivity of Sydney funnel-web spider antivenom: neutralization of the in vitro toxicity of other Australian funnel web (*Atrax* and *Hadronyche*) spider venoms. *Toxicon.* 2002;40(3):259–266.

41. Dieckmann J, Prebble J, McDonogh A, et al. Efficacy of funnel-web spider antivenom in human envenomation by *Hadronyche* species. *Med J Aust.* 1989;151:706–707.

42. Bennett RG, Vetter RS. An approach to spider bites: erroneous attribution of dermonecrotic lesions to brown recluse or hobo spider bites in Canada. *Can Fam Physician.* 2004;50:1098–1101.

43. Vetter RS, Barger DK. An infestation of 2,055 brown recluse spiders (Araneae: Sicariidae) and no envenomations in a Kansas home: implications for bite diagnoses in nonendemic areas. *J Med Entomol.* 2002;39:948–951.

44. Majeski JA, Durst GG. Necrotic arachnidism. *South Med J.* 1976;69:887.

45. Pauli I, Puka J, Gubert IC, et al. The efficacy of antivenom in loxoscelism treatment. *Toxicon.* 2006;48:123–137.

46. Singletary EM, Rochman AS, Bodmer JCA, et al. Envenomations. *Med Clin North Am.* 2005;89:1195–1224.

47. Saucier JR. Arachnid envenomation. *Emerg Med Clin North Am.* 2004;22:405–422.

48. Sofer S. Scorpion envenomation. *Intensive Care Med.* 1995;21(8):626–628.

49. Gwee MCE, Nirthanan S, Khoo HE, et al. Autonomic effects of some scorpion venoms and toxins. *Clin Exp Pharmacol Physiol.* 2002;29(9):795–801.

50. Crest M. Kaliotoxin, a novel peptidyl inhibitor of neuronal BK-type Ca^{++}-activated K^+ channels characterized from *Androctonus mauretanicus mauretanicus* venom. *J Biol Chem.* 1992;267:1640–1647.

51. Garcia-Calvo M, Leonard RJ, Novick J, et al. Purification, characterization, and biosynthesis of margatoxin, a component of *Centruroides margaritatus* venom that selectively inhibits voltage-dependent potassium channels. *J Biol Chem.* 1993;268:18866–18874.

52. Jenkinson DH. Potassium channels: multiplicity and challenges. *Br J Pharm.* 2006;147:S63–S71.

53. Bosmans F, Tytgat J. Voltage-gated sodium channel modulation by scorpion α-toxins. *Toxicon.* 2007;49:142–158.

54. Gordon D. A new approach to insect pest control: combination of neurotoxins interacting with voltage sensitive sodium channels to increase selectivity and specificity. *Invert Neurosci.* 1997; 3:103–116.

55. Gordon D, Karbat I, Ilan N, et al. The differential preference of scorpion α-toxins for insect or mammalian sodium channels: implications for improved insect control. *Toxicon.* 2007;49: 452–472.

56. Gueron M, Ilia R, Margulis G. Arthropod poisons and the cardiovascular system. *Am J Emerg Med.* 2000;18:708–714.

57. Bahloul M, Rekik N, Chabchoub I, et al. Neurological complications secondary to severe scorpion envenomation. *Med Sci Monit.* 2005;11:CR196–CR202.

58. Ismail M. The scorpion envenoming syndrome. *Toxicon.* 1994; 33:825–858.

59. Dehisa-Devila M, Alagon AC, Possani LD. Biology and distribution of scorpions of medical importance. In: Meier J, White J, eds. *Handbook of Clinical Toxicology of Animal Venoms and Poisons.* Boca Raton, Fla: CRC Press. 1995:239–258.

60. Curry SC, Vance MV, Ryah PJ, et al. Envenomation by the scorpion *Centruroides sculpturatus. J Toxicol Clin Toxicol.* 1985;21:417–449.

61. Hamed MI. Treatment of the scorpion envenoming syndrome: 12-years experience with serotherapy. *Int J Antimicrob Agents.* 2003;21:170–174.

62. Abroug F, Elatrous S, Nouira S, et al. Serotherapy in scorpion envenomation: a randomized control trial. *Lancet.* 1999;354:906–909.

63. Biswal N, Bashir RA, Murmu UC, et al. Outcome of scorpion sting envenomation after a protocol guided therapy. *Indian J Pediatr.* 2006;73:577–582.

64. Sofer S, Gueron M. Vasodilators and hypertensive encephalopathy following scorpion envenomation in children. *Chest.* 1990;97: 118–120.

65. Gupta V. Prazosin: a pharmacological antidote for scorpion envenomation. *J Trop Pediatr.* 2006;52:150–151.

66. Al-Asmari AK, Al-Seif AA, Hassen MA, et al. Role of prazosin on cardiovascular manifestations and pulmonary edema following severe scorpion stings in Saudi Arabia. *Saudi Med J.* 2008;29: 299–302.

67. Foex B, Wallis L. Best evidence topic report: Scorpion envenomation—does administration of antivenom alter outcome? *Emerg Med J.* 2005;22:195.

68. Foex B, Wallis L. Best evidence topic report: Scorpion envenomation—does antivenom reduce serum venom concentrations? *Emerg Med J.* 2005;22:195–197.

69. Dehesa-Davila M, Possani LD. Scorpionism and serotherapy in Mexico. *Toxicon.* 1994;32:1015–1018.

70. Masina S, Broady KW. Tick paralysis: development of a vaccine. *Int J Parasitol.* 1999;29:535–541.

71. Centers for Disease Control and Prevention. Tick paralysis: Washington, 1995. *MMWR.* 1996;45:325–326.

72. Grattan-Smith PJ, Morris JG, Johnston HM, et al. Clinical and neurophysiological features of tick paralysis. *Brain.* 1997;20: 1975–1987.

73. Dworkin MS, Shoemaker PC, Anderson DE Jr. Tick paralysis: 33 human cases in Washington state, 1946–1996. *Clin Infect Dis.* 1999;9:1435–1439.

74. Aeschlimann A, Freyvogel TA. Biology and distribution of ticks of medical importance. In: Meier J, White J, eds. *Handbook of Clinical Toxicology of Animal Venoms and Poisons.* Boca Raton, Fla: CRC Press; 1995:177–203.

75. Greenstein P. Tick paralysis. *Med Clin North Am.* 2002;86: 441–446.

76. Centers for Disease Control and Prevention. Cluster of tick paralysis cases: Colorado, 2006. *MMWR.* 2006;55:933–935.

77. Erasmus LD. Regional tick paralysis: sensory and motor changes caused by a male tick, genus *Hyalomma. S Afr Med J.* 1952;26:985–987.

78. Rose I. A review of tick paralysis. *Can Med Assoc J.* 1954;70: 175–176.

79. Kaire GH. Isolation of tick paralysis toxin from *Ixodes holocyclus. Toxicon.* 1966;4:91–97.

80. Cooper BJ, Spence I. Temperature-dependent inhibition of evoked acetylcholine release in tick paralysis. *Nature.* 1976; 263:693–695.

81. Wright IG, Stone BF, Neish AL. Tick (*Ixodes holocyclus*) paralysis in the dog: induction of immunity by injection of toxin. *Aust Vet J.* 1983;69:69–70.

82. Stone BF, Neish AL. Tick-paralysis toxoid: an effective immunizing agent against the toxin of *Ixodes holocyclus. Aust J Exp Biol Med Sci.* 1984;62(Pt 2):189–191.

83. Felz MW, Smith CD, Swift TR. A six-year-old girl with tick paralysis. *N Engl J Med.* 2000;342:90–94.

84. Foster B. A tick in the auditory meatus. *Med J Aust.* 1931;1: 15–16.

85. Miller MK. Massive tick (*Ixodes holocyclus*) infestation with delayed facial nerve palsy. *Med J Aust.* 2002;176:254–265.

86. Vedanarayanan V, Sorey WH, Subramony SH. Tick paralysis. *Semin Neurol.* 2004;24:181–184.

87. Libersat F. Wasp uses venom cocktail to manipulate the behavior of its cockroach prey. *J Comp Physiol A Neuroethol Sens Neural Behav Physiol.* 2003;189:497–508.

88. Eberhard W. Spider manipulation by a wasp larva. *Nature.* 2000;406:255–256.

89. Kutsukake M, Shibao H, Nikoh N, et al. Venomous protease of aphid soldier for colony defense. *Proc Natl Acad Sci USA.* 2004;101:11338–11343.

90. Schmidt JO. Biochemistry of insect venoms. *Ann Rev Entomol.* 1982;27:339–368.

91. Vetter RS, Visscher PK, Camazine S. Mass envenomations by honey bees and wasps. *West J Med.* 1999;170:223–227.

92. Joint Task Force on Practice Parameters, American Academy of Allergy, Asthma and Immunology, American College of Allergy, Asthma and Immunology. Allergen immunotherapy: a practice parameter. *Ann Allergy Asthma Immunol.* 2003; 90(1 Suppl 1):1–40.

93. Balderrama N, Nunez F, Guerrieri F, Giurfa M. Different functions of two alarm substances in the honeybee. *J Comp Physiol A.* 2002;188:485–491.

94. Lamprecht I, Schmolz E, Schricker B. Pheromones in the life of insects. *Eur Biophys J.* 2008;37:1083–1278.

95. Likkitanasombut P, Witoonpanich R, Viranuvatti K. Encephalomyeloradiculopathy associated with wasp sting. *J Neurol Neurosurg Psychiatry.* 2003;74:134–139.

96. Bernhard JH. Studies of 400 hymenoptera stings in the United States. *J Allergy Clin Immunol.* 1973;52:259–264.

97. Meier J. Biology and distribution of hymenopterans of medical importance, their venom apparatus and venom composition. In: Meier J, White J, eds. *Handbook of Clinical Toxicology of Animal Venoms and Poisons.* Boca Raton, Fla: CRC Press; 1995:331–348.

98. Palma MS. Insect venom peptides. In: Kastin A, ed. *Handbook of Biologically Active Peptides.* San Diego: Elsevier; 2006:409–417.

99. Piek T. Neurotoxic kinins from wasp and ant venoms. *Toxicon.* 1991;29:139–149.

100. Konno K, Hisada M, Itagaki Y, et al. Isolation and structure of pompilidotoxins, novel peptide neurotoxins in solitary wasp venoms. *Biochem Biophys Res Commun.* 1998;250: 612–616.

101. Konno K, Palma MS, Hitara IY, et al. Identification of bradykinins in solitary wasp venoms. *Toxicon.* 2002;40:309–312.

102. Sahara Y, Gotoh M, Kono K, et al. A new class of neurotoxin from wasp venom slows inactivation of sodium current. *Eur J Neurosci*. 2000;12:1961–1970.

103. Gale AN. Insect-sting encephalopathy. *BMJ*. 1982;284:20–21 (and follow-up discussions).

104. Reisman RE. Unusual reactions to insect stings. *Curr Opin Allergy Clin Immunol*. 2005;5:355–358.

105. Brumlick J. Myasthenia gravis associated with wasp sting. *JAMA*. 1976;235:2120–2121.

106. Hira HS, Mittal A, Kumar SA, et al. Myasthenia gravis and acute respiratory muscle paralysis following wasp sting. *Indian J Chest Dis Allied Sci*. 2005;47:197–198.

107. Means ED, Barron KD, Van Dyne BJ, et al. Nervous system lesions after sting by yellow jacket: a case report. *Neurology*. 1973;23:881–890.

108. Creange A, Saint-Val C, Guillevin L, et al. Peripheral neuropathies after arthropod stings not associated with Lyme disease: a report of five cases and review of the literature. *Neurology*. 1993;43:1483–1488.

109. Light WC, Reisman RE, Shimizu M, et al. Unusual reactions following insect sting: clinical features and immunologic analysis. *J Allergy Clin Immunol*. 1977;59:391–397.

110. Boz C, Velioglu S, Ozmenoglu M. Acute disseminated encephalomyelitis after bee sting. *Neurol Sci*. 2003;23:313–315.

111. Agarwal V, Dcruz S, Sachdev A, et al. Quadriparesis following wasp sting: an unusual reaction. *Indian J Med Sci*. 2005;59:117–119.

112. Caldwell ST, Schuman SH, Simpson WM. Fire ants: a continuing community health threat in South Carolina. *J SC Med Assoc*. 1999;95:231–235.

113. deShazo RD, Butcher BT, Banks WA. Reactions to the stings of the imported fire ant. *N Engl J Med*. 1990;323:462–466.

114. Williams DF, deShazo RD. Biological control of fire ants: an update on new techniques. *Ann Allergy Asthma Immunol*. 2004;93:15–22.

115. Howell G, Butler J, deShazo RD, et al. Cardiodepressant and neurologic actions of *Solenopsis invicta* (imported fire ant) venom alkaloids. *Ann Allergy Asthma Immunol*. 2005;94:380–386.

116. Yi GB, McClendon D, Desaiah D, et al. Fire ant venom alkaloid, isosolenopsin A, a potent and selective inhibitor of neuronal nitric oxide synthase. *Int J Toxicol*. 2003;22:81–86.

117. Piek T. Neurotoxins from venoms of the hymenoptera: twenty-five years of research in Amsterdam. *Bomp Biochem Physiol C*. 1990;96:223–233.

118. Pluzhnikov K, Nosyreva E, Shevchenko L, et al. Analysis of ectatomin action on cell membranes. *Eur J Biochem*. 1999;262:501–506.

118a. deShazo RD, Williams DF, Moak ES. Fire ant attacks on residents in health care facilities: A report of two cases. *Ann Intern Med*. 1999;131:424–429.

119. Koya S, Crenshaw D, Agarwal A. Rhabdomyolysis and acute renal failure after fire ant bites. *J Gen Intern Med*. 2007;22:145–147.

120. Fox RW, Lockey RF, Bukantz SC. Neurologic sequelae following the imported fire ant sting. *J Allergy Clin Immunol*. 1982;70:120–124.

121. Candiotti KA, Lamas AM. Adverse neurologic reactions to the sting of the imported fire ant. *Int Arch Allergy Immunol*. 1993;102:417–420.

122. Kemp SF, deShazo RD, Moffitt JE, et al. Expanding habitat of the imported fire ant *(Solenopsis invicta)*: a public health concern. *J Allergy Clin Immunol*. 2000;105:683–691.

123. Haddad V Jr, Cardoso JLC, Moraes RHP. Description of an injury in a human caused by a false tocandira (*Dinoponera gigantean*, Perty, 1833) with a revision on folkloric, pharmacological and clinical aspects of the giant ants of the genera *Paraponera* and *Dinoponera* (sub-family Ponerinae). *Rev Inst Med Trop Sao Paulo*. 2005;47:235–238.

124. Bequaert JC. Medical report of the Hamilton Rice 7th expedition to the Amazon, in conjunction with the department of tropical medicine of Harvard University, 1924–1925. In: *Contributions from the Harvard Institute for Tropical Biology and Medicine*. no. 4. Cambridge: Harvard University Press; 1926:250–253.

125. Weber NA. The sting of an ant. *Am J Trop Med*. 1937;17:765–768.

126. Klotz JH, deShazo RD, Pinnas JL, et al. Adverse reactions to ants other than imported fire ants. *Ann Allergy Asthma Immunol*. 2005;95:418–425.

127. deShazo RD, Kemp SF, deShazo MD, et al. Fire ant attacks on patients in nursing homes: an increasing problem. *Am J Med*. 2004;116:843–846.

128. Ouzounellis T. Some notes on quail poisoning. *JAMA*. 1970;211:1186–1187.

129. Grivetti LE, Rucker RB. Human poisoning by European migratory quail *Coturnix coturnix*. Dumbacher and Daly (Conveners). *J Ornith*. 1994;135:409.

130. Bartram S, Boland W. Chemistry and ecology of toxic birds. *Chembiochem*. 2001;2:809–811.

131. Giannopoulos D, Voulioti S, Skarelos A, et al. Quail poisoning in a child. *Rural Remote Health*. 2006;6:564.

132. Escalante P, Daly JW. Alkaloids in extracts of feathers of the red warbler. Dumbacher and Daly (Conveners). *J Ornith*. 1994;135:410.

133. Dumbacher JP, Wako A, Derrickson SR, et al. Melyride beetles *(Choresine)*: a putative source for the batrachotoxin alkaloids found in poison-dart frogs and toxic passerine birds. *Proc Natl Acad Sci USA*. 2004;101:15857–15860.

134. Aparicio R, Onate JM, Arizcun A, et al. Epidemic rhabdomyolysis due to the eating of quail: a clinical, epidemiological, and experimental study. *Med Clin (Barc)*. 1999;112:143–146.

135. Conn H. How do you like your quail prepared? *Am J Gastroent*. 2001;96:2790–2792.

136. Papapetropoulos T, Hadziqiannis S, Ouzounellis T. On the pathogenetic mechanism of quail myopathy. *JAMA*. 1980;244:2263–2264.

137. Musumeci O, Aguennouz M, Cagliani R, et al. Calpain 3 deficiency in quail eater's disease. *Ann Neurol*. 2004;55:146–147.

138. Dumbacher JP, Beehler BM, Spande TF, et al. Homobatrachotoxin in the genus *Pitohui*: Chemical defense in birds? *Science*. 1992;258:799–801.

139. Dumbacher JP, Spande TF, Daly JW. Batachotoxin alkaloids from passerine birds: a second toxic bird genus *(Ifrita kowaldi)* from New Guinea. *Proc Natl Acad Sci USA*. 2000;97:12970–12975.

140. Weldon PJ. Avian chemical defense: toxic birds not of a feather. *Proc Natl Acad Sci USA*. 2000;97:12948–12949.

141. Wilson A. *American Ornithology, or The Natural History of the Birds of the United States*. vol 3. New York: Collins & Co; 1829:18–23.

142. Bloom K, Grivetti LE. The mysterious history of partridge poisoning. *J Hist Med Allied Sci*. 2001;56:68–76.

143. Papadimitriou A, Hadjiggeorgiou GM, Tsairis P, et al. Myoglobinuria due to quail poisoning. *Eur Neurol*. 1996;36:142–145.

144. Tsironi M, Andriopoulos P, Xamodraka E, et al. The patient with rhabdomyolysis: have you considered quail poisoning? *CMAJ*. 2004;171:325–326.

145. Dufton MJ. Venomous mammals. *Pharmacol Ther*. 1992;53:199–215.

146. Kita M, Nakamura Y, Okumura Y. Blarina toxin, a mammalian lethal venom from the short-tailed shrew *Blarina brevicauda*:

isolation and characterization. *Proc Natl Acad Sci USA*. 2004; 101:7542–7547.

147. Krane S, Itagaki Y, Nakanishi K, et al. "Venom" of the slow loris: sequence similarity of prosimian skin gland protein and Fel d 1 cat allergen. *Naturwissenschaften*. 2003;90:60–62.

148. Grant TR, Temple-Smith PD. Field biology of the platypus *(Ornithorhynchus anatinus):* historical and current perspectives. *Phil Trans R Soc Lond B.* 1998;353:1081–1091.

149. Kourie JI. A component of platypus *(O. anatinus)* venom forms slow-kinetic cation channels. *J Membr Biol.* 1999;172:37–45.

150. de Plater GM, Milburn PJ, Martin RL. Venom from the platypus, *Ornithorhychus anatinus,* induces a calcium-dependent current in cultured dorsal root ganglion cells. *J Neurophysiol.* 2001;85:1340–1345.

151. Torres AM, Wang X, Fletcher JI, et al. Solution structure of a defensin-like peptide from platypus venom. *Biochem J.* 1999; 341:785–794.

152. Torres AM, de Plater GM, Doverskog M, et al. Defensin-like peptide-2 from platypus venom: member of a class of peptides with a distinct structural fold. *Biochem J.* 2000;348:649–656.

153. Martin CJ, Tidswell F. Observations on the femoral gland of *Ornithorhynchus* and its secretions, together with an experimental enquiry concerning its supposed toxic action. *Proc Linn Soc NSW.* 1894;9:471–500.

154. Fenner PJ, Williamson JA, Myers D. Platypus envenomation: a painful learning experience. *Med J Aust.* 1992;157:829–832.

155. Tonkin MA, Negrine J. Wild platypus attacks in the antipodes: a case report. *J Hand Surg.* 1994;19:162–164.

156. Barroso E, Hidaka AS, dos Santos AX, et al. Centipede stings notified by the "Centro de Informacoes Toxicologicas de Belem" over a 2-year period. *Rev Soc Bras Med Trop.* 2001; 34:527–530.

157. Gomes A, Datta A, Sarangi B, et al. Isolation, purification, and pharmacodynamics of a toxin from the venom of the centipede *Scolopendra subsinipes dehaani* Brandt. *Indian J Exp Biol.* 1983;21:203–207.

158. Noda N, Yashiki Y, Nakatani T, et al. A novel quinoline alkaloid possessing a 7-benzyl group from the centipede *Scolopendra subsinipes. Chem Pharm Bull.* 2001;49:930–931.

159. Rates B, Bemquerer MP, Richardson M, et al. Venomic analysis of *Scolopendra viridicornis nigra* and *Scolopendra angulata* (Centipede, *Scolopendromorpha):* shedding light on venoms from a neglected group. *Toxicon.* 2007;49:810–826.

160. Stankiewicz M, Hamon A, Benkhalifa R, et al. Effects of a centipede venom fraction on insect nervous system, a native *Xenopus* oocyte receptor on an expressed *Drosophila* muscarinic receptor. *Toxicon.* 1999;37:1431–1445.

161. Ren Y, Houghton P, Hider RC. Relevant activities of extracts and constituents of animals used in traditional Chinese medicine for central nervous system effects associated with Alzheimer's disease. *J Pharm Pharmacol.* 2006;58:989–996.

162. Bhagirath T, Chingtham B, Mohen Y. Venom of a hill centipede *Scolopendra viridicornis* inhibits growth of human breast tumor in mice. *Indian J Pharmacol.* 2006;38:291–292.

163. Balit CR, Harvey MS, Waldock JM, et al. Prospective study of centipede bites in Australia. *J Toxicol Clin Toxicol.* 2004;42: 41–48.

163a. Bush SP, King BO, Norris RL, Stockwell SA. Centipede envenomation. *Wilderness and Environmental Medicine.* 2008;12: 93–99.

164. Mohri S, Sugiyama A, Saito K, et al. Centipede bites in Japan. *Cutis.* 1991;47:189–190.

165. Logan JL, Ogden DA. Rhabdomyolysis and acute renal failure following the bite of the giant desert centipede *Scolopendra heros. West J Med.* 1985;142:549–550.

166. Ozsarac M, Karcioglu O, Ayrik C, et al. Acute coronary ischemia following centipede envenomation: case report and review of the literature. *Wilderness Environ Med.* 2004;15:109–112.

167. Guerrero APS. Centipede bites in Hawai'i: A brief case report and review of the literature. *Hawaii Med J.* 2007;66: 125–127.

168. Wang IK, Hsu SP, Chi CC, et al. Rhabdomyolysis, acute renal failure, and multiple focal neuropathies after drinking alcohol soaked with centipede. *Ren Fail.* 2004;26:93–97.

168a. Pineda EV. A fatal case of centipede bite. *J Med Assoc.* 1923;3:59–61.

169. Remington CL. The bite and habits of a giant centipede *(Scolopendra subspinipes)* in the Philippine Islands. *Am J Trop Med.* 1950;30:453–455.

169a. Serinken M, Erdur B, Sener S, et al. A case of mortal necrotizing fasciitis of the trunk resulting from a centipede (Scolopendra Moritans) bite. *The Internet Journal of Emergency Medicine.* 2005, Vol 2.

170. Acosta M, Cazorla D. Centipede *(Scolopendra* sp) envenomation in a rural village of semi-arid region from Falcon State, Venezuela. *Rev Invest Clin.* 2004;56:712–715.

171. Bush SP, King BO, Norris RL, et al. Centipede envenomation. *Wilderness Environ Med.* 2001;12:93–99.

172. Dar NR, Raza N, Rehman SB. Millipede burn at an unusual site mimicking child abuse in an 8-year-old girl. *Clin Pediatr.* 2008:47:490–492.

173. Hendrickson RG. Millipede exposure. *Clin Toxicol.* 2005;43: 211–212.

174. Hudson BJ, Parsons GA. Giant millipede "burns" and the eye. *Trans R Soc Trop Med Hyg.* 1997;91:183–185.

175. Diaz J. The evolving global epidemiology, syndromic classification, management, and prevention of caterpillar envenoming. *Am J Trop Med Hyg.* 2005;72:347–357.

176. Carrijo-Carvalho LC, Chudzinski-Tavassi AM. The venom of the *Lonomia* caterpillar: an overview. *Toxicon.* 2007;49: 741–757.

177. White J. Bites and stings from venomous animals: a global overview. *Ther Drug Monitor.* 2000;22:65–68.

178. Chippaux JP. Snake bites: appraisal of the global situation. *Bull World Health Organ.* 1998;76:515–524.

179. Warrell DA. WHO/SEARO guidelines for the clinical management of snake bite in the South-East Asia region. *Southeast Asian J Trop Med Public Health.* 1999;30:1–85 (Suppl 1).

180. Agrawal PN, Aggarwal AN, Gupta D, et al. Management of respiratory failure in severe neuroparalytic snake envenomation. *Neurol India.* 2001;49:25–28.

181. McNamee D. Tackling venomous snake bites worldwide. *Lancet.* 2001;357:1680.

182. Juckett G, Hancox JG. Venomous snakebites in the United States: management review and update. *Am Fam Physician.* 2002;65:1367–1374.

183. Potter LT. Snake toxins that bind specifically to individual subtypes of muscarinic receptors. *Life Sci.* 2001;68:2541–2547.

184. Yee JSP, Afifiyan F, Donghui M, et al. Snake postsynaptic neurotoxins: gene structure, phylogeny and applications in research and therapy. *Biochimie.* 2003;86:137–149.

185. Schiavo G, Matteoli M, Montecucco C. Neurotoxins affecting neuroexocytosis. *Physiol Rev.* 2000;80:717–766.

186. Anderson AJ, Harvey AL, Mbugua PM. Effects of fasciculin 2, an anticholinesterase polypeptide from green mamba venom, on neuromuscular transmission in mouse diaphragm preparations. *Neurosci Lett.* 1985;54:123–128.

187. Wollberg Z, Shabo-Shina R, Intrator N, et al. A novel cardiotoxic polypeptide from the venom of *Atractoaspis engaddensis* (burrowing asp): cardiac effects in mice and isolated rat and human heart preparations. *Toxicon.* 1988;26:525–534.

188. Warrell DA. Clinical toxicology of snakebite in Africa and the Middle East/Arabian peninsula. In: Meier J, White J, eds. *Handbook of Clinical Toxicology of Animal Venoms and Poisons.* Boca Raton, Fla: CRC Press; 1995:433–478.

189. Yap CH, Ihle BU. Coagulopathy after snake envenomation. *Neurology.* 2003;61:1788.

190. Isbister GK, Little M, Cull G, et al. Thrombotic microangiopathy from Australian brown snake *(Pseudonaja)* envenoming. *Intern Med J.* 2007;37:523–528.

191. Sutherland SK, Coulter AR, Harris RD. Rationalization of first aid measures for elapid snakebite. *Lancet.* 1979;1:183–186.

192. Bawaskar HS, Bawaskar PH. Evenoming by the common krait *(Bungarus caeruleus)* and Asian cobra *(Naja naja):* Clinical manifestations and their management in a rural setting. *Wilderness Environ Med.* 2004;15:257–266.

193. Mars M, Hadley GP, Aitchinson JM. Direct intracompartmental pressure measurement in the management of snakebites in children. *S Afr Med J.* 1991;80:227–228.

194. Strimple PD, Tomassoni AJ, Otten EJ, et al. Report on envenomation by a Gila monster *(Heloderma suspectum)* with discussion of venom apparatus, clinical findings, and treatment. *Wilderness Environ Med.* 1997;8:111–116.

195. Fry BG, Vidal N, Norman JA, et al. Early evolution of the venom system of lizards and snakes. *Nature.* 2006;439:584–588.

196. Utaisincharoen P, Mackessy SP, Miller RA, et al. Complete primary structure and biochemical properties of gilatoxin, a serine protease with kallikrein-like and angiotensin-degrading activities. *J Biol Chem.* 1993;268:21975–21983.

197. Alagon A, Possani LD, Smart J, et al. Helodermatine, a kallikrein-like, hypotensive enzyme from the venom of *Heloderma horridum horridum* (Mexican beaded lizard). *J Exp Med.* 1986;164:1835–1845.

198. Morrissette J, Kratzschmar J, Haendler B, et al. Primary structure and properties of helothermine, a peptide toxin that blocks ryanodine receptors. *Biophys J.* 1995;68:2280–2288.

199. Nobile M, Noceti F, Prestipino G, et al. Helothermine, a lizard venom toxin, inhibits calcium current in cerebellar granules. *Exp Brain Res.* 1996;110:15–20.

200. Mebs D. Clinical toxicology of helodermatidae lizard bites. In: Meier J, White J, eds. *Handbook of Clinical Toxicology of Animal Venoms and Poisons.* Boca Raton, Fla: CRC Press; 1995:361–366.

201. Cantrell FL. Envenomation by the Mexican beaded lizard: a case report. *J Toxicol Clin Toxicol.* 2003;41:241–244.

202. Hooker KR, Caravati EM. Gila monster envenomation. *Ann Emerg Med.* 1994;24:731–735.

203. Albritton DC, Parrish HM, Allen ER. Venenation by the Mexican beaded lizard *(Heloderma horridum):* report of a case. *SD J Med.* 1970;23:9–11.

204. Miller M. Comment on Gila monster envenomation. *Ann Emerg Med.* 1995;25:720.

205. Isidore of Seville. Etymologies. *Book 12.* 7th century AD;4:36.

206. Bradley SG, Klika LJ. A fatal poisoning from the Oregon rough-skinned newt *(Taricha granulosa). JAMA.* 1981;246:247.

207. Mosher HS, Fuhrman FA, Buchwald HD, et al. Tarichatoxin–tetrodotoxin: a potent neurotoxin. *Science.* 1964;144:1100–1110.

208. Hanifin CT, Brodie ED III, Brodie ED Jr. Tetrodotoxin levels of the rough-skin newt, *Taricha granulosa,* increase in long-term captivity. *Toxicon.* 2002;40:1149–1153.

209. Hanifin CT, Brodie ED III, Brodie ED Jr. Tetrodotoxin levels in eggs of the rough-skinned newt, *Taricha granulosa,* are correlated with female toxicity. *J Chem Ecol.* 2003;29:1729–1739.

210. Davis W. The ethnobiology of the Haitian zombi. *J Ethnopharmacol.* 1983;9:85–104.

211. Yasumoto T, Kao CY. Tetrodotoxin and the Haitian zombie. *Toxicon.* 1986;24:747–749.

212. Yotsu M, Iorizzi M, Yasumoto T. Distribution of tetrodotoxin, 6-epitetrodotoxin, and 11-deoxytetrodotoxin in newts. *Toxicon.* 1990;28:238–241.

213. Geffeney S, Brodie ED Jr, Ruben PC, Brodie ED III. Mechanisms of adaptation in a predator–prey arms race: TTX-resistant sodium channels. *Science.* 2002;297:1336–1339.

214. Bodie ED III, Feldman CR, Hanifin CT, et al. Parallel arms races between garter snakes and newts involving tetrodotoxins as the phenotypic interface of coevolution. *J Chem Ecol.* 2005; 31:343–356.

215. Yoshida S, Matsuda Y, Samejima A. Tetrodotoxin-resistant sodium and calcium components of action potentials in dorsal root ganglion cells of the adult mouse. *J Neurophysiol.* 1978; 41:1096–1106.

216. Daly JW, Spande TF, Garraffo HM. Alkaloids from amphibian skin: a tabulation of over eight-hundred compounds. *J Nat Prod.* 2005;68:1556–1575.

217. Kozorog M. Salamander brandy: "a psychedelic drink" between media myth and practice of home alcohol distillation in Slovenia. *Anthropology of East Eur Rev.* 2003;21:epub.

218. King BR, Hamilton RJ, Kassutto Z. "Tail of newt": an unusual ingestion. *Pediatr Emerg Care.* 2000;16:268–269.

219. Isbister GK, Son J, Wang F, et al. Puffer fish poisoning: a potentially life-threatening condition. *Med J Aust.* 2002;177: 650–653.

220. Kellaway CH. Animal poisons. *Annu Rev Biochem.* 1939;8: 541–556.

221. Lawrence DT, Dobmeier SG, Bechtel LK, et al. Food poisoning. *Emerg Med Clin North Am.* 2007;25:357–373.

222. Weil AT, Davis W. *Bufo alvarius:* a potent hallucinogen of animal origin. *J Ethnopharmacol.* 1994;41:1–8.

223. Xie JT, Dey L, Wu JA, et al. Cardiac toxicity of resibufogenin: electrophysiological evidence. *Acta Pharmacol Sin.* 2001;22: 289–297.

224. Oka K, Kantrowitz JD, Spector S. Isolation of morphine from toad skin. *Proc Natl Acad Sci USA.* 1985;82:1852–1854.

225. Marki F, Witkop B. The venom of the Columbian arrow poison frog *Phyllobates bicolor. Experientia.* 1963;19:329–376.

226. Daly JW, Spande TF, Garraffo HM. Alkaloids from amphibian skin: a tabulation of over eight-hundred compounds. *J Nat Prod.* 2005;68:1556–1575.

227. Hitt M, Ettinger DD. Toad toxicity. *N Engl J Med.* 1986; 314:1517.

228. Keomany S, Mayxay M, Souvannasing P, et al. Toad poisoning in Laos. *Am J Trop Med Hyg.* 2007;77:850–853.

229. Kwan T, Paiusco AD, Kohl L. Digitalis toxicity caused by toad venom. *Chest.* 1992;102:949–950.

230. Yei CC, Deng JF. Toad or toad cake intoxication in Taiwan: report of four cases. *J Formos Med Assoc.* 1993;92 (Suppl 3): S135–S139.

231. Barry TL, Petzinger G, Zito SW. GC/MS comparison of the West Indian aphrodisiac "love stone" to the Chinese medication "chan su": bufotenine and related bufadienolides. *J Forensic Sci.* 1996;41:1068–1073.

232. Gowda RM, Cohen RA, Khan IA. Toad venom poisoning: resembling to digoxin toxicity and therapeutic implications. *Heart.* 2003;89:e14.

233. Daly JW, Witkop B. Batrachotoxin, an extremely active cardio- and neurotoxin from the Colombian arrow poison frog *Phyllobates aurotaenia. Clin Toxicol.* 1971;4:331–342.

234. Brubacher JR, Ravikumar PR, Bania T, et al. Treatment of toad venom poisoning with digoxin-specific Fab fragments. *Chest.* 1996;110:1282–1288.

CHAPTER 44 ••••

Neurotoxic Pesticides

David A. Jett and Jason R. Richardson

ANTICHOLINESTERASE INSECTICIDES

Anticholinesterase pesticides inhibit the hydrolytic enzyme acetylcholinesterase (AChE; BC 3.1.1.7). The most common of these are esters of phosphoric or phosphorothioic acid. Commonly referred to as the organophosphates (OPs), this group is a large, chemically diverse class that includes more than 200 compounds containing one of a dozen or more different organophosphorus esters. Most are insecticides, but there are OP and carbamate herbicides and fungicides that are relatively nontoxic to humans. Several subclasses of OPs include the phosphorothionates (e.g., diazinon and chlorpyrifos), phosphorothionothiolates (e.g., malathion), and phosphoramidothiolates (e.g., methamidophos; Figure 44-1). Related to the OP insecticides are the organophosphorus nerve gases developed for chemical warfare during World War II. These include the highly toxic VX and sarin (see Figure 44-1). Another important class of pesticides is the carbamates, which are carbamic acid esters with an anticholinesterase mode of action that is similar to that of the OPs. These compounds are used as insecticides, fungicides, and herbicides. They possess the RNC(O)−, RNC(O)S−, or RNC(S)S− moieties (see Figure 44-1) and inhibit cholinesterases by way of their carbamoyl and thiocarbamoyl structure.

Toxicology

The anticholinesterase pesticides can be absorbed through the skin, through the gut, or by inhalation. They undergo extensive biotransformation, resulting in more toxic or less toxic metabolites. The oxidative, reductive, and hydrolytic (Phase I), as well as conjugation (Phase II) reactions are catalyzed by various enzyme systems, most notably the cytochrome P450 and glutathione-related system, respectively. Some species differences in the toxicity of OPs are related to differences the ability of particular species to metabolize the parent compounds into nontoxic forms. Not all OPs require bioactivation; for example, OP nerve agents and some insecticides are bioactive in the parent form. OP insecticides are effective because of their ability to phosphorylate and deactivate AChE. This enzyme is also carbamylated by carbamate pesticides that produce similar effects. In mammalian systems, the acute toxicity of OP and carbamate insecticides is derived from this anticholinesterase activity and subsequent parasympathomimetic effects. AChE is an essential hydrolytic enzyme found in the central nervous system (CNS) and the autonomic systems of the peripheral nervous system, as well as at all neuromuscular junctions. OPs and other anticholinesterases acylate the enzyme at the esteratic site, as does its substrate, the neurotransmitter acetylcholine (ACh). A major difference

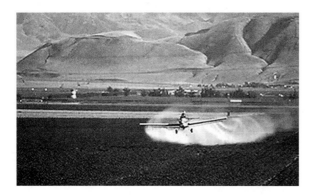

 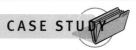
between the OPs and the carbamates is the rate of de-phosphorylation or decarbamoylation of the inhibited enzyme. The carbamates are largely reversible because of a fast rate of deacylation, whereas the rate is so slow with OPs that they are considered irreversible; consequently, they require more extensive medical intervention.

AChE is also found in red blood cells and is sometimes used as a clinical biomarker for exposure to these compounds. Another related molecule that binds OPs and carbamates is butyrylcholinesterase (BChE; BC 3.1.1.8). It is found in myelin, liver, and plasma, where its physiological function is poorly understood but may serve as a scavenger of toxic compounds.[3,4] Inhibition of AChE alters cholinergic neurotransmission by preventing the hydrolysis of the ACh. This leads to an accumulation of ACh in the synaptic cleft and overstimulation, followed by desensitization of ACh receptors on cell surfaces. Some OPs and carbamates also interact with another enzyme termed *neuropathy target esterase*. This is believed to be the initiating event for the development of a delayed polyneuropathy called *organophosphate-induced delayed neurotoxicity* (OPIDN).[5]

The acute and chronic toxicity of OPs has been studied extensively in laboratory animal models and in occupationally exposed humans; this has been reviewed elsewhere.[6] Some OPs can be transferred to the fetus via the placenta and are teratogenic, causing various abnormalities such as growth retardation, micromelia, and axial skeletal problems, and this may have serious implications for the health of children exposed to low to moderate levels.[6,7] These studies and evidence of extensive human exposures in some areas have led to concern that public health may be adversely affected by their extensive commercial and residential use. Some of the most widely used pesticides, such as parathion and chlorpyrifos, have been banned from use because of their toxicity to humans. Effects on the developing CNS have been demonstrated in animals and include anencephaly, stunted growth of various brain structures, altered cholinergic and glutamatergic neurochemistry, and regional brain histopathology. OPs are also believed to act as immunosuppressants, primarily through alteration of macrophage function.[6] Some toxicity may be modified with continuous exposure. Tolerance to OPs develops as a result of

 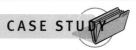

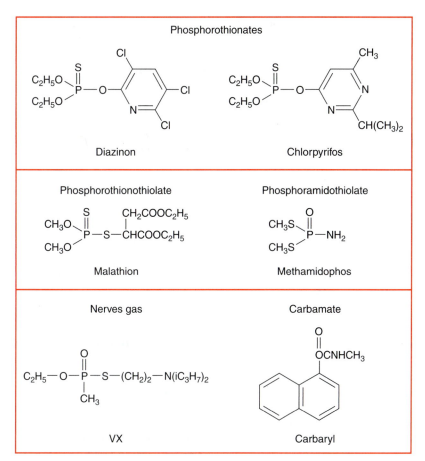

Figure 44-1. Typical organophosphate and carbamate insecticides and nerve gases.

Clinical Presentation and Public Health

Most cases of acute poisoning from anticholinesterase pesticides are from suicide attempts. Signs of acute intoxication by these compounds depend on the severity of exposure, and they reflect their anticholinesterase activity at muscarinic and nicotinic cholinergic synapses. The muscarinic effects are primarily parasympathomimetic and are manifested in the lung, gastrointestinal system, sweat glands, salivary glands, lacrimal glands, cardiovascular system, pupils, and bladder. With some OPs, pancreatitis may occur and lead to fatality, often without any pain or other indications. Other effects on the sympathetic nervous system and somatic motor nerves are a result of overstimulation of nicotinic cholinergic receptors. The mnemonic SLUD, for salivation, lacrimation, urination, and defecation, has been used to describe acute effects of OP insecticides. Another mnemonic in the diagnosis of anticholinesterases that incorporates more of the hallmark signs of intoxication is DUMBELS, for diarrhea, urination, miosis, bronchospasm, emesis, lacrimation, and

salivation (Figure 44-2). Other muscarinic effects include tightness in the chest, wheezing, rhinitis, dyspnea, increased bronchial secretions, pulmonary edema, cyanosis, nausea, tenesmus, sweating, and blurred vision. Other nicotinic effects are muscular twitching and fasciculations, weakness, cramps, and pallor. Some muscarinic and nicotinic effects may be antagonistic in nature. Stimulation of muscarinic receptors causes bradycardia and a fall in blood

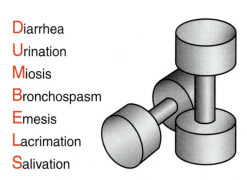

Diarrhea
Urination
Miosis
Bronchospasm
Emesis
Lacrimation
Salivation

Figure 44-2. Signs and symptoms of organophosphate toxicity.

pressure, whereas nicotinic effects include tachycardia and elevation of pressure.

Chronic neurological sequelae may result from acute OP poisoning, possibly due to the initiation of neurodegenerative processes by excitotoxic responses. There is some evidence that Gulf War veterans and victims of the terrorist attacks in Japan may have suffered long-term effects from exposures to nerve agents and pesticides.[8,9] Chronic exposures may result in two distinct syndromes, OPIDN and one that results in symptoms that are intermediate between OPIDN and acute effects. The intermediate syndrome appears between the appearance of signs of acute poisoning and the onset of delayed polyneuropathies associated with OPIDN. It is characterized by respiratory paresis and motor cranial nerve weakness and can lead to death from respiratory failure. OPIDN is related not to inhibition of AChE but rather to inhibition of neuropathy target esterase. Consequently, respiratory muscles are spared, but flaccid weakness and atrophy of distal limbs, spasticity, and ataxia are diagnostic of a delayed sensorimotor polyneuropathy.[10] Asymptomatic OP neurotoxicity resulting from chronic low-level exposures is not well understood. These are more subtle effects that are revealed by testing using specific intellectual and personality scales. Many neuropsychological effects of low-level exposure appear to involve the cognitive processes that underlie learning and memory. Some people exposed to these compounds may experience memory loss even in the absence of overt toxicity or significant cholinesterase inhibition.

The diagnosis of acute poisoning from anticholinesterases is based on the presence of the compounds or metabolites in available biological samples, inhibition of AChE, cholinergic signs of intoxication, and response to treatment with atropine and 2-PAM. It should be noted that the use of oximes is contraindicated in cases of poisoning by carbamate or dimethylorganophosphates because of the rapid rate of reactivation of the carbamylated and dimethoxyphosphorylated AChE. Furthermore, certain carbamates complexed with oximes can actually form a more toxic moiety. Thus, in cases in which the poisoning agent is not known, it may be prudent to limit treatment to atropine. Diazepam is also recommended for reducing anxiety in mild poisoning cases, while it functions to treat muscle fasciculations and convulsions in more severe cases. Other benzodiazepines such as midazolam are being studied as possible treatments for OP-induced convulsions and seizures.

The diagnosis of chronic poisoning from laboratory data is more difficult because of the uncoupling of chronic toxicity to AChE inhibition. AChE inhibition is present in the intermediate syndrome of OP poisoning but not with OPIDN. The inhibition of lymphocyte neurotoxic esterase is a good predictor of OPIDN that may appear some 2 to 3 weeks after laboratory analysis.[10] Laboratory analysis of AChE activity can be determined in red blood cells, and BChE can be determined in plasma, but it does not always correlate well with AChE. The cholinesterase reactivator 2-PAM can be used in confirmatory tests for the presence of anticholinesterases.[11] It is also recommended that a test for signs of pancreatitis be conducted. Tests include imaging ultrasound and computerized tomography scan, as well as serum or urine analysis for pancreatic enzymes.

ORGANOCHLORINE INSECTICIDES

The organochlorine (OC) insecticides (also called chlorinated hydrocarbons) are neurotoxic and have several other harmful effects related to their estrogenic properties. They were banned from use in the United States in the 1970s. This was due primarily to evidence that these compounds have carcinogenic properties and their ability to accumulate and cause harmful effects in wildlife. This was best described in the famous book *Silent Spring* by Rachael Carson. Insect resistance to many compounds played a much less publicized role in the decline in use of OC insecticides. Currently there is debate as to the global cost of tougher regulations on these compounds relative to their beneficial role in controlling insectborne diseases such as malaria. DDT is a major part of programs to eradicate mosquito larvae and is still used as a human delousing agent and as an inexpensive agricultural insecticide in some parts of the world. Several methods of classification may be used to describe the OC insecticides, and a more extensive review of their toxicology is presented elsewhere.[13] One structural classification includes the dichlorodiphenylethanes, most notably DDT; the

---

CASE STUDY

A 13-month-old boy was found with an open bottle of Kwell lotion (1% lindane), with some contents in his mouth and on his clothes.[12] The child vomited twice and had a generalized tonic–clonic seizure before being transported to the hospital. After having another seizure in the hospital, he was given phenobarbital, underwent gastric lavage, and was given activated charcoal. His respiratory effort diminished, and he was intubated. Urinalysis results were normal, and his blood lindane concentrations were 0.32 µg/mL 4 hours after ingestion, and 0.02 µg/mL 20 hours after ingestion. The child was extubated 8 hours later, and his condition improved over the next 2 days, at which time he was discharged.

cyclodienes (e.g., dieldrin); and the cyclohexanes (e.g., lindane; Figure 44-3). The toxicity of DDT and analogues such as methoxychlor highly depend on slight differences in chemical structure. The cyclodienes are extremely toxic as a group, and they have diverse chemical structure and toxicity, as seen with the caged structures of mirex and chlordecone and the aldrin–dieldrin isomers.[14] The cyclohexanes are among the oldest synthetic insecticides, and many are isomers of hexachlorocyclohexane. Lindane is the y-isomer (see Figure 44-3).

Toxicology

The OCs are absorbed readily by the body and stored for extended periods in adipose tissues. DDT is poorly absorbed through the skin and has a relatively good safety record with manufacturers and applicators. However, the cyclodienes and cyclohexanes have resulted in several fatalities because they are more readily absorbed through the skin. Although banned by the U.S. Environmental Protection Agency in 2006 for agricultural use, lindane is used topically to treat scabies and in shampoo to combat lice in cases for which alternative treatments are either not well tolerated or ineffective. It should be noted that lindane exposure has resulted in serious illness and deaths when used improperly. DDT is oxidized and conjugated to water-soluble metabolites that are excreted in urine or by dehydrochlorination and reductive dechlorination to other, less toxic metabolites. The primary urinary metabolite in humans is dideoxyadenosine, or DDA (bis[p-chlorophenyl]acetic acid). One of the more important metabolites is dichlorodiphenyldichloroethylene, or DDE (1,1-dichloro-2,2-bis[p-chlorophenyl]ethylene) because it may be stored in adipose tissues for decades. The putative link between this compound and breast cancer in humans has not been well supported; however, the role of DDE in human disease has not been dismissed and is still under investigation.[15] The highly toxic and persistent cyclodienes undergo various metabolic reactions that may result in more toxic compounds. For example, chlordane can be metabolized to heptachlor and then to heptachlor epoxide, each more toxic than its precursor. Aldrin is rapidly metabolized to dieldrin in humans, and lindane is metabolized to numerous water-soluble metabolites, but the β-isomer of hexachlorohexane is resistant to metabolism and persistent in human tissue. The metabolism of OCs is relatively slow compared with that of other pesticides, partly because of the complex ring structure and extent of chlorination. The slow metabolism, high lipid solubility, and persistence in adipose tissue are why the OCs are still of concern to health-care professionals.

The OC insecticides are acutely neurotoxic. The mechanism of action is best understood where they interfere with neurotransmission at the level of the nerve synapse. DDT interferes with the function of sodium channels by prolonging the falling phase of the action potential, leading to repetitive firing of the nerve impulse.[14] This, along with an interaction with axonal ATPases and calmodulin, causes hyperexcitability. The mechanism of toxicity for the cyclodienes and cyclohexanes is by interference with γ-aminobutyric acid (GABA) neurotransmission through inhibition of GABA receptors and blockage of voltage-gated chloride channels. The OC insecticides can be divided into two groups based on their mode of action: tremorogenic compounds that act on sodium channels (e.g., DDT and related compounds) and convulsant compounds that act on GABA receptors (cyclodienes and lindane).

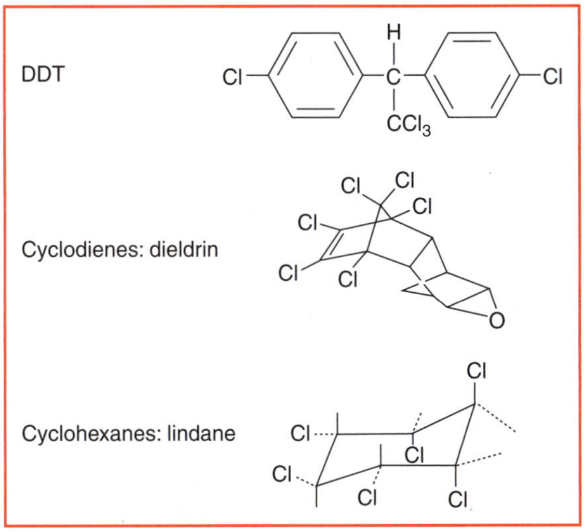

Clinical Presentation and Public Health

The signs and symptoms of poisoning from OC insecticides are outlined in Figure 44-4. The signs from acute exposure are due to the alteration of ion channels causing neuronal hyperexcitability. Hallmark signs and symptoms of OC exposure differ somewhat between the tremorogenic DDT and the convulsant lindane and cyclodiene class, but there is some significant overlap (see Figure 44-4). Other signs of DDT exposure include numbness and, in rare cases, convulsions. Acute effects in addition to those listed in Figure 44-4 include hearing whistling noises, seeing colored lights, visual impairment, giddiness, headache preceding mixed-type seizures, confusion, and speech difficulties. The cyclodienes, including dieldrin, chlordane, and the once widely used toxaphene, may also cause hypothermia, anorexia, epigastric pain, and vomiting. Seizures from acute OC exposure may be delayed and may not occur for as long as 6 to 8 months after exposure.

Figure 44-3. Typical organochlorine insecticides.

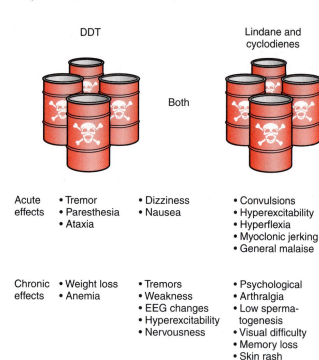

Figure 44-4. Signs and symptoms of organochlorine insecticide poisoning.

Chrysanthemum. The pyrethrins have been used as insecticides for more than a century, but large-scale agricultural and home use has been facilitated by efforts over the past few decades to synthesize less expensive analogues with better stability in the environment. The synthetic pyrethroids have remarkable knockdown insecticidal properties and have retained some of the chemical properties that made the pyrethrins virtually nontoxic to mammals. The chemical structure of pyrethroids is somewhat similar to that of pyrethrins except that the sites most vulnerable to metabolism and photolysis have been replaced. The general structure of pyrethroids resembles that of pyrethrins, which are composed of esters of two carboxylic acids, chrysanthemic acid and pyrethric acid (Figure 44-5). Many different compounds have been synthesized based on this structure, and the structure–activity relationship for the pyrethroids indicates that the overall molecule, rather than certain active moieties, is what determines activity.[14]

Toxicology

The pyrethroids are among the least toxic pesticides to mammals. Systemic toxicity of these compounds is usually associated with oral or inhalation exposures. Absorption through the skin is minimal. However, many

Chronic exposure to OCs is of particular importance because of their long half-lives in human adipose tissues. In addition to the tremors, weight loss, and anemia caused by prolonged exposure to DDT (see Figure 44-4), a DDT analogue, dicofol, may cause headache, blurred vision, numbness, and other psychological changes and cognitive deficits.[10] Other chronic signs of lindane and cyclodiene exposure are headache, dizziness, myoclonic jerking, chest pain, ataxia, loss of coordination, and slurred speech. Chlordecone (Kepone) was studied extensively after industrial workers in Hopewell, Virginia, were exposed through poor industrial hygiene.[16] Typical signs of cyclodiene exposure such as ocular flutter, hepatomegaly, and splenomegaly were noted to appear 30 days after initial exposure, and they persisted for several months after termination.[14] Cholestyramine was found to be an effective antidote for poisoning with Kepone in these industrial workers by enhancing the rate of excretion of the compound.

PYRETHROID INSECTICIDES

Like many insecticides, the pyrethroids target the nervous systems of insects so that rapid incapacitating and killing function is maximized. The botanical pyrethroid insecticides are synthetic analogues of pyrethrins extracted from pyrethrum flowers of the genus

CASE STUDY

A 44-year-old woman who had been using cans of pyrethroid insecticides almost every day for 3 years in an unventilated room experienced tongue numbness, nausea, and rhinitis while using the insecticides.[20] After 2 years, she had difficulty lifting heavy objects with her left arm, and her symptoms steadily worsened over the next 8 months. Three months before admission to the hospital, she developed slurred speech, gait disturbance, and generalized muscle weakness. On admission, neurological examination revealed dysarthria, nasal voice, and dysphagia with fasciculations and moderate muscle weakness. Sensory and autonomic systems were all normal. Nerve conduction studies showed decreased compound muscle action potentials amplitudes, and motor evoked potentials revealed prolonged central conduction time. Two months after cessation of pesticide use, her motor weakness partially ameliorated and fasciculation in all four limbs ceased. A subclinical hypothyroidism seen on admission had also improved, and 7 months after cessation of pesticide use, no exacerbation was apparent.

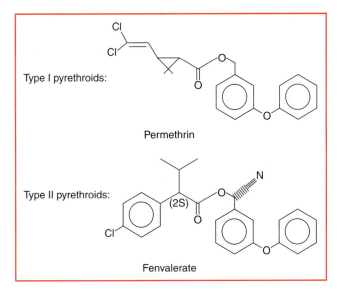

Type I pyrethroids:

Permethrin

Type II pyrethroids:

(2S)

Fenvalerate

Figure 44-5. Typical pyrethroid insecticides.

characterized by choreoathetosis (C) and salivation (S). The CS syndrome may also produce an increase in coarse whole-body tremors, but they progress to sinuous writhing and seizures. In humans, these two syndromes are not well defined, probably because of the low mammalian toxicity of pyrethroids relative to other classes of pesticides. Some clinical manifestations of exposure to natural pyrethrins include rhinitis, sneezing, cough, and other asthma-like symptoms related to an allergic reaction in sensitized patients. A reaction to dermal exposure to pyrethroids may result in cutaneous paresthesia, which has been observed with pyrethrins along with Type I and II pyrethroids. To date, there has been little evidence to suggest that environmental exposures to pyrethroids produce chronic toxicity. However, laboratory studies have demonstrated that developing animals are more sensitive to the toxic effects of pyrethroids, raising the possibility that children may be uniquely vulnerable to pyrethroids. In fact, the number of pyrethrin- and pyrethroid-related poisoning incidents in children has been increasing in the last few years,[21] and children in day-care centers have been reported to be exposed to several pyrethroid pesticides.[22]

reported occupational and home poisonings are due to allergic reactions to dermal exposures accompanied by rashes and paresthesia. The metabolism of pyrethroids is extensive, primarily because of the numerous sites for Phase I hydroxylation, rapid ester cleavage, and posthydroxylation Phase II conjugation. These metabolic reactions usually render the parent compound nontoxic. In a few cases, such as with some bromine-containing compounds, bioactivation may occur after Phase I metabolism. Like the OP and the OC pesticides, the pyrethroids are nerve poisons. In fact, the pyrethroids and DDT have remarkably similar effects on voltage-gated sodium channels. The action of pyrethroids on sodium channels causes repetitive neuronal discharge and the neuronal hyperexcitability characteristic of nerve excitants. The molecular mechanisms of action of pyrethroids may be complex. These compounds interfere with the function of voltage-gated calcium channels and calcium homeostasis, and they alter the function of chloride channels and GABA receptors at higher concentrations.

Clinical Presentation and Public Health

Two distinct classes of pyrethroid insecticides have been identified based on specific sets of symptoms they produce in laboratory rats. The T syndrome, or Type I poisoning, is characterized primarily by tremor and results from exposure to compounds without the α-cyano substituent. Acute symptoms are virtually indistinguishable from DDT intoxication. Other related symptoms in laboratory animals observed with Type I pyrethroids are aggression, restlessness, muscle twitches, hyperexcitability, incoordination, and prostration. The Type II pyrethroids possess the α-cyano group and produce the CS syndrome

OTHER PESTICIDES

Herbicides are the most widely used pesticides in the world. There are many chemical classes of herbicides, ranging from botanicals such as nicotine and rotenone to carbamates such as propham and the chlorphenoxy compounds, including the infamous defoliant Agent Orange made from a 50:50 ratio of the butyl esters of 2,4-dichlorophenoxyacetic acid and 2,4,5-trichlorophenoxyacetic acid. Before more rigid guidelines for the manufacture of 2,4,5-trichlorophenoxyacetic acid were instituted, a major contaminant found in this herbicide was dioxin (2,3,7,8-tetrachlorodibenzo-p-dioxin). Most herbicides are not particularly neurotoxic and, by design, are more toxic to plants than to animals. Some complaints from patients exposed to chlorphenoxy herbicides include headache, dizziness, weakness, and fatigue.

The rodenticides represent a large and chemically diverse class of pesticides. Both organic and inorganic compounds are used in the United States. Most human exposures to rodenticides in the United States are to the anticoagulant compounds such as warfarin, a compound isolated from spoiled sweet clover. The discovery of warfarin resistance in rats led to development of the superwarfarins (e.g., brodifacoum) and new, longer-acting anticoagulants (e.g., diphacinone). Several cases of human exposures to other, structurally dissimilar, rodenticides are reported annually. Two examples of highly toxic rodenticides are fluoroacetate and strychnine. Because these compounds are designed to kill mammals, they can be dangerous to humans and some may even be agents that pose a threat from deliberate and intentional use to cause harm. Most rodenticides do not target the nervous system, but strychnine is a CNS stimulant because of its antagonizing effects on GABA receptors in the brain and glycine receptors in the spinal cord. A hyperresponsiveness (muscle spasms) to minor stimuli is characteristic of strychnine poisoning. Sodium monofluoroacetate ("1080") may produce renal failure and degeneration and atrophy of tissues within the CNS. In severe cases, this may progress to seizure and coma.

PESTICIDE EXPOSURES AND NEUROLOGICAL DISEASE

Historically, most emphasis on the neurotoxic effects of pesticides has been relegated to neurological symptoms following high level acute exposures. However, recent interest has focused on the possibility that longer-term lower-level exposures to pesticides may be involved in the development of persistent neurological deficits and several neurological diseases including Parkinson's disease, Alzheimer's disease, and Amyotrophic Lateral Sclerosis.[23] Several studies have identified pesticide exposure as a risk factor for Parkinson's disease (PD; for review see Hatcher et al.[23]). Other studies have demonstrated that drinking well-water and living in a rural setting, both of which may increase exposure to agricultural pesticides, increase the risk of developing PD. Nevertheless, the majority of the epidemiological studies have not identified specific agents and there is little experimental evidence available to corroborate these epidemiological findings. Sanchez-Ramos and coworkers[19] demonstrated that the presence of the organochlorine dieldrin in post-mortem brain tissue was significantly associated with the diagnosis of PD. This observation has recently been confirmed by Corrigan and associates, who demonstrated elevated levels of dieldrin and lindane in post-mortem samples of substantia nigra taken from patients with Parkinson's disease.[18] However, both of these studies suffered from relatively small sample sizes (>20).

Unfortunately, there are much fewer data with regards to pesticide exposure as a potential risk factor for Alzheimer's disease (AD). Santibanez et al.[25] reviewed several of the epidemiological studies that have looked at environmental risk factors for AD and concluded that of the six studies that explored the possible relationship between pesticide exposure and AD, there was sufficient evidence from prospective design studies to conclude there was a significant relationship between pesticide exposure and risk of AD. For example, Baldi and co-workers[26] found an adjusted risk ratio of 2.39 for AD in men occupationally exposed to pesticides. However, these studies suffered from lack of identification of specific pesticides as many of the epidemiological studies do with regards to neurodegenerative disease. However, in the study cited above by Fleming and co-workers, p, p-DDT was more likely to be found in AD brain than PD or control samples.

With regards to ALS, there are relatively few data regarding the role of pesticides as an etiological factor. Pall and co-workers described a single case report concerning a 59-year-old man who experienced the onset of ALS two weeks following high-dose exposure to permethrin.[27] This single case report was followed by another report from Doi and co-workers[20] reporting the development of motor neuron disease resembling ALS following chronic inhalation of pyrethroid pesticides. Fonseca and coworkers[28] described two Brazilian farmers that worked together diagnosed with ALS and demonstrating high blood levels of organochlorine pesticides (aldrin, lindane, heptachlor). Using data from a large case-control study, McGuire and co-workers[29] found an association between exposure to agricultural chemicals and risk of ALS. However, the odds ratios were relatively low (1.5–2.8). More recently, research has focused on potential gene-environment interactions in the development of ALS.[30,31] Taken in concert, the current data available in the literature suggests that long-term exposures to a variety of pesticides may significantly contribute to neurological disease. However, much more study is needed with regards to the identification of specific pesticides that may be involved. Additionally, much more study is needed in the emerging area of gene-pesticide interactions with regards to risk for neurological disease.

REFERENCES

1. Futagami K, Otsubo K, Nakao Y, et al. Acute organophosphate poisoning after disulfoton ingestion. *J Toxicol Clin Toxicol.* 1995;33:151–155.
2. Solomon GM, Moodley J. Acute chlorpyrifos poisoning in pregnancy: a case report. *Clin Toxicol (Phila).* 2007;45:416–419.
3. Broomfield CA, Maxwell DM, Solana RP, et al. Protection by butyrylcholinesterase against organophosphorus poisoning in nonhuman primates. *J Pharmacol Exp Ther.* 1991;259:633–638.
4. Mikami LR, Wieseler S, Souza RL, et al. Five new naturally occurring mutations of the BCHE gene and frequencies of 12 butyrylcholinesterase alleles in a Brazilian population. *Pharmacogenet Genomics.* 2008;18:213–218.
5. Weiner ML, Jortner BS. Organophosphate-induced delayed neurotoxicity of triarylphosphates. *Neurotoxicology.* 1999;20:653–673.
6. Gupta R, ed. *Toxicology of Organophosphate and Carbamate Compounds.* New York: Elsevier Academic Press; 2006.
7. Jett DA, Lein PJ. Non-cholinesterase mechanisms of central and peripheral neurotoxicity: muscarinic receptors and other targets.

In: Gupta R, ed. *Toxicology of Organophosphate and Carbamate Compounds*. New York: Elsevier; 2006:233–246.

8. Hoffman A, Eisenkraft A, Finkelstein A, et al. A decade after the Tokyo sarin attack: a review of neurological follow-up of the victims. *Mil Med*. 2007;172:607–610.

9. Yamasue H, Abe O, Kasai K, et al. Human brain structural change related to acute single exposure to sarin. *Ann Neurol*. 2007;61:37–46.

10. Ellenhorn MJ, Schonwald S, Ordog G, Wasserberger J. *Ellenhorn's Medical Toxicology: Diagnosis and Treatment of Human Poisoning*. Baltimore: Williams & Wilkins; 1997:1663.

11. Flanagan RJ, Braithwaite RA, Brown SS, et al. *Basic Analytical Toxicology*. Geneva: World Health Organization; 1995:225.

12. Aks SE, Krantz A, Hryhrczuk DO, et al. Acute accidental lindane ingestion in toddlers. *Ann Emerg Med*. 1995;26:647–651.

13. Costa LG, Giordano G, Guizzetti M, Vitalone A. Neurotoxicity of pesticides: a brief review. *Front Biosci*. 2008;13:1240–1249.

14. Chang LW, Dyer RS. *Handbook of Neurotoxicology*. New York: Marcel Dekker; 1995:1103.

15. Safe S. Endocrine disruptors and human health: is there a problem. *Toxicology*. 2004;205:3–10.

16. Huff JE, Gerstner HB. Kepone: a literature summary. *J Environ Pathol Toxicol*. 1978;1:377–395.

17. Corrigan FM, Murray L, Wyatt CL, Shore RF. Diorthosubstituted polychlorinated biphenyls in caudate nucleus in Parkinson's disease. *Exp Neurol*. 1998;150:339–342.

18. Corrigan FM, Wienburg CL, Shore RF, et al. Organochlorine insecticides in substantia nigra in Parkinson's disease. *J Toxicol Environ Health A*. 2000;59:229–234.

19. Fleming L, Mann JB, Bean J, et al. Parkinson's disease and brain levels of organochlorine pesticides. *Ann Neurol*. 1994;36:100–103.

20. Doi H, Kikuchi H, Murai H, et al. Motor neuron disorder simulating ALS induced by chronic inhalation of pyrethroid insecticides. *Neurology*. 2006;67:1894–1895.

21. Power LE, Sudakin DL. Pyrethrin and pyrethroid exposures in the United States: a longitudinal analysis of incidents reported to poison centers. *J Med Toxicol*. 2007;3:94–99.

22. Morgan MK, Sheldon LS, Croghan CW, et al. An observational study of 127 preschool children at their homes and daycare centers in Ohio: environmental pathways to *cis-* and *trans-*permethrin exposure. *Environ Res*. 2007;104:266–274.

23. Kamel F and Hoppin JA. Association of pesticide exposure with neurologic dysfunction and disease. *Environ Health Perspect*. 2004;112(9): 950–958.

24. Hatcher JM, Pennell KD, and Miller GW. Parkinson's disease and pesticides: a toxicological perspective. *Trends Pharmacol Sci*. 2008;29(6):322–329.

25. Santibanez M, Bolumar F, and Garcia AM. Occupational risk factors in Alzheimer's disease: a review assessing the quality of published epidemiological studies. *Occup Environ Med*. 2007;64(11):723–732.

26. Baldi I, Lebailly P, Mohammed-Brahim B, et al. Neurodegenerative diseases and exposure to pesticides in the elderly. *Am J Epidemiol*. 2003;157(5):409–414.

27. Pall HS, Williams AC, Waring R, and Elias E. Motoneurone disease as manifestation of pesticide toxicity. *Lancet*. 1987;2(8560):685.

28. Fonseca RG, Resende LA, Silva MD, and Camargo A. Chronic motor neuron disease possibly related to intoxication with organo chlorine insecticides. *Acta Neurol Scand*. 1993;88(1):56–58.

29. McGuire V, Longstreth WT, Jr, Nelson LM, et al. Occupational exposures and amyotrophic lateral sclerosis. A population-based case-control study. *Am J Epidemiol*. 1997;145(12):1076–1088.

30. Morahan JM, Yu B, Trent RJ, and Pamphlett R. Genetic susceptibility to environmental toxicants in ALS. *Am J Med Genet B Neuropsychiatr Genet*. 2007;144B(7): 885–890.

31. Qureshi MM, Hayden D, Urbinelli L, et al. Analysis of factors that modify susceptibility and rate of progression in amyotrophic lateral sclerosis (ALS). *Amyotroph Lateral Scler*. 2006;7(3): 173–182.

Carbon Monoxide

Leon Prockop

INTRODUCTION

Carbon monoxide (CO) intoxication is one of the most common types of poisoning in the modern world and a leading cause of death by poisoning in the United States, including intentional suicides and unintentional exposures from home heating, automobile exhaust, and smoke inhalaton.[1–6] When not fatal, a spectrum of encephalopathy ranges from reversible dysfunction to severe irreversible dementia.[7] Other features may include a parkinsonian syndrome[8,9] and a delayed neuropsychiatric syndrome.[10–12] Statistics on acute, nonfatal CO encephalopathy and the delayed CO-induced neuropsychiatric syndrome are imprecise. Sequelae of low-level exposure may be misdiagnosed or overlooked.[4,6,13]

CO is a tasteless, odorless, nonirritating but highly toxic gas. Because of these properties and because it often lacks a unique clinical signature, CO is difficult to detect and can mimic other common disorders. Therefore, the true incidence of CO poisoning is unknown and many cases probably go unrecognized. CO has been termed "the unnoticed poison of the 21st century."[14] An environmental CO exposure is suggested when more than one person, animals, or both are affected; by a history of fire, presence of fireplace or combustion appliances, or occupation; and by the relation of symptoms to a possible exposure.[5,14]

CO is a byproduct of the incomplete combustion of hydrocarbons.[15] Common sources include motor vehicle exhaust exposure in a poorly ventilated garage or areas close to garages and combustion appliances (e.g., heating units) in which partial combustion of oils, coal, wood, kerosene, and other fuels generate CO. A common scenario is that of a heating unit used only occasionally and not well maintained. Retrograde flow can occur in residential, occupational, or institutional settings in the presence of pressure problems and chimney or equipment malfunction. CO poisoning with immediate deaths may occur during a building fire or from fuel-powered generators and heaters, especially in poorly ventilated spaces. The latter causes are often reported during winter storms, hurricanes, earthquakes or other disasters after a power outage has occurred.

Endogenous sources of CO include the heme degradation to bile pigments, catalyzed by heme oxygenases.[16]

Constitutive and inducible isoforms (heme oxygenase-1, heme oxygenase-2) of the enzyme are known. Endogenously produced CO serves as a signaling molecule involved in multiple cellular functions, such as inflammation, proliferation, and apoptosis. CO, like nitric oxide, is a recently defined gaseous neurotransmitter in the central nervous system (CNS). Endogenous and exogenous sources of CO are contained in Table 1.

The fatal effects of CO exposure are well recorded in past and recent history. For example, the ancient Greeks and Romans used CO to execute criminals. The deaths of two Byzantine emperors was related to CO produced by the burning of coal in braziers, the usual method of indoor heating then.[17] In World War II, wood used widely as fuel caused many cases of acute or chronic CO poisoning.[18] An article published in 2005 reported the death of one person among nine exposed to CO accidentally because of a faulty apartment house heating unit.[19]

CO was first prepared by the French chemist Joseph-Marie-François de Lassone in 1776. Because it burned with a blue flame, he mistakenly thought it to be hydrogen. In 1880, William Cruikshank identified it as a compound containing carbon and oxygen. In the middle of the 19th century, Claude Bernard recognized that CO causes hypoxia by interaction with hemoglobin (Hb). He poisoned dogs with the gas, noticing the scarlet appearance of their blood. Toward the end of the 19th century, John Scott Haldane demonstrated that a high partial pressure of oxygen can counteract the interaction between Hb and CO despite the high affinity for this interaction.[20]

PATHOPHYSIOLOGY

CO binds rapidly to Hb, leading to the formation of carboxyhemoglobin (COHb). The oxygen-carrying capacity of the blood decreases, causing tissue hypoxia. COHb is red, which explains the "cherry-like" discoloration of victims. CO diffuses from the alveoli to the blood in the pulmonary capillaries across the alveolocapillary membrane that is composed of pulmonary epithelium, the capillary endothelium, and their fused basement membrane. CO is taken up by Hb at such a high rate that the partial pressure of CO in the capillaries stays low. Therefore, the CO transfer is diffusion limited. The affinity of Hb for CO is 210 times its affinity for oxygen. CO easily displaces oxygen from Hb. On the other hand, COHb liberates CO slowly. In the presence of COHb, the dissociation curve of the remaining hyperbaric oxygen (HBO) shifts to the left, further decreasing the amount of the oxygen released. The amount of COHb formed depends on the duration of exposure to CO, the concentration of CO in the inspired air, and the alveolar ventilation.[21]

CO toxicity is caused by impaired oxygen delivery and use, leading to cellular hypoxia. Body organs with poorly developed anastomotic vessels, high metabolic activity, or both, such as the heart and areas of the brain, are especially vulnerable to CO toxic damage. At least several pathophysiological effects occur. The relative contributions of each to resulting damage remains somewhat controversial[22]:

1. Inhalation of CO replaces oxygen on the Hb molecule, leading to a relative anemia. The body requires 5 mL of oxygen dissolves per 100 mL of blood; the remaining 3 mL of oxygen per 100 mL blood (3 vol%) comes from the release of oxygen from Hb. Impairment of oxyhemoglobin formation by CO results in cellular hypoxia.
2. COHb impairs the release of oxygen from Hb by increasing oxygen binding to Hb. The result is a shift of the oxyhemoglobin dissociation curve to the left, which reduces unloading of oxygen in the tissues.
3. CO bind to cytochrome oxidase in vitro; however, the affinity of oxygen for cytochrome oxidase is so much greater than that of CO that in vivo binding

Table 1: Sources of Carbon Monoxide
ENDOGENOUS
Normal heme catabolism by heme oxygenase
Increased in hemolytic anemia or sepsis
EXOGENOUS
Incomplete combustion of carbonaceous fossil fuel
Propane-powered vehicles, e.g., forklifts, ice-skating rink resurfacers
Gas-powered furnaces, ovens, fireplaces
House fires
Heaters
Automobile exhaust
Boat exhaust
Indoor grills
Camp stoves
Cigarette smoke

of CO to cytochrome oxidase may be small. Inhibition of cellular respiration may explain the poor correlation of toxicity to COHb in blood levels and justify the use of hyperbaric oxygen.

4. CO saturates myoglobin in three times higher concentration than skeletal muscle. The resultant myocardial depression and hypotension cause ischemia and potentiate the hypoxia induced by impaired oxygen delivery.

Because of increased accumulation in fetal blood, the human fetus is especially vulnerable to CO poisoning. Furthermore, the fetal Hb dissociation curve lies to the left of the adult curve, resulting in greater tissue hypoxia at similar COHb levels. Neonates are even more susceptible, since fetal Hb constitutes 20% of the total at 3 months. Acute nonlethal maternal intoxication may cause fetal death or permanent neurological sequelae.[23–25] Likewise, children may be especially vulnerable to acute and delayed effects of CO poisoining.[26]

The Normal COHb level for nonsmokers is less than 2% and for smokers is 5% to 13%. The Expert Panel on Air Quality Standard of the World Health Organization (WHO) in 1994 reported that blood COHb levels between 2.5% and 4% decrease the short-term maximal exercise duration in young healthy men. Decreased exercise duration because of increased chest pain and in patients with ischemic hearts occurred at levels from 2.7% to 4.1%. Levels between 2% and 20% can cause effects on visual perception, as well as on audition, motor, and sensory motor functions and behavior. Therefore, ambient air CO levels that produce blood COHb levels below 2.5% are recommended. The COHb levels depend not only on the CO level in ambient air but also on the duration of exposure. According to WHO guidelines, exposures to levels of ambient air carbon dioxide in parts per million (ppm) should conform to the following durations of exposure: 87.1 ppm (100 mg/m³) for 15 minutes; 52.3 ppm (60 mg/m³) for 30 minutes; 26.1 ppm (30 mg/m³) for 60 minutes; 8.7 ppm (10 mg/m³) for 80 minutes.[27] Any exposure to ambient air with CO levels greater than 100 ppm is dangerous to human health.[7,28,29]

At equilibration, atmospheric CO levels of 50, 100, and 200 ppm produce average COHb levels of 8%, 16%, and 30% respectively.[30] Perceptible clinical effects occur with a 20-hour exposure to concentrations as low as 0.01% (100 ppm). The industrial exposure limit, expressed as threshold limit value, is 35 ppm for an 8-hour day, allowing for a maximum COHb of 5% during an 8-hour period, assuming normal activity. The ceiling concentration to which a worker may be transiently exposed without changing the COHb level is 200 ppm.

CLINICAL FINDINGS

Because of their high metabolic rate, the brain and the heart are most susceptible to CO toxicity. The clinical symptoms of CO poisoning are often nonspecific and can mimic various common disorders. The severity ranges from mild flulike symptoms to coma and death. About 50% of exposed people may develop weakness, nausea, confusion, and shortness of breath. Less often, abdominal pain, visual changes, chest pain, and loss of consciousness occur. Tachycardia and tachypnea develop to compensate from cellular hypoxia and cardiac output increases initially. Some potential complications of CO poisoning are contained in Table 2. Responses to cellular hypoxia vary depending on the premorbid condition of victims; those with underlying lung and heart diseases have little tolerance to even mild hypoxia. Hypoxia leads to increased intracranial pressure and cerebral edema, which is partly responsible for decreased level of consciousness, seizures, and coma. The classic cherry-red discoloration of the skin and cyanosis are rarely seen.[5,15,20] Varying degrees of cognitive impairment have been reported.[10–12,19,31]

Headache is one of the most common presenting features of CO poisoning: it occurs in 84% of the victims and has been described as predominantly frontal, dull, sharp, continuous, throbbing, and intermittent in patients with a mean COHb level of 21.3% (+9.3%).[32] There is not clear correlation between pain intensity and COHb levels.[32] Some have reported tightness across the forehead at COHb levels of 10% to 20%, throbbing in the temples at 20% to 30%, and severe headache at 30% to 40%. Headaches, generalized weakness, fatigue, and sleepiness are part of the vague symptomatology observed in subjects with COHb levels below 20%. Headache is a frequent complaint not only with acute but also with chronic CO poisoning. Dizziness is a frequent companion of headache and can be seen in about 92% in victims of CO poisoning. In one report, 76% of 38 victims reported weakness with COHb levels greater than 30% to 40%.[33] Chest pain as a symptom of myocardial ischemia can occur without underlying coronary artery disease. For example, 3 weeks after accidental exposure to CO, 34% of Swiss soldiers had chest pain.[34] Cerebellar atrophy by magnetic resonance imaging (MRI) criteria and signs of cerebellar dysfunction have been reported.[35]

The delayed neuropsychiatric syndrome, also named "delayed neurological sequelae", may occur in patients from 3 to 240 days after acute CO exposure and poses especially difficult diagnostic and therapeutic problems. Rarely this syndrome may present years after exposure.[35a] Even those victims without neurological and psychiatric symptoms immediately after an exposure accident may demonstrate features of delayed impairment ranging from subtle abnormalities such as personality changes or

Table 2:   Potential Complication of Carbon Monoxide Poisoning

NEUROLOGICAL AND/OR PSYCHIATRIC	
Death	Coma
Stupor	Agitation
Confusion	Mutism
Leukoencephalopathy	Muscular rigidity
Parkinsonism	Personality change
Dystonia and chorea	Behavioral disorder
Seizures	Psychosis
Dementia	Urinary incontinence
Ataxia	Fecal incontinence
Peripheral neuropathy	Headache
CARDIOVASCULAR	
Angina	Arrhythmia
Tachycardia	Heart block
ST segment change	Myocardial infarction
Hypotension	
PULMONARY	
Edema	Hemorrhage
OPHTHALMOLOGICAL	
Retinal hemorrhage	Cortical blindness
Decreased visual acuity	Papilledema
Decreased light sensitivity	Paracentral scotomas
Retrobulbar neuritis	
VESTIBULAR AND AUDITORY	
Central hearing loss	Vertigo
Tinnitus	Auditory nystagmus
GASTROINTESTINAL	
Vomiting	Hepatic necrosis
Diarrhea	Melena

DERMATOLOGICAL	
Bullae	Cyanosis
Alopecia	Sweat gland necrosis
Pallor	Erythematous patches
MUSCULOSKELETAL	
Rhabdomyolysis	Myonecrosis
RENAL	
Myoglobinuria	Proteinuria
METABOLIC	
Lactic acidosis	Hypocalcemia
Diabetes insipidus	Polycythemia
Hyperglycemia	
FETAL	
Death	Psychomotor retardation
Cerebral atrophy	Seizures
Microcephalus	Spasticity
Low birth weight	

mild cognitive deficit to severe dementia, gait disturbance, impaired coordination with cerebellar dysfunction, psychosis, parkinsonism, mutism, and fecal and urinary incontinence. Some authors report a "characteristic symptom triad" of mental deterioration, urinary incontinence, and gait disturbances in both humans and experimental animals.[10,11,36] Urinary incontinence in children and adults has been reported as an especially distressing complication of CO poisoning.[10,26,36–39]

CO encephalopathy may cause several behavioral functional impairments, including alterations in attention, executive function, verbal fluency, motor abilities, visuospatial skills, learning, short-term memory, and mood and social adjustment. Formal neuropsychological testing usually confirms these impairments.[28,39a]

DIAGNOSIS

Diagnosis of CO poisoning requires a high level of suspicion. Epidemiological history with information about other affected individuals or pets, as well as circumstances

503

suggestive of possible exposure, is of paramount importance. Ambient air CO levels should be obtained as soon as possible after the exposure. Because the half-life of COHb is 4 to 5 hours, a victim's COHb level should also be obtained as soon as possible.

Physicians who deal with CO intoxication should be aware that pulse oximetry is a colorimetric method, unreliable for the diagnosis of CO intoxication since it cannot distinguish oxyhemoglobin from COHb. Therefore, the pulse oximeters overestimate arterial oxygenation in patients with severe CO poisoning. Accurate assessment of arterial oxygenation in patients with severe CO poisoning can currently be performed only by analysis of arterial blood with a laboratory CO oximetry. High-flow oxygen should be administered to all patients suspected of significant CO exposure until direct measurement of CO levels can be performed, regardless of pulse oximetry readings.[40]

For clinical purposes, automated spectrophotometric CO-oximeter device are recommended. Spectrophotometry measures light intensity as a function of color and can differentiate the wavelengths of oxyhemoglobin and COHb. With an acceptable accuracy for COHb saturation levels above 5%, the device can simultaneously estimate total Hb and the percentage oxyhemoglobin and COHb. Gas chromatography, a more sensitive method, can be used for low-level exposure and for postmortem blood samples.[41,42]

CARDIAC EFFECTS

Even though this chapter focuses upon the toxic effects of CO on the brain, some discussion of its toxic cardiac effects is important, especially because cardiac stress may shed light on brain effects. CO binds to the intracellular myoglobin of the myocardium and impairs the oxygen supply to the mitochondria. This negatively affects the oxidative phosphorylation and, consequently, the energy source of heart muscle. Patients with underlying cardiac conditions are at risk for death from arrhythmias, and fatal heart attacks can occur. Henry et al. studied mortality risk in patients with moderate to severe CO poisoning. In those at low risk for cardiovascular diseases, 37% suffered acute myocardial injury and 38% of them were dead within 7.6 years. The mortality rate was three times higher than the United States expected by age and sex.[43]

After CO exposure, angina attacks, arrhythmias, and increased level of cardiac enzymes often occur. This has led to a search for morphological changes that could be attributed to CO, especially because the myocardium binds more CO than skeletal muscle. Ultramicroscopic lesions have been reported, but the relative roles of general tissue hypoxia and specific CO toxicity are unknown.

In addition to the COHb effects, binding of CO to cytochromes is significant and is thought to be responsible for the cytotoxic phenomena. Combined ultrastructural and cytochemical studies have enabled differentiation among toxic, hypoxic, and mixed alteration. The marked decrease in cytochrome oxidase in experimental studies suggests a direct toxic effect.[44]

Myocardial injury with ischemic changes on electrocardiogram (ECG) and elevated cardiac biomarkers were found in 37% of 230 patients with moderate to severe CO poisoning, with 5% in-hospital mortality.[45] Therefore, patients admitted to the hospital with CO poisoning should have a baseline ECG and serial cardiac enzymes. Myocardial fiber necrosis was described in a 26-year-old patient with accidental CO poisoning and blood concentration of COHb of 46.6%.[46] Electron microscopy of left ventricular biopsies of a 25-year-old woman with functional evidence of cardiac failure after acute CO poisoning, and otherwise normal myocardial perfusion showed slight ultrastructural changes in the myocytes, large glycogen deposits, and swollen mitochondria. The preceding changes have been thought to be signs of impaired energy metabolism of the myocardial cells.[47] In the rat heart, CO causes vasodilatation and increased coronary flow that are not mediated by simple hypoxia.[48] CO exposure in the fetal period in rats causes myocyte hyperplasia and cardiomegaly. This cellular response is sustained through the early neonatal period in animals exposed to CO both in utero and postpartum.[49] Although hemorrhages and areas of necrosis in the heart, mostly in the septum and the papillary muscles, were described with CO poisoning as early as 1865, only a few human cases of acute, fatal CO intoxication, with small foci of coagulation necrosis, have been reported.[50,51]

Cardiac function must be monitored closely by ECG, two-dimensional echocardiogram, and cardiac enzymes. Patients with underlying cardiac disorders, whose reserves are impaired at baseline, are at higher risk than are normal individuals. Cardiac arrest and sudden cardiac death can be expected. Chest pain due to myocardial ischemia or infarction is a consequence of decreased oxygen supply to the cardiac muscle. Features of ischemia, as well as other abnormalities, such as tachycardia, bradycardia, atrial and ventricular fibrillation, premature ventricular contractions, and conduction abnormalities, can be easily detected on ECG. Noninvasive devices that can be used to screen firefighters and victims and can estimate the COHb levels in the exhaled alveolar breath have been suggested.[11] A noninvasive, high-resolution method of measuring COHb fraction using expiratory gas analysis in patients without evidence for pulmonary edema or atelectasis has been found to have accuracy equivalent to that of CO oximetry.[40–42]

OTHER TOXIC MECHANISMS

Investigations suggest other mechanisms of CO-mediated toxicity. One hypothesis is that CO-induced tissue hypoxia may be followed by reoxygenation injury to the CNS. Hyperoxygenation facilitates the production of partially reduced oxygen species, which in turn can oxidize essential proteins and nucleic acids, resulting in typical reperfusion injury. In addition, CO exposure has been shown to cause lipid preoxygenation, i.e., degradation of unsaturated fatty acids leading to reversible demyelination of CNS lipids. CO exposure also creates substantial oxidative stress on cells, with production of oxygen radicals resulting from the conversion of xanthine dehydrogenase to xanthine oxidase.[52]

Acute disturbances of brain function predominate in acute CO intoxication, ranging from transient confusion to severe dementia and death. As stated, delayed neurological effects also occur. Tissue hypoxia is the end result of intoxications with CO and many other physical and chemical agents. Some brain regions are sensitive to hypoxic damage, including the cerebral cortex, particularly its second and third layers; the white matter; the basal nuclei; and the Purkinje cells of the cerebellum. Attempts have been made to relate this "selective vulnerability" to the cause of the hypoxia, but the nature and distribution of the lesions appear to depend on the severity, suddenness, and duration of the oxygen deprivation, as well as on its mechanism (hypoxemia or ischemia), rather than on its cause. Regions with relatively poor vascularization and "watershed" areas between two sources of blood supply, such as the globus pallidus, may be more vulnerable, especially during periods of hypotension. The effects of hypoxia on the brain, therefore, do not reflect it cause, and neither the character of the lesions nor the areas affected are regarded as pathognomonic for CO.

NEUROPATHOLOGY

The neuropathology of CO toxicity has been well described in postmortem studies by Lasprele and Fardeau.[53]

Lesions can be separated into four categories: multifocal necrosis, multifocal necrosis involving the cortex, myelinopathy with discrete globus pallidus and cortical lesions, and white matter lesions. When bilateral globus pallidus damage occurs, it is usually asymmetrical. It can extend anteriorly, superiorly, or into the internal capsule. Occasionally, a small linear focus of necrosis at the junction of the internal capsule and the internal nucleus of the globus pallidus was noted. Less commonly, hemorrhages in the hippocampus were seen.

Relatively spared were the hypothalamus, walls of the third ventricle, thalamus, striatum, and brainstem. In acute cases, petechial hemorrhages of the white matter involved in particular the corpus callosum; in cases surviving more than 48 hours, there is multifocal necrosis involving the globus pallidus, hippocampus, pars reticularis of the substantia nigra, laminar necrosis of the cortex, and loss of Purkinje cells in the cerebellum, along with white matter lesions. The typical pallidal lesions are well-defined, bilateral globus pallidus macroscopic infarctions, usually asymmetrical, extending anteriorly, superiorly, or into the internal capsule. Occasionally, only a small linear focus of necrosis is found at the junction of the internal capsule and the internal nucleus of the globus pallidus. CO intoxication usually spares the hypothalamus, walls of the third ventricle, thalamus, striatum, and brainstem. Myelin damage ranges from discrete, perivascular foci in corpus callosum, internal–external capsule and optic tracts usually seen in comatose patients who died within 1 week to extensive periventricular demyelination and axonal destruction observed in comatose subjects with longer survival, sometimes leading to formation of plaques of demyelination.

NEUROIMAGING

A distinct constellation of brain and MRI abnormalities appears premortem and in those surviving exposure. It includes globus pallidus lesions, white matter changes, and diffuse low-density lesions throughout the brain. In general, computerized tomography (CT) and magnetic resonance neuroimaging findings reflect the neuropathological changes described by Laspresle and Fardeau (Figures 45-1 to 45-4).

Differences between neuroimaging findings and neuropathological findings include findings of MRI thalamic lesions.[54] Although some authors suggest that CT findings correlate with long-term outcome after CO poisoning,[55] others questions their prognostic value. However, the database that correlates patient outcome to serial CT, MRI, or both types of studies is limited.[56,57]

Tom et al.[58] reported neuroimaging studies in 18 patients with CO toxicity, age 19 to 70 years (mean 35.6 years). CO exposure occurred by four routes: suicide attempt with car exhaust, 44%; portable heater, 33%; smoke inhalation, 17%; and hotel heating systems, 6%. COHb levels on hospital admission ranged from 1.9% to 40% (mean 18.49%). The most common findings were low-density lesions in the globus pallidus, deep white matter changes, generalized edema, and low-density lesions in the mesial temporal lobes

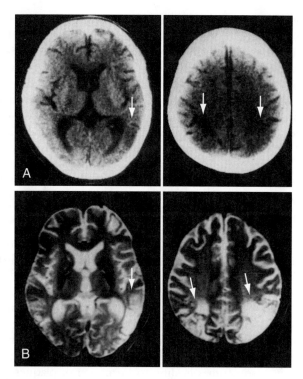

Figure 45-1. Brain computerized tomography (CT) and magnetic resonance imaging (MRI) scans in the same patient. *(A)* CT findings. The arrows show low-density areas. *(B)* T$_2$-weighted MRI. Cortical areas are more affected than the subcortical areas. (Murata S, Asaba H, Hiraishi K, et al. Magnetic resonance imaging findings on carbon monoxide intoxication. *J Neuroimaging.* 1993;3:128–131.)

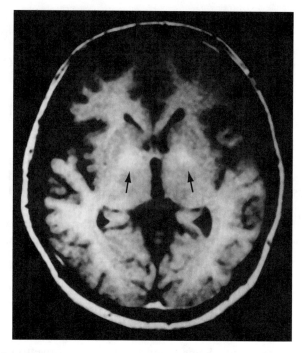

Figure 45-2. T$_1$-weighted magnetic resonance imaging. High-signal regions are seen in both globi pallidi *(arrows)*. (Murata S, Asaba H, Hiraishi K, et al. Magnetic resonance imaging findings on carbon monoxide intoxication. *J Neuroimaging.* 1993;3:128–131.)

(Figures 45-3 to 45-6). In 5 patients, multiple CT findings appeared acutely; however, those patients did not have higher COHb levels than those with less prominent CT findings. A typical noncontrasted CT scan (see Figure 45-4) showed bilateral low-density lesions in the globus pallidus with calcification, cortical atrophy, enlargement of the quadrigeminal cistern, and left choroid plexus calcification. Overall the most common positive findings were low-density lesions in the globus pallidus (7 of 18 patients, 39%) and deep white matter changes (5 patients, 28%). Six brain CT scans showed no acute changes. Tom et al.[58] provided representative CT or magnetic resonance images in this series. A 24-year-old man accidentally exposed to CO was admitted to the hospital with a COHb of 24%. The brain CT scan showed only low-density lesions in the globus pallidus bilaterally without generalized edema, deep white matter changes, or low-density lesions in the mesial temporal lobes. Brain MRI was obtained 7 days later. The T$_1$-weighted transaxial (see Figure 45-3A) and coronal views (see Figure 45-3B) showed globus pallidus hemorrhages bilaterally. A 49-year-old woman accidentally exposed to CO was admitted to the hospital

with a COHb of 13.7%. Noncontrasted brain CT (see Figure 45-6) showed bilateral low-density lesions in the globus pallidus, cortical atrophy, and enlargement of the quadrigeminal cistern. A 30-year-old man suffered accidental CO exposure with COHb of only 1.9%. His T$_2$-weighted brain magnetic resonance image (see Figure 45-5) showed hyperintense bilateral deep white matter changes. Brain CT showed low-density lesions in the globus pallidus. He was in persistent coma. A 41-year-old woman inhaled CO in a suicide attempt, attaining a 33.7% COHb. A noncontrasted brain CT scan demonstrated a finding consistent with generalized edema with effacement of the cortical suprasella and quadrigeminal cistern. There was also attenuation within the quadrigeminal, ambient, and suprasella cisterns representing subarachnoid hemorrhage (see Figure 45-6). She died.

In this series of 18 patients, 4 died. None of them showed globus pallidus lesions on CT. However, 2 suffered generalized edema, 1 had deep white matter changes, and 1 had low-density lesions in the mesial temporal lobe. Both patients in coma had globus pallidus lesions and deep white matter changes. One also

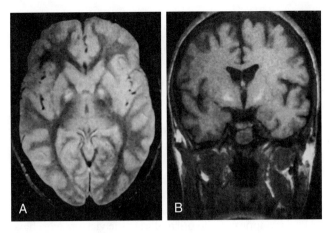

Figure 45-3. *(A)* Proton density brain magnetic resonance imaging (MRI), transaxial view, shows bilateral hemorrhage in the globus pallidus. *(B)* T$_1$-weighted brain MRI, coronal view. (Tom T, Abedon S, Clark RI, Wong W. Neuroimaging characteristics in carbon monoxide toxicity. *J Neuroimaging.* 1996:161–166.)

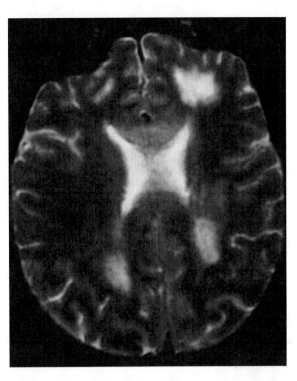

Figure 45-5. T$_2$-weighted brain magnetic resonance image showing bilateral hyperintense white matter lesion, most prominent in the left frontal lobe. (Tom T, Abedon S, Clark RI, Wong W. Neuroimaging characteristics in carbon monoxide toxicity. *J Neuroimaging.* 1996:161–166.)

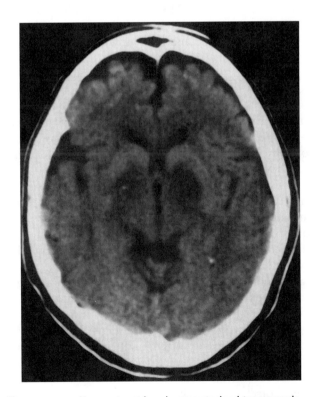

Figure 45-4. Noncontrast head computerized tomograph showing bilateral low-density lesions of the globus pallidus with calcification *(right)*, enlargement of the quadrigeminal cistern, and choroid plexus calcification *(left)*. (Tom T, Abedon S, Clark RI, Wong W. Neuroimaging characteristics in carbon monoxide toxicity. *J Neuroimaging.* 1996:161–166.)

had low-density lesions in the mesial temporal lobes. Tom et al.[58] concluded the following:

1. Advanced age, method of exposure (i.e., whether intentional or accidental), and severity of COHb levels did not predict neuroimaging or clinical outcomes.
2. Although CT findings always predicted clinical courses in this patient population, negative CT findings usually were associated with a good outcome.
3. Because 17 of the 18 patients received HBO therapy, the data cannot be used to assess the value of this therapy and the prevention of CT findings.

Gotoh et al. obtained sequential brain MRI studies in two patients 4 days, 1 month, 2 months, and 4 months after CO exposure.[57] The serial changes were coagulation necrosis with surrounding edema, decrease in lesion size and edema in both patients, and development of gliotic tissue and evidence of neovascularization. MRI offered the best prognostic index at the 1– to 2-month mark. Brain MRI and changes in the level of consciousness in one of the patients are depicted in Figure 45-7. In 19 patients, Jones et al.[59] reported CT findings similar

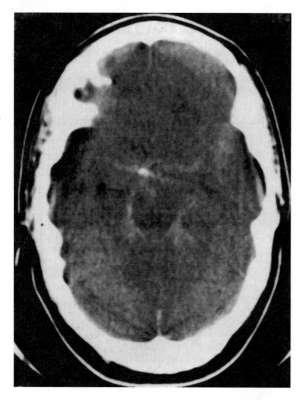

Figure 45-6. Noncontrasted heat computerized tomography scan showing generalized edema evidenced by effacement of the sulci, as well as the quadrigeminal, ambient, and suprasellar cisterns whose effacement represents subarachnoid hemorrhage. (Tom T, Abedon S, Clark RI, Wong W. Neuroimaging characteristics in carbon monoxide toxicity. *J Neuroimaging.* 1996:161–166.)

to those noted by Tom et al.[58] The mean COHb level of these patients was 35%. There were no direct relationships among age, admission COHb level, and neuroimaging abnormalities.

Diffusion-weighted brain MRI shows white matter high-signal intensities consistent with restricted diffusion in the acute CO poisoning. Follow-up MRI performed 16 days later reveals disappearance of white matter lesions, suggesting the white matter can be more sensitive to hypoxia than gray matter in the acute phase.[60]

T_2-weighted brain MRI shows increased signal intensity bilaterally in the putamen and the caudate nucleus, as well as high-signal intensity in the globus pallidus.[61] Initially, unilateral low attenuation areas in the right putamen, globus pallidus, and thalamus were observed on CT in a patient after CO exposure, followed by transient bilateral appearance on subsequent CT examination. Hemorrhagic infarction of the right putamen and ischemic lesions in both thalami were visualized on MRI 2 weeks later.[62] Diffusion-weighted MRI in a case of

CO poisoning revealed pallidoreticular damage and delayed leukoencephalopathy characterized by a restricted water diffusion pattern in the early stage. Diffusion-weighted brain MRI is more sensitive than brain CT and is useful for early identification of the effects of acute CO poisoning.[63,64]

Brain MRI changes after CO poisoning are variable and reflect the neuropathological lesions. Most unconscious patients present with abnormalities of globus pallidus or the entire lentiform nucleus (globus pallidus and putamen), putamen alone, caudate nucleus, thalamus, periventricular and subcortical white matter, cerebral cortex hippocampus, and cerebellum. Brain CT and MRI may appear to be normal in some victims who have suffered CO brain damage.[58,64] Previously unreported brain MRI findings in CO poisoning included a bilateral diffuse high signal in the centrum semiovale and bilateral high-intensity lesions in the anterior thalami.[65] Extensive bilateral cerebellar white matter signal change, with sparing of the overlying cortex, consistent with demyelination was reported 6 years previously after CO poisoning.[35]

In a study of patients with severe CO intoxication, coma on admission, and normobaric 100% oxygen, persistent changes on the MRI were found 1 to 10 years after exposure independently of the neuropsychiatric findings. T_2-weighted and fluid-attenuated inversion recovery (FLAIR) images showed bilateral symmetrical hyperintensity of the white matter, more often involving the centrum semiovale, with relative sparing of the temporal lobes and anterior parts of the frontal lobes. There was also atrophy of the cerebral cortex, cerebellar hemispheres, vermis, and corpus callosum, as well as T_1 hypointensities and T_2 and FLAIR hyperintensities in the globus pallidus.[66]

Kim et al.[11] studied the delayed effects of CO on the cerebral white mater 25 to 95 days after the exposure, with initial recovery followed by relapse of neuropsychiatric symptoms. T_2-weighted images, diffusion-weighted images, and FLAIR sequences demonstrate bilateral, diffuse, and confluent lesions in the periventricular white matter and centrum semiovale; more prominent changes were present in the frontal lobes than elsewhere. The effects of CO poisoning in acute stages can be evaluated by diffusion-weighted images on brain MRI.[11] A restricted water diffusion pattern in the globus pallidus and substantia nigra can be seen.[63]

Cerebral edema occurs early. Clinical status and outcome correlate with diffuse white matter changes.[62] Long term (25 years) after CO exposure, MRI has demonstrated symmetrical globus pallidus and white matter changes in most patients.[67] Temporal, parietal, and occipital lobes are usually affected with asymmetrical cortical and subcortical lesions.[68]

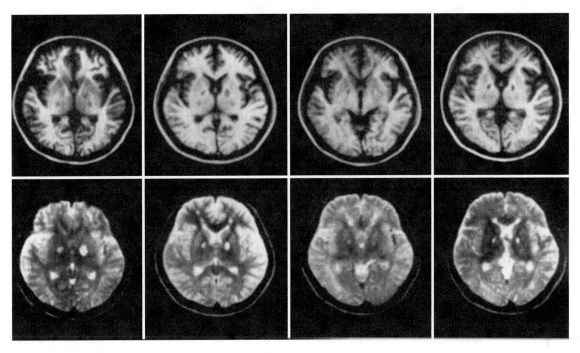

Figure 45-7. Changes in the level of consciousness and the magnetic resonance images of a 20-year-old woman acutely exposed to carbon monoxide. The disappearance of the lesions in the cerebral white matter coincided with amelioration of the patient's clinical neurological condition. The globus pallidus lesions, which became obscure on magnetic resonance images 2 months after exposure, reappeared on the magnetic resonance images 4 months after the incident. *(A)* The T_1-weighted images 4 days after exposure demonstrating areas of hypointensity in the globus pallidus bilaterally; areas appear hyperintense on the T_2-weighted images. *(B)* The T_1-weighted images 1 month after exposure still show distinct, but diminished, areas of hypointensity in the globus pallidus bilaterally. In addition, areas of abnormal signal intensity are seen in the subcortical white matter; areas are more clearly seen and appear hyperintense on T_2-weighted images. *(C)* The T_1- and T_2-weighted images 2 months after exposure showing diminution of the lesions in the globus pallidus and the subcortical white matter. *(D)* The T_1- and T_2-weighted images 4 months after exposure showing distinct lesions in the globus pallidus bilaterally. (Gotoh M, Kuyama H, Asari S, Ohmoto T, Akioka T, Lai, MY. Sequential changes in MR images of the brain in acute carbon monoxide poisoning. *Comput Med Imaging Graph.* 1993;17:55–59.)

Magnetic resonance spectroscopy (MRS) examines brain metabolites. The major resonances of MRS are N-acetyl aspartate (NAA), choline, and creatine. NAA is located within neurons and is a specific neuronal and axonal marker. Choline is part of the membrane constituent phosphatidyl choline. Based on previous studies of demyelinating brains, choline increases are due to an increase in phosphatidyl choline, which in turn is due to demyelination or gliosis. The NAA decreases in the demyelinated white matter presumably represent axonal and neuronal loss.[69] MRS provides evidence for CO-induced brain damage, including decreased NAA that can be found in the basal ganglia and elsewhere.[70]

Proton magnetic resonance spectroscopy (^{1}H-MRS) is a noninvasive method that can provide biochemical information about brain tissues. In early CO poisoning ^{1}H-MRS studies showed a persistent increase in choline related to progressive demyelination. In irreversible injury, lactate appears and NAA decreases.[70] ^{1}H-MRS studies of frontal lobe white matter revealed increases in the choline-containing compounds, and reductions of NAA in all cases. Normalization of the findings was found in a subclinical case. In two cases with akinetic mutism, presenting increased lactate was noted to persist. These results indicate the ^{1}H-MRS is a useful indicator in the clinical evaluation of patients with the interval form of CO poisoning when compared to MRI, electroencephalogram, and N-isopropyl-p-[123]iodoamphetamine single-photon emission computed tomography (SPECT).[71]

Kamada et al.[72] reported that MRS in patients with delayed sequelae of CO exposure precisely reflects the severity of symptoms. With severe clinical dysfunction, marked lowering of the NAA-to-creatine ratio and a slightly increased choline-to-creatine ratio are noted, with subsequent return of the NAA- and choline-to-creatine ratios to normal with clinical improvement. ^{1}H-MRS appears to be superior to conventional radiological examinations in CO poisoning.

Differential Diagnosis on Neuroimaging

The globus pallidus CT and MRI findings are common in but not pathognomonic of CO toxicity. Other diseases may mimic CO toxicity. Bilateral basal ganglia lesions similar to those described in CO poisoning are also present in Leigh's disease and in Hallervorden-Spatz disease. Basal ganglia infarcts and lesions can also appear in other metabolic disorders (e.g., propionic academia). Basal ganglia hamartomas associated with neurofibromatosis may appear similar to the lesions seen in CO toxicity.[68] Prockop[73] reported a young man suffering occupational exposure to mixed volatile organic compounds. He suffered cerebral edema documented by CT scan and later developed bilateral globus pallidus lesions almost identical to those noted in CO toxicity. Likewise, white matter hyperintensities are not pathognomonic of CO toxicity but are sometimes seen in healthy aging individuals.[74] They occur more often and to a greater degree in cerebrovascular insufficiency, i.e., hypoxia, ischemia, or both. As such, these white matter hyperintensities are often considered markers of cerebral ischemia. However, white matter hyperintensities, especially of the centru semiovale regions, are significantly associated with CO induced cognitive impairments.

OTHER BIOCHEMICAL MARKERS OF CARBON MONOXIDE POISONING

Very high levels of S100B protein, a structural astroglial protein in the astroglia, have been found in patients who died; elevated levels have been found in unconscious patients; and normal levels have been found in those without loss of consciousness. It was proposed that S100B protein levels could be used as a biochemical marker of brain injury in CO poisoning.[75] However, Rasmussen et al. failed to find significant increase in blood concentrations of neuron-specific enolase and S100 protein and found no correlation with level of consciousness in CO poisoning.[76]

Overall, brain CT, MRI, and MRS, as well as neuropsychological testing, are useful tools in diagnosis of CO toxicity and its severity. In addition, positron emission tomography and SPECT may provide additional information.[77,78]

TREATMENT

Tissue hypoxia is the major outcome of CO intoxication. Therefore, based on chemical and pathophysiological data, oxygen is the "natural antidote."[79] Since the clinical signs and symptoms of CO toxicity are nonspecific, all suspected victims should be treated with oxygen inhalation immediately after blood is drawn for COHb content. Individual responses to similar levels of CO exposure vary widely, ranging from death, to a parkinsonian syndrome, to mild or moderate intellectual impaiment.[19] Therefore, immediately after securing the airway and adequate ventilation, administration of normobaric oxygen is the cornerstone of therapy, reducing the half-life of COHb from a mean of 5 hours (range 2 to 7 hours) to about 1 hour. HBO at 2.5 atmospheres reduces it to 20 to 30 minutes and has other benefits, at least in animal models. For example in rat brains, it prevents lipid peroxidation and leukocyte adherence to brain microvascular endothelium while accelerating regeneration of inactivated cytochrome oxidase. Therefore, usually at 2.5 to 3 atmospheres absolute for 90 to 120 minutes, it is considered the treatment of choice for those who present with syncope, coma, or seizure; a focal neurological deficit; or COHb greater than 25% (15% in pregnancy).[80–85]

In theory, normobaric oxygen should be the treatment for the least severely poisoned patients, reserving HBO therapy for severe intoxications. However, there are problems with this policy: (1) COHb levels do not correlate with the clinical severity of CO poisoning. (2) There is no universally accepted severity scale of CO poisoning, although loss of consciousness and neurological deficits generally indicate severe poisoning. (3) All victims of CO poisoning are at risk for delayed neuropsychological sequelae. Therefore, in general, the following approach is appropriate: (1) Patients with presumed CO poisoning should be placed on 100% oxygen. (2) Patients with severe poisoning must receive HBO regardless of COHb level. (3) Pregnant women must be treated with HBO irrespective of signs and symptoms. (4) In patients with lesser degrees of poisoning, careful evaluation is advised before deciding that 100% normobaric oxygen for more than 6 hours is the adequate therapy.[79] Administration of more than one course of HBO for those who remain in coma is controversial. There are several practical considerations because not all treatment facilities, e.g., hospital emergency rooms, can measure COHb or administer HBO. For example, in one recent study, only 44% of acute care hospitals had the capability of measuring COHb.[86]

HBO is 100% oxygen at two to three times the atmospheric pressure at sea level. The oxygen tension in the arteries increases to about 2000 mm Hg and that of the tissues—to almost 400 mm Hg. The pressure is expressed in multiples of the atmospheric pressure, which is 1 at sea level. At sea level, the blood oxygen concentration is 0.3 mL/dL. At 100% oxygen at ambient (normobaric) pressure, the amount of the dissolved oxygen in the blood increases fivefold to 1.5 mL/dL. At 3 atmospheres, the dissolved-oxygen content reaches 6 mL/dL. HBO decreases the bubble formation in the blood and replaces inert gases with oxygen, which is rapidly taken up and used by the tissues. HBO can be bactericidal or bacteriostatic, or it can suppress toxin production, increasing tissues resistance against infections. HBO is more effective than normobaric oxygen in promoting collagen formation and angiogenesis and thus can facilitate wound healing. HBO inhibits neutrophil adherence to the walls of the ischemic vessels, which decreased free radical production, vasoconstriction, and tissue destruction.

HBO is commonly delivered in a monoplace chamber or less often in a multioccupant chamber. The duration of a single treatment for CO poisoning is about 45 minutes. HBO with oxygen pressures of up to 3 atmospheres for a maximum of 120 minutes is safe. Adverse effects include reversible myopia, cataract, tracheobronchial symptoms, self-limited seizures, and barotraumas to the middle ear, cranial sinuses, and rarely teeth or lungs. Claustrophobia can be an issue in monoplace chambers. Despite the conflicting results from the literature regarding the effect of HBO versus normobaric oxygen, Tibbles and Edelsberg[84] determined that patients with severe CO poisoning should receive at least one HBO treatment at 2.5 to 3.0 atmospheres because this therapy is the fastest method of treatment of the potentially reversible life-threatening effects.

The treatment of a patient with CO poisoning should not be based solely on the COHb levels. The clinical manifestations, COHb levels, and importantly, the patient's underlying medical history should be taken into account. In patients with suspected CO poisoning, 100% oxygen should be given immediately by a mask. The goal is to raise the PaO_2 levels, decrease the half-life of CO, and facilitate its dissociation from Hb, thus allowing oxygen to attach to the freed binding sites. Strict bed rest should be provided, since it decreases oxygen demand and consumption. Patients with respiratory distress and decreased level of consciousness should be intubated and ventilated. Chest radiographs, blood lactate levels, and arterial blood gases should be performed in the emergency department. Headache improved before HBO treatment in 72%, resolving entirely in 21%. Of those with residual headache, pain improved with hyperbaric oxygen in 97%, resolving entirely in 44%.

Even though deaths from CO poisoning have decreased in the United States in recent years, the total burden, including fatal and nonfatal cases, has not significantly changed.[87]

Juurlink et al.[88] analyzed available data from six randomized controlled trials involving nonpregnant adults acutely poisoned with CO. At 1 month follow-up after treatment, symptoms possibly related to CO poisoning were present in 34.2% not of those treated with HBO, compared with 37.2% not treated with HBO.[88] They found no evidence that unselected use of HBO in the treatment of acute CO poisoning reduces the frequency of neurological symptoms at 1 month. Because of insufficient

evidence, they recommend further research for defining the role of HBO in treatment of CO poisoning. Five years later, the same group examined the evidence for the effectiveness of the HBO for prevention of neurological sequelae in patients with acute CO poisoning. *Four out of six trials found no benefit of HBO for the reduction of neurological sequelae, while two others found HBO beneficial.* The authors conclude that the existing randomized trials have not been able to establish reduction of neurological sequelae with the administration of HBO to patients with CO poisoning.[89]

Close monitoring of serum pH and lactic acid levels is required, since anaerobic metabolism in the presence of tissue hypoxia generates lactic acidosis. Acidosis below 7.15 pH should be treated with sodium bicarbonate. Caution has to be exercised with the administration of sodium bicarbonate because carbon dioxide, a byproduct of its metabolism, could lead to respiratory acidosis and has to be eliminated by proper ventilation.

CONCLUSION

CO, a highly toxic gas produced by incomplete combustion of hydrocarbons, is a relatively common cause of damage to humans. Because CO is tasteless and odorless and its clinical symptoms and signs are nonspecific, human toxicity is often overlooked. The brain and the heart may be severely affected after exposure to COHb levels exceeding 20%. Such damage occurs because the affinity of Hb for CO is 210 times higher than for oxygen. Hypoxic damage in the brain predominates in the cerebral cortex, cerebral white matter, and basal ganglia, especially the globus pallidus. Diagnosis requires clinical acumen and a high index of suspicion, often combined with epidemiological data, a careful clinical examination, analysis of ambient air CO and patient COHb levels, cardiological evaluations including ECG, and neurological evaluations including brain imaging (CT, MRI, MRS) and neuropsychological testing. SPECT and positron emission tomography may also be useful. Although immediate oxygen breathing is sometimes an adequate treatment, HBO treatment is favored. Subsequently, only symptomatic therapy is available for sequelae occurring in the course of long-term follow-up evaluations. An especially perplexing and unresolved issue is establishment of therapy or therapies to prevent the development of long-term sequelae in victims, e.g., the delayed neuropsychiatric syndrome and neurological dysfunction in children exposed to CO while they were in utero.

Because prevention is the best treatment, our society should be on high alert in its attempts to prevent cases of CO poisoning.

REFERENCES

1. Hardy KR, Thom SR. Pathophysiology and treatment of carbon monoxide poisoning. *J Toxicol Clin Toxicol.* 1994;32:613–629.

2. Centers for Disease Control and Prevention. Deaths from motor-vehicle-related unintentional carbon monoxide poisoning: Colorado 1996, New Mexico 1980–1995, and United States 1979–1988. *MMWR.* 1996;45:1029–1032.

3. Cobb N, Etzel RA. Unintentional carbon monoxide–related deaths in the United States, 1979–1988. *JAMA.* 1991;266:659–663.

4. Abelsohn A, Sanborn MD, Jessiman BJ, Weir F. Identifying and managing adverse environmental health effects: VI. Carbon monoxide poisoning. *CMAJ.* 2002;166:1685–1690.

5. Kao LW, Nanagas KA. Carbon monoxide poisoning. *Emerg Med Clin North Am.* 2004;22:985–1018.

6. Prockop LD, Chichkova R. Carbon monoxide intoxication: An environmental updated review. In: Román GC, Reis J, Defer G, Prockop L, eds. Special Issue on Environmental Neurology. *J Neurol Sci.* 2007; 262:122–130.

7. Mimura K, Harada M, Sumiyoshi S, et al. Long-term follow-up study on sequelae of carbon monoxide poisoning: serial investigation 33 years after poisoning. *Seishin Shinkeigaku Zashi.* 1999;101:592–618.

8. Klawans HL, Stein RW, Tanner CM, Goetz CG. A pure parkinsonian syndrome following acute carbon monoxide intoxication. *Arch Neurol.* 1982;39:302–304.

9. Sohn YH, Jeong T, Kim HS, Im JH, Kim JS. The brain lesion responsible for parkinsonism after carbon monoxide poisoning. *Arch Neurol.* 2000;57:1214–1218.

10. Choi S. Delayed neurological sequelae in carbon monoxide intoxication. *Arch Neurol.* 1982;40:433–435.

11. Kim JH, Chang KH, Song IC, et al. Delayed encephalopathy of acute carbon monoxide intoxication: diffusivity of cerebral white matter lesions. *Am J Neuroradiol.* 2003;24:1592–1597.

12. Min SK. A brain syndrome with delayed neuropsychiatric sequelae following acute carbon monoxide intoxication. *Acta Psychiatry Scand.* 1986;73:80–86.

13. Candura SM, Fonte R, Finozzi E, et al. Indoor pollution: a report of 2 clinical cases of occult carbon monoxide poisoning. *G Ital Med Lav.* 1993;15:1–4.

14. Carbon Monoxide: The Unnoticed Poison of the 21st Century. Proceedings of Satellite Meeting: International Union of Toxicology, 8th International Congress of Toxicology. Universite de Bourgogne, Dijon, France; 1998.

15. Wikipedia contributors. Carbon Monoxide. Available at: http://en.wikipedia.org/wiki/Carbon_monoxide_poisoning. Accessed 2008.

16. Ryter SW, Alam J, Choi AM. Heme oxygenase-1/carbon monoxide: from basic science to therapeutic applications. *Physiol Rev.* 2006;86(2):583–650.

17. Lascaratos JG, Marketos SG. The carbon monoxide poisoning of two Byzantine emperors. *J Toxicol Clin Toxicol.* 1998;36(1–2):103–107.

18. Tvedt B, Kjuus H. Chronic CO poisoning: use of generator gas during the Second World War and recent research. *Tidsskr Nor Laegeforen.* 1997;117(17):2454–2457.

19. Prockop LD. Carbon monoxide brain toxicity: clinical, magnetic resonance imaging, magnetic resonance spectroscopy, and neuropsychological effects in 9 people. *J Neuroimaging.* 2005;15(2):144–149.

20. Chance BC, Erecinska M, Wanger M. Mitochondrial responses to carbon monoxide toxicity. *Ann NY Acad Sci.* 1970 Oct 5;174(1):193–204.

21. Tomaszewski C. Carbon monoxide. In: Ford MD, Delaney KA, Ling LS, Erickson T, eds. *Clinical Toxicology.* Philadelphia: WB Saunders; 2001:57–667.

22. Ellenhorn MJ, Schonwald S, Ordog G, Wasserberger J, eds. *Respiratory Toxicology in Ellenhorn's Medical Toxicology.* 2nd ed. Philadelphia: Williams & Wilkins; 1997:1448–1531.

23. Longo LD. The biological effects of carbon monoxide on the pregnant woman, fetus, and newborn infant. *Am J Obstet Gynecol.* 1997;129:69–103.

24. Cramer CR. Fetal death due to accidental maternal carbon monoxide poisoning. *J Toxicol Clin Toxicol.* 1982;19: 297–301.

25. Margulies JL. Acute carbon monoxide poisoning during pregnancy. *Am J Emerg Med.* 1986;4:515–519.

26. Kim JK, Coe CJ. Clinical study on carbon monoxide intoxication in children. *Yonsei Med J.* 1987;28:266–273.

27. Department of the Environment. Expert Panel on Air Quality Standard. London: Her Majesty's Stationery Office, 1994.

28. White RF, Feldman RG, Proctor SP. Neurobehavioral effects of toxic exposure. In: White RF, ed. *Clinical Syndrome in Adult Neuropsychology: The Practitioner's Handbook.* New York: Elsevier; 1992:1–51.

29. Townsend CL, Maynard RI. Effects on health of prolonged exposure to low concentrations of carbon monoxide. *Occup Environ Med.* 2002;59(10):708–711.

30. Peterson JE, Steward RD. Absorption and elimination of carbon monoxide by active young men. *Arch Environ Health.* 1970;21:165–171.

31. Handa PK, Tai DY. Carbon monoxide poisoning: a five year review at Tan Tock Seng Hospital, Singapore. *Ann Acad Med Singapore.* 2005;34(10):611–614.

32. Hampson NB, Hampson LA. Characteristics of headache associated with acute carbon monoxide poisoning. *Headache.* 2002;42(3):220–223.

33. Choi IS. Carbon monoxide poisoning: systemic manifestations and complication. *J Korean Med Sci.* 2001;16(3):253–261.

34. Henz S, Maeder M. Prospective study of accidental carbon monoxide poisoning in 38 Swiss soldiers. *Swiss Med Wkly.* 2005;135(27–28):398–408.

35. Durak AC, Coskun A, Yikilmaz A, Erdogan F, Mavili E, Guven M. Magnetic resonance imaging findings in chronic carbon monoxide intoxication. *Acta Radiol.* 2005;46:322–327.

35a. Prockop, LD. Unpublished data, 2008.

36. Ginsberg MD, Myers RE, McDonagh BF. Experimental carbon monoxide encephalopathy in the primate: II. Clinical aspects, neuropathology, and physiologic correlation. *Arch Neurol.* 1974;30:209–216.

37. Cohen RE. Behavioral treatment of incontinence in a profoundly neurologically impaired adult. *Arch Phys Med Rehabil.* 1986;67(12):883–884.

38. Kwon, OY, Chung SP, Ha YR, Yoo IS, Kim SW. Delayed postanoxic encephalopathy after carbon monoxide poisoning. *Emerg Med J.* 2004;21:250–251.

39. Hu MC, Shiah IS, Yeh CB, Chen HK, Chen CK. Ziprasidone in the treatment of delayed carbon monoxide encephalopathy. *Prog Neuropsychopharmacol Biol Psychiatry.* 2006;30:755–757.

39a. Chambers CA, Hopkins RO, Weaver LK, Kay C. Cognitive and affective outcomes of more severe compared to less severe carbon monoxide poisoning. *Brain Injury.* 2008;22(5):387–395.

40. Hampson NB. Pulse oximetry in severe carbon monoxide poisoning. *Chest.* 1998;114(4):1036–1041.

41. Bozeman WP, Hampson NB. Pulse oximetry in CO poisoning: additional data. *Chest.* 2000;117(1):295–296.

42. Widdop B. Analysis of carbon monoxide. *Ann Clin Biochem.* 2002;39(Pt 4):378–391.

43. Henry CR, Satran D, Lindgren B, Adkinson C, Nicholson CI, Henry TD. Myocardial injury and long-term mortality following moderate to severe carbon monoxide poisoning. *JAMA.* 2006;295(4):398–402.

44. Somogyi E, Balogh I, Rubanyi G, Sotonyi P, Szegedi L. New findings concerning the pathogenesis of acute carbon monoxide (CO) poisoning. *Am J Forensic Med Pathol.* 1981;2(1):31–39.

45. Satran D, Henry CR, Adkinson C, Nicholson CI, Bracha Y, Henry TD. Cardiovascular manifestations of moderate to severe carbon monoxide poisoning. *J Am Coll Cardiol.* 2005;3;45(9): 1513–1516.

46. Kumazawa T, Watanabe-Suzuki K, Seno H, Ishii A, Suzuki O. A curious autopsy case of accidental carbon monoxide poisoning in a motor vehicle. *Leg Med (Tokyo).* 2000;2(3):181–185.

47. Tritapepe L, Macchiarelli G, Rocco M, et al. Functional and ultrastructural evidence of myocardial stunning after acute carbon monoxide poisoning. *Crit Care Med.* 1998;26(4):797–801.

48. Lin H, McGrath JJ. Responses of the working rat heart to carbon monoxide. *Physiol Behav.* 1989;46(1):81–84.

49. Clubb FJ Jr, Penney DG, Baylerian MS, Bishop SP. Cardiomegaly due to myocyte hyperplasia in prenatal rats exposed to 200 ppm carbon monoxide. *J Mol Cell Cardiol.* 1986;18(5):477–486.

50. Anderson RF, Allensworth DC, DeGroot WJ. Myocardial toxicity from carbon monoxide poisoning. *Ann Intern Med.* 1967;67(6):1172–1182.

51. Fineschi V, Agricola E, Baroldi G, et al. Myocardial findings in fatal carbon monoxide poisoning: a human and experiment morphometric study. *Int J Legal Med.* 2000;113(5):276–282.

52. Ernst A, Zibrak JD. Current concepts: Carbon monoxide poisoning. *N Engl J Med.* 1998;339(22):1603–1608.

53. Lasprele J, Fardeau M. The central nervous system and carbon monoxide poisoning: II. Anatomical study of brain lesions following intoxication with carbon monoxide (22 cases). *Prog Brain Res.* 1967;24:31–74.

54. Tuchman RF, Moser FG, Moshe SL. Carbon monoxide poisoning: bilateral lesions in the thalamus on MR imaging of the brain. *Pediatr Radiol.* 1990;20(6):478–479.

55. Sawada Y, Ahashi N, Maenura K, et al. Computerized tomography as an indication of long–term outcome after carbon monoxide poisoning. *Lancet.* 1980;1:783–786.

56. Murata S, Asaba H, Hiraishi K, et al. Magnetic resonance imaging findings on carbon monoxide intoxication. *J Neuroimaging.* 1993;3:128–131.

57. Gotoh M, Kuyama H, Asari S, Ohmoto T, Akioka T, Lai, MY. Sequential changes in MR images of the brain in acute carbon monoxide poisoning. *Comput Med Imaging Graph.* 1993;17:55–59.

58. Tom T, Abedon S, Clark RI, Wong W. Neuroimaging characteristics in carbon monoxide toxicity. *J Neuroimaging.* 1996:161–166.

59. Jones JS, Lagasse J, Zimmerman G. Computed tomographic findings after acute carbon monoxide poisoning. *Am J Emerg Med.* 1994;12:448–451.

60. Sener RN. Acute carbon monoxide poisoning: diffusion MR imaging findings. *Am J Neuroradiol.* 2003;24(7):1475–1477.

61. Ferrier D, Wallace CJ, Fletcher WA, Fong TC. Magnetic resonance features in carbon monoxide poisoning. *Can Assoc Radiol J.* 1994;45(6):466–468.

62. Schils F, Cabay JE, Flandroy P, Dondelinger RF. Unusual CT and MRI appearance of carbon monoxide poisoning. *JBR-BTR.* 1999;82(1):13–15.

63. Kinoshita T, Sugihara S, Matsusue E, Fujii S, Ametani M, Ogawa T. Pallidoreticular damage in acute carbon monoxide poisoning: diffusion-weighted MR imaging findings. *AJNR Am J Neuroradiol.* 2005;26(7):1845–1848.

64. O'Donnell P, Buxton PJ, Pitkin A, Jarvis LJ. The magnetic resonance imaging appearances of the brain in acute carbon monoxide poisoning. *Clin Radiol.* 2000;55(4):273–280.

65. Mascalchi M, Petruzi P, Zampa V. MRI of cerebellar white matter damage due to carbon monoxide poisoning: case report. *Neuroradiology.* 1996;38(Suppl 1):S73–S74.

66. Kawada N, Ochiai N, Kuzuhara S. Diffusion MRI in acute carbon monoxide poisoning. *Intern Med.* 2004;43(7):639–640.

67. Inagaki T, Ishino H, Seno H, Umegae N, Aoyama T. A long-term follow-up study of serial magnetic resonance images in patients with delayed encephalopathy after acute carbon monoxide poisoning. *Psychiatry Clin Neurosci.* 1997;51(6):4213.

68. Prockop LD, Naidu KA. Brain CT and MRI findings after carbon monoxide toxicity. *J Neuroimaging.* 1999;9(3):175–181.

69. Van Zijl PCM, Barker PB. Magnetic resonance spectroscopy and spectroscopic imaging for the study of brain metabolism. *Ann NY Acad Sci.* 1997;820:75–96.

70. Murata T, Itoh S, Koshino Y, et al. Serial proton magnetic resonance spectroscopy in a patient with the interval form of carbon monoxide poisoning. *J Neurol Neurosurg Psychiatry.* 1995;58:100–103.

71. Murata T, Kimura H, Kado H, et al. Neuronal damage in the interval form of carbon monoxide determined by serial diffusion-weighted magnetic resonance imaging plus 1H-magnetic resonance spectroscopy. *J Neurol Neurosurg Psychiatry.* 2001;71(2):250–253.

72. Kamada K, Houkin K, Aoki T, et al. Cerebral metabolic changed in delayed carbon monoxide sequelae studied by proton MR spectroscopy. *Neuroradiology.* 1994;36(2):104–106.

73. Prockop LD. Neuroimaging in neurotoxicology. In: L Chang, ed. *Handbook of Neurotoxicology.* New York. M Dekker, 1995. 753–763.

74. Frazeka F, Schmidt R, Offenbacker H, et al. Prevalence of white matter and periventricular magnetic resonance hyperintensity in asymptomatic volunteers. *J Neuroimaging.* 1991:1:27–30.

75. Brvar M, Mozina H, Osredkar J, et al. S100B protein in carbon monoxide poisoning: a pilot study. *Resuscitation.* 2004;61(3):357–360.

75a. Parkinson RB, Hopkins RO, Cleavinger LK, et al. White matter hyperintensities and neuropsychological outcome following carbon monoxide poisoning. *Neurology.* 2002;58:1525–1532.

76. Rasmussen LS, Poulsen MG, Christiansen M, Jansen EC. Biochemical markers from brain damage after carbon monoxide poisoning. *Acta Anaesthesiol Scand.* 2004;48(4):469–473.

77. Tengvar C, Johansson B, Sorensen J. Frontal lobe and cingulated cortical metabolic dysfunction in acquired akinetic mutism: a PET study of the interval form of carbon monoxide poisoning. *Brain Inj.* 2004;18(6):615–625.

78. Gale SD, Hoskins RO, Weaver LK, Bigler ED, Booth EJ, Blatter DD. MRI, quantitative MRI, SPECT, and neuropsychological findings following carbon monoxide poisoning. *Brain Inj.* 1999;13(4):229–243.

79. Elkharrat D. Indications of Normobacic and Hyperbaric Oxygen Therapy in Acute CO intoxication. Proceedings of Satellite Meeting: International Union of Toxicology, 8th International Congress of Toxicology. International Congress of Toxicology. Dijon, France, July 3–4, 1998.

80. Tibbles PM, Perotta PL. Treatment of carbon monoxide poisoning: a critical review of human outcome studies comparing normobaric oxygen with hyperbaric oxygen. *Ann Emerg Med.* 1994;24:269–276.

81. Weaver LK, Hopkins RO, Larson-Lorh V, Howe S, Haberstock D. Double blind, controlled, prospective, randomized clinical trial (RCT) in patients with acute carbon monoxide (CO) poisoning: outcome of patients tested with normobaric oxygen or hyperbaric oxygen (HBO$_2$), an interim report. *Undersea Hyperb Med.* 1995;22(Suppl):14.

82. Thom SR, Taber RI, Mediguren II, Clark JM, Hardy KR, Fisher AB. Delayed neuropsychological sequelae after carbon monoxide poisoning: prevention by treatment with hyperbaric oxygen. *Ann Emerg Med.* 1995;25:479–486.

83. Van Meter KW, Weiss L, Harch PE, et al. Should the pressure be off or on with use of oxygen in the treatment of carbon monoxide poisoned patients? *Ann Emerg Med.* 1994;24:283–288.

84. Tibbles PM, Edelsberg JS. Hyperbaric-oxygen therapy. *N Engl J Med.* 1996;334:1642–1648.

85. Weaver LK, Hopkins RO, Chan KJ, et al. Hyperbaric oxygen for acute carbon monoxide poisoning. *N Engl J Med.* 202;347:1057–1067.

86. Hampson NB, Scott KL, Zmaeff JL. Carboxyhemoglobin measurement by hospitals: implications for the diagnosis of carbon monoxide poisoning. *J Emerg Med.* 2006;31(1):13–16.

87. Hampson NB. Trends in the incidence of carbon monoxide poisoning in the United States. *Am J Emerg Med.* 2005;23(7):838–841.

88. Juurlink DN, Stanbrook MB, McGuigan MA. Hyperbaric oxygen for carbon monoxide poisoning. *Cochrane Database Syst Rev.* 2000;(2):CD002041.

89. Juurlink DN, Buckley NA, Stanbrook MB, Isbister GK, Bennett M, McGuigan MA. Hyperbaric oxygen for carbon monoxide poisoning. *Cochrane Database Syst Rev.* 2005;(1):CD002041 [review].

Cyanide

Michael R. Dobbs

INTRODUCTION

Cyanide is a lethal toxic agent that can occur naturally and is widely used in industries around the world, including printing, agriculture, photography, and manufacturing of paper and plastics. Each year, more than 300,000 tons of cyanide are produced in the United States.

Hydrogen cyanide is now listed under schedule 3 of the Chemical Weapons Convention, indicating that it is a potential weapon with large-scale industrial use. Because of this designation, plants that produce significant amounts of cyanide must declare this and are subject to inspection by the Organisation for the Prohibition of Chemical Weapons.

Cyanides may be gases, liquids, or solids. At room temperature, hydrogen cyanide is a colorless or pale blue liquid. It is volatile and easily forms explosive mixtures with air. In addition, cyanide may be dissolved into solvents to form liquids such as cyanogen chloride. Solids are typically salts made up of sodium, potassium, or calcium with the cyano group.

CHEMICAL PROPERTIES

Cyanides are usually stored in their liquid state. However, hydrogen cyanide (Figure 46-1) is a colorless gas at temperatures above 78°F. It has a faint, bitter, almond-like odor, which nearly 40% of people cannot smell. It is flammable and potentially explosive.

The salts, potassium cyanide and sodium cyanide, are white powders. In damp air, these powders may have a slight almond odor because they hydrolyze into hydrogen cyanide.

People may be environmentally exposed to cyanide through inhalation of hydrogen cyanide vapor, contact with cyanide solutions or salts and absorption through the skin or eyes, or ingestion of cyanide solutions or salts. For hydrogen cyanide gas to be harmful to humans, high concentrations of it must be contained in a confined space. Otherwise, the highly volatile gas typically disperses before it can do significant harm.

Cyanide vapor can ignite and explode. The density of hydrogen cyanide is less than air; thus, the safest place to breathe in an area contaminated with hydrogen cyanide

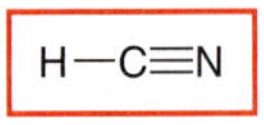

$$H—C≡N$$

Figure 46-1. Chemical structure of hydrogen cyanide.

is probably at the lowest point in the room. Still, cyanide vapor can easily reach high concentrations in all parts of an enclosed space.

MECHANISM OF ACTION

Cyanide has a high affinity for ferric iron (Fe^{3+}), such as found in cytochrome c oxidase—an important enzyme in the electron transport chain. Cyanide binds and irreversibly inhibits cytochrome c oxidase in mitochondria. This results in a shutdown of cellular respiration, soon followed by cellular death (Figure 46-2). Cyanide readily diffuses through cell walls, which is why onset of symptoms occurs so quickly. Small amounts of cyanide are metabolized to thiocyanate through endogenous rhodanese and then excreted in the urine.

As a cellular poison, cyanide affects all cells throughout the body, but the central nervous system and heart are particularly sensitive. The mechanism of death in most cases of cyanide poisoning is central apnea, in which cyanide depresses the respiratory center in the brain.

Common Sources of Exposure

Environmental Sources

Hydrogen cyanide gas is produced in blast furnaces, gas works, and coke ovens. Cyanide is also found in combustion products of x-ray film, wool, silk, nylon, paper, nitriles, rubber, urethanes, polyurethane, and other synthetics. Along with carbon monoxide, it is a common cause of fatalities in industrial and domestic fires.[1–5]

Those involved in certain occupations such as healthcare and select laboratory workers are at a higher relative risk for suicidal ingestion of cyanides from cyanide salt

solids. This is from proximity to cyanide salts found in some hospital or research laboratories.

Low-Level Sources

Cigarette smoke contains cyanide, and smokers' cyanide levels are significantly higher than those of nonsmokers.

Cyanogenetic glycosides, naturally occurring compounds, are found in foods such as almonds, fruit pits, and cassava beans. The most clinically significant of these compounds is amygdalin (Laetrile; Figure 46-3). This is found in apple seeds, peach pits, cherry pits, plum pits, and almond kernels.

Amygdalin has caused deaths in both children and adults when taken in excessive quantities.[6] An endogenous enzyme in the seeds converts amygdalin into glucose, benzaldehyde, and hydrogen cyanide. This enzyme is released when the seeds are crushed and moistened, especially in an alkaline solution such as in the duodenum. Amygdalin has also been investigated as a cancer treatment and has been reported to cause cyanide toxicity when ingested in "vitamin supplements."[7]

Iatrogenic: Sodium Nitroprusside

Cyanide is formed in vivo when nitroprusside is administered intravenously, typically for difficult-to-control hypertension, and particularly when therapy is prolonged or exceeds the maximum recommended dose.[8,9]

Sodium nitroprusside remains an important intravenous medication for difficult-to-control hypertension. In neurology, it is often used in the acute stroke patient with hypertension. The breakdown of nitroprusside in the body leads to dissociation into the components cyanide and nitric oxide. Cyanide is then metabolized to thiocyanate through liver rhodanese and excreted. In patients with normal renal function, mean elimination half-time for thiocyanate is 3 days. It is much longer in patients with renal insufficiency. Accumulation of cyanide is more common in infusions of sodium nitroprusside exceeding 2 μg/kg/min. Concomitant administration of sodium thiosulfate can be helpful to prevent cyanide toxicity in patients undergoing high rates of infusion

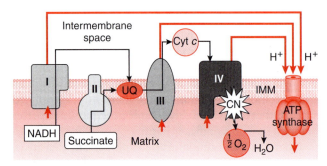

Figure 46-2. Cyanide mechanism of action.

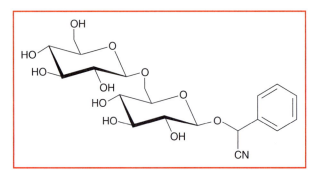

Figure 46-3. Chemical structure of amygdalin (Laetrile).

with sodium nitroprusside. Thiocyanate itself can be toxic, especially in renally impaired patients. Thiocyanate concentrations in patients on nitroprusside for long periods should not be allowed to exceed 0.1 mg/mL. Thiocyanate can be removed easily by hemodialysis. Lactic acidosis and cardiovascular instability in someone undergoing sustained infusion of sodium nitroprusside is highly suggestive of cyanide poisoning.[10]

CLINICAL SYMPTOMS

Symptoms vary depending on the dose, route, and speed of administration; the chemical form of the cyanide; and other factors, including the gender, age, weight, and general physical condition of the exposed person. Typically, symptoms present almost immediately and progress rapidly from skin color changes and rapid breathing to seizures, cessation of breathing, and cardiac arrest. With inhalation of high concentrations, death can occur within minutes (Table 1). The symptoms may be slower to develop for lower concentrations of cyanide gas or for oral or skin exposures.

To the bystander, the only observed signs may be sudden collapse of the victim. The patient who presents with sudden collapse and unresponsiveness always has the possibility of cyanide intoxication in the differential diagnosis, especially if the individual has no other pertinent medical history. This is obviously a diagnostic challenge.

Low Concentrations (Nonlethal)

Signs of acute cyanide poisoning in low concentrations include the following:

- Anxiety
- Hyperventilation
- Headaches, dizziness, and vomiting
- Flushed or "cherry red" skin

Table 1: Progression of Lethal Cyanide Intoxication

Time from Exposure	Symptoms
15 seconds	Hyperpnea
30 seconds	Seizures
3–5 minutes	Breathing ceases
6–8 minutes	Death

Symptoms improve when victims are removed from the cyanide source. Cyanide liquid on the skin or in the eyes may cause irritation and swelling at the exposed site. In addition, this exposure can lead to systemic effects as cyanide is absorbed into the body.

High Concentrations (Inhalation)

Signs of acute cyanide poisoning in high concentrations include the following:

- Hyperventilation (often the first sign, appearing within a few seconds after massive inhalation)
- Loss of consciousness (after as little as 30 seconds)
- Seizures and convulsions (after as little as 30 seconds)
- Muscle rigidity including opisthotonus and trismus
- Cherry-red skin and membranes from higher-than-usual oxygen concentrations in venous blood; cyanosis sometimes occurs
- Metabolic acidosis
- Cessation of breathing
- Decerebrate posturing
- Dilated pupils
- Asystole and death

DIFFERENTIAL DIAGNOSIS

At initial assessment, it may be difficult to distinguish cyanide exposure from organophosphate intoxication (although generally organophosphorus compounds cause pupillary miosis and create more secretions than does cyanide) and carbon monoxide exposure. Cyanide-induced coma patients often show dilated pupils.[7] Carbon monoxide patients typically have normal pupils.[11–13] Seizures are relatively rare in carbon monoxide victims compared to in cyanide victims and are common in organophosphate intoxication. Seizures have been reported as common with carbon monoxide poisoning, but in a prospective study of 629 carbon monoxide patients only 18 seizures were witnessed (2.9%)[14] (Table 2).

The clinician should also consider exposure to hydrogen sulfide, carbon monoxide exposure, ethylene glycol (antifreeze) ingestion, and other less common intoxications. It is critical to know the patient's history.

LABORATORY TESTING

Although laboratory tests can be performed to measure cyanide levels in an exposed person, they are generally not available in time to guide acute treatment.

Table 2: Comparison of Cyanide, Carbon Monoxide, and Organophosphate Intoxications

Signs and Symptoms	Cyanide	Carbon Monoxide	Organophosphates
Headache	+	+	−
Increased secretions	−	−	+ + +
GI disturbances	+	+ +	+ + +
Confusion	+	+ +	+ +
Loss of consciousness	+ (sustained)	+ (transitory)	+
Seizures	+ +	?	+ + +
Dizziness	+	+ +	+
Coma	+	+	+
Pupils	Dilated or normal	Normal	Constricted (miosis)
Hypotension	+	+	+ / −
Cardiac arrhythmia	+ +	+ +	+
Lactic acidosis	+ +	+ +	+ / −

GI, gastrointestinal.
+, typically present; −, absent or atypical;
+ + and + + +, very common.

They are reliable, however, in assessing cyanide levels and can be used for confirmation. The following can be assessed:

- Red blood cell cyanide level—Mild toxicity is observed at cyanide concentrations of 0.5 to 1.0 μg/mL. Concentrations of 2.5 μg/mL and higher are associated with coma, seizures, and death.
- Arterial and venous blood gases—Cyanide toxicity is characterized by a normal arterial partial pressure of oxygen and an abnormally high venous partial pressure of oxygen, that is, a lowered arteriovenous oxygen gradient.
- Serum chemistries and lactate level—Cyanide poisoning is classically associated with high-anion-gap metabolic acidosis and an elevated serum lactate level.
- Carboxyhemoglobin level—The carboxyhemoglobin level may be used to exclude carbon monoxide poisoning, especially in smoke inhalation victims. Be aware that an elevated carboxyhemoglobin does not exclude concomitant exposure to cyanide, which is common in fires that also generate carbon monoxide. (See also Chapter 45.)

TREATMENT

There are three basic goals for cyanide management:

1. Prevent further contamination
2. Provide supportive therapies
3. Remove cyanide from the cell with antidotes

Decontamination

The likelihood of exposed people spreading cyanide to others through direct contact or off-gassing of vapors depends on whether the agent was a gas or liquid. Gas disperses quickly, and those exposed to it self-decontaminate simply by exposure to fresh air. Liquid can be spread through direct contact or off-gassing of vapors.

Therefore, general decontamination procedures should be practiced when dealing with a mass dispersal of a cyanide agent. However, do not delay lifesaving measures such as securing and maintaining the airway, instituting artificial ventilation, or administering cyanide antidotes. Decontamination of liquid cyanide, as long as

Box 1   Cyanide in a Mass-Casualty Situation

Cyanide gas release may involve multiple casualties needing lifesaving treatment. This could occur in a large fire (industrial or domestic) or a deliberate release from a terrorist attack.

If a patient is exhibiting symptoms of cyanide poisoning, take the following steps:

1. Remove the victim from the contaminated area.
2. Remove the victim's clothing.
3. Wash with soap and water.
4. Give amyl nitrite perles in a bag ventilator until the IV with sodium nitrite is ready.[*]
5. Prepare an IV with 300 mg (10-cc amp) of sodium nitrite and administer for more than 5 minutes.
6. Monitor blood pressure carefully to check for hypotension.
7. Administer vasopressor drugs if hypotension is severe.
8. Monitor methemoglobin levels if possible and ensure they stay below 35% to 40% (the range at which methemoglobin itself causes oxygen-carrying deficits).
9. Add 12.5 mg (50-cc amp) of sodium thiosulfate to the IV.
10. Provide oxygen if the patient is unconscious and bag-mask ventilate.
11. Check airways frequently and ensure they are open.
12. Administer IV bicarbonate as needed, titrating to effect and the serum bicarbonate level.
13. Administer fluids via IV as necessary.
14. Consider diazepam to control seizures in unconscious victims.[†]

If the patient is not exhibiting symptoms of cyanide poisoning, take the following steps:

1. Remove the victim from the contaminated area.
2. Remove the victim's clothing.
3. Administer oxygen and IV fluids as necessary.
4. Observe the victim for development of symptoms.
5. Do not administer antidotes without a laboratory confirmation unless cyanide exposure is strongly suspected.

If after 4–6 hours the victim has still not shown any symptoms of cyanide poisoning, discharge the patient with instructions to seek medical attention if symptoms develop.

For protection against cyanide in a contaminated area, each responder should wear a positive-pressure self-contained breathing apparatus and chemical protective clothing.

When working with decontaminated patients in uncontaminated areas, each responder should wear butyl or neoprene gloves and apron and chemical splash goggles.

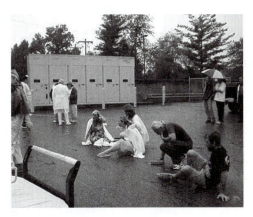

Exposure "victims" from a mock disaster drill waiting for triage and treatment. (Courtesy of author.)

---

[*]An alternative and possibly superior therapy to nitrites is hydroxocobalamin.
[†]For unconscious patients, be sure to begin treatment as you are decontaminating them.

the prehospital provider is protected from exposure, can usually wait if necessary until after immediate lifesaving treatment.

These steps apply in almost all situations involving contamination:

1. Remove patients from the contaminated area as quickly as possible.
2. Remove the patients' clothing.
3. Wash the patients with soap and water.

Support

Appropriate supportive steps depend on the injury. In a severe intoxication, secure and maintain the airway. Assure adequate ventilation, and institute artificial ventilation as needed. Administer oxygen to help restore oxidative phosphorylation in cells and allow normal return to metabolism. Administer bicarbonate to help reduce the acidity of body fluids. Administer intravenous fluids to help keep the patient hydrated and the fluid balance stable.

Oxygen

Oxygen therapy is a mainstay of the treatment of cyanide poisoning and, for many patients, may be all that is needed. Oxygen (normobaric) therapy should be started as soon as is possible.

Hyperbaric Oxygen

Hyperbaric oxygenation may be a useful adjunct to both hydroxocobalamin and nitrite therapies (described in the next section). However, it needs to be studied further before being definitively recommended. Hyperbaric oxygen may work by competitively displacing cyanide from cytochrome oxidase.[12] In the case of a mixed gas inhalation, carbon monoxide may be effectively displaced from hemoglobin and allow higher levels of nitrite to be used.

Hyperbaric oxygen therapy should not be used to replace the antidote treatments or to delay antidote treatment in most cases. Hyperbaric oxygen therapy is unlikely to be available in the event of a terrorist attack with cyanide, since most chambers have the capacity for a few patients at the maximum.[15]

Specific Therapies

Several antidotes are available for the treatment of cyanide intoxication. This includes the nitrites, sodium thiosulfate, and hydroxocobalamin, all of which are approved for use in the United States. I recommend treating moderate to severe cases of cyanide poisoning with antidotes. However, it should be noted that many cases of cyanide intoxication recover without antidotal therapy.[16–18]

Nitrites and Thiosulfate

Cyanide has a strong affinity for the Fe^{3+} in methemoglobin. Amyl nitrite and sodium nitrite are therefore administered to convert hemoglobin (which contains ferrous iron, Fe^{2+}) to methemoglobin (with its Fe^{3+}). The methemoglobin combines with the cyanide, releasing the cytochrome oxidase and normalizing cellular oxygen metabolism.

The clinician must monitor blood pressure carefully when administering nitrites because they can cause significant orthostatic hypotension with the potential for shock and death. Nitrite-induced methemoglobinemia could also cause a potentially fatal reduction in oxygen-carrying capacity of the blood.

To complete the removal of cyanide from the body, sodium thiosulfate is administered. Thiosulfate reacts irreversibly with cyanide in a reaction catalyzed by rhodanese and produces thiocyanate, which is excreted through the kidneys in the urine.

Note that amyl nitrite is given via inhalation but that both sodium nitrite and sodium thiosulfate must be given intravenously. Early establishment of intravenous access is therefore paramount.

In 1972, Way et al. showed that nitrite increases the median lethal dose of potassium cyanide in mice from 11 mg/kg to 21 mg/kg. Adding thiosulfate leads to an increase in the median lethal dose to 52 mg/kg.[19]

Oxygen therapy is believed to maximize the therapeutic effects of nitrites and thiosulfate.

Hydroxocobalamin

Hydroxocobalamin has been used for decades to treat acute cyanide poisoning in Europe and was approved for use in France in 1996. The simple mechanism of action is that hydroxocobalamin binds cyanide and forms nontoxic cyanocobalamin, which is excreted in urine.

Hydroxocobalamin was recently approved in the United States for use as a component of the Cyanokit. Cyanokit (containing the drug hydroxocobalamin, intravenous tubing, and a sterile spike for reconstituting the drug product with saline) may be used in the United States and other countries for the treatment of known or suspected cyanide poisoning. In cyanide-poisoned adult dogs, the use of Cyanokit resulted in reduced whole-blood cyanide concentration by approximately 55% by the end of treatment. Survival was significantly improved compared with placebo. Because hydroxocobalamin does not interfere with oxygen-carrying capacity of blood, it may be a superior therapy compared to nitrites. This may be especially important in cases of possible carbon monoxide intoxication. It is believed that it takes at least 5 g of hydroxocobalamin administered intravenously over 10 minutes to neutralize a lethal dose of cyanide in adults.[20] It does not cause hypotension or methemoglobinemia and may therefore be reasonably given to victims before confirming cyanide exposure.

In a small retrospective study of 14 cyanide-intoxicated human patients, adverse events that may have been caused by hydroxocobalamin were reported in 8 patients (57%). Reported events included chromaturia (red urine [Figure 46-4; see color plate]; $n = 5$), pink-to-red skin discoloration ($n = 3$), increase in heart rate ($n = 1$), and elevated blood pressure ($n = 1$). In that same study, hydroxocobalamin (total dose 5 to 20 g) was given as first-line antidotal therapy beginning a mean of 3.1 hours (3.2 standard deviation, median 2.1 hours, range 0.3 to 12) after cyanide exposure. Seventy-one percent of patients survived.[21] The reddish, discolored urine may be confused with rhabdomyolysis or intravascular hemolysis, and it can interfere with glucose and bilirubin measurements.[22] Thiosulfate may also be given with hydroxocobalamin.

Age-related Considerations

For the same environmental concentration of cyanide, a child may receive larger doses than adults. This is because children have a greater lung surface area–to–body weight ratio and an increased minute volume–to–weight ratio.

When treating children, use a lower dose of sodium nitrite, 0.33 mL of the 10% solution per kilogram of body weight, to avoid lethal methemoglobin levels.

Chronic Effects in Survivors of Acute Exposure

A syndrome of delayed striatal degeneration with parkinsonism and dystonia is described in some survivors of acute cyanide intoxication. Acute cyanide poisoning affects the cerebral structures with the highest oxygen requirement, including the basal ganglia, the cerebral cortex, and the sensorimotor cortex. Magnetic resonance imaging is the method of choice for depicting the extent and structure of lesions in the cyanide-sensitive regions of the brain. Pseudolaminar necrosis of the cerebral cortex and hemorrhagic necrosis in the basal ganglia are characteristic chronic findings following acute cyanide intoxication.[23] This is similar to chronic effects found in survivors of acute carbon monoxide intoxication.

Chronic, Low-Level Exposures

Intake of cassava, which contains cyanogenetic glycosides, in the setting of protein–calorie malnutrition can cause neurodegenerative disorders such as tropical ataxic neuropathy,[24] which is a syndrome with sensory neuropathy, sensory gait ataxia, optic atrophy, and hearing loss. The upper motor neuron disease konzo may also be linked to thiocyanate exposure from bitter cassava roots.[25] (See also Chapter 53.)

CONCLUSION

Cyanide agents are lethal chemicals that impair and kill quickly. Cyanide is an important industrial chemical in the United States and abroad and is therefore readily available to terrorists. Moreover, it can be rapidly effective when released into enclosed spaces by terrorists. Cyanide inhibits cellular oxygen metabolism and energy production, killing a severely exposed individual in minutes. The central nervous system, because of high oxygen demand, is particularly sensitive to cyanide. The duration of effects is brief, and if exposure is not severe, an individual may recover quickly from inhaled cyanide when removed from the contaminated area. The three goals of cyanide management are to prevent further contamination, provide support, and remove cyanide from the cell with antidotes. Oxygen should always be administered to cyanide victims. Acceptable antidotes include a combination of amyl nitrite, sodium nitrite, and sodium thiosulfate. Another option is hydroxocobalamin with or without thiosulfate.

ACKNOWLEDGMENTS

Thanks to Roger Humphries, M.D., Associate Professor of Emergency Medicine at the University of Kentucky, for review and advice on this chapter.

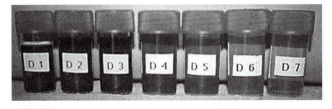

Figure 46-4. Discoloration of urine induced by a 10-g dose of hydroxocobalamin in a patient with normal renal function (patient 13). Urine samples from 7 days (D1–D7) are shown (see color plate). (Borron SW, Baud FJ, Mégarbane B, Bismuth C. Hydroxocobalamin for severe acute cyanide poisoning by ingestion or inhalation. *Am J Emerg Med.* 2007;25(5):551–558.)

REFERENCES

1. Lowry WT, Juarez L, Petty CS, Roberts B. Studies of toxic gas production during actual structural fires in the Dallas area. *J Forensic Sci.* 1985;30:59–72.
2. Alarie Y. The toxicity of smoke from polymeric materials during thermal decomposition. *Am Rev Pharm Toxicol.* 1985;25:325–347.

3. Anderson RA, Harland WA. Fire deaths in the Glasgow area: III. The role of hydrogen cyanide. *Med Sci Law*. 1982;22:35–37.

4. Levine MS, Radford MPH, Radford EP. Occupational exposures to cyanide in Baltimore fire fighters. *J Occup Med*. 1978;20:53–56.

5. Montgomery R, Reinhart CF, Terril JB. Comments on fire toxicity. *Comb Toxicol*. 1975;2:179–212.

6. Sadoff L, Fuchs J, Hollander J. Rapid death associated with Laetrile ingestion. *JAMA*. 1978;239:1532.

7. O'Brien B, Quigg C, Leong T. Severe cyanide toxicity from "vitamin supplements." *Eur J Emerg Med*. 2005;12(5):257–258.

8. Atkins D. Cyanide toxicity following nitroprusside-induced hypotension. *Can Anaesth Soc J*. 1977;24:651–660.

9. Vesey CJ, Cole PV, Simpson PJ. Cyanide and thiocyanate concentrations following sodium nitroprusside infusion in man. *Br J Anaesth*. 1976;48:651–659.

10. Cottrell JE, Casthely P, Brodie JD, Patel K, Klein A, Turndorf H. Prevention of nitroprusside-induced cyanide toxicity with hydroxocobalamin. *N Engl J Med*. 1978;298:809–811.

11. Meigs JW, Hughes JP. Acute carbon monoxide poisoning: an analysis of one hundred five cases. *AMA Arch Ind Hyg Occup Med*. 1952;6:344–356.

12. Bour H, Tutin M, Pasquier P. The central nervous system and carbon monoxide poisoning: I. Clinical data with reference to 20 fatal cases. *Prog Brain Res*. 1967;24:1–30.

13. Thompson N, Henry JA. Carbon monoxide poisoning: poisons unit experience over five years. *Hum Toxicol*. 1983;2:335–338.

14. Raphael JC, Elkharrat D, Jars-Guincestre MC, et al. Trial of normobaric and hyperbaric oxygen for acute carbon monoxide intoxication. *Lancet*. 1989;2:414–419.

15. Kindwall EP. Carbon monoxide and cyanide poisoning. In: Davis JC, Hunt TK, eds. *Hyperbaric Oxygen Therapy*. Bethesda, Md: Undersea Medical Society; 1977:177–190.

16. Graham DL, Laman D, Theodore J, Robin ED. Acute cyanide poisoning complicated by lactic acidosis and pulmonary edema. *Arch Intern Med*. 1977;137:1051–1055.

17. Brivet F, Delfraissy JF, Duche M, Bertrand P, Dormont J. Acute cyanide poisoning: recovery with non-specific supportive therapy. *Intensive Care Med*. 1983;9:33–35.

18. Saincher A, Swirsky N, Tenenbein M. Cyanide overdose: survival with fatal blood concentration without antidotal therapy. *J Emerg Med*. 1994;12:555–557.

19. Way JL, End E, Sheehy MH, et al. Effects of oxygen on cyanide intoxication: IV. Hyperbaric oxygen. *Toxicol Appl Pharmacol*. 1972;22:415–421.

20. Houeto P, Hoffman JR, Imbert M, Levillain P, Baud FJ. Relation of blood cyanide to plasma cyanocobalamin concentration after a fixed dose of hydroxocobalamin in cyanide poisoning. *Lancet*. 1995;346:605–608.

21. Borron SW, Baud FJ, Mégarbane B, Bismuth C. Hydroxocobalamin for severe acute cyanide poisoning by ingestion or inhalation. *Am J Emerg Med*. 2007;25(5):551–558.

22. Baud FJ. Cyanide: critical issues in diagnosis and treatment. *Hum Exp Toxicol*. 2007;26:191–201.

23. Rachinger J, Fellner FA, Stieglbauer K, Trenkler J. MR changes after acute cyanide intoxication. *Am J Neuroradiol*. 2002;23:1398–1401.

24. Osuntokun BO. Cassava diet, chronic cyanide intoxication and neuropathy in Nigerian Africans. *World Rev Nutr Diet*. 1981;36:141.

25. Spencer PS. Food toxins, AMPA receptors, and motor neuron diseases. *Drug Metab Rev*. 1999;31:561.

Neurotoxic Plants

Brent Furbee

INTRODUCTION

Each year, hundreds of thousands of exposures to toxic plants occur around the world. Most of these exposures are of minimal toxicity largely because they involve pediatric ingestions that are of low quantity. The more serious poisonings usually involve adults who have mistaken a plant for a food source or who have deliberately consumed it for its medicinal or toxic properties, such as hallucinogens or abortifacients.

A poor correlation exists between taxonomy and toxicity. Members of the same family of plants may have different toxic effects or, sometimes, no toxicity. Not infrequently, a single plant may contain several different toxins. In this discussion, plants are grouped by their toxins rather than on the basis of their taxonomy.

Plant identification is often a difficult. If a specimen is available, local nurseries may be of help in identification. Poison centers are usually a good starting point in the identification of plants and management of their ingestion. Most centers have botanical consultants and other resources that can assist in plant exposures. Few antidotes exist for plant exposures, and treatment is usually supportive.

ACONITINE

Members of the *Aconitum* genus grow throughout the world. Exposures are commonly associated with the overzealous consumption of herbal preparations containing aconitine. Although fatal poisonings have been reported, aconitine is still readily available at many nutrition or herbal medicine stores.

Plants

Aconitum exposures are primarily to *Aconitum napellus* (monkshood; Figure 47-1) and *Aconitum vulparia* (wolfsbane). Several species are also used in herbal preparations, including *Aconitum carmichaeli* ("chuanwu") and *Aconitum kusnezoffii* ("caowu").[1] The latter two appear to account for more fatalities than ingestion of monkshood. *Delphinium* species (larkspur) have similar toxicity.[2]

Location

A. napellus and *A. vulparia* grow in meadow areas of the mountainous areas from Arizona into Canada. *Aconitum* species are cultivated as perennial ornamentals. *Delphinium*

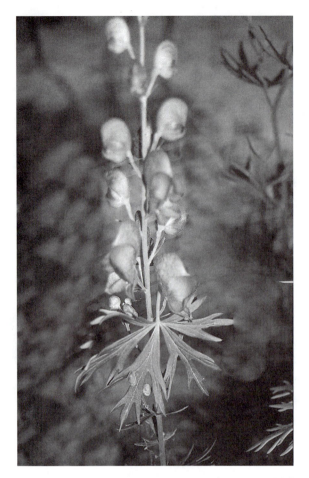

Figure 47-1. Aconitine. *Aconitum napellus* (see color plate).

species are found throughout the United States and Canada, where they are also grown as ornamentals.

Description

Aconitum plants grow to 3 to 4 feet. The leaves are palmately divided into five lobes, which are divided into narrow segments. Flowers, which are dark blue to purple or purple and white, are composed of five petal-like sepals, one of which covers the top of the flower. The latter forms a hoodlike structure over the flower, hence the name. These plants, although perennial, dry up and appear dead soon after the onset of summer heat.

Toxic Parts

All parts of *Aconitum* plants are toxic, with toxicity greatest in roots and decreasing through flowers, through leaves, and to the lowest toxicity in stems.[3]

Mechanism of Toxicity

Like grayanotoxins and veratrum alkaloids, aconitine effects its toxicity through action on sodium channels. Aconitine appears to increase sodium entry into muscle, nerve, baroreceptors, and Purkinje fibers to produce a positive inotropic effect, enhanced vagal tone, neurotoxicity, and increased automaticity and torsade de pointes.[4] During late repolarization of the Purkinje fiber (late phase 4), aconitine attaches to a limited number of the sodium channels and increases Na^+ influx,[5-7] causing late (or delayed) afterdepolarizations and increased automaticity (e.g., premature ventricular beats). However, aconitine-induced sodium accumulation may also lead to early afterdepolarization during late phase 2 or early phase 3 of the action potential. These early afterdepolarizations produce lengthening of the QT interval and are thought to explain reports of torsade de pointes in patients poisoned with aconitine.[5,7-9] Bifascicular ventricular tachycardia, a dysrhythmia most often associated with digitalis toxicity, has also be reported in patients poisoned with aconitine.[10]

Clinical Presentation

Most case reports of aconitine poisoning have come from ingestion of herbs containing aconitine.[1,11] Following exposure, onset of symptoms has been reported in one series of cases to occur between 3 minutes to 2 hours, with a median of 30 minutes.[9] Symptoms may persist for 30 hours.[12] Neurological complaints include initial visual impairment, dizziness, limb paresthesias, weakness,[13] and ataxia.[3] Coma may follow. Chest discomfort, dyspnea, tachycardia, and diaphoresis may also occur.[13] Hyperglycemia, hypokalemia, bradycardia (with hypotension), atrial and nodal ectopic beats, supraventricular tachycardia, bundle branch block, intermittent bigeminy, ventricular tachycardia, ventricular fibrillation, and asystole have been reported.[3,5,13,14] Death is usually due to ventricular arrhythmia.[13,15] Ingestion of delphinium root has also resulted in ventricular dysrhythmias and cardiac arrest.[2,13,15]

Laboratory Studies

The presence of aconitine has been demonstrated by high-performance liquid chromatography at autopsy.[15]

Management

Neurological complaints related to aconitine require supportive care. The paramount concern is management of lethal arrhythmias. Ventricular tachycardia has failed to respond to several antiarrhythmic agents, including lidocaine, disopyramide, bretylium, amiodarone, potassium, and phenytoin. Tai et al. reported successful use of flecainide following lidocaine failure in a single case.[10] Yeih et al. reported successful use of amiodarone following lidocaine failure in a case report.[16] No antiarrhythmic agents have demonstrated clear superiority. In animal studies, Adaniya et al. demonstrated the ability of magnesium to suppress early afterdepolarizations and polymorphic ventricular tachycardia.[5] It should be noted that while some authors[17] differentiate between polymorphic ventricular tachycardia and torsade de pointes, Adaniya et al. seem to use the two terms interchangeably.[5]

ANTHRACENONES

Toxicity of *Karwinskia humboldtiana* was first reported by Clavijero in 1769.[5a] In 1917, Castillo-Najera reported poisoning in 106 soldiers of whom 20% died. [5b] Autopsies indicated peripheral nerve damage. Since that time, the consumption of berries of tullidora also known as coyotillo has been reported to cause paralysis. More recently, with ventilatory support, death occurs considerably less often. The plant is also toxic to sheep, goats, hogs, birds, and cattle.[18]

Plants

Toxic exposure of *Karwinskia* species (Figure 47-2) most often involves *K. humboldtiana* and less often involves *Karwinskia mollis*, *Karwinskia parvifolia*, *Karwinskia johnstonii*, *Karwinskia rzedowskii*, and others.

Location

Karwinskia species is found throughout Mexico, in the southern United States (primarily southwest Texas and southern California), in Central America, in Caribbean countries, and in northern Columbia. In Mexico, plants are found in areas of scrub vegetation at altitudes under 1000 meters above sea level with a dry climate.[19]

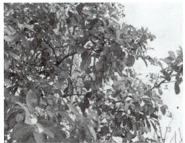 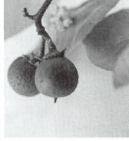

Figure 47-2. Anthracenones. *Karwinskia* species.

Description

Karwinskia species have several common names, among which coyotillo and tullidora are the most used. It is an evergreen shrub growing from 3 to 21 feet in height. It has deeply veined, oblong, smooth edged, dark green leaves up to 7 inches long. The leaves have an opposite attachment to the stem. The fruit is a small berry that is green to red to black (mature) and about 1 centimeter in diameter.

Toxic Parts

Highest concentration of *Karwinskia* toxin is in the seeds of the berry. The fruit is most toxic when unripe.

Mechanism of Toxicity

Several toxins classified as anthracenones have been identified. T-544 is thought to be the cause of paralysis. T-496 causes diarrhea, and T-514 causes hepatic and pulmonary damage in animal models.[20] Axonal swelling has been observed in humans and is thought to be secondary to Schwann cell injury.[21] Wheeler and Camp described uncoupling of oxidative phosphorylation as a result of application of *Karwinskia* extracts.[22] Thus, decreasing adenosine triphosphate production[23] and the formation of reactive oxygen species appear to be responsible for the cellular damage.

Clinical Presentation

Ingestion of multiple *Karwinskia* berries may initially produce vomiting and diarrhea in some cases. Onset of a distal, ascending flaccid paralysis begins within 2 to 3 weeks and may progress to bulbar paralysis that can be fatal in the absence of respiratory support. Symptoms are symmetrical with absent tendon reflexes. Surviving patients usually have full recovery if complications such as anoxia do not occur. The latency period between ingestion and onset of symptoms makes this a difficult diagnosis that is compounded because it occurs most often in children. Differential diagnosis includes Guillain-Barré syndrome and poliomyelitis.[18,24] Pulmonary hemorrhage and renal failure may occur. About 40 cases are reported each year in Mexico, with up to five fatalities annually.[24]

Laboratory Studies

Bermudez et al. described the use of thin-layer chromatography to identify the *Karwinskia* toxins in the blood of patients with acute flaccid paralysis.[24a] Electromyography demonstrates a peripheral polyneuropathy with segmental demyelinization. Cerebrospinal fluid is normal. Sural nerve biopsy has demonstrated demyelinization without inflammatory infiltrate or axonal degeneration.

Management

Supportive care and physical rehabilitation are the only therapies for anthracenone exposure. With ventilatory support, patients can survive, and most recover within a year. A few patients are left with residual effects.

ANTICHOLINERGICS

Numerous plants and mushrooms exhibit anticholinergic properties. The best known of these are the members of the Solanaceae family. Of the anticholinergic plants, the genera *Atropa*, *Datura*, and *Hyoscyamus* produce hyoscyamine (atropine). Other members of this group produce scopolamine. The members of both groups are listed here, but for this discussion *Datura* species are the primary focus because they account for more hospitalizations than the other plants.

The first recorded *Datura* poisoning occurred in 1676 during the Bacon Rebellion, when soldiers under Captain John Smith made a salad of *Datura stramonium* leaves and began to hallucinate. The name "Jamestown weed" was given to this plant, and its name has been corrupted over the years to "Jimson weed."

Plants

Anticholinergic properties are found in *Atropa belladonna* (deadly nightshade), *Datura meteloides* (sacred datura; Figure 47-3), *Datura stramonium* (Jimson weed), *Datura arborea* (trumpet lily), *Datura candida*, *Datura suaveolens* (angel trumpet), other *Datura* species, *Hyoscyamus niger* (henbane), *Lycium barbarum* (matrimony vine), and *Mandragora officinarum* (mandrake).

Location

D. meteloides is a perennial southwestern plant that grows well in desert areas. *D. stramonium* grows as an annual on recently disturbed ground throughout the United States. It is often found in soybean fields.

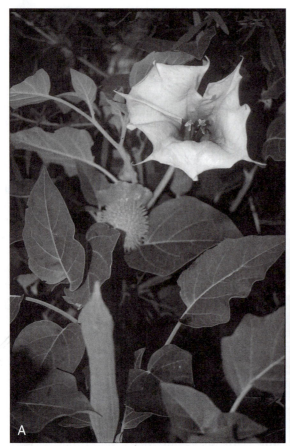

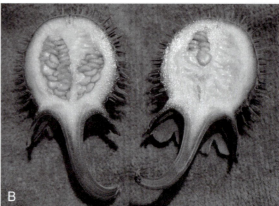

Figure 47-3. Anticholinergics. *(A) Datura meteloides* (see color plate). *(B) Datura metalloids* seed pod (see color plate).

Description

D. meteloides is a stout bushy plant with thick stems. The large leaves are oval with wavy edges. The foliage has a pungent odor. Seeds are found in spiney pods about 1.5 inches long. The flowers are 6 to 8 inches long and white with purple edges. *D. stramonium* is similar to *D. meteloides;* Jimson weed has a dark purple stem and is a taller plant.

Toxic Parts

The entire *Datura* plant is toxic. The flowers, fruits, and seeds are especially toxic.

Mechanism of Toxicity

The members of the genus *Datura* contain varying amounts of hyoscyamine and scopolamine. Young plants tend to contain mostly scopolamine, but as they mature, hyoscyamine predominates. The toxicity of these compounds results from competitive blockade of acetylcholine at peripheral and central muscarinic receptors.

Clinical Presentation

Onset of anticholinergic symptoms is usually within 30 to 60 minutes of ingestion and may last for 24 to 48 hours. Both central and peripheral syndromes may be seen. Levy described 27 cases in which every patient had altered mental status and mydriasis.[25]

Central Anticholinergic Syndrome

Central nervous system (CNS) excitation often manifests as agitation and hallucinations. CNS depression and coma may follow. Hallucinations are generally visual but may be auditory. Speech has a characteristic mumbling quality and is often incomprehensible. Patients often answer questions with appropriate one-word answers, but if prompted (and able) to speak in sentences, the fragmented speech pattern becomes obvious. Undressing behavior is not uncommon.

Peripheral Anticholinergic Syndrome

Tachycardia and mydriasis are common findings of peripheral anticholinergic syndrome. Flushed skin may be more difficult to detect. Fever is occasionally noted. Bowel sounds may be depressed or absent but are usually persist. Bladder motility may be decreased as well. Although dry mucous membranes may be associated with hyperventilation, dry axillae, in association with the other signs, indicate anticholinergic poisoning and help distinguish it from increased adrenergic activity.

Datura accounts for many admissions to critical care units each year. Although children are occasionally poisoned, most exposure occurs in patients who have ingested seeds or a tea brewed from the seeds in an attempt to induce hallucinations. Death is rare and may occur more as the result of impaired judgment than direct toxicity. A few death reports do seem to indicate potentially fatal toxicity in high-dose exposures.[26,27] Petechial hemorrhages of the endocardium and hyperemia and edema of the lungs were reported in both cases.

Laboratory Studies

Atropine may be detected by radioimmunoassay, gas chromatography–mass spectrometry, thin-layer chromatography,[28] and liquid chromatography. Scopolamine has been analyzed in plasma and urine by radioreceptor assay and gas chromatography–mass spectrometry.[29]

Management

Anticholinergic decontamination is best accomplished with the administration of activated charcoal if the ingestion has occurred within the previous 2 hours. The recommended dose of activated charcoal is 0.5 to 1g/kg in children or 25 to 100g in adults. Tachycardia rarely requires treatment. Patients should be monitored for urine output and bladder distention. A nasogastric tube should be inserted in patients with decreased gut motility. Hypotension should be treated with intravenous isotonic fluids. Dopamine may be used if hypotension persists after the patient's intravascular volume has been restored, but this is unusual. The combination of impaired diaphoresis with agitation may lead to severe hyperthermia, which must be aggressively treated with sedation or paralysis and active cooling. Rhabdomyolysis is common and explains renal failure and other complications seen in severe *Datura* toxicity. Because of their anticholinergic activity, phenothiazines and diphenhydramine should be avoided. Haloperidol does not appear to be effective for resolution of central anticholinergic effects.[30] Benzodiazepines are, on the other hand, effective in the treatment of agitation.

Several authors have advocated the use of intravenous physostigmine for patients with central anticholinergic effects.[25,30,31] Physostigmine inhibits acetylcholinesterase, thus increasing the amount of acetylcholine available to the muscarinic receptors. While benzodiazepines may be used to sedate agitated patients, physostigmine may restore the patient's level of consciousness to its baseline. It is particularly helpful in differentiating anticholinergic poisoning from other causes of altered mental status. It should not be used unless peripheral anticholinergic signs accompany a clinical picture of central anticholinergic poisoning. Seizure activity, bradycardia, heart blocks, and asystole have followed use of physostigmine.[32,33] Potential benefit should be weighed against risk before use.

CARDIAC GLYCOSIDES

The medicinal properties of the cardiac glycosides were known to the ancient Egyptians, as well as the Romans, who used it as an emetic, heart tonic, and diuretic.[34] In 1785, William Withering published *An Account of the Foxglove and Some of Its Medical Uses: With Practical Remarks on Dropsy and Other Diseases,* thus popularizing its use.[34a] In 1890, Sir Thomas Fraser introduced *Strophanthus* and its digitalis-like effects. Worldwide, these plants have been used as abortifacients; in the treatment of leprosy, venereal disease, and malaria; and as a suicide agent.[35] More than 200 naturally occurring cardiac glycosides have been identified to date. *Digitalis* species ingestion is seldom reported. *Convallaria majalis* (lily of the valley) exposures are associated with minimal morbidity and, in a recent review of 10 years of data from regional poison centers, have had no associated mortality.[36] Of the many plants containing cardiac glycosides, *Nerium oleander* is responsible for the greatest number of toxic exposures each year.[37]

Plants

Plants known to contain cardiac glycosides include *Digitalis purpurea, Digitalis lanata* (foxglove; Figure 47-4A), *Nerium oleander* (oleander; Figure 47-4B), *Strophanthus gratus* (ouabain), *Thevetia peruviana* species (yellow oleander); *Convallaria majalis* (lily of the valley), *Urginea maritima,* and *Urginea indica* (squill). Other plants thought to contain cardiac glycosides are *Asclepias* (milkweed), *Calotropis* (crown flower),[38] *Euonymus europaeus* (spindle tree), *Cheiranthus* and *Erysimum* (wall flower), and *Hellaborus niger* (henbane).

Toxic Parts

All parts of plants containing cardiac glycosides are toxic. Seeds are said to contain more glycoside than other parts of the plant.

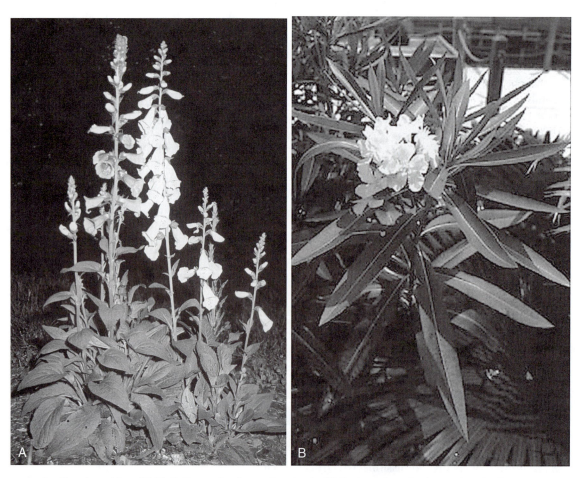

Figure 47-4. Cardiac glycosides. *(A) Digitalis* species (see color plate). *(B) Nerium oleander* (see color plate).

Location

Oleander is a native of the Mediterranean and Asia but grows in tropical and subtropical areas around the world. It is grown as an ornamental across the southern part of the United States. It does not tolerate freezing temperatures. *Digitalis spp.* and *Convallaria majalis* may be found throughout North America.

Description

N. oleander can grow to 30 feet. The leaves are leathery and have a lanceolate shape. They may be six or more inches long in mature plants. *Thevia peruviana* is a small tree with similarly shaped but smaller leaves. Its flowers are yellow-orange. All parts of these plants, including the seeds, are toxic.

Mechanism of Toxicity

The glycoside toxin attaches to the α subunit of the Na$^+$/K$^+$-ATPase pump to inhibit its action. Because this pump exchanges intracellular sodium ions for extracellular potassium ions, inhibition leads to an overall increase in intracellular sodium ions. Rises in intracellular sodium concentration result in secondary rises in intracellular calcium levels, explaining the positive inotropic effect of cardiac glycosides. In toxic amounts, the rises in intracellular sodium and calcium depolarize the cell following repolarization to cause late afterdepolarizations and increased automaticity typical of cardiac glycoside poisoning. Depolarization of baroreceptors innervated by the ninth cranial nerve triggers afferent reflexes, which increase vagal tone and produce bradycardia and heart blocks.[39] Severe poisoning results in hyperkalemia as the ability to pump potassium into the muscle is curtailed.

Neurotoxicity is also thought to occur as a result of Na$^+$/K$^+$-ATPase pump inhibition. Marx et al.[39a] proposed that this occurred in both neurons and astrocytes. While this would directly affect impulse transmission of neurons, the effect on astrocytes might also adversely affect neuronal activity. A major function of the astrocyte is to take up glutamate and convert it to glutamine, which in turn, is converted to both glutamate and γ-aminobutyric acid (GABA). Inhibition of the glutamate transporter GLT-1 would lead to an increase of the excitatory neurotransmitter, glutamate, and a decrease in the inhibitory GABA. Excitotoxicity would occur, eventually leading to neuronal and astrocyte death.[40] Evidence also indicates that serotonergic transmission may play a role.[41] It should be noted that significant interspecies variation occurs in physiological response to cardiac glycosides. Rodents, for example, tend to be resistant to cardiac effects, while neurotoxicity is more apparent than in humans. Care should be taken in extrapolating from rodent studies to humans.[42,43]

Clinical Presentation

Gastrointestinal irritation is common with ingestion of cardiac glycosides, particularly *N. oleander* or *T. peruviana*. The latter was studied as a potential antiarrhythmic agent in the 1930s but was not marketed because it caused more gastrointestinal irritation than digitalis.[44] Saravanapavananthan et al. reviewed 170 cases of *T. peruviana* ingestion and found that vomiting was the most common presenting complaint (68.2%).[45] Other symptoms are shown in Table 1.

Electrocardiographic effects have occurred in up to 61.8% of patients in one study.[45] They include, in order of frequency, atrioventricular block, bradycardia, T wave changes, ST depression, ventricular ectopy, and atrial ectopy. PR prolongation, QT shortening, and P or T wave flattening may also occur.[46] Hyperkalemia is reported in more serious acute poisonings.[46–48] Normal or decreased serum potassium levels are commonly found in chronic poisoning if renal function is normal.

Neurological affects have occurred with plant ingestions and are similar to those associated with therapeutic use of digitalis. Visual abnormalities include scotomas, hazy vision, flickering halos, and yellow–green–tinted vision (chromatopsia).[49,50] Nonspecific symptoms such as malaise, fatigue, drowsiness, restlessness, and agitation have all been reported.[51] While vague symptoms occur at lower doses, more severe symptoms are often associated with cardiotoxicity. CNS depression may occur as a direct effect of the toxin[48] but is often associated with bradycardia and hypotension. Death has been reported.[45,46]

Although rare, neuropsychiatric changes are also observed. They are associated with high-dose exposures. Delirium, hallucinations, and psychosis have been reported and may occur early.[51–53] The administration of digoxin immune Fab therapy has been reported to result in rapid reversal.[53]

Table 1: Relative Frequency of Signs and Symptoms Associated with Oleander Poisoning	
Symptom	**Percentage (%)**
Dizziness	35.9
Diarrhea	38.0
Abdominal pain	5.9
Pain or numbness in tongue, throat, lips	4.1
No symptoms	12.9

Laboratory Studies

Osterloh et al. described cross-reactivity of oleander glycosides on radioimmunoassay for digoxin.[47] The test may serve as confirmation of the presence of cardiac glycosides; however, clinical symptoms are more indicative of toxicity. Postmortem serum concentrations are known to increase and do not predict the premortem levels.[46]

Management

In general, management of cardiac glycoside toxicity from plants is the same as for digitalis toxicity. Airway control and other basic life support measures are the first concern. Gastric decontamination with activated charcoal should follow those measures. The recommended dose of activated charcoal is 0.5 to 1g/kg in children or 25 to 100g in adults. Hyperkalemia may be treated with such agents as insulin and dextrose infusions or sodium bicarbonate infusion. Ventricular tachyarrhythmias may be managed with lidocaine, and bradyrhythmias may respond to atropine or ventricular pacing. Large doses of Fab-antidigoxin antibodies correct both rhythm and hyperkalemia in dogs poisoned by oleander.[54] Shumaik et al. reported the use of digoxin-specific Fab fragments in the treatment of a 37-year-old man who had ingested *N. oleander* leaves.[55] Other reports of their use have supported those findings.[48,56]

CICUTOXIN

The first reports of toxic effects from *Cicuta* species occurred in 1697. Stockbridge reported the first case of poisoning in the United States in 1814.[57] In a review of deaths reported to poison centers between 1986 and 1996, Krenzelok et al. found reports of 19 deaths. Of these, *Cicuta* species accounted for more deaths than did any other plant.[58] Exposure to *Cicuta* and *Oenanthe* species may be accidental, as in most pediatric cases, but more commonly, the fatal cases involve misidentification of the plant as a foodstuff or as a hallucinogen.

Plants

Cicutoxin is found in *Cicuta maculata* (water hemlock) and *Cicuta douglasii* (western water hemlock; Figure 47-5). The related oenanthotoxin is found in *Oenanthe crocata* (hemlock water dropwort).

Location

Water hemlock grows in the eastern half of the United States and Canada. *C. douglasii* grows in the western United States. *O. crocata* is considered to be a European plant but is reported to have been transplanted into the Washington, DC, area.[59] These plants are found in or immediately adjacent to water. They are most often

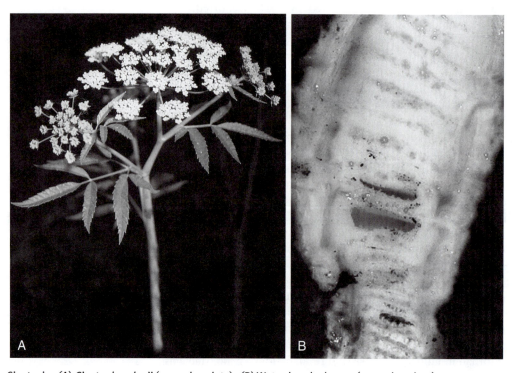

Figure 47-5. Cicutoxin. *(A) Cicuta douglasii* (see color plate). *(B)* Water hemlock root (see color plate).

encountered in lakes or streams but may be found in marshy areas.

Description

Plants of the *Cicuta* and *Oenanthe* species are generally found growing out of the water or close enough for their roots to make contact with the water. Both varieties form a low-growing bush that may be 3 to 4 feet tall. Stems are hollow and have a carrot-like odor. Flowers, which occur during the summer months, are small and white in flat-topped clusters or umbels. Leaves are compound and toothed. Both plant species have thick whitish roots that, when sliced sagittally, possess transverse stripes. The stripes may form small chambers late in the growing season. The roots have been mistaken for wild carrots. They are 5 to 6 inches long and white, and when cut they have a strong carrot-like odor. Although the roots are characterized as having transverse chambers, they are often solid. Roots of *Oenanthe* species are also said to secrete a yellowish sap when cross sectioned.[60] Water hemlock bears a striking resemblance to other umbellifores, which are nontoxic. *Heracleum lanatum* (cow parsnip) and *Daucus carota* (Queen Anne's lace) may be distinguished by their location and physical differences in the stem. Mistaking a toxic member of the Apiaceae family for a nontoxic one has been a fatal error for numerous foragers over the years.[61–64] Almost yearly, one to two deaths are reported to poison centers in the United States due to the ingestion of these plants.

Toxic Parts

All parts of plants of the *Cicuta* and *Oenanthe* species are toxic, especially the roots.

Mechanism of Toxicity

Although nausea and vomiting are considered to be the most consistent findings, seizure activity followed by cardiac arrest is the common sequence in fatal cicutoxin or oenanthotoxin exposures.[65] An exact mechanism for the proconvulsant activity of cicutoxin has not been determined. Starreveld and Hope suggested that seizure activity might be due to cholinergic overstimulation of the reticular formation or basal ganglia.[66] Nelson et al. performed a series of experiments in mice to explore the efficacy of anticholinergic agents in the prevention of cicutoxin-induced seizures. They found that anticholinergic agents failed to protect the animals while pretreatment with cholinergic agents did not appear to lower the seizure threshold.[67]

By 1979, a more appealing theory for cicutoxin's proconvulsant activity had arisen. Carlton et al. suggested that cicutoxin is structurally similar to picrotoxin, an indirect antagonist at GABA$_A$ receptors.[68] GABA receptors serve as ion channels to allow the passage of chloride ions into the neuron. This hyperpolarizes the neuron moving it away from its threshold for firing. Many anticonvulsants such as the benzodiazepines and barbiturates act as indirect agonists at the GABA receptor. By preventing the action of GABA, picrotoxin hyperpolarizes the neuron, moving it closer to its threshold for firing. If cicutoxin acts on the GABA receptor at the picrotoxin site, seizure activity would be expected as it is with picrotoxin. This would also be consistent with Nelson's findings that seizures were better controlled in animals treated with diazepam or barbiturates than with other agents.[67,69]

Clinical Presentation

Case reports of *Cicuta* species[61,65,66,70–72] and *Oenanthe* species[60,73–76] ingestions are similar in presentation. Ingestion is followed by nausea, vomiting, and diaphoresis. While these signs and symptoms have led some authors to speculate about increased cholinergic activity as the mechanism for seizure activity,[66] the frequent reports of mydriasis[70–72] detract from this theory. The initial convulsion often occurs within the first hour. Repeated convulsions, with intermittent lethargy, ensue for the next several hours. Fatalities usually occur within about 10 hours and are almost invariably associated with repeated seizure activity. *O. crocata* poisoning has been estimated to be 70% fatal in one small series.[75]

Rhabdomyolysis and renal failure have been reported.[68] Although some toxins may cause rhabdomyolysis directly, the presence of prolonged seizure activity that was reported in this patient may well be the etiology.

Laboratory Studies

Although clinically useful means of determining cicutoxin or oenanthotoxin are not available, methods of identification are described by King et al. for the latter.[74] These methods included ultraviolet absorption, thin-layer chromatography, high-performance liquid chromatography, and mass spectrometry, which may be useful for later confirmation of exposure.

Management

Asymptomatic patients should be given activated charcoal and observed for 4 hours after ingestion. If no cicutoxin or oenanthotoxin symptoms occur, they may be released. The recommended dose of activated charcoal is 0.5 to 1g/kg in children or 25 to 100g in adults. This should be given orally or through a nasogastric tube. Activated charcoal should not be given to a comatose patient until the patient's airway is protected.

Symptomatic patients often arrive after seizures have occurred. The patient's airway should be secured first. Diazepam or phenobarbital are most appropriate for seizure control and should be used aggressively. Phenytoin has no clear role in management of cicutoxin-induced seizures. Because of vomiting and, occasionally, diarrhea, fluid replacement is often required. Creatine phosphokinase should be monitored because of the possibility of rhabdomyolysis. In addition to maintaining urine output, urine alkalinization may be beneficial patients with rhabdomyolysis.[77] Hemodialysis plus charcoal hemoperfusion has been performed in one case[36]; however, clearance of cicutoxin was not measured and the favorable outcome is consistent with many of the cases managed without extracorporeal elimination.[71] At this time, hemodialysis or hemoperfusion have not been shown to be beneficial. Seizure control and supportive care are the most effective therapies.

GRAYANOTOXINS

Rhododendrons and azaleas were introduced into Europe from Asia in the mid-1700s to early 1800s. Both are parts of the 500 to 1000 natural species with numerous hybrids. Exact species identification can be difficult. The toxic components of this genus vary, and their presence in a given plant is difficult to predict. Although ingestion of leaves, flowers, or nectar or use of the leaves in the production of tea produces toxicity, most poisonings result from consuming honey made from nectar collected from these plants. Honey poisonings are less common today because honey from several sources is combined before marketing. The earliest description of poisoning by these plants appears in the anabasis, a description of the unsuccessful military expedition of Cyrus the Younger to overthrow Artaxerxes II (401 to 400 BC). The following is an account of the incident that took place in what is now northeastern Turkey on the coast of the Black Sea:

> The number of bee hives was extraordinary, and all of the soldiers that ate of the honey combs lost their senses, vomited, and were affected with purging, and none of them was able to stand upright; such as had eaten only a little were like men greatly intoxicated, and such as had eaten much were like mad men and some like persons at the point of death. They lay upon the ground, in consequence, in great numbers, as if there had been a defeat; and there was general dejection. The next day, no one of them was found dead; and they recovered their senses about the same hour they had lost them on the preceding day.

Several other accounts of the toxicity of "mad honey" are available.[78]

Plants

Grayanotoxins are found in *Rhododendron* species (rhododendrons, azaleas; Figure 47-6), *Kalmia angustifolia* (sheep laurel), *Kalmia latifolia* (mountain laurel), and *Pieris* species *(Andromeda)*. Grayanotoxin I may also be found in honey made from the nectar of these plants.

Location

Native to the temperate parts of the world, rhododendrons are grown widely as ornamentals. *Rhododendron occidentale*, *Rhododendron macrophyllum*, and *Rhododendron albiflorum* are of special interest on the West Coast in the production of honey. Reports of contaminated honey have also occurred in the eastern United States, where rhododendrons as well as *K. latifolia* and *K. angustifolia* may serve as a source of grayanotoxin.

Description

Rhododendron leaves are evergreen, oblong, and leathery and have a smooth margin. They appear in whorls about the branch. Because of the many species, the leaf size is variable but generally ranges from 1 to 5 inches. The flowers are white to pink (rhododendrons) and white, pink, magenta, crimson, or orange (azaleas).

Toxic Parts

The entire rhododendron plant is toxic.

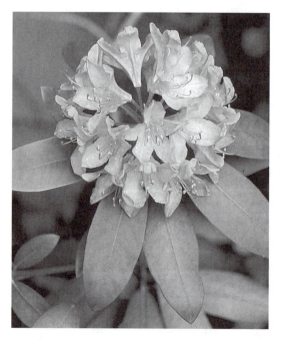

Figure 47-6. Grayanotoxins. *Rhododendron* species (see color plate).

Mechanism of Toxicity

In 1955, it was discovered that the members of the Ericaceae family contained structurally similar compounds that were responsible for their toxicity. These compounds, which were formerly known as andromedotoxin, acetylandromedol, and rhodotoxin, are now termed grayanotoxin I.[79] Grayanotoxin II and III are toxic derivatives of grayanotoxin I. Animal studies initially indicated that these toxins were capable of producing respiratory depression, bradycardia, hypotension, and seizure activity.[80] Subsequent studies in squid axons have shown that grayanotoxin I acts by attaching to the sodium channels of cell membranes and changing both open and closed channels to a modified open state. This increases sodium conductance dramatically and leads to cellular depolarization.[81,82] It appears that a single molecule of grayanotoxin is sufficient to activate a sodium channel.[83] This effect is thought to explain, in part, the CNS and cardiac manifestations of grayanotoxin poisoning. Masutani et al. noted in their study of grayanotoxin effects on frog skeletal muscle that grayanotoxin appears to contain four hydroxyl groups essential for its biological activity. These are also present in veratridine (false and white hellebore), batrachotoxin (poison dart frog), and aconitine (monkshood).[84]

The increases in intracellular sodium concentrations in the heart, baroreceptor cells, and brain cells mimic the effects of cardiac glycosides to produce increased automaticity, enhanced vagal tone (heart blocks, bradyrhythmias, etc.), and CNS changes. Because Na+/K+-ATPase is not inhibited, hyperkalemia is notably absent.

Clinical Presentation

While most grayanotoxin exposures are of little consequence,[85] serious cardiotoxicity has been reported. Vomiting, loss of consciousness, and seizure were observed in a 27-year-old female who had ingested 75 mL of honey she had purchased in Turkey. She was hypotensive and bradycardic. Her only laboratory abnormality was a mild leukocytosis. Dysrhythmias included sinus node arrest, atrioventricular-escape beats, second-degree atrioventricular block, and intraventricular conduction block. The patient recovered after insertion of a cardiac pacemaker.[86]

Laboratory Studies

Thin-layer chromatography has been used to identify grayanotoxin compounds.[87]

Management

Initial grayanotoxin management should include the administration of activated charcoal if the ingestion has occurred within the last 2 hours. The recommended dose of activated charcoal is 0.5 to 1g/kg in children or 25 to 100g in adults. Supportive care is usually sufficient for management. Significant bradycardia may be treated with atropine or cardiac pacemaker. Although experimental agents such as tetrodotoxin[88] have been used to reverse the effects of grayanotoxin I, no clinically available antidote exists. Lidocaine or other sodium channel–blocking antiarrhythmics (group I) would seem appropriate for ventricular arrhythmias.

LATHYRISM

As far back as Hippocrates, the toxicity of a diet of *Lathyrus sativus* was known to cause illness in animals and people. In fact, in the early 1800s, Francisco Goya painted *Gracias a la Almorta (Thanks to the Grasspea)* depicting a woman dispensing bowls of the legumes to the people surrounding her. As has occurred over the years, war had produced a need for alternative sources of cereals and flour. While intermittent ingestion of *Lathyrus* species did not cause illness, the need for frequent consumption resulted in two forms of illness, neurolathyrism and osteolathyrism. In 1942, 1200 Romanian Jewish males were interred in a German forced-labor camp where they received a diet of approximately 400 grams of grass peas a day. By December of that year, 800 of the inmates were showing signs of spastic paraparesis.[89] Seyle is credited for coining the terms neurolathyrism to describe the disorder of the nervous system and osteolathyrism to denote the connective tissues.[90] In the mid-1950s, β-aminopropionitrile had been identified as the toxic component of *Lathyrus odoratus* causing bone lesions and aneurysms in animals. In 1964, Rao et al. reported the isolation of β-N-oxalyl-L-α,β-diaminopropionic acid, also known as β-oxalyamino-L-alanine (L-BOAA). In the last 50 years, most cases have been found in Bangladesh, India, China, Chile, Ethiopia, and Nepal.[89,91]

Plants

Lathyrism primarily results from *L. sativus* exposure (Figure 47-7); however, other implicated species include *Lathyrus cicera, Lathyrus ochrus,* and *Lathyrus clymenum. Lathyrus odoratus* (sweet pea), a common ornamental, has been reported to cause osteolathyrism.

Location

While the *Lathyrus* genus may grow worldwide, cases of lathyrism are usually confined to Bangladesh, India, China, Chile, Ethiopia, and Nepal. There are 60 species of *Lathyrus*. In the United States, *L. sativus* grows in California, Oregon,

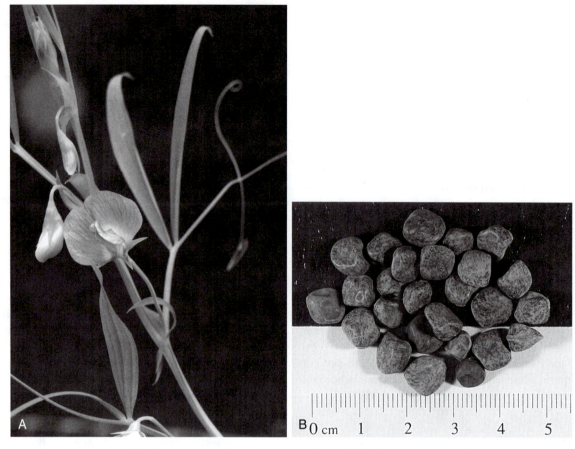

Figure 47-7. *Lathyrus* species *(A) Lathyrus sativus* flower (see color plate). *(B) Lathyrus sativus* seeds (see color plate).

Maryland, and Washington, DC. All states in the United States have some species of *Lathyrus*.[92]

Description

Lathyrus is a low-growing vine with small blue flowers producing approximately 1 centimeters long. It is drought resistant, which contributes to its use in times of famine.

Toxic Parts

Toxicity is primarily in the *Lathyrus* seeds. Of interest, efforts have been under way to produce a toxin-free cultivar of *L. sativus*.[93]

Mechanism of Toxicity

Lathyrism is a disease of the upper motor neurons. The primary injury is degeneration of the corticospinal tract. Swelling of the anterior horn cells and diminished Nissl substance with Hirano bodies were reported by Streifler et al.[94] At a cellular level, it appears that L-BOAA acts on non-*N*-methyl-d-aspartate receptors such as a-amino-3-hydroxy-5-methyl-isoxazole-4-propionic acid or kainic acid receptors. Both ion channel receptors allow the influx of sodium ions, leading to membrane depolarization. Calcium ion influx causes long-term changes in synaptic connections and leads to cellular degeneration. Initial changes may be reversible but become permanent if exposure is not stopped.

Clinical Presentation

Onset of lathyrism symptoms is often associated with heavy exertion. Leg weakness is the most common initial complaint. Neurological signs include increased deep tendon reflexes of the knee and ankle, sustained patellar clonus, bilateral extensor plantar reflexes, and spasticity of lower extremity adductors and extensors.[89] Drory et al. conducted a nearly 50-year follow-up study of eight randomly selected men from the Wapniarka forced-labor camp mentioned earlier.[95] The patients had spastic paraparesis and scissors gait requiring aid from one or two canes. Tendon reflexes in the lower extremities were increased, and bilateral extensor plantar reflexes were evident. Upper limbs were normal, and sensory deficits were absent. All nerve conduction velocities were normal. Electromyography studies showed abnormalities of the lower limbs in five of the eight patients, but the authors speculated that some changes may have been due to aging. They found widespread neurogenic pathology in the lower limb muscles of two of the eight patients.[95]

Spencer et al. studied lathyrism in a population of Ethiopians between 1988 and 1990. They estimated the prevalence to be from 1 to 75 per 10,000 population. Men were affected 2.6 times more often than women. Onset of symptoms occurred between 1 to 6 months of regular grass pea consumption.[89] Haque et al. found a prevalence rate of 14 per 10,000 in two northwestern districts of Bangladesh.[96]

Osteolathyrism presents as bone pain and deformity usually found as a separate population but occasionally found in those suffering from neurolathyrism.[97] The primary toxin appears to be β-aminopropionitrile. Dawson et al. found that semicarbazide, thiosemicarbazide, and aminoacetonitrile may also induce bony deformities with lysyl oxidase, a cofactor.[98] Cohn and Streifler described clinical signs including the absence of ossification centers of the ischial tuberosities and ileac crest, as well as bowing and thickening of the femoral shaft. Before that, osteolathyrism had been considered a separate entity from neurolathyrism.[99]

Laboratory Studies

Diagnostic studies of lathyrism are not clinically available. Diagnosis is based upon physical examination, history of exposure, and exclusion of other neuropathies.

Management

Beyond removal of exposure, treatment of lathyrism is supportive. Many patients improve after exposure ends, but most have some permanent sequelae, including permanent spastic paraplegia.

NICOTINE AND RELATED COMPOUNDS

The pyridine and piperidine alkaloids—nicotine, coniine, anabasine, cystisine, arecoline, lobeline, and many others—have a similar mechanism of action. Plants containing these alkaloids are widely distributed today but are thought to have originated in South America. *Nicotiana rustica*, which contains up to 18% nicotine, is thought to have been the first tobacco export from the New World. Much more potent than *Nicotiana tabacum* (0.5% to 9% nicotine), it is still smoked in Turkey and serves as a source for commercial nicotine production.[100] *N. tabacum* is planted throughout the southeastern United States as the source of cigar and cigarette

tobacco. Because the toxicity of smoked tobacco has been widely discussed elsewhere, only dermal and gastrointestinal absorption is addressed in this chapter. Small quantities of nicotine are also found in plants from the Solanaceae family, such as tomatoes, potatoes, and eggplant. This is of little consequence in terms of poisoning.[101,102] Several of the *Nicotiana* and *Lobelia* species are cultivated as flowering plants. Of the uncultivated plants in this group, *Nicotiana glauca* (tree tobacco) and *Conium maculatum* (poison hemlock) are the most common sources of poisoning.

Plants

Plants containing nicotine include *N. tabacum* (tobacco; Figure 47-8A), *N. glauca* (tree tobacco; Figure 47-8B), *Nicotiana trigonophylla* (desert tobacco), and *Nicotiana attenuata* (coyote tobacco). Coniine is primarily found in *C. maculatum* (poison hemlock; Figure 47-8C). *Aethusa cynaprium* (fool's parsley) contains coniine. Lobeline and lobelamine are found in *Lobelia inflata* (indian tobacco), *Lobelia cardinalis*, and other *Lobelia* species. *Laburnum anagyroides* (golden chain tree), *Sophora secundiflora* (mescal bush bean), *Sophora tomentosa* (necklace pod *Sophora*), and *Gymnocladus dioicus* (Kentucky coffee bean) all contain cystisine. *Areca catechu* (betel palm or betel nut) contains arecoline.[100]

Location

Conium maculatum

Poison hemlock grows throughout the United States and southern Canada except in desert regions. It is often found along roadways or railroads.

Nicotiana glauca

Tree tobacco is common from the southeast to the southwest of the United States, where it may grow to 10 feet or higher. It grows in the desert but is commonly found along ditches in those areas. Where water is more plentiful, it has a wider range.

Description

Conium maculatum

The biennial *C. maculatum* may reach 10 feet in height. The leaves are pinnately divided three to four times and have a fernlike appearance similar to parsley, for which it is sometimes mistaken. The flower is umbrella shaped and strikingly similar to that of *D. carota* (Queen Anne's lace) or *Cicuta* species (water hemlock). The stem is hollow and has red to purple speckles along its length. The crushed stems are said to smell like mouse urine; however, that observation is extremely subjective and should not be used to identify the plant. Its taproot is

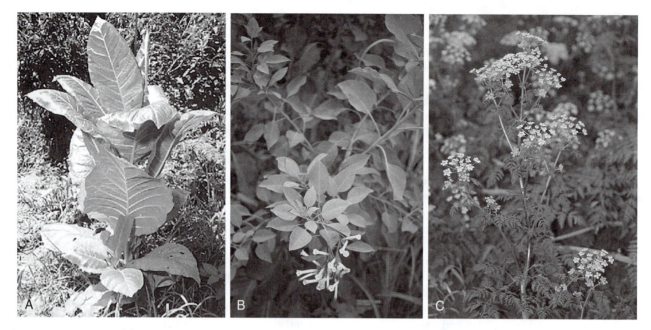

Figure 47-8. Nicotine. *(A) Nicotiana tabacum. (B) Nicotiana glauca.* Coniine. *(C) Conium maculatum.*

occasionally mistaken for parsnip. This plant is reputed to be the source of poison used in the execution of Socrates.[69]

Nicotiana glauca

Early *N. glauca* growth has a shrublike appearance and may be mistaken for collard greens due to the grayish cast of the green leaves. The leaves are oval with a smooth margin and a rubbery texture, and they grow up to 6 inches in length. The flowers are approximately 2 inches long by ½ inch wide and bright yellow with a tubular shape.

Toxic Parts

All parts of both *C. maculatum* and *N. glauca* are poisonous. The seeds and roots of *C. maculatum* are especially toxic.

Mechanism of Toxicity

Nicotine, coniine, anabasine, lobeline, and related pyridine and piperidine alkaloids cause similar toxicity. Their primary action is activation and then blockade of nicotinic acetylcholine receptors. Activation of nicotinic receptors in the cortex, thalamus, interpeduncular nucleus, and other locations in the CNS accounts for coma and seizures. Nicotine has been shown to enhance fast excitatory neural transmission in the CNS by triggering presynaptic cholinergic receptors, which increase presynaptic calcium and stimulate both cholinergic and glutamatergic transmission.[103] Nicotinic receptor activation facilitates the release of many neurotransmitters, including acetylcholine, norepinephrine, dopamine, serotonin, and β-endorphins.[104]

Activation of nicotinic receptors at autonomic ganglia produces varied effects in the sympathetic and parasympathetic nervous system. These most commonly include nausea, vomiting, diarrhea, bradycardia, tachycardia, and miosis.[105] Nicotine alkaloids act as depolarizing neuromuscular blocking agents and produce fasciculations and paralysis.

Clinical Presentation

Ingestion or dermal exposure to nicotine and related compounds can result in any or all of the signs and symptoms listed in Table 2.

Although rare, severe poisonings do occur.[106] One of the more commonly reported poisonings results from the ingestion of cigarettes. The ingestion of a single cigarette is enough to cause symptoms in a small child. Smolinske et al. reported that 3 severely poisoned children had ingested a minimum of 1.4 mg/kg and 25 asymptomatic children ingested less than 1 mg/kg.[107] Curry et al. reported nine cases of ingestion of *N. glauca*, which had been mistaken for collard and turnip greens.[108] Three fatalities occurred. Symptoms included leg cramps, paresthesias, dizziness, and headache. Onset was within 1 hour, and resolution in the surviving patients ranged from 3 to several hours.[108] Mellick et al. reported two cases of *N. glauca* ingestion resulting in

Table 2: Muscarinic and Nicotinic Effects of Nicotine and Related Compounds

Muscarinic	Nicotinic
Salivation	Weakness
Lacrimation	Fasciculations
Urination	Paralysis
Gastroenteric cramping	Tachycardia
Emesis	Coma
Miosis	Seizures
Bronchospasm	
Bradycardia	

neuromuscular blockade and eventual complete recovery.[109] Frank et al. reported a *C. maculatum* ingestion in a 4-year-old child that resulted in miosis, vomiting, and coma. The onset of symptoms was 30 minutes after ingestion, with resolution in about 9 hours.[110] Drummer et al. reported three fatalities from *C. maculatum*.[102] Foster et al. reported the accidental ingestion of *C. maculatum* by a 14-year-old child that resulted in respiratory failure, asphyxia, and eventual death and that another child who ingested a smaller amount of the same *C. maculatum* plant had symptoms of nausea, malaise, and tingling of the extremities and survived.[111] The 2002, the American Association of Poison Control Centers annual report described a 13-year-old child who developed ascending paralysis, a seizure, and then death after ingestion of *C. maculatum* that was mistaken for parsley.[112]

Green tobacco sickness commonly occurs in the tobacco-growing states. Workers handling leaves can absorb nicotine through the skin. It occurs almost exclusively in workers who are cropping leaves from the plant.[105] Symptoms comprise nausea, vomiting, diarrhea, diaphoresis, and weakness, which usually resolve with symptomatic treatment.

The use of betel quid which is popular in India, Southeast Asia, and the East Indies,[100] has been reported in people who have immigrated to the United States from those countries. The quid is a betel nut wrapped in a betel vine leaf and smeared with a paste of burnt lime.[113] It contains arecoline and several other cholinergic pyridine alkaloids.

Rhabdomyolysis has been reported from the ingestion of *C. maculatum*, although the reports are somewhat confusing in that "hemlock poisoning" is attributed to exposure to both *Cicuta* and *Conium* species.[114,115]

Laboratory Studies

Nicotine, coniine, and other alkaloids may be measured in urine by various methods, including gas chromatography,[29] mass spectrometry,[102] and thin-layer chromatography.[116]

Management

Activated charcoal should be administered for ingestions of nicotine and related alkaloids have occurred in the previous 2 hours. The recommended dose of activated charcoal is 0.5 to 1g/kg in children or 25 to 100g in adults. Because vomiting is a common symptom, ipecac administration is not indicated, and lavage of plant materials is probably not as effective as the administration of activated charcoal. In patients with dermal exposure, as in the case of green tobacco sickness, the skin should be thoroughly washed with soap and water. Atropine may be used to block muscarinic symptoms such as bronchospasm, vomiting, diarrhea, or bradycardia. There is no standard dose in this situation, and the amount given should be titrated to reverse muscarinic symptoms without inducing anticholinergic toxicity. Convulsions are best treated with benzodiazepines or barbiturates. Nicotinic symptoms such as weakness, fasciculations, or paralysis cannot be reversed, but supportive care is generally sufficient to manage the patient, with some patients requiring ventilatory support. No clinically useful antidotes have been found for the nicotinic effects. Patients should be monitored for rhabdomyolysis and its subsequent renal impairment. Due to the usual rapid onset of symptoms, patients who present and remain asymptomatic and who are not suicidal may be released after 4 hours of observation.

VERATRUM ALKALOIDS

Veratrum alkaloids are found in the various species of *Veratrum* and *Zigadenus* throughout the United States and in parts of Canada. Historically, these plants have been used as sources of medicines and insecticide. Their toxicity was noted in sneezing powders, made from pulverized roots of these plants. Inhalation or ingestion has resulted in several signs and symptoms, including hypotension or bradyrhythmia. Teratogenicity in farm animals, particularly sheep, has been widely reported.

Plants

Veratrum alkaloids are found in *Veratrum album* (white hellebore; Figure 47-9A), *Veratrum californicum* (corn lily, skunk cabbage), *Veratrum viride* (false hellebore), and *Zigadenus* species (death camus; Figure 47-9B).[117,118]

Location

V. viride is found in Canada and the eastern United States from New England to Georgia. Related species are found in western United States *(V. californicum)*, Alaska and Europe *(V. album)*, and Asia *(Veratrum japonicum)*.[119] False hellebore tends to grow in low-lying, swampy areas, while white hellebore is found in alpine meadows.[79]

Description

Veratrum plants are tall (2 to 7 feet) perennial herbs. Broad, longitudinally plicated leaves are spirally arranged on a stout stem. White to yellowish-green pedicellate flowers line the terminal 30 to 60 centimeters of the stem. These plants also contain a highly seeded fruit.[79]

Zigadenus is a genus of the lily family. It is found throughout the United States and Canada. Flowers are pale yellow, pink, or white. The leaves are long, thin, and grasslike. The root is a bulb, which is similar in appearance to and often mistaken for wild onion. *Zigadenus*, however, lacks an onion-like odor.[117,120]

Toxic Parts

The entire veratrum plant contains toxic veratrum alkaloids; however, the bulb and flowers most commonly cause poisoning. Fruit seeds and leaves rarely cause human toxicity.

Mechanism of Toxicity

The veratrum alkaloids, which are chemically similar to steroids, include protoveratrine, veratridine, and jervine.[119] These agents were introduced in the 1950s as antihypertensive agents; however, they were found to have a narrow therapeutic index and their use was discontinued.[119,121] Of these steroidal alkaloids, veratridine is the most potent.[83] The primary activity of these compounds is to attach to voltage-sensitive sodium channels in conductive cells and increase sodium permeability, raising intracellular sodium concentration like grayanotoxins. Veratrine affects only a limited number of the sodium channels, but those so affected reactivate 1000 times more slowly than the unaffected channels (i.e., slow recovery). These alkaloids also appear to block inactivation of sodium channels and change the

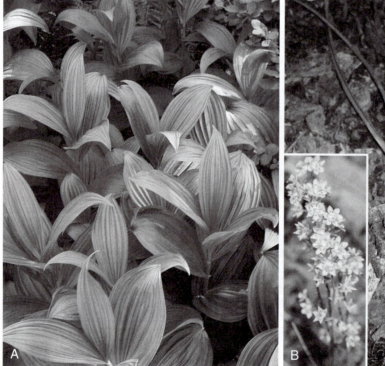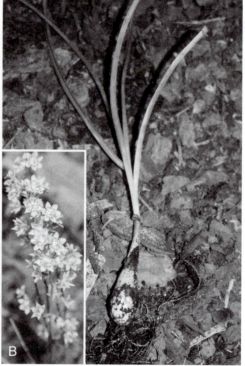

Figure 47-9. Veratrum. *(A) Veratrum* species. *(B) Zigadenus* species.

activation threshold of the sodium channels so that some remain open even at their resting potential.[83] Again, the rise in intracellular sodium concentrations leads to increased automaticity, enhanced vagal tone without hyperkalemia, and occasional neurotoxicity. High doses given to animals result in cardiac arrest.[6]

Clinical Presentation

Poisoning with veratrum alkaloids most typically occurs after accidental ingestion of the plant secondary to confusion with an edible species.[119] Toxicity also results from inhalation of sneezing powders prepared from pulverized white hellebore root.[122] Nausea and vomiting are most commonly seen after ingestion of the veratrum alkaloids. Clinically significant bradycardia and hypotension are also generally seen. Other reported toxic effects have included abdominal pain and distention, salivation, respiratory depression, yellow or green scotomata, paresthesias, increased muscle tone, rigors, and rarely, seizures.[119,121,124] Various electrocardiogram changes have also been reported with veratrum poisoning. Marinov et al. reported a characteristic electrocardiogram pattern in 10 of 12 patients poisoned with *V. album* that included PR and QT interval shortening, ST segment depression, T wave morphology changes, and bundle branch block.[125] Quatrehomme et al. noted nausea and vomiting followed by hypotension. In contrast to the observations of Marinov and colleagues, Quatrehomme and colleagues reported QT prolongation.[126]

Characteristic facial deformities (cyclopia, cleft lip and palate, microphthalmia) and limb defects (bowed fibulae, shortened tibia, excessive flexure of the knees) occur in offspring of pregnant sheep who ingest plants containing veratrum alkaloids. Jervine and other steroidal alkaloids found in the *Veratrum* species are responsible for these birth defects.[127]

Laboratory Studies

No clinically useful laboratory studies confirm veratrum alkaloid exposure.

Management

Initial management following veratrum alkaloid exposure should include the administration of activated charcoal if the ingestion has occurred within the last 2 hours. The recommended dose of activated charcoal is 0.5 to 1g/kg in children or 25 to 100g in adults. Bradycardia usually responds to atropine administration. Hypotension may or may not respond to the atropine. Crystalloid fluids or vasopressors such as dopamine have been used to support blood pressure. Symptoms generally resolve in 24 to 48 hours or less, and deaths are rare.[119]

REFERENCES

1. Chan TYK, Chan JCN, Tomlinson B, et al. Chinese herbal medicines revisited: a Hong Kong perspective. *Lancet*. 1993;342:1532–1534.

2. Tomassoni AJ, Snook CP, McConville BJ, et al. Recreational use of delphinium: an ancient poison revisited [abstract]. *J Toxicol Clin Toxicol*. 1996;34(5):598.

3. Fatovich DM. Aconite: a lethal Chinese herb. *Ann Emerg Med*. 1992;21(3):309–311.

4. Chan TYK, Tse LLK, Chan J, Aconitine poisoning due to Chinese herbal medicines: a review. *Vet Hum Toxicol*. 1994;36(5):452–455.

5. Adaniya H, Hayami H, Hiraoka M, Effects of magnesium on polymorphic ventricular tachycardias induced by aconitine. *J Cardiovasc Pharmacol*. 1994;24:721–729.

5a. Clavijero FX. Historia de la antigua o Baja Clifornia, 3rd ed. Mexico: Editorial Porrua. 1990.

5b. Castillo-Najera F. Contribución al estudio de la parálisis tóxica. un envenenamiento colectivo con tullidora. In: Memoria del V Congreso Medico Mexicano. Mexico: Direccion de Talleres Garaficaos 1920:240–244.

6. Penner JP, Aubin M. Effects of aconitine and veratrine on the isolated perfused heart of the common eel (*Anguilla anguilla* L.). *Comp Biochem Physiol*. 1984;77C(2):367–369.

7. Sawanobori T, Hirano Y, Hiraoka M. Aconitine-induced delayed afterdepolarization in frog atrium and guinea pig papillary muscles in the presence of low concentrations of Ca^{++}. *Jpn J Physiol*. 1987;37:59–79.

8. Leichter D, Danilo P, Boyden P, A canine model of torsade de pointes. *PACE*. 1988;11:2235–2245.

9. Tai YT, But PPH, Young K, et al. Cardiotoxicity after accidental herb-induced aconite poisoning. *Lancet*. 1992;340:1254–1256.

10. Tai YT, Lau CP, But PPH, et al. Bidirectional tachycardia induced by herbal aconite poisoning. *PACE*. 1992;15:831–839.

11. Chan TYK. Aconitine poisoning: a global perspective. *Vet Hum Toxicol*. 1994;36(4):326–328.

12. Chan TYK, Critchley JAJH. The spectrum of poisonings in Hong Kong: an overview. *Vet Hum Toxicol*. 1994;36(2):135–137.

13. But PPH, Tai YT, Young K. Three fatal cases of herbal aconite poisoning. *Vet Hum Toxicol*. 1994;36(3):212–215.

14. Chan TYK. Aconitine poisoning following the ingestion of Chinese herbal medicines: a report of eight cases. *Aust NZ J Med*. 1993;23:268–271.

15. Dickens P, Tai YT, But PPH, et al. Fatal accidental aconitine poisoning following ingestion of Chinese herbal medicine: a report of two cases. *Forensic Sci Intl*. 1994;67:55–58.

16. Yeih DF, Chiang FT, Huang SK. Successful treatment of aconitine-induced life-threatening ventricular tachyarrhythmia with amiodarone. *Heart*. 2000;84(4):E8.

17. Jackman WM, Friday KJ, Anderson JL, et al. The long QT syndrome: a critical review, new clinical observations and a unifying hypothesis. *Prog Cardiovasc Dis*. 1988;31(2):115–172.

18. Ocampo-Roosens LV, Ontiveros-Nevares PG, Fernandez-Lucio O. Intoxication with buckthorn (*Karwinskia humboldtiana*): report of three siblings. *Pediatr Dev Pathol*. 2007;10(1):66–68.

19. Nava ME, Castellanos JL, Castaneda ME. Geographical factors in the epidemiology of intoxication with *Karwinskia* (tullidora) in Mexico. *Cad Saude Publica*. 2000;16(1):255–260.

20. Bermudez MV, Gonzalez-Spencer D, Guerrero M, et al. Experimental intoxication with fruit and purified toxins of buckthorn (*Karwinskia humboldtiana*). *Toxicon*. 1986;24(11–12):1091–1097.

21. Salazar-Leal ME, Flores MS, Sepulveda-Saavedra J, et al. An experimental model of peripheral neuropathy induced in rats by

Karwinskia humboldtiana (buckthorn) fruit. *J Peripher Nerv Syst.* 2006;11(3):253–261.

22. Wheeler MH, Camp BJ. Inhibitory and uncoupling actions of extracts from *Karwinskia humboldtiana* on respiration and oxidative phosphorylation: Life sciences. 2. Biochemistry. *Gen Mol Biol.* 1971;10(1):41–51.

23. Jaramillo-Juarez F, Rodriguez-Vazquez ML, Munoz-Martinez J, et al. The ATP levels in kidneys and blood are mainly decreased by acute ingestion of tullidora *(Karwinskia humboldtiana)*. *Toxicon.* 2005;46(1):99–103.

24. Martinez HR, Bermudez MV, Rangel-Guerra RA, et al. Clinical diagnosis in *Karwinskia humboldtiana* polyneuropathy. *J Neurol Sci.* 1998;154(1):49–54.

24a. Bermudez de Rocha MV, Lozano Melendez FE, Salazar Leal ME, et al. Familial poisoning with Karwinskia humboldtiana. *Gaceta Medica de Mexico* 1995;131(1):100–106.

25. Levy R. Jimson seed poisoning: a new hallucinogen on the horizon. *JACEP.* 1977;6(2):58–61.

26. Michalodimitrakis M. Discussion of "*Datura stramonium:* a fatal poisoning." *J Forensic Sci.* 1984:961–962.

27. Ulrich RW, Bowerman DL, Levisky JA, *Datura stramonium:* a fatal poisoning. *J Forensic Sci.* 1982;27(4):948–954.

28. Smith EA, Meloan CE, Pickell JA, et al. Scopolamine poisoning from homemade "moon flower" wine. *J Anal Toxicol.* 1991;15(4):216–219.

29. Baselt RC, Cravey RH. *Disposition of Toxic Drugs and Chemicals in Man.* vol 4. Foster City, Calif: Chemical Toxicology Institute; 1995:682.

30. Ramakrishnan SS. Pitfalls in the treatment of Jimson weed intoxication. *Am J Psychiatry.* 1994;151(9):1396–1397.

31. Hanna JP, Schmidley JW, Braselton WE. *Datura* delirium. *Clin Neuropharmacol.* 1992;15(2):109–113.

32. Litovitz TL, Clark LR, Soloway RA. 1993 annual report of the American Association of Poison Control Centers Toxic Exposure Surveillance System. *Am J Emerg Med.* 1994;12(5): 546–584.

33. Pentel P, Peterson C. Asystole complicating physostigmine treatment of tricyclic antidepressant overdose. *Ann Emerg Med.* 1980;9:588.

34. Gilman A, Rall T, Nies A, et al. *Goodman and Gilman's The Pharmacological Basis of Therapeutics.* New York: Macmillan; 1990:814.

34a. Silverman ME. William Withering and an account of the Foxglove. *Clin Cardiol.* 1989;12(7):415–418.

35. Langford SD, Boor PJ. Oleander toxicity: an examination of human and animal toxic exposures. *Toxicology.* 1996;109:1–13.

36. Knutsen OH, Paszkowski P. New aspects in the treatment of water hemlock poisoning. *Clin Toxicol.* 1984;22(2):157–166.

37. Shaw D, Pearn J. Oleander poisoning. *Med J Aust.* 1979; 2:267–269.

38. Radford DJ, Gillies AD, Hinds JA, et al. Naturally occurring cardiac glycosides. *Med J Aust.* 1986;144:539–540.

39. Ayachi S, Brown A. Hypotensive effects of cardiac glycosides in spontaneously hypertensive rats. *J Pharmacol Exp Ther.* 1980;213:520.

39a. Marx J, Pretorius E, Bornman MS. The neurotoxic effects of prenatal cardiac glycoside exposure: a hypothesis. *Neurotoxicol Teratol* 2006;28(1):135–143.

40. Marx J, Pretorius E, Bornman MS. The neurotoxic effects of prenatal cardiac glycoside exposure: a hypothesis. *Neurotoxicol Teratol.* 2006;28(1):135–143.

41. Gaitonde BB, Joglekar SN. Mechanism of neurotoxicity of cardiotonic glycosides. *Br J Pharmacol.* 1977;59(2):223–229.

42. Gupta RS, Chopra A, Stetsko DK. Cellular basis for the species differences in sensitivity to cardiac glycosides (digitalis). *J Cell Physiol.* 1986;127(2):197–206.

43. Langer GA. Interspecies variation in myocardial physiology: the anomalous rat. *Environ Health Perspect.* 1978;26:175–179.

44. Middleton WS, Chen KK. Clinical results from oral administration of thevetin, a cardiac glycoside. *Am Heart J.* 1936;11:75–88.

45. Saravanapavananthan N, Ganeshamoorthy J. Yellow oleander poisoning: study of 170 cases. *Forensic Sci Intl.* 1988;36:247–250.

46. Haynes BE, Bessen HA, Wightman WD. Oleander tea: herbal draught of death. *Ann Emerg Med.* 1985;14(4):350–353.

47. Osterloh J, Herold S, Pond S. Oleander interference in the digoxin radioimmunoassay in a fatal ingestion. *JAMA.* 1982;247:1596–1597.

48. Safadi R, Levy I, Amitai Y, et al. Beneficial effect of digoxin-specific Fab antibody fragments in oleander intoxication. *Arch Intern Med.* 1995;155:2121–2125.

49. Butler VP, Jr., Odel JG, Rath E, et al. Digitalis-induced visual disturbances with therapeutic serum digitalis concentrations. *Ann Intern Med.* 1995;123(9):676–680.

50. Closson RG. Visual hallucinations as the earliest symptom of digoxin intoxication. *Arch Neurol.* 1983;40(6):386.

51. Shear MK, Sacks MH. Digitalis delirium: report of two cases. *Am J Psychiatry.* 1978;135(1):109–110.

52. Eisendrath SJ, Sweeney MA. Toxic neuropsychiatric effects of digoxin at therapeutic serum concentrations. *Am J Psychiatry.* 1987;144(4):506–507.

53. Varriale P, Mossavi A. Rapid reversal of digitalis delirium using digoxin immune Fab therapy. *Clin Cardiol.* 1995;18(6):351–352.

54. Clark RF, Selden B, Curry SC. Digoxin-specific Fab fragments in the treatment of oleander toxicity in a canine model. *Ann Emerg Med.* 1991;20(10):1073–1077.

55. Shumaik G, Wu AW, Ping AC. Oleander poisoning: treatment with digoxin-specific Fab antibody fragments. *Ann Emerg Med.* 1988;17(7):732–735.

56. Bartell S, Anchor A. Use of digoxin-specific antibody fragments in suicidal oleander toxicity [abstract]. *J Toxicol Clin Toxicol.* 1996;34(5):600.

57. Stockbridge J. Account of the effect of eating, a poisonous plant called *Cicuta maculata. Boston Med Surg J.* 1814;3:334–337.

58. Krenzelok EP, Jacobsen TD, Aronis JM. Hemlock ingestions: the most deadly plant exposures [abstract]. *J Toxicol Clin Toxicol.* 1996;34(5):601–602.

59. Lampe KF, McCann MA. *The AMA Handbook of Poisonous and Injurious Plants.* Chicago: Chicago Review Press; 1985:124.

60. Mitchell M, Routledge PA. Poisoning by hemlock water dropwort. *Lancet.* 1977;1:423–424.

61. Applefeld JJ, Caplan ES. A case of water hemlock poisoning. *JACEP.* 1979;8(10):401–403.

62. Centers of Disease Control and Prevention. Water hemlock poisoning: Maine, 1992. *MMWR.* 1994;43(13):229–231.

63. Litovitz TL, Felberg L, Skoloway RA, et al. 1994 annual report of the American Association of Poison Control Centers Toxic Exposure Surveillance System. *Am J Emerg Med.* 1995;13(5): 551–597.

64. Withers LM, Cole FR, Nelson RB. Water-hemlock poisoning [letter]. *New Engl J Med.* 1975;281:566–567.

65. Landers D, Seppi K, Blauer W. Seizures and death on a white river float trip: report of water hemlock poisoning. *West J Med.* 1985;142:637–640.

66. Starreveld E, Hope CE. Cicutoxin poisoning (water hemlock). *Neurology.* 1975;25(August):730–734.

67. Nelson RB, North DS, Kaneriya M, et al. The influence of biperiden, benztropine, physostigmine and diazepam on the convulsive effects of *Cicuta douglasii. Proc West Pharmacol Soc.* 1978;21:137–139.

68. Carlton BE, Tufts E, Girard DE. Water hemlock poisoning complicated by rhabdomyolysis and renal failure. *Clin Toxicol.* 1979;14(1):87–92.

69. Nelson RB, Cole FR. The convulsive profile of *Cicuta douglasii* (water hemlock). *Proc West Pharmacol Soc.* 1976;19:193–197.

70. Costanza DJ, Hoversten VW. Accidental ingestion of water hemlock: report of two patients with acute and chronic effects. *Calif Med.* 1973;119(May):78–82.

71. Egdahl A. A case of poisoning due to eating poison-hemlock (*Cicuta maculata*). *Arch Int Med.* 1911;7:348–356.

72. Robson P. Water hemlock poisoning. *Lancet.* 1965;2:1274–1275.

73. Ball MJ, Flather ML, Forfar JC. Hemlock water dropwort poisoning. *Postgrad Med J.* 1987;63:363–365.

74. King LA, Lewis MJ, Parry D, et al. Identification of oenanthotoxin and related compounds in hemlock water dropwort poisoning. *Hum Toxicol.* 1985;4:355–364.

75. Mitchell MI, Routledge PA. Hemlock water dropwort poisoning: a review. *Clin Toxicol.* 1978;12(4):417–426.

76. Mutter L. Poisoning by western water hemlock. *Can J Public Health.* 1976;67:368.

77. Curry SC, Chang D, Conner D. Drug- and toxin-induced rhabdomyolysis. *Ann Emerg Med.* 1989;18:1068–1084.

78. Lampe KF. Rhododendrons, mountain laurel, and mad honey. *JAMA.* 1988;259(13):2009.

79. Frohne D, Pfander HJ. *A Colour Atlas of Poisonous Plants: A Handbook for Pharmacists, Doctors, Toxicologists, and Biologists.* London: Solfe Publishing; 1983:152–154.

80. Moran NC, Dresel PE, Perkins ME, et al. The pharmacological actions of andromedotoxin, an active principle from *Rhododendron maximum. J Pharmacol Exp Ther.* 1954;110:415–432.

81. Seyama I, Narahashi T. Modulation of sodium channels of squid nerve membranes by grayanotoxin I. *J Pharmacol Exp Ther.* 1981;219:614–624.

82. Yakehiro M, Yamamoto S, Baba N, et al. Structure–activity relationship for D-ring derivatives of grayanotoxin in the squid giant axon. *J Pharmacol Exp Ther Toxicol.* 1993;265(3):1328–1332.

83. Catterall WA. Neurotoxins that act on voltage-sensitive sodium channels in excitable membranes. *Ann Rev Pharmacol Toxicol.* 1980;20:15–43.

84. Masutani T, Seyama I, Narahashi T, et al. Structure–activity relationship for grayanotoxin derivatives in frog skeletal muscle. *J Pharmacol Exp Ther.* 1981;217:812–819.

85. Klein-Schwartz W, Litovitz T. Azalea toxicity: an overrated problem? *Clin Toxicol.* 1985;23(2–3):91–101.

86. Gossinger H, Hruby K, Haubenstock A. Cardiac arrhythmias in a patient with grayanotoxin-honey poisoning. *Vet Hum Toxicol.* 1983;25(5).

87. Clarke EGC, Humphries DJ, King T. *Animal and Plant Toxins.* Müchen: Goldmann; 1973.

88. Narahashi T, Seyama I. Mechanism of nerve membrane depolarization caused by grayanotoxin I. *J Physiol.* 1974;242:471–487.

89. Spencer PS. Food toxins, AMPA receptors, and motor neuron diseases. *Drug Metab Rev.* 1999;31(3):561–587.

90. Selye H. Lathyrism. *Rev Can Biol.* 1957;16(1):1–82.

90a. Rao SLN, Adiga PR, Sarma PS. The isolation and characterization of b-N-Oxalyl-L-α,β-Diaminopropionic acid: a neurotoxin from the seeds of *Lathyrus sativus. Biochem.* 1964;3(3):432–436.

91. Ludolph AC, Spencer PS. Toxic models of upper motor neuron disease. *J Neurol Sci.* 1996;139 (Suppl):53–59.

92. Hurst S. USDA, NRCS. 2009. The PLANTS Database (http://plants.usda.gov/). National Plant Data Center, Baton Rouge, LA 70874-4490 USA. Accessed February 14, 2009.

93. Mehta SL, Santha IM: Development of regeneration protocols to exploit somaclonal variations in *Lathyrus sativus* for developing toxin free cultivars. In: Jaiwal PK, Singh RP (eds). *Improvement Strategies of Leguminosae Biotechnology–Focus on Biotechnology,* Vol. 10A. New York:Springer 2003, 291–299.

94. Streifler M, et al. The central nervous system in a case of neurolathyrism. *Neurology.* 1977;27(12):1176–1178.

95. Drory VE, Rabey MJ, Cohn DF. Electrophysiologic features in patients with chronic neurolathyrism. *Acta Neurol Scand.* 1992;85(6):401–403.

96. Haque A, Hossain M, Wouters G, et al. Epidemiological study of lathyrism in northwestern districts of Bangladesh. *Neuroepidemiology.* 1996;15(2):83–91.

97. Haque A, Hossain M, Lambein F, et al. Evidence of osteolathyrism among patients suffering from neurolathyrism in Bangladesh. *Nat Toxins.* 1997;5(1):43–46.

98. Dawson DA, Rinaldi AC, Poch G. Biochemical and toxicological evaluation of agent–cofactor reactivity as a mechanism of action for osteolathyrism. *Toxicology.* 2002;177(2–3):267–284.

99. Cohn DF, Streifler M. Intoxication by the chickling pea (*Lathyrus sativus*): nervous system and skeletal findings. *Arch Toxicol.* 1983;6(Suppl):190–193.

100. Kunkel DB. Tobacco and friends. *Emerg Med.* 1985:142–158.

101. Domino E, Hornbach E, Demana T. The nicotine content of common vegetables. *New Engl J Med.* 1993;329(6):437.

102. Drummer OH, Roberts AN, Bedford PJ, et al. Three deaths from hemlock poisoning. *Med J Aust.* 1995;162:592–593.

103. McGehee DS, Heath MJS, Gelber S, et al. Nicotine enhancement of fast excitatory synaptic transmission in CNS by presynaptic receptors. *Science.* 1995;269:1692–1696.

104. Benowitz NL. Pharmacology of nicotine: addiction and therapeutics. *Annu Rev Pharmacol Toxicol.* 1996;36:597–613.

105. Hipke ME. Green tobacco sickness. *South Med J.* 1993;86(9):989–992.

106. Litovitz TL, Normann SA, Veltri JC. 1985 annual report of the American Association of Poison Control Centers National Data Collection System. *Am J Emerg Med.* 1986;4(5):427–458.

107. Smolinske SC, Spoerke DG, Spiller SK, et al. Cigarette and nicotine chewing gum toxicity in children. *Hum Toxicol.* 1988;7:27–31.

108. Curry S, Bond R, Kunkel D. Acute nicotine poisonings after ingestions of tree tobacco. *Vet Hum Toxicol.* 1988;30(4):369.

109. Mellick LB, Makowski T, Mellick GA, et al. Neuromuscular blockade after ingestion of tree tobacco (*Nicotiana glauca*). *Ann Emerg Med.* 1999;34(1):101–104.

110. Frank BS, Michelson WB, Panter KE, et al. Ingestion of poison hemlock (*Conium maculatum*). *West J Med.* 1995;163:573–574.

111. Foster PF, McFadden R, Trevino R, et al. Successful transplantation of donor organs from a hemlock poisoning victim. *Transplantation.* 2003;76(5):874–876.

112. Watson WA, Litovitz TL, Rodgers GC, et al. 2002 annual report of the American Association of Poison Control Centers Toxic Exposure Surveillance System. *Am J Emerg Med.* 2003;21(5):353–421.

113. Taylor RFH, Al-Jarad N, John LME, et al. Betel-nut chewing and asthma. *Lancet.* 1992;339:1134–1136.

114. Rizzi D, Basile C, Di Maggio A, et al. Rhabdomyolysis and acute tubular necrosis in coniine (hemlock) poisoning [letter]. *Lancet.* 1989:1461–1462.

115. Scatizzi A, Di Maggio A, Rizzi D, et al. Acute renal failure due to tubular necrosis caused by waildfoul-mediated hemlock poisoning. *Ren Fail.* 1993;15(1):93–96.

116. Cromwell BT. The separation, micro-estimation and distribution of the alkaloids of hemlock (*Conium maculatum* L.). *Biochem J.* 1956;64:259–266.

117. Heilpern KL. *Zigadenus* poisoning. *Ann Emerg Med.* 1995;25(2):259–262.

118. Wagstaff DJ, Case AA. Human poisoning by *Zigadenus. Clin Toxicol.* 1987;25(4):361–367.

119. Jaffe AM, Gephardt D, Courtemanche L. Poisoning due to ingestion of *Veratrum viride* (false hellebore). *J Emerg Med.* 1990;8:161–167.

120. Schmutz EM, Hamilton LB. *Plants That Poison*. 1st ed. Flagstaff, Ariz: Northland Publishing; 1979:175.

121. Crummet D, Bronstein D, Weaver Z. Accidental *Veratrum viride* poisoning in three "ramp" foragers. *NC Med J*. 1985;46(9):469–471.

122. Fogh A, Kulling P, Wickstrom E. Veratrum alkaloids in sneezing-powder a potential danger. *J Toxicol Clin Toxicol*. 1983;20(2):175–179.

123. Kulig K, Rumack BH. Severe veratrum alkaloid poisoning [abstract]. *Vet Hum Toxicol*. 1982;24(4):294.

124. Nelson DA. Accidental poisoning by *Veratrum japonicum*. *JAMA*. 1954;156(1):33–35.

125. Marinov A, Koev P, Mircher N. Electrocardiographic studies in patients with acute hellebore *(Veratrum album)* intoxication. *Vulr Boles (Bulgaria)*. 1987;26:36–39.

126. Quatrehomme G, Bertrand F, Chauvet C, et al. Intoxication from *Veratrum album*. *Hum Exp Toxicology*. 1993;12(2):111–115.

127. Keeler RF, Binns W. Teratogenic compounds of *Veratrum californicum* (Durand): comparison of cyclopian effects of steroidal alkaloids from the plant and structurally related compounds from other sources. *Teratology*. 1968;1:5–10.

Radiation

L. Cameron Pimperl

INTRODUCTION

Radiation injury in the nervous system presents an uncommon problem with a complex clinical picture. The mechanisms of radiation injury are still poorly understood, but much progress has been made in recent years to attempt to more precisely define the pathophysiology of radiation injury to the nervous system, and this in turn produces a better potential for rational therapeutic intervention.

This chapter first addresses the details of the pathophysiology of radiation injury to the nervous system, with consideration of the historical context that forms the basis for past clinical experience. Emerging paradigms for explaining the complex processes at the cellular and molecular level are then described, with possible opportunities for therapeutic intervention.

A discussion of the sources of radiation injury follows, with an overview of some experiences with accidental exposures, as well as planned exposures due to medical procedures and treatment. Finally, clinical scenarios of radiation injury are individually described, with specific suggestions for therapy. There is limited clinical experience with many of these therapeutic options, so experimental results in animals are discussed in some detail. In some cases, experimental results have been quickly applied to clinical studies, so much of this experience in animal models may in fact be implemented in humans in the near future.

WHAT IS RADIATION?

Radiation in general refers to energy propagated through space in the form of waves and particles and includes both nonionizing and ionizing radiation. Nonionizing radiation includes visible light, ultraviolet light, infrared light, low-energy electromagnetic fields, microwaves, and radiofrequency energy (radio waves). Ionizing radiation includes x-rays, gamma-rays, cosmic rays, and particulate radiation such as electrons, protons, neutrons, or heavy ions. Most of the discussion here focuses on the effects of ionizing radiation.

HEALTH EFFECTS OF RADIATION

Nonionizing Radiation and Health Effects

There is more limited injury associated with nonionizing radiation, including the possible risk of carcinogenesis and some potential for noncancer health risks, than with ionizing radiation. Only ultraviolet radiation has been unequivocally accepted to increase cancer risk, particularly for skin cancer but possibly for brain tumors as well.[1] Low-energy electromagnetic field radiation (e.g., associated with electrical transmission lines) is considered a possible causative agent for leukemia and cancer of the brain,[2] as well as possibly related to neurodegenerative diseases such as amyotrophic lateral sclerosis and Alzheimer's disease, although this evidence is considered weak.[3] Concern for cell phone usage as a potential causative agent for central nervous system (CNS) malignancy has resulted in great interest in this question. A recent study found no such association.[4] Other possible nervous system effects of cell phone usage need further study.[5] Other health effects of nonionizing radiation include injury from laser light and heating from microwave radiation and radiofrequency energy.

Of greater clinical significance is the impact of ionizing forms of radiation.

Ionizing Radiation and Health Effects

Ionizing radiation interacts with living tissue by displacing electrons from atoms, generating molecules that have potential to cause injury as they interact with other molecules and cellular structures. Injury to DNA produces the main biological effects, including consequences in cells ranging from severe injury with rapid cell death, to mutations that lead to later reproductive death, to mutations potentially producing malignancy in somatic cells or inherited genetic abnormalities in germ cells. Counterbalanced against this attack is the organism's response to injury, in some cases successfully mitigating or repairing the injury and in other cases exacerbating the injury.

The net result of this interplay between injury and repair varies in relation to many risk variables, some of which are listed in Table 1. Some of these factors are relevant only to the therapeutic use of radiation. Radiation is useful therapeutically when the net balance of these factors yields a significantly greater probability of benefit versus injury. This chapter focuses on the injury associated with radiation, but it is worth noting that radiation has been used for therapeutic benefit for more than 100 years, has saved the lives of vast numbers of patients, and has eased the suffering of many more. This discussion of radiation injury is broad to include in principle all potential exposures to radiation, both therapeutic and otherwise. More detail is known of the experiences from therapeutic applications, but nuclear accidents and intentional exposure from nuclear weapons also contribute to the body of data. The clinician potentially may be faced with any of these problems, as well as new concerns related to radiological terrorism.

The concept of radiation *dose* is important, since generally most risks are greater for higher radiation doses. Dose refers to the amount of energy absorbed by tissue per unit mass and has been described in units called rads or currently as Gray, abbreviated Gy. The centiGray (cGy) is 1/100th of a Gray and is the same as 1 rad. To account for varying biological effects of different forms of ionizing radiation, a unit called the Sievert (Sv) is employed to indicate the "equivalent dose." For purposes of this discussion, 1 Gy is accepted as indicating the same dose as 1 Sv.

When radiation is used therapeutically, it is commonly delivered over many days, usually with a portion (or *fraction*) of the total dose given once each day. Typically, the size of the fraction given each day is 180 to 200 cGy, and this is called *conventional fractionation*. Because many aspects of radiation injury depend on the amount of radiation given with each fraction, it is important to understand both the total amount of radiation delivered over a course of therapy and the way in which the dose was fractionated over the time course of the overall treatment. In some circumstances, multiple fractions are given each day *(hyperfractionation)*, and a certain total dose may be delivered over a shorter-than-typical amount of time *(accelerated fractionation)*. Other circumstances may require the dose to be given only once each day but in larger-than-conventional fraction sizes *(hypofractionation)*. Each of these approaches produces different risks of injury, so it is important to know more about a course of radiation treatment than just "the dose," which is presumed to refer only to the total dose.

PATHOLOGY AND PATHOPHYSIOLOGY OF RADIATION INJURY TO THE NERVOUS SYSTEM

Pathology

The nervous system exhibits a particular array of responses to injury, and radiation injury can produce numerous components of these responses. However,

Table 1: Factors that Increase the Risk of Permanent Radiation Injury

Exposure-related Factors	Host Factors
Higher total dose	Hypertension
Higher dose per fraction	Diabetes
Larger treated volume	Ataxia telangiectasia
Concurrent chemotherapy	Connective tissue diseases
Brachytherapy (in the brain)	Vascular disease

the morphological changes resulting from radiation injury are not unique. Although no pathognomonic microscopic changes occur, radiation injury demonstrates a distinct tendency to affect white matter preferentially. Generally, gray matter is not affected in the absence of coexisting white matter injury. In the classic microscopic picture, demyelination and necrosis are commonly associated with white matter injury irrespective of the cause, including radiation injury. Effects on vasculature and glial cells are variable, and the specific roles of vascular injury versus oligodendroglial cell injury (causing demyelination) create controversy regarding pathogenesis.[6] Because of this prevalence of vascular changes and demyelination in radiation injury, much study has focused on the impact of radiation on vascular cells and oligodendrocytes, often to try to demonstrate how the relative contribution of injury to each of these populations subsequently produces necrosis. This issue is discussed further later in this chapter.

An excellent discussion with illustrations of the morphology associated with radiation injury in the nervous system can be found in Fajardo et al.[7] Very high doses of radiation can cause direct neuronal cell injury, often as part of the acute radiation syndrome after whole-body exposure. Nonlethal doses can produce gliosis and demyelination. Vascular injury can compromise the blood–brain barrier (BBB) and lead to edema. Further vascular injury can impair circulation, leading to ischemia and necrosis.[7]

Commonly, the spectrum of radiation changes in the nervous system are divided into three categories based on a consistent relationship to time of appearance after initial exposure. These are described as (1) acute (or early), (2) subacute (also called intermediate or early delayed), and (3) delayed (or late delayed). Some of these pathological features are described in Table 2.

These morphological changes are similar for the brain, spinal cord, and peripheral nerves, although typically higher doses of radiation have been considered necessary to produce peripheral nerve injury, where dense fibrotic changes are notable.[8]

Each of these time-related categories is associated with a typical set of potential clinical sequelae, which are discussed in detail later. Importantly, the severity of pathological changes does not correlate closely with the severity of clinical morbidity, and this is particularly true for cognitive deficits in which there may be no abnormal morphology.[9–11]

Pathophysiology

The basic array of cellular and molecular responses to injury in the nervous system provides a canvas on which to illustrate the complexity of the pathophysiology of

Table 2: Pathological Features of Radiation Injury

Category	Time Frame after Irradiation	Pathological Changes
Acute (early)	Before 6 months	Shallow sulci, flattened convolutions, edema, mass effect, focal demyelination, dilated blood vessels, platelet–fibrin thrombi, perivascular collections of mononuclear cells
Subacute (intermediate or early delayed)	6–9 months	Diffuse demyelination, necrosis in some cases
Delayed (late delayed)	More than 12 months	Widened sulci, dilated ventricles, necrosis, myelin destruction, hemorrhagic exudates, occlusion of capillaries, endothelial cell loss, vasogenic edema, calcifications, ischemic infarcts

radiation injury. Primary cellular responses can include cell death, membrane injury, excitatory amino acid release, cationic fluxes, and induction of expression of certain genes. Cytokines generated in this way can assist with repair or may exacerbate injury. Many injury processes involve reactive oxygen species and oxidative stress. The interplay of cell death, oxidative injury, and repair via products from inductions in gene expression culminates in the net effect of the injury. Irradiation can be demonstrated to be active in each of these three realms.[12,13]

Emerging Understanding of Molecular Processes

Historically, much research into radiation injury to the nervous system has focused on identifying which cell type was the primary target of radiation effect. The nature of morphological changes identified on microscopic examination and imaging studies has produced much interest in the role of the vascular endothelial cell and the oligodendrocyte. In recent years, further research has added a great deal of information related to the role of other cell types. Also, interest has been directed toward the role of individual molecular processes and the interplay among various cells via cytokines and growth factors.

Vascular Injury Is More Important

Vascular abnormalities in blood vessels including dilation, wall-thickening, and endothelial cell changes are well documented after radiation. Early changes of increased vascular permeability can occur within days after irradiation.[7,14] The development of vascular changes that could later lead to necrosis generally takes longer, in some studies more than 20 weeks.[15,16] Areas of decreased blood vessel density and endothelial cell loss are felt to indicate relative ischemia that could precipitate necrosis.[12,15,17,18]

However, necrosis due to irradiation has also been described in the absence of vascular changes.[19,20] In addition, the cell type that would seem most likely to be affected by ischemia and hypoxia is the neuron,[21] located in the gray matter, which does not typically develop necrosis before white matter necrosis. These points argue against radiation necrosis being purely due to vascular injury. On the other hand, studies using a vasculature-specific treatment called boron neutron capture show how doses deposited only in the immediate vicinity of blood vessels clearly confirm that severe vascular injury alone can produce necrosis.[12,13,22,23] Therefore, significant vascular injury is sufficient, but not necessary, to cause necrosis.

The role of vascular mechanisms of nervous system injury has produced broad efforts to characterize as precisely as possible the details of these mechanisms, with the possibility of targeting specific features of these mechanisms for therapeutic gain. The general oxidative stress produced by vascular injury from radiation includes the production of reactive oxygen species and cytokines leading to progressive inflammatory injury.[24–27]

An emerging understanding of the role of vascular endothelial growth factor (VEGF) further emphasizes the importance of vascular injury in radiation-induced pathology.[28] After CNS irradiation, endothelial cell loss produces compromise of the BBB, leading to increased production of VEGF.[25,26,29–32] VEGF then contributes to further injury to the BBB before ultimately turning on angiogenesis.[28]

Myelin Injury Is More Important

Another hallmark of radiation injury to nervous tissue is demyelination, which has produced much attention on the oligodendrocyte as the target cell of radiation-related injury. Research in rats has resulted in the identification of a progenitor cell to the mature oligodendrocyte[33] and has demonstrated that irradiation leads to the loss of these progenitor cells.[34–36] Consequently, mature oligodendrocytes are not replaced as they are lost, and demyelination results. A link between oxidative stress and production of reactive oxygen species causing myelin injury has been reported, with the suggestion that the structure of the myelin membrane may make it particularly vulnerable to reactive oxygen species.[37] These lines of evidence are consistent with the known tendency for radiation to preferentially affect white matter. However, there is no clear correlation between demyelination, which can occur early, and later development of white matter necrosis.

Are Both Important?

An obvious conclusion would seem to be that injury to the oligodendrocyte and to the endothelial cell plays a role in radiation-induced injury. Focus on these two cell types and their function has been a natural consequence of the observed morphological and functional changes associated with irradiation, but evolving evidence suggests that a broader interpretation of pathophysiology involving the whole nervous system is needed. All cell types in the nervous system need to be considered, with broader attention to the intercellular communication among different cell types. Interactions among all cell types are important in the normal physiology of nervous tissue; clearly these interactions must be assumed to be important in pathophysiology as well.[12]

Role of Astrocytes

There is evidence of dose-dependent increases in astrocyte populations after irradiation in rat and mouse models,[38] and astrocytes have clear roles in regulating the number and function of oligodendrocytes, maintaining the BBB, regulating angiogenesis, and protecting other cell types from oxidative injury.[39–44]

Role of Microglia

Increases in the number of microglia after irradiation occur,[19,38,45–47] and their response to injury could be relevant to the overall nervous system tissue response.

Role of Neurons

Clinical evidence supports direct neuronal toxicity from radiation in the absence of necrosis; long-term cognitive impairment after irradiation is well documented.[48–52] Animal models have also demonstrated alterations in brain electrical activity after irradiation.[53,54] Neuronal cell death has been demonstrated in vitro after irradiation, generally via apoptosis.[55–57] However, in vivo, the neuron seems to be protected from cell death after clinically typical doses of radiation, perhaps due to the protective effect of astrocytes.[12,56] Effects on gene expression have been demonstrated in neurons after irradiation,[56,58–60] producing a spectrum of possible mechanisms whereby irradiation can induce functional alterations in neuronal function.

Neural stem cells are becoming better understood as potential targets for radiation injury. The subependymal region and the subgranular zones of the dentate gyrus have been demonstrated to contain neural stem cells,[61–64] and some evidence suggests these cells may be recruited to assist with repair after tissue injury.[62,65] These cells appear to migrate to other parts of the brain and can differentiate into both neurons and glial cells.[61,63,64] The generation of new neurons, or *neurogenesis,* may play a role in memory and learning.[66,67] These neural stem cells are dose dependently reduced in number by irradiation,[68–75] as illustrated nicely by the work at the Brain Tumor Research Center at University of California, San Francisco (Figures 48-1 and 48-2; see color plates). In this work, Mizumatsu et al. demonstrated an adverse impact on neurogenesis at doses of radiation as low as 2 Gy.[76] This radiation-induced impact on neurogenesis has been shown to affect cognitive function.[72,77,78]

This impact on neurogenesis could potentially impair an important mechanism of repair after radiation injury and adversely affect cognitive functions such as memory and learning. The fascinating possibility of manipulating these cells could provide an important tool for investigating repair processes and perhaps even lead to potential therapeutic approaches. Early studies of manipulating the microenvironment of these cells to mitigate radiation injury has shown some promise,[79–81] for example, using antioxidants such as superoxide dismutase and catalase mimetics.[82,83] Tetracyclines and ceftriaxone have demonstrated protective effects in neuron cell cultures, presumably due to antioxidant and antiexcitotoxic amino acid activities, respectively.[84]

Other Diseases That Can Mimic Radiation Injury in the Nervous System

Aspects of other diseases affecting the CNS can produce similar morphological and clinical impact to radiation injury.

Alzheimer's Dementia
Demyelination can occur in Alzheimer's dementia, together with diminished cerebral perfusion and altered cerebral metabolism.[85] These changes are commonly seen in irradiated patients, and there is some preliminary evidence of lowering of acetylcholine and choline acetyltransferase in the brains of irradiated developing mice,[86] a common pattern seen in Alzheimer's disease patients.

Multiple Sclerosis
Multiple sclerosis can be associated with radiographic findings similar to radiation injury,[87] but differentiation from radiation injury can often be made based on clinical grounds.[88]

SOURCES OF RADIATION EXPOSURE

Exposure of the nervous system to radiation can occur from various sources, including environmental sources and medical sources. Environmental sources can include low-level exposures from continuous sources in the environment, accidental exposures due to nuclear accidents, and intentional exposures due to the use of weapons containing radioactive material. Exposure due to radioactive weapons has in the past only been associated with the use of atomic bombs by the United States. After the bombing of Hiroshima and Nagasaki, the United States and the former Soviet Union built massive stockpiles of weapons that continue to provide the possibility of large-scale exposure of large populations to the effects of radiation. Other countries have developed nuclear weapons as well, making the potential risk even larger. In addition, the possibility of radiological terrorism in the form of "dirty bombs" has recently become a significant concern, as poorer entities seek the ability to intimidate others with what is a psychologically powerful weapon.

The interest here is specifically related to the effects on the nervous system to radiation, and the relevance of this information is particularly poignant in the current geopolitical environment.

Environmental Sources

Environmental sources of radiation exposure include cosmic rays, radon, manmade contributions from nuclear facilities, and industries that use radionuclides. The average radiation dose across the planet for each person is estimated to be 2.4 mSv annually from natural sources, with additional small contributions from nuclear facilities of less than 0.2 μSv per year on average.[89] Small additional contributions have occurred in the past from atmospheric nuclear weapons testing and near nuclear weapons installations and certain industrial facilities using radionuclides. Contributions from radon are known to vary dramatically with location, and there is mounting concern about the contribution to lung cancer causation by radon since contaminated dust particles are inhaled and can deposit a significant dose in the bronchial epithelium. The clinical impact of these low-level exposures from environmental sources, and the occupational exposures related to workers in the nuclear industry, is the subject of much research. This research has focused primarily on the question of cancer causation, and the impact on other human diseases is currently not well understood. Although controversial to some, it is generally believed that small incremental increases in cancer risk are associated even with very small doses of radiation, that there is no threshold dose below which there is no risk, and that risk increases linearly with increasing dose.[90]

Medical Sources

Radiation exposure due to medical procedures can be much higher than exposure due to environmental sources, particularly with the use of therapeutic doses of

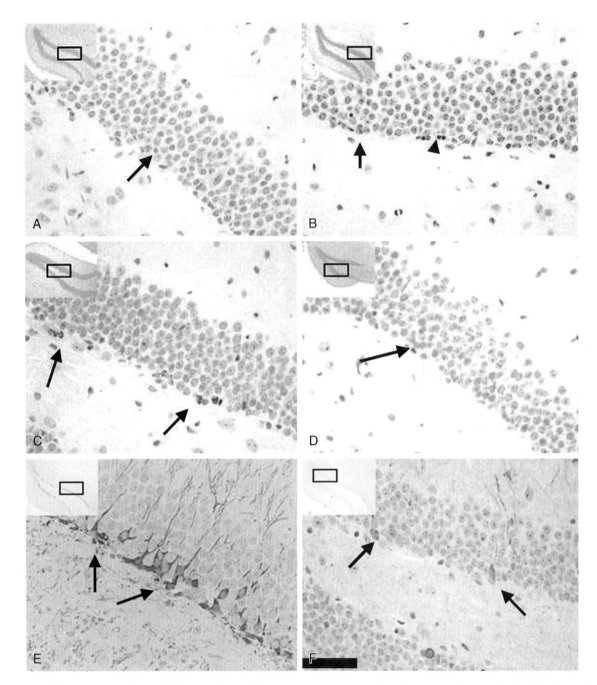

Figure 48-1. Photomicrographs depicting specific cellular responses in mouse dentate gyrus before irradiation *(A, C, and E)* and either 12 hours *(B)* or 48 hours *(D and E)* after 10 Gy. Panels include apoptosis *(A and B)*, proliferating cells (Ki-67; *C and D)*, and immature neurons (Dcx; *E and F)*. The SGZ is a narrow band of cells between the hilus *(H)* and granule cell layer. Apoptotic nuclei are characterized by TUNEL *(arrows, A and B)* or dense chromatin or nuclear fragmentation *(arrowhead, B)*. Although an occasional apoptotic nucleus was seen in tissues from unirradiated mice *(A)*, a significant increase in apoptosis was seen in the SGZ 12 hours after irradiation *(B)*. Proliferating Ki-67-positive cells *(arrows, C)* are spread out within the SGZ in tissues from unirradiated animals; only an occasional Ki-67-positive cell was found after 10 Gy *(D)*. Dcx-positive cells are highly concentrated in the SGZ and lower regions of the granule cell layer of unirradiated mice *(arrows, E)*. After 10 Gy, there are substantially fewer Dcx-positive cells *(F; scale bar = 50 μm)*. All micrographs are ×40. The inset in each panel is a low-power image (×10) of the dentate gyrus; black boxes are the areas photographed at ×40 (see color plate). TUNEL, terminal deoxynucleotidyl transferase–mediated biotin 2′-deoxyuridine 5′-triphosphate nick end labeling. (Mizumatsu S, Monje ML, Morhardt DR, et al. Extreme sensitivity of adult neurogenesis to low doses of x-irradiation. *Can Res.* 2003;63:4021–4027.)

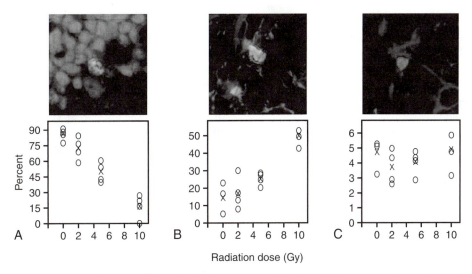

Figure 48-2. Two months after irradiation, cell fate in the dentate gyrus is altered by low to moderate doses of x-rays. Confocal images *(top)* were used to quantify the percentage of BrdUrd-positive cells that coexpressed mature cell markers. Proliferating cells were labeled with BrdUrd (red or orange stain in confocal images), and 3 weeks later, the relative proportion of cells adopting a recognized cell fate was determined as a function of radiation dose *(bottom)*. Neurons (green cells in *A, top*), oligodendrocytes (green cells in *B, top*), and astrocytes (blue cells in *C, top*) were labeled with antibodies against neuron-specific nuclear protein (NeuN), neuron-glial antigen 2 (NG2), and glial fibrillary acidic protein (GFAP) respectively. Each confocal image shows a double-labeled cell. The production of new neurons *(A, bottom)* was reduced dose dependently ($p < 0.001$), whereas there was no apparent change in the production of GFAP with dose *(C, bottom)*. In contrast, the percentage of BrdUrd-positive cells adopting an oligodendrocyte fate *(B, bottom)* appeared to increase, particularly after 10 Gy. In the graphs, each circle represents the value from an individual animal; each X represents the mean value for a given dose group (see color plate). BrdUrd, bromodeoxyuridine. (Mizumatsu S, Monje ML, Morhardt DR, et al. Extreme sensitivity of adult neurogenesis to low doses of x-irradiation. *Can Res.* 2003;63:4021–4027.)

radiation to control malignancy. In therapeutic cases, doses may range from about 500 cGy to 7000 cGy or more, with varying tissues and volumes treated depending on clinical indication. Risks vary widely as well for both carcinogenesis and other clinical sequelae, which are discussed later. Exposure from diagnostic procedures is much lower, in the range of about 0.1 to 12 mSv per imaging procedure. This is felt to produce a small potential risk of carcinogenesis, with multiple studies per year producing a lifetime risk of carcinogenesis on the order of the risk of being killed in a traffic accident at some point in one's life in the United States.[90] In some instances, much higher exposures occur in conjunction with higher-risk procedures involving fluoroscopy, and these risks tend to be more comparable to those associated with therapeutic radiation, including noncancer risks such as severe soft-tissue toxicity.

Nuclear Accidents and Nuclear Weapons

Even greater radiation exposure has been seen associated with nuclear accidents and the bombing of Hiroshima and Nagasaki,[89,91] with people close by accumulating doses producing dramatic clinical sequelae, including acute radiation syndrome (discussed later). Farther from

these events, varying degrees of lower levels of exposure occurred, producing additional carcinogenesis events that have been studied extensively, to produce the overall dose–response data for carcinogenesis over a range of doses.[90] Neurological development disorders including mental retardation, seizure disorders, and poor school performance have been noted in individuals exposed prenatally in Japan.[92–94]

The specter of the dirty bomb from a terrorist attack has become a serious concern in recent years. By definition, this is a bomb designed to disperse radioactive material with the intention of causing panic. Significant exposure from what would likely be a small amount of radioactive material is unlikely. Individuals close to the bomb (perhaps within a few city blocks) may receive more significant exposure, depending on the dispersal mechanism, but clinically significant exposure is not felt to be likely.[95]

GENERAL THERAPEUTIC CONSIDERATIONS

Specific clinical scenarios are discussed in the next section, with therapeutic options for brain, spinal cord, and peripheral nervous system injury. Still, some principles to radiation injury potentially apply to most of these clinical scenarios due to the common mechanisms for radiation injury in different parts of the nervous system. Much of this data has been accumulated from animal studies, with limited clinical experience in many areas. However, some therapies have been rapidly transitioned from animal studies to human clinical cases.

The inflammatory response due to radiation can be moderated by indomethacin in experimental studies.[96] Angiotensin converting enzyme (ACE) inhibitors may play a role here as well,[30,97–99] given the proinflammatory qualities of the angiotensin system.[27,100–104] 3-hydroxy-3-methylglutaryl–coenzyme A reductase inhibitors, commonly called *statins,* have antiinflammatory properties and antioxidant properties[105–107] and increase neurogenesis, with consequent neurological function improvement after injury.[108,109] Protection from radiation-induced impairment of neurogenesis has recently been demonstrated.[27] Superoxide dismutase mimetics are being studied for their ability to reduce oxidative stress in the brain after injury.[110–112] VEGF inhibitors have shown potential for reduction in brain injury in early studies,[113,114] including a preliminary clinical experience after irradiation.[115]

CLINICAL SCENARIOS

Acute Radiation Syndrome

Whole-body exposures to radiation can produce effects in multiple organ systems, including the nervous system. A poorly understood effect of whole-body doses greater than about 50-100 Gy is called the cerebrovascular syndrome, with death occurring within 24 to 48 hours after exposure. Lower doses may cause death via effects on other organ systems, but at these very high dose levels the cerebrovascular characteristics overwhelm the patient rapidly before the other two major acute radiation syndromes (gastrointestinal and hematopoietic). The cerebrovascular syndrome occurs with whole-body exposures at dose levels greater than 50-100 Gy, but much higher doses are required to cause death if the cranium alone is irradiated. Postmortem studies show extensive endothelial cell injury, perivascular hemorrhage, and edema within the CNS.[116,117]

The effects on the CNS at lower whole-body doses can be demonstrated by the impact on electrophysiological, behavioral, and biochemical processes. Induction of proinflammatory cytokines within the CNS after irradiation has been demonstrated and may be implicated in the systemic response that leads to injury in other organs.[118]

Therapy for the Acute Radiation Syndrome

At doses high enough to cause the cerebrovascular syndrome, supportive care is appropriate in this universally and rapidly fatal situation. Lower doses of whole-body exposure may be associated with some chance of survival, and estimation of the dose is necessary to guide management. For this purpose, lymphocytes are obtained from the patient's peripheral blood and examined for certain DNA abnormalities that are specific for given known dose levels. Bone marrow transplants have been used with variable success at certain dose levels. Generally, these patients have been exposed during nuclear accidents, and 24-hour consultative support for these patients is provided by the U.S. Department of Energy's Radiation Emergency Assistance Center/Training Site at (865) 576-1005.[117] This organization also provides valuable training on how to establish an institutional program for radiological decontamination in the emergency setting.

Acute Injury from Nervous System Irradiation (During and Within a Few Weeks of Exposure)

Brain

Common acute neurological sequelae of brain irradiation include fatigue, hearing loss due to fluid in the middle ear, and symptoms of cerebral edema. The symptoms associated with cerebral edema can include headaches, nausea, vomiting, dysequilibrium, and focal symptoms related to the area involved by tumor.

Therapy for Acute Injury in the Brain These symptoms are commonly prevented or controlled with the judicious use of corticosteroids, often requiring high doses that necessitate concurrent prophylaxis against gastric bleeding (e.g., with acid lowering agents), although this is controversial. The likelihood of having more difficulty controlling symptoms is increased with large tumor masses and preexisting significant edema. Consideration for surgical removal of large dominant metastases should be given before radiotherapy if the clinical condition of the patient otherwise supports operative therapy. With primary brain tumors, maximal surgical resection of the tumor is generally considered of primary importance to the overall treatment plan, and debulking large masses that are not completely resectable can be helpful in reducing the likelihood of poorly controlled cerebral edema. Other options for control of cerebral edema in the future may include corticotropin-releasing factor,[119] bevacizumab,[115] AZD2171,[120] and cyclooxygenase-2 inhibitors.[121]

Seizures can occur as focal or generalized manifestations of brain injury by tumor and may be more likely to occur with the additional disturbance introduced by radiotherapy. Anticonvulsants are commonly used to prevent seizures in patients presenting with a seizure but may not be indicated as prophylaxis in patients who have not had a seizure.[122] However, there is evidence of benefit for prophylaxis in the early postoperative period in patients undergoing surgery.[123]

Spinal Cord

Acute problems associated with irradiation of the spinal cord are generally seen only in cases of preexisting spinal canal or cord compromise because of spinal cord encroachment by tumor, preirradiation surgical manipulation, or severe degenerative disease producing severe canal compromise. Exacerbation of preexisting edema by radiation is generally preventable.

Therapy for Acute Injury in the Spinal Cord

Corticosteroids are used both to reduce existing spinal cord edema and to mitigate any edema introduced by irradiation. Again, gastric prophylaxis may be prudent with high-dose steroid use.

Peripheral Nervous System

The peripheral nervous system is not commonly known to demonstrate acute symptoms either during or shortly after radiotherapy.

Early-Delayed or Subacute Injury from Nervous System Irradiation (1 to 6 Months after Irradiation)

Brain

Occasionally, symptoms associated with early demyelination may be observed, such as gait disturbances and dysequilibrium. More commonly, demyelination is incidentally noted on posttreatment imaging, demonstrable by magnetic resonance imaging with increased T_2-signal intensity over large volumes of the brain.

A *somnolence syndrome* has been described primarily in children, with onset within 1 to 2 months after radiotherapy. This common condition has been reported to occur in as many as 40% to 60% of irradiated children.[48,124,125] Typical symptoms include severe drowsiness, anorexia, irritability, nausea, apathy, and dizziness.

Persistent edema with associated symptoms can continue into this time frame, often due to continued effect by an incompletely controlled tumor.

Therapy consists of symptom control and supportive care.

Leukoencephalopathy

Multiple areas of white matter injury, cerebral atrophy, and mineralizing microangiopathy can characterize this entity. Patients present with severe symptoms of spasticity, ataxia, lethargy, seizures, and motor deficits. The risk substantially increases with the use of methotrexate, commonly in children with acute lymphoblastic leukemia. The risk is particularly significant in patients with

overt CNS leukemia as opposed to the risk from treatment in the prophylactic setting.[126]

Therapy for Leukoencephalopathy

Ventriculoperitoneal shunting has been advocated for hydrocephalus with leukoencephalopathy.[127] These patients have a generally poor prognosis, and considerable supportive care is often required.

Spinal Cord

Demyelination within the spinal cord is thought to be the cause of the Lhermitte sign, which is commonly seen when long lengths of spinal cord are irradiated. The sign is elicited with flexion of the neck, producing a sensation of electric shock down the spine and sometimes into the extremities. There is no known relationship between the Lhermitte sign and the later possible development of radiation myelopathy.

Therapy for Subacute Injury in the Spinal Cord

The Lhermitte sign is self-limited, with no specific intervention required other than reassurance to the patient. Other demyelinating diseases such as multiple sclerosis can be associated with this sign.

Peripheral Nervous System

Subacute phenomena related to the peripheral nervous system are not typically described, other than extension of the electric-shock sensation from the spinal cord into the extremities as part of the Lhermitte sign.

Late-Delayed Injury from Nervous System Irradiation (Greater Than 6 Months after Irradiation)

Radiation Carcinogenesis in the Nervous System

A historical discussion of the data supporting radiation-induced tumors in the nervous system has been published previously.[94] These tumors may be benign or malignant and are probably not significantly different in their behavior from their non-radiation-induced counterparts. They are treated in essentially the same way as well, with appropriate consideration to the limitations posed by prior irradiation. They may in some cases be best treated with radiation, with the long latency period of 10 to 20 years allowing abundant time for sufficient recovery from radiation effects in many cases.

Brain

Radiation Necrosis

Radiation necrosis was described as a consequence of radiation therapy more than 50 years ago.[128–132] Typically, radiation necrosis involves a focal radiographic lesion. Some describe a diffuse radiation necrosis,[133] while others describe perhaps the same pattern as necrotizing leukoencephalopathy. Focal lesions tend to occur in the region of the tumor (or in the immediately surrounding high-radiation-dose region), particularly with modern localized radiation.

Imaging for Radiation Necrosis Differentiation of recurrent tumor from radiation necrosis can be difficult, and many imaging modalities have been employed for this purpose:

Magnetic resonance imaging (MRI). MRI continues to be a mainstay in imaging of the nervous system, and some describe specific MRI features of radiation necrosis,[134] but the limitations of conventional MRI

in this disease have led to the use of other imaging techniques, including positron emission tomography, thallium single-photon emission computed tomography, magnetic resonance spectroscopy, magnetic resonance diffusion-weighted imaging, and perfusion-sensitive MRI.[133] The conventional MRI features generally involve irregularly enhancing masses intermixed with areas of low signal suggesting necrosis. Figures 48-3 and 48-4 illustrate the MRI features of radiation necrosis.

Magnetic resonance spectroscopy (MRS). MRS uses imaging characterization of chemical metabolites in areas of interest, with relative levels of certain metabolites (particularly N-acetyl aspartate and choline) generating spectra that are indicative of

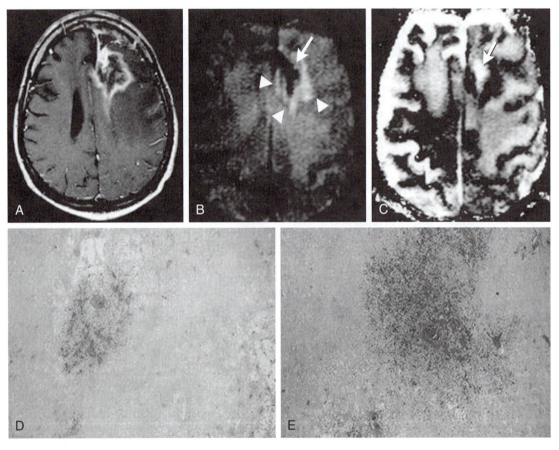

Figure 48-3. Images obtained in a 54-year-old man with biopsy-proven radiation necrosis after receiving radiation and chemotherapy for anaplastic oligodendroglioma. *(A)* Gadolinium-enhanced T$_1$-weighted image shows an irregular ring-enhancing lesion with mass effect. *(B)* Diffusion-weighted image obtained at the same level as panel A shows a mixed signal intensity pattern *(arrowheads),* with marked hypointensity *(arrow),* which is typical for radiation necrosis. Radiation necrosis may have various signal intensity patterns on diffusion-weighted images, reflecting the development of necrosis. Marked diffusion-weighted imaging hypointensity is probably attributable to liquefactions in late-stage necrosis. *(C)* Apparent diffusion coefficient (ADC) map, which corresponds to panel B, shows a mixed signal intensity (SI) pattern, with a markedly high ADC value *(arrow).* *(D and E)* Histopathological specimens (hematoxylin and eosin, ×20, *D,* and ×40, *E*) show total parenchymal necrosis with hemorrhage. No evidence of viable tumor cells was found (see color plate). (Asao C, Korogi Y, Kitajima M, et al. Diffusion-weighted imaging of radiation-induced brain injury for differentiation from tumor recurrence. *Am J Neuroradiol.* 2005;26:1455–1460.)

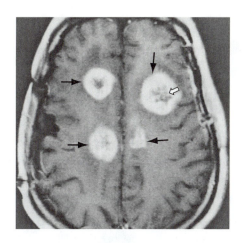

Figure 48-4. Autopsy-proven radiation necrosis within both cerebral hemispheres simulating multiple metastases, tumefactive multiple sclerosis, or both in a 30-year-old man who underwent subtotal resection of a multicentric, nonenhancing anaplastic astrocytoma in the right parietal lobe and left anterior temporal lobe, followed by whole-brain accelerated radiation therapy (60 Gy) and chemotherapy. A postcontrast transverse T_1-weighted spin–echo image (500/17) obtained 17 months after radiation therapy shows multiple enhancing masses *(solid arrows)* within the frontal lobe white matter simulating metastases. Central soap bubble–like areas of necrosis *(open arrow)* were seen within the masses. Autopsy revealed no evidence of tumor, and the histopathological findings showed extensive areas of radiation necrosis that corresponded to the multiple enhancing lesions identified by magnetic resonance imaging. (Kumar AJ, Leeds NE, Fuller GN, et al. Malignant gliomas: MR imaging spectrum of radiation therapy–and chemotherapy-induced necrosis of the brain after treatment. *Radiology.* 2000;217:377–384.)

necrosis, tumor, or normal brain tissue. This technique has proven useful in the identification of radiation necrosis.[135–139]

Perfusion-sensitive MRI. A relative difference in the rate of contrast enhancement occurring in tumor tissue versus treatment effects has produced interest in the perfusion-sensitive MRI technique.[140,141]

Diffusion-weighted MRI. In radiation necrosis, diffusion coefficients are expected to be different from areas of cellular tumor, so the diffusion-weighted MRI technique has been used to differentiate the two.[142,143] Figures 48-3 and 48-5 illustrate how this approach can help differentiate between radiation necrosis (Figure 48-3; see color plate) and recurrent tumor (Figure 48-5; see color plate).

Positron emission tomography (PET). PET produces images of relative metabolic activity in different tissues. Areas of active tumor demonstrate a high signal, indicating high metabolic activity, while areas of necrosis demonstrate a low signal due to low metabolic activity.[144–150]

Thallium single-photon emission computed tomography (SPECT). Another nuclear medicine technique capitalizing on metabolic differences between regions of necrosis and active tumor, thallium SPECT has shown some ability to differentiate between high- and low-grade tumors.[151] It has also shown utility in differentiating between tumor and radiation necrosis,[152] although some reports indicate poor specificity.[153–155]

Which Is Best? Different institutions have different preferences for these various imaging options. PET, thallium SPECT, and MRS are perhaps more commonly used and have been compared, with varying conclusions about which is best.[156–159] In practice, given institutions have their own preference based on technical preferences, as well as cost considerations.

Clinical Picture of Radiation Necrosis Doses of 50 to 60 Gy to partial brain volumes probably produce necrosis in 0.1% to 5% of patients, with conventional fractionation,[124,160–162] although it can be argued that the incidence data are based on limited reporting and that the incidence may be higher as a result of frequent lack of tissue evaluation. In addition, the incidence data available may be based partly on a radiographic impression of necrosis that can be difficult to differentiate from the radiographic appearance of tumor recurrence or progression.[87,133,163] The risk is probably increased with chemotherapy, and chemotherapy when given without radiation has been associated with cerebral necrosis.[164–166]

Higher rates of radiation necrosis are reported in some series associated with other-than-conventional fractionation and doses, as seen in Kumar et al.'s experience with patients treated with accelerated hyperfractionation and concurrent chemotherapy as part of a research protocol.[134] The rate of 24% commonly quoted from this report[87,133,163] of histologically examined specimens included both "pure" radiation necrosis and "predominantly" radiation necrosis. This raises significant questions when malignant gliomas often contain areas of necrosis and when a desired effect of radiation treatment is in fact necrosis of tumor tissue. The widely appreciated infiltrative growth pattern of malignant gliomas and the need to target these tumor extensions with radiotherapy produce a complex scenario for coexisting tumor-produced necrosis and therapy-induced necrosis of both tumor tissue and normal brain tissue. The primary goal of Kumar et al. was to characterize the radiographic correlates of pathologically documented necrosis. In practice, the patient is treated as the clinical condition warrants regardless of the etiology of the imaging findings, and tissue confirmation of the etiology may or may not be pursued if conservative management is felt to be appropriate.

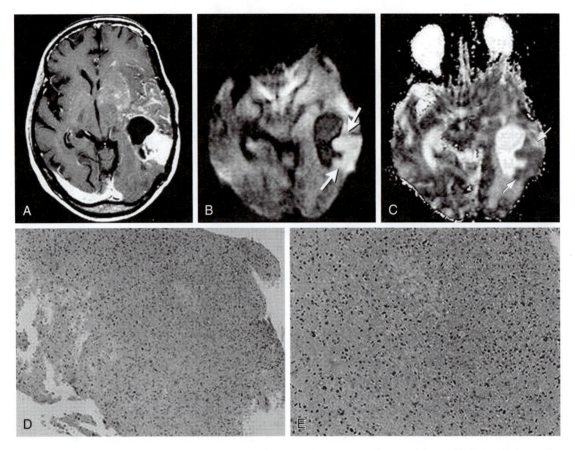

Figure 48-5. Images obtained in a 53-year-old woman with biopsy-proven tumor after receiving radiation and chemotherapy for anaplastic astrocytoma. *(A)* Gadolinium-enhanced T₁-weighted image shows a ring-enhancing lesion with a solid enhancing component in the left temporal lobe. Multiple patchy enhancements with mass effect are also seen in the left basal ganglia and insula, suggestive of tumor infiltration. *(B)* Diffusion-weighted image obtained at the same level as that of panel A shows the solid enhancing component of predominant hyperintensity *(arrows)*, which usually represents densely packed tumor cells. *(C)* ADC map, which shows the relatively low apparent diffusion coefficient value of the lesion *(arrows)*. *(D* and *E)* Histopathological specimens (hematoxylin and eosin, ×20, *D,* and ×80, *E)* show tumor tissues with increased cellular density corresponding to anaplastic astrocytoma. No evidence of necrotic tissue was found (see color plate). (Asao C, Korogi Y, Kitajima M, et al. Diffusion-weighted imaging of radiation-induced brain injury for differentiation from tumor recurrence. *Am J Neuroradiol.* 2005;26:1455–1460.)

The latency period between irradiation and clinical presentation of necrosis is typically 1 to 3 years.[13,167] The latency can be shortened by increasing the dose,[168] particularly the dose per fraction, e.g., with radiosurgery and with interstitial brachytherapy.[169,170]

The clinical picture often involves symptoms of mass effect and can involve severe focal neurological abnormalities related to the size and location of the lesion. Electroencephalogram abnormalities have been observed as well.[161] The clinical course varies from self-limited to relentlessly progressive and even recurrent after surgical resection. Although this entity unquestionably causes significant clinical morbidity and even potentially death, there is some suggestion that survival in patients with glioblastoma may be better in those who develop radionecrosis.[169,171,172]

Therapy for Radiation Necrosis Surgical debulking may be required for symptoms not controlled with conservative treatment, of which the mainstay is corticosteroids. When the diagnosis of radiation necrosis is established, often the patient is already on steroids to control symptoms of mass effect. Consideration for increasing the dose of steroids can be given, as well as the addition of anticoagulant and antiplatelet therapy.[133,173] An important part of this treatment approach is gastrointestinal prophylaxis to address the combined risk of high-dose steroids and anticoagulant therapy.

Hyperbaric oxygen has also been used with limited effect.[174–177] Cyclooxygenase-2 inhibitors have shown possible usefulness in the treatment of radiation necrosis.[121] Drugs that increase blood flow and limit reperfusion injury have shown promise in the rat model.[178]

Targeting VEGF has been hypothesized as a therapeutic option. Endothelial cell injury as the result of radiation produces elevated levels of VEGF as discussed earlier, and promising preliminary results have been seen with the use of the VEGF monoclonal antibody bevacizumab, as illustrated in Figure 48-6.[115]

Multiple studies in rats have investigated the use of amifostine as a radioprotective agent. Varying degrees of benefit (and in some cases no benefit) were seen with differing amifostine doses and radiotherapy schedules in protecting against endpoints including vascular damage, necrosis, and death.[179-182] Additional animal data suggest a role for anti-inflammatory medications used prophylactically.[183-188] Growth factors shown in animals to protect against nervous system damage from radiation include insulin-like growth factor-1, fibroblast growth factor, platelet-derived growth factor, and carbamylated erythropoietin.[189-192]

Cognitive Impairment Much literature has been generated on the subject of cognitive impairment

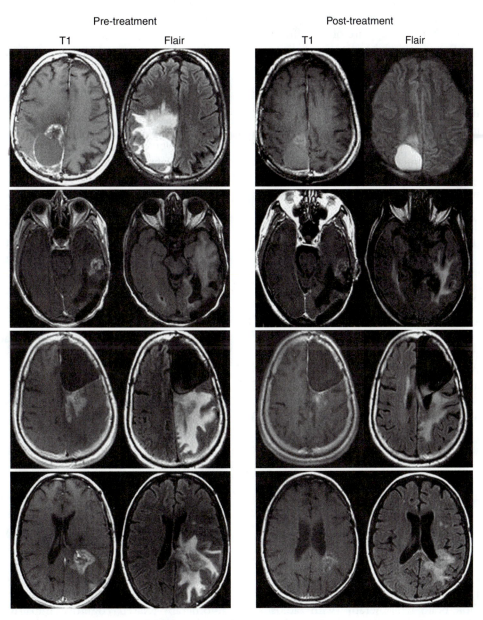

Figure 48-6. Axial gadolinium-enhanced T_1-weighted and fluid-attenuated inversion recovery images of four selected patients (from top to bottom, patients 1, 2, 3, and 5) with radiation necrosis obtained before and after bevacizumab treatment. (Gonzalez J, Kumar AJ, Conrad CA, Levin VA. Effect of bevacizumab on radiation necrosis of the brain. *Int J Radiat Oncol Biol Phys.* 2007;67[2]:323–326.)

associated with radiation therapy to the brain. Some of this literature, particularly older reports, must be interpreted with caution due to outdated treatment techniques that may increase the risk of impairment. Perhaps the most common limitation to accurate delineation of radiation-induced complications in the literature is the variability in confirming the absence of recurrent tumor as the primary cause of symptoms. This is particularly important in the CNS, where tumor control is commonly elusive.

In addition to the cognitive effects associated with brain radiotherapy, many cancer patients are treated with chemotherapy, and chemotherapy may have its own adverse cognitive effects.[193] As with radiotherapy-related effects, the effects of chemotherapy are often difficult to define due to lack of pretreatment baseline data,[193] as well as several other methodological problems present in published studies.[194] Other factors contributing to cognitive decline in brain tumor patients include the common use of corticosteroids and anticonvulsants.[195–198]

Differences in treatment volume undoubtedly play a major role as well. Irradiation of the entire brain is a common approach to treating metastatic disease of the brain and in prophylaxis therapy. Although a great deal of literature has been built on the adverse effects of whole-brain radiotherapy on cognitive function, many of the studies do not report baseline cognitive function before irradiation. Long-term survivors of prophylactic cranial irradiation in small-cell lung cancer represent an oft-studied clinical group, and often long-term cognitive decline in these patients is used as the strongest evidence for an adverse impact due to irradiation. In two randomized studies addressing the effectiveness of irradiation in these patients, baseline cognitive tests were performed and then followed as part of the study design. In both the irradiated and the nonirradiated groups, cognitive deficits were identified at baseline. Cognitive decline was seen in both groups of patients, with no difference seen in the irradiated and non-irradiated groups over 1 to 2 years.[199,200] This period of observation may have been too short to discriminate a difference between the two groups.

In patients treated with whole-brain radiotherapy for clinically overt brain metastases, much of the concern for adverse cognitive effects arises from a study published in 1989 reporting on 12 patients treated with higher daily fraction sizes than are currently used, with cases selected from two large cohorts, producing an incidence of 1.9% to 5.1%.[201] The only randomized data addressing this issue showed no difference in neurological toxicity (including limited neurocognitive evaluation) in patients treated with whole-brain radiotherapy (with radiosurgery boost) versus radiosurgery alone.[202] Concern for neurocognitive impairment with whole-brain radiation is often used by advocates of radiosurgery alone in the management of limited brain metastases.[203–205]

Cognitive decline does appear to be common in patients with brain tumors, even though the relative contribution of brain irradiation continues to be debatable. An important contributing factor to cognitive decline in these patients is injury due to the malignancy itself. An analysis of patients treated with radiosurgery for brain metastases, with the goal of avoiding toxicity expected from whole-brain irradiation, showed that patients treated in this way had a high frequency of symptomatic recurrence within the brain, often associated with neurological deficits.[206] In high-grade glioma patients, typically treated with partial brain irradiation, decline in cognitive function in irradiated patients has been shown to precede radiographically apparent tumor progression, with stability in cognitive function seen in patients who continue to demonstrate tumor control.[207] Others support the important impact of tumor progression on cognitive decline and, at least in short-term follow-up, note the absence of decline due to the radiotherapy itself.[208,209]

Children clearly have greater sensitivity than do adults for the adverse effects of radiation on neurocognitive function. Data for children treated for tinea capitis demonstrated a small degree of neurocognitive impairment even with very low doses of radiation to the brain, with a mean dose to neural tissue of only 150 cGy.[210–212] A large volume of literature supports neurocognitive impairment in children treated prophylactically for acute lymphoblastic leukemia with modest doses in the range of 2400 cGy in conventional fractionation, particularly associated with methotrexate treatment.[213–215] In these patients, memory deficits, diminished mental processing speed, and difficulty acquiring new knowledge have been described.[216–218] Others note poorer academic achievement, greater psychological stress, and poorer self-image.[219] Impairment has been more severe in children treated for CNS tumors, requiring higher doses than acute lymphoblastic leukemia prophylaxis, most dramatically for children younger than 3 years and when larger volumes are treated.[217,219]

Imaging correlates of cognitive injury from radiation include the use of MRS, with some reporting MRS abnormalities in patients with cognitive dysfunction[220,221]; others did not identify an association.[222] It has been suggested that MRS abnormalities may be a more sensitive measure of radiation injury than typical cognitive testing.[223]

Therapy for Radiation-induced Cognitive Impairment

Several possible approaches toward treating or preventing radiotherapy-related cognitive impairment have been proposed. Excluding the portions of the brain that are thought to be the source for stem cells (the hippocampus) from the radiation treatment volume has been considered.[224] The use of drugs that affect the renin–angiotensin system are another possibility.[99] Drugs that reduce cerebral ischemic damage or that reduce delayed radiation injury in other organs may represent additional possibilities.[225]

Donepezil, a reversible acetylcholinesterase inhibitor used in the treatment of Alzheimer's dementia, was studied in a phase II trial to assess the impact on cognitive functioning, mood, and quality of life in primary brain tumor patients treated with radiation. Improvements in each of these areas were noted in this preliminary study, and a Phase III trial is planned.[85] In animal studies, the ACE inhibitor ramipril has recently been shown to limit the impact of radiation on neurogenesis in the dentate gyrus.[98] A particularly intriguing possibility is the use of neurogenesis manipulation to repair radiation injury.[226]

Another agent showing potential benefit in preventing cognitive decline is motexafin gadolinium, with prolongation of time to neurological progression and neurocognitive decline in patients with brain metastases treated with radiation.[209] Hyperbaric oxygen has been studied in humans as a treatment for cognitive impairment with limited success.[227]

Pediatric patients have shown cognitive improvements with neurocognitive remediation approaches.[228] Cognitive behavioral therapy and some drug therapy are being offered to these patients, although the underlying mechanisms are poorly understood.[193]

Optic Neuropathy and Retinopathy

Retinopathy can occur following radiation,[229] and the risk is increased with hypertension, diabetes, and chemotherapy.[230] Radiation doses in excess of 6000 cGy and higher than conventional fraction sizes predispose to this complication.[230] I have observed this complication in doses as low as 2400 cGy in conventional fractionation in a patient treated for Grave's ophthalmopathy (Pimperl, unpublished data).

Optic neuropathy and other cranial neuropathies are generally rare with modern careful planning incorporating computerized tomography and MRI. Optic neuropathy is particularly dependent on fraction size and has been one of the key clinical entities in the driving force to avoid large fraction sizes in irradiation of the CNS. Cases generally are seen only with total doses greater than 5000 cGy with conventional fractionation,[231] and some report no instances of clinically significant optic neuropathy below 6000 cGy.[232] The time of onset is generally greater than about 1 year, but a case has been reported with onset as early as 3 months.[233] Visual loss is often rapidly progressive. MRI can show areas of focal discrete enhancement along the optic nerve. A dramatic case of radiation necrosis involving the optic nerves, chiasm, and tracts associated with accelerated hyperfractionation and concurrent chemotherapy was included in the report of Kumar et al.[134]

Therapy for Optic Neuropathy Experimental studies in rats have demonstrated a favorable impact on optic neuropathy with the use of the ACE inhibitor ramipril.[30,97] Intravitreal instillation of bevacizumab has shown benefit in a clinical case report.[234]

Endocrine Dysfunction

Irradiation of the hypothalamus and pituitary gland can lead to endocrine abnormalities, with hypothyroidism, hypogonadism, and hyperprolactinemia being common in some studies[235,236] and probably underdiagnosed.[235]

Spinal Cord

Radiation Myelopathy

Radiation myelopathy is rare at doses below 5000 cGy, and the dose required to produce a 5% risk of causing this dreaded complication is probably near 6000 cGy[6,237] with conventional fractionation. If other-than-conventional fraction sizes are used, the dose levels required to produce this risk are different, and in practice there are well-defined methods to adjust prescribed doses accordingly to maintain a low risk. In general, radiation oncologists are conservative in this area and tend to keep spinal cord doses below 5000 or even below 4500 cGy in conventional fractionation,[237] with the result that this complication is rarely seen in modern practice. In cases of metastatic disease to the spine, larger fraction sizes are commonly used, with acceptable risk when appropriate adjustment for total dose is made.[238] Although once strongly avoided, retreatment of the spinal cord with radiation after adequate recovery has been supported by extensive animal data[6] and with evolving clinical experience.[239] Risk of injury is felt to be greater in patients treated with concurrent chemotherapy and perhaps with diseases such as hypertension, diabetes, and vascular disease. Risk is likely increased with prior trauma due to severe extrinsic tumor compression and vascular compromise, surgical manipulation, and tumors intrinsic to the spinal cord.

Patients may present with any combination of motor and sensory deficits related to the level of spinal cord injury. Similar symptoms can be produced from other causes, most commonly due to tumor progression. The latency period for radiation myelitis is generally greater than 6 months but may be shorter with larger doses per fraction. MRI may show low T_1-signal intensity, a high T_2-signal, cord swelling, and areas of enhancement.[240] The MRI features may not be consistent with the clinical picture in some cases.[241] Pathological features include varying combinations of vascular and myelin injury. Some report predominantly vascular findings,[242] while there is at least one report in humans of myelin injury in the absence of vascular injury.[243] Ultimately, the diagnosis may be challenging to differentiate from other causes of myelopathy.[88]

Therapy for Radiation Myelopathy Commonly, corticosteroids are used to decrease cord edema. Hyperbaric oxygen has been used with mixed results.[175,244] Its use has been advocated on the basis of poor alternatives in this difficult situation.[245] Heparin and warfarin have been used successfully.[173,246] The outcome in radiation myelopathy is typically poor,[88] particularly in cases with complete cord transection.[6] Somewhat better results have been reported with incomplete transection.[243]

Peripheral Nervous System

Plexopathy is unlikely below doses of 60 Gy in conventional fractionation. Typical symptoms range from paresthesias to complete sensory and/or motor deficits in the involved extremity. The presence of pain is suggestive of tumor recurrence, although radiation-induced plexopathy can also be associated with pain.

Brachial Plexopathy
Brachial plexopathy is an uncommon sequela of treatment for breast cancer and Hodgkin's disease.[247–249] Lymphedema is often coexisting, with paresthesias and progressing motor deficits distal to the injury. The presence of pain may be more suggestive of malignancy than radiation injury, although pain can occur in both. Lower plexus involvement usually suggests malignancy, since most cases of radiation plexopathy involve the upper plexus. The latency is as long as several years or as short as a few months.[247,250,251] Imaging findings may include thickening and enhancement of the plexus without an associated mass on MRI, and a low T_2-signal differentiates this entity from tumor infiltration, which generally involves a high T_2-signal.[252] Both tumor infiltration and radiation plexopathy can demonstrate some degree of enhancement with gadolinium, making this component of imaging less useful in differentiating the two.[253]

Therapy for Brachial Plexopathy A small randomized trial investigating the impact of hyperbaric oxygen in brachial plexopathy showed no benefit over the control group.[254] Heparin and warfarin have been used with some success.[173]

Sacral Plexopathy
Radiotherapy for pelvic malignancies rarely produces sacral plexopathy.[255,256] The clinical picture is analogous to that of brachial plexopathy, with similar importance of differentiating between radiation injury and recurrent tumor.[257,258]

Peripheral Neuropathy
Peripheral neuropathy beyond the named plexuses is rarely reported as a consequence of radiation therapy.[259] Paresthesias are presumably related to demyelinating injury. Radiation-induced fibrosis can cause chronic neuropathic pain.[260] Symptom-directed therapy is appropriate.

CONCLUSION

Radiation-induced nervous system injury presents a challenging diagnostic and therapeutic picture to the clinician. Understanding of the basic underlying mechanisms is rapidly evolving, and novel therapeutic approaches are being investigated both in animals and in clinical studies. Potential exposure of the nervous system to radiation comes from various sources, including the medical application of radiation for therapeutic purposes, as well as various generally low-level environmental exposures. Therapeutic options for common radiation injury scenarios are limited, although intense research has produced several possibilities for the future.

REFERENCES

1. Karipidis KK, Benke G, Sim MR, et al. Occupational exposure to ionizing and non-ionizing radiation and risk of glioma. *Occup Med (Lond)*. 2007;57(7):518–524.
2. International Agency for Research on Cancer. Non-ionizing radiation: I. Static and extremely low-frequency (ELF) electric and magnetic fields. vol 80. France: World Health Organization; 2002.
3. Ahlbom A, Cardis E, Green A, et al. Review of the epidemiologic literature on EMF and health. *Environ Health Perspect*. 2001;109(Suppl 6):911–933.
4. Schüz J, Jacobsen R, Olsen JH, et al. Cellular telephone use and cancer risk: an update of a nationwide Danish cohort. *J Natl Cancer Inst*. 2006;98:1707–1713.
5. Zhao T-Y, Zou S-P, Knapp PE. Exposure to cell phone radiation up-regulates apoptosis genes in primary cultures of neurons and astrocytes. *Neurosci Lett*. 2007;412(1):34–38.
6. Schultheiss TE, Kun LE, Ang KK, Stephens LC. Radiation response of the central nervous system. *Int J Radiat Oncol Biol Phys*. 1995;31(5):1093–1112.
7. Fajardo LF, Berthrong M, Anderson RE. *Radiation Pathology*. New York: Oxford University Press; 2002:351–363.
8. Gillette EL, Mahler PA, Powers BE, et al. Late radiation injury to muscle and peripheral nerves. *Int J Radiat Oncol Bio Phys*. 1995;31:1309–1318.
9. Butler RW, Hill JM, Steinherz PG, et al. Neuropsychological effects of cranial irradiation, intrathecal methotrexate, and systemic methotrexate in childhood cancer. *J Clin Oncol*. 1994;12:2621–2629.
10. Abayoma OK. Pathogenesis of irradiation-induced cognitive dysfunction. *Acta Oncol*. 1996;35:659–663.
11. Crossen J, Garwood D, Glasein E, et al. Neurobehavioral sequelae of cranial irradiation in adults: a review of radiation-induced encephalopathy. *J Clin Oncol*. 1994;12(3):627–642.
12. Tofilon PJ, Fike JR. The radioresponse of the central nervous system: a dynamic process. *Radiat Res*. 2000;153:357–370.
13. Nieder C, Andratschke N, Astner ST. Experimental concepts for toxicity prevention and tissue restoration after central nervous system irradiation. *Radiat Oncol*. 2007;2(23).
14. Nordal RA, Wong CS. Molecular targets in radiation-induced blood–brain barrier disruption. *Int J Radiat Oncol Biol Phys*. 2005;62(1):279–287.

15. Calvo W, Hopewell JW, Reinhold HS, Yeung TK. Time- and dose-related changes in the white matter of the rat brain after single doses of x-rays. *Br J Radiol.* 1988;61:1043–1052.

16. Reinhold HS, Calvo W, Hopewell JW, van den Berg AP. Development of blood vessel–related radiation damage in the fimbria of the central nervous system. *Int J Radiat Oncol Biol Phys.* 1990;18:37–42.

17. Ljubimova NV, Levitman MK, Plotnikova ED, Eidus LK. Endothelial cell population dynamics in rat brain after local irradiation. *Br J Radiol.* 1991;64:934–940.

18. Hopewell JW, van der Kogel AJ. Pathophysiological mechanisms leading to the development of late radiation-induced damage to the central nervous system. *Front Radiat Ther Oncol.* 1999;33:265–275.

19. Schultheiss TE, Stephens LC. Permanent radiation myelopathy. *Br J Radiol.* 1992;65:737–753.

20. Mastaglia FL, McDonald WI, Watson JV, Yogendran K. Effects of x-radiation on the spinal cord: an experimental study of the morphological changes in central nerve fibres. *Brain.* 1976;99:101–122.

21. Lutz PL. Mechanisms for anoxic survival in the vertebrate brain. *Annu Rev Physiol.* 1992;54:601–618.

22. Morris GM, Coderre JA, Bywaters A, et al. Boron neutron capture irradiation of the rat spinal cord: histopathological evidence of a vascular-mediated pathogenesis. *Radiat Res.* 1996;146:313–320.

23. Coderre JA, Morris GM, Micca PL, et al. Late effects of radiation on the central nervous system: role of vascular endothelial damage and glial stem cell survival. *Radiat Res.* 2006;166:495–503.

24. Logan A, Berry M. Transforming growth factor β1 and basic fibroblast growth factor in the injured CNS. *Trends Pharmacol Sci.* 1993;14:337–343.

25. Tsao MN, Li YQ, Lu G, et al. Upregulation of vascular endothelial growth factor is associated with radiation-induced blood–spinal cord barrier disruption. *J Neuropathol Exp Neurol.* 1999;58:1051–1060.

26. Chiang CS, Hong JH, Stadler A, et al. Delayed molecular responses to brain irradiation. *Int J Radiat Biol.* 1997;72:45–53.

27. Kim JH, Brown SL, Jenrow KA, Ryu S. Mechanisms of radiation-induced brain toxicity and implications for future clinical trials. *J Neurooncol.* 2008. online prepublication.

28. Ljubimova N, Hopewell JW. Experimental evidence to support the hypothesis that damage to vascular endothelium plays the primary role in the development of late radiation-induced CNS injury. *Br J Radiol.* 2004;77:488–492.

29. Robbins MEC, Zhao W. Chronic oxidative stress and radiation-induced late normal tissue injury: a review. *Int J Radiat Biol.* 2004;80:251–259.

30. Kim JH, Brown SL, Kolozsvary A, et al. Modification of radiation injury by ramipril, inhibitor of angiotensin-converting enzyme, on optic neuropathy in the rat. *Radiat Res.* 2004;161:137–142.

31. Li Y-Q, Ballinger JR, Nordal RA, et al. Hypoxia in radiation-induced blood–spinal cord barrier breakdown. *Cancer Res.* 2001;61(8):3348–3354.

32. Nordal RA, Nagy A, Pintilie M, Wong CS. Hypoxia and hypoxia-inducible factor-1 target genes in central nervous system radiation injury: a role for vascular endothelial growth factor. *Clin Cancer Res.* 2004;10:3342–3353.

33. Raff M, Miller R, Noble M. A glial progenitor cell that develops in vitro into an astrocyte or an oligodendrocyte depending on culture medium. *Nature.* 1983;303:390–396.

34. Van der Maazen RW, Kleiboer BJ, Verhagen I, van der Kogel AJ. Irradiation in vitro discriminates between different O-2A progenitor cell subpopulations in the perinatal central nervous system of rats. *Radiat Res.* 1991;128:64–72.

35. Van der Maazen RW, Verhagen I, Kleiboer BJ, van der Kogel AJ. Radiosensitivity of glial progenitor cells of the perinatal and adult rat optic nerve studied by an in vitro clonogenic assay. *Radiother Oncol.* 1991;20:258–264.

36. Van der Maazen RWM, Kleiboer BJ, Berhagen I, van der Kogel AJ. Repair capacity of adult rat glial progenitor cells determined by an in vitro clonogenic assay after in vitro or in vivo fractionated irradiation. *Int J Radiat Biol.* 1993;63:661–666.

37. Smith KJ, Kapoor R, Felts PA. Demyelination: the role of reactive oxygen and nitrogen species. *Brain Pathol.* 1999;9:69–92.

38. Chiang CS, McBride WH, Withers HR. Radiation-induced astrocytic and microglial responses in mouse brain. *Radiother Oncol.* 1993;29:60–68.

39. Schroeter ML, Mertsch K, Giese H, et al. Astrocytes enhance radical defence in capillary endothelial cells constituting the blood–brain barrier. *FEBS Lett.* 1999;449:241–244.

40. Wilson JX. Antioxidant defense of the brain: a role for astrocytes. *Can J Physiol Pharmacol.* 1997;75:1149–1163.

41. Iwata-Ichikawa E, Kondo Y, Miyazake I, et al. Glial cells protect neurons against oxidative stress via transcriptional up-regulation of the glutathione synthesis. *J Neurochem.* 1999;72:2334–2344.

42. Ijichi A, Sakuma S, Tofilon PJ. Hypoxia-induced vascular endothelial growth factor expression in normal rat astrocyte cultures. *Glia.* 1995;14:87–93.

43. Hong-Brown LQ, Brown CR. Cytokine and insulin regulation of β₂ macroglobulin, angiotensinogen and hsp70 in primary cultured astrocytes. *Glia.* 1994;12:211–218.

44. Janzer RC, Raff MC. Astrocytes induce blood–brain barrier properties in endothelial cells. *Nature.* 1987;325:253–257.

45. Schultheiss TE, Stephens LC, Maor MH. Analysis of the histopathology of radiation myelopathy. *Int J Radiat Oncol Biol Phys.* 1988;14:27–32.

46. Mildenberger M, Beach TB, McGeer EG, Ludgate CM. An animal model of prophylactic cranial irradiation: histologic effects at acute, early and delayed stages. *Int J Radiat Oncol Biol Phys.* 1990;18:1051–1060.

47. Nakagawa M, Bellinzona M, Seilhan TM, et al. Microglial responses after focal radiation-induced injury are affected by α-difluoromethylornithine. *Int J Radiat Oncol Biol Phys.* 1996;36:113–123.

48. Dropcho E. Central nervous system injury by therapeutic irradiation. *Neurol Clin.* 1991;9(4):969–988.

49. Duffner P, Cohen M. Long-term consequences of CNS treatment for childhood cancer: II. Clinical consequences. *Pediatr Neurol.* 1991;7(4):237–242.

50. Einhorn L. The case against prophylactic cranial irradiation in limited small cell lung cancer. *Semin Radiat Oncol.* 1995;5(1):57–60.

51. Ahles T, Silberfarb P, Herndon J, et al. Psychologic and neuropsychologic functioning of patients with limited small-cell lung cancer treated with chemotherapy and radiation therapy with or without warfarin: a study by the cancer and leukemia group B. *J Clin Oncol.* 1998;16(5):1954–1960.

52. Senzer N. Rationale for a phase III study of erythropoietin as a neurocognitive protectant in patients with lung cancer receiving prophylactic cranial irradiation. *Semin Oncol.* 2002;12(3):47–52.

53. Gangloff H, Haley TJ. Effects of x-irradiation on spontaneous and evoked brain electrical activity in cats. *Radiat Res.* 1960;12:694–704.

54. Pellmar TC, Lepinski DL. Gamma radiation (5–10 Gy) impairs neuronal function in the guinea pig hippocampus. *Radiat Res.* 1993;136:255–261.

55. Enokido Y, Araki T, Tanaka S, et al. Involvement of p53 in DNA strand break-induced apoptosis in post-mitotic CNS neurons. *Eur J Neurosci.* 1996;8:1812–1821.

56. Noel F, Tofilon PJ. Astrocytes protect against x-ray-induced neuronal toxicity in vitro. *Neuroreport.* 1998;9:1133–1137.

57. Gobbel GT, Bellinzona M, Vogt AR, et al. Response of post-mitotic neurons to x-irradiation: implications for the role of DNA damage in neuronal apoptosis. *J Neurosci.* 1998;18:147–155.

58. Chiang CS, McBride WH. Radiation enhances tumor necrosis factor-α production by murine brain cells. *Brain Res.* 1991;566:265–269.

59. Moore AH, Olschowka JA, Williams JP, et al. Regulation of prostaglandin E2 synthesis after brain irradiation. *Int J Radiat Oncol Biol Phys.* 2005;62:267–272.

60. Hayakawa K, Borchardt PE, Sakuma S, et al. Microglial cytokine gene induction after irradiation is affected by morphologic differentiation. *Radiat Med.* 1997;15:405–410.

61. Morshead CM, Reynolds BA, Craig CG, et al. Neural stem cells in the adult mammalian forebrain: a relatively quiescent subpopulation of subependymal cells. *Neuron.* 1994;13:1071–1082.

62. Morshead CM, van der Kooy D. In vivo clonal analyses reveal the properties of endogenous neural stem cell proliferation in the adult mammalian forebrain. *Development.* 1992;125:2251–2261.

63. Gage FH, Ray J, Fisher LJ. Isolation, characterization and use of stem cells from the CNS. *Annu Rev Neurosci.* 1995;18:159–192.

64. Gritti A, Parati EA, Cova L, et al. Multipotential stem cells from the adult mouse brain proliferate and self-renew in response to basic fibroblast growth factor. *J Neurosci.* 1996;16:1091–1100.

65. Doetsch F, Garcia-Verdugo JM, Asvarez-Buylla A. Cellular composition and three-dimensional organization of the subventricular germinal zone in the adult mammalian brain. *J Neurosci.* 1997;17:5046–5061.

66. Gould E, Beylin A, Tanapat P, et al. Learning enhances adult neurogenesis in the hippocampal formation. *Nat Neurosci.* 1999;2:260–265.

67. Van Praag H, Christie BR, Sejnowski TJ, Gage FH. Running enhances neurogenesis, learning, and long-term potentiation in mice. *Proc Natl Acad Sci USA.* 1999;96:13427–13431.

68. Hopewell JW, Cavanath JB. Effects of x-irradiation on the mitotic activity of the subependymal plate of rats. *Br J Radiol.* 1972;45:461–465.

69. Cavanagh JB, Hopewell JW. Mitotic activity in the subependymal plate of rats and the long-term consequences of x-irradiation. *J Neurosci.* 1972;15:471–482.

70. Hubbard BM, Hopewell JW. Quantitative changes in cellularity of the rat subependymal plate after x-irradiation. *Cell Tissue Kinet.* 1980;13:403–413.

71. Andres-Mach M, Rola R, Fike JR. Radiation effects on neural precursor cells in the dentate gyrus. *Cell Tissue Res.* 2008;331(1):251–262.

72. Fike JR, Rola R, Limoli CL. Radiation response of neural precursor cells. *Neurosurg Clin N Am.* 2007;18(1):115–127.

73. Monje M, Palmer T. Radiation injury and neurogenesis. *Curr Opin Neurol.* 2003;16:129–134.

74. Giedzinski E, Rola R, Fike JR, Limoli CL. Efficient production of reactive oxygen species in neural precursor cells after exposure to 250 MeV protons. *Radiat Res.* 2005;164(4 Pt 2):540–544.

75. Rola R, Sarkissian V, Obenaus A, et al. High-LET radiation induces inflammation and persistent changes in markers of hippocampal neurogenesis. *Radiat Res.* 2005;164(4 Pt 2):556–560.

76. Mizumatsu S, Monje ML, Morhardt DR, et al. Extreme sensitivity of adult neurogenesis to low doses of x-irradiation. *Can Res.* 2003;63:4021–4027.

77. Madsen TM, Kristjansen PE, Bolwig TG, et al. Arrested neuronal proliferation and impaired hippocampal function following fractionated brain irradiation in the adult rat. *Neuroscience.* 2003;119:635–642.

78. Raber J, Rola R, LeFevour A, et al. Radiation-induced cognitive impairments are associated with changes in indicators of hippocampal neurogenesis. *Radiat Res.* 2004;162:39–47.

79. Limoli CL, Giedzinski E, Baure J, et al. Altered growth and radiosensitivity in neural precursor cells subjected to oxidative stress. *Int J Radiat Oncol Biol Phys.* 2006;82(9):640–647.

80. Limoli CL, Giedzinski E, Baure J, et al. Redox changes induced in hippocampal precursor cells by heavy ion irradiation. *Radiat Environ Biophys.* 2007;46(2):167–172.

81. Fan Y, Liu Z, Weinstein PR, et al. Environmental enrichment enhances neurogenesis and improves functional outcome after cranial irradiation. *Eur J Neurosci.* 2007;25(1):38–46.

82. Rola R, Zou Y, Huang TT, et al. Lack of extracellular superoxide dismutase (EC-SOD) in the microenvironment impacts radiation-induced changes in neurogenesis. *Free Radic Biol Med.* 2007;42(8):1131–1145.

83. Limoli CL, Giedzinski E, Buare J, et al. Using superoxide dismutase/catalase mimetics to manipulate the redox environment of neural precursor cells. *Radiat Prot Dosimetry.* 2006;122(1–4):228–236.

84. Tikka T, Usenius T, Tenehumen M, et al. Tetracycline derivatives and ceftriaxone, a cephalosporin antibiotic, protect neurons against apoptosis induced by ionizing radiation. *J Neurochem.* 2001;78:1409–1414.

85. Shaw EG, Rosdhal R, D'Agostino RB, et al. Phase II study of donepezil in irradiated brain tumor patients: effect on cognitive function, mood and quality of life. *J Clin Oncol.* 2006;24(9):1415–1420.

86. Dimberg Y, Vazquez M, Soderstrom S, et al. Effects of x-irradiation on nerve growth factor in the developing mouse brain. *Toxicol Lett.* 1997;90:35–43.

87. Cross NE, Glantz MJ. Neurologic complications of radiation therapy. *Neurol Clin N Am.* 2003;21:249–277.

88. De Seze J, Stojkovic T, Breteau G, et al. Acute myelopathies: clinical, laboratory and outcome profiles in 79 cases. *Brain.* 2001;124:1509–1521.

89. Scientific Committee on the Effects of Atomic Radiation. 2000 Report. New York: United Nations; 2000:2–17.

90. National Research Council Committee. Health Risks from Exposure to Low Levels of Ionizing Radiation: Beir VII—Phase II. Executive Summary. Washington, DC: National Academies Press; 2006.

91. Scientific Committee on the Effects of Atomic Radiation. 2000 Annex J. New York: United Nations; 2000:451–466.

92. Otake M, Yoshimaru H, Schull W. Severe Mental Retardation among the Prenatally Exposed Survivors of the Atomic Bombing of Hiroshima and Nagasake: A Comparison of the T65DR and DS86 Dosimetry Systems. Hiroshima: Radiation Effects Research Foundation; 1987:TR 16–87.

93. Dunn K, Yoshimaru H, Otake M, et al. Prenatal exposure to ionizing radiation and subsequent development of seizures. *Am J Epidemiol.* 1990;131(1):114–123.

94. Pimperl LC. Radiation as a nervous system toxin. *Neurol Clin.* 2005;23:571–597.

95. United States Nuclear Regulatory Commission. Fact Sheet on Dirty Bombs. Washington; DC: Office of Public Affairs; March 2003.

96. Monje ML, Mizumatsu S, Fike JR, et al. Irradiation induces neural precursor-cell dysfunction. *Nat Med.* 2003;8:955–962.

97. Ryu S, Kolozsvary A, Jenrow KA, et al. Mitigation of radiation-induced optic neuropathy in rats by ACE inhibitor ramipril: importance of ramipril dose and treatment. *J Neurooncol.* 2007; 82:119–124.

98. Jenrow K, Liu J, Kolozsvary A, et al. Ramipril mitigates radiation-induced impairment of dentate gyrus neurogenesis. Abstract 4132. 13th International Congress of Radiation Research, July 8-12, 2007, San Francisco.

99. Robbins MEC, Diz DI. Pathogenic role of the rennin-angiotensin system (RAS) in modulating radiation-induced late effects. *Int J Radiat Oncol Biol Phys.* 2006;64:6–12.

100. Liu YH, Yang XP, Sharov VG, et al. Effects of angiotensin-converting enzyme inhibitors and angiotensin II type 1 receptor antagonists in rats with heart failure: role of kinins and angiotensin II type 2 receptors. *J Clin Invest.* 1997;99:1926–1935.

101. Nakajima M, Hutchinson HG, Fujinaga M, et al. The angiotensin II type 2 (AT2) receptor antagonizes the growth effects of the AT1 receptor antagonizes the growth effects of the AT1 receptor: gain-of-function study using gene transfer. *Proc Natl Acad Sci USA.* 1995;92:10663–10667.

102. Griendling KK, Minieri CA, Ollerenshaw JD, et al. Angiotensin II stimulates NADPH and NADPH oxidase activity in cultured vascular smooth muscle cells. *Circ Res.* 1994;74:1141–1148.

103. Mehta JL, Hu B, Chen J, et al. Pioglitazone inhibits LOX-1 expression in human coronary artery endothelial cells by reducing intracellular superoxide radical generation. *Arterioscler Thromb Vasc Biol.* 2003;23:2203–2208.

104. Tojo A, Onozato ML, Kobayashi N, et al. Angiotensin II and oxidative stress in Dahl salt-sensitive rat with heart failure. *Hypertension.* 2002;40:834–839.

105. Haendeler J, Hoffman J, Zeiher A, et al. Antioxidant effects of statins via S-nitrosylation and activation of thioredoxin in endothelial cells. *Circulation.* 2004;110:856–861.

106. Shishehbor MH, Brennan ML, Aviles RJ, et al. Statins promote potent systemic anti-oxidant effects through specific inflammatory pathways. *Circulation.* 2003;108:426–431.

107. Diomede L, Albani D, Sottocorno M, et al. In vivo anti-inflammatory effect of statins is mediated by non-sterol mevalonate products. *Arterioscler Throm Vasc Biol.* 2001; 21:1327–1332.

108. Lu D, Goussev A, Chen J, et al. Atorvastatin reduces neurological deficit and increases synaptogenesis, angiogenesis, and neuronal survival in rats subjected to traumatic brain injury. *J Neurotrauma.* 2004;21:21–32.

109. Lu D, Qu C, Goussev A, et al. Statins increase neurogenesis in the dentate gyrus, reduce delayed neuronal death in the hippocampal CA3 region, and improve spatial learning in rat after traumatic brain injury. *J Neurotrauma.* 2007;24:1132–1146.

110. Imaizumi S, Woolworth V, Fishman RA, et al. Liposome-entrapped superoxide dismutase reduces cerebral infarction in cerebral ischemia in rats. *Stroke.* 1990;21:1312–1327.

111. He YY, Hsu CY, Ezrin AM, et al. Polyethylene glycol–conjugated superoxide dismutase in focal cerebral ischemia–reperfusion. *Am J Physiol.* 1993;265:H252–H256.

112. Liu R, Liu IY, Bi X, et al. Reversal of age-related learning deficits and brain oxidative stress in mice with superoxide dismutase/catalase mimetics. *Proc Natl Acad Sci USA.* 2003;100:8526–8531.

113. Van Bruggen N, Thigbodeaux H, Palmer JT, et al. VEGF antagonism reduces edema formation and tissue damage after ischemia/reperfusion injury in the mouse brain. *J Clin Invest.* 1999;104:1613–1620.

114. Winkler F, Kozin SV, Tong RT, et al. Kinetics of vascular normalization by VEGFR2 blockade governs brain tumor response to radiation: role of oxygenation, angiopoietin-1, and matrix metalloproteinases. *Cancer Cell.* 2004;6:553–563.

115. Gonzalez J, Kumar AJ, Conrad CA, Levin VA. Effect of bevacizumab on radiation necrosis of the brain. *Int J Radiat Oncol Biol Phys.* 2007;67(2):323–326.

116. Fajardo LF, Berthrong M, Anderson RE. *Radiation Pathology.* New York: Oxford University Press; 2002:43–51.

117. Hall EJ. *Radiobiology for the Radiologist.* 5th ed. Philadelphia: Lippincott Williams & Wilkins; 2000:124–135.

118. Gourmelon P, Marquette C, Agay D, et al. Involvement of the central nervous system in radiation-induced multi-organ dysfunction and/or failure. *BJR Suppl.* 2005;27: 62–68.

119. Tjuvajev J, Uehara H, Desai R, et al. Corticotropin-releasing factor decreased vasogenic brain edema. *Cancer Res.* 1996; 56:1352–1360.

120. Batchelor TT, Sorensen AG, di Tomaso E, et al. AZD2171, a pan-VEGF receptor tyrosine kinase inhibitor, normalizes tumor vasculature and alleviates edema in glioblastoma patients. *Cancer Cell.* 2007;11:83–95.

121. Khan RB, Krasin MJ, Kasow K, Leung W. Cyclooxygenase-2 inhibition to treat radiation-induced brain necrosis and edema. *J Pediatr Hematol Oncol.* 2004;26(4):253–255.

122. Sirven JI, Wingerchuk DM, Drazkowski JF, et al. Seizure prophylaxis in patients with brain tumors: a meta-analysis. *Mayo Clin Proc.* 2004;79(12):1489–1494.

123. Temkin NR. Antiepileptogenesis and seizure prevention trials with antiepileptic drugs: meta-analysis of controlled trials. *Epilepsia.* 2001;42(4):515–524.

124. Anscher M, Green D, Kneece S, et al. Radiation injury of the brain and spinal cord. In: Wilkins R, Rengachary S, eds. *Neurosurgery Update II: Vascular, Spinal Pediatric, and Function Neurosurgery.* New York: McGraw-Hill; 1991:42–49.

125. Eiser C. Intellectual abilities among survivors of childhood leukaemia as a function of CNS irradiation. *Arch Dis Child.* 1978; 54(5):391–395.

126. Halperin EC, Constine LS, Tarbell NJ, et al. *Pediatric Radiation Oncology.* Philadelphia: Lippincott Williams & Wilkins; 1999: 457–537.

127. Perrini P, Scollato A, Cioffi F, et al. Radiation leukoencephalopathy associated with moderate hydrocephalus: intracranial pressure monitoring and results of ventriculoperitoneal shunting. *Neurol Sci.* 2002;23:237–241.

128. Russell DS, Wilson CW, Tansley K. Experimental radionecrosis of the brain in rabbits. *J Neurol Neurosurg Psychiatry.* 1949; 12:187.

129. Arnold A, Bailey P. Alterations in the glial cells following irradiation of the brain in primates. *Arch Path.* 1954;57:383.

130. Davidoff LM, Dyke CG, Elsberg CA, Tarlov IM. The effect of radiation applied directly to the brain and spinal cord. Experimental investigations on the *Macacus rhesus* monkeys. *Radiology.* 1938;31:451.

131. Lowenberg-Scharenberg K, Bassett RC. Amyloid degeneration of the human brain following x-ray therapy. *J Neuropath Exp Neurol.* 1950;9:93.

132. Lampert P, Tom MI, Rider WD. Disseminated demyelination of the brain following CO60 (Gamma) radiation. *Arch Path.* 1959; 68:322.

133. Giglio P, Gilbert MR. Cerebral radiation necrosis. *Neurologist.* 2003;9:180–188.

134. Kumar AJ, Leeds NE, Fuller GN, et al. Malignant gliomas: MR imaging spectrum of radiation therapy- and chemotherapy-induced necrosis of the brain after treatment. *Radiology.* 2000; 217:377–384.

135. Dowling C, Noworolski SM, Bollen AW, et al. Preoperative proton MR spectroscopic imaging of brain tumors: correlation with histopathologic analysis of resection specimens. *Am J Neuroradiol.* 2001;22:604–612.

136. Lin A, Blum LS, Mamelak AN. Efficacy of proton magnetic resonance spectroscopy in clinical decision making for patients with suspected malignant brain tumors. *J Neurooncol.* 1999;45(1):69–81.

137. Wald LL, Nelson SJ, Day MR, et al. Serial proton magnetic resonance spectroscopy imaging of glioblastoma multiforme after brachytherapy. *J Neurosurg.* 1997;87(4):525–534.

138. Hall WA, Martin A, Liu H, Truwit CL. Improving diagnostic yield in brain biopsy: coupling spectroscopic targeting with real-time needle placement. *J Magn Reson Imaging.* 2001;13(1):12–15.

139. Rock J, Scarpace L, Hearshen D, et al. Associations among magnetic resonance spectroscopy, apparent diffusion coefficients, and image-guided histopathology with special attention to radiation necrosis. *Neurosurgery.* 2004;54(5):111–1117; discussion, 1117–1119.

140. Sugahara R, Korogi Y, Tomiguchi S, et al. Posttherapeutic intra-axial brain tumor: the value of perfusion-sensitive contrast-enhanced MR imaging for differentiating tumor recurrence from nonneoplastic contrast-enhancing tissue. *Am J Neuroradiol.* 2000;21:901–909.

141. Hazle JD, Jackson EF, Schomer DF, Leeds NE. Dynamic imaging of intracranial lesions using fast spin–echo imaging: differentiation of brain tumors and treatment effects. *J Magn Reson Imaging.* 1997;7(6):1084–1093.

142. Tsui EY, Chan JH, Ramsey RG, et al. Late temporal lobe necrosis in patients with nasopharyngeal carcinoma: evaluation with combined multi-section diffusion-weighted and perfusion weighted MR imaging. *Eur J Radiol.* 2001;39(3):133–138.

143. Asao C, Korogi Y, Kitajima M, et al. Diffusion-weighted imaging of radiation-induced brain injury for differentiation from tumor recurrence. *Am J Neuroradiol.* 2005;26:1455–1460.

144. Doyle WK, Budinger TF, Valk PE, et al. Differentiation of cerebral radiation necrosis from tumor recurrence by 18F FDG and 82 Rb positron emission tomography. *J Comput Assist Tomogr.* 1987;11(4):563–570.

145. Patronas NJ, DiChio G, Brooks RA, et al. Work in progress: 18F fluorodeoxyglucose and positron emission tomography in the evaluation of radiation necrosis of the brain. *Radiology.* 1982;144:885–888.

146. Valk PE, Budinger TF, Levin VA, et al. PET of malignant cerebral tumors after interstitial brachytherapy: demonstration of metabolic activity and correlation with clinical outcome. *J Neurosurg.* 1988;69(6):830–838.

147. Ricci PE, Karis JP, Heiserman JE, et al. Differentiating recurrent tumor from radiation necrosis: time for reevaluation of positron emission tomography. *Am J Neuroradiol.* 1998;19(3):407–413.

148. Thompson TP, Lunsford LD, Kondziolka D. Distinguishing recurrent tumor and radiation necrosis with positron emission tomography versus stereotactic biopsy. *Stereotact Funct Neurosurg.* 1999;73(1–4):9–14.

149. Chao ST, Suh JH, Raja S, et al. The sensitivity and specificity of FDG PET in distinguishing recurrent brain tumor from radionecrosis in patients treated with stereotactic radiosurgery. *Int J Cancer.* 2001;96(3):191–197.

150. Sonoda Y, Kumabe T, Takahashi T, et al. Clinical usefulness of ^{11}C-MET PET and 201 T_1 SPECT for differentiation of recurrent glioma from radiation necrosis. *Neurol Med Chir.* 1998;38(6):342–347.

151. Black KL, Hawkins RA, Kin KT, et al. Use of thallium-201 SPECT to quantitate malignancy grade of gliomas. *J Neurosurg.* 1989;71:342–346.

152. Kline JL, Noto RB, Glantz M. Single-photon emission CT in the evaluation of recurrent brain tumor in patients treated with gamma knife radiosurgery or conventional radiation therapy. *Am J Neuroradiol.* 1996;17(9):1681–1686.

153. Moody EB, Hodes JE, Walsh JW, et al. Thallium-avid cerebral radiation necrosis. *Clin Nucl Med.* 1994;19(7):611–613.

154. Yoshii Y, Moritake T, Suzuki K, et al. Cerebral radiation necrosis with accumulation of thallium 201 on single-photon emission CT. *Am J Neuroradiol.* 1996;17(9):1773–1776.

155. De Vries B, Taphoorn MJ, van Isselt JW, et al. Bilateral temporal lobe necrosis after radiotherapy: confounding SPECT results. *Neurology.* 1998;51(4):1183–1834.

156. Yoshino E, Imahori Y, Ohmori Y, et al. Irradiation effects on the metabolism of metastatic brain tumors: analysis by positron emission tomography and 1H-magnetic resonance spectroscopy. *Stereotact Funct Neurosurg.* 1996;66(Suppl 1):240–259.

157. Buchpiguel CA, Alavi JB, Alavi A, Kenyon LC. PET versus SPECT in distinguishing radiation necrosis from tumor recurrence in the brain. *J Nucl Med.* 1995;36:159–164.

158. Kahn D, Follett KA, Bushnell DL, et al. Diagnosis of recurrent brain tumor: value of 201 T_1 SPECT vs fluorodeoxyglucose PET. *Am J Roentgenol.* 1994;163(6):1459–1465.

159. Stokkel M, Stevens H, Taphoorn M, Van Rijk P. Differentiation between recurrent brain tumor and post-radiation necrosis: the value of 201 T_1 SPECT versus 18F-FDG PET using a dual-headed coincidence camera-a pilot study. *Nucl Med Commun.* 1999;20:411–417.

160. Marks J, Wong J. The risk of cerebral radionecrosis in relation to dose, time and fractionation: a follow-up study. *Prog Exp Tumor Res.* 1985;29:210–218.

161. Martins A, Johnston J, Henry J, et al. Delayed radiation necrosis of the brain. *J Neurosurg.* 1977;47:336–345.

162. Soffietti R, Sciolla R, Giordana MT, et al. Delayed adverse effects after irradiation of gliomas: clinicopathological analysis. *J Neurooncol.* 1985;3(2):187–192.

163. Ruben JD, Dally M, Bailey M, et al. Cerebral radiation necrosis: incidence, outcomes, and risk factors with emphasis on radiation parameters and chemotherapy. *Int J Radiat Oncol Biol Phys.* 2006;65(2):499–508.

164. Asada Y, Kohga S, Sumiyoshi A, et al. Disseminated necrotizing encephalopathy induced by methotrexate therapy alone. *Acta Pathol Jpn.* 1988;38(10):1305–1312.

165. Burger PC, Kamenar E, Schold SC, et al. Encephalomyelopathy following high-dose BCNE therapy. *Cancer.* 1981;48:1318–1327.

166. Dropcho EJ. Neurotoxicity of cancer chemotherapy. *Semin Neurol.* 2004;24:419–426.

167. Keime-Guibert F, Napolitano M, Delattre J-Y. Neurological complications of radiotherapy and chemotherapy. *J Neurol.* 1998;245(11):695–708.

168. Kamiro T, Kassell NF, Thai QA, et al. Histological changes in the normal rat brain after gamma irradiation. *Acta Neurochir.* 1996;138(4):451–459.

169. Gutin PH, Prados MD, Phillips TL, et al. External irradiation followed by an interstitial high-activity iodine-125 implant "boost" in the initial treatment of malignant gliomas: NCOG study 6G-82-2. *Int J Radiat Oncol Biol Phys.* 1991;21:601–606.

170. Wowra B, Schmitt HP, Sturm V. Incidence of late radiation necrosis with transient mass effect after interstitial low-dose rate radiotherapy for cerebral gliomas. *Acta Neurochir.* 1989;99(3–4):104–108.

171. Floyd NS, Woo SY, Teh BS, et al. Hypofractionated intensity-modulated radiotherapy for primary glioblastoma multiforme. *Int J Radiat Oncol Biol Phys.* 2004;58:721–726.

172. Forsyth PA, Kelly PJ, Cascino TL, et al. Radiation necrosis or glioma recurrence: is computer-assisted stereotactic biopsy useful? *J Neurosurg.* 1995;82:436–444.

173. Glantz MJ, Burger PC, Friedman AH, et al. Treatment of radiation-induced nervous system injury with heparin and warfarin. *Neurology.* 1994;44(11):2020–2027.

174. Chuba PJ, Aronin P, Bhambhani K, et al. Hyperbaric oxygen therapy for radiation induced brain injury in children. *Cancer.* 1997;80:2005–2012.

175. Hart GB, Mainous EG. The treatment of radiation necrosis with hyperbaric oxygen (OHP). *Cancer.* 1976;37(6):2580–2585.

176. Kohshi K, Imada H, Nomoto S, et al. Successful treatment of radiation-induced brain necrosis by hyperbaric oxygen therapy. *J Neurol Sci.* 2003;209(1–2):115–117.

177. Leber KA, Eder HG, Kovac H, et al. Treatment of cerebral radionecrosis by hyperbaric oxygen therapy. *Stereotact Funct Neurosurg.* 1998;70:229–236.

178. Hornsey S, Myers R, Jenkinson T. The reduction of radiation damage to the spinal cord by post-irradiation administration of vasoactive drugs. *Int J Radiat Oncol Biol Phys.* 1990;18(6):1437–1442.

179. Alaoui F, Pratt J, Trocheri S, et al. Acute effects of irradiation on the rat brain: protection by glutamate blockade. *Eur J Pharmacol.* 1995;276(1):55–66.

180. Guelman LR, Zubilete MAZ, Rios H, Zieher LM. WR-2721 (amifostine, Ethyol®) prevents motor and morphological changes induced by neonatal X-irradiation. *Neurochem Int.* 2003;42(5):385–391.

181. Lamproglou I, Djazouli K, Boisserie G, et al. Radiation-induced cognitive dysfunction: the protective effect of ethyol in young rats. *Int J Radiat Oncol Biol Phys.* 2003;57(4):1109–1115.

182. Nieder C, Price RE, Rivera B, et al. Effects of insulin-like growth factor-1 (IGF-1) and amifostine in spinal cord re-irradiation. *Strahlenther Onkol.* 2005;181:691–695.

183. Hong JH, Chiang CS, Campbell IL, et al. Induction of acute phase gene expression by brain irradiation. *Int J Radiat Oncol Biol Phys.* 1995;33:619–626.

184. Kondziolka D, Mori Y, Martinez AJ, et al. Beneficial effects of the radioprotectant 21-aminosteroid U-74389G in a radiosurgery rat malignant glioma model. *Int J Radiat Oncol Biol Phys.* 1999;44:179–184.

185. Monje ML, Toda H, Palmer TD. Inflammatory blockade restores adult hippocampal neurogenesis. *Science.* 2003;302:1760–1765.

186. Tanaka J, Fujita H, Matsuda S, et al. Gluco-corticoid- and mineralocorticoid receptors in microglial cells: the two receptors mediate differential effects of corticosteroids. *Glia.* 1997;20:23–37.

187. Zhao W, Payne V, Tommasi E, et al. Administration of the peroxisomal proliferators-activated receptor gamma agonist pioglitazone during fractionated brain irradiation prevents radiation-induced cognitive impairment. *Int J Radiat Oncol Biol Phys.* 2007;67:6–9.

188. Yuan H, Gaber MW, McColgan T, et al. Radiation-induced permeability and leukocyte adhesion in the rat blood–brain barrier: modulation with anti-ICAM-1 antibodies. *Brain Res.* 2003;969:59–69.

189. Andratschke NH, Nieder C, Price RE, et al. Modulation of rodent spinal cord radiation tolerance by administration of platelet-derived growth factor. *Int J Radiat Oncol Bio Phys.* 2004;60:1257–1263.

190. Erbayraktar S, de Lanerolle N, de Lotbiniere A, et al. Carbamylated erythropoietin reduces radiosurgically induced brain injury. *Mol Med.* 2006;12:74–80.

191. Nieder C, Andratschke N, Price RE, Ang KK. Evaluation of insulin-like growth factor-1 for prevention of radiation-induced myelopathy. *Growth Factors.* 2005;23:15–18.

192. Nieder C, Price RE, Rivera B, et al. Experimental data for insulin-like growth factor-1 and basic fibroblast growth factor in prevention of radiation myelopathy. *Strahlenther Onkol.* 2002;178:147–152. (Original in German.)

193. Schagen SB, Vardy J. Cognitive dysfunction in people with cancer. *Lancet Oncol.* 2007;8:852–853.

194. Vardy J, Rourke S, Tannock IF. Evaluation of cognitive function associated with chemotherapy: a review of published studies and recommendations for future research. *J Clin Oncol.* 2007;25(17):2455–2463.

195. Klein M, Heimans JJ, Aaronson NK, et al. Effect of radiotherapy and other treatment-related factors on mid-term to long-term cognitive sequelae in low-grade gliomas: a comparative study. *Lancet.* 2002;360:1361–1368.

196. Hall RCW, Popkin M, Kirkpatrick B. Tricyclic exacerbation of steroid psychosis. *J Nerv Ment Dis.* 1978;166(10):738–742.

197. Hall RCW, Popkin M, Stickney S, et al. Presentation of "steroid psychosis." *J Nerv Ment Dis.* 1979;167:229–236.

198. Lupien SJ, McEwen BS. The acute effects of corticosteroids on cognition: integration of animal and human model studies. *Brain Res Rev.* 1997;24(1):1–27.

199. Arriagada R, Le Chevalier T, Borie F, et al. Prophylactic cranial irradiation for patients with small-cell lung cancer in complete remission. *J Natl Cancer Inst.* 1995;87(3):183–190.

200. Gregor A, Cull A, Stephens RJ, et al. Prophylactic cranial irradiation is indicated following complete response to induction therapy in small cell lung cancer: results of a multicentre randomised trial. *Eur J Cancer.* 1997;33(11):1752–1758.

201. DeAngelis LM, Delattre J-Y, Posner JB. Radiation-induced dementia in patients cured of brain metastases. *Neurology.* 1989;39:789–796.

202. Aoyama H, Shirato H, Tago M, et al. Stereotactic radiosurgery plus whole-brain radiation therapy vs stereotactic radiosurgery alone for treatment of brain metastases. *JAMA.* 2006;295(21):2483–2491.

203. Amendola B, Wolf A, Coy S, et al. Gamma knife radiosurgery in the treatment of patients with single and multiple brain metastases from carcinoma of the breast. *Cancer J.* 2000;6(2):88–92.

204. Flickinger J. Radiotherapy and radiosurgical management of brain metastases. *Curr Oncol Rep.* 2001;3(6):484–489.

205. Sneed P, Lamborn K, Forstner J, et al. Radiosurgery for brain metastases: is whole brain radiotherapy necessary? *Int J Radiat Oncol Biol Phys.* 1999;43(3):549–558.

206. Regine WF, Huhn JL, Patchell RA, et al. Risk of symptomatic brain tumor recurrence and neurologic deficit after radiosurgery alone in patients with newly diagnosed brain metastases: results and implications. *Int J Radiat Oncol Biol Phys.* 2002;52(2):333–338.

207. Brown PD, Jensen AW, Felten SJ, et al. Detrimental effects of tumor progression on cognitive function of patients with high-grade glioma. *J Clin Oncol.* 2006;24(34):5427–5433.

208. Torres IJ, Mundt AJ, Sweeney PJ, et al. A longitudinal neuropsychological study of partial brain radiation in adults with brain tumors. *Neurology.* 2003;60:1113–1118.

209. Meyers CA, Smith JA, Bezjak A. Neurocognitive function and progression in patients with brain metastases treated with whole-brain radiation and motexafin gadolinium: results of a randomized phase III trial. *J Clin Oncol.* 2004;22(1):157–165.

210. Ron E, Modan B, Floro S, et al. Mental function following scalp irradiation during childhood. *Am J Epidemiol.* 1982;116(1)149–160.

211. Ron E, Modan B, Boice J Jr. Mortality after radiotherapy for ringworm of the scalp. *Am J Epidemiol.* 1988;127(4):713–725.

212. Werner A, Modan B, Davidoff D. Doses to brain, skull and thyroid following x-ray therapy for tinea capitis. *Phys Med Biol.* 1968;13(2):247–258.

213. Mulhern R, Wasserman A, Fairclough D, et al. Memory function in disease-free survivors of childhood acute lymphocytic leukemia given CNS prophylaxis with or without 1800 cGy cranial irradiation. *J Clin Oncol.* 1988;6(2):315–320.

214. Waber D, Tarbell N, Kahn C, et al. The relationship of sex and treatment modality to neuropsychologic outcome in childhood acute lymphoblastic leukemia. *J Clin Oncol.* 1992;10(5): 810–817.

215. Waber D, Tarbell N, Fairclough D, et al. Cognitive sequelae of treatment in childhood acute lymphoblastic leukemia: cranial radiation requires an accomplice. *J Clin Oncol.* 1995;13(10): 2490–2496.

216. Iuvone L, Mariotti P, Colosimo C, et al. Long-term cognitive outcome, brain computed tomography scan, and magnetic resonance imaging in children cured for acute lymphoblastic leukemia. *Cancer.* 2002;95(12):2562–2570.

217. Mulhern R, Hancock J, Fairclough D, et al. Neuropsychological status of children treated for brain tumors: a critical review and integrative analysis. *Med Pediatr Oncol.* 1992;20:181–191.

218. Meadows A, Massari D, Fergusson J, et al. Declines in IQ scores and cognitive dysfunctions in children with acute lymphocytic leukaemia treated with cranial irradiation. *Lancet.* 1980;2(8254):1015–1028.

219. Syndikus I, Tait D, Ashley S, et al. Long-term follow-up of young children with brain tumors after irradiation. *Int J Radiat Oncol Biol Phys.* 1994;30(4):781–787.

220. Chan Y, Roebuck D, Yuen M, et al. Long-term cerebral metabolite changes on proton magnetic resonance spectroscopy in patients cured of acute lymphoblastic leukemia with previous intrathecal methotrexate and cranial irradiation prophylaxis. *Int J Radiat Oncol Biol Phys.* 2001:50(3):759–763.

221. Virta A, Patronas N, Raman R, et al. Spectroscopic imaging of radiation-induced effects in the white matter of glioma patients. *Magn Reson Imaging.* 2000;18(7):851–857.

222. Davidson, A, Tait D, Payne G, et al. Magnetic resonance spectroscopy in the evaluation of neurotoxicity following cranial irradiation for childhood cancer. *Br J Radiol.* 2000;73:421–424.

223. Movsas B, Li BSY, Babb JS, et al. Quantifying radiation therapy–induced brain injury with whole-brain proton MR spectroscopy: initial observations. *Radiology.* 2001;221:327–331.

224. Barani IJ, Benedict SH, Lin PS. Neural stem cells: implications for the conventional radiotherapy of central nervous system malignancies. *Int J Radiat Oncol Biol Phys.* 2007;68:324–333.

225. Healy J. Mitigating radiation-induced cognitive impairment. *Lancet Oncol.* 2007;8(12):1055–1056.

226. Emsley JG, Mitchell BD, Kempermann G, Macklis JD. Adult neurogenesis and repair of the adult CNS with neural progenitors, precursors, and stem cells. *Prog Neurobiol.* 2005;75(5):321–341.

227. Hulshof M, Stark NM, van der Kleij A, et al. Hyperbaric oxygen therapy for cognitive disorders after irradiation of the brain. *Strahlenther Onkol.* 2002;178(4):192–198.

228. Butler RW, Copeland DR. Attentional processes and their remediation in children treated for cancer: a literature review and the development of a therapeutic approach. *J Int Neuropsychol Soc.* 2002;8:115–124.

229. Thompson GM, Migdal CS, Whittle RJ. Radiation retinopathy following treatment of posterior nasal space carcinoma. *Br J Ophthalmol.* 1983;67:609–614.

230. Gupta A, Dhawahir-Scala F, Smith A, et al. Radiation retinopathy: case report and review. *BMC Ophthalmol.* 2007;7(6).

231. Young WC, Thornton AF, Gebarski SS, Cornblath WT. Radiation-induced optic neuropathy: correlation of MR imaging and radiation dosimetry. *Radiology.* 1992;185:904–907.

232. Parsons JT, Bova FJ, Fitzgerald CR, et al. Radiation optic neuropathy after megavoltage external-beam irradiation: analysis of time-dose factors. *Int J Radiat Oncol Biol Phys.* 1994;30(4): 755–763.

233. McClellan RL, Gammal TE, Kline LB. Early bilateral radiation-induced optic neuropathy with follow-up MRI. *Neuroradiology.* 1995;37(2):131–133.

234. Finger PT. Anti-VEGF bevacizumab (Avastin) for radiation optic neuropathy. *Am J Ophthalmol.* 2007;143(2):335–338.

235. Arlt W, Hove U, Muller B, et al. Frequent and frequently overlooked: treatment-induced endocrine dysfunction in adult long-term survivors of primary brain tumors. *Neurology.* 1997;49:498–506.

236. Constine LS, Wolff PD, Cann D, et al. Hypothalamic-pituitary dysfunction after radiation for brain tumors. *N Engl J Med.* 1993;328:87–94.

237. Fowler JF, Bentzen SM, Bond SJ, et al. Clinical radiation doses for spinal cord: the 1998 international questionnaire. *Radiother Oncol.* 2000;55:295–300.

238. Maranzano E, Bellavita R, Floridi P, et al. Radiation-induced myelopathy in long-term surviving metastatic spinal cord compression patients after hypofractionated radiotherapy: a clinical and magnetic resonance imaging analysis. *Radiother Oncol.* 2001;60:281–288.

239. Ryu S, Gorty S, Kazee AM, et al. "Full dose" reirradiation of human cervical spinal cord. *Am J Clin Oncol.* 2000;23(1):29–31.

240. Wang PY, Shen WC, Jan JS. MR imaging in radiation myelopathy. *Am J Neuroradiol.* 1992;13(4):1049–1055.

241. Maddison P, Southern P, Johnson M. Clinical and MRI discordance in a case of delayed radiation myelopathy. *J Neurol Neurosurg Psychiatry.* 2000;69(4):563–564.

242. Okada S, Okeda R. Pathology of radiation myelopathy. *Neuropathology.* 2001;21(4):247–265.

243. Lengyel Z, Rékó G, Majtényi K, et al. Autopsy verifies demyelination and lack of vascular damage in partially reversible radiation myelopathy. *Spinal Cord.* 2003;41:577–585.

244. Calabrò F, Jinkins JR. MRI of radiation myelitis: a report of a case treated with hyperbaric oxygen. *Eur Radiol.* 2000;10(7): 1079–1084.

245. Feldmeier JJ, Hampson NB. A systematic review of the literature reporting the application of hyperbaric oxygen prevention and treatment of delayed radiation injuries: an evidence-based approach. *Undersea Hyperb Med.* 2002;29(1):4–30.

246. Liu CY, Yim BT, Wozniak AJ. Anticoagulation therapy for radiation-induced myelopathy. *Annals Pharmacother.* 2001;35(2):188–191.

247. Olsen NK, Pfeiffer P, Johannsen L, et al. Radiation-induced brachial plexopathy: neurological follow-up in 161 recurrence-free breast cancer patients. *Int J Radiat Oncol Biol Phys.* 1993;26(1):43–49.

248. Powell S, Cooke J, Parsons C. Radiation-induced brachial plexus injury: follow-up of two different fractionation schedules. *Radiother Oncol.* 1990;18(3):213–220.

249. Gosk J, Rutowski R, Reichert P, Rabczynski J. Radiation-induced brachial plexus neuropathy: aetiopathogenesis, risk factors, differential diagnostics, symptoms and treatment. *Folia Neuropathol.* 2007;45(1):26–30.

250. Kori SH, Foley KM, Posner JK. Brachial plexus lesions in patients with cancer: 100 cases. *Neurology.* 1989;39:45–50.

251. Wilburn AJ. Brachial plexus. In: Dyck PJ, Thomas PK, eds. *Peripheral Neuropathy.* 3rd ed. Philadelphia: Saunders; 1993:911–950.

252. Glazer HS, Lee JKT, Levitt RG, et al. Radiation fibrosis: differentiation from recurrent tumor by MR imaging: work in progress. *Radiology.* 1985;156:721–726.

253. Wittenberg KH, Adkins MC. MR imaging of nontraumatic brachial plexopathies: frequency and spectrum of findings. *Radiographics.* 2000;20:1023–1032.

254. Pritchard J, Anand P, Broome J, et al. Double-blind randomized phase II study of hyperbaric oxygen in patients with radiation-induced brachial plexopathy. *Radiother Oncol.* 2001;58: 279–286.

255. Georgiou A, Grigsby Perez C. Radiation-induced lumbosacral plexopathy in gynecologic tumors: clinical findings and dosimetric analysis. *Int J Radiat Oncol Biol Phys.* 1993;26(3): 479–482.

256. Stryker J, Sommerville K, Perez R, et al. Sacral plexus injury after radiotherapy for carcinoma of cervix. *Cancer.* 1990;66(7): 1488–1492.

257. Ebner F, Kressel HY, Mintz MC, et al. Tumor recurrence versus fibrosis in the female pelvis: differentiation with MR imaging at 1.5 T. *Radiology.* 1988;166:333–340.

258. Thomas JE, Cascino TL, Earle JD. Differential diagnosis between radiation and tumor plexopathy of the pelvis. *Neurology.* 1985;35:1–7.

259. Mendes D, Nawalker R, Eldar S. Post-irradiation femoral neuropathy: a case report. *J Bone Joint Surg Am.* 1991;73(1): 137–140.

260. Portenoy RK, Lesage P. Management of cancer pain. *Lancet.* 1999;353:1695–1700.

NEUROTOXIC ENVIRONMENTS AND CONDITIONS

CONTENTS

CHAPTER 49

Thermal Injury of the Nervous System

Joseph R. Berger and Michael R. Dobbs

INTRODUCTION

The hypothalamus is critical for the control of body temperature. Ablation experiments indicate that neither the cortex nor the thalamus is necessary for thermoregulation. Lesional experiments in animals indicate that the anterior hypothalamus, chiefly, the preoptic area, leads to dissipation of body heat via vasodilation, sweating, and increased rates. The posterior regions of the hypothalamus are responsible for heat generation and conservation, including vasoconstriction and shivering. Firing rates of cells within the hypothalamus are altered with changes in body temperature. In general, mechanisms that raise body temperature are regarded as adrenergic (sympathetic) and those that lower it are regarded as cholinergic (parasympathetic).

The human body has a thermostatic set point between 37.0°C and 37.2°C that it attempts to tenaciously maintain.[1] Thermoregulation above these levels is driven by intracranial temperatures; thermoregulation for temperatures below these levels is not. For instance, lowering intracranial temperatures by 0.5°C did not result in increased heat generation provided that skin temperatures were held above 33°C. On the other hand, heat generation is greatly augmented when skin temperatures are below 33°C. These findings suggest that the hypothalamus has a heat receptor only and that afferent pathways conduct skin temperature to the hypothalamus, signaling an increase in heat generation.[1] However, these findings contradict those of Sherrington, who observed shivering in animals whose spinal cord had been transected, suggesting that there is a central thermosensitive mechanism for cooling.[2] Other studies have also revealed evidence for central therma dector for cold, as well as heat.

The maintenance of body temperature requires a fine balance between heat generation and heat loss. The processes leading to both are tightly regulated by several physiological processes that include both chemical and physical heat transfer. Body heat generation is chiefly generated by the metabolism of food. At rest, respiration and circulation are responsible for approximately 10% of body heat production, brain and muscle metabolism for 20% each, and abdominal viscera for about 50%. The contribution of muscle metabolism increases with exercise. Muscles are exquisitely important in temperature regulation because their activity can be rapidly increased or decreased to adjust to need.

As with other physical objects, heat elimination from the body is effected by three fundamental mechanisms: radiation, vaporization, and convection. Approximately 60% of body heat is eliminated via radiation, the process of transferring heat from warmer to cooler bodies.

Vaporization occurs as a consequence of evaporation of water from the skin and respiratory passages. Vaporization accounts for about 20% to 27% of total body heat loss. Convection, which is the loss of heat to air circulating over the body and respiratory passages, accounts for about 12% to 15% of heat loss. When the ambient temperature exceeds the body's core temperature, sweat evaporation is the most important mechanism by which heat is dissipated.[3] Every 1.7 mL of sweat that is vaporized results in dissipation of 1 kcal of heat energy; therefore, the body can eliminate up to 600 kcal of heat energy per hour.[4]

Fever-causing substances are referred to as pyrogens, of which there are both exogenous and endogenous forms. The pyrogens affect neurons in the preoptic area of the anterior hypothalamus.[5] When the heat load is excessive and heat stroke supervenes, the body's defense is to shift its thermoregulatory set point upward, which detrimentally decreases demand for cutaneous blood flow and increases blood flow to vital organs.[6]

In cold conditions, two mechanisms predominate, namely, a reduction of blood flow to the skin and an increase in muscle activity. Initially, with respect to the latter, the number of action potentials in muscles rises without evident activity. Then, with an increasing need to generate body heat, the number of muscle contractions increase, ultimately resulting in shivering. The remarkable ability of the body to regulate skin blood flow is critical for heat dissipation as well. Studies have revealed that the volume of circulation of the skin can be altered as much as 100-fold in some regions of the body.[7] An increase of skin and respiratory passage blood flow increases heat loss. Visible sweating typically occurs when the ambient temperature exceeds 31°C.

HYPERTHERMIA

Heatstroke

Heatstroke was first documented in 24 BC by the Romans but was not demonstrated to result in multiorgan dysfunction until 1946.[8] Heatstroke is classified as either classical, occurring as a consequence of environmental factors, or exertional. People at the extremes of age are predisposed to classical heatstroke—children due to their small surface area, lower rate of sweating, and poor acclimatization and the elderly due to failure of heat regulation.[9] Certain medications may contribute to the development of heatstroke, including antipsychotic medication, amphetamine-like drugs, antidopaminergics, and anticholinergics. These drugs may act directly on temperature sensors.

The disorder typically develops suddenly after the core body temperature has exceeded 40.6°C. Manifestations include extreme fatigue, headache, heavy perspiration, or hot dry skin which may become pale or bluish if cardiac failure occurs, facial erythema, nausea, vomiting, diarrhea, disorientation, vertigo, and uncoordinated movements.[10] Examination usually shows constricted pupils, areflexia, and even loss of brainstem reflexes if the patient is comatose. The plantar responses may be extensor or equivocal.[11] Among the observed acute neurological abnormalities are encephalopathy, altered level of consciousness, and convulsions.[11] Complex automatic movements, such as chewing, swallowing, and lip smacking; body shivering; and rarely, a pancerebellar syndrome and hemiparesis may be observed.[11] Rhabdomyolysis may occur and result in myoglobinuric renal failure. Laboratory abnormalities sometimes observed with heatstroke include elevated creatine kinase, hypophosphatemia, and elevated uric acid. Heatstroke must be distinguished from heat exhaustion, which is a milder illness that occurs from dehydration and salt depletion. In this entity, the body temperature is more than 37°C but less than 40°C. It is characterized by mental status changes and varying degrees of organ failure (Figure 49-1).

In addition to heatstroke, similar neurological complications of hyperthermia may attend malignant hyperthermia (MH), the neuroleptic malignant syndrome (NMS), the serotonin syndrome (SS). In addition, severe elevations in body temperature may occur with various brain insults, including brainstem hemorrhage.[12]

Malignant Hyperthermia

MH was initially described in 1960 as an inherited disorder of skeletal muscle that predisposed affected individuals to hyperthermia, hypermetabolism, and skeletal muscle rigidity following exposure to general anesthetics.[13] The disorder results from abnormalities in the channels that regulate the duration and amplitude of calcium efflux from the sarcoplasmic reticulum, referred to as the ryanodine receptor, located on chromosome 19q13.1.[14] More than 90 mutations have been discovered in this gene, and at least 25 are causal for MH.[15] Abnormalities in the CACNA1S gene, which is responsible for the L-type voltage gated calcium channel α subunit, has also been associated with malignant hyperthermia.[15a] The estimated incidence of this disorder is 1:10,000 to 1:50,000, and approximately 1:1600 people develop features of MH following exposure to general anesthetics.[16] Exposure to offending agents, typically volatile anesthetics or depolarizing muscle relaxants, results in muscle contracture, tachycardia, hyperthermia, rhabdomyolysis, myoglobinuria, and metabolic acidosis. Mortality rates exceed 80% in untreated patients but are 5% in those treated. Dantrolene sodium, which prevents intracellular calcium release in the myocyte through action on the ryanodine receptor of calcium channels, is an effective intravenous antidote.[16a]

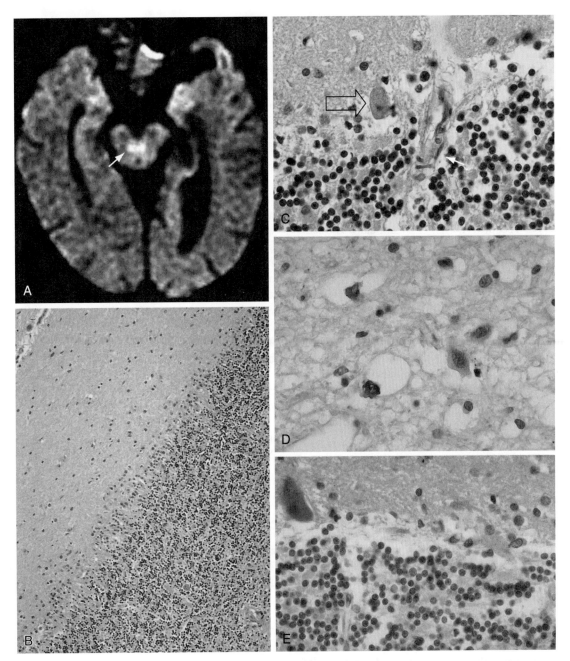

Figure 49-1. *(A)* Magnetic resonance imaging performed 12 days after heatstroke; axial diffusion showing an increased signal *(arrow)* in the central tegmentum of the midbrain at the anterior aspect of the periaqueductal gray matter, corresponding to Wernekinck's commissure (see color plate). *(B)* Cerebellar cortex showing complete loss of Purkinje cells with proliferation of Bergmann glia. Note that the granule cells and molecular layers are relatively spared (hematoxylin and eosin, ×100). *(C)* In situ end labeling in the cerebellar cortex showing that one remaining Purkinje cell with pyknotic nucleus and homogenized cytoplasm is not stained *(large empty arrow),* whereas an endothelial cell serving as internal controls is stained *(thin arrow;* Apoptag kit, ×400). *(D)* In situ end labeling in the centromedian nucleus of the thalamus showing positivity of the nuclei of remaining neurons; cellular remnants within vacuoles are also positively stained (Apoptag kit, ×400). *(E)* Immunostaining for heat shock protein 70 in the cerebellar cortex showing positively stained astrocytes of Bergmann glia around a necrotic Purkinje cells (avidin–biotin complex, peroxidase–antiperoxidase technique, ×400). (Bazille C, Megarbane B, Bensimhon D, et al. Brain damage after heatstroke. *J Neuropathol Exp Neurol.* 005;64[11]:970–975.)

Neuroleptic Malignant Syndrome and Serotonin Syndrome

NMS and SS are characterized by hyperthermia, muscular rigidity, and altered level of consciousness. NMS occurs with the use of neuroleptics, and was first recognized in 1956 after the introduction of phenothiazine. NMS develops in 30% of affected individuals within 48 hours of initiation of the drug and within 7 days in 66% of cases.[16b] The SS occurs chiefly with serotoninergic antidepressants (Figure 1). The pathogenesis of the NMS is poorly understood;[17] however, an association exists with the Taq1 polymorphisms of dopamine D2 receptor gene.[17a] SS appears to result from overstimulation of the 5 hydroxytryptamine receptors (1A and 2).[18] SS is characterized by mental, autonomic and neurological features typically occurring within 24 hours of the start of the offending therapy or after overdose.[18a] Definitive diagnosis of NMS requires the presence of elevated temperature and diffuse muscle rigidity coupled with two of the following: autonomic instability, changes in mental status, leukocytosis, and elevated creatine kinase levels. Mortality rates of 10% are seen in the untreated patient. The principal form of treatment is removal of the offending agent. Bromocriptine and dantrolene are sometimes used.

Neurological Consequences of Hyperthermia

Long-term neurological sequelae have been reported to occur in approximately 20% of heatstroke victims[10]; however, this percentage seems excessive and prompt and appropriate treatment has reduced both complications and mortality. The latter is currently below 10%[11] but is significantly higher if treatment is delayed for more than 2 hours.[10] Most reported experiences have been case reports or small series. In July 1995, Chicago suffered an intense heat wave that resulted in 600 excess deaths, 2200 excess emergency department visits, and a large number of people suffering near-fatal heatstroke. In a series of 58 patients with heatstroke that occurred during that heat wave, 100% had multiorgan dysfunction with neurological impairment, 53% had severe renal insufficiency, 45% had disseminated intravascular coagulation, and 10% had respiratory distress.[19] Of the patients in the series, 78% experienced mild to severe long-term neurological consequences.[19] In a smaller series from Wisconsin during the same heat wave, a persistent neurological sequelae was seen in only 2 of 11 patients; both suffering a pancerebellar syndrome.[20] Physicians in Saudi Arabia have had a unique experience with heatstroke resulting from the hajj, the pilgrimage to Mecca, during which millions of unacclimated Moslems visit the desert kingdom.[11] Despite these reports, permanent neurological consequences of heatstroke are indeed rare and younger patients may be more resistant to ill aftereffects. For instance, in one study of 21 young adults suffering heatstroke, neither permanent neurological nor permanent psychological complications were detected at follow-up.[21] Permanent injury of cranial and peripheral nerves from systemic hyperthermia has not been reported.

The most common neurological consequences of heatstroke include cerebellar ataxia, encephalopathy, and parkinsonism. There are isolated case reports of cerebellar syndrome with downbeat nystagmus,[22,23] an isolated ataxic dysarthria,[24] parkinsonism, central pontine myelinolysis,[25] Bickerstaff brainstem encephalitis,[26] Klüver-Bucy syndrome,[27] focal hemispheric findings,[28] transverse myelopathy,[29] flaccid quadriplegia with anhydrosis, and sphincter dysfunction secondary to damage to the anterior horn cells and spinal cord autonomic neurons.[30] A unique syndrome referred to as hemorrhagic shock encephalopathy has been observed in infants ranging in age from 3 to 140 weeks. This unusual entity that has been attributed to heatstroke.[31]

The neurological complications of NMS parallel those of heatstroke, including reports of cerebellar ataxia and progressive cerebellar atrophy.[32,33] Global encephalopathy[34] and pyramidal and extrapyramidal disorders have also been reported as neurological sequelae following NMS.[35]

Mechanisms of Injury

During the acute phase response to thermal injury, interleukins, in particular IL-1 and IL-6, play a major role and mediate the systemic inflammatory response. Their elaboration results in increased antiinflammatory acute phase proteins that inhibit reactive oxygen species and release proteolytic enzymes. Tumor necrosis factor-α is needed to mediate the fever, promote leukocytosis, and prevent muscle catabolism.[10] Subsequently, heat shock proteins are expressed as heat stress progresses. Heat shock protein 72 is the primary protein that accumulates in the brain and produces a state of transient tolerance to the heat stress; however, it appears to be effective only with sublethal thermal injury.[4] The critical thermal maximum in humans is body temperature between 41.6°C and 42°C for 45 minutes to 8 hours, but beyond 49°C to 50°C, cellular necrosis occurs in 5 minutes.[4]

Most authorities ascribe the neurological complications arising from heatstroke to the accompanying arterial hypotension, reduction in cerebral perfusion pressure, and resulting cerebral ischemic damage,[36,37] although neuronal damage may result from hyperthermia itself or as a consequence of other heat-related physiological disorders, such as metabolic disturbances, disseminated intravascular coagulation[38] and hypernatremia.[39] Hyperpyrexia by itself causes enzymatic denaturation of the cell, liquefaction of cellular membranes, and mitochondrial damage.[40] The precise mechanism of brain injury with hyperthermia remains uncertain. Studies in the rat model of heatstroke reveal an increase in free radicals, particularly hydroxyl radicals and superoxide anions; higher lipid peroxidation; lower enzymatic antioxidant defenses; and higher proxidants.[41] High extracellular levels for the monoamines, dopamine, serotonin, and norepinephrine, as well as for IL-1, IL-6, and tumor necrosis factor-α, have been detected.[42] Nitric oxide (NO) is also significantly increased in the cerebellum and the cortex in rats dying from hyperthermia.[43] High concentrations of circulating cytokines following heatstroke may induce NO release from the vascular walls and its subsequent diffusion across the blood–brain barrier.[44] NO has been implicated in N-methyl-d-aspartate-mediated neurotoxicity and hypoxic ischemic damage.[45] Dopamine is released from the striatum during heatstroke,[46] and levels nearly three times baseline have been reported in the rat model.[47] High levels of serotonin release with heatstroke have been detected in the anterior hypothalamus, striatum, and frontal cortex, and pharmacological depletion of serotonin prolongs survival in the animal model.[48] Local cerebral glucose usage decreases, as does cerebral perfusion.[49]

Quantitative measurements of neurotransmitters in three patients dying from hyperthermia have revealed depletion of hypothalamic noradrenalin in the hypothalamus and moderate to severe loss of choline acetyltransferase.[50]

Neuroradiology

In the acute phase of heatstroke, loss of gray–white differentiation on computed tomography of the brain has been proposed as a sensitive marker of severe brain injury.[51] Magnetic resonance imaging studies may show pathology that predominates in the cerebellum, the striatum, and the white matter. The cerebellum often appears to receive the brunt of the insult. Over time, cerebellar atrophy develops and may be progressive in nature over 1 or more years.[52,53] Despite evidence of progressive cerebellar atrophy, clinical symptoms may continue to improve.[54] Lesions in the white matter are generally irregular and patchy. Symmetrical increased signal intensity of the paraventricular thalamus and external capsule and the cerebellum on T_1- and T_2-weighted images has been reported.[55]

Radiological studies may reveal evidence of venous or arterial infarction as a consequence of heat-induced disseminated intravascular coagulation.[56]

Neuropathology of Hyperthermia

The pathology of heatstroke has been rarely reported. A detailed neuropathological study of three elderly patients who suffered heatstroke during a heat wave in France revealed that each had a severe diffuse loss of Purkinje cells associated with heat shock protein 70 expression by Bergmann glia.[57] As in situ labeling was negative in surviving Purkinje cells, the mechanism of cell death was not thought to be apoptosis. Cerebellar afferent pathways were affected, including the superior cerebellar peduncles, superior cerebellar decussation, and dentatothalamic tracts. Neuronal death in the dentate nuclei and centromedian nuclei of the thalamus was attributed to deafferentiation.[57] Vascular congestion of the brain and brain edema were observed in a child dying from heatstroke.[58]

Treatment of Hyperthermia

The fundamentals of hyperthermia treatment are treat the underlying etiology of the condition, cool the patient, and prevent or treat the complications that arise from the insult. The goal is to decrease core temperature to less than 38.9°C within 30 minutes, ideally reducing the core temperature by 0.2°C/min.[8] Cooling measures may be either external or internal. Evaporative cooling is the safest measure and includes cooling the patient with large fans after covering the patient's body with a wet sheet or spraying tepid water over the undressed patient. Cold-water immersion or the application of a cooling blanket may result in complications, chiefly from vasoconstriction, but both forms are widely used. Internal cooling is achieved with iced gastric lavage, iced peritoneal lavage, or cardiopulmonary bypass; however, it is rarely used and is associated with complications such as water intoxication. Antipyretics do not decrease core temperature, and aspirin should be avoided because it can worsen existing coagulopathies. In patients being treated for heatstroke, shivering can be treated with phenothiazines, benzodiazepines, or nondepolarizing muscle relaxants. Overshoot hypothermia should be avoided.

Dehydration and electrolyte imbalances need to be corrected as well. The total free water deficit needs to be corrected slowly to avoid central pontine myelinolysis. Half of the water deficit should be corrected over the first 3 to 6 hours. Hypotension may need pharmacological treatment if fluid repletion is insufficient in raising the blood pressure. The patient should be monitored for seizures and cardiac arrhythmias.

Several experimental therapeutic approaches have been studied. Hyperthermia has been demonstrated to decrease basal ganglia dopamine levels in rat[59] and rabbit[60] models. Hypervolemic hemodilution with the maintenance of mean arterial pressure has been beneficial in the animal model.[46] Pretreatment with conventional hydroxyl radical scavengers increases survival time in the animal model.[41] L-arginine p-nitroanilide has been demonstrated to suppress the elevation of NO following hyperthermia[42] and may hold therapeutic potential. DL-tetrahydropalmatine pretreatment has also demonstrated a neuroprotective effect in heatstroke.[61] The administration of IL-1 receptor antagonist also improves survival in the animal model.[47] Hyperbaric oxygen in the rat model of heatstroke has been shown to ameliorate cerebral ischemic damage and improve survival.[62] Other experimental therapies that are effective in the animal model are naloxone[63] and ketanserin.[64] None of these experimental measures have been adopted for use in humans.

HYPOTHERMIA

Peripheral Hypothermia

There has been little written about cold injury of the nervous system. Hypothermia with temperatures between 33° and 35° C. will often exhibit incoordination, slowed movements,[65] and mild confusion.[66] When core body temperatures fall below 32° C., shivering stops and dysarthria, cognitive slowing, amnesia, and ataxia are observed.[66] Irrational behavior, such as, paradoxical undressing which has been reported in up to 20 to 50% of mountain climbers affected by severe hypothermia.[67] This may be attributed to hypothalamic injury or paradoxical vasodilation when skin vessels lose their vasomotor tone. Cold exposure may damage the peripheral nervous system. Following both frostbite and a non-freezing cold injury such as trench foot, patients may complain of numbness, dysesthesias, and neuropathic pain in the affected extremities. These symptoms arise as a consequence of cold injury to the peripheral nerves and may occur in the absence of either frostbite or trench foot. In one study of Himalayan climbers,[68] 8 (4.8%) of 165 European mountaineers experienced these symptoms without preceding frostbite or trench foot. The affected climbers complained of a "corky" sensation in their feet, with superimposed severe lancinating pain.[68] Damage to both large- and small-nerve fibers has been demonstrated with clinical sensory testing, including two-point discrimination and pressure, vibration, and thermal thresholds.[69] Immunohistochemical studies of terminal cutaneous nerve fibers showed decreased numbers but an increase in staining for von Willebrand factor, indicating increased vascularity; the investigators proposed that myelinated and unmyelinated nerve damage

was the consequence of a cycle of ischemia and reperfusion.[69] Treatment with carbamazepine or similar drugs may be helpful in alleviating the discomfort, and the outcome may be favorable, with resolution over the course of several months.[68]

Systemic Hypothermia

Systemic hypothermia is defined as core body temperatures below 35°C. Hypothermia is often employed to protect the central nervous system. Neurological complications arise as a consequence of the effect of hypothermia on physiological processes, such as blood coagulation and cardiac conduction.

REFERENCES

1. Benzinger TH, Pratt AW, Kitzinger. The thermostatic control of human metabolic heat production. *Proc Natl Acad Sci USA.* 1961;47:730.
2. Sherrington CS. Notes on temperature after spinal transection, with some observations on shivering. *J Physiol.* 1924;58:405.
3. Robinson S, Robinson AH. Chemical composition of sweat. *Physiol Rev.* 1954;34:202–220.
4. Bouchama A, Knochel JP. Heat stroke. *N Engl J Med.* 2002; 346(25):1978–1988.
5. Vaughn LK, Veale WL, Cooper KE. Antipyresis: its effect on mortality rate of bacterially infected rabbits. *Brain Res Bull.* 1980;5(1):69–73.
6. Attia M, Khogali M, El-Khatib G, et al. Heat stroke: an upward shift of temperature regulation set point at an elevated body temperature. *Int Arch Occup Environ Health.* 1983;53(1):9–17.
7. Burton AC. Range and variability of blood flow in human fingers and vasomotor regulation of body temperature. *Amer J Physiol.* 1939;127:437.
8. Grogan H, Hopkins PM. Heat stroke: implications for critical care and anaesthesia. *Br J Anaesth.* 2002;88(5):700–707.
9. Kunihiro A, Foster J: Heat exhaustion and heat stroke. emedicine from Webmed. http://emedicine.medscape.com/article/770413-overview. Accessed March 11, 2009.
10. Yeo TP. Heat stroke: a comprehensive review. *AACN Clin Issues.* 2004;15(2):280–293.
11. Yaqub B, Al Deeb S. Heat strokes: aetiopathogenesis, neurological characteristics, treatment and outcome. *J Neurol Sci.* 1998;156(2):144–151.
12. Kitanaka C, Inoh Y, Toyoda T, et al. Malignant brainstem hyperthermia caused by brainstem hemorrhage. *Stroke.* 1994;25(2):518–520.
13. Denborough MA, Lovel RH. Anesthetic deaths in a family. *Lancet.* 1960;2:45.
14. Brandom BW. Genetics of malignant hyperthermia. *ScientificWorldJournal.* 2006;6:1722–1730.
15. Rosenberg H, Davis M, James D, et al. Malignant hyperthermia. *Orphanet J Rare Dis.* 2007;2:21.
15a. Monnier N, Procaccio V, et al. Malignant-hyperthermia susceptibility is associated with a mutation of the alpha 1-subunit of the human dihydropyridine-sensitive L-type voltage-dependent calcium-channel receptor in skeletal muscle. *Am J Hum Genet* 1997;60(6):1316–1325.

16. Donnelly AJ. Malignant hyperthermia. Epidemiology, pathophysiology, treatment. *AORN J*. 1994;59(2):393–395, 398–400, 403–405.

16a. Nelson TE, Lin M, Zapata-Sudo G, Sudo RT. Dantrolene sodium can increase or attenuate activity of skeletal muscle ryanodine receptor calcium release channel. Clinical implications. *Anesthesiology*. 1996;84(6):1368–1379.

16b. Caroff SN and Mann SC. Neuroleptic malignant syndrome. *Med Clin North Am* 1993;77(1):185–202.

17. Murray JB. Neuroleptic malignant syndrome. *J Gen Psychol*. 1987;114(1):39–46.

17a. Mihara K, Kondo T, et al. Relationship between functional dopamine D2 and D3 receptors gene polymorphisms and neuroleptic malignant syndrome. *Am J Med Genet B Neuropsychiatr Genet* 2003;117B(1):57–60.

18. Sternbach H. The serotonin syndrome. *Am J Psychiatry*. 1991; 148(6):705–713.

18a. Birmes P, Coppin D, et al. Serotonin syndrome: a brief review. *CMAJ* 2003;168(11):1439–1442.

19. Dematte JE, O'Mara K, Buescher J, et al. Near-fatal heat stroke during the 1995 heat wave in Chicago. *Ann Intern Med*. 1998; 129(3):173–181.

20. Dixit SN, Bushara KO, Brooks BR. Epidemic heat stroke in a Midwest community: risk factors, neurological complications and sequelae. *Wis Med J*. 1997;96(5):39–41.

21. Royburt M, Epstein Y, Solomon Z, Shemer J. Long-term psychological and physiological effects of heat stroke. *Physiol Behav*. 1993;54(2):265–267.

22. Van Stavern GP, Biousse V, Newman NJ, Leingang JC. Downbeat nystagmus from heat stroke. *J Neurol Neurosurg Psychiatry*. 2000;69(3):403–404.

23. Deleu D, El Siddig A, Kamran S, et al. Downbeat nystagmus following classical heat stroke. *Clin Neurol Neurosurg*. 2005; 108(1):102–104.

24. Manto MU. Isolated cerebellar dysarthria associated with a heat stroke. *Clin Neurol Neurosurg*. 1996;98(1):55–56.

25. McNamee T, Forsythe S, Wollmann R, Ndukwu IM. Central pontine myelinolysis in a patient with classic heat stroke. *Arch Neurol*. 1997;54(8):935–936.

26. Uzawa A, Mori M, Tamura N, et al. Bickerstaff brainstem encephalitis after heat stroke. *J Neurol*. 2006;253(4):533–534.

27. Pitt DC, Kriel RL, Wagner NC, Krach LE. Klüver-Bucy syndrome following heat stroke in a 12-year-old girl. *Pediatr Neurol*. 1995;13(1):73–76.

28. Rav-Acha M, Shuvy M, Hagag S, et al. Unique persistent neurological sequelae of heat stroke. *Mil Med*. 2007;172(6): 603–606.

29. Lin JJ, Chang MK, Sheu YD, et al. Permanent neurologic deficits in heat stroke. *Zhonghua Yi Xue Za Zhi (Taipei)*. 1991; 47(2):133–138.

30. Delgado G, Tunon T, Gállego J, Villanueva JA. Spinal cord lesions in heat stroke. *J Neurol Neurosurg Psychiatry*. 1985; 48(10):1065–1067.

31. Bacon CJ, Hall SM. Haemorrhagic shock encephalopathy syndrome in the British Isles. *Arch Dis Child*. 1992;67(8):985–993.

32. Lee S, Merriam A, Kim TS, et al. Cerebellar degeneration in neuroleptic malignant syndrome: neuropathologic findings and review of the literature concerning heat-related nervous system injury. *J Neurol Neurosurg Psychiatry*. 1989;52(3):387–391.

33. Fujino Y, Tsuboi Y, Shimoji E, et al. Progressive cerebellar atrophy following acute antidepressant intoxication. *Rinsho Shinkeigaku*. 2000;40(10):1033–1037.

34. Labuda A, Cullen N. Brain injury following neuroleptic malignant syndrome: case report and review of the literature. *Brain Inj*. 2006;20(7):775–778.

35. Pelletier J, Habib M, Pellissier JF, et al. Neurologic sequelae of the neuroleptics–lithium combination: role of hyperthermia. *Rev Med Interne*. 1991;12(3):187–191.

36. Shih CJ, Lin MT, Tsai SH. Experimental study on the pathogenesis of heat stroke. *J Neurosurg*. 1984;60(6):1246–1252.

37. Lin MT, Lin SZ. Cerebral ischemia is the main cause for the onset of heat stroke syndrome in rabbits. *Experientia*. 1992; 48(3):225–227.

38. Mustafa KY, Omer O, Khogali M, et al. Blood coagulation and fibrinolysis in heat stroke. *Br J Haematol*. 1985;61(3):517–523.

39. Ayus JC, Arieff AI. Features and outcomes of classic heat stroke. *Ann Intern Med*. 1999;130(7):613; author reply, 614–615.

40. Shibolet S, Coll R, Gilat T, Sohar E. Heatstroke: its clinical picture and mechanism in 36 cases. *Q J Med*. 1967;36(144):525–548.

41. Chang CK, Chang CP, Liu SY, Lin MT. Oxidative stress and ischemic injuries in heat stroke. *Prog Brain Res*. 2007;162:525–546.

42. Lin MT. Heatstroke-induced cerebral ischemia and neuronal damage. Involvement of cytokines and monoamines. *Ann NY Acad Sci*. 1997;813:572–580.

43. Canini F, L Bourdon, Cespuglio R, Buguet A. Voltametric assessment of brain nitric oxide during heatstroke in rats. *Neurosci Lett*. 1997;231(2):67–70.

44. Clark IA, Rockett KA, Cowden WB. Possible central role of nitric oxide in conditions clinically similar to cerebral malaria. *Lancet*. 1992;340(8824):894–896.

45. Wada K, Chatzipanteli K, Busto R, Dietrich WD. Role of nitric oxide in traumatic brain injury in the rat. *J Neurosurg*. 1998;89(5):807–818.

46. Chang CK, Chien CH, Chou HL, Lin MT. The protective effect of hypervolemic hemodilution in experimental heatstroke. *Shock*. 2001;16(2):153–158.

47. Chiu WT, Kao TY, Lin MT. Increased survival in experimental rat heatstroke by continuous perfusion of interleukin-1 receptor antagonist. *Neurosci Res*. 1996;24(2):159–163.

48. Kao TY, Lin MT. Brain serotonin depletion attenuates heatstroke-induced cerebral ischemia and cell death in rats. *J Appl Physiol*. 1996;80(2):680–684.

49. Chang L, Huang Y, Lin M. Local cerebral glucose utilization decreases after heatstroke onset in rats. *Neurosci Lett*. 2001; 308(3):206–208.

50. Kish SJ, Kleinert R, Minauf M, et al. Brain neurotransmitter changes in three patients who had a fatal hyperthermia syndrome. *Am J Psychiatry*. 1990;147(10):1358–1363.

51. Szold O, Reider-Groswasser II, Ben Abraham R, et al. Gray–white matter discrimination—a possible marker for brain damage in heat stroke? *Eur J Radiol*. 2002;43(1):1–5.

52. Biary N, Madkour MM, Sharif H. Post-heatstroke parkinsonism and cerebellar dysfunction. *Clin Neurol Neurosurg*. 1995;97(1):55–57.

53. Albukrek D, Bakon M, Moran DS, et al. Heat-stroke-induced cerebellar atrophy: clinical course, CT and MRI findings. *Neuroradiology*. 1997;39(3):195–197.

54. Mohapatro AK, Thomas M, Jain S, et al. Pancerebellar syndrome in hyperpyrexia. *Australas Radiol*. 1990;34(4):320–322.

55. McLaughlin CT, Kane AG, Auber AE. MR imaging of heat stroke: external capsule and thalamic T_1 shortening and cerebellar injury. *AJNR Am J Neuroradiol*. 2003;24(7): 1372–1375.

56. Aoki K, Yoshino A, Ueda Y, et al. Severe heat stroke associated with high plasma levels of plasminogen activator inhibitor 1. *Burns*. 1998;24(1):74–77.

57. Bazille C, Megarbane B, Bensimhon D, et al. Brain damage after heat stroke. *J Neuropathol Exp Neurol*. 2005;64(11):970–975.

58. Ohshima T, Maeda H, Takayasu T, et al. An autopsy case of infant death due to heat stroke. *Am J Forensic Med Pathol*. 1992;13(3):217–321.

59. Chou YT, Lai ST, Lee CC, Lin MT. Hypothermia attenuates circulatory shock and cerebral ischemia in experimental heatstroke. *Shock.* 2003;19(4):388–393.

60. Chou YT, Chen JC, Liu RS, et al. Dopamine overload visualized in the basal ganglia of rabbit brain during heatstroke can be suppressed by hypothermia. *Neurosci Lett.* 2005;375(2):87–90.

61. Chang CK, Chueh FY, Hsieh MT, Lin MT. The neuroprotective effect of DL-tetrahydropalmatine in rat heatstroke. *Neurosci Lett.* 1999;267(2):109–112.

62. Tsai HM, Gao CJ, Li WX, et al. Resuscitation from experimental heatstroke by hyperbaric oxygen therapy. *Crit Care Med.* 2005; 33(4):813–818.

63. Panjwani GD, Mustafa MK, Muhailan A, et al. Effect of hyperthermia on somatosensory evoked potentials in the anaesthetized rat. *Electroencephalogr Clin Neurophysiol.* 1991;80(5):384–391.

64. Lee-Chiong TL Jr, Stitt JT. Heatstroke and other heat-related illnesses. The maladies of summer. *Postgrad Med.* 1995;98(1):26–28, 31–33, 36.

65. Cheung SS, Montie DL, et al. Changes in manual dexterity following short-term hand and forearm immersion in 10 degrees C water. *Aviat Space Environ Med* 2003;74(9):990–993.

66. Sterba JA. Field management of accidental hypothermia during diving. Washington, D.C., Department of Navy. 1990,1–90.

67. Wedin B, Vanggaard L, et al. "Paradoxical undressing" in fatal hypothermia. *J Forensic Sci* 1979;24(3):543–553.

CHAPTER 50

Neurological Effects in Electrical Injury

Mary Capelli-Schellpfeffer

INTRODUCTION

Most employees work on, near, or with electricity every day. While often unnoticed, proximity to the flow of electrical charges, or current, can transition activity from harmless to harmful across short time and spatial dimensions. U.S. data from 1992 to 2002 note 3378 workers died from on-the-job electrical injuries and 46,598 workers were nonfatally injured.[1] Lightning-related electrical injuries are not included in these figures. Data on nonoccupational electrical injuries are not systematically tracked; however, electrical injuries from products (e.g., extension cords, household appliances, and electronic weapons), as well as in medical, home, school, and recreational environments, affect thousands more annually.

In most occupational exposures, the source of electricity is attributable to commercially generated 50- to 60-Hz alternating current power delivery. However, as suggested in Table 1, devices that leverage the advantages of the electromagnetic spectrum to do work can result in electrical exposures across frequency and energy ranges. For example, injury can result with exposures to radiofrequency sources, such as radiofrequency antennas, or capacitive coupling with sources of changing magnetic gradients, like diagnostic magnetic resonance imaging devices.[2] Electrical exposures to direct current sources also can produce injury, for example, with maintenance of photovoltaics (solar cells), operation of transportation systems like electric trains, or research activities in energy laboratories.

The hazards associated with electricity use are uniquely challenging: Because electrical energy's presence saturates daily life in a silent, odorless, and invisible manner, people are routinely cognitively desensitized to the physical potency of electrical energy's fundamental nature. The remainder of this chapter discusses the occupational trauma mechanisms and neurological effects with regard to power frequency electrical energy generated, transmitted, or distributed in electrical installations and used in the function of electrical components.

Electrical energy has the potentially destructive capability of a highly flammable, explosive, and deadly chemical, as illustrated in Figure 50-1 (see color plate). Even though it is not common to think of this analogy, just as a chemical's containment can be breached, so can power frequency electrical energy's restraint within its engineered conducting path be unintentionally faulted by installation or component operation or by human error. Figure 50-1 shows video-captured images from two staged high-voltage laboratory testing examples of

Table 1: Electromagnetic Radiation Exposure Sources

Electromagnetic Spectrum	Commercial Source Examples
Radio	Radiofrequency towers
Microwave	Microwave ovens
Infrared	Fast-food heating lamps
Visible	Lightbulbs
Ultraviolet	Tanning beds
X-rays	Medical and dental equipment
Gamma-rays	Particle accelerators

industrial electrical accidents. In the top sequence, a mannequin worker stands in front of a 480-V electrical panel holding a screwdriver. The bottom sequence has a mannequin worker in an aerial bucket with extremities extended in simulated work action at an overhead power line installation.

The first frame of each sequence demonstrates the initial electrical failure event, when an electric current flows at the testing start. At this point in the sequence, electric shock is the hazard, with current flow from the equipment to the test mannequin's nearby tools or body. In the second frame of the Figure 50-1 sequences, the staged tests show electrical arcing subsequent to the electrical failure in the first frame. The electric current is flowing through conductors and through the arcs. The arcs are supplied energy from the test laboratories' electrical systems. Ionized air conducts electric current while

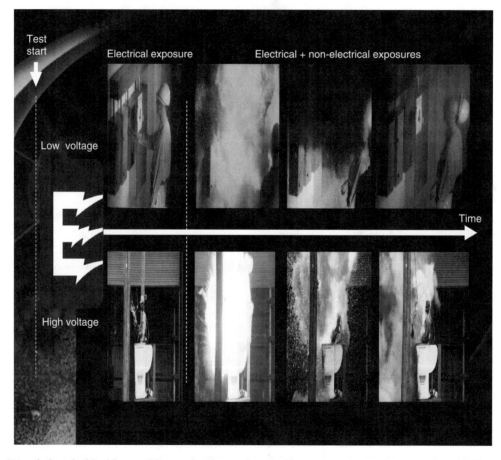

Figure 50-1. Staged electrical incidents with mannequin employees. The top sequence shows an electrical incident staged as a maintenance employee at a low-voltage (480 V) installation.[3] Peak monitored temperature exceeded 225°C within 10 msec at the mannequin's hand and at 120 msec at the neck. Peak pressure estimate was at 2160 lb/ft² and a 141.5-dB sound. Cooling of the hand to 70°C required more than 2500 msec. The bottom sequence was staged as a high-voltage (>1000 V) illustration of a line worker in a bucket at an overhead cable, with video images courtesy of ConEd frame captured for visual comparison (see color plate).

metals are vaporized, leading to a complex event wherein electrical energy is transformed and transferred to the surrounding space in electrical, thermal, acoustic, mechanical, and radiation (ultraviolet, infrared) forms. The third frame of the Figure 50-1 sequences suggests the intensively explosive, thermal, and radiating nature of the resulting electrical "fireballs" by their shape, brightness, and dimension. The last frame shows the destructive results.

ELECTRICITY AS A TOXIC EXPOSURE

The nature of power frequency electrical energy's unrestrained interaction with the surrounding environment is governed by physics. The principles of electrochemical and electromechanical energy balance and release can be adopted from the chemical and toxicology literature to conceptualize electrical hazard parameters.[4] The toxicity of electricity can be described using terms familiar from material safety data sheet (MSDS) formats common to hazard materials (HAZMAT) notices, including, for electricity, the chemical nature and ingredients, flash point, explosivity, threshold limit, and lethal dose. In this way, common industrial electrical language can be placed into the context of MSDS terms.

Chemical Nature and Ingredients

The chemical nature of electricity in commercial and industrial conductors is electrons, the charge carriers in copper, iron, aluminum, and other metals. Where electricity is conducted in nonmetals, for example, fuel cells, the chemical charge carrier may be active in solution.

Flash Point

The chemical parameter of flash point can be recognized with electricity as the dielectrical breakdown characteristic of the power frequency electrical source. In safety practice, as a rough rule, equipment is designed to allow 1 inch of space for each 1000-V electrical force to reduce the chance for "flash" or electrical arcing.

Explosivity

Just as concentrated gases like oxygen in a small space can be detonated to explode, high power density in small geometric spaces can exceed the installation's ratings. For example, the potential ignition of 1 MW 50- to 60-Hz electrical power is roughly equivalent to the potential ignition of one stick of dynamite (approximately ⅓-pound TNT equivalent).

Threshold Limit

The toxicity threshold limit of power frequency electrical energy exposure is the fractional amount of current that may flow from a voltage source to an exposed employee which may result in a potentially harmful biological effect. Considering Table 2, a source current at 6 to 30 mA is consistent with a threshold limit.

Lethal Dose

The lethal dose of power frequency electrical energy can be considered as the current exposure that interferes with the human body's breathing, the electrical conduction patterns in the heart, or both. As a result of exposure to less than 1/10th of 1 ampere current flow (0.1 A) at a 110-V electrical force, respiratory function can be disrupted, with subsequent impairment of brain

Table 2: Effects of a 50- to 60-Hz Electric Current on the Body (<600 V)

Source Current[*]	Neuromuscular Response
1 mA	Perception of faint tingling.
5 mA	Perception of possibly disturbing but not painful slight shock.
6–12 mA (F)[†] 9–30 mA (M)[†]	Painful shock associated with loss of muscular control. Inability to release forceful grip or relax contracted muscles may occur.
50–150 mA	Perception of extremely painful shock, respiratory paralysis, and severe muscle contraction.
1000–4300 mA (1–4.3 A)	Ventricular fibrillation due to interference from an extraphysiological electrical source with cardiac conduction, muscle contraction, and neural damage. Death is likely.
10,000 mA (10 A)	Cardiac arrest and severe burns occur. Death is probable.
15,000 mA (15 A)	Lowest overcurrent at which a typical electrical circuit protector (fuse, breaker) operates.

[*]One milliamp (mA) is 1/1000th of one ampere (A).
[†]Differences in female (F) and male (M) responses are related to average difference in total body muscle and fat content.
Adapted from NIOSH[5] and DOL[6] based on research by Dalziel[7,8] and the presentation by Lee.[9]

and other vital organ oxygenation. As suggested again by Table 2, with a 1- to 4.3-A current exposure without intervention, death is likely.

INCIDENT HISTORY IN OCCUPATIONAL ELECTRICAL INJURY

The incident history in occupational electrical injury raises clinical suspicion for the patient's possible exposures. Once incident features are fully appreciated, the clinician can place into context the patient's neurological complaints, past medical history, review of symptoms, and physical findings, including neurological examination. To identify relevant incident facts, suggested questions for the incident history are included in Table 3. Both fatal and nonfatal injury events share three characteristics:

1. The unintentional exposure of the affected person to electrical energy
2. Compliance failure in at least one aspect of electrical design, installation, policies, procedures, practice, or personal protection
3. Energy transfer to the exposed individual in some combination of electrical, thermal, radiation, acoustic (pressure), mechanical, light, and kinetic forms

Lee and Dougherty note that in the extra-low-frequency range (0 to 1 kHz) relevant to commercially available power sources, the body's dissociated ions are the most important charge carriers, and passage of current during an electric shock is mediated at the source–body interface by electrochemical reactions.[10]

Under accidental conditions, the dose or amount of total energy transferred to an individual involved in an unintended electrical exposure can be conceptualized by considering how efficient the coupling between the source and the individual is during the energy release. This "efficiency" is partly a function of current, exposure duration, distance from the source, barriers used, surface area of the body exposed, and material properties of biological tissues, including the following:

- Conductance
- Impedance
- Resistance
- Absorbance of human "biomaterials," i.e., the water, lipids, fats, proteins, and minerals that constitute the body

Other factors include ambient conditions (e.g., confined space, humid or wet surfaces, or hazardous location), the employee's position in the electrical circuit (i.e., parallel or series relationship to the circuit), and the protection afforded by nearby equipment (e.g., grounding) and personal gear, such as voltage-rated gloves or insulated boots.

Table 3: Questions Relevant to Electrical Incident History
1. What was the voltage and current of the electrical source?
2. Did the electrical source touch your body?
3. Did the current "jump" to you?
4. How did you break away from the electrical source?
5. Were there other hazards in the area?
6. Were you working in a confined space or on a ladder?
7. Were you equipped with protective earplugs, glasses, clothing, gloves, or boots?
8. Were you wearing any jewelry, a cell phone, or metal tools?
9. Did you see a flash of light?
10. Did you hear a pop, crack, or boom?
11. Did you feel heat or see fire?
12. Was there an explosion?

Finally, considering the electrical system, the amount of current flow is also a function of the protective mechanical and electronic equipment engineered into the system's electrical coordination, such as current-interrupting devices (i.e., electronic controllers, fuses, breakers, or other switching equipment). The more quickly these devices respond, the less time that current will be available to produce injury and destruction. The longer it takes a current-interrupting device to operate, the longer the amount of time that will be available for current to flow with damaging consequences. If current-interrupting devices fail to operate, or if the duration for operation is long enough for the shock event to escalate, then the electrical charges flowing through installation and adjacent materials will more likely be able to cross an air gap via dielectric breakdown, again referred to as arcing. A highly dynamic thermal environment can result.

With completion of the incident history, the clinician may anticipate the possibility that the patient has sustained a nonuniform electrical exposure (i.e., electric shock propagated over or through the body's biomaterials) or a nonuniform electrical exposure complicated by cooccurrent energy exposures from thermal, radiation, acoustic, and mechanical releases (including blast, shrapnel, and equipment disintegration).

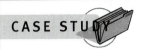

CASE STUDY

While presumably working on deenergized equipment, a 37-year-old electrician reached into a transformer box with a metal wrench in his ungloved dominant right hand and contacted an electrical installation surface energized with 4160 V while standing on the second step of a wooden ladder.[11] He immediately felt a shock in his right hand and arm, with pain and the smell of burning flesh. He was unable to let go of the wrench and lost his balance, falling from the ladder and landing on his feet. No blow to the head or loss of consciousness occurred. Ambulance transport to the nearest hospital and an emergency medical evaluation followed. Full-thickness burns at right fingers 3 and 4 and over the radial right elbow were noted associated with decreased right elbow extension. Additional testing showed a normal electrocardiogram. Emergency orthopedic exploration at the right upper extremity demonstrated 60% disruption of the right triceps tendon. Repair was done with discharge at 24 hours after the injury. Within 48 hours of the electrical exposure, the patient presented for burn center evaluation and treatment with severe right upper extremity pain and swelling associated with sensory loss at right fingers 2 and 4, as well as complications at his surgical wound. Laboratory studies for fractionated skeletal muscle creatinine kinase and lactate dehydrogenase were elevated. Diagnostic imaging included abnormalities on technetium–pyrophosphate scan and magnetic resonance imaging. Electrophysiological studies included refractory period spectroscopy and nerve conduction studies and demonstrated decreased peak action potential amplitudes compared to the unaffected left extremities. Surgery and pain management followed. Subsequent rehabilitative care included psychiatric and neuropsychiatric evaluation and treatment.

TRAUMA CONSEQUENCES IN ELECTRICAL INCIDENTS

Researchers have understood since Haddon's pioneering publications in the mid-20th century that all injuries share an energy damage process.[12] In an occupational electrical fatality, the electrical incident results in sufficient energy transfer from the work environment to the person—via electrical, mechanical, radiation, acoustic, or pressure exposure—in such ways and amounts as to result an unrecoverable destructive effect. Nonfatal electrical events result from sublethal exposures.

An electric "burn" injury can have multiple causes, including tissue destruction from electroporation of cellular membranes or direct electrical effects on proteins,[10] thermal injury from ohmic heating by current or conduction from ignited materials and structures, ultraviolet radiation (e.g., corneal "flash burn," "ground glass" eye, welder's flash, and photokeratitis), infrared radiation (e.g., corneal or retinal burns and cataract), and chemical reactions by molten metals.

While burns may or may not be present, additional physical findings in electrical injury may include laceration wounds, traumatic amputation, fracture dislocations, impaired neuromuscular function, or edema.

As suggested by the case study, the physical examination, supported by laboratory studies for the serum markers of muscle damage (e.g., serum enzymes and urine myoglobin), provides correlative information for radiology and electrophysiology diagnostic studies. Even when external wounds are not observed, a high degree of clinical suspicion of occult neurological injury is advised. Magnetic resonance imaging and nuclear medicine examination can evaluate nervous system structural damage and identify fractures, local tissue edema, and focal areas of inflammation. Central nervous system findings may include infarction or hemorrhage.[13]

With regard to electrophysiology diagnostic studies, muscle weakness, easy fatigue, endurance loss, paralysis, or pain are indications for electromyography and peripheral nerve conduction studies (sensory and motor). Further evaluation may be needed with peripheral nerve refractory period spectroscopy and magnetic resonance spectroscopy. Additional complaints like history of loss of consciousness or seizures, headache, impaired memory, attentional problems, personality changes, or cognitive changes may be evaluated by electroencephalography.[14]

When documented at the scene or through initial evaluation and treatment, an electrical injury patient's loss of consciousness may be attributable to direct electrical effects on the brain or indirect effects. Indirect effects may include oxygen deficiency related to respiratory paralysis with simultaneous muscle contraction or cardiac insufficiency with arrhythmia. Secondary causal explanations for loss of consciousness may include oxygen deficiency (related to oxygen consumption by combustion or to a hypoxic confined space) or blunt force trauma from fall, shrapnel, or blast effects.

A history of temporary or persistent hearing change, tinnitus, or memory change related to verbal communication are indications for auditory evoked potentials. Visual acuity changes or visual disturbances are indications for visual evoked potentials. Cardiac rhythm disturbances, syncope, chest pain, and easy fatigue are indications for electrocardiography.

REHABILITATIVE CONSIDERATIONS

Functional impairment following electrical injury is well known. The most comprehensive review of a large workforce's experience tracked the outcomes of 2080 electrical injury survivors over a 19-year period. Of these, 515 patients, or 25%, were noted to have postinjury complications, including 63% burn related, with amputations in 5%; 18% neuropsychiatric, 12% sensory; 5% orthopedic; and 1% cardiovascular.[15] Sense organ disorders included vision-related changes, auditory sequelae, and anosmia. In 59 of the 515 patients, disability was considered serious, with impairment rating from 31% to 100%.

Even when functional and neuropsychological impairments are resolved, if posttraumatic seizure or syncope conditions complicate an electrical injury patient's recovery and rehabilitation, there may be significant occupational implications. These sequelae may disqualify an employee for safety-sensitive work, such as driving trucks, commercial vehicles, cranes, forklifts, or tractors; flying; operating or maintaining energy installations (such as gas pipelines, steam generators, or refineries); and working on or near moving parts, above or below ground level, or in construction.

REFERENCES

1. Cawley JC, Homce GT. Trends in electrical injuries. 2006 Philadelphia IEEE IAS PCIC Conference Proceedings, Sept 11–Oct 15, 2006; Paper No. PCIC-PH-03, pp. 1–14.
2. Patterson T, Stecker MM, Netherton BL. Mechanisms of electrode induced injury: II. Clinical experience. *Am J Electroneurodiagnostic Technol.* 2007;47(2):93–113.
3. Jones R, Liggett DP, Capelli-Schellpfeffer M, et al. Staged tests increase awareness of arc-flash hazards in electrical equipment. *IEEE Trans Ind Appl Soc.* 2000;36(2):659–667.
4. Capelli-Schellpfeffer M. Creating electrical hazard awareness with communication using MSDS and labeling. IEEE Industrial and Commercial Power Systems Technical Conference Record, May 2–6, 2004. IEEE Catalog Number 03CH37555, pp. 163–166.
5. National Institute for Occupational Safety and Health. *Electrical Safety: Safety and Health in Electrical Trades—Student Manual.* DHHS (NIOSH) Pub. No. 2002-123. Cincinnati, Ohio: NIOSH; 2002.
6. Department of Labor. *Controlling Electrical Hazards.* Washington, DC: U.S. Department of Labor, Occupational Safety and Health Administration; 1997.
7. Dalziel CF. Effect of frequency on let-go currents. *Trans Am Inst Elect Engr.* 1943;62:745–750.
8. Dalziel CF. Threshold 60-cycle fibrillating currents. *AIEE Trans III Power Apparatus Syst.* 1960;79:667–673.
9. Lee RL. Electrical safety in industrial plants. *Am Soc Safety Eng J.* 1973;18(9):36–42.
10. Lee RC, Dougherty W. Electrical injury: mechanisms, manifestations, and therapy. *IEEE Trans Dielect Elect Insulat.* 2003;10(5):810–819.
11. Chico M, Capelli-Schellpfeffer M, Kelley KM, et al. Management and coordination of postacute medical care for electrical trauma survivors. *Ann NY Acad Sci.* 1994;888:334–342.
12. Haddon W Jr. Energy damage and the ten countermeasure strategies. *J Trauma.* 1973;13(4):321–331.
13. Cherington M. Central nervous system complications of lightning and electrical injuries. *Semin Neurol.* 1995;15:233–240.
14. Danielson JR, Capelli-Schellpfeffer M, Lee RC. Upper extremity electrical injury. *Hand Clinics.* 2000;16(2):225–234.
15. Gourbiere E, Corbut JP, Bazin Y. Functional consequence of electrical injury. *Ann NY Acad Sci.* 1994;720:259–271.

CHAPTER 51

Neurological Complications of Submersion and Diving

Des Gorman

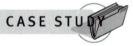

CASE STUDY

A 30-year-old man dives alone to a depth of 20 m of seawater onto a sandy sea bed and collects shellfish for 45 minutes before swimming back to the surface. He uses a self-contained underwater breathing apparatus (SCUBA) and breathes compressed air. He has only a short swim to his boat and climbs onboard. The dive has been uneventful except for some minor difficulties during the descent, when he had to use forceful valsalva maneuvers to eliminate a sense of pain and fullness in his right ear. He feels tired, but otherwise well, and puts his diving gear away before pulling up his anchor. Immediately after recovering the anchor, he feels lightheaded. Within minutes he is incapacitated by a sense of spinning; he feels as though his head is turning clockwise. He starts his outboard motor and tries to head to shore but has an equally sudden worsening of this rotational sense and is unable to stand and steer. His boat goes into an uncontrolled circling. His situation is seen by people on a nearby boat, who, after some good boat handling, come alongside and take control of the injured diver's boat. He is eventually taken ashore. He is severely incapacitated and vomits often.

The issues to consider are what are the possible causes of this diver's vertigo and what should be done about it by way of first aid and definitively.

INTRODUCTION

For reasons that include secondary gain, humans are greatly attracted to the ocean, lakes, and rivers, and many engage in underwater recreations and occupations.[1] The practice of underwater diving is ancient. Alexander the Great used divers in military roles, and the aboriginal women of Tasmania, Australia, have dived, using breath-hold techniques, to collect abalone for tens of millennia. This human aquatic attraction is not easily rationalized, especially given the consequent and unavoidable hazards for a species that is best described as a highly adapted air-breathing terrestrial mammal. Although some human physiology is similar to that of diving mammals, most of us are "a long way from the primeval slime," and the "diving reflex" is not a human characteristic. Putting aside the Jacques Cousteau–inspired romanticism of *e mare a mare,* returning to "Mother Ocean" is not natural, and it is only the "physiological fluke" of the relatively low pulmonary artery pressure (PAP) that allows prolonged human diving underwater, breathing compressed gases, without a neurological stroke syndrome of some sort resulting. Sadly, for the communities concerned, and in much the same way as for Sherpa children in relation to working at high altitudes, the children of the Australian aboriginal diver women and those of the Japanese and Korean Ama divers are no more aquatically adapted than your children or mine.

This chapter focuses on the neurological consequence of submersion and especially that of diving. The important subject of drowning is not discussed, and you are referred to a relevant symposium publication for further information.[2] This is not to depreciate the significance of drowning; it is the oft-final lethal event in many situations in which consciousness is impaired in the water. About 5% of those who suffer a cerebral arterial gas embolism (CAGE) die because of brainstem involvement and cardiorespiratory arrest; many more die by drowning during the period of interrupted brain–blood flow, which follows bubble release into the arterial system. The latter causes only a transient loss of brain function, although a relapse some time later is common.[3] The problem is that the otherwise short-lived impairment occurs for someone in a nonrespirable environment.

The chapter also does not consider the effect of submersion and diving on preexisting neurological disease. This is too extensive a subject for this review and includes phenomena as varied as experiencing increasingly frequent and severe migraines by the many divers who are migraineurs, diving per se precipitating convulsions in susceptible individuals, unexpectedly losing consciousness due to hypoglycemia in insulin-dependent diabetic divers, and suffering catastrophic sequelae by divers with cerebral palsy from what to an "able-bodied" diver would have been a self-limiting and or easily treated episode of decompression illness (DCI) affecting the spinal cord.

To simplify the subject, the chapter is divided into those phenomena that transiently impair neural function, such as gas toxicities and inert gas narcosis (IGN), and those that usually resolve but do have the potential for sustained impairment, such as DCI and CAGE.

TRANSIENT IMPAIRMENT

In addition to the obvious problem of becoming cold, immersion in water has a plethora of less self-evident physiological effects; for example, the effect of gravity on blood distribution is essentially mitigated, and there is a sequential centralization of blood, a resulting impairment of pulmonary compliance, a decrease in antidiuretic hormone production, a diuresis, and a loss of blood volume. Prolonged immersion can be fatal during a subsequent rescue because of a sudden return of gravity to a person who has, out of the water, depleted blood volume.[4] This problem is well recognized in space travel. The importance of this observation, in a neurological context, is that DCI causes an impairment of microcirculations and a reperfusion injury, and divers are already hemoconcentrated before any viable bubbles are formed.[5]

Submersion also results in hyperbaria. The submersed person is subject to an ambient pressure that is the sum of the atmospheric pressure and the water pressure. The water pressure is a product of depth and density. With the exception of polar seas and a few famous high-salinity oceans, every 10 m of seawater (msw) depth exerts a pressure roughly equivalent to that due to the Earth's atmosphere at sea level. Because fluids are relatively incompressible, the pressure acting on the submersed person is transmitted through their tissues. This is reasonably well described by Pascal's principle and is analogous to the physical basis of hydraulics. The small extent to which fluids can be compressed can become a problem and does at great depth when neural membrane compression causes, at least partly, high-pressure neurological syndrome (HPNS).[6,7] However, more commonly, it is the relative stability of compressed fluids that can result in tissue damage in the body and does so at any fluid–gas interface, as the gas space is, by contrast, relatively compressible. Gas volumes, ignoring Van de Waal's intermolecular forces and the humidification and warming of inspired gases, are inversely proportional to ambient pressure (Boyle's law). The resulting tissue injuries are collectively known as barotrauma and are common in divers descending and ascending in the ocean.[8] Nondivers recognize the problem because it affects their middle ears and facial sinuses in aircraft. The degree of injury is actually determined not by the pressures per se, as evidenced by the protection against lung inflation injuries during a decompression in the water when the chest is girdled to limit expansion.[9]

Hyperbaria also causes an increase in alveolar gas tensions. In general accordance with Dalton's law, a gas partial pressure is a product of the relevant fraction of the gas mix and the ambient pressure. Gases then diffuse from the alveoli of a submersed person's lung along the partial pressure gradient to arterial blood, and to tissues and venous blood, until equilibrium is established at the alveolar gas tension. The time it takes to achieve this balance is determined by the perfusion of the tissue concerned, the rate at which the gas diffuses into and through the tissue, and the solubility of the gas in question in blood and the tissue. Gas solubility in a fluid is also directly linearly related to gas partial pressure and hence ambient pressure (Henry's law). Changes in temperature have a profound and complicated effect on these gas kinetics as has been demonstrated by significant increases in the rate of overt DCI in diving operations when nothing else happened other than the divers being kept warmer underwater. Any subsequent decompression can result in tissue gas tensions exceeding ambient pressure, and bubbles may both form and survive. The process is well understood at a qualitative but not at a quantitative level, which is a problem in designing a program, known as a decompression schedule, to allow a submersed person to return to the surface of the ocean without becoming unwell.[10] The physics here are daunting, and only more intrepid readers are referred to an interactive consideration of the Gibb's free energy formulation and La Place's law.[11] The fate of these "survivor" bubbles are discussed later in this chapter in the section on DCI.

Neurological function and especially alertness, concentration, and higher cognitive functions are variously, but reversibly, impaired in a submersed person, particularly in a deep diver. The constitutive problems in this context, in alphabetical order, include carbon dioxide (CO_2) and monoxide (CO) toxicities, HPNS, hypoxia, IGN, and oxygen (O_2) toxicity,

Carbon-based Gas Toxicities

Combustion and metabolism result in CO_2 and CO production, although CO poisoning is due to exogenously acquired gas.

Hypercarbia is an important problem in diving.[8] Not only is CO_2 directly toxic, it also increases the risk of a significant DCI, worsens IGN, and predisposes a diver to central nervous system O_2 toxicity.[12] Care is taken then in diving systems to eliminate CO_2. In most situations, CO_2 tensions do not increase because the gas is highly soluble in plasma, the gas is buffered in venous blood by hemoglobin, and in most people, the ventilation rate is determined by CO_2 levels. A small group of people is relatively insensible to CO_2; these people present as divers who have slow rates of breathing gas consumption, and they often attract attention because of recurrent headaches and nausea when diving or because they have had an O_2 toxic convulsion. Hypoventilation is another typical cause of hypercarbia in divers, either deliberate hypoventilation, which is known as skipbreathing, or nondeliberate hypoventilation as a result of a nonsensible increase in CO_2 set points to reduce the work of breathing, which in diving is largely gas density dependent and hence ambient pressure dependent. The other common causes of hypercarbia are failure of CO_2 removal systems in diving apparatus in which gas is recycled and system failure because of actual or effective dead space in diving systems allowing CO_2 accumulation.

The complex biology and toxicology of CO are not addressed in detail in this chapter. This gas is both an endogenous gaseous neurotransmitter and an exogenous poison. It is anesthetic and causes a DCI-like delayed immune-mediated neuropathy, which might be preventable by hyperbaric oxygen (HBO)—again, in much the same way as DCI can be treated. Extraordinarily, one of the many ways in which we have shown that the brain might be protected against CO-induced hypoxemia is via the cortical neuronal production of CO itself and nitric oxide to cause preferential perfusion of the cortex at the expense of the white matter. Refer for more detail to some recent reviews of CO biology and toxicology[13,14] and to a recent excellent randomized controlled clinical trial of HBO in the treatment of CO poisoning, which was published in the *New England Journal of Medicine*.[15] Divers using air sources contaminated with compressor exhaust fumes have presented with persistent confusion and, sometimes, a transient loss of consciousness, which often developed late in a dive or upon surfacing. The receiving physician has similarly been confused, and the distinction between CO poisoning and both CAGE and DCI can be difficult. The common treatment brings some professional comfort.

High-Pressure Neurological Syndrome

The compression of neural membranes to cause at least some features of HPNS has already been mentioned. This syndrome is not a simple gas toxicity, as is seen by it being manifest in animals breathing liquids. The effect is mitigated by the use of an anesthetic, and vice versa. The first signs of HPNS are usually only evident at depths below 150 msw and include problems in coordination and tremor. At depths greater than 300 msw, higher functions are progressively impaired and electroencephalogram studies show microsleep. Convulsions and death are the endpoint, although the limits of human exposure are yet to be determined. Divers breathing both O_2–helium (He) mixes, usually with a nitrogen (N_2) admixture to alleviate some effects of HPNS, and O_2–hydrogen (H_2) mixes have been able to dive successfully to depths greater than 600 msw. At such pressures, metabolic rates increase and divers complain of persistent fatigue. Exercise responses are limited. Temperature sensitivity is altered, and blood cell survival is reduced. Simply, human physiology is profoundly impaired, all be it reversibly.[6,7,16] Notwithstanding these effects, the psychology of deep diving is more limiting for many of us.

Hypoxia

The insidious problem of hypoxia in diving was first noted in military divers using gas-recirculating apparatus in the late 19th century. The problem of such divers suddenly losing consciousness as they neared the surface after a dive was "solved" by the famous physiologist, John Haldane. He showed that in these diving sets O_2 content would fall if divers were working so hard that they were consuming O_2 faster than it was being supplied. The problem would not manifest at depth because the elevated ambient pressure would be such that the alveolar O_2 tension would still be adequate for normal blood oxygenation. For example, normoxia can be achieved at a depth of 30 msw for a diver who has an alveolar O_2 fraction as low as 4%. The conundrum is that divers do not suffer any hypoxia as long as they do not try to surface. During any subsequent decompression, the ambient pressure will decrease, as will the O_2 partial pressure in accordance with Dalton's law, and somewhere near the surface hypoxia will suddenly and dramatically onset.[8]

This mechanism of hypoxia is not seen in open circuit–demand diving systems but is a known complication of breath-hold diving, where it is accurately and colloquially known as "shallow water blackout." The likelihood of such a blackout increases with the duration of the breath-hold, as can be achieved by hyperventilating before diving to lower CO_2 tensions, and is more likely in a diver who is working hard.[8]

Inert Gas Narcosis

By 1930, the utility of divers using compressed air for deep work was found to be reduced by two related phenomena. The first was an intoxication, the so-called rhapsody of the deep,[6,8,16] and the second was due to the work of breathing an increasingly dense gas. Eventually, N_2 was blamed for both. Diving schedules for the use of O_2–He mixes were introduced into the U.S. Navy in 1939, and during World War II the Swede Arnie Setterstrom dived to 150 msw using an O_2–H_2 gas mix.

The narcotic effect of gases is most closely related to their lipid solubility—hence the attraction of He and H_2. Just over 30 years after the U.S. Navy adopted its first O_2–He diving practices, Hans Keller first dived to 300 msw in a dive that proved lethal for two of his companions. Through this dive he "discovered" HPNS, which, ironically, meant some breathing gas lipid solubility would become desirable again.

IGN is an invariable and unavoidable consequence of submersion. Its effects are not well explained by physical effects alone[6]; are unpredictable even in an individual; are influenced by anxiety, work, and being in the ocean; and are made worse by any hypercarbia. There is also an unpredictable interaction with any central nervous system–active drug and alcohol. A colleague invented the "Martini law," comparing increments of depth for a diver breathing compressed air with glasses of martinis. The law was amusing but was always fanciful as the impairment is not that easily predicted. Most incidents and accidents in diving, as in any human occupation, are the result of human error.[17] In this context, IGN is a usual and major contributor.

Oxygen Toxicity

Humans are well able to manage the products of O_2 metabolism, but not in hyperbaric conditions.[12] If a gas mix of greater than 60 kPa of O_2 is breathed long enough, the total lung capacity is reduced. When the forced vital capacity is about 75% of normal for that person, dyspnea is experienced; eventually, irreversible interstitial lung injury will accrue. This is pulmonary O_2 toxicity and is known as the Lorraine-Smith effect.

If the mix contains O_2 at a tension greater than 100 kPa, then convulsions may ensue, usually after a noticeable aura. This is often lethal for divers and literally and figuratively agitates the marine animals and fish. It is known as the Paul Bert effect and results in quite restrictive diving practices; for example, the use of a mix that results in an O_2 tension of 160 kPa is limited to a maximum acceptable diving duration of 30 minutes. There are extraordinary day-to-day and person-to-person variations in convulsion threshold. The threshold is greatly lowered by hypercarbia and, to a lesser extent, by work, being in the ocean, anxiety, the use of some drugs, fever, and so on. The only good news is that should the diver survive the experience, there is little risk of convulsion-related sequelae, and there is no evidence of an increased risk of other forms of epilepsy.

PERSISTENT AND POTENTIALLY DISABLING IMPAIRMENT

The process of bubble formation in submersion was briefly described in an earlier section. Bubbles form first in favorable conditions, such as in "vacuums" between tissue planes, and in crevices and surface defects, where the effect of surface tension pressures are reduced. Anyone who has carefully observed bubbles forming in a glass of beer and or champagne has noticed that the bubbles form on the wall of the glass and not in the fluid itself. Bubbles also form first in areas in which gas tensions exceed ambient pressure; that is, bubbles form in tissues and venous blood but rarely in arterial blood, which is just as well. Most bubbles do not last long, at least partly because of surface tension pressures, but survival in this context is facilitated by coalescence and by the bubble absorbing surfactants onto its surface.

Most tissue bubbles remain in tissue but are not innocent, as explained in the section on DCI, whereas, venous bubbles travel with blood flow to the right side of the heart to be trapped in the pulmonary arteries and to resolve first by diffusion of the gases into the alveolus and then by expiration. The physiological fluke cited earlier is this process of pulmonary bubble "filtering." This is a process that avoids arterial bubbles and, in turn, stroke syndromes. The trapping occurs because the PAP is overcome by surface tension pressures acting on the proximal interface of bubbles at the bifurcations of arterioles. By contrast, the greater systemic arterial pressure is such that few arterial bubbles trap. My colleagues and I, as well as other researchers, have been able to recover more than 80% of the volume of gas emboli injected into a carotid artery of animals from jugular vein air traps within 5 minutes of the injection.[5,18,19]

The pulmonary filtration is not without consequence: The alveolar–blood vessel interface is damaged and takes hours to repair. As a result, fluid leaks into the alveolus. PAP increases after almost any compressed gas dive, right heart pressures increase as a consequence of this afterload, and significant right-to-left shunts may arise through anatomical defects such as a patent foramen ovale, which is a predictable and actual risk factor for neurological DCI. In addition, central venous pressures increase, perhaps to the point where venous drainage of the thoracic spinal cord is impaired, causing a form of spinal DCI, which is almost refractory to treatment. If the rate of pulmonary gas embolism exceeds the rate at which bubbles resolve by diffusion, then a ventilation–perfusion mismatch arises and the person becomes dyspneic. This is known as pulmonary DCI or, colloquially, as the "chokes" and is the usual lethal form of DCI in humans. This contrasts with many animal species in which a consumptive coagulopathy is a common feature of lethal DCI. Humans show a fall in platelets and a rise in fibrin-degradation products after diving, but the rheological effect is usually minor and the treatment of divers who have a DCI with antiplatelet agents has consequently been somewhat unrewarding.[5,20]

Decompression Illness

It is probable that almost any dive underwater involving the breathing of compressed gases results in persistent bubble formation.[10,11] It is just as probable that any such bubbles cause disease by both biochemical and mechanical means.[5] The onset of recognizable disease is usually within the first few hours after the causative dive is complete, and first symptoms arising more than a day later are rare unless a further decompression to altitude has occurred and or there has been some other unusual intervention such as a nitrous oxide–based anesthetic. We reported one diver whose DCI was onset by such an exposure to nitrous oxide 19 days after diving, which also indicates possible bubble survival times.[21] It is not advisable for anyone who has dived underwater breathing compressed gases to fly, even in pressurized aircraft, or to travel overland to more than 300 m above sea level within 24 hours of diving. The "safe" time for someone who has been treated for DCI to fly after that treatment is anyone's guess, but a week is a conservative minimum.

The hydrophobic bubble surface activates an inflammatory response, platelets, and other coagulation factors; deranges blood lipoproteins; and activates white blood cells, especially polymorphonuclear leucocytes (PMNLs), which then become rigid, bind to endothelial cells, and crawl out of the circulation (diapedesis).[22] The exiting PMNLs damage lipids and, in the nervous system, alter brain proteins antigenically such that a harmful glial-based inflammatory response occurs (Figure 51-1). Bubbles also strip the surfactant water proofing from endothelial cells, which causes a fluid loss from the circulation (Figure 51-2).[23] This is exaggerated by both the preexisting hemoconcentration consequent to immersion and the action of inflammatory mediators, such as the kinins. The hematocrit is a good measure of the severity of DCI, as is urine output.

Bubbles forming in noncompliant tissues, such as the fatty marrow of long bones; in tendons; and in the white matter of the spinal cord can cause compressive injury (Figure 51-3).

Different gases have a different potential to cause DCI. Using the mean PAP increase as a marker, the relative disease risk in one animal study was 1.0 for N_2, 0.7 for He, and 0.3 for O_2. The risk for CO_2 is very low.[5]

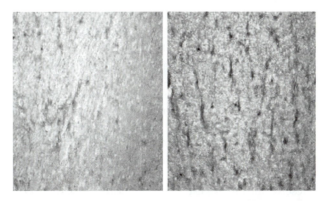

Figure 51-1. A photomicrograph showing glial activation in periventricular white matter in response to polymorphonuclear leukocyte–mediated injury to brain lipids. Glial fibrillary acidic protein staining for glia show as darkened cells (control animal, *left*).

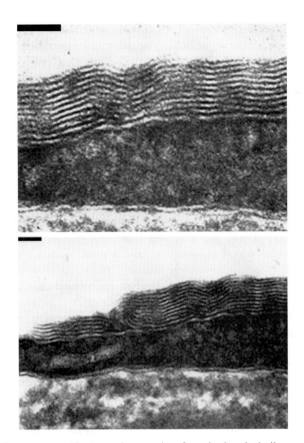

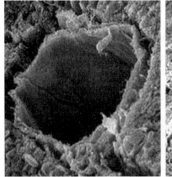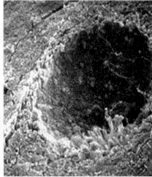

Figure 51-3. Electron micrographs of spinal cord white matter. Blood vessel *(left)*; bubble cavity secondary to decompression illness and compression of adjacent white matter *(right)*. (Courtesy of Professor Brain Hills.)

Figure 51-2. Electron micrographs of cerebral endothelia. Precerebral arterial gas embolism *(top)*; postcerebral arterial gas embolism *(bottom;* bar = 50 nm). (Courtesy of Professor Brain Hills.)

It also follows from this discussion, that DCI is not an unusual state and perhaps should be seen as an inevitable consequence of compressed gas diving. Thus, conservative diving practice is useful to mitigate rather than to prevent DCI. The outcome of this disease varies from no discernable effect at one extreme, and perhaps even from a state of elevated comfort, to death at the other. Thus, the concept of DCI is perhaps best considered as a categorical outcome imposed on a spectrum of disease. This imposition is arbitrary and susceptible to biases in both directions of the spectrum. This accounts for variable reported rates of disease and in treatment exhibition. The incidence of a DCI syndrome in which there is a demonstrable neurological deficit in a modern recreational diver is about 1 in every 1000 dives. Far more common is a malaise syndrome, which includes low-grade fever, and both polymyalgia and polyarthralgia. These symptoms are usually self-limiting. The long-term outcome of this syndrome is uncertain, and the role of intervention is controversial.[24] Of note is that the number needed to harm for the recompression of an injured diver in a recompression chamber is extremely high if only permanent somatic sequelae are considered. The

downside of intervention for a self-limiting malaise syndrome is more to do with disabling illness beliefs.

More localized pain can arise as referred pain from a neural injury (e.g., girdle pain in a diver who has an injured spinal cord) and from long-bone infarction; pain can also arise if bubbles in tendons compress nociceptive c-fibers and $\alpha\delta$-fibers. Bubbles formed in joints are painless.

Nervous system injury is both multifactorial and usually multifocal.[20] A clumsy and ataxic gait is often seen and may arise from a concurrent and interactive injury to the extrapyramidal pathways, the inner ear, the dorsal columns of the spinal cord, and the peripheral nerves of the legs. Proteus was a sea god capable of various forms, and it is appropriate then that we describe the clinical condition of DCI as genuinely protean.

The mechanisms of injury include arterial embolism of the brain, which is described later, and tissue-based disease states, which vary from the immune-mediated neuropathy cited earlier, to venous hemorrhagic infarction of the thoracic spinal cord secondary to extensive pulmonary gas embolism, to bubbles in spinal cord white matter compressing adjacent structures and vessels.[5] The spinal cord is not subject to air embolism as the distribution of bubbles in the arteries is determined by their buoyancy and by blood flow. Almost all arterial bubbles in an upright diver consequently embolize one middle cerebral artery.

Some common foci, such as the inner ear, are unexpected. The common syndromes involve the dorsal columns of the spinal cord, to cause imbalance, and the innervation of the bladder, to cause oliguria or anuria. A common presentation in the context of the latter is a history of small, frequent voids. Both the central and the peripheral nervous systems can be involved and often are in a patchy fashion. Parasthesias are common, whereas pyramidal motor disorders are not. A loss of higher functions is also common, and sequelae of depressed mood and impaired cognition are found in almost half of all divers who were treated for DCI 1 month after their discharge from hospital.[24]

Effective treatment of the neurological syndromes is based on a mixed mechanical and biochemical disease model.[5,20] First aid consists of breathing as close to 100% O₂ as possible, fluid loading with crystalloids, and bladder catheterization, if indicated. If brain involvement is suspected, there may also be a role for lignocaine infusion.[25] The latter is based on two randomized controlled clinical trials in patients undergoing open heart surgery, in whom the number needed to treat to prevent one brain injury is five (Figure 51-4). Although solid emboli may account for the 5% to 7% of patients who have a

stroke, a combined effect of hypotension and CAGE is a better explanation of the 40% to 60% of open heart surgery patients who suffer other forms of brain injury.

Any benefit from lignocaine is likely to result from an inhibition of PMNL diapedesis from the circulation, a lowering of blood viscosity, a stabilization of ischemic cell membranes and reduced ion flux, and a reduction in cerebral metabolic rate. Definitive treatment of a neurological DCI is based on recompression to reduce gas volumes, which increases the surface tension pressures acting on the bubble, increases the gradient for gas elimination from the bubbles, reduces the surface area of the bubble available for tissue interaction and local compressive effects, and promotes the redistribution of any bubbles trapped in blood vessels. HBO also repairs any hypoxia, and, if the dose is close to 300 kPa, inhibits the cyclic guanosine monophosphate regulation of PMNL-binding glycoproteins and hence diapedesis. The detail of recompression therapy is also beyond the scope of this chapter; you are invited to consult one of several good reviews in this context.[20]

Most divers need two or three recompressions to control their symptoms. It may take as long as a month for the disordered physiology to recover fully, and this is considered a suitable time to stand down from diving. The gold standard of follow-up is clinical assessment, which should include a collateral history. None of the many investigations available have satisfactory sensitivity or specificity. Any form of sequelae is generally considered a contraindication to any further compressed gas diving.[20,24]

Cerebral Arterial Gas Embolism

Bubbles may be introduced into arterial blood accidentally, as in divers; iatrogenically, as in cardiac surgery; and by criminal acts. This brief review is constrained to accidental arterial gas embolism in divers. Such embolism can arise from venous bubbles gaining access into the arterial system or from a lung injury, which causes a bronchopulmonary vein fistula.[9,19]

Venous bubbles can become "arterialized" if the PAP is high enough to "pump" them through to the pulmonary veins or if right heart pressures are high enough to cause significant shunting of bubble-rich venous blood through a patent foramen ovale, etc., into the arterial circulation.[5] Both mechanisms depend on large amounts of pulmonary gas embolism and cause a stroke syndrome some time after the diver has left the water and often after a period of dyspnea. By contrast, arterial emboli arising from a pulmonary injury, usually barotrauma of ascent, almost invariably cause a sudden stroke on or shortly after surfacing. The incidence of such an injury is about 1 in every 60,000 ascents in novices; the risk is doubled in asthmatics.[26] About 25% present with a pneumothorax,

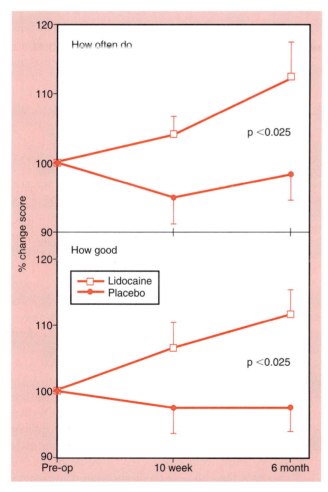

Figure 51-4. Sequential group mean percentage change scores for lignocaine- and placebo-treated cardiac surgical patient groups in two subscales of the Memory Assessment Clinics Self-Report Inventory before and after surgery. Data are mean ± standard error of mean. (Mitchell SJ, Pellett O, Gorman DF. Cerebral protection by lidocaine during cardiac operations. *Ann Thoracic Surg.* 1999;67:1117–1124.)

gas in the mediastinum and neck tissues, or both; about 70% present with a CAGE; and only about 5% present with concurrent evidence of a lung injury and a CAGE.[3,5,18,22,27–29] The typical pulmonary injury is not known, but it is thought that the major etiology is a shearing injuring between adjacent areas of lung of differing compliance. Predictably, then, lung function testing by spirometry is poorly predictive of risk as it does not convey any sense of pulmonary tissue heterogeneity.[30] Bubbles in the pulmonary veins float into the heart and to the upper surface of the aorta. They are then carried with blood flow into one middle cerebral artery to largely pass through the arterioles and to be literally sucked through the capillaries because of the relatively greater venous caliber.[18,19] Thus, the natural history is for a stroke (bubble passage), recovery within 5 to 30 minutes (bubble redistribution into the veins), and then relapse in the next few hours (reperfusion injury and an immune-mediated neuropathy; Figure 51-5).[3,22,28,29] This triphasic history is seen in at least 60% of divers who suffer a CAGE; sometimes, and again somewhat mysteriously, the relapse involves the spinal cord.[31] The most common initial stroke syndrome, however, is a sudden loss of consciousness, which can lead to drowning.

Of the remaining divers who have brain gas embolism, 35% or so do not recover from the stroke without treatment (bubbles trapped and or neurons shut down); the remainder die immediately (presumably because of brainstem embolism). The first aid and definitive treatment is as for DCI except that there are good reasons to stop anyone who has suffered a CAGE from sitting or standing up. Systemic hypotension must be avoided. For about 5 hours or more after a CAGE, and as a consequence of direct endothelial injury (see Figure 51-2), cerebral autoregulation is lost and perfusion is passively determined by blood pressure. Hypotension also promotes bubble trapping, which is clearly undesirable. Over the years, much effort has been expended trying to prevent and or treat brain edema without logic or success.[20] The issue here is the quality of perfusion.

Large intravenous doses of steroids work as long as they are administered before the embolism.[20]

Any episode of pulmonary barotrauma is considered a contraindication to further diving.[32]

CONCLUSION

Regardless of water depth, apparatus chosen, gases used, and, so on; environmental factors exist and interact to render divers confused. Humans underwater are variously narcotized, intoxicated, sensory deprived and overloaded, and neurologically crushed. There is a consequent compelling argument for keeping diving practices

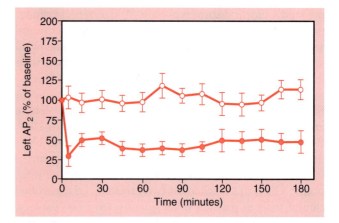

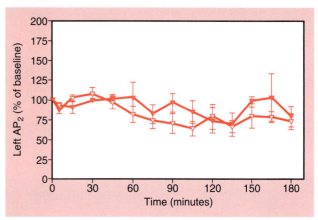

Figure 51-5. Graph of mean ± standard error of mean amplitude of P_2 wave of left cortical somatosensory evoked response as a percentage of preinfusion mean in air embolized *(filled symbols)* and control *(open symbols)* groups of animals. Untreated group *(top)*; leukocyte-depleted animals *(bottom)*. (Helps SC, Gorman DF. Air embolism of the brain in rabbits pretreated with mechlorethamine. *Stroke.* 1991;22:351–354.)

simple in such a dense and nonrespirable environment and for the adoption and application of well-practiced and pragmatic emergency drills.

Diseases caused by bubbles in divers are common. Fortunately, based on acute symptoms, few require treatment and even fewer suffer any impairment. An important caveat exists here, however, due to the unknown effect of aging and the related radiological-based concern about the effect of diving on brain function. Among even those divers who have not had a recognizable episode of DCI, magnetic resonance imaging–apparent white matter periventricular brain infarction is significantly more common than in nondivers.[5,20] The risk is even greater in those who have had a DCI and independently in those who have a patent foramen ovale. The unknown is the likelihood that these bright spots on a scan will be associated with a loss of function, such as premature dementia. Historical cohorts of occupational divers are too small and heavily confounded by smoking and alcohol drinking habits to answer the question. The large number of recreational divers recruited during the peak of sport diving fashionability in the 1980s and 1990s might prove more instructive.

It is unlikely that the human attraction to the ocean and to underwater diving will be susceptible to a simple sociological explanation. It is, however, inevitable that this attraction is hazardous and sometimes injurious. The rationale for a careful and cautious risk-related approach to diving is hopefully self-evident.

CASE STUDY

Vertigo in divers can be due to causes seen in people who have not been diving, such as Ménière's disease. If it is assumed that a diver has no past history of vertigo, then diving-related causes need to be given priority in the differential diagnosis. Vertigo can be a result of a DCI, inner ear barotrauma, middle ear barotrauma when cold water floods the middle ear after a tympanic membrane rupture, and unequal venting of a middle ear during the early phases of a decompression (alternobaric vertigo). Vertigo can also be positional.

Some of these diagnoses are able to be excluded immediately. First, in this case study, caloric vertigo due to cold water was impossible because the diver was in the boat at the time the vertigo developed. Second, by definition, this vertigo could be neither alternobaric nor positional. The differential diagnosis was then between DCI and inner ear barotrauma. This is an important and difficult differentiation in that a diver who has an injured inner ear may well be harmed by hyperbaric treatment. Concurrent inner ear barotrauma and DCI do occur and require such measures as tympanotomy so that the diver does not have to valsalva.

Inner ear involvement is common in DCI but not in isolation if compressed air is breathed. The problem here is that severe vertigo is such an overwhelming experience that other symptoms are not recognized or reported. However, this story was almost pathognomonic of inner ear barotrauma, that is, the sudden onset of vertigo with straining and a sudden pressure wave along the cochlear duct into the middle ear. In this case, the strain was caused by the act of recovering the anchor. The antecedent history of ear problems during the descent would be such that the middle ear would have been congested and any damping of the inner ear by the oval and round window would have been reduced and or lost.

The diver needed to be kept still. An audiogram was necessary because profound deafness is an indication for a referral to an ear, nose, and throat surgeon. Most divers recover well in response to several days of strict bed rest. Most inner ear barotrauma does not need surgery because most cases do not involve an accessible and repairable oval or round window fistula.

Because the ambulance personnel were uncertain of the diagnosis, the diver was given 100% O_2 to breathe by way of a sealing mask and a reservoir bag and was given intravenous normal saline. This is the first aid for DCI but, at the least, does inner ear barotrauma no harm. By the time the diver arrived at the nearest hospital, which had a hyperbaric unit, he was free of any signs of neurological disease outside his inner ear. He had a right-sided pan-frequency sensorineural hearing loss of 35 to 50 dB. On this basis, conservative treatment was chosen and was successful. After 72 h in bed, his vertigo had resolved completely, his balance was normal, and his hearing was restored. Given the recurrent nature of this injury, he was strongly advised not to dive again.

REFERENCES

1. Gorman DF. An essay on the hazards of human life in the ocean. *SPUMS J.* 2003;33(4):199–202.
2. Bierens JLM, ed. *Handbook on Drowning.* Berlin: Springer; 2006.
3. Stonier JC. A study in prechamber treatment of cerebral air embolism patients by a first provider at Santa Catalina Island. *Undersea Biomed Res.* 1985;12(Suppl):58.
4. Golden FS, Hervey GR, Tipton MJ. Circum-rescue collapse: collapse, sometimes fatal, associated with rescue of immersion victims. *J R Nav Med Serv.* 1991;77(3):139–149.
5. Francis TJR, Gorman DF. Pathogenesis of the decompression disorders. In: Bennett PB, Elliott DH, eds. *The physiology and medicine of diving.* 4th ed. London: Baillière-Tindall; 1993:454–480.
6. Rostain JC, Balon N. Recent neurochemical basis of inert gas narcosis and pressure effects. *Undersea Hyperb Med.* 2006;33(3):197–204.
7. Talpalar AE, Grossman Y. CNS manifestations of HPNS: revisited. *Undersea Hyperb Med.* 2006;33(3):205–210.
8. Edmonds CW, Lowry C, Pennefather J, Walker R. *Diving and Subaquatic Medicine.* 4th ed. London: Arnold; 2002.
9. Gorman DF, Mitchell S. A history of cerebral arterial gas embolism research: key publications. *SPUMS J.* 1998;29(1):34–39.
10. Hill L. *Caisson sickness, and the physiology of work in compressed air.* London E. Arnold, 1912.
11. Hills BA. *Decompression sickness: The biophysical basis of prevention and treatment.* New York: John Wiley and Sons, 1977.
12. Donald KW. *Oxygen and the diver.* United Kingdom: Harley Swan: The Spa Ltd., 1992.

13. Gorman DF, Drewry A, Huang YL, Sames C. The clinical toxicology of carbon monoxide. *Toxicology.* 2003;187:25–38.

14. Gorman DF, Huang YL, Williams C. Early evidence of a regulated response to hypoxaemia in sheep that preserves the brain cortex. *Neurosci Lett.* 2006;394:174–178.

15. Weaver LK, Hopkins RO, Chan KJ, et al. Hyperbaric oxygen for acute carbon monoxide poisoning. *New Engl J Med.* 2002;347(14):1057–1067.

16. Brubakk A, Neuman T, eds. *Bennett and Elliotts' Physiology and Medicine of Diving.* 5th ed. London: Elsevier Science Health Science; 2007.

17. Reason J. *Human Error.* Cambridge, UK: Cambridge University Press; 1990.

18. Gorman DF, Browning DM, Parsons DW, Traugott FM. The distribution of arterial gas emboli in the pial circulation. *SPUMS J.* 1987;17(3):101–116.

19. Van Allen CM, Hrdina LS, Clark J. Air embolism from the pulmonary vein: a clinical and experimental study. *Arch Surg.* 1929;19:567–599.

20. Moon RE, Gorman DF. Treatment of the decompression disorders. In: Bruback A, Newman T, eds. *The Physiology and Medicine of Diving.* 5th ed. London: Saunders; 2003:600–650.

21. Acott CJ, Gorman DF. Decompression illness and nitrous oxide anaesthesia in a sports diver. *Anaesth Intensive Care.* 1992;20(2):249.

22. Helps SC, Gorman DF. Air embolism of the brain in rabbits pre-treated with mechlorethamine. *Stroke.* 1991;22:351–354.

23. Hills BA. *The biology of surfactant.* Cambridge: Cambridge University Press, 1988.

24. Gorman DF, Edmonds CW, Parsons DW, et al. Neurologic sequelae of decompression sickness: a clinical report. In: Bove AA, Bachrach AJ, Greenbaum LJ Jr, eds. *Underwater and Hyperbaric Physiology IX.* Bethesda, Md: Undersea and Hyperbaric Medical Society; 1987:993–998.

25. Mitchell SJ, Pellett O, Gorman DF. Cerebral protection by lidocaine during cardiac operations. *Ann Thoracic Surg.* 1999;67:1117–1124.

26. Gorman DF, Richardson D. The SPUMS Workshop on emergency ascent training. *SPUMS J.* 1993;23:236–239.

27. Gorman DF. Cerebral arterial gas embolism as a consequence of pulmonary barotrauma. In: Desola J, ed. *Diving and Hyperbaric Medicine.* Barcelona: European Undersea Biomedical Society; 1984:347–368.

28. Helps SC, Parsons DW, Reilly PL, Gorman DF. The effect of gas emboli on rabbit cerebral blood flow. *Stroke.* 1990;21:94–99.

29. Helps SC, Meyer-Witting M, Reilly PL, Gorman DF. Increasing doses of intracarotid air and cerebral blood flow in rabbits. *Stroke.* 1990;21:1340–1345.

30. Brooks GJ, Pethybridge RJ, Pearson RR. Lung Function Reference Values for FEV1, FEV1/FVC Ratio and FEF75-85 Derived from the Results of Screening 3788 Royal Navy Submariners and Submarine Candidates by Spirometry. EUBS Paper No. 13, Aberdeen: European Undersea Biomedical Society; 1988.

31. Gorman DF, Sames C, Drewry A, Bodicoat S. A case of type 3 DCS with a radiologically normal spinal cord. *Intern Med J.* 2006;36(3):193–196.

32. Elliott D, Gorman D, Haller V, Walker R, Williams G. Fitness to dive. *SPUMS J.* 2001;31(3):168–174.

CHAPTER 52

Neurological Complications of High Altitude

Sundeep Dhillon

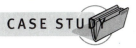

CASE STUDY

A normally fit, experienced climber was found collapsed and unable to move at 5900 m in the Himalaya. He had a mild gastrointestinal disorder the day before making this ascent from Advanced Base Camp at 5600 m. His climbing experience included an ascent of Aconcagua, in Argentina, which at 6959 m is the highest mountain outside the Himalaya. His colleagues, believing he had succumbed to high-altitude cerebral edema, radioed for help. Two doctors and six Sherpas from a medical research expedition were sent to assist.

Consider the causes of acute collapse and loss of consciousness in this high-altitude environment and the diagnosis and treatment of each.

INTRODUCTION

Mankind probably evolved in the tropics at sea level. Advances in technology, especially clothing and housing, have allowed humans to colonize a range of environments, including austere ones. There are, however, many environments in which acute exposure makes the individual prone to illness. As far as high altitude is concerned, the unacclimatized lowlander can become ill at altitudes as low as 1500 m. Conversely, some individuals have, after a period of acclimatization, climbed Mount Everest (8848 m) without supplemental oxygen. Predicting who will fare well at altitude and who will suffer is almost impossible; there is no reliable sea level test. Previous performance at altitude is a reasonable but not reliable predictor of future performance.

Of all the systems in the body, the central nervous system (CNS) is the most dependent on adequate perfusion, glucose, and oxygen. The most common form of altitude illness, acute mountain sickness (AMS) presents after subacute exposure (as opposed to the acute effects of hypoxia described in Chapter 54) and is most likely a mild cerebral edema. High-altitude cerebral edema (HACE) lies at the other end of the spectrum and is distinguished from severe AMS by ataxia and clouding of consciousness. The other main disease of altitude is high-altitude pulmonary edema (HAPE), which is due to hypoxemia and may be confused with HACE. This chapter describes the terrestrial high-altitude environment and the common conditions (AMS, HACE, HAPE) encountered. Consideration is also given to the acute and long-term neurological sequelae of high-altitude exposure.

According to UN estimates, 45.6 million people live at altitudes above 2500 m, 13.2 million above 3500 m, and 4.1 million above 4500 m.[1] The two regions of the world with the largest high-altitude populations are the South American Andes and the Tibetan plateau (Himalaya and Karakorum). It is estimated that between 10 million and 17 million people live at more than 2500 m in the Andes and that more than 50,000 people in Peru reside above 4000 m. Lhasa (3658 m) in Tibet has more than 130,000 inhabitants. Other areas of the world with significant high-altitude populations include Central and North America (Rockies), Europe (Alps), Russia (Caucuses), Africa (Tanzania, Kenya, Uganda, Somalia, and South Africa), and Indonesia.[2]

DEFINITIONS

No universally accepted definition of high altitude exists. Pollard and Murdoch[3] use the definitions in Table 1, which are based on changes in physiology. There is considerable individual variation, with some individuals suffering from rapid ascent to 2000 m. Commercial aircraft are pressurized to around 2500 m, and people with preexisting medical conditions may suffer from this degree of hypoxia. Most people suffer with rapid ascent above 3000 m. Most attitude-related illness is seen at the relatively modest altitudes of 2500 to 3500 m due to the large number of people making rapid ascents for recreational purposes (mainly skiing).

High-Altitude Environment

The high-altitude environment places considerable stress on the body, mainly due to hypobaric hypoxia. As far as the atmosphere is concerned, the only area of interest is the troposphere where all weather phenomena take place. Its average upper limit is 10,000 m, varying from 6000 m over the polar regions to 19,000 m over the equator. The following factors should be considered.

Barometric Pressure

Barometric pressure does not decrease linearly since the upper atmosphere compresses the lower atmosphere. If the temperature in the troposphere remained constant this would result in an exponential decrease, but since the temperature decreases with altitude the barometric pressure falls faster than the exponential relationship. As the proportion of oxygen in the troposphere remains constant at 21%, the inspired oxygen concentration is directly related to barometric pressure. While the International Civil Aviation Organization Standard Atmosphere is used in aviation, it does not accurately predict the barometric pressure on the world's highest peaks. The barometric pressure also varies with season (higher in summer) and latitude (higher over the equator). The Model Atmosphere better describes this situation. Both can be found at medicine.ucsd.edu/phys/convert.html. The water vapor pressure at body temperature is 47 mm Hg irrespective of altitude. This figure, which accounts for humidification in the upper airways, must be deducted to get the inspired partial

Table 1:	High-Altitude Definitions	
Description	**Altitude (in meters)***	**Comments**
Low altitude	<1500	Altitude has no effect on healthy individuals.
Intermediate altitude	1500–2500	Arterial oxygen saturation remains above 90%. Altitude illness is possible, especially with preexisting disease.
High altitude	2500–3500	Altitude illness is common in healthy individuals with rapid ascent above 2500 m.
Very high altitude	3500–5800	Arterial oxygen saturation falls below 90%, especially with exertion or exercise. Altitude illness is common even with gradual ascent.
Extreme altitude	>5800	Limit of permanent human habitation. Progressive deterioration with increased length of stay eventually outstrips acclimatization. People show marked difficulty at rest.

*1 m = 3.281 feet; 1 foot = 0.305 m.
Pollard AJ, Murdoch DR. *The High Altitude Medicine Handbook*. 3rd ed. Oxford: Radcliffe Medical Press; 2003.

pressure of oxygen. At sea level, this accounts for around 6% of the total barometric pressure, increasing to 19% on the summit of Everest. As a rule of thumb, the inspired partial pressure of oxygen is 149 mm Hg at sea level, 78 mm Hg at 5000 m (around the height of Everest Base Camp), and 42 mm Hg near the Everest summit (8848 m).[2]

Humidity

Absolute humidity is the amount of water vapor in the air, and it decreases with altitude. A climber working hard can easily dehydrate in cold, high environments as exhaled breath is fully saturated with water.

Temperature

Within the troposphere, temperature falls linearly with increasing altitude (1°C drop for every 150 m of altitude gained). In a mountainous environment, little heat is stored by the ground and the main source of heat is radiant energy from the sun. Ultraviolet radiation increases by about 4% every 300 m, increasing the risk of sunburn, snow blindness, and skin cancer. Reflected heat can result in temperatures exceeding 40°C, but when the sun is not visible, the temperature can plummet within minutes. Hence, both heat and cold illnesses can occur on the same day.

Wind Chill

The effect of wind on exposed flesh is more relevant than the actual air temperature. The apparent temperature on exposed skin is known as the wind chill and is determined by the ambient air temperature and the wind speed (Table 2).

Acclimatization

Sudden exposure to the summit of Mount Everest (8848 m) would be akin to loss of pressure in a commercial aircraft at a cruising altitude. Consciousness would be lost within a few minutes, followed rapidly by death. Yet, some people have managed to reach the summit of Mount Everest without supplemental oxygen. This is only possible due to a series of physiological changes, collectively known as acclimatization. This is a poorly understood process that starts within hours and continues for months with the aim of increasing oxygen delivery. There is considerable individual variation in the speed and degree of acclimatization. Acclimatization is only possible up to an altitude of around 5000 m. Above this altitude, high-altitude deterioration sets in such that permanent human inhabitation is not possible. Climbers wishing to go higher must balance acclimatization against deterioration or use supplemental oxygen. Unlike adaptation taking place over generations, which has provided permanent genetic advantages for the high-altitude residents of South America and Asia, the effects of acclimatization are rapidly lost by lowlanders on return to lower altitude.

The most important initial compensation is an increase in the rate and depth of ventilation, which can be detected at altitudes as low as 1500 m. The resting heart

Table 2: Windchill Index Chart

Wind Speed (km/hr)	Air Temperature (Celsius)																
	0	-1	-2	-3	-4	-5	-10	-15	-20	-25	-30	-35	-40	-45	-50	-55	-60
6	-2	-3	-4	-5	-7	-8	-14	-19	-25	-31	-37	-42	-48	-54	-60	-65	-71
8	-3	-4	-5	-6	-7	-9	-14	-20	-26	-32	-38	-44	-50	-56	-61	-67	-73
10	-3	-5	-6	-7	-8	-9	-15	-21	-27	-33	-39	-45	-51	-57	-63	-69	-75
15	-4	-6	-7	-8	-9	-11	-17	-23	-29	-35	-41	-48	-54	-60	-66	-72	-78
20	-5	-7	-8	-9	-10	-12	-18	-24	-30	-37	-43	-49	-56	-62	-68	-75	-81
25	-6	-7	-8	-10	-11	-12	-19	-25	-32	-38	-44	-51	-57	-64	-70	-77	-83
30	-6	-8	-9	-10	-12	-13	-20	-26	-33	-39	-46	-52	-59	-65	-72	-78	-85
35	-7	-8	-10	-11	-12	-14	-20	-27	-33	-40	-47	-53	-60	-66	-73	-80	-86
40	-7	-9	-10	-11	-13	-14	-21	-27	-34	-41	-48	-54	-61	-68	-74	-81	-88
45	-8	-9	-10	-12	-13	-15	-21	-28	-35	-42	-48	-55	-62	-69	-75	-82	-89
50	-8	-10	-11	-12	-14	-15	-22	-29	-35	-42	-49	-56	-63	-69	-76	-83	-90
55	-8	-10	-11	-13	-14	-15	-22	-29	-36	-43	-50	-57	-63	-70	-77	-84	-91
60	-9	-10	-12	-13	-14	-16	-23	-30	-36	-43	-50	-57	-64	-71	-78	-85	-92
65	-9	-10	-12	-13	-15	-16	-23	-30	-37	-44	-51	-58	-65	-72	-79	-86	-93
70	-9	-11	-12	-14	-15	-16	-23	-30	-37	-44	-51	-58	-65	-72	-80	-87	-94
75	-10	-11	-12	-14	-15	-17	-24	-31	-38	-45	-52	-59	-66	-73	-80	-87	-94
80	-10	-11	-13	-14	-16	-17	-24	-31	-38	-45	-52	-60	-67	-74	-81	-88	-95
85	-10	-11	-13	-14	-16	-17	-24	-31	-39	-46	-53	-60	-67	-74	-81	-89	-96
90	-10	-12	-13	-15	-16	-17	-25	-32	-39	-46	-53	-61	-68	-75	-82	-89	-96
95	-10	-12	-13	-15	-16	-18	-25	-32	-39	-47	-54	-61	-68	-75	-83	-90	-97
100	-11	-12	-14	-15	-16	-18	-25	-32	-40	-47	-54	-61	-69	-76	-83	-90	-98
105	-11	-12	-14	-15	-17	-18	-25	-33	-40	-47	-55	-62	-69	-76	-84	-91	-98
110	-11	-12	-14	-15	-18	-18	-26	-33	-40	-48	-55	-62	-70	-77	-84	-91	-99

0 to -10 Low   -10 to -25 Moderate   -25 to -45 Cold   -45 to -59 Extreme   -60 Plus very Extreme

Wikipedia. Windchill Chart. Available at: http://upload.wikimedia.org/wikipedia/en/0/02/Windchill_chart.GIF.

rate increases and the maximum heart rate decreases. At extreme altitude the two converge so that exercise capacity is severely limited. Hypoxia-induced erythropoiesis results in polycythemia with increased hematocrit and hemoglobin concentrations.

Central Nervous System at Altitude

The CNS is exquisitely sensitive to both acute and subacute hypoxia and is unable to either acclimatize or adapt to high altitude. It therefore depends on the process of acclimatization to function normally.

Historical Vignette

The first manned balloon flight took place in Paris in 1783. Shortly afterward, early balloonists were exposed to the effects of hypobaric hypoxia in their quest to ascend to ever-higher altitudes. The following is from a review by Doherty.[4]

On September 5, 1862, James Glaisher and Henry Coxwell, two well-respected aeronauts with at least 25 documented scientific balloon ascents, took off from Wolverhapton, England. They took with them in their open basket barometers, thermometers, hygrometers, a compass, a watch, scissors, a magnifying lens, note-taking equipment, ballast, a bottle of brandy, and six pigeons. They ascended to an estimated altitude above 29,000 feet (8000 m) in about 48 minutes (Figure 52-1).

At 18,000 feet, Coxwell began panting for breath. Glaisher noted the following at 26,000 feet:

> I could not see the fine column of the mercury in the wet-bulb thermometer; nor the hands of the watch, nor the fine divisions on any instrument.

At 29,000 feet, he recorded the following:

> I laid my arm upon the table, possessed of its full vigour; but on being desirous of using it, I found it powerless— it must have lost its power momentarily; trying to move the other arm, I found it powerless also. Then I tried to shake myself, and succeeded, but I seemed to have no limbs. In looking at the barometer, my head fell over my left shoulder; I struggled, and shook my body again, but could not move my arms. Getting my head upright, for an instant only, it fell on my right shoulder; and then I fell backwards, my back resting against the side of the car, and my head on its edge. In this position my eyes were directed to Mr. Coxwell in the ring. When I shook my body I seemed to have full power over the muscles of the back, and considerably so over those of the neck, but none over either my arms or my legs. As in the case of the arms, all muscular power was lost in an instant from my back and neck. I dimly saw Mr. Coxwell, and endeavored to speak, but could not; in an instant intense darkness overcame me, so that the optic nerve lost power suddenly, but I was still conscious, with as active

a brain as at the present moment while writing this. I thought I had been seized with asphyxia, and believed I should experience nothing more, as death would come unless we speedily descended: other thoughts were entering my mind when I suddenly became unconscious, as on going to sleep. I cannot tell anything of the sense of hearing: as no sound reaches the ear to break the perfect stillness and silence of regions between six and seven miles from the Earth.

He further states:

> No inconvenience followed my insensibility; and when we dropped it was in a country where no conveyance of any kind could be obtained, so I had to walk between seven and eight miles.

Glaisher and Coxwell threw four of the six pigeons they brought with them out of the basket at various altitudes. The remaining two landed with them: one was dead.

Doherty insists that the neurological symptoms described are more consistent with decompression illness than with hypoxia, a position backed by Rodway,[5] who claims that the symptoms are consistent with the cerebral form of decompression sickness seen in aviators and cites neurological examples from U.S. Air Force chamber studies. West,[6] an expert on high-altitude hypoxia, does not agree with this position.

Unfortunately, detailed clinical examination notes from this episode do not exist, but you can refer to the original texts and references, along with Chapter 54. Further discussion on the neurological complications of high altitude follows a description of the common high-altitude illnesses.

HIGH-ALTITUDE ILLNESSES

Ascending to high altitude too rapidly can result in a range of disorders that may be life threatening. They are best prevented using a gentle ascent profile that allows plenty of time to acclimatize. There is great individual variation, and some people are susceptible to the effects of high altitude even with an extremely conservative ascent profile. Awareness, early recognition, and prompt treatment of high-altitude illnesses are thus paramount.

The main illnesses encountered at high altitude are AMS (mild cerebral edema), HACE, and HAPE. A range of neurological and other disorders may also occur.

Acute Mountain Sickness

AMS is a self-limiting illness that affects normally healthy individuals who ascend too rapidly to altitude. Symptoms usually develop within 8 to 24 hours of arrival at a new altitude, worsening over the next 2 days and

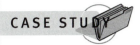

CASE STUDY

Four teenage members of a youth expedition were attempting Kilimanjaro in Tanzania (5895 m). Setting off late from the park entrance (1600 m), the group reached Mandara Hut (2740 m) in just under 3 hours. After a poor night's sleep, all four complained of a headache, loss of appetite, and tiredness the following morning. All were assumed to have AMS and were treated with a combination of ibuprofen (400 mg every 8 hours) and acetazolamide (125 mg every 12 hours). Following 2 days rest at the same altitude, the group was able to continue and all successfully reached the summit.

usually resolving by the fifth day, provided no further height has been gained. The symptoms may reappear with further ascent.

Epidemiology

The incidence of AMS depends on the rate of ascent, the altitude, and how the disease is defined. People can be affected at altitudes as low as 2000 m. On reaching the Himalayan Rescue Association post in Pheriche (4343 m), 43% of trekkers were found to be suffering from AMS. The incidence was higher (49%) in people who had flown to Lukla (2800 m) than in those that had walked all the way from lower altitudes (31%).[7] Among lowland pilgrims who ascended to a holy lake at 4300 m over 2 days, the incidence was 68%.[8] Previous experience to altitude and knowledge of AMS seem to reduce the incidence.

There are varying scoring systems for AMS, which leads to difficulties in defining the incidence. The most widely accepted system is the consensus from the hypoxia meetings in Lake Louise in 1991 and 1993 (Table 3).

Clinical Presentation

The symptoms of AMS are varied. The commonest ones are those used in the Lake Louise AMS scoring system (headache, nausea, vomiting, lethargy, fatigue, loss of appetite, and poor sleep). None are specific, and other conditions such as dehydration, hypothermia, exhaustion and viral infections are also common, but AMS must be excluded at altitude, especially if there has been a recent height gain.

Pathophysiology and Mechanisms

The mechanisms underlying AMS are still under investigation, but a mild vasogenic cerebral edema is thought to be likely. This is similar to HACE, and a fuller explanation is given in the section on HACE and in Figure 52-3 in that section.

Clinical Course

Most cases of AMS resolve spontaneously within 1 to 3 days if no further ascent is made. AMS is a risk factor for both HACE and HAPE, and if there are any symptoms of either of these, then descent, specific treatment, or both should be initiated immediately.

Treatment

Often, no specific treatment is required. While descent to a lower altitude is the definitive treatment for all forms of altitude illness, this is often not feasible or practicable. Rest at the same altitude often relieves the symptoms of AMS.[9] Further ascent while symptomatic is contraindicated. Simple analgesics (aspirin, acetaminophen, ibuprofen) and antiemetics can be used to treat headache and nausea, but they are often ineffective and lack controlled trials.

Acetazolamide (Diamox) is a carbonic anhydrase inhibitor that increases renal bicarbonate excretion. The resulting metabolic acidosis stimulates respiration. The treatment dose is 250 mg every 8 hours, which improves arterial oxygen saturation and decreases periodic breathing with its accompanying dramatic drop in oxygen saturation.[10] Dexamethasone relieves symptoms of AMS but has no effect on oxygenation, periodic breathing, or other physiological parameters. It can be used as an adjunct to descent and acetazolamide. Oxygen is often not available, is not always effective, and delays acclimatization.

A portable hyperbaric chamber (Gamow, Certec, portable altitude chamber) operated by a foot pump can simulate a descent of many thousands of meters within a few minutes by increasing the pressure within the bag. Its use is limited to altitudes where constant pumping (to remove carbon dioxide) can be maintained. The beneficial effects seem to last up to 10 hours, which may be enough to provide a window for safe descent. Patients suffering from HAPE may not tolerate lying down due to increased hypoxia, in which case the head should be elevated by 30 degrees. Patients with HACE may be too uncooperative to be placed inside.

Prevention

The rate of ascent is the most important modifiable factor in preventing high-altitude illness. Above 3000 m, people should ascend no more than 300 m per day with a rest day every 3 days. This may be irritatingly slow for some members of the team, but it provides an opportunity for everyone to acclimatize. Even with this gradual ascent profile, approximately 50% are not protected.[11] A survey found that the incidence of AMS decreased by 19% for every additional

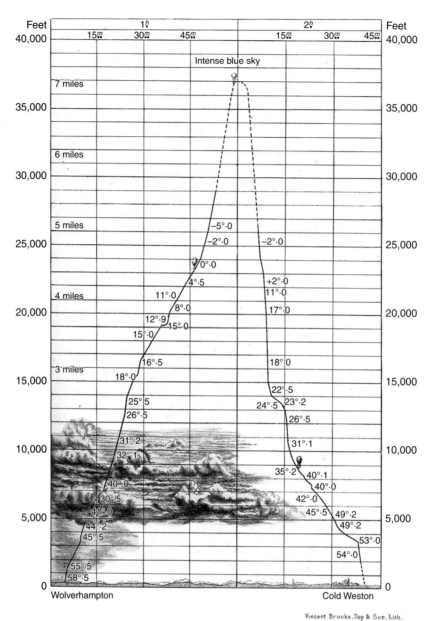

Path of the Balloon in its ascent from Wolverhampton to
Cold Weston near Ludlow.

5ᵗʰ September 1862.

Figure 52-1. Path of Glaisher and Coxwell's 1862 balloon ascent. (Glaisher J, Flammarion C, de Fonvielle W, Tissandier G. *Travels in the Air*. Philadelphia: JB Lippincott; 1871.)

day spent between Lukla (2804 m) and Pheriche (4243 m).[12] Sometimes, it is not possible to camp within a 300-m altitude gain of the previous night's camp. In these situations, an extra night before the extra height gain is required. It is the sleeping altitude that matters, so it is acceptable to carry supplies higher (say 500 m) provided the climber descends to a camp at a lower altitude (300 m or less above the previous night's camp)— "climb high, sleep low."

Acetazolamide is an effective prophylaxis against AMS in susceptible individuals or when a large height gain is unavoidable. The recommended dose varies from 125 mg at night to 250 mg twice daily. It is most effective if taken for a few days before ascending above 3000 m.

Table 3:   The Lake Louise Acute Mountain Sickness Scoring System

	SELF-ASSESSMENT*			
1.	Headache	0	No headache
		1	Mild headache
		2	Moderate headache
		3	Severe incapacitating headache
2.	Gastrointestinal symptoms	0	No gastrointestinal symptoms
		1	Poor appetite or nausea
		2	Moderate nausea or vomiting
		3	Severe incapacitating nausea or vomiting
3.	Fatigue or weakness	0	Not tired or weak
		1	Mild fatigue or weakness
		2	Moderate fatigue or weakness
		3	Severe incapacitating fatigue or weakness
4.	Dizziness or lightheadedness	0	Not dizzy
		1	Mild dizziness
		2	Moderate dizziness
		3	Severe incapacitating dizziness
5.	Difficulty sleeping	0	Slept as well as usual
		1	Did not sleep as well as usual
		2	Woke many times; poor night's sleep
		3	Could not sleep

CLINICAL ASSESSMENT

6.	Change in mental status	0	No change in mental status
		1	Lethargy or lassitude
		2	Disorientated or confused
		3	Stupor or semiconscious
		4	Coma
7.	Ataxia (heel–toe walking)	0	No ataxia
		1	Balancing maneuvers

Table 3: The Lake Louise Acute Mountain Sickness Scoring System—cont'd

		2	Steps off the line
		3	Falls down
		4	Unable to stand
8.	Peripheral edema	0	None
		1	One location
		2	Two or more locations
FUNCTIONAL SCORE			
	Overall, if you had any of these symptoms, how did they affect your activities?	0	No reduction in activity
		1	Mild reduction
		2	Moderate reduction
		3	Severe reduction (e.g., bed rest)

*For a diagnosis of acute mountain sickness, headache and at least one other symptom must be present with a combined score of at least 3 (sum of all answers).

Adapted from Roach RC, Bärtsch P, Hackett PH, Oelz O. The Lake Louise acute mountain sickness scoring system. In: Sutton JR, Houston CS, Coates G, eds. *Hypoxia and Mountain Medicine.* Burlington, Vt: Queen City Printers; 1993:272–274.

High-Altitude Cerebral Edema

HACE is the other end of the spectrum of cerebral altitude illness. It can be rapidly life threatening and may be difficult to distinguish from AMS. In an excellent review, Hackett and Roach[13] define it as "a condition occurring in persons who have recently arrived at high altitude, usually secondary to acute mountain sickness or high-altitude pulmonary edema, and marked by disturbances of consciousness that may progress to deep coma, psychiatric changes of varying degree, confusion, and ataxia of gait." Recognizing the difficult distinction between severe AMS and HACE, they suggest that HACE is clinically an encephalopathy, whereas AMS is not.

Epidemiology

HACE is usually preceded by AMS and sometime HAPE. While it is rare below 3000 m (the lowest reported altitude is 2100 m[14]), it can occur in apparently well-acclimatized climbers at more than 7000 m, where it may be particularly dangerous.[15] The incidence reported in the literature varies (due to differences in definition and clinical diagnosis) from 1% among trekkers in Nepal between 4243 and 5500 m (increasing to 3.4% in

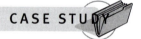

CASE STUDY

A previously fit mountaineer fell behind his companions while ascending the Lhotse Face on Everest between 6400 m and Camp 3 at 7100 m. He had a proven pedigree at high altitude, having climbed Cho Oyu (8201 m) the previous year. For a few days before the ascent, he had been suffering from an upper respiratory tract infection. By the time he arrived at Camp 3, he was exhausted, clumsy, apathetic, and withdrawn, and he had slurred speech. He was unable to pass urine. A diagnosis of HACE was made, and he was treated with intravenous dexamethasone and oxygen. By the morning he had improved considerably and was able to descend with assistance. He continued to improve rapidly over the next few days but abandoned his summit attempt on medical advice. His concurrent upper respiratory illness was thought to have tipped him into HACE by increasing his hypoxemia.

those already suffering from AMS)[7] to 31% among Vedic pilgrims to a holy lake in Nepal at 4300 m.[8] This is far higher than any other study and may reflect the large numbers of lowland pilgrims ascending from 2000 to 4300 m in 2 days and then spending the night there. In the same study, 68% of pilgrims developed AMS. HACE is less common than either AMS or HAPE, with young males possibly at increased risk from continuing to ascend while symptomatic, but no age, sex, ethnic group, or high-altitude resident is immune.

HACE and HAPE may occur concurrently, making the diagnosis of HACE difficult since the hypoxemia produced by HAPE may lead to hypoxic cerebral dysfunction. Postmortem examination of HAPE victims reveals that 50% of them also had HACE.[13] Among 52 HAPE patients in the French Alps, 13% had stupor or coma.[16] In the Colorado Rockies, 14% of 150 patients with HAPE also had HACE.[17] Conversely, 11 of 13 patients with HACE in the Colorado Rockies also had HAPE.[18]

Clinical Presentation

> "If the patient seems mildly drunk at altitude they have cerebral edema."[15]

HACE usually develops in individuals suffering from AMS more than 24 to 36 hours, but the speed of progression varies and may be as little as a few hours. The risk factors are the same as for AMS, with the Vedic pilgrim study highlighting the importance of the rate of ascent.

Symptoms of HACE include headache, loss of appetite, nausea, vomiting, and photophobia. Physical performance decreases dramatically and is replaced by lethargy, withdrawal, and irritability. This may lead to bizarre and inappropriate behavior (e.g., removing protective clothing and gloves) and hallucinations. Untreated the clouding of consciousness develops into coma and eventually death.

In a series of HACE patients ($n = 44$) by Dickinson,[19] disturbance of consciousness and ataxia were the cardinal distinguishing features of HACE. Ataxia was present in 48 of 66 patients with HACE (72.7%) in a series from construction workers along the Qinghai-Tibetan Railway.[20] Ataxia may initially be tested by heel–toe walking but later becomes truncal such that the patient cannot sit up. The mechanism of ataxia is unknown but may be due to hypoxic cerebellar dysfunction rather than cerebral edema. Other common neurological features are shown in Table 4. Note that almost any neurological presentation is possible (Dickinson also reported abducens nerve palsies, anisocoria, visual field loss, speech difficulty, hearing loss, and flapping tremor).

The signs and symptoms are nonspecific, and a range of differential diagnoses must be considered, especially if there is a lack of response to treatment. The following factors favor an alternate diagnosis: onset of illness after 3 days at a stable altitude, abrupt onset, trauma, focal neurological signs, high fever, and a stiff neck.[13] A detailed history and careful examination are essential to avoid the wrong diagnosis. Differential diagnoses to be considered are given in Table 5. Given the association between HACE and HAPE, a chest radiograph or pulse oximetry in the field should be undertaken, with low spot oxygen saturation being sufficient to mandate treatment for HAPE. All but the mildest cases should be evacuated to a hospital.

Imaging is not essential for the diagnosis, but evidence of cerebral edema can usually be found on computerized tomography scanning (attenuation of signal, particularly in the white matter, with corresponding loss of sulci and gyri). T_2-weighted or diffusion-weighted magnetic resonance imaging (MRI) is more diagnostic, especially as the resolution may lag behind clinical improvement. Typically intense signals in the white matter are seen, especially the splenium and corpus callosum (Figure 52-2).

Pathophysiology

Hypoxia increases microvascular permeability and extravascular fluid. Together, these two factors suggest that the cerebral edema is vasogenic in origin—that is, due to increased permeability of the blood–brain barrier. This is consistent with the images seen on MRI, where no gray matter edema is seen.[21] The time course of the development and resolution of cerebral edema also suggest a vasogenic origin. Post-postmortem studies have confirmed gross cerebral edema, along with petechial hemorrhages and various thromboses that are not seen on imaging, suggesting that these are terminal events.[19]

Table 4: Neurological Features in HACE
Symptom
Disturbance of consciousness
Ataxia
Retinal hemorrhages
Papilledema
Urinary retention or incontinence
Abnormal plantar reflexes
Abnormal limb tone and power
HACE, high-altitude cerebral edema.

Table 5: Differential Diagnoses of HACE	
Acute psychosis	Hypoglycemia
Brain tumor	Hyponatremia
Carbon monoxide poisoning	Hypothermia
Central nervous system infection	Ingestion of drugs, alcohol, or toxins
Cerebrovascular bleed or infarct	Migraine
Cerebrovascular spasm	Seizure disorder
Diabetic ketoacidosis	Transient ischemic attack
HACE, high-altitude cerebral edema.	

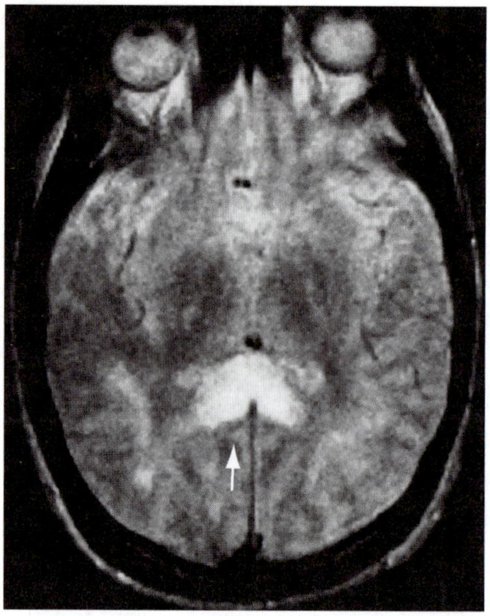

Figure 52-2. Magnetic resonance image of a patient with high-altitude cerebral edema. An increased T_2-signal in the splenium of the corpus callosum (arrow) indicates edema. (Auerbach PS. *Wilderness Medicine.* 5th ed. Philadelphia: Mosby Elsevier; 2007.)

Mechanisms

Vasogenic edema could result from mechanical factors disrupting the blood–brain barrier (capillary hypertension), biochemical mediators affecting permeability, or both. The list of potential chemical mediators of cerebral vascular leak in cerebral edema includes bradykinin, histamine, arachidonic acid, oxygen and hydroxyl free radicals, and inducible nitric oxide synthase–generated nitric oxide.[13] Severinghaus[22] proposed that vascular endothelial growth factor (VEGF) may play a role in HACE. Normally, VEGF is expressed during angiogenesis and increases capillary permeability. Severinghaus and colleagues found that hypoxia induces expression of VEGF in mice. This was blocked by a VEGF-specific antibody. Furthermore, dexamethasone is effective at preventing angiogenesis and appears to block VEGF expression in hypoxia-induced cerebral edema. Recently, free VEGF was measured among 19 volunteers during acute ascent to 4300 m. There was a correlation between free VEGF and AMS symptoms,[23] implying that in response to hypoxia VEGF attempts to initiate angiogenesis: vascular permeability is increased as part of this process.

The Tight-Fit Hypothesis

Ross[24] first proposed the "tight-fit" hypothesis to account for what he described as the "random nature of cerebral mountain sickness," i.e., the difficulty in predicting which individuals are likely to suffer from the effects of high altitude. His proposal was that individuals with a more compliant cerebrospinal fluid system (larger ventricles and more cerebral atrophy) would tolerate more hypoxic cerebral edema than those with less compliant systems and would thus be protected against a rise in intracranial pressure (ICP).

A remarkable experiment was undertaken in 1985 to examine this hypothesis. Brian Cummins, a Bristol-based neurosurgeon, implanted ICP monitoring devices in three climbers on the British Himalayan Mountaineering Expedition to Kishtwar. The devices made 776 separate readings between sea level and 16,500 feet (5030 m). There are no other published reports of invasive ICP monitoring at altitude, and given the current ethical requirements for research, this unique study is unlikely to be repeated.

Sadly, Cummins died in 2003 believing that all his data had been lost shortly after his return from the Himalaya in a car fire. Mark Wilson (neuroscience lead for Caudwell Xtreme Everest) recently wrote to Cummins' wife asking for any pictures from the expedition. His wife found all of the data in the attic, which Wilson has analyzed and submitted for publication.[25] In addition to the ICP monitoring, computerized tomography scans were performed on the team members ($n = 10$) and analyzed by an independent neuroradiologist and neurologist, who were asked to rate the ventricle size as small, normal, or large. Daily symptom scores obtained by interview and a self-assessment were both correlated inversely with ventricular size—i.e., those with the largest ventricles had the least symptoms of high-altitude illness. The largest ventricles were seen in the oldest climbers, in keeping with age-related atrophy. In the three subjects undergoing ICP monitoring, the pressures were normal at all altitudes and during exercise and breath holding except for the climber with the smallest ventricles, who suffered greatly from the altitude. His pressures were found to be normal while still (14 mm Hg), but even minimal exertion (head turning) increased the pressure significantly (24 mm Hg). This trend was exaggerated with exercise (51 mm Hg while undertaking a push-up).

A summary of the proposed mechanisms of AMS and HACE is given in Figure 52-3.

Clinical Course

Untreated HACE can be rapidly fatal, especially once coma has developed. Early recognition and treatment usually result in rapid recovery; conversely, a delay in treatment usually results in slower recovery. Average

recovery times in a series of nine patients was 2.4 weeks, with a average hospital stay of 5.6 days.[21] Ataxia is often present at discharge and is commonly the last symptom to resolve.

Treatment

Like all altitude illnesses, the mainstay of treatment of HACE is descent to a lower altitude and oxygen. A portable hyperbaric chamber is useful if descent is prolonged or dangerous due to weather, darkness, lack of personnel, etc. The degree of descent and the time to recovery with HACE are no greater or longer than with AMS or HAPE. Although no controlled trials have been undertaken in humans, steroids (dexamethasone) are used with good effect. The usual dose is 8 mg IV/IM/PO stat followed by 4 mg every 6 hours. Patients in a coma must be managed appropriately. Loop diuretics, hypertonic saline, mannitol, and oral glycerol have all been used, but no controlled trials exist to support their use, especially in the prehospital setting.

Prevention

Prevention of all altitude illnesses is based on a gradual, graded ascent. Since HACE seems to occur more often in people suffering from AMS and HAPE, avoidance of these illnesses is vital. At extreme altitude, HACE may present suddenly, and climbers ascending to these heights should seek advice from a physician familiar with high-altitude illnesses on the early recognition and treatment of HACE. Prophylactic use of dexamethasone to prevent HACE at high altitude is fraught with dangers and cannot be recommended.

High-Altitude Pulmonary Edema

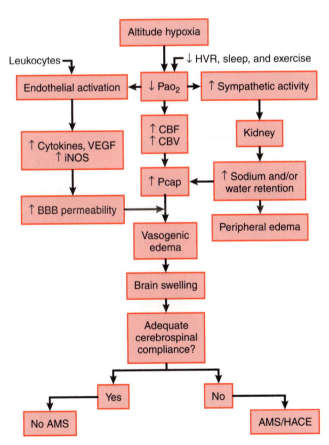

Figure 52-3. Proposed pathophysiology of acute mountain sickness and high-altitude cerebral edema. BBB, blood–brain barrier; CBF, cerebral blood flow; CBV, cerebral blood volume; HVR, hypoxic ventilatory response; iNOS, inducible nitric oxide synthase; Pcap, capillary pressure; VEGF, vascular endothelial growth factor. (Auerbach PS. *Wilderness Medicine.* 5th ed. Philadelphia: Mosby Elsevier; 2007.)

> **CASE STUDY**
>
> On descending from the summit of Aconcagua in Argentina (6962 m), a young female climber became increasingly tired and breathless. On arriving back at Camp 2 (5700 m), she began to cough up blood-stained sputum and complained of pain in her chest. On examination, at rest she was found to have a respiratory rate of 44, a heart rate of 142, and an arterial oxygen saturation of 65%. A diagnosis of HAPE was made, and 20 mg of nifedipine, slow release, were given. With her friends carrying her equipment, she was able to descend to Base Camp (4200 m). The following morning she was evacuated by helicopter to the local hospital. After 2 days of treatment, she was given the "all clear" and discharged home.

Epidemiology

HAPE may be preceded by AMS and occurs in association with HACE as described earlier. As with all altitude illnesses, the incidence varies with rate of ascent. Hackett and Rennie[7] reported an incidence of 2.5% among trekkers in Nepal, whereas Menon[26] reported an incidence of 0.75% among Indian soldiers flown to Leh (3500 m). An incidence of up to 10% has been reported with rapid ascent to 4500 m. It can occur in high-altitude residents after a stay at lower altitudes and, like HACE, may affect apparently well-acclimatized climbers who make rapid ascents to 7000 m. There is an increased risk with viral upper respiratory tract infections.[3]

Clinical Presentation

Subclinical pulmonary edema probably occurs in most people at altitude due to hypoxic pulmonary vasoconstriction coupled with microvascular leak. Menon[26] managed a series of 101 patients with HAPE. The frequency of symptoms is shown in Table 6. Dyspnea on exertion, reduced exercise tolerance, and prolonged recovery are usually the earliest signs.

The earliest signs are basal crackles, tachycardia (70 out of 101 patients in Menon's series[26]), tachypnea, and cyanosis. The raised pulmonary artery pressure produces a right ventricular heave and prominent second pulmonary sound in 50% of patients. The temperature is mildly raised

(0.8°C) in 70% of patients. Raised jugular venous pressure, raised systemic blood pressure, and dependent edema have been reported in Menon's series[26] 15 patients had confusion and amnesia. It is not clear whether this was due to hypoxia or concurrent cerebral edema.

Figure 52-4 shows the typical radiological features of mild and severe HAPE.

The electrocardiogram usually shows a tachycardia. P pulmonale and right axis deviation may be present, consistent with increased right ventricular strain. Partial pressure of oxygen and oxygen saturation are decreased even when adjusted for altitude. Cardiac catheter studies reveal a normal wedge pressure but raised pulmonary artery pressure, with both systolic and diastolic pressures approaching those of the systemic circulation.[2]

Pathophysiology

Certain individuals are more susceptible to HAPE. Undoubtedly, there is genetic susceptibility. Current research suggests that the following characteristics may be involved: smaller lung volumes, blunted ventilatory response to hypoxia, and exaggerated hypoxic pulmonary vasoconstriction, perhaps mediated by nitric oxide and other factors.[2] A proposed mechanism is given in Figure 52-5.

Mechanisms

Postmortem studies reveal a patchy hemorrhagic edema. The pulmonary capillaries are congested and may contain fibrin clots. The alveoli are filled with fluid that contains macrophages, polymorphs, and erythrocytes.[19] Recent studies have confirmed a lack of inflammatory processes and the presence of a protein-rich edema fluid consistent with transcapillary leak.[2]

Clinical Course

Untreated death from HAPE usually occurs within a few hours. With rapid descent recovery takes 1 to 2 days, but individuals can continue to deteriorate and even die, especially if HACE is also present.[19]

Treatment

Treatment of HAPE involves immediate descent (if possible) and supplemental oxygen (if available). Nifedipine has been successfully used to treat HAPE. The dose from one study is 10 mg sublingually followed by 20 mg every 6 hours thereafter. Despite continued exercise at 4559 m, this resulted in better oxygenation and clearing of symptoms.[27] Nevertheless, descent must be the first option. If there is any evidence of HACE, this must be treated concurrently with HAPE by using dexamethasone.

Phosphodiesterase inhibitors (via their action on nitric oxide), dexamethasone, hydralzine, phentolamine, diuretics, antibiotics, digoxin, morphine, and positive

Table 6: Symptoms of High-Altitude Pulmonary Edema in 101 Cases	
Symptom	**No. of Cases**
Breathlessness	84
Chest pain	66
Headache	63
Nocturnal dyspnea	59
Dry cough	51
Hemoptysis	39
Nausea	26
Insomnia	23
Dizziness	18

Adapted from Menon ND. High-altitude pulmonary edema: a clinical study. *N Engl J Med* 1965;273:66–73.

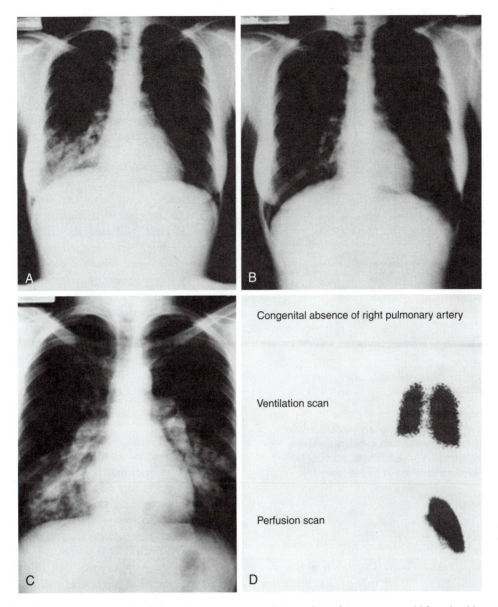

Figure 52-4. *(A)* Radiograph demonstrating high-altitude pulmonary edema (HAPE) in a 29-year-old female skier at 2450 m. *(B)* Same patient 1 day after descent and oxygen therapy, showing rapid improvement. *(C)* Typical bilateral pulmonary infiltrates in severe HAPE. *(D)* Ventilation–perfusion scans from a patient after recovery from HAPE demonstrating congenital lack of right pulmonary artery. (Auerbach PS. *Wilderness Medicine.* 5th ed. Philadelphia: Mosby Elsevier; 2007.)

end-expiratory pressure have all been used to treat HAPE with varying results.[2]

Prevention

A slow ascent protects against all altitude illnesses. There is some evidence that young men are more susceptible to HAPE, possibly because they are often keen to be at the front of a group and compete with one another. There is anecdotal evidence that exercise at altitude increases the risk of HAPE (increased cardiac output against leaky pulmonary capillaries). The Indian Army has considerable experience of altitude illness and claims great success with a policy of enforced rest for new arrivals at 3000 m for 3 weeks.[28]

People who have suffered an episode of HAPE remain susceptible to HAPE (usually around the same altitude as the original episode). Further ascent is inadvisable, but if unavoidable nifedipine may be used prophylactically. There is some evidence that inhaled salmeterol (125 μg twice daily) may also be effective. Prophylaxis against HAPE should not be a substitute for graded ascent.

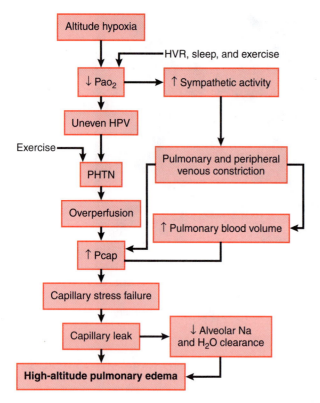

Figure 52-5. Proposed pathophysiology of high-altitude pulmonary edema (HAPE). HPV, hypoxic pulmonary vasoconstriction; HVR, hypoxic ventilatory response; Pcap, capillary pressure; PHTN, pulmonary hypertension. (Auerbach PS. *Wilderness Medicine.* 5th ed; Philadelphia: Mosby Elsevier; 2007.)

Chronic Mountain Sickness

Chronic mountain sickness (CMS) is found in all populations that have lived at altitude for many years. With the exception of Han Chinese immigrants in Tibet, it is not a disease of lowlanders. It was first recognized in 1925 in Peru by Carlos Monge and is also known as Monge's disease. Its incidence increases with altitude and age. It is characterized by excessive erythrocytosis with hematocrits exceeding 80% (CMS), which predominates in the Andes, and in some cases high-altitude pulmonary hypertension, which is more common in Asia. It improves with descent to lower altitudes.[2]

High-Altitude Pulmonary Hypertension

Hypoxia causes pulmonary hypertension. In the fetus, this diverts blood from the nonfunctioning lung through the ductus arteriosis. After birth, it is thought that this improves ventilation-to-perfusion ratios in underperforming lung (e.g., pneumonia) since the hypoxic vasoconstriction diverts blood to well-ventilated areas of the lung. At high altitude, there is hypoxic vasoconstriction throughout the whole lung, resulting in pulmonary hypertension. This pulmonary hypertension is present in high-altitude residents and is accompanied by muscularization of the pulmonary arterioles. The pulmonary hypertension can eventually result in right heart failure.

More commonly, high-altitude pulmonary hypertension affects newborn infants at altitude, particularly Han Chinese immigrants in Tibet, where the condition has been called subacute infantile mountain sickness.[29] The condition was fatal within weeks, and postmortems revealed massive medial hypertrophy of pulmonary arteries and arterioles, along with excessive hypertrophy and dilatation of the right ventricle and pulmonary trunk.

Ananad[30] described cardiomegaly, pericardial effusion, dependent edema, and elevated pulmonary pressures in 21 soldiers who spent nearly 2 years above 5800 m. The pulmonary artery pressures increased from 26 mm Hg at rest to 40 mm Hg with exercise. All of the soldiers recovered rapidly with descent to low altitude. Other treatments for high-altitude residents who do not have the option of descent include nifedipine and sildenafil.[2]

OTHER PROBLEMS OF HIGH ALTITUDE (NONNEUROLOGICAL)

Various other disorders occur at high altitude. Cold- and heat-related injuries may occur, and a dry, nonproductive cough and cold-induced rhinorrhea are almost ubiquitous in the dry, cold air. Peripheral edema may occur with or without symptoms of altitude illness. There is anecdotal evidence that infections are more common, may predispose to altitude illnesses (e.g., HAPE), and are slow to resolve. Above 5000 m, high-altitude deterioration eventually outstrips any benefit from acclimatization. Gastrointestinal diseases may result from assuming glacial water is clean or not boiling water long enough. The temperature at which water boils decreases with barometric pressure; therefore, water must be boiled longer. Fresh snow may hide the site of a previous camp toilet, and care must be taken to select appropriate water sources and ensure the water is clean. Alluvial deposits in glacial water may lead to gastrointestinal discomfort and mild upset. Anxiety about developing any of the preceding diseases can it itself become disabling.[3]

OTHER NEUROLOGICAL PROBLEMS OF HIGH ALTITUDE

Various neurovascular disorders that fall outside the definition of AMS have been identified at high altitude (Table 7).[31]

Table 7: Neurovascular Disorders at High Altitude
• Transient ischemic attacks and strokes or cerebrovascular accidents
• Migraine
• Cerebral venous thrombosis
• Subarachnoid hemorrhage
• Seizure disorders, including epilepsy
• High-altitude syncope
• Space-occupying lesions
• Transient global amnesia
• Delirium at high altitude
• Cranial nerve palsies
• Possible coagulation problems
• Opthalmological problems
Adapted from Basnyat B, Wu T, Gertsch JH. Neurological conditions at altitude that fall outside the usual definition of altitude sickness. *High Alt Med Biol.* 2004;5(2):171–179.

In a review of the literature, 16 cerebrovascular accidents at altitude are described. All were male, and 14 were lowland climbers (the other 2 were Sherpas). The signs included hemiparesis (mainly on the right), dysphasia, decreased level of consciousness, headache, visual disturbance, numbness, motor weakness, diplopia, right lateral rectus palsy, and possibly migraine. Of the patients 2 died, the fate of 1 is unknown and 13 recovered. There is an impression that these events resolve within 24 hours and are more likely to be transient ischemic attacks than ischemic strokes. This is consistent with transient ischemic attacks observed in chamber studies at low barometric pressure.[2]

A series of 30 Indian Army personnel were admitted to hospital with strokes after a stay at high altitude. Most had ischemic arterial strokes, but 2 had central venous thromboses.[32] Thrombosis is common at altitude due to increased hematocrit, dehydration, cold, and lack of movement (e.g., confined to a tent in a storm).

Migraine is common at sea level, and headache (due to AMS) is common at altitude. Anecdotal reports suggest that altitude may be a trigger for migraine, which is consistent with reports from acute hypoxic exposure in pressure chambers.[31]

Transient loss of memory and confusion, without motor or sensory dysfunction, can occur in the absence of other high-altitude disorders and has been called high-altitude global amnesia. Litch and Bishop[33] describe two subjects at moderate altitude (3750 and 4400 m) who were disorientated in space and person and unable to remember autobiographical episodes. The disorder resolved rapidly with descent. I experienced this during a medical research expedition. One of my colleagues developed marked cerebral desaturation at the end of a maximal exercise test at 5600 m. He was left with headache, confusion, and a nominal aphasia, which resolved over 48 hours.

Any cranial nerve palsy is possible, but the most commonly reported is the VIth (abducens) nerve, which supplies the lateral rectus. Typically, nerve palsy occurs occur in isolation without evidence of AMS or HACE and resolves spontaneously. The resulting diplopia may persist for weeks or months.[34]

Six cases of transient cortical blindness have been reported at altitudes around 4300 m. There was no evidence of other altitude illnesses and no retinal hemorrhages. The episodes lasted between 20 minutes and 24 hours (with intermittent normal vision). This is thought to be due to the direct effect of hypoxia on the visual cortex, which is also seen in acute exposure in a chamber.[35]

Retinal hemorrhages are common at altitude, occurring in 30% to 35% of trekkers at 5000 m. They are usually asymptomatic (unless the macula is involved, when sudden painless visual field defects can occur) and self-limiting (some cases of scotomata have not resolved). Features on fundoscopy are disc hyperemia, vascular engorgement, and tortuosity of vessels. They are thought to be more common in individuals suffering from AMS, following rapid ascent, at higher altitudes, after coughing or straining, and during the first few days at altitude (the risk period for AMS). There is no specific treatment, although descent is usually advised if there is a visual field defect.[3]

Sleep is almost universally impaired at altitude, with difficulty falling asleep, frequent waking, unpleasant dreams, and a sense of poor unrefreshing sleep in the morning often reported, despite spending many hours apparently sleeping soundly. There is a reduction in both slow-wave sleep and rapid eye movement sleep. This is accompanied by periodic breathing (Cheyne-Stokes respiration) with apneic pauses lasting 10 to 15 seconds, followed by increased depth and rate of ventilation. Marked desaturation occurs during the periods of apnea.[36] Supplemental oxygen (even at low flow rates of 1 L/min) can eliminate apneic periods, reduce periodic breathing, and increase the arterial oxygen saturation. The mechanism of periodic breathing is thought to be central (via chemoreceptors) rather than due to airway obstruction. In essence, hyperventilation washes out carbon dioxide and ventilation ceases until the level of carbon dioxide rises sufficiently to trigger ventilation again. Periodic breathing is uncommon in native highlanders; this is thought to be secondary to a blunted hypoxic ventilatory response and to be a useful adaptation to prevent nocturnal desaturation. Lowlanders at altitude, particularly those who acclimatize well, tend to have a brisk hypoxic ventilatory response (i.e., they increase their rate and depth of ventilation markedly in response to hypoxia), which helps wash out the carbon dioxide and trigger periodic breathing.[2]

Acetazolamide (250 mg at night) is effective at reducing periodic breathing and improving nocturnal arterial oxygen saturation.[7] There is conflicting evidence on the usefulness of benzodiazepines in improving sleep at altitude, but zolpidem improved sleep in a chamber study.[2] There is insufficient evidence to recommend anything other than acetazolamide or supplemental oxygen (or descent) to improve sleep at altitude.

Sleep deprivation affects mental performance, with higher functions being the most vulnerable. Problem-solving skills and initiative are particularly impaired. The same effect is seen in people at high altitude, and sleep deprivation may confound the effects of hypoxia on the brain.[2]

NEUROPSYCHOLOGICAL IMPAIRMENT AT HIGH ALTITUDE

Hypoxia causes cerebral vasodilatation, whereas hypocapnia causes cerebral vasoconstriction. These two factors compete to determine cerebral blood flow. Cerebral blood flow combined with the arterial oxygen saturation determines brain oxygenation. Given the degree of hypoxia seen at altitude and the brain's dependence on oxygen, it is not surprising that neuropsychological derangement is seen following both acute and subacute exposure to hypoxia. Slow learning of complex mental tasks, impaired reaction times, hand–eye coordination, and higher functions such as memory and language have all been reported. In mountaineering, particularly with ascents above 8000 m without supplemental oxygen, persistent defects are found on neuroimaging and formal neuropsychological testing. Lowlanders with a strong hypoxic ventilatory drive (who tend to perform better at high altitude) have the most residual impairment. This paradox is explained by the hypocapnia caused by increased ventilation, which in turn causes cerebral vasoconstriction and reduced oxygen delivery, compounding cerebral hypoxia.[2]

The lowest altitude at which psychometric disturbances can be detected is widely debated. Learning of complex tasks has been shown to be impaired at 1524 and 2440 m, leading partly to pressure to reduce the cabin altitude of new commercial aircraft from 2500 to 1800 m. Shift workers commuting to high-altitude mines and telescopes have been investigated, and there is a suggestion of transient psychometric impairment, but these studies are confounded by the symptoms of AMS.[2] The lowest altitude at which memory dysfunction has been observed is 3500 m.[37] The psychomotor effects of altitude are probably due to the effects of hypoxia on the brain. Anxiety and fatigue (centrally mediated) also play a part, and research to date has been unable to separate the contribution of each.

Psychomotor efficiency was measured in 25 Indian soldiers who spent 2 years at an altitude of 4000 m. The soldiers were given hand–eye coordination and speed tests performed at sea level and after 1, 10, 13, 18, and 24 months at altitude. Psychomotor efficiency declined steadily over the first 10 months at altitude and improved over the following months as a result of acclimatization, but it never reached sea level values.[38] A subanalysis of the results showed that accuracy increased significantly during the first 10 months, but there was little improvement in speed.

Higher mental functions (e.g., language, cognition, and flexibility) are affected by hypoxia. As far as language is concerned, errors in verbal fluency and aphasia have been reported above 6400 m, but no long-term impairment has been reported after returning to lower altitudes. Reductions in cognitive flexibility (the ability to jump from one learned concept to another) have been repeatedly reported above 2500 m, and there is a general feeling of reduced confidence in performing cognitive and memory tasks.[39]

Climbers at altitude often rate their own performance as poor, even through there is no objective evidence to support this. The same applies to hours of sleep, with climbers reporting much less sleep than they actually get.

Mountaineers exhibit less neuroticism, less social conformity, greater emotional stability, and more sensation-seeking behavior than controls.[40]

Hallucinations have been commonly reported at altitude. One study of world-class mountaineers reported a nearly 90% incidence of hallucinations, mainly visual and auditory, along with the sense of having another companion (particularly if the climber was alone).[41] It is difficult to distinguish the various contributions of hypoxia, hypothermia, hypoglycemia, stress, sensory, and social deprivation or the experience of danger to these experiences.

Neurological Investigations

Electroencephalographic studies of eight world-class mountaineers (repeated ascents above 8000 m without supplementary oxygen) revealed chronic anomalies in two climbers in their frontal and temporal electroencephalogram activity measured months after their last ascent.[42]

High-intensity signals were detected on MRI in five out of nine subjects after ascending above 8000 m without supplementary oxygen. These were predominantly in the periventricular areas (leukoaraiosis), posterior parietal cortex, and occipital white matter.[43] In a controlled study of 21 lowland mountaineers, 61% showed signs of cortical atrophy and high-density signals (mainly in the periventricular regions of the posterior horns of the lateral ventricles) after an average stay of 445 hours above 7000 m and 56.5 hours above 8000 m. No abnormalities were detected in controls or seven world-class Sherpas.[44]

Leukoaraiosis is associated with corticosubcortical injury and widening of the Virchow-Robin spaces containing the perforating vessels of the middle cerebral artery. Leukoaraiosis (in the absence of ventricular enlargement) also is associated with a slowing down in complex mental processes as seen in early dementia.[39] This is similar to the "acute organic brain syndrome" described by the Polish climber and psychiatrist Ryn. The syndrome persisted for several weeks after returning to low altitude.[45]

Positive emission tomography studies of regional glucose metabolism in six U.S. Marines after 63 days at altitude (3181 to 6157 m) demonstrated a reduction in brain activity in the frontal lobes, the left occipital lobe, and the right thalamus.[46] Conversely, there was a bilateral increase in cerebellar activity. No abnormalities were detected in Sherpas whose regional glucose metabolism was similar to that of lowlanders.[47]

Mechanisms

During hypoxia, whole human brain oxygen consumption remains constant; therefore, cerebral blood flow has to increase. Although oxygen consumption remains constant, glucose usage and lactate production increase except in severe hypoxemia. The hippocampus, white matter, superior colliculus, and lateral geniculate are especially sensitive to hypoxia. Brain tissue energy markers (ATP/ADP/AMP) are close to normal levels, even during hypoxia comparable to 8000-m altitude. Both ion flux (especially calcium and potassium) and neurotransmitter metabolism are deranged in hypoxia, with accumulation of free radicals causing further injury. It is unclear whether this is due to hypoxia itself or a secondary effect. The α-portion of hypoxia-inducible factor 1α (HIF-1α) acts as a transcription factor for several growth factors, including VEGF stimulating angiogenesis and vascular remodeling to increase capillary density and therefore oxygen delivery (see the HACE section earlier). Research in cerebral ischemia suggests that inhibition of proline hydroxylation, which rapidly inactivates HIF-1α, may provide a useful therapeutic adjunct for the treatment of stroke.[2]

LONG-TERM NEUROLOGICAL IMPAIRMENT

In 1981, 21 members of the American Medical Research Expedition to Everest were subjected to a battery of psychological tests (Halstead-Reitan battery, repeatable cognitive–perceptual–motor battery, selective reminding test, and the Wechsler memory scale) before, immediately after (in Kathmandu), and 12 months after the expedition (not all tests were repeated). The main findings are presented in Table 8. Verbal learning and memory declined significantly during the expedition (Wechsler memory scale). Language errors also increased, and the degree of aphasia was significantly related to the maximum altitude gained by the climber. Finger tapping speed (number of times a lever could be pressed in 10 seconds) decreased significantly. The criterion for this test was five measurements on each hand, with a difference of less than five taps between trials. All subjects managed this preexpedition, but immediately afterward, 15 out of 20 subjects could not maintain motor speed. A year later, 13 out of 16 subjects still could not reach the criterion.[48]

Along with the persistent electroencephalogram changes noted earlier, the same investigators described persistent cognitive impairment (reduced ability to concentrate, short-term memory, and cognitive flexibility).[42]

CONCLUSION

Rapid ascent to altitude may result in illness in otherwise healthy individuals due to hypobaric hypoxia. This subacute hypoxic exposure triggers various poorly understood responses, collectively called acclimatization. Increases in the rate and depth of ventilation and erythropoiesis are the most important. Acclimatization rates and the maximum altitude that can be reached vary enormously among individuals and depend on various factors (genetics, hypoxic ventilatory response, previous performance at altitude, etc.), of which the rate of ascent is the most important modifiable factor.

AMS is common and is a self-limiting benign condition. HACE is a rare but life-threatening disease at the other end of the spectrum of cerebral mountain sickness. Both AMS and HACE are thought to be caused by vasogenic cerebral edema. HAPE is caused by a combination of hypoxic pulmonary vasoconstriction and increased capillary permeability. The resulting hypoxemia may be confused with HACE, and all altitude illnesses may coexist. The definitive treatment for all altitude illnesses is descent, although supplemental oxygen, portable hyperbaric chambers, and medicines (acetazolamide, dexamethasone, and nifedipine) are also used. A gradual ascent profile is

Table 8: Psychomotor Function at Altitude

Performance	Before	After	Follow-up
IMPROVED			
Tactual performance test (right hand)	4.68 ± 1.56	3.86 ± 1.46	
Category test	24.29 ± 15.46	11.05 ± 8.39	
WORSENED			
Finger tapping test (right hand)	53.71 ± 4.07	45.40 ± 6.18	48.40 ± 6.60
Finger tapping test (left hand)	47.65 ± 4.60	42.45 ± 5.96	41.73 ± 5.23
Criterion (right)	1.00 ± 0	0.14 ± 0.36	0.27 ± 0.46
Criterion (left)	1.00 ± 0	0.14 ± 0.36	0.13 ± 0.35
Wechsler Memory Scale			
Short-term verbal recall	18.12 ± 1.90	15.90 ± 2.15	17.13 ± 2.20
Trials to criterion	1.24 ± 0.44	2.40 ± 1.54	2.27 ± 0.70
Long-term verbal recall	16.35 ± 2.91	12.70 ± 3.78	14.50 ± 2.85
Aphasia screening test	0.59 ± 0.79	1.25 ± 1.25	0.47 ± 0.52

Mean results ± standard error comparing performance before, immediately afterward (Kathmandu), and after 12 months from the American Medical Research Expedition to Everest in 1981.

Adapted from Townes BD, Hornbein TF, Schoene RB, Sarnquist FH, Grant I. Human cerebral function at extreme altitude. In: West JB, Lahiri S, eds. *High Altitude and Man.* Bethesda, Md: American Physiological Society; 1984:32–36.

the best form of prevention, although in some instances the same medicines may be used prophylactically.

The CNS is exquisitely sensitive to hypoxia, and a large variety of often unpredictable neurological symptoms and illnesses can result. Some, such as strokes, are made worse by the body's acclimatization (increased hematocrit). Many are transient and self-limiting, but others may persist.

Neuropsychological function is impaired at altitude and partially recovers with extended stay at moderate altitude. Residual effects have been demonstrated up to a year after returning to low altitude and are confirmed with MRI and positron emission tomography studies. The same effects have not been demonstrated in native highland populations in South America and Asia who have adapted over many generations. Maladaptations in the form of an excessive hematocrit and pulmonary hypertension are the CMSs that affect native highlanders.

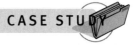

CASE STUDY

This case is a real-life scenario that took pace during the Caudwell Xtreme Everest research expedition to Cho Oyu (Tibet) in 2006. The case report has been submitted to *Stroke*.[49]

The differential diagnosis of collapse at high altitude includes hypoxia, hypothermia, and hypoglycemia. First aid treatment of any collapse involves treating all three—namely, getting the casualty to shelter, insulating from the elements (cold and wind), rewarming, and if conscious, giving hot, sugary drinks. Oxygen is rarely available except on expeditions to the highest mountains, but it should be administered if available.

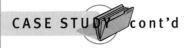

CASE STUDY cont'd

Returning to the collapsed climber—once the two doctors arrived, they discovered a dense right hemiplegia, right-sided neglect, and profound dysphasia with loss of gag reflex. The climber was commenced on oxygen, given dexamethasone at 4 mg IV stat, and then evacuated by stretcher on foot over rough glacial terrain from 5900 to 5600 m (Advanced Base Camp), where he was warmed and given intravenous fluids, oxygen, and aspirin. He was made nil by mouth, and a urinary catheter was inserted. Pressure areas were protected, and hourly neurological observations, blood pressure, heart rate, oxygen saturation, and urine output were recorded.

Transcranial Doppler (TCD) revealed normal flow in the right middle cerebral artery but absent flow in the left middle cerebral artery. Cerebral near-infrared spectroscopy revealed a regional oxygen saturation of 70% (normal) on the right but only 55% on the left, consistent with an ischemic cerebrovascular accident (Figure 52-6).

The team was not in a position to administer thrombolysis but attempted continuous TCD overnight, because there is some evidence that continuous TCD with or without thrombolysis may help clot breakdown by direct action on fibrin polymers.[50,51] If 12-O-tetradecanoylphorbol-13-acetate is administered at the same time, it is thought that this molecular breakdown increases the surface area for the drug to work.[52]

In the morning, the patient had improved—some power had returned to his right leg, and his speech could be understood. He was evacuated by stretcher to 4900 m and then by road to 1300 m, where he was evacuated by helicopter after spending a night at 2300 m. He was subsequently flown back to North America for definitive treatment.

Figure 52-7 is a single slice of the computerized tomography performed in Canada confirming an ischemic area within the left middle cerebral artery lenticulostriate branches (deep perforator) territory.

As this is the first case report of the use of ultrasound in the diagnosis (and possibly treatment) of ischemic stroke at altitude, it is difficult to assess any impact of the continuous TCD.

The causes of cerebral events at high altitude remain multifactorial but unclear. Undoubtedly, hypobaric hypoxia itself has a toxic effect on the CNS. Anything other than a short exposure (e.g., a cable car ride) initiates erythropoiesis, which increases the hematocrit, with a correspondingly exponential rise in blood viscosity and the tendency toward thrombotic strokes. Hypoxia itself is also thought to induce a prothrombotic state.[28]

Dehydration is common at altitude due to increased ventilatory losses in the dry air, further contributing to a sluggish circulation. In this case, the climber's gastrointestinal upset may have exaggerated this. Other risk factors for increased thrombosis at altitude include decreased physical activity and cold. Women taking certain types of oral contraceptive pill are more prone to

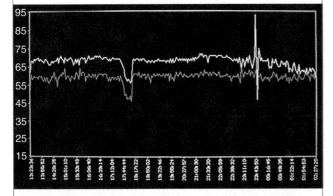

Figure 52-6. Near-infrared spectroscopy monitoring of cerebral regional oxygen saturations. Blue is left (ischemic) cortices; white is right (normal) cortices. (Courtesy of Mark Wilson and Caudwell Xtreme Everest.)

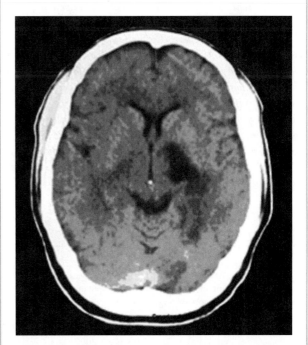

Figure 52-7. Single-slice computerized tomography confirming left middle cerebral artery (deep perforator territory) ischemia. (Courtesy of Mark Wilson and Caudwell Xtreme Everest.)

Continued

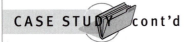

CASE STUDY cont'd

thrombosis, particularly if there are other risk factors (e.g., family history or smoking). This risk is almost certainly increased at altitude.

Further consideration of women, children, the elderly, and those with preexisting medical conditions at altitude is outside the scope of this chapter, but more information is available in the texts listed in the References section.

Acknowledgments and Funding

Caudwell Xtreme Everest (CXE) is a research project coordinated by the Centre for Altitude, Space and Extreme Environment Medicine, University College London, United Kingdom. The aim of CXE is to conduct research into hypoxia and human performance at high altitude to improve understanding of hypoxia in critical illness. Membership, roles, and responsibilities of the CXE Research Group can be found at www.caudwell-xtreme-everest.co.uk/team. The research was funded from various sources, none of which are public. Entrepreneur John Caudwell, whose name the expedition carries, donated £500,000 specifically to support the research. BOC Medical, now part of Linde Gas Therapeutics, generously supported the early research and continues to do so. Lilly Critical Care, The London Clinic (a private hospital), Smiths Medical, Deltex Medical, and The Rolex Foundation have also donated money to support the research and logistics. All monies were given as unrestricted grants. Specific research grants were awarded by the Association of Anaesthetists of Great Britain and Ireland, the UK Intensive Care Foundation, and the Sir Halley Stuart Trust. The CXE volunteers who trekked to Everest Base Camp also kindly donated to support the research.

REFERENCES

1. Huddleston B, Ataman E, Fè de'Ostiane L. Towards a GIS-based Analysis of Mountain Environments and Populations. Working Paper 10. Rome: Food and Agriculture Organization of the United Nations; 2003.
2. West JB, Schoene RB, Milledge JS. *High Altitude Medicine and Physiology.* 4th ed. London: Hodder Arnold; 2007.
3. Pollard AJ, Murdoch DR. *The High Altitude Medicine Handbook.* 3rd ed. Oxford: Radcliffe Medical Press; 2003.
4. Doherty MJ. James Glaisher's 1862 account of balloon sickness: altitude, decompression injury, and hypoxemia. *Neurology.* 2003;60:1016–1018.
5. Rodway GW. Limb paralysis and visual changes during Glaisher and Coxwell's 1862 balloon ascent to over 8800 m. *High Alt Med Biol.* 2007;8:3 256–259.
6. West JB. Paralysis and blindness during a balloon ascent to high altitude. *High Alt Med Biol.* 2004;5:453–456.
7. Hackett PH, Rennie D. The incidence, importance and prophylaxis of acute mountain sickness. *Lancet.* 1976;2:1149–1154.
8. Basnyat B, Subedi D, Sleggs J, et al. Disoriented and ataxic pilgrims: an epidemiological study of acute mountain sickness and high altitude cerebral edema at a sacred lake at 4300 m in the Nepal Himalayas. *Wilderness Environ Med.* 2000;11(2):89–93.
9. Bärtsch P, Merki B, Maggiorini M, Kayser B, Oelz O. Treatment of acute mountain sickness by simulated decent: a randomised controlled trial. *BMJ.* 1993;306:1098–1101.
10. Grissom CK, Roach RC, Sarnquist FH, Hackett PH. Acetazolamide in the treatment of acute mountain sickness: clinical effects on gas exchange. *Ann Intern Med.* 1992;116:461–465.
11. Murdoch DR. How fast is too fast? Attempts to define a recommended ascent rate to prevent acute mountain sickness. *ISMM Newsletter.* 1999;9:2–6.
12. Basnyat B, Leomaster J, Litch JA. Everest or bust: a cross sectional, epidemiological survey of acute mountain sickness at 4234 m in the Himalaya. *Aviat Space Environ Med.* 1999;70:867–873.
13. Hackett PH, Roach RC. High altitude cerebral edema. *High Alt Med Biol.* 2004;5:136–146.
14. Dickinson J. Severe acute mountain sickness. *Postgrad Med.* 1979;55:454–458.
15. Clarke C. High altitude cerebral oedema. *Int J Sports Med.* 1988;9:170–174.
16. Gabry AL, Ledoux X, Mozziconacci M, Martin C. High altitude pulmonary edema at moderate altitude. (2400 m; 7870 feet): a series of 52 patients. *Chest.* 2003;123(1):49–53.
17. Hultgren HN, Honigman B, Theis K, Nicholas D. High altitude pulmonary edema at a ski resort. *West J Med.* 1996;164(3):222–227.
18. Yarnell PR, Heit J, Hackett PH. High altitude cerebral edema (HACE): the Denver/Front Range experience. *Semin Neurol.* 2000;20(2):209–217.
19. Dickinson JG. High altitude cerebral edema: cerebral acute mountain sickness. *Semin Respir Med.* 1983;5:151–158.
20. Wu T, Ding S, Liu J, et al. Ataxia: an early indicator in high altitude cerebral edema. *High Alt Med Biol.* 2006;7:275–280.
21. Hackett PH, Yarnell PR, Hill R, Reynard K, Heit J, McCormick J. High altitude cerebral edema evaluated with magnetic resonance imaging: clinical correlation and pathophysiology [see comments]. *JAMA.* 1998;280(22):1920–1925.
22. Severinghaus JW. Hypothesis: angiogenesis cytokines in high altitude cerebral oedema. *Acta Anaesthesiol Scand Suppl.* 1995;107:177–178.
23. Tissot van Patot MC, Leadbitter G, Keyes LE, Bendrick-Peart J, Beckey VE, Hackett PH. Greater free plasma VEGF and lower soluble VEGF receptor-1 in acute mountain sickness. *J Appl Physiol.* 2005;98:1626–1629.
24. Ross RT. The random nature of cerebral mountain sickness. *Lancet.* 1985;1(8435):990–901.
25. Wilson MH, Milledge JS. Direct measurement of intracranial pressure at altitude and correlation of ventricular size with acute mountain sickness: Brian Cummin's results from the 1985 Kishtwar expedition. *Neurosurgery.* 2008;63(5):970–974.
26. Menon ND. High altitude pulmonary edema: a clinical study. *N Engl J Med.* 1965;273:66–73.
27. Oelz O, Maggiorini M, Ritter M, et al. Nifedipine for high altitude pulmonary oedema. *Lancet.* 1989;2:1241–1244.
28. Clarke C. Acute mountain sickness: medical problems associated with acute and subacute exposure to hypobaric hypoxia. *Postgrad Med J.* 2006;82(973):748–753.

29. Sui GJ, Lui YH, Cheng XS, et al. Subacute infantile mountain sickness. *J Pathol.* 1988;155:161–170.

30. Ananad IS, Malhotra RM, Chandrashekar Y, et al. Adult subacute mountain sickness: a syndrome of congestive heart failure in man at very high altitude. *Lancet.* 1990;335:561–565.

31. Basynat B, Wu TY, Gertsch JH. Neurological conditions at altitude that fall outside the definition of altitude illness. *High Alt Med Biol.* 2004;5:171–179.

32. Jha SK, Anand AC, Sharma V, Kumar N, Adya CM. Stroke at high altitude: Indian experience. *High Alt Med Biol.* 2002;3:21–27.

33. Litch JA, Bishop RA. High altitude global amnesia. *Wilderness Exp Med.* 2000;11:25–28.

34. Murdoch DR. Lateral rectus palsy at high altitude. *J Wilderness Med.* 1994;5:179–181.

35. Hackett PH, Hollingshead KF, Roach RB, et al. Cortical blindness in high altitude climbers and trekkers: a report of six cases. In: Sutton JR, Houston CS, Coates G, eds. *Hyoxia and Cold.* New York: Praeger; 1987:536.

36. Salvaggio A, Insalaco G, Marrone O, et al. Effects of high-altitude periodic breathing on sleep and arterial oxyhaemoglobin saturation. *Eur Respir J.* 1998;12:408–413.

37. Shukitt-Hale B, Stillmannn MJ, Welch DI, Levy A, Devine JA, Lieberman HR. Hypobaric hypoxia impairs spatial memory in an elevation-dependent fashion. *Behav Neural Biol.* 1994,62.244–253.

38. Sharma VM, Malhotra MS, Baskaran AS. Variations in psychomotor efficiency during prolonged stay at altitude. *Ergonomics.* 1975;18:511–516.

39. Virués-Ortega J, Buela-Casal G, Garrido G, Alcázar B. Neuropsychological functioning associated with high-altitude exposure. *Neuropsychol Rev.* 2004;14:197–224.

40. Freixanet M. Personality profile of subjects engaged in high physical risk sports participants. *Pers Individ Dif.* 1991;12:1087–1093.

41. Brugger P, Regard M, Landis T, Oelz O. Hallucinatory experiences in extreme altitude climbers. *Neuropsychiatry Neuropsychol Behav Neurol.* 1999;12:67–71.

42. Regard M, Oelz O, Brugger P, Landis T. Persistent cognitive impairment in climbers after repeated exposure to extreme altitude. *Neurology.* 1989;39:210–213.

43. Garrido E, Segura R, Capdevilla A, Aldomá J, Rodriguez FA, Javierre C, et al. New evidence from magnetic resonance imaging of brain changes after climbs at extreme altitude. *Eur J Appl Physiol.* 1995;70:477–481.

44. Garrido E, Segura R, Capdevilla A, Pujol J, Javierre C, Ventura JL. Are Himalayan sherpas better protected against brain damage associated with extreme altitude climbs? *Clin Sci.* 1996;90:81–85.

45. Ryn Z. Psychopathology in mountaineering: mental disturbance under high altitude stress. *Int J Sports Med.* 1988;9:163–169.

46. Hochachka PW, Clark CM, Matheon GO, et al. Effects on regional brain metabolism of high-altitude hypoxia: a study of 6 U.S. marines. *Am J Physiol.* 1999;277:314–319.

47. Hochachka PW, Clark CM, Monge C, et al. Sherpa brain glucose metabolism and defense adaptations against chronic hypoxia. *J Appl Physiol.* 1996;81:1355–1361.

48. Townes BD, Hornbein TF, Schoene RB, Sarnquist FH, Grant I. Human cerebral function at extreme altitude. In: West JB, Lahiri S, eds. *High Altitude and Man.* Bethesda, Md: American Physiological Society; 1984:32–36.

49. Wilson MH, Levett D, Dhillon S, et al. High altitude stroke diagnosed in the field using portable ultrasound. *Stroke.* Submitted.

50. Alexandrov AV. Ultrasound identification and lysis of clots. *Stroke.* 2004;35: (11 Suppl 1):2722–2725.

51. Cintas P, Le Traon AP, Larrue V. High rate of recanalization of middle cerebral artery occlusion during 2-MHz transcranial color-coded Doppler continuous monitoring without thrombolytic drug. *Stroke.* 2002;33(2):626–628.

52. Daffertohofer M, Fatar M. Therapeutic ultrasound in ischemic stroke treatment: experimental evidence. *Eur J Ultrasound.* 2002;16(1–2):121–130.

53. Roach RC, Bärtsch P, Hackett PH, Oelz O. The Lake Louise acute mountain sickness scoring system. In: Sutton JR, Houston CS, Coates G, eds. *Hypoxia and Mountain Medicine.* Burlington, Vt: Queen City Printers; 1993:272–274.

FURTHER READING

Auerbach PS. *Wilderness Medicine.* 5th ed. Philadelphia: Mosby Elsevier; 2007.

Medex. Travel at High Altitude. Available at: http://www.medex.org.uk. Accessed July 1, 2008.

CHAPTER 53

Neurological Complications of Malnutrition

Redda Tekle Haimamot

PROTEIN–CALORIE MALNUTRITION

In the developed world, malnutrition no longer plays a significant role in the causation of neurological disorders except in consumers of excessive alcoholic beverages. In the context of low-income countries, however, the problem is quite common. Sections of populations in these countries suffer from both general malnutrition and deficiencies of micronutrients. The problem predominantly affects children. Undernourished children may be thin and "wasted." When growth is retarded, the child becomes "stunted." There are two clinical conditions associated with severe malnutrition in early children. Deficiency of protein without calorie malnutrition results in kwashiorkor. When the deficiency involves both protein and energy, the condition is referred to as marasmus. Infections tend to precipitate both conditions. Kwashiorkor arises when a child is weaned on a traditional low-protein diet after prolonged breastfeeding. It is commonly encountered between 1 and 4 years of age. In kwashiorkor, the child is anorexic and anemic. There is failure in growth, muscle wasting, and edema from hypoalbuminemia. Skin and hair change their texture. Associated vitamin A deficiency causes xerophthalmia and keratomalacia.

In contrast to kwashiorkor, marasmus occurs in infants younger than 1 year. It is caused by early weaning extending over 2 years due to economical reasons and pregnancy, coupled with inadequate and unbalanced artificial feeding. Marasmic infants are underweight, with wasting of subcutaneous fat and muscles. These changes give affected children an old appearance. They often have watery diarrhea and signs of avitaminosis (stomatitis, cheilosis, keratomalacia).

These types of malnutrition cause neurological complications, particularly in children. The nervous system is susceptible to the adverse effects of malnutrition during the early stages of its development, i.e., in utero and early infancy. When serious and prolonged, the nutritional insult has long-term effects on intellectual development of the affected child.[1-3] Malnourished children are weak, indifferent, and apathetic and tend to be irritable and restless. They are often uninterested in their surroundings and do not communicate with people around them. There is clumsiness in repetitive motor tasks and impaired intellectual functions.[4,5] The related cognitive development further causes learning disability, poor performance at school, and behavioral problems.[6,7] Protein malnutrition has also been documented to cause muscle pain and wasting, hypotonia, and hyporeflexia.[8]

Food supplementation is the cornerstone of management of the malnourished child. However, special attention should be paid to how these children are treated. Their dysfunctional gastrointestinal system is initially unable to handle a normal diet. A protein-rich bland and digestible diet is preferred during the early stages of the nutritional rehabilitation. However, even the high-protein supplementation should be built up gradually. Multivitamin and mineral supplementation is mandatory, and early treatment of infections is crucial. Children exposed to chronic malnutrition require special guidance and stimulation at home and at school to improve their cognitive development and intellectual performance.[9] While these approaches address the individual cases, it should be emphasized that the problem of general malnutrition is a major global concern that calls for political leaders and international agencies to urgently seek and design strategies to enhance economical development to reduce and possibly prevent poverty. This particularly applies to low-income countries that are vulnerable to crop failures and famine.

VITAMIN DEFICIENCIES AND NEUROLOGICAL COMPLICATIONS

Vitamin deficiency is common in some populations, especially in low-income countries, due to the nonavailability or poor content of vitamins in traditional staple diets. Excessive alcohol intake results in thiamine deficiency, which is commonly encountered in the developed world. Significant neurological complications are seen in the deficiencies of thiamine (vitamin B_1), niacin (vitamin B_3), pyridoxine (vitamin B_6), and cobalamin (vitamin B_{12}) and folate. These deficiencies are dealt with individually.

Thiamine (Vitamin B_1)

Thiamine is mainly found in legumes, liver, pork, nuts, germ of cereals, and yeast. Little is available in dairy products and green vegetables. Alcoholic beverages have very low or no content of this vitamin. Thiamine is lost with cooking. The vitamin is not stored in the body; hence, deficiencies develop over a short period.

Extreme deficiency of vitamin B_1 causes a clinical condition known as beriberi, which is characterized by a combination of cardiomyopathy, peripheral neuropathy, and/or encephalopathy. Pins-and-needles sensations in the legs signal the onset of neuropathy. There may also be tenderness in muscles, which subsequently develop weakness and wasting. This causes difficulties in walking. The cerebral form of thiamine deficiency is manifested as Wernicke's encephalopathy and Korsakoff's psychosis. The two conditions are commonly encountered among excessive alcohol consumers. They are therefore discussed in detail, together with the management of thiamine deficiency, under the toxic nutritional disorders section dealing with alcohol.

Cuban Epidemic Neuropathy

From 1992 to 1993, an epidemic involving more than 50,000 people occurred in Cuba. The affected subjects presented initially with chronic fatigue, sleep disturbance, irritability, and lack of concentration with poor memory. These symptoms were followed by signs of optic neuropathy (centrocecal scotoma), sensorineural deafness, dorsolateral myelopathy, and polyneuropathy, predominantly sensory. The cause of the disorder was found to be deficiency of the B complex vitamins, especially thiamine, accompanied by a lack of sulfur-containing amino acids. These deficiencies were associated with the excess consumption of cane sugar due to food shortage and unbalanced diet. Treatment with a vitamin B complex brought about dramatic response.[10,11]

Niacin (Vitamin B_3)

Meat, fish, whole grain cereals (with the bran), and pulses are rich in niacin. Although cooking does not destroy the vitamin, it could be lost with the cooking water if discarded. Niacin is synthesized in the body from the amino acid tryptophan. The medical condition resulting from the deficiency of this amino acid is similar to that of niacin deficiency. Niacin deficiency is commonly seen in rural communities of African countries, where the diet is composed of mainly maize. Niacin and tryptophan deficiencies cause pellagra, a clinical condition with the three important features of dermatitis, diarrhea, and dementia. Pellagra is also seen in the genetic inborn error of tryptophan metabolism known as Hartnup's disease. The neurological complications associated with mild deficiency are irritability, depression, and lack of concentration. More severe forms develop delirium acutely and dementia in the chronic state. Treatment includes the administration of nicotinamide (niacin) 500 mg po daily for 7-10 days, then 50-100 mg daily until symptoms have ameliorated. This should be supplemented with a vitamin complex and a high-protein diet. The major preventive measure for this condition is vitamin fortification of the maize diet.

Pyridoxine (Vitamin B_6)

The main sources of vitamin B_6 are whole grain cereals, liver, peanuts, and banana. Dietary deficiency is rare. However, infants on artificial feeding deficient in vitamin B_6 develop convulsions. Peripheral neuropathy is associated with isoniazid therapy for tuberculosis. Isoniazid causes its toxicity on the nervous system through the disturbance of the pyridoxine metabolism because the administration of the drug leads to an increased excretion of the vitamin through the urine. Treatment is effective with the administration of pyridoxine orally in the daily dose of 50 to 100 mg.

Cobalamin (Vitamin B₁₂) and Folate Deficiencies

Vitamin B_{12} is found in meat and other animal food stuffs. Besides inadequate dietary intake, vitamin B_{12} deficiency is associated with malabsorption from the gastrointestinal tract. A rigid vegetarian diet also leads to a deficiency state with overt clinical manifestations. Vitamin B_{12} deficiency causes megaloblastic anemia and subacute combined degeneration of the spinal cord. The pathological changes in the spinal cord consist of degeneration in the posterior and lateral columns. Neurological symptoms are manifested initially by a symmetrical, painful paresthesia of the lower limbs, followed by ataxia of gait. Sensory deficits range from tactile hypoesthesia and hypalgesia to complete analgesia. Position and vibration sensations are grossly affected. Dementia may also occur in some cases. The polyneuropathy is found in 75% of the cases. Pyramidal signs are elicited. The tendon jerks are absent at the ankle and the knee. Treatment includes two parenteral doses of 1000 μg of hydroxocobalamin during the first week followed by a similar 1000-μg dose weekly for four weeks.

Folate is available in vegetables and animal food stuffs. It is destroyed by cooking. Like vitamin B_{12}, folate deficiency causes megaloblastic anemia, with neurological signs of posterior column and pyramidal tract affection. Neuropathy is found in 20% to 60% of the affected individuals. In addition to these complications, neural tube defects such as myelomeningocele have been documented in babies born to folate-deficient mothers. The fortification of cereals (wheat) has proven to be an effective preventive measure.[12]

MINERAL DEFICIENCIES

The two trace elements whose deficiencies are well documented to cause neurological complications include iodine and iron. In addition, calcium deficiency leads to seizures in early childhood, proximal myopathy in adults, and tetany at all ages. Although rare, deficiencies of zinc, magnesium, and cobalt have been reported to also cause neurological deficits.

Iodine Deficiency

Iodine deficiency is a worldwide nutritional problem involving 130 countries, and well more than 1 billion people are at risk. It causes goiter, hypothyroidism, abortions, and increased perinatal mortality. Affected children have feeding problems and fail to achieve normal developmental milestones. Congenital hypothyroidism known as cretinism has different manifestations. The severe type is associated with mental retardation, spastic paraplegia, dwarfism, and bulbar signs. The bulbar and pyramidal signs may be absent is the less severe form. In the mild form, deafness may be the only sign. Cretins have coarse puffy faces, a large protruding tongue, and an umbilical hernia. The preventive measure of iodine deficiency is iodinization of salt, which has proven effective and successful in many countries where iodine deficiency is an endemic problem. Encouraging declines of iodine-deficiency states have been recorded throughout the world with the interventional program.

Iron Deficiency

Liver, fish, and meat are rich in iron. In low-income countries, iron-deficiency anemia is common. The causes include blood loss through multiple pregnancies and poor obstetric services, as well as parasitic infections such as hookworm, schistosomiasis, and malaria. Children with iron-deficiency anemia are physically weak and mentally apathetic. The anemia affects their cognitive function and learning ability. Iron-deficiency anemia is corrected with the treatment of infections and iron supplementation. Blood loss is prevented through better obstetrics services and effective family planning.

TOXIC NUTRITIONAL DISORDERS

Neurological Disorders Caused by Alcohol

Depending on the extent and duration of consumption, alcohol causes various damages to the nervous system, both central and peripheral. The damages may be the direct toxic effects of the alcohol, as well as structural changes that are a consequence of the associated malnutrition, particularly vitamin deficiency; notably, thiamine is in short supply in alcohol beverages. The chronic alcoholic often depends on alcoholic beverages as the source of calorie requirement and hence suffers from additional protein malnutrition. In developing countries, clinicians do not see as many alcohol-caused neurological complications as in the developed world. The explanation is related to economical factors. Due to low incomes, few people in developing countries can afford to be chronic consumers of alcohol. The following neurological complications are seen in long-term alcohol consumers.

Wernicke's Encephalopathy

The clinical manifestations of Wernicke's encephalopathy include varying levels disturbance of mental state, ocular muscle paresis, nystagmus, autonomic dysregulation, and cerebellar signs in the form of ataxia. It is commonly caused by thiamine deficiency in a person with chronic alcoholism and malnutrition. The disease occurs acutely, mainly during abstinence. However, it is also seen in beriberi caused by nutritional deficiency of vitamin B_1. Wernicke's encephalopathy is a medical emergency that requires urgent administration of high-dose intravenous thiamine. Delay in treatment could lead to Korsakoff's psychosis. Treatment is started with 50 mg of intravenous and 50 mg of intramuscular thiamine. Thereafter, 50 mg of intramuscular thiamine are given until the patient is able to eat normally.

Korsakoff's Psychosis

The clinical entity of Korsakoff's psychosis is also referred to as amnestic-confabulatory psychosis characterized by retrograde and anterograde amnesia. Confabulation may be witnessed early at onset and during recovery. The cause of the disease is thiamine deficiency. Response of the psychosis to thiamine therapy is not as dramatic as with Wernicke's encephalopathy. This may be due the permanent structural neurological damage, as seen in neuropathological examination, which reveals symmetrical hemorrhagic spongiform lesions in the thalamus, the hypothalamus, and the floor of the fourth ventricle.

Cerebellar Atrophy

Alcohol-related cerebellar atrophy predominantly affects men (10:1). It is more common than Wernicke's encephalopathy. Clinically affected people demonstrate marked ataxia of stance and gait (worse on eye closure) and nystagmus. Neuropathology reveals atrophy of the anterior and middle cerebellum.

Polyneuropathy

The polyneuropathy complication is characterized by insidious onset of progressive symptoms of pain, paresthesias, night muscular cramps, and coldness in the feet (distal to proximal) affecting the legs and later the arms. Pain can be elicited by pressure on muscles and superficial nerves. The leg muscles show wasting and atrophy, and the affected person has difficulty walking. Polyneuropathy is found in 30% of alcoholics. However, twice as many cases affected by the neuropathy may be discovered through electrophysiological investigations. Abstention from alcohol and well-balanced diet results in dramatic improvement of the neuropathy depending on the clinical stage of the complication. Thiamine with folate and vitamin B complex supplements should also be administered orally.

Neurological Disorder Caused by *Lathyrus sativus* Consumption

Lathyrism has been known since the time of Hippocrates (460 to 377 BC). Although this neurological disorder has in the past occurred in epidemics in North Africa, the Middle East, Asia, and the Indian subcontinent, it is now only endemic in Ethiopia, India, and Bangladesh. The earliest accurate descriptions of the disease come from India through Sleeman in 1844[13] and Acton in 1922.[14] The toxic properties of *Lathyrus* flour were recognized in Europe as early as 1671 by the Duke of Wurthemberg, but it was only in the 1960s that investigators in India firmly established the direct causative relationship of excessive consumption of grass pea or chickling pea (*L. sativus*). The most direct confirmation that *L. sativus* was responsible for human lathyrism came from the unfortunate experience of Romanian Jews interned in a German forced labor camp in the Ukraine. They developed the disease after being maintained on a daily diet of 400 g of grass pea cooked in saltwater with 200 gm of barley bread.[15] Prisoners who consumed less of the grass pea (200 g per day) did not develop the disease. The emergence of new cases ceased with the discontinuation of the grass pea diet in the camp. From the same camp, there was also indirect evidence that malnutrition did not significantly contribute to the manifestation of the disease. It appears that excessive consumption plays a major role in toxicity.

Murti[16] and Rao[17] independently isolated the neurotoxic amino acid, β-N-oxalyl-α, β-diaminopropionic acid (ODAP or β-N-oxalylamino-L-alanine), the suspected culprit of neurolathyrism. The legume grass pea (*L. sativus*) is a hardy crop that is drought and waterlogging resistant and can withstand pest and weeds. At times of food shortage, it may provide the entire diet of communities. In times of plenty, it is mixed with other cereals like rice and wheat. The seeds and fodder are also used an animal feed. Epidemiological studies have shown that most people develop lathyrism after consuming grass pea consisting of more than 30% of their daily diet for more than 3 months. Men are affected more often than women.

Knowledge of the neuropathology of lathyrism is rather limited. Few postmortem examinations have been performed on cases of lathyrism because most patients are poor and die at home in remote regions and in endemic countries where there are religious and cultural prohibitions on postmortems. The few published reports indicate that the neuropathological findings of human lathyrism are dominated by symmetrical axonal degeneration and crossed and uncrossed pyramidal tracts in the thoracic, lumbar, and sacral spinal cord.[18,19] In addition, loss of pyramidal cells in the region of the motor cortex controlling the leg is noted in an early study of the pathology of the brain in human lathyrism.[20] Primary neuronal degeneration, with secondary loss of cortical motor axons, is consistent with the neurotoxic action of ODAP, the culpable agent in grass pea.

Lathyrism is characterized by the sudden onset of severe spastic paraparesis associated with adductor spasm in the worst cases, as well as exaggerated deep tendon reflexes, extensor plantar response, and ankle clonus (Figures 53-1 and 53-2). Distal lower limb objective sensory deficits to pinprick and light touch are uncommon. Reversible urinary frequency and urgency, nocturnal erection, and ejaculation have been reported in victims of lathyrism. Mental status, speech, and cranial nerve function are intact. Cerebellar signs are not detected. All ages are affected. However, more than 80% of affected individuals are younger than 40 years. Males are affected more commonly (2.5:1) and more severely than females. The severity of the paraparesis can be graded using a system based on the mobility support they use. They include no stick, one stick, two sticks, and crawler stages. The first two stages are found in 90% of the affected cases.[21]

Important myelopathies that come into the differential diagnosis of lathyrism include konzo, tropical spastic paraparesis (TSP) and HTLV-1-associated myelopathy (HAM). TSP is a slowly progressive spastic paraparesis with an insidious onset. Unlike lathyrism, cases of TSP commonly complain of sensory and autonomic disturbances, including incontinence and impotence.[22] The same applies to HAM.[23] Lack of excessive grass pea consumption rules out lathyrism in doubtful cases. The other spastic paraparesis that has similar clinical setting and manifestations is konzo, caused by excessive and exclusive consumption of insufficiently processed cassava (*Manihot esculenta*). The dietary history helps differentiate between konzo and lathyrism, and the two conditions exist in different geographical isolates. However, the clinical and pathological similarities of the two diseases present an investigatory challenge in neurotoxicology. Additional conditions to be considered in the differential diagnosis are motor neuron disease (amyotrophic lateral sclerosis), cord compression, and other myelopathies, including those caused by human immunodeficiency virus. There are no specific investigations

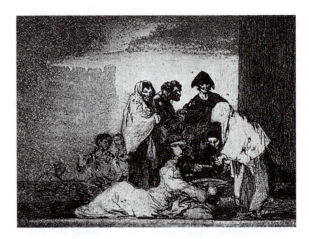

Figure 53-2. Goya (1746–1828), *Thanks to the grasspea*. This aquatint depicts the grass pea as a famine food. Note the woman lying on the floor, already crippled from its effects.

or biomarkers for lathyrism. A detailed dietary history and the exclusion of other conditions mentioned earlier are the hallmarks of the diagnosis. Lathyrism is an irreversible condition for which there are no known cures once it is established.

Neurological Disorders Caused by Cyanide Toxicity

Konzo

Konzo is the local word in the Kwango area in the Bandundu province of the Democratic Republic of the Congo, formerly known as Zaire. Konzo means "tied or bound legs," which lends a descriptive picture to the spastic paraparesis caused by the toxic effects of cyanide present in cassava consumed without proper processing.[24] Cassava (*M. esculenta*) is a starchy root crop that constitutes the major source of dietary energy for nearly half the populations of sub–Saharan Africa. It provides food security in times of drought and famine. The major use of cassava is for human consumption. It has also many industrial applications.

Cassava is a perennial plant that has the agricultural advantages of giving high yield per unit area of land and being drought resistant. It also does not require high-quality soil and has flexibility in planting and harvesting times. Cassava roots are rich in carbohydrates. The protein content is lower than that of cereals, legumes, and other root and tuber crops such as yams and potatoes. Vitamins are low in cassava. In communities where cassava is cultivated as the only source of diet, there is a high prevalence of protein energy malnutrition among preschool children, pregnant women, and lactating mothers.

Cassava contains cyanogenic glucosides. High content of the glucoside correlates to the bitter taste of fresh

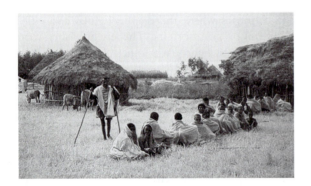

Figure 53-1. Lathyrism cases gathered for evaluation in village in northern Ethiopia. The person standing is a two stick case.

roots. Glucoside is hydrolyzed to cyanohydrin and hydrogen cyanide through the endogenous enzymatic action of linamarase. In the absence of complete processing, cyanogens are not removed effectively, resulting in the accumulation of cyanide. Grating and moist formation are the most important steps of cassava processing, which ensure the reduction of cyanogen content. The insufficient processing of the bitter form of cassava, combined with low intake of sulfur, results in neural damage manifested as sudden onset spastic paraparesis with a scissor gait (Figure 53-3). The condition predominantly affects children and women. Blurring of vision and dysarthria have been reported in some patients. Neurological examination reveals pyramidal signs of exaggerated reflexes and upgoing plantar response in the lower limbs. In a few cases, pyramidal signs have been elicited in the upper limbs. There are no sensory deficits or cerebellar signs. Depending on the severity of the paraparesis, the clinical state is described as mild, moderate, or severe. The mild and subclinical forms may be difficult to diagnose. Some investigators have reported repeated attacks of the paraparesis, which tend to be worse than the initial one. There is no treatment for konzo other than supportive physical rehabilitation. This neurological disorder has occurred as epidemic in Mozambique,[25,26] Democratic Republic of the Congo,[24,27] Central African Republic,[28] and Tanzania.[29,30]

Konzo has clinical similarities to lathyrism, TSP, and HAM. Dietary history is important in the diagnosis of the condition.

Tropical Ataxic Polyneuropathy

Tropical ataxic polyneuropathy has been reported from tropical and subtropical countries including Nigeria, Senegal, Mozambique, and Tanzania. It has also been seen among prisoners of war. Variability of symptoms and signs has been observed among affected patients. However, the common manifestations encountered in this slowly progressive chronic disorder were bilateral optic atrophy, sensorineural deafness, posterior column myelopathy, and polyneuropathy. Both sexes are affected equally. The neuropathy is manifested with painful paresthesia, numbness, and burning sensation in the legs, which are also weak and wasted. There is blurring of vision, as well as tinnitus and deafness. Posterior column damage of the spinal cord results in ataxia of gait. The cause of this disorder is believed to be related to protein malnutrition associated with deficiency of sulfur-containing amino acids in a population exposed to chronic cyanide toxicity due to the consumption of a monotonous cassava diet.[31–33] The myelopathy of tropical ataxic polyneuropathy is often confused with konzo because both conditions have been attributed to cyanide toxicity through the consumption of insufficiently processed cassava. There are suggestions that cases of tropical ataxic polyneuropathy are exposed to a low cyanide level over a long period as compared to konzo victims who develop paraparesis after consumption of high doses over shorter periods.

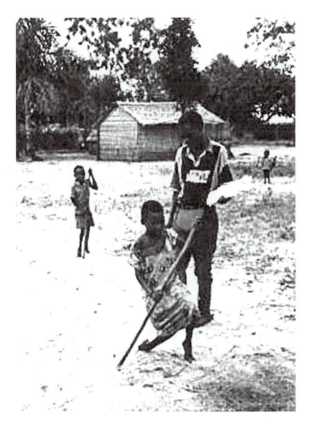

Figure 53-3. Konzo-affected children in a village in the Democratic Republic of the Congo (formerly Zaire). The children have spastic scissor gait and use one stick.

REFERENCES

1. Galler JR, Ramsey F, Salt P, Archer E. The long-term effects of early kwashiorkor compared with marasmus: I. Physical growth and sexual maturation. *J Pediatr Gastroenterol Nutr.* 1987;6: 841–846.
2. Grantham-McGregor S, Ani C. Cognition and undernutrition: evidence for vulnerable period. *Forum Nutr.* 2003;56:272–275.
3. Grantham-McGregor S, Baker-Henningham H. Review of the evidence linking protein and energy to mental development. *Public Health Nutr.* 2005;8:1191–1201.
4. Galler JR, Ramsey F, Salt P, Forde V. The long-term effect of early kwashiorkor and marasmus: intellectual performance. *J Pediatr Gastroenterol Nutr.* 1987;6:847–854.
5. Sigman M. Cognitive abilities of Kenyan children in relation to nutrition, family characteristics and education. *Child Dev.* 1989;60:1463–1474.
6. Galler JR, Ramsey F, Solimano G. The influence of early malnutrition on subsequent development: III. Learning disability as a sequel of malnutrition. *Pediatr Res.* 1984;18:309–313.

7. Galler JR, Ramsey F, Solimano G. A follow-up study of the influence of early malnutrition on subsequent development: VI. Home and classroom behaviour. *J Am Acad Child Adolesc Psychiatry*. 1989;28:254–261.

8. Chopra JS, Dhand UK, Mehta S, Bakshi V, Rana SV, Mehta J. Effect of protein calorie malnutrition on peripheral nerves. A clinical, electrophysiological and histopathological study. *Brain*. 1986;109:307–323.

9. Grantham-McGregor SM, Schofield W, Powel C. Development of severely malnourished children who received psychosocial stimulation: six years follow-up. *Pediatrics*. 1987;79:247–254.

10. McCarthy M. Cuban neuropathy. *Lancet*. 1994;343:844.

11. Roman GC. Epidemic neuropathy in Cuba: a plea to end the United States economic embargo on a humanitarian basis. *Neurology*. 1994;44:1784–1786.

12. Eichholzer M, Tonz O, Zimmerman R. Folic acid: a public health challenge. *Lancet*. 2006;367:1352–1361.

13. Sleeman WH. *Rambles and Recollections of an Indian Official*. vol. 1. London: Hatchard and Sons; 1844.

14. Acton HW. An investigation into the causation of lathyrism in man. *Ind Med Gaz*. 1922;57:241–247.

15. Kessler A. Lathyrismus. *Monatsschr Psychiatr Neurol*. 1947;113:345–376.

16. Murti VVS. Neurotoxic compounds of seeds of *Lathyrus sativus*. *Phytochemistry*. 1964;3:73–78.

17. Rao SLN. Isolation and characterization of β-N-oxalyl-α, β-diaminopropionic acid (ODAP): a neurotoxin from the seeds of *Lathyrus sativus*. *Biochemistry*. 1964;3:432–436.

18. Buzzard EF, Greenfield JG. *Pathology of the Nervous System*. London: Constable; 1921:232.

19. Streifler M, Cohn DF, Hirano A. The central nervous system in a case of neurolathyrism. *Neurology*. 1977;27:1176–1178.

20. Filimonoff IN. Zur pathologisch-anatomischen charakteristik des Lathyrismus. *Z Gesamte Neurol Psychiatr*. 1926;105:75–92.

21. Tekle-Haimanot R, Kidane Y, Wuhib E, et al. Lathyrism in rural central Ethiopia: a highly prevalent neurotoxic disorder. *Int J Epid*. 1990;19:664–672.

22. Gessain A, Gout O. Chronic myelopathy associated with human T-lymphotropic virus type I (HTLV-I). *Ann Intern Med*. 1992;117:933–946.

23. Osame M. HAM/TSP: global review and WHO-diagnostic guidelines. In: Chopra JS, Jagannathan K, Sawhney IMS, eds. *Advances in Neurology*. Amsterdam: Excerpta Medcia; 1990:265–271.

24. Banea M, Poulter N, Rosling H. Shortcuts in cassava processing and risk of dietary cyanide exposure in Zaire. *Food Nutr Bull*. 1992;14:137–143.

25. Ministry of Health Mozambique. Mantakassa: an epidemic of spastic paraparesis associated with chronic cyanide intoxication in a cassava stable area of Mozambique: I. Epidemiology and clinical and laboratory findings in patients. *Bull World Health Organ*. 1984;62:477–484.

26. Ministry of Health Mozambique. Mantakassa: an epidemic of spastic paraparesis associated with chronic cyanide intoxication in a cassava stable area of Mozambique: II. Nutritional factors and hydrocyanic content of cassava products. *Bull World Health Organ*. 1984;62:485–492.

27. Tylleskär T, Banea M, Bikangi N, Fresco L, Persson LA, Rosling H. Epidemiological evidence from Zaire for dietary aetiology of konzo, an upper motor neuron disease. *Bull World Health Organ*. 1991;69:581–590.

28. Tylleskär T, Legue F, Peterson S, Kpizingui E, Stecker P. Konzo in the Central Africa Republic. *Neurology*. 1994;44:959–961.

29. Howlett WP, Brubaker GR, Mlingi N, Rosling H. Konzo: an epidemic upper motor neuron disease studied in Tanzania. *Brain*. 1990;113:223–235.

30. Mlingi N, Poulter N, Rosling H. An outbreak of acute intoxications from consumption of insufficiently processed cassava in Tanzania. *Nutr Res*. 1992;12:677–687.

31. Osuntokun BO. An ataxic neuropathy in Nigeria, a clinical, biological and electrophysiological study. *Brain*. 1968;91:215–248.

32. Osuntokun BO. Cassava diet, chronic cyanide intoxication and neuropathy in Nigerian Africans. *World Rev Nutr Diet*. 1981;36:141–173.

33. Osuntokun BO, Aladetoyinbo A, Bademosi O. Vitamin B nutrition in the Nigerian tropical ataxic neuropathy. *J Neurol Neursurg Psychiatry*. 1985;48:154–156.

CHAPTER 54

The Neurology of Aviation and Space Environments

Michael S. Jaffee

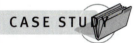

CASE STUDY

A 28-year-old military pilot has a witnessed episode of loss of consciousness in a centrifuge while training to deal with increased G-forces. There are associated myoclonic jerks with this episode. When he loses consciousness, he releases his hand brake, which automatically slows the centrifuge, and he regains consciousness without any prolonged postepisode confusion. Two weeks later, he has a witnessed loss of consciousness when he is out to dinner with his friends. Witnesses describe tonic–clonic jerks and 10 to 15 minutes of confusion following the event. History is consistent with a seizure. Workup reveals normal head magnetic resonance imaging and normal routine and sleep-deprived electroencephalogram. The only provoking factor appears to be some sleep deprivation.

This chapter reviews the pathophysiology of the first event and issues to think about when considering a waiver following the second event. This patient desires to travel to another city to get a second medical opinion. Thus, attention is also given in this chapter to considerations when considering clearance to travel as a passenger on a commercial airline.

INTRODUCTION

Clinical neurology is the study of disease and dysfunction of the nervous system in our normal environment. Our normal environment is considered 1 atmosphere (atm) of pressure and has a gaseous composition of 21% oxygen and 78% nitrogen.

Aerospace neurology focuses on the function of a normal nervous system exposed to environmental conditions other than those encountered in our normal standard conditions. Clinical considerations in these environments include the toxic effects of changes in atmospheric pressure, acceleration, and gravity. These environmental factors enter into considerations of safety when evaluating both aviators and potential passengers with neurological disease. This chapter provides an overview of the environmental factors encountered in aviation and space environments that are most implicated in neurological dysfunction. Following a review of the environmental factors, some consideration is given to neurological evaluation of both aviators and patients who are potential passengers on commercial flights.

ENVIRONMENTAL FACTORS

The aviation and space environments have unique factors related to neurological dysfunction; there also are features shared between the aviation and the underwater environments (Table 1). Environmental factors unique to the aviation environment are hypoxia and acceleration. Common environmental factors that affect the aviation and underwater environments are the effects of pressure and decompression. A unique factor of the underwater environment is the effect of gases at depth, and this is covered in Chapter 51. The distinguishing feature of the space environment is microgravity.

Aviation Environment

There are several environmental factors that affect the nervous system at altitude in the aviation environment. These factors include decreased oxygen, acceleration, mechanical vibration, and effects of motion on the vestibular system.

Hypoxia is considered an oxygen deficiency at the tissue level. This deficiency may be caused by any number of abnormalities that affect uptake, transport, or use of oxygen. The central nervous system (CNS) is thought to be particularly vulnerable to deficiencies in oxygenation. Four types of hypoxia have been recognized: histotoxic, hyperemic, stagnant, and hypoxic.[1]

Table 1: Environmental Factors Related to Neurological Dysfunction

Factor	Environment		
	Aviation	Underwater	Space
Hypoxia (gas at decreased pressure)	x		
Acceleration	x		
Pressure changes (gradual)	x	x	
Decompression (rapid change)	x	x	
Gases at depth (gases at increased pressure)		x	
Microgravity			x

Histotoxic hypoxia results from the inability of a cell to use delivered oxygen. This condition is usually due to dysfunction or the cytochrome oxidase system such as from the toxin cyanide. Hyperemic hypoxia is a decrease in oxygen use due to a reduction in oxygen-carrying capacity such as in anemia. Carbon monoxide poisoning causes this form of hypoxia due to its competitive blockade or hemoglobin oxygen-binding sites and by shifting the oxygen dissociation curve to the left, making it more difficult to release peripheral oxygen to tissues. Stagnant hypoxia is decreased oxygen use due to inadequate blood flow systemically or locally. In normal environments, this type of hypoxia would be seen in clinical settings of shock. In the aviation environment, stagnant hypoxia can be a result of pooled blood from acceleration forces or seen as a complication of decompression sickness (DCS).

Hypoxic hypoxia, the most common cause or hypoxia clinically and in the aviation environment, is a deficiency in alveolar oxygenation. In the normal clinical setting, this condition is most commonly due to a ventilation–perfusion mismatch. With increasing altitude, there are associated decreases in both air pressure and air density. With the decrease in pressure, there are associated decreases in partial pressures or the gases of the environment. At any altitude, the ratio or the gaseous components of air remains the same: 78% nitrogen and 21% oxygen. The total amount of oxygen we breathe is determined by the partial pressure of oxygen. Because the partial pressure of oxygen decreases with increasing altitude, the body and nervous system have less total oxygen available, which creates a risk of complications of decreased oxygen (hypoxia).

In general, hypoxic hypoxia from altitude becomes clinically important whenever a human exceeds 10,000 feet in altitude. The CNS is usually the most sensitive organ to hypoxia and the first to manifest symptoms. Symptoms may include visual changes such as tunnel vision or blurred vision, fatigue, drowsiness, and headache. Clinical signs include confusion, behavioral changes, loss of coordination, and eventually, unconsciousness. An important consideration in aviation is the effect that hypoxia has on performance. Many studies have documented the decreased effective performance time of individuals exposed to hypoxic conditions. The onset of these symptoms is often so gradual and subtle that aviators may not recognize their own decrease in cognitive performance. To enable pilots to understand their own signs and symptoms of hypoxia, they are exposed to an altitude chamber and the condition of hypoxia during their training. This contingency must be considered because there is always a risk of mechanical failure at altitude.[2]

"Time of useful consciousness" is the time from first exposure to an environment of decreased oxygen to when useful function is lost. It is not the time to unconsciousness but is the time until the individual is incapable of taking proper corrective action. Time of useful consciousness becomes shorter with exertion and with increasing altitudes.[1]

Treatment of hypoxic hypoxia is administration of 100% oxygen. If an oxygen system was already being used at the onset of symptoms, then a different source of oxygen should be used or the concentration should be increased. If the altitude is greater than 40,000 feet, then the oxygen must be administered under pressure. If the hypoxia cannot successfully be managed, then the aircraft should descend to an altitude below 10,000 feet. Recovery of hypoxia symptoms is usually immediate with proper oxygenation, but symptoms such as headache and fatigue can persist.[2]

Pressurized cabins are used on many aircraft to prevent hypoxia and the need for oxygen supplementation. Commercial flights often fly at an altitude of approximately 40,000 feet, with the aircraft cabins usually pressurized to between 5000 and 7000 feet. Military cabins that are pressurized are usually maintained at 8000 feet. Pressurization to sea level is not cost effective. Pressurization is achieved by drawing in external air and delivering it, compressed, to the cabin. The outflow is controlled to maintain a positive ambient pressure.[3]

Acceleration

Acceleration is the rate of change of velocity with time and occurs when the speed, direction of motion, or both of a body alters.[4] Physiological responses to acceleration are determined by its magnitude and by the duration and direction of its action. The magnitude is measured in multiples of the acceleration due to gravity (g).[5] Duration is classified as being long or short, the time division between the two being arbitrarily set at 1 second.[3] The direction is defined by a system of anatomical axes. Pilots of civilian and military aircraft are exposed to $+gz$ at all times during G-force maneuvers because they sit upright in the flight deck. This notation refers to acceleration forces going from head to toe ("eyeballs down").[5]

The primary acute limitation to exposure to 1gz is the response of the CNS. The main symptoms are loss of vision and loss of consciousness due to decreased perfusion to the retina and brain as blood is forced toward the feet and away from the brain. The first vision lost is peripheral; it is followed by central vision, leading to a visual blackout. This is usually prelude to G-force-induced loss of consciousness (GLOC).[4]

Autoregulation controls cerebral blood flow during normal conditions. During G-force, flow is maintained by a combination of autoregulation and the siphon effect. A pressure gradient is established between the afferent carotid arterial system and the efferent jugular venous system. This pressure differential is able to maintain cerebral blood flow with very low cerebral perfusion pressures by way of the siphon effect. Blood flow to the cerebellum and brainstem are maintained even when flow is diminished to higher cerebral centers.[5]

GLOC results when blood flow to the nervous system is reduced below the critical level necessary to support conscious function. This result is a normal response to transient G-force-induced CNS ischemia. On average, there is a total time of 15 seconds of unconsciousness, followed by a period of confusion and disorientation of 12 to 15 seconds.[6] Surveys by the U.S. Air Force and the U.S. Navy indicate that the pilot population of the fighter airframes report about a 12% to 14% incidence of GLOC.[7]

Myoclonic jerks are often seen in association with GLOC. Centrifuge observational studies suggest that they occur in 70% of cases of GLOC. Research using electroencephalogram recordings demonstrates that during GLOC, δ-activity but not epileptiform activity has been observed, even when GLOC is associated with myoclonic jerks.[4]

Pressure

Human tissue is mostly composed of incompressible fluid. The gas-filled spaces of the body such as the lungs, sinuses, middle ear, and intestines are vulnerable to changes in pressure that can occur during ascent or descent. These gas-filled spaces of the body are governed by the gas laws: Boyle's, Dalton's, and Henry's.[8]

Various forms of barotrauma occur with tissue damage when a gas-filled body space fails to equalize its internal pressure to accommodate changes in ambient pressure. These forms are governed primarily by Boyle's law, which states that at a constant temperature the volume of a gas varies inversely with the applied pressure. Therefore, as pressure increases, volume decreases; conversely, when pressure decreases, volume expands.[8,9] There is a common pathophysiology to these "squeezes": engorgement of the mucosal lining, swelling, fluid buildup, and finally, hemorrhage into the space.[3]

Problems When Going from Higher to Lower Pressure (Increasing Altitude in Aviation and Ascent to Water Surface When Diving)

Middle ear—Middle ear barotrauma is one of the most common injuries. These symptoms are prevented by repeated maneuvers such as the valsalva or Frenzel maneuver that force exhalation against a pinched nose to keep the eustachian tube open, which allows pressure equalization of the middle ear.[10]

Sinus block—On occasion, a branch of a cranial nerve can be affected. Maxillary sinus barotraumas of ascent have been associated with compression of the infraorbital branch of the trigeminal nerve, causing facial numbness.[8]

Inner ear squeeze—Tinnitus, vertigo, and decreased hearing are the typical symptoms of increased pressure affecting the inner ear (otic barotraumas). These symptoms may be indistinguishable from inner ear DCS, but the timing of symptoms and flight or dive profile may help clarify.

External ear squeeze—External ear pain can be associated with increasing pressures.

Problems When Going from Lower to Higher Pressure (Decreasing Altitude in Aviation and Diving Deeper Underwater)

Barodontalgia—Pain in a tooth can be a cause of facial pain. This pain is due to irritation of circulation in an already diseased pulp or to an increase in pressure in the air space behind a filling or deposit of caries.[3]

Alternoharic vertigo—The alternoharic form of vertigo arises when there is a sudden and unilateral pressure difference between the inner and the middle ears. It usually arises after attempts are made at equalization with the Valsalva maneuver.[10]

Pulmonary embolism and its sequelae, including cerebral air embolism—Lungs expand in response to increased pressure, and when unable to vent, the pressure may be high enough to rupture alveoli and release air into the interstitial space. This air can go into one of four places: the mediastinum, the subcutaneous tissue, the pleura of the lungs (pneumothorax), or the pulmonary veins through which the air bubbles can travel to the arterial circulation and cause an arterial gas embolism (AGE) that affects the cerebral or cardiac vasculature. An AGE that affects the cardiac vessels is known as AGE type I and accounts for 5% of cases. AGE accounts for 40% of the caseload at active emergent dive centers in the United States. An AGE that affects the cerebral vasculature is known as AGE type II and accounts for 95% of cases. The differential diagnosis of cerebral AGE is DCS, and the treatment is the same: hyperbaric recompression.[8,11,12]

"Reverse" ear squeeze—In severe cases, the increase in middle ear pressure can cause reversible weakness of the facial nerve and Bell's palsy.[11]

Expansion of gas in the intestine—Intestinal gas expansion can cause abdominal discomfort and increased flatulence.

Decompression Sickness

DCS is a result of the release of inert gas bubbles into the bloodstream and tissues after a reduction in ambient pressure. The bubbles causing DCS are usually formed of nitrogen. When in an environment of increased pressure such as at altitude with aviation or diving at depth, the partial pressures of gases in a breathing mixture increase in proportion to the increase in ambient pressure

in accordance with Dalton's law, which states that the total pressure equals the sum of partial pressures of each gas in the mixture. Oxygen is actively metabolized; however, nitrogen is inert and becomes dissolved until saturation. Henry's law relates this saturation to ambient pressure by stating that at a constant temperature the amount of a given gas that will dissolve in a liquid is directly proportional to the partial pressure of that gas in contact with the liquid. During decompression, the increased level of nitrogen equilibrates by diffusing out of body tissues. The amount of dissolved nitrogen exceeds the body's ability to offload the nitrogen, and the nitrogen comes out of solution as bubbles and enters the bloodstream and tissues.[8,13]

Many factors affect nitrogen bubble formation. For aviation-related DCS, these factors include higher altitude (most commonly cited minimum altitude is 25,000 feet), time at altitude, faster rate of ascent, and exercise during altitude. Factors that increase the risk of DCS in both aviation and diving environments include recent injury, age greater than 40 years, gender (women have a three to four times greater risk), and presence of a patent foramen ovale.[14]

DCS symptoms have been classically grouped into type I and type II. Type I DCS includes joint pain and symptoms involving the skin and lymphatics. Type II DCS comprises serious symptoms or signs involving the nervous system (central or peripheral) or the cardiorespiratory system. Type II DCS usually requires rapid treatment.[8]

The nitrogen bubbles cause neurological dysfunction by mechanical effects that include nerve compression, vascular stenosis, or obstruction leading to distal ischemia. There are blood–bubble interface effects that include activation of inflammatory pathways and platelet aggregation produced by venous bubbles, with a release of vasoactive substances causing vasoconstriction.[14]

Cerebral DCS most often involves the arterial circulation, whereas spinal cord DCS involves obstruction of venous drainage and the formation of bubbles within the parenchyma of the spinal cord.[8]

Inner ear DCS presents with acute vertigo, nausea, emesis, nystagmus, and tinnitus. Spinal cord DCS usually presents with a partial myelopathy that localizes to the thoracic cord. Pathological features within the cord include hemorrhagic infarcts, edema, bubble defects, axonal degeneration, and demyelination.[13]

Cerebral DCS can present with an alteration in consciousness, weakness, headache, gait disturbance, fatigue, diplopia, or visual loss. The examination may show focal signs such as hemiparesis, aphasia, gait ataxia, or hemianopsia. The pathological features of cerebral DCS are similar to those of spinal DCS, although usually not as pronounced. In addition, hyalinized vessels and lacune formation have been noted.[8]

The diagnosis of neurological DCS is primarily clinical. Magnetic resonance imaging demonstrates abnormalities only 30% to 55% of the time. These abnormalities are best seen on T_2-weighted images showing high-signal lesions suggestive of ischemia, edema, and swelling. These lesions do not enhance with contrast.[8]

Initial management consists of basic and advanced cardiac life support, 100% oxygen, hydration, and transport to a hyperbaric recompression facility. The definitive treatment is hyperbaric therapy using the U.S. Navy protocol. This consists of initial recompression to 60 feet with 100% oxygen for 60 minutes. The patient is then decompressed to 30 feet for two additional periods each of breathing pure oxygen and air. Hyperbaric recompression therapy reduces bubble size and increases the nitrogen gradient to expedite off-gassing. Most cases of neurological DCS that receive prompt recompression therapy have a good recovery.[13]

Differences between hypobaric (altitude) and hyperbaric (diving) DCS according to Stepanek[14] include (1) smaller nitrogen load with altitude exposure; (2) different bubble dynamics (slower release of bubbles with altitude exposure, even with the same pressure differential); (3) generally less severe symptomatology with altitude exposure; (4) different spectrum of clinical manifestations, even though there is significant overlap (altitude: cerebral > spinal; diving: spinal > cerebral); (5) inherent recompression with altitude exposure; and (6) gas density and composition (bigger role for water vapor, oxygen, and carbon dioxide at altitude).

Space Neurology

The main aspects of the space environment that affect the nervous system are microgravity and various space hygiene issues (e.g., radiation, toxicology, and life support).[19] Gravity provides the CNS with a fundamental reference for estimating spatial orientation and coordinating movements in the terrestrial environment. Key developmental processes in mammals (e.g., locomotion) require gravity stimuli.[20]

Microgravity affects many systems of the body. Changes include redistribution of fluid and electrolytes, cardiac deconditioning, red blood cell alterations, immune system dysfunction, skeletal muscle atrophy, bone demineralization, and gastrointestinal tract adaptations. The effects most relevant to neurology are the associated neurovestibular disturbances.[21]

Neurovestibular Factors

There are two main varieties of neurovestibular adaptation. The first includes vestibular reflex phenomena such as postural and movement illusions, sensations of rotation, nystagmus, vertigo, and dizziness.[20]

The second form of neurovestibular adaptation is space motion sickness (SMS). SMS is due to the neurovestibular adaptation to microgravity. Symptoms that are similar to motion sickness include malaise, loss of appetite, and somnolence. There are differences between SMS and motion sickness, especially with autonomic symptoms. In SMS, there is rarely sweating, nausea, or pallor. Vomiting is usually episodic, sudden, and brief.[21]

Onset of SMS ranges from minutes to hours after entering the microgravity environment and then usually resolves within 48 and 72 hours. There are two theories regarding the etiology of SMS. One is the fluid shift theory, in which SMS is caused by biochemical and biomechanical effects on the vestibular receptors. The prevailing theory involves sensory conflict that is a result of an adaptive increase in otolith crystals and an increase in hair cells and synapses.[22] There is no correlation between SMS and prior motion sickness in astronauts.

Early literature quoted the incidence of SMS as being 40% to 50%. A more recent study reported that the incidence of SMS during a first shuttle flight was 67%.[23] Antiemetic injections have been the treatment of choice and are thought to produce a 50% reduction in symptoms. Future pharmacological interventions may include anticonvulsants, CNS stimulants such as modafinil, 5-hydroxytryptamine (5-HT$_3$) agonists, and calcium channel blockers.

Just as adaptation occurs when going from 1 g to a microgravity environment, there is more adaptation required when astronauts return to Earth. This process involves going from a microgravity environment to being exposed to high G-forces during reentry and then a 1-g environment. Symptoms include ataxia and decreased coordination.[24] These symptoms are thought to be due to changes in Purkinje cell morphology.[25]

In addition, there have been reports of flashbacks of the vestibular symptoms experienced after return to Earth. These episodes have varied from 4 days to 2 months later.[20]

Decompression Risks in Space

Decompression is primarily a risk to astronauts during extravehicular activities. The typical extravehicular mobility unit (or space suit) is pressurized to less than 30% of the spacecraft to facilitate mobility without significant decompressive effects. There is also a risk during launch and reentry.[26] The 1971 Soyuz 11 accident attributed the deaths of all three crewmembers to decompression that occurred due to a faulty pressure equalization valve during reentry.

Other Neurology Issues of Space

The most common neurological symptom reported by astronauts is headache, which has been reported by 67% of astronauts. Other neurological consequences include impaired cognitive performance (i.e., "space dementia") and impaired autonomic function. Neurological complaints account for the most common reasons for taking medications in space. These reasons are SMS (30%), headache (20%), sleeplessness (15%), back pain (10%), and constipation (<10%).[21]

Back pain has been a chronic complaint of many astronauts. Although dull and localized to the low back, it is thought to have a different pathophysiology than the common back pain seen at 1 g. Back pain in microgravity is thought to be due to stretching of the anterior and posterior spinous ligaments, which results in approximately 7 cm of increased height at 0 g.[27]

AVIATOR WAIVERS

The military and the Federal Aviation Administration (FAA) both stratify their medical certifications into three categories.

FAA categories include the following:

- Class 1 certificates are required of pilots of commercial airliners and are only valid for a 6-month period.
- Class 2 certificates are for commercial, nonairline duties such as charter and corporate pilots. The certificate is valid for 1 year of commercial duties.
- Class 3 certificates are for private pilot duties and are valid for 3 years if the pilot is under the age of 40 and 2 years for those 40 years and older.[23]

Military examinations include the following:

- Class I qualifies for selection into flight training.
- Class II qualifies flight-training students and rated officers for continued flying duties. This includes qualifying physician applicants for flight surgeon training.
- Class III qualifies individuals for nonrated duties such as flight crew.[24]

Aerospace consultants are often required to evaluate aviators or astronauts who have a neurological problem to determine whether they should be granted a waiver. In general, these considerations include course of the disorder (static, progressive, or paroxysmal), potential for sudden incapacitation that may compromise safety, predictability of course of the disorder, ability to monitor disease, and potential adverse effects of medications. Consideration of waivers for military and civilian pilots and astronauts who have neurological conditions can sometimes be clinically challenging. The decision is made based on a risk estimate, keeping in mind that an aviator who is in control of an aircraft may have a medical incident that could lead to an adverse outcome not only for the aviator but also for other individuals who may be passengers, crew, or part of unanticipated collateral damage in the event of a mishap.

In the U.S. Air Force, the following criteria must be met for any waiver:

1. Not pose a risk of sudden incapacitation
2. Pose minimal potential for subtle performance decrement, particularly with regard to the higher senses
3. Be resolved or be stable and be expected to remain so under the stresses of the aviation environment
4. If the possibility of progression or recurrence exists, the first symptoms or signs must be easily detectable and not pose a risk to the individual or the safety of others
5. Cannot require exotic tests, regular invasive procedures, or frequent absences to monitor for stability or progression
6. Must be compatible with the performance of sustained flying operations in austere environments[25]

Because of the risks, the medical standards for aviators are often higher than those used for continued service for a nonaviator. Each branch of the military has its own published aeromedical standards and guidelines; each branch also has its own system for consideration of waivers. In general, there are two kinds of waiver considerations. One is for initial flying clearance before training. Considerations include cost of training and avoiding early withdrawal, as well as consideration of ability to serve a normal duration for career. The other type of waiver consideration occurs for aviators who were already trained and qualified before they developed their neurological condition. Considerations include training costs and experience already gained. In other words, these are aviators who had been qualified based on a Flying Class II examination. Several subcategories can be applied for those who qualify for a waiver. These include the following:

- Flying Class IIA qualifies rated officers for duty in low-G aircraft (tanker, transport, bomber)
- Flying Class IIB qualifies rated officers for duty in nonejection seat aircraft
- Flying Class IIC qualifies rated officers for aviation duty as specified with any special remarks[27]

Some challenging conditions include evaluation of aviators with headaches, traumatic brain injury, and herniated disks.

Civilian aviators have their medical clearances provided by certified FAA medical examiners. These decisions are guided by Title 14 of the Code of Federal Regulations, Part 67.[23] To maintain an FAA medical certificate, there can be no established history or diagnosis of the following:

1. Epilepsy (Of note: 10 years must pass from a single seizure, and risk factors must also be taken into consideration.)
2. A disturbance of consciousness without satisfactory medical explanation of the cause
3. A transient loss of control of nervous system function without satisfactory medical explanation of the cause
4. No other seizure disorder or neurological condition that the federal air surgeon, based on the case history and appropriate qualified medical judgment, finds that the person is unable to safely perform the duties of a class 1 pilot[23]

PATIENTS WITH NEUROLOGICAL CONDITIONS

One challenge often faced by the clinician is the patient who is being managed for a neurological condition and desires clearance to fly on a commercial aircraft. According to a 2002 review analyzing 2042 medical incidents, neurological conditions were the No. 1 category for passenger in-flight incidents on commercial airline flights, accounting for 31% of all incidents.[28] The overall likelihood of a serious incident in flight is quite low; only 0.01% of all flights are affected. These in-flight neurological incidents included dizziness or vertigo, which accounted for the highest number, followed by seizure, headache, and cerebrovascular symptoms. Contributing factors included cabin pressurization, turbulence, and hypoxemia. Cabin pressurization on commercial flights is roughly equivalent to 6000 to 8000 feet above sea level, which results in a lower alveolar oxygenation level of 59 to 76.8 mm Hg.[29]

Of those incidents that required the pilot to divert, neurological conditions were second, accounting for 34% of medical diversions. (Cardiovascular conditions accounted for 35% of medical diversions.)[26] There were no in-flight neurological incidents that resulted in death. These results have been further supported by other studies and findings to include a report from the FAA's Civil Aeromedical Institute.[30]

The most common neurological symptoms resulting in diversion include seizures and dizziness or vertigo. The overall likelihood of diversion for an in-flight neurological problem was 17%. However, the likelihood of diversion was highest for loss of consciousness or syncope (71%), non-alcohol-induced confusion (66%), cerebrovascular symptoms (23.8%), and seizures (23.6%).[26] The main rationale for the diversions that were done in

context of loss of consciousness/syncope was the flight crew concern that there was a serious medical emergency requiring immediate attention. Although most cases of dizziness/vertigo did not result in diversion, the cases that did were because the flight crew thought that a loss of consciousness was imminent.[26]

There are currently no official American Academy of Neurology guidelines regarding clearing neurology patients for commercial air travel. The commercial airlines have their own recommended guidelines. The main reference to neurological conditions in these guidelines includes stating that having had a stroke or neurosurgical procedure within prior 2 weeks of flight is considered a relative contraindication. Additional medical counseling that can be provided to neurological patients includes suggesting that patients with chronic neurological conditions avoid alcoholic beverages and adhere to medication compliance. For pain conditions and chronic headache syndromes, carrying additional abortive analgesic medications would be advised. Seizure disorder patients can be advised to carry additional dosages of their antiepileptic drugs. Careful consideration should be given to the timing of medication changes, perhaps waiting until after travel so as to avoid potential complications.[31]

CONCLUSION

Aspects of different environments can have adverse effects on normal, healthy nervous systems. A background in the toxic effects of an abnormal environment on the nervous system can be used to make better clinical judgments when considering effects of exposing someone with an abnormal nervous system to such environmental stressors.

REFERENCES

1. Fisher P. High altitude respiratory physiology. In: O'Brien D, ed. USAF Flight Surgeons Guide. 4th ed. San Antonio: USAF School of Aerospace Medicine; 1996.
2. Pickard J. Atmosphere and respiration. In: DeHart R, Davis J, ed. Fundamentals of Aerospace Medicine. 3rd ed. Philadelphia: Lippincott Williams & Wilkins; 2002:19–38.
3. Harding R, Mills J. Aviation medicine. BMJ. 1988;2:30–43.
4. Burton R, Whinnery J. Biodynamics. In: DeHart R, Davis J, ed. Fundamentals of Aerospace Medicine. 3rd ed. Philadelphia: Lippincott Williams & Wilkins; 2002:122–153.
5. Eldridge L, Northrup S. Effects of acceleration. In: O'Brien D, ed. USAF Flight Surgeons Guide. 4th ed. San Antonio: USAF School of Aerospace Medicine; 1996.
6. Whinnery J, Whinnery A. Acceleration-induced loss of consciousness. Arch Neurol. 1990;47:764–776.
7. Morrissette K, McGowan D. Further support for the concept of an GLOC syndrome: a survey of military high-performance aviators. Aviat Space Environ Med. 2000;71:496–499.

8. Newton H. Neurological complications of scuba diving. *Am Fam Physician*. 2001;63:2211–2218.

9. Pennefather J. Physics and physiology. In: Edmond C, Lowry C, Pennefather J, et al., ed. *Diving and Subaquatic Medicine*. 4th ed. London: Arnold; 2002:11–22.

10. Martin L. *Scuba Diving Explained: Questions and Answers on Physiology and Medical Aspects*. Flagstaff, Ariz: Best Publishing; 1997.

11. Dick APK, Massey EW. Neurologic presentation of decompression sickness and air embolism in sport divers. *Neurology*. 1985;35:667–671.

12. Walker R. Pulmonary barotraumas. In: Edmonds C, Lowry C, Pennefather J, et al., ed. *Diving and Subaquatic Medicine*. 4th ed. London: Arnold; 2002:137–150.

13. Rudge F, Zwart B. Effects of decreased pressure: decompression sickness. In: O'Brien D, ed. *USAF Flight Surgeons Guide*. 4th ed. San Antonio: USAF School of Aerospace Medicine; 1996.

14. Stepanek J. Decompression sickness. In: DeHart R, Davis J, ed. *Fundamentals of Aerospace Medicine*. 3rd ed. Philadelphia: Lippincott Williams & Wilkins; 2002:67–98.

15. Locke J. Space environments. In: DeHart R, Davis J, ed. *Fundamentals of Aerospace Medicine*. 3rd ed. Philadelphia: Lippincott Williams & Wilkins; 2002:245–270.

16. Clark J. Neurological effects of space flight: adaptation, maladaptation, and readaptation. Presented at the 2004 Aerospace Medicine in Space Operations Course at USAF School of Aerospace Medicine, San Antonio.

17. Martin G. Space medicine. In: O'Brien D, ed. *USAF Flight Surgeons Guide*. 4th ed. San Antonio: USAF School of Aerospace Medicine; 1996.

18. Deleted in proof.

19. Davis J, Vanderploeg JM, Santy PA, et al. Space motion sickness during 24 flights of the space shuttle. *Aviat Space Environ Med*. 1988;59:1185–1189.

20. Paloski WH, Black FO, Reschke MF, et al. Vestibular ataxia following shuttle flights: effects of microgravity on otolith-mediated sensorimotor control of posture. *Am J Otol*. 1993;14:9–17.

21. Newberg A. Changes in the central nervous system and their clinical correlates during long-term spaceflight. *Aviat Space Environ Med*. 1994;65:562–572.

22. Wing PC, Tsang IK, Susak L, et al. Back pain and spinal changes in microgravity. *Orthop Clin North Am*. 1991;22:255–262.

23. Federal Aviation Administration. Federal Aviation Regulations. Title 14: Code of Federal Regulations. Part 67: Medical Standards and Certification. Springfield, Va: National Technical information Service; August 1996.

24. Air Force Flight Surgeons Guide.

25. Air Force Instruction 48-123. Air Force Electronic Publishing Library. Accessed June 5, 2006.

26. Conkin, J. Evidence-based Approach to the Analysis of Serious Decompression Sickness with Application to EVA Astronauts. NASA Technical Report 210196. Houston, TX, NASA; 2001.

27. Yoho, R. Air Force Medical Standard. Aerospace Medicine Primary Course. Brooks City-Base, San Antonio: USAF School of Aerospace Medicine.

28. Sirven J, Claypool DW, Sahs KL, et al. Is there a neurologist on this flight? *Neurology*. 2002;58:1739–1744.

29. AMA Commission on Emergency Medical Services. Medical aspects of transportation aboard commercial aircraft. *JAMA*. 1982;247(7):1007–1011.

30. Federal Aviation Administration. In-flight Medical Care: An Update. Publication DOT/FAA/AM-97/2. Springfield, Va: National Technical Information Service; 1997.

31. Sirven, J. Syllabus to "Can I Fly?" Course presented at American Academy of Neurology Annual Meeting. Spring 2007, Boston.

SECTION 6

NEUROLOGICAL WEAPONS AND WARFARE

CONTENTS

CHAPTER 55

Neurobiological Weapons

Peter J. Osterbauer and Michael R. Dobbs

INTRODUCTION

Biological warfare has been employed since ancient times[1–5] and continues to be a threat today. Biological weapons can be highly potent, relatively simple to acquire or produce, challenging to detect before exacting a significant toll, and stable under extreme conditions.[6–8] Technological advances enabling the addition of virulence factors and treatment-resistant mechanisms by means of genetic manipulation pose an additional focus of concern.[9,10] Much has been written on the various aspects of biological warfare and its implications for public health and safety. The purpose of this chapter is to provide a comprehensive summary of the most significant biological agents from a neurological perspective.

Various methods exist for the deployment of such agents (Figure 55-1), and there are many potential routes of infection (Table 1). Release of microscopic infectious particles in aerosol form is perhaps the most likely route for most organisms (Figure 55-2).[7] This is an attractive option because it can be accomplished using simple, inexpensive technology, such as standard spraying devices available in the garden section of any store.[7,11] Depending on weather conditions, the infective particles may remain suspended in the air for several hours, thereby increasing their infective capability (Figure 55-3).[11]

Some believe that contamination of food and water supplies would be the easiest manner of biological attack.[12] Others argue that, in most cases, the amount of agent necessary to make a significant impact renders this form of deployment impractical.[7,13]

Dissemination using bombs or missiles is another option; however, the effectiveness of this method is limited for several reasons. With such a method, much of the agent is driven into the ground on impact and much is destroyed by the ensuing explosion. Of the portion that is deployed, particle size can vary widely, and disbursement can be limited and unpredictable.[7,17]

This chapter represents a revision and update of previously published material (Neurobiological weapons. *Neurol Clin.* 2005;23[2]:599–621). This material appears courtesy of the permission of the editor, Michael R. Dobbs, MD.

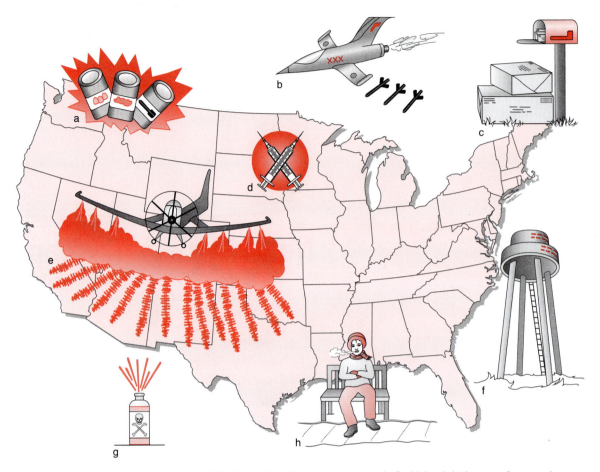

Figure 55-1. There are many ways to deploy biological and toxic weapons, several of which might be easy for terrorists to accomplish: *(A)* contamination of food supplies; *(B)* bombs or missiles; *(C)* contamination of mail items; *(D)* direct injection; *(E)* spraying of aerosolized toxin; *(F)* contamination of water supplies; *(G)* setting off small canisters of aerosolized toxin; and *(H)* infiltration of contagious people. (Osterbauer PJ, Dobbs MR. Neurobiological weapons. *Neurol Clin.* 2005;23:599–621.)

Recognition of a biological attack is crucial for beginning effective treatment of exposed victims and to prevent further affliction. This can be difficult, however, because the signs and symptoms caused by such agents often are nonspecific and can be confused easily with those of many common illnesses.[1,11] The fundamental concept in differentiating a naturally occurring epidemic from the intentional release of a biological agent lies in recognition of epidemiological patterns.[15,16] Clues suggesting a biological attack include peculiar clustering of illness[17]; unusual age distribution of seemingly common illnesses, such as a chickenpox-like outbreak in adults[17]; a rapid, rather than gradual, rise in incidence of a suspicious illness[11]; or an increased incidence in illness and death in pets or other animals.[18] Maintaining a high level of suspicion is mandatory.[19]

Treatment of illness resulting from a biological attack involves stabilization and supportive care, although more specific treatments are available in some instances. Prevention of illness sometimes can be achieved by active immunization; vaccines are available for prophylaxis against some of the more likely agents.[20–22] This, however, is not always possible or practical. Passive immunization of exposed individuals is another viable treatment option, offering the advantages of low toxicity and high specificity.[23] Antibiotics and antiviral agents also are effective in some cases. Various other novel treatment options are under investigation, such as high-affinity toxin antagonists,[24] topical application of organism-specific lytic enzymes to contaminated mucous membranes,[25] and development of generic treatments based on common pathways shared by several agents.[26]

ANTHRAX

General Characteristics

A well-known disease of herbivorous animals, anthrax is considered by many to be an ideal biological weapon. Historically, it probably dates back to the time of the

Table 1:   Potential Routes of Infection

Biological Agent	Inhalation	Ingestion	Direct Contact	Person to Person	Other
Botulism	+	+	+	−	
VEEV	+	+	+	−	+[a]
Anthrax	+	+	+	+	
Smallpox	+	−	+	+	
Anatoxin-a	−	+	+	−	
Mycotoxin	+	+	+	+[b]	
Ricin	+	+	−	−	+[c]
Tetrodotoxin	−	+	+	−	
Saxitoxin	−	+	+	−	
Q fever	+	−	−	−	
Tularemia	+	+	+	−	+[d]

*A negative indicator does not suggest that the agent cannot be transmitted in the manner indicated, only that it is less likely.

[a]Can be transmitted by a mosquito vector.

[b]Can be by direct contact.

[c]Transmissible by injection.

[d]Can be transmitted by the bite of an infected animal or insect.

VEEV, Venezuelan equine encephalitis virus.

Osterbauer PJ, Dobbs MR. Neurobiological weapons. *Neurol Clin.* 2005;23:599–621.

biblical plagues of ancient Egypt.[27–31] Anthrax also holds a distinguished position in medical history as the prototype disease for Koch's postulate and the target of the first vaccine developed by Pasteur that contained attenuated live organisms.[32] The largest documented outbreak of human infection occurred in 1979 near a Soviet military microbiology facility in Sverdlovsk.[29,32] Deliberate release of anthrax spores in October and November 2002 led to 18 confirmed, and 4 suspected, cases of the disease in the United States.[29,31–33]

Clinical anthrax is acquired by infection with spores of the gram-positive organism, *Bacillus anthracis*. The anthrax spores are hearty and can survive in severe environmental conditions for years or even decades,[8,19,25,30,31] making *B. anthracis* the most environmentally hardy known biological warfare agent.[28] The spores are simple and inexpensive to produce, can be stored almost indefinitely, are highly infective, and carry a morbidity rate of 65% to 80% if treatment is not initiated promptly.[8] It is estimated that the controlled, uniform release of 50 kg

of aerosolized *B. anthracis* over a population of 5 million would produce approximately 100,000 deaths.[34]

Although heat resistant, the spores can be inactivated in water if maintained at a temperature of 95°C for 25 minutes. They can also be removed by various methods of filtration, provided the filtration pores are smaller than 1 μm. Formaldehyde, sodium hypochlorite, free chlorine solution (10,000 mg/L), autoclaving, ethylene oxide, hydrogen peroxide, ultraviolet irradiation, boiling, and 2% glutaraldehyde are all effective means of destroying the spores on contaminated surfaces.[19,28] Thorough decontamination of all exposed areas is critical for the prevention of secondary aerosolization and further spread of disease.

Potential Methods of Deployment

Weaponized anthrax can be produced as an insoluble, liquid slurry or as a dry powder.[8] The former is easier to manufacture; however, it is not as stable as the dry form

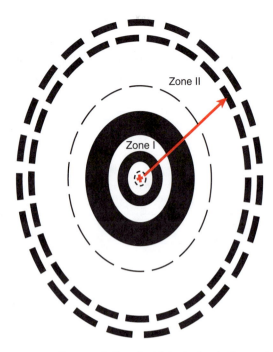

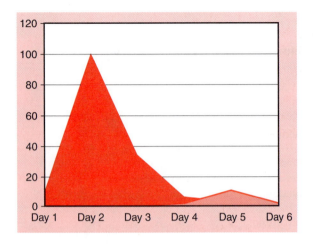

Figure 55-3. A typical epidemic curve for a point-source outbreak, as is usual for Venezuelan equine encephalitis. The flulike cases *(black)* are followed days later by a few cases of fulminant encephalitis. (Osterbauer PJ, Dobbs MR. Neurobiological weapons. *Neurol Clin.* 2005;23:599–621.)

Figure 55-2. Characteristics of a biological or toxic agent cloud released from a single point source (X). The cloud is seen in black. The arrow emphasizes movement outward over time from the point of release. Direction of movement and time to dispersal depend on wind conditions. In zone I, for the first few hours, the cloud remains intact. The cloud grows in width and length over time until it begins to break up in zone II. (Osterbauer PJ, Dobbs MR. Neurobiological weapons. *Neurol Clin.* 2005;23:599–621.)

and is more difficult to disburse effectively.[8] The dry form requires fine milling to a state that the powder is easily and rapidly dispersed through the air. The most likely method of deployment is via aerosolization of dry spores.[8,27,29,35] This form of deployment carries the additional risk of secondary aerosolization if the infected area is not decontaminated properly, resulting in a sustained risk of exposure.[25,35]

Ingestion of spore-contaminated water is known to cause infection in animals. A similar susceptibility in humans can be inferred, and it is known that human ingestion of spore-contaminated foods results in illness.[19,36] Contamination of food and water supplies, therefore, is within the realm of possibility[19,36]; however, colonies are only thought to remain viable in water for 24 hours.[29]

Clinical Aspects

Infection is accomplished by ingestion, inhalation, or absorption of the spores through mucous membranes and breaks in skin. Three main forms of illness, therefore, are emphasized: pulmonary, cutaneous, and gastrointestinal.[25,27,29,31] Inhaled spores are transported to

pulmonary lymph nodes by alveolar macrophages. Subsequent germination within the lymph nodes leads to a massive release of bacteria and toxins into the bloodstream.[29,30] Germination typically occurs within 2 to 5 days but may require as long as 60 days in some cases.[29]

Serious neurological manifestations, such as headaches, mental status changes, impaired visual acuity, and visual field defects can occur, regardless of the manner in which the disease is acquired.[25] The most deadly neurological manifestation is hemorrhagic meningitis, which can disseminate from the pulmonary (or other) forms of the disease and has a mortality of nearly 100%.[29] Cerebrospinal fluid in such cases reveals an elevated leukocyte count, which can be greater than 500/mL; elevated protein, which can be greater than 0.4 g/dL; and typically an elevated erythrocyte count.[25,29] Gram stain and culture are usually positive as well for gram-positive bacilli.[29] Contrast-enhanced computerized tomography of the brain would be expected to show diffuse leptomeningeal enhancement, as well as intracerebral and subarachnoid hemorrhages.[29]

Mortality rates of up to 20% for the cutaneous form, 60% to 80% for the gastrointestinal form, and 90% to 99% for the pulmonary form make prompt treatment essential.[29,30] The recommended antibiotic regimen for pulmonary anthrax is ciprofloxacin or doxycycline, plus clindamycin and rifampin.[37] Doxycycline and clindamycin exhibit poor cerebrospinal fluid penetration; therefore, the addition of rifampin is crucial for the prevention and treatment of neurological manifestations.[25,37]

In the case of a biological attack, resistance to penicillins and tetracyclines should be assumed until proven otherwise by susceptibility testing.[35] *B. anthracis* may produce cephalosporinase, rendering treatment with cephalosporins ineffective.[29] Empirical postexposure prophylaxis with ciprofloxacin or doxycycline is recommended and should be continued for 60 days.[29]

A preexposure vaccine, consisting of an initial series of six doses, followed by yearly boosters, is available and seems to be effective against pulmonary and cutaneous infection.[25] Vaccination currently is not recommended for the public.[31] Adverse effects associated with the vaccine include fever, chills, myalgia, arthralgia, nausea, and possibly rheumatoid arthritis.[38]

BOTULINUM NEUROTOXIN

General Characteristics

Clostridium botulinum, an anaerobic, gram-positive bacillus, produces botulinum neurotoxin (BoNT), which is considered to be one of the deadliest substances known. The estimated lethal dose of the toxin for a 70-kg person is only 70 μg if ingested or 0.7 to 0.9 μg if inhaled.[25] It is technically possible for a single gram of toxin to kill more than 1 million people.[44,45] BoNT is 15,000 times more lethal than the highly potent chemical agent VX and 100,000 times more lethal than sarin.[11]

The Japanese used this toxin as a weapon in World War II, when their biological warfare unit (unit 731) fed *C. botulinum* cultures to prisoners of war in Manchuria with lethal results. The United States was also researching BoNT as a weapon during World War II. Out of concern that Nazi Germany had weaponized BoNT, more than 1 million doses of botulinum toxoid vaccine were prepared for allied troops in preparation for the D-Day invasion.

After the Biological and Toxin Weapons Convention in 1972, the United States halted work on BoNT and other biological weapons, but other entities did not.[44,46] The former Soviet Union tested weaponized BoNT at Aralsk-7 on the Aral Sea. Iraq had weaponized massive amounts of BoNT before the Gulf War.[44] The Aum Shinrikyo cult released BoNT by aerosol at least three times in Japan between 1990 and 1995. These attacks failed, apparently because of poor microbiological technique.[44,46]

There are seven subtypes of BoNT (A through G), each defined by its absence of cross-neutralization with the others.[11,44] The toxins are proteins contained within spores produced by the *C. botulinum* organism.[11,47] They employ similar mechanisms of action, with essentially the same clinical effects.[11]

Naturally acquired botulism is contracted by ingesting food that has been contaminated with the spores; however, the spores can be aerosolized for use as a potential weapon.[47] The toxin is absorbed readily by gastrointestinal

or respiratory epithelium.[43] It is not known to penetrate intact skin.[25]

Despite its deadly nature, BoNT is destroyed easily by heat. A temperature of 80°C for 30 minutes, or 85°C for 5 minutes, effectively denatures the protein, inactivating the toxin.[19,44] Direct sunlight can deactivate toxin within 1 to 3 hours.[19,46] Simple exposure to open air can deactivate toxin within 12 hours.[19,46] Decontamination of exposed objects can be accomplished by washing them in a 0.5% sodium hypochlorite solution.[6]

These time estimates presume optimal conditions. The actual degradation rate depends on the size of particles released and the ambient atmospheric conditions of the area. The estimated rate of decay of aerosolized toxin is less than 1% to 4% per minute.[44,46] It could, therefore, take up to 2 days for significant inactivation to occur.[44] Botulism is not known to be contagious, making standard precautions sufficient when caring for exposed individuals.[6]

Understanding the mechanism of action of BoNT necessitates a brief review of the physiology of the neuromuscular junction. As a nerve impulse reaches the presynaptic terminal of the neuromuscular junction, vesicles containing the neurotransmitter acetylcholine (ACh) fuse with the presynaptic membrane, triggering exocytosis of the neurotransmitter molecules into the synaptic cleft, where they then bind with muscle cell receptors, resulting in muscle contraction. Within the presynaptic membranes are complexes of soluble N-ethylmaleimide-sensitive factor attachment protein receptor (SNARE), which act to facilitate fusion of the ACh-containing vesicles with the presynaptic membrane.[49] It is these SNARE proteins that are targeted, and cleaved, by BoNT. Cleavage of these proteins prevents the vesicles from fusing with the membrane, thereby preventing ACh from being released into the synaptic cleft, ultimately inhibiting muscle contraction.[11,25,49]

Potential Methods of Deployment

Aerolization of preformed BoNT is presumed to be the most likely means of deployment in a warfare scenario.[48,50] The toxin is colorless, odorless, and most likely tasteless, making contamination of food supplies possible.[44] Because of its susceptibility to deactivation by heat, it is only of concern in foods that are not heated thoroughly. Because an acidic environment would deactivate the toxin, it is also more commonly expected in foods that have a lower acid content, such as vegetables.[44]

The toxins are inactivated readily by most standard water treatments, such as chlorination, aeration, and even filtration with charcoal, to some extent.[19,44,46,50] For this reason, contamination of water supplies, although possible, would be more difficult to accomplish. Such a large amount of toxin would be required for any significant amount of contamination to occur that it virtually renders this form of deployment useless. No instances of waterborne botulism have been documented.[44,46,50] The toxin could remain stable for several days, however, in beverages or untreated water supplies.[44,50] Water purification devices using reverse osmosis can eradicate the toxin.[50]

Clinical preparations of BoNT type A are not likely to be used in an attack. A standard vial contains only 0.3% of the estimated lethal inhalational dose and 0.005% of the estimated lethal oral dose, making use of this form both expensive and impractical.[44]

Clinical Aspects

The clinical features of botulism are similar, regardless of the manner in which it is contracted. Onset of symptoms, however, may vary with the route of absorption.[11,25,47] Incubation time is approximately 12 to 36 hours for foodborne botulism and approximately 24 to 72 hours for the inhaled form.[46,47] Clinical onset is dose dependent and can begin anywhere from 2 hours to 8 days after exposure.[11,25]

Cranial nerves are preferentially affected, making bulbar symptoms such as ptosis, blurred vision, diplopia, dysarthria, dysphonia, and dysphagia some of the earliest and most prominent indications of exposure.[11,25,46] A symmetrical, descending paralysis of skeletal muscles follows, which can quickly lead to respiratory failure. Ascending weakness has not been reported; this information can aid in the differential diagnosis.[47]

Gastrointestinal symptoms can sometimes precede neurological symptoms if the toxin is ingested. This, however, is believed to be caused by other bacterial metabolites in the food and may not manifest if purified toxin is used.[44,46] Dermatological abnormalities have not been described in association with botulism.[51]

Physical examination may reveal mydriasis, dry mucous membranes, depressed or absent gag reflex, cranial nerve palsies, and even orthostatic hypotension.[11,25,44] Since the toxin does not penetrate the blood–brain barrier, mental status generally is unaffected. Patients can, however, appear lethargic and have difficulty communicating because of diffuse muscle and bulbar weakness.[6,44] Deep tendon reflexes are intact in the beginning but diminish gradually over days.[11,44] Sensory changes are usually not seen.[44]

Electrophysiological studies, if obtained, are expected to show normal nerve conduction velocities, normal sensory nerve conduction, small motor unit potentials, and incremental response to repetitive stimulation at 50 Hz.[44,46] Cerebrospinal fluid and brain imaging studies are normal.[25,46]

Initial diagnosis of botulism is by clinical recognition. A symmetrical, descending, flaccid paralysis with significant bulbar palsies in an afebrile patient with an intact mental status is the characteristic clinical picture.[11,44] Laboratory findings are generally nonspecific and of limited value in the acute setting.[6,11] Antibodies do not develop because the amount of toxin required to initiate a clinical response is not large enough to generate an immunological response.[6,11] A mouse bioassay is available to detect BoNT in serum, stool, gastric aspirate, or food.[6,11,44,52–54] It has been suggested, however, that aerosolized toxin may not be detectable in serum or stool.[11]

The differential diagnosis of botulism includes myasthenia gravis, tick paralysis, pontine infarction, diphtheria, and Guillain-Barré syndrome.[11,25,46] The edrophonium (Tensilon) test may be transiently positive in botulism, limiting its usefulness in differentiating botulism from myasthenia gravis.[11,46] It has been suggested that, in the United States, botulism is more likely to cause a cluster of acute cases of flaccid paralysis than Guillain-Barré syndrome or poliomyelitis.[44]

Initial treatment of botulism should, as in all cases of urgent treatment, focus on the basics of maintaining airway, breathing, and circulation. Mechanical ventilation should be initiated if vital capacity falls below 15 mL/kg or negative inspiratory force below 20 centimeters of water.[25] Placement of a nasogastric tube should also be considered to help prevent aspiration. Contaminated wounds should be surgically debrided.[46] In cases of ingested toxin, activated charcoal should be administered until antitoxin is available.[46]

With regard to specific treatment, a trivalent equine antitoxin is available from the Centers for Disease Control and Prevention.[11,25,44,47] This antitoxin is active against types A, B, and E, the three most common forms of foodborne toxin.[11,25] Because this antitoxin is derived from horse serum, skin testing for serum sensitivity should be considered before it is administered. Diphenhydramine and epinephrine should also be available during administration of the antitoxin to manage possible hypersensitivity reactions or anaphylaxis.[48]

A human-derived antitoxin is also effective against BoNT types A and B. It is available from the California State Health Department for treatment of patients in whom the equine-derived antitoxin is contraindicated or who experience an adverse reaction to the trivalent antitoxin. Although unable to reverse existing symptoms, the antitoxins may be able to stabilize the deficits and stop progression.[25,46] Animal studies suggest that, if administered before clinical effects appear, antitoxin might prevent symptoms from occurring.[11]

A heptavalent antitoxin has been developed but is not available at this time to the public.[11,25,47] A pentavalent toxoid (types A through E) is available through the Centers for Disease Control for active immunization but is in limited supply.[6,11] It is used to vaccinate high-risk laboratory workers and members of the military.[44] The toxoid is administered subcutaneously at 0, 2, and 12 weeks. This administration schedule produces antibody in 83% of individuals. If an additional, fourth dose is given, antibody production rises to 100%. Annual booster doses are recommended. The pentavalent toxoid provides no protection against toxin types F and G; therefore, if toxin strains F and G are used in an attack, the vaccine would prove useless. Fortunately, however, strains of *C. botulinum* that produce toxins type F and G are difficult to grow in large quantities, making them less likely to be used as weapons.[55]

Guanidine hydrochloride was formerly given to botulism patients as adjunctive therapy and believed to be of some benefit in recovery.[45,46] Puggiari and Cherington reported benefit in 39 of 52 treated cases.[45] A double-blind crossover study of 14 patients with BoNT type A intoxication, however, showed no benefit.[46] Faich et al, in 1971, reported the lack of beneficial effects from guanidine hydrochloride in their series of four patients who had type A BoNT intoxication.[47] Roblot et al.[48] suggest that guanidine is most beneficial in patients who have type B botulism intoxication, particularly when symptoms are mild. They report, in their series, 29 patients treated with guanidine alone and 35 patients treated with guanidine and antitoxin. Of their patients, 2 showed mild signs of intolerance to guanidine.[46] Treatment with guanidine hydrochloride is not considered standard of care for botulism.

Antibiotics are of no use because illness is produced by preformed toxin, not by the bacterium itself.[6] Recovery from botulism occurs only by the sprouting of new axons and may require up to a year or longer.[25,46,49]

SMALLPOX

General Characteristics

Smallpox is a potentially devastating disease caused by variola, a DNA virus of the orthopoxvirus family.[56] It has been used as an agent of biological warfare since the French and Indian wars in the mid-1700s, when Native Americans were given contaminated blankets by British soldiers.[56] The disease was declared eradicated in 1980 by the World Health Organization, with the last known case having occurred in 1977.[11,56–58] It is well known that remnants of this virus have been retained for research purposes at two World Health Organization laboratories: one in the United States and one in the former Soviet Union.[11,56,59]

The orthopoxvirus family constitutes one of the largest and most complex of all viruses.[56] Other members of this family include cowpox, monkeypox, camelpox, and vaccinia.[56,60] Although each of these has the capacity to be transmitted between individuals, only smallpox is believed to do so readily.[56]

Variola virus first invades mucosal cells of the respiratory system. It then migrates to regional lymph nodes, where it begins to multiply. After 3 to 4 days, an asymptomatic viremia develops as the virus is carried to the bone marrow, spleen, and other lymph nodes, where further replication takes place. After another 3 to 4 days, infected leukocytes transport the virus to the dermis and oropharyngeal mucosa, where neighboring cells are invaded, producing the characteristic skin lesions.[46,56] From there, the virus particles are released into the environment, enabling them to infect others by droplet exposure or by direct contact with infected people or contaminated fomites.[11,46,56] Thus far, no animal vector is known, humans being the only recognized reservoir.[11,61]

The extent of the threat posed by an outbreak of smallpox is debated. Although recent studies suggest that smallpox transmission may not be as rapid and far reaching as once believed,[58,62] it has been categorized as a Class A bioterrorism threat by the Centers for Disease Control.[63]

Potential Methods of Deployment

Given its capacity for infectivity in droplet form, aerosol release is most likely in an attack situation. Another conceivable scenario is infiltrating crowded areas with infected individuals. Strategic placement of contaminated fomites is a possible approach, although this method is less likely, given its lower propensity for transmission.

Clinical Aspects

The course of illness that follows variola infection is well described and fairly predictable. The typical sequence begins with an asymptomatic period of 7 to 17 days (characteristically 12 to 14 days) after the initial exposure.[56] The patient then experiences an abrupt onset of fever, rigors, headache, backache, and malaise.[11,56] Delirium also manifests during this phase in approximately 15% of patients.[11]

Within 2 to 3 more days, a maculopapular rash begins to develop centrifugally, affecting the oropharyngeal mucosa, face, and upper extremities before spreading to the trunk.[11,56] This lesional pattern is one characteristic that helps distinguish variola from varicella. In the latter condition, lesions are more profuse on the trunk than on the extremities.[11,56] The lesions produced by variola tend to present in approximately the same stage of development. In contrast, varicella lesions typically form in waves, with a new group appearing every few days, resulting in lesions in various stages of development. A few days after the lesions appear, they begin to crust over, forming scabs. As the scabs fall off, deep, pitting scars form in their place. This residual scarring is another characteristic unique to variola.[56]

The greatest period of infectivity occurs during the first week in which the patient becomes symptomatic.[56] From that point on, the smallpox victim is considered contagious until all the scabs have separated.[11,46] A caveat, however, is that some people can be asymptomatic carriers, shedding infectious virions without ever manifesting the disease themselves.[11] For this reason, during a known smallpox outbreak, prompt identification and isolation of exposed individuals, whether or not they are symptomatic, is crucial.[11]

Prevention of further disease spread is one of the most important aspects of management. All current and potential exposure victims, including the initial exposure victim and all people in his or her household, should be isolated immediately. Everyone with whom he or she had face-to-face contact since the time of exposure should also be quarantined.[56]

Vaccination within 4 days of exposure has been shown to prevent, or at least attenuate, symptomatic illness.[56] Treatment otherwise is supportive. One aspect that bears mentioning from a neurological standpoint is a complication from the vaccine itself. An estimated 1 in 300,000 primary vaccinees acquires postvaccinal encephalitis, with a mortality rate of 25%.[56] A constellation of headache, meningismus, fever, drowsiness, and vomiting that presents 8 to 15 days after vaccination is the characteristic clinical picture. A spastic paralysis occurs as well in some cases. No specific treatment exists other than supportive care, and the reaction can result in seizure, coma, or death.[56]

ANATOXIN-A

General Characteristics

Anatoxin-a, also known as "very fast death factor," is a bicyclical amine produced by *Anabaena flos-aquae*. This filamentous, freshwater bacterium is found in pond scum worldwide.[19,64,65] Two mechanisms of action are used by this toxin. First, it acts as an ACh agonist, stimulating muscle contraction by binding to postsynaptic ACh receptors. Unlike ACh, however, anatoxin-a is not released from the receptor, which results in continuous contraction of the affected muscle.[65] Second, it inhibits acetylcholinesterase, which leads to an increase of the neurotransmitter within the synaptic cleft. The combined effect causes paralysis, resulting in death if respiratory muscles are affected.[65]

Potential Methods of Deployment

Specific information regarding the use of this toxin as an agent of biological warfare is limited. One possible route of deployment is through contamination of water supplies, because many standard methods of water decontamination, including chlorination and carbon filtration, are poorly effective at best.[19] Nonetheless, the toxin is converted to a nontoxic form in water within several days.[19]

Clinical Aspects

When ingested by animals, anatoxin-a is known to produce staggering, gasping, and convulsions. This is followed within minutes to hours by death, resulting from respiratory arrest.[19] Similar symptoms are expected in humans. Symptoms mimicking organophosphate poisoning, such as miosis, excess oral and lacrimal secretions, and muscle fasciculations, are anticipated.[65] Onset of symptoms is within 5 minutes of exposure.[65] Currently, no antidote is known for treatment of antitoxin-a exposure. Animal models suggest that pretreatment with pralidoxime and physostigmine may be effective.[65] Supportive care, including mechanical ventilation if necessary, is the primary focus of treatment.

RICIN

General Characteristics

Ricin, a toxin obtained from the bean of the castor plant, has been known for centuries.[19,46,50,66] It consists of an A-chain and a B-chain linked by a disulfide bond.[49,50,66] Both chains are necessary for cytotoxicity to occur. The B-chain binds to cell surface receptors, triggering internalization of the ricin molecule by the cell membrane.[49,50,66] Once inside the cell, the A-chain enzymatically inactivates ribosomes. This inhibits DNA replication and protein synthesis, in turn causing cellular necrosis.[49,50,66] Ricin is inactivated by heat. A temperature of 80°C for 10 minutes or 50°C for approximately 1 hour is sufficient for neutralization of the toxin.[19]

Potential Methods of Deployment

Historically, ricin has been used to assassinate individuals rather than as a weapon of mass destruction.[1,19,66] Dispersion of the toxin could occur by means of aerosol, droplet, or injection.[66] Theoretically, it can be used to contaminate food or water supplies; however, the large quantity required to produce a substantial effect makes this method of deployment impractical.[49,50] Because a considerable amount of aerosolized toxin is required to exact a significant toll on a large population, its use in this manner is believed limited.[19]

Clinical Aspects

Clinical manifestations depend on the route of exposure but generally are secondary to necrosis of the affected tissue. Ingestion of the toxin results in necrosis of gastrointestinal epithelium and local hemorrhage, with subsequent hepatic, splenic, and renal necrosis.[19,49] Necrosis of upper and lower respiratory epithelium, leading to tracheitis, bronchitis, bronchiolitis, and interstitial pneumonia, occurs if the toxin is inhaled.[49,66]

Tissue damage begins within 8 to 12 hours; however, symptoms may not appear for 12 to 24 hours.[19] Death from ricin toxin is dose dependent and occurs 36 to 72 hours after inhalation.[49] Injection of the toxin produces the most severe symptoms, with the central nervous system affected soon after injection, leading to convulsions and decreased heart function.[19]

Diagnosis is by clinical suspicion, although testing for specific antigens and immunohistochemical properties of exposed tissues can be accomplished.[49,66] Currently, no specific treatment exists for ricin toxicity except for general supportive care.[49,50,66] Vaccine development is, however, under way.[49,50]

TULAREMIA

General Characteristics

Francisella tularensis is a nonmotile, aerobic, facultative intracellular, gram-negative coccobacillus most commonly associated with zoonoses in rural areas.[11,46,67] Although five subspecies of the organism can be found in the Northern Hemisphere, only two, *F. tularensis* subspecies *tularensis* and *F. tularensis* subspecies *holarctica*, are known to cause disease in humans.[68] Introduction of only 10 to 50 organisms is sufficient to cause illness, making *F. tularensis* one of the most infectious bacteria known.[11,46,67] It was first studied as a potential biological warfare agent in the 1930s and is considered a prime candidate for such because of its high rate of infectivity and its significant capability to cause disease.[67]

Potential Methods of Deployment

The most likely method of deployment is via aerosol, although contamination of food and water sources also is possible.[11,67] Human-to-human transmission has not been documented.[46] The organism is destroyed by heat (55°C for 10 minutes) or standard disinfectant solutions, such as 10% bleach.[11,69]

Clinical Aspects

The expected presentation of inhaled, or typhoidal, tularemia is similar to that of an atypical pneumonia, with abrupt onset of constitutional symptoms and a nonproductive cough.[46,67] A local, suppurative skin lesion with subsequent spread to regional lymph nodes characterizes the ulceroglandular form of the disease, which would be anticipated from direct inoculation of the organism to exposed skin or mucous membranes.[11,46,67] Neurological manifestations of meningitis or encephalopathy are rare and expected to occur only with widespread dissemination of the organism sufficient to cause sepsis.[46,67]

Initial diagnosis of deliberate infection is difficult because of the nonspecific symptoms. A rapid test involving fluorescent-labeled antibodies to the organism is available if the diagnosis is suspected.[67] Definitive diagnosis is by culture of oropharyngeal specimens or fasting gastric fluid. Rarely is it isolated from blood.[67] Various other methods, such as enzyme-linked immunoassay, polymerase chain reaction, and antigen detection assays can be used[67]; however, these are more likely to be employed retrospectively.

Recommended treatment is a 10-day course of streptomycin or gentomycin.[11,46,55,67] Alternatives are doxycycline, chloramphenicol, or ciprofloxacin.[11,55,67] Use of alternative medications is associated with considerable potential for relapse, however; thus, an extended course of treatment, 14 to 21 days, is required.[11,55] Postexposure prophylaxis with a 14-day course of doxycycline or ciprofloxacin is shown effective if initiated within 24 hours of exposure.[11,55] A novel, intranasal treatment method is also being explored.[70] A live, attenuated vaccine exists but is not recommended for use by the public.[11,67]

TRICHOTHECENE MYCOTOXINS

General Characteristics

Trichothecene mycotoxins, the best known of which is T-2 toxin, are produced by the *Alternaria, Fusarium, Myrotecium, Trichoderma, Aspergillus, Claviceps, Penicillium,* and *Stachybotrys* species of fungi.[19,46,66,71] These toxins have tremendous potential for weaponization. They are resistant to high temperatures, autoclaving, and ultraviolet light; are fairly simple to obtain; and can be lethal within minutes at proper doses.[19,46,66] They are believed to be as potent as the mustard gases but are more readily absorbed through the skin.[19]

Given their lipophilic nature, tricothecenes are quickly absorbed by cell membranes. This property leads to rapid onset of symptoms.[66] The toxins are highly soluble in organic solvents.[66] They inhibit protein synthesis by interfering with ribosomal peptidyl transferase, with subsequent failure of protein translation.[19,66] They can secondarily affect DNA.[66] They are implicated in disrupting electron transport within mitochondria and in enhancing lipid peroxidation of cell membranes.[19]

Potential Methods of Deployment

Infection is by ingestion, inhalation, or absorption through skin or mucous membranes.[19,66] The toxins, therefore, can be deployed by several methods. They are believed responsible for the "yellow rain" poisonings in Southeast Asia and Afghanistan in the 1970s and 1980s.[66,71]

Clinical Aspects

Although the principal symptoms of T-2 toxicity are cutaneous (blistering and necrosis) and respiratory (epistaxis, cough, and dyspnea), the toxin can affect the central nervous system, with generalized symptoms of lethargy and incoordination.[6,19] Diagnosis is difficult but should be considered if clinical signs and symptoms consistent with tricothecene toxicity occur in the setting of exposure to a yellowish-colored mist or smoke. A rapid diagnostic test currently is not available; however, antigens to toxin metabolites can be detected in blood, feces, and urine for up to 1 month after exposure.[46,66]

Treatment of T-2 toxicity is by decontamination and supportive care. Decontamination of skin is accomplished by washing thoroughly with soap and water. Decontamination of exposed surfaces can be achieved with a 1% sodium hypochlorite solution with sodium hydroxide.[6,66] Although no human studies have been performed, treatment with corticosteroids has shown promise in animal models, as has gastric infusion with superactivated charcoal with magnesium sulfate.[6,46]

VENEZUELAN EQUINE ENCEPHALITIS VIRUS

General Characteristics

There have, as yet, been no reported uses of viruses as modern biological weapons. However, potential exists for the use of viral pathogens as agents of bioterrorism, as suggested by the history of biological warfare. As late as the late 1980s, the Soviet Union had been developing viral pathogens for potential use as biological weapons. One pathogen in which they had particular interest was Venezuelan equine encephalitis virus (VEEV), one of many RNA-containing viruses that cause various mosquito-transmitted diseases.

VEEV is an alphavirus that causes an epidemic zoonosis normally limited to the tropical and subtropical Americas. Although several arboviral encephalitic agents might be exploited as weapons, many factors make VEEV a likely choice as a bioterrorism agent. First, it has high infectivity coupled with a low infectious dose. Second, no specific treatment exists for the disease caused by VEEV infection. Finally, few people are vaccinated against infection by the virus.

Immediate recognition of the involvement of VEEV in a bioterrorism attack may be difficult. In nature, Venezuelan equine encephalitis epidemics are easily recognizable by the large numbers of equines succumbing to the disease. Because a deliberate aerosol release would likely occur indoors or in areas remote from livestock, however, dead equines may not be a useful barometer for recognition of an attack with VEEV.

The most significant indicator of a deliberate VEEV release would be a human case occurring anywhere outside of the tropical or subtropical Western Hemisphere. Such a sentinel event would require an immediate and detailed investigation. Because of a 1- to 6-day incubation period, covert release of VEEV does not have an immediate effect on public health. The time course of VEEV-associated disease may therefore have an impact on identification of VEEV as a bioterrorism agent.

Clinical Aspects

VEEV typically causes a bimodal illness in humans (see Figure 55-3), with an initial, severe, flulike illness in nearly everyone exposed, followed several days later by potentially deadly encephalitis in a few patients.[48] While only about 1% of adult cases and 4% of pediatric cases progress to encephalitis, the mortality rate of those that do is 20%.[72,73]

Potential Methods of Deployment

The use of infected vectors would be highly unpredictable and logistically difficult to accomplish; therefore, attacks involving VEEV would likely be carried out using aerosolized viral particles. Studies of VEEV infection using animal models suggest that aerosolized VEEV is highly neurotropic and accesses the central nervous system through the olfactory epithelium.[74] Given this information, it is reasonable to expect increased numbers of encephalitis cases in attacks involving aerosolized viral particles.

Diagnosis is accomplished by polymerase chain reaction detection of the virus in cerebrospinal fluid.[73] Preventative and postexposure options are limited. Vaccines have been shown, in limited studies, to have protective efficacy.[75] An inactivated vaccine is available for laboratory personnel at high risk of exposure.[73] Live attenuated vaccines are under development.[73]

Treatment of the disease subsequent to infection is limited to supportive care. In severe cases, prophylactic, anticonvulsant drugs should be considered. Pegylated interferon-α results in improved survival in mice,[76] but implications of these results for humans are unclear. Studies also suggest that interferon-γ may be useful in treatment.[73] More research is needed to find effective therapies for this and other viral encephalitides, especially in light of the potential for the use of VEEV and other viral pathogens as agents of bioterrorism.

TETRODOTOXIN

General Characteristics

Widely recognized as the deadly substance produced by fugu, or puffer fish, tetrodotoxin works at the level of the cell membrane. The toxin binds tightly to voltage-gated sodium channels, blocking the influx of sodium necessary for conduction of action potentials.[77] It affects peripheral nerves, both motor and sensory, and causes depression of medullary respiratory and vasomotor centers.[78] The lethal human dose is believed 1 to 2 mg by ingestion.[19]

Potential Methods of Deployment

Tetrodotoxin most likely would be used to contaminate food or water supplies. It is soluble in water that is slightly acidic, and is not affected significantly by extremes of temperature.[19] Chlorine readily inactivates the toxin under acidic (pH < 3) and alkalinic (pH > 9) conditions.[19]

Clinical Aspects

Initial symptoms of oral numbness, gastrointestinal distress, anxiety, headache, and mild peripheral weakness begin to appear within 10 minutes to 4 hours of ingestion. This is followed by an ascending, generalized paralysis, hypotension, convulsions, and cardiac arrhythmias. Death occurs in 4 to 6 hours secondary to respiratory failure.[19,78] Distressingly, the victim may remain conscious, although paralyzed, until just before death.

No specific treatment is known for tetrodotoxin poisoning; treatment is supportive. Empirical gastric lavage with activated charcoal and administration of anticholinergic agents may be beneficial; however, insufficient data are available to assess adequately the efficacy of these options.[78]

SAXITOXIN

General Characteristics

Saxitoxin is produced by the dinoflagellates *Gonyaulax*, *Alexandrium*, *Gymnodinium*, and *Pyrodinium*.[19,69,80] Similar to tetrodotoxin, saxitoxin binds to voltage-gated sodium channels within cell membranes, inhibiting membrane depolarization and blocking proliferation of action potentials.[69,81] Because this toxin molecule is not a protein, it is more stable in extremes of temperature and pH.[19,82] It has a lethal human dose of approximately 0.2 mg for the average adult and is approximately 1000 times more toxic than the chemical warfare agent sarin.[69]

Clinical Aspects

Clinical manifestations of oral numbness, gastrointestinal distress, vertigo, tachycardia, and headache occur within approximately 30 minutes of saxitoxin ingestion.[19] Symptoms may include incoordination, dysarthria, and respiratory distress.[69,83] Death secondary to respiratory failure can occur within 1 to 24 hours.[19] Data regarding routes of exposure are limited; however, inhalation is believed to produce the most severe effects.[19] No antidote exists for saxitoxin toxicity, making supportive care the only available means of treatment.

Q FEVER

General Characteristics

Q fever is a febrile zoonosis associated with exposure to infected sheep, cattle, goats, or other livestock.[11] It is caused by the obligate intracellular coccobacillus, *Coxiella burnetii*.[11,84] Its usefulness as a biological warfare agent comes from its sporelike form, which is resistant to heat and desiccation, allowing it to persist in an area for weeks or even months.[11] This form can be distributed for miles by wind[11] and is highly infective, with as few as one organism necessary to produce disease (range 1 to 100).[84] Decontamination of exposed surfaces is by saturation with 5% hydrogen peroxide or 70% ethyl alcohol for 30 minutes.[84]

Clinical Aspects

The actual illness caused by *C. burnetii* is mild compared with that caused by many agents discussed previously. Even without treatment, mortality and chronic morbidity are low.[11] Flulike symptoms with or without cough are characteristic.[11] Neurological symptoms of severe, retrobulbar headache, meningitis, and encephalitis are reported in up to one-fourth of patients with Q fever.[85]

Standard treatment of Q fever is a course of tetracycline or doxycycline, although macrolide antibiotics can be used.[11] Use of a fluoroquinolone should be considered in cases of Q fever meningitis.[86] Treatment is continued until the patient has been afebrile for 1 week.[84] Postexposure prophylaxis with a 5-day course of tetracycline or doxycycline can be efficacious if initiated within 8 to 12 days of exposure.[84] Effective vaccines have been developed but are under investigation in the United States.[11,84]

Table 2: Neurologic Symptoms and Signs

Biological Agent	Headache or Meningitis	Vision Change	Incoordination	Paralysis	Encephalopathy	Sensory Symptoms	Seizure	Miscellaneous
Botulism	−	+[a,b]	+	+[c]	−	−	−	Normal CSF
VEEV	+	+/−	−	−	+	−	+/−	
Anthrax	+	+[d,f]	−	−	+/−	−	+/−	Possible hemorrhagic meningitis
Smallpox	+	−	−	+/−[e]	+/−	−	+/−	
Anatoxin-a	−	−	+	+[f]	−	−	+/−	Possible hypercholinergic symptoms
Mycotoxin	−	−	+	−	+	−	−	
Ricin	−	−	−	−	−	−	+[g]	
Tetrodotoxin	+	−	+	+[h]	+	+[i]	+	Can affect central nervous system respiratory centers
Saxitoxin	+	−	+	+	−	+[i]	+	
Q fever	+	−	−	−	+	−	−	
Tularemia	+/−	−	−	−	+/−	−	−	

Abbreviations: +, sign/symptom is known to be associated with respective agent; −, sign/symptom typically is not seen with infection by respective agent, or a definite association has not yet been documented.

[a]Blurring.
[b]Diplopia.
[c]Bulbar/descending.
[d]Visual field defect.
[e]Spastic.
[f]Flaccid.
[g]More likely if injected.
[h]Ascending.
[i]Perioral paresthesias.

+, sign or symptom is known to be associated with the respective agent; −, sign or symptom typically is not seen with infection by the respective agent, or a definite association has not yet been documented; CSF, cerebrospinal fluid; VEEV, Venezuelan equine encephalitis virus.
Osterbauer PJ, Dobbs MR. Neurobiological weapons. *Neurol Clin.* 2005;23:599–621.

Table 3: Nonneurological Symptoms and Signs

Biological Agent	Fever	Flu-like Symptoms	Gastrointestinal	Pulmonary	Cardiac	Cutaneous
Botulism	−	−	+	+[a]	−	−
VEEV	+	+	+	+	−	−
Anthrax	+	+	+	+	−	+[b]
Smallpox	+	+	+	+	−	+[c]
Anatoxin-a	−	−	−	+[a]	−	−
Mycotoxin	−	−	+	+	−	+[d]
Ricin	+	+	+[e]	+	+[f]	−
Tetrodotoxin	−	−	+	+[g]	+	−
Saxitoxin	−	−	+	+	+	−
Q fever	+	+	+[h]	+	|[i]	
Tularemia	+	+	−	+	−	+

[a]If respiratory muscles are affected.
[b]Nontender, pruritic papules.
[c]Centrifugal pattern, affecting face and extremities more than trunk. Also with late scarring.
[d]Severe blistering and necrosis.
[e]Hemorrhagic.
[f]More likely if injected.
[g]Works centrally by affecting central nervous system respiratory centers.
[h]Possible mild hepatitis.
[i]Can produce chronic endocarditis.
+, sign or symptom is known to be associated with the respective agent; −, sign or symptom typically is not seen with infection by the respective agent, or a definite association has not yet been documented; VEEV, Venezuelan equine encephalitis virus.
Osterbauer PJ, Dobbs MR. Neurobiological weapons. *Neurol Clin.* 2005;23:599–621.

CONCLUSION

Biological warfare is a potential threat on the battlefield and in daily life. It is vital for neurologists and other health-care practitioners to be familiar with biological and toxic agents that target the nervous system. Most illnesses caused by biological warfare agents are not commonly considered neurological diseases; however, many of these agents may present with headache, meningitis, or mental status changes, in addition to fever and other symptoms and signs (Tables 2 and 3). A neurologist may therefore be consulted to aid in diagnosis. Given the incubation time of many biological agents and their protean manifestations, it is likely that health-care workers will be on the front lines in the event of a bioterrorist attack. A proactive stance is a must.

REFERENCES

1. Christopher GW, Cieslak TJ, Pavlin JA, et al. Biological warfare: a historical perspective. *JAMA.* 1997;278:412–417.
2. Jacobs MK. The history of biological warfare and terrorism. *Dermatol Clin.* 2004;22:231–246.
3. Lesho ME, Dorsey MD, Bunner D. Feces, dead horses, and fleas: evolution of the hostile use of biological agents. *West J Med.* 1998;168:512–516.
4. Ongradi J. Microbial warfare and bioterrorism. *Orv Hetil.* 2002;143:1935–1939.
5. Wheelis M. Biological warfare at the 1346 siege of Caffa. *Emerg Infect Dis.* 2002;8:971–975.
6. Blazes DL, Lawler JV, Lazarus AA. When biotoxins are tools of terror: early recognition of intentional poisoning can attenuate effects. *Postgrad Med.* 2002;112:89–92, 95–96, 98.
7. Simon JD. Biological terrorism: preparing to meet the threat. *JAMA.* 1997;278:428–430.

8. Ziliniskas RA. Iraq's biological weapons: the past as future? *JAMA*. 1997;278:418–425.

9. Daly MJ. The emerging impact of genomics on the development of biological weapons: threats and benefits posed by engineered extremophiles. *Clin Lab Med*. 2001;21:619–629.

10. Whitby S, Millett P, Dando M. The potential for abuse of genetics in militarily significant biological weapons. *Med Confl Surviv*. 2002;18:157–160.

11. Franz DR, Jahrling PB, Friedlander AM, et al. Clinical recognition and management of patients exposed to biological warfare agents. *JAMA*. 1997;278:399–411.

12. Khan AS, Swerdlow DL, Juranek DD. Precautions against biological and chemical terrorism directed at food and water supplies. *Public Health Rep*. 2001;116:3–14.

13. Burrows WD, Renner SE. Biological warfare agents as threats to potable water. *Environ Health Perspect*. 1999;107:975–984.

14. Cieslak TJ, Christopher GW, Kortepeter MG, et al. Immunization against potential biological warfare agents. *Clin Infect Dis*. 2000;30:843–850.

15. Atlas RM. The medical threat of biological weapons. *Crit Rev Microbiol*. 1998;24:157–168.

16. Berns KI, Atlas RM, Cassell G, et al. Preventing the misuse of microorganisms: the role of the American Society of Microbiology in protecting against biological weapons. *Crit Rev Microbiol*. 1998;24:273–280.

17. CDC. Recognition of illness associated with the intentional release of a biologic agent. *MMWR*. 2001;50:893–897.

18. Tjaden JA, Lazarus AA, Martin GJ. Bacteria as agents of biowarfare: how to proceed when the worst is expected. *Postgrad Med*. 2002;112:57–60.

19. Horn JK. Bacterial agents used for bioterrorism. *Surg Infect*. 2003;4:281–287.

20. Greenfield RA, Bronze MS. Current therapy and the development of therapeutic options for the treatment of diseases due to bacterial agents of potential biowarfare and bioterrorism. *Curr Opin Investig Drugs*. 2004;5:135–140.

21. Hassani M, Patel MC, Pirofski LA. Vaccines for the prevention of diseases caused by potential bioweapons. *Clin Immunol*. 2004;111:1–15.

22. Casadevall A. Passive antibody administration (immediate immunity) as a specific defense against biological weapons. *Emerg Infect Dis*. 2002;8:833–841.

23. Paddle BM. Therapy and prophylaxis of inhaled biotoxins. *J Appl Toxicol*. 2003;23:139–170.

24. Fischetti VA. Novel method to control pathogenic bacteria on human mucous membranes. *Ann NY Acad Sci*. 2003;987:207–214.

25. Martin CO, Adams HP. Neurological aspects of biological and chemical terrorism: a review for neurologists. *Arch Neurol*. 2003;60:21–25.

26. Hepburn MJ, Purcell BK, Paragas J. Pathogenesis and sepsis caused by organisms potentially used as biologic weapons: opportunities for targeted intervention. *Curr Drug Targets*. 2007;8(4):519–532.

27. Wenner KA, Kenner JR. Anthrax. *Dermatol Clin*. 2004;22:247–256.

28. Kenar L, Ortatatli M, Yaren H, et al. Comparative sporicidal effects of disinfectants after release of a biological agent. *Mil Med*. 2007;172(6):616–621.

29. Zajkowska J, Hermanowska-Szpakowicz T. Anthrax as a biological warfare weapon. *Med Pr*. 2002;53:167–172.

30. Schuch R, Nelson D, Fischetti VA. A bacteriologic agent that detects and kills *Bacillus anthracis*. *Nature*. 2002;418:884–889.

31. Atlas RM. Responding to the threat of bioterrorism: a microbial ecology perspective—the case of anthrax. *Int Microbiol*. 2002;5:161–167.

32. Sternbach G. The history of anthrax. *J Emerg Med*. 2003;24:463–467.

33. Bartlett JG, Inglesby TV Jr, Borio L. Management of anthrax. *Clin Infect Dis*. 2002;35:851–858.

34. Hendrickson RG, Hedges JR. Introduction: what critical care practitioners should know about terrorism agents. *Crit Care Clin*. 2005;21:641–652.

35. Whitby M, Ruff TA, Street AC, et al. Biological agents as weapons: II. Anthrax and plague. *Med J Aust*. 2002;176:605–608.

36. Erickson MC, Kornacki JL. *Bacillus anthracis*: current knowledge in relation to contamination of food. *J Food Prot*. 2003;66:691–699.

37. Gilbert DN, Moellering RC Jr, Sande MA. In: *The Sanford Guide to Antimicrobial Therapy*. 33rd ed. Hyde Park, NY: Antimicrobial Therapy; 2003:46.

38. Vasudev M, Zacharisen MC. New-onset rheumatoid arthritis after anthrax vaccination. *Ann Allergy Asthma Immunol*. 2006;97(1):110–112.

39. Arnon SS, Schechter R, Inglesby TV, et al. Botulinum toxin as a biological weapon: medical and public health management. *JAMA*. 2001;285:1059–1071.

40. Gill MD. Bacterial toxins: a table of lethal amounts. *Microbiol Rev*. 1982;46:86–94.

41. Manoj K, Currie B, Kvetan V. Bioterrorism: preparing for the impossible or the improbable. *Crit Care Med*. 2005;4(1):S75–S80.

42. Berg J, Chandrasoma S, Yang I, et al. Learning about bioterrorism and chemical warfare: medical students explore key threats. *West J Med*. 2002;176:58–60.

43. Robinson RF, Nahata MC. Management of botulism. *Ann Pharmacother*. 2003;37:127–131.

44. Anonymous. Drugs and vaccines for biological weapons. *Med Lett Drugs Ther*. 2001;46:25–34.

45. Puggiari M, Cherington M. Botulism and guanidine: ten years later. *JAMA*. 1978;240:2276–2277.

46. Kaplan JE, Davis LE, Narayan V, et al. Botulism type A and treatment with guanidine. *Ann Neurol*. 1979;6:69–71.

47. Faich GA, Graebner RW, Sato S. Failure of guanidine therapy in botulism A. *N Engl J Med*. 1971;285:773–776.

48. Roblot P, Roblot F, Fauchere JL, et al. Retrospective study of botulism in Poitiers, France. *J Med Microbiol*. 1994;40(6):379–384.

49. Greenfield RA, Brown BR, Hutchins JB, et al. Microbiological, biological, and chemical weapons of warfare and terrorism. *Am J Med Sci*. 2002;323:326–340.

50. Villar RG, Elliott SP, Davenport KM. Botulism: the many faces of botulinum toxin and its potential for bioterrorism. *Infect Dis Clin North Am*. 2006;20:313–327.

51. Cieslak TJ, Talbot TB, Harstein BH. Biological warfare and the skin: I. Bacteria and toxins. *Clin Dermatol*. 2002;5:138–141.

52. Leggiadro RJ. The threat of biological terrorism: a public health and infection control reality. *Infect Control Hosp Epidemiol*. 2000;21:53–57.

53. Robinson-Dunn B. The microbiology laboratory's role in response to bioterrorism. *Arch Pathol Lab Med*. 2002;126:291–294.

54. Burda AM, Sigg T. Pharmacy preparedness for incidents involving weapons of mass destruction. *Am J Health Syst Pharm*. 2001;43:87–89.

55. Ellison DH. *Handbook of Chemical and Biological Warfare Agents*. Boca Raton, Fla: CRC Press; 2000.

56. Henderson DA, Inglesby TV, Bartlett JG, et al. Smallpox as a biological weapon: clinical and public health management. *JAMA*. 1999;281:2127–2137.

57. Beeching NJ, Dance DA, Miller AR, et al. Biological warfare and bioterrorism. *BMJ*. 2002;324:336–339.

58. Pennington H. Smallpox and bioterrorism. *Bull World Health Organ*. 2003;81:762–767.

59. Breman JG, Henderson DA. Poxvirus dilemmas—monkeypox, smallpox, and biologic terrorism. *N Engl J Med*. 1998;339:556–559.

60. Georges AJ. Biohazards due to orthopoxvirus: should we re-vaccinate against smallpox? *Med Trop.* 1999;59(4 Pt 2):483–487.

61. Slifka MK, Hanifin JM. Smallpox: the basics. *Dermatol Clin.* 2004;22:263–274.

62. Eichner M, Dietz K. Transmission potential of smallpox: estimates based on detailed data from an outbreak. *Am J Epidemiol.* 2003;158:110–117.

63. Whitley RJ. Smallpox: a potential agent of bioterrorism. *Antiviral Res.* 2003;57:7–12.

64. Aronstam RB, Witkop B. Anatoxin-a interactions with cholinergic synaptic molecules. *Proc Natl Acad Sci USA.* 1981;78:4639–4643.

65. Fact Sheets on Chemical and Biological Warfare Agents. CBWInfo.com, Ver 2.1. September 2002. Available at: http://www.cbwinfo.com/Biological/Toxins/AnatoxinA.html. Accessed September 4, 2004.

66. Henghold WB. Other biologic toxin bioweapons: ricin, staphylococcal enterotoxin B, and tricothecene mycotoxins. *Dermatol Clin.* 2004;22:257–262.

67. Dennis DT, Inglesby TV, Henderson DA, et al. Tularemia as a biological weapon: medical and public health management. *JAMA.* 2001;285:2763–2773.

68. McLendon MK, Apicella MA, Allen LA. *Francisella tularensis:* taxonomy, genetics, and immunopathogenesis of a potential agent of biowarfare. *Annu Rev Microbiol.* 2006;60:167–185.

69. Strichartz G. Structural determinants of the affinity of saxitoxin for neuronal sodium channels. *J Gen Phys.* 1984;84:281–305.

70. Pammit MA, Budhavarapu VN, Klose EK, et al. Intranasal interleukin-12 treatment promotes antimicrobial clearance and survival in pulmonary *Francisella tularensis* subsp. *novicida* infection. *Antimicrob Agents Chemother (Bethesda).* 2004;48(12):4513–4519.

71. Etzel RA. Mycotoxins. *JAMA.* 2002;287:425–427.

72. Paredes A, Alwell-Warda K, Weaver SC, et al. Structure of isolated nucleocapsids from Venezuelan equine encephalitis virus and implications for assembly and disassembly of enveloped virus. *J Virol.* 2003;77:659–664.

73. Pappas G, Panagopoulou P, Christou L, et al. Category B potential bioterrorism agents: bacteria, viruses, toxins, and foodborne and waterborne pathogens. *Infect Dis Clin North Am.* 2006;20:395–421.

74. Steele KE, Davis KJ, Stephan K, et al. Comparative neurovirulence and tissue tropism of wild-type and attenuated strains of Venezuelan equine encephalitis virus administered by aerosol in C3H/HeN and BALB/c mice. *Vet Pathol.* 1998;35:386–397.

75. Bronze MS, Huycke MM, Machado LJ, et al. Viral agents as biological weapons and agents of bioterrorism. *Am J Med Sci.* 2002;323:316–325.

76. Lukaszewski RA, Brooks TJ. Pegylated interferon is an effective treatment for virulent Venezuelan equine encephalitis virus and has profound effects on the host immune response to infection. *J Virol.* 2000;74:5006–5015.

77. Oda K, Araki K, Totoki T, Shibasaki H. Nerve conduction study of human tetrodotoxication. *Neurology.* 1989;39:743–745.

78. Benzor T. Toxicity, Tetrodotoxin: August 5, 2004. Available at: http://www.emedicine.com/emerg/topic576.htm#section~bibliography. Accessed September 25, 2004.

79. Edwards N. Saxitoxin: From Food Poisoning to Chemical Warfare. Available at: http://www.bris.ac.uk/Depts/Chemistry/MOTM/stx/saxi.htm. Accessed September 4, 2004.

80. Gallacher S, Flynn KJ, Franco JM, et al. Evidence for production of paralytic shellfish toxins by bacteria associated with *Alexandrium* spp. (Dinophyta) in culture. *Appl Environ Microbiol.* 1997;63:239–245.

81. Narahashi T. Chemicals as tools in the study of excitable membranes. *Physiol Rev.* 1971;51:813–889.

82. Cheng HS, Chua SO, Hung JS, et al. Creatine kinase MB elevation in paralytic shellfish poisoning. *Chest.* 1991;99:1032–1033.

83. Hunter B. Paralytic shellfish poisoning: a growing problem. *Consumer Res Mag.* 1992;75:8–9.

84. Rosenbloom M, Leikin JB, Vogel SN, et al. Biological and chemical agents: a brief synopsis. *Am J Ther.* 2002;9:5–14.

85. Dupuis G, Petite J, Olivier P, et al. An important outbreak of human Q fever in a Swiss alpine valley. *Int J Epidemiol.* 1987;16:282–287.

86. Gilbert DN, Moellering RC Jr, Sande MA. ***. In: *The Sanford Guide to Antimicrobial Therapy.* 33rd ed. Hyde Park, NY: Antimicrobial Therapy; 2003:48.

CHAPTER 56

Nerve Agents

Jonathan Newmark

Nerve agents, the deadliest of the classical warfare agents, primarily function as acetylcholinesterase inhibitors and cause a rapidly progressive cholinergic crisis. Because of the speed of symptom onset, treatment must be rendered emergently, most likely by first responders. Neurologists should familiarize themselves with the pathophysiology and treatment principles for the syndromes caused by nerve agents, not only to assist with the hospital care of these patients but also to serve as resources to their local medical communities in preparation for chemical terrorism. Because nerve agents injure the nervous system, nonneurologists have a right to expect neurologists to have mastered these principles.

INTRODUCTION

The organophosphonate nerve agents are the deadliest of the classical chemical warfare agents. Since terrorists have a proven interest in these compounds, it behooves neurologists to know something about them and about the acute treatment of patients exposed to them.[1]

The nerve agent sarin was used in two recent terrorist attacks in Japan.[2] Data have also become available on the battlefield use of these agents by Iraq in 1984 to 1987.[3] In the aftermath of the terrorist attacks of 2001, emphasis has been placed upon familiarity with the principles of recognition and treatment of casualties of agents of terrorist interest.

HISTORY

The nerve agents are extremely toxic relatives of organophosphate insecticides, which have been used in agriculture since the early 20th century. The first three, tabun, sarin, and soman, were invented in Nazi Germany between 1938 and 1944. Tabun and sarin were weaponized by the German military.[4] Germany never used her tabun and sarin weapons in World War II, for reasons still debated today. During the Cold War, the United States and Soviet Union maintained large stockpiles of nerve agents but refrained from their use.

Nerve agents were not used on the battlefield until 1984, when Iraq turned to the chemical arm to achieve victory against Iran. Iraq had invaded Iran in 1981, but Iraq's invasion bogged down against the numerically superior Iranian defenders. From 1984 to 1987, Iraq used sulfur mustard, and the nerve agents sarin and tabun, against Iranian soldiers; Iraq later used these against Iranian cities.[5–7] Infamously, in 1988 Iraq used chemical weapons, probably nerve agents, against Iraqi Kurdish civilians in the al-Anfal campaign, most notably at Halabja.[8] There were anywhere from 45,000 to 100,000 Iranian chemical casualties in the war, of whom the majority appear to have been caused by nerve agents. Only recently have data from these patients begun to appear in the open literature.[3]

The United States has fought two wars with Iraq, in 1991 and beginning in 2003. In neither war were chemical weapons used, but Iraq's incontestable record of their use played a role in justifying these wars. In 1995, Iraq admitted to the United Nations its possession of nerve agents, as well as other chemical and biological weapons. A full accounting of the quantities admitted by Iraq has not been made.

In May 2004, two U.S. soldiers serving in Iraq were exposed to liquid sarin contained in a round that formed part of an improvised explosive device (IED). The round was most likely an old one from the Saddam Hussein era, and whoever placed it in the IED may not have known that it contained sarin. These two men are the only battlefield nerve agent casualties in U.S. history. Interestingly, they made the diagnosis themselves, presented promptly for care, and did well clinically, showing that U.S. military training on recognizing signs and symptoms is effective.

The Japanese religious cult Aum Shinrikyo (Divine Truth) used the nerve agent sarin twice in terrorist attacks. In 1994, the cult rigged up a spray tank on a vehicle that circled the apartment house in the city of Matsumoto, Japan, that served as temporary quarters for judges about to render an adverse judgment against the cult in Land Court. The judges survived this attack, but seven people died and there were almost 300 casualties. Six months later, in March 1995, the cult released sarin liquid in a 30% pure solution on three subway trains converging on Kasumigaseki Station, which sits under several government ministries in central Tokyo. Twelve people died and 5500 people sought medical attention, of whom only about 1000 were symptomatic. Several of the physicians who cared for these patients have published their experiences.[9] The accounts by patients, transcribed by novelist Haruki Murakami, are also highly recommended for insights into how people going about their daily business experience chemical terrorism.[10]

The United States signed the Chemical Weapons Convention in 1995, and it came into force in 1997.

Under its terms, all nations possessing certain chemical weapons, including nerve agents, agreed to destroy their stockpiles. Nerve agents, unlike anthrax and other biological agents, cannot simply be burned in the open but must be chemically destroyed in specially designed facilities. The United States has completed the destruction of its former overseas stockpile, originally housed in Okinawa and Germany, at a specially built plant on Johnston Atoll in the Pacific Ocean. The so-called continental stockpile of chemical warfare agents, maintained at eight sites in the United States, is gradually being destroyed at onsite plants. Rarely, cases of nerve agent poisoning occur among workers at the six sites housing old nerve agent munitions. These sites were located at Tooele, Utah; Umatilla, Oregon; Anniston, Alabama; Newport, Indiana; Pine Bluff, Arizona; and Richmond, Kentucky. The largest stockpile, at Tooele, has already been destroyed. The convention gives the United States 10 years to destroy all of its chemical munitions. The United States and Russia have successfully petitioned the Organization for the Prevention of Chemical Weapons, which oversees the convention, for permission to extend this deadline.

Iraq is the only country to have used nerve agents in warfare. It is not known how many other countries have clandestine programs involving these agents. Al-Qaeda and other terrorist groups have expressed interest in these agents. U.S. forces captured literature on nerve agents in Al-Qaeda sites in Afghanistan after the 2001 invasion.

PHYSICAL CHARACTERISTICS

Chemical weapons have both common chemical names and two-letter North Atlantic Treaty Organization (NATO) codes. The classical military nerve agents include tabun (GA), sarin (GB), soman (GD), cyclosarin (GF), and VX. Their structures are shown in Figure 56-1.

All classical nerve agents are liquids at standard temperature and pressure. The term "nerve gas" is wrong and arises from a historical misunderstanding. The first chemical warfare agents, World War I agents such as chlorine and phosgene, were true gases at standard temperature and pressure. As a result, popular accounts have tended to call all subsequently developed chemical weapons "poison gas." Clinicians must remember the liquid nature of nerve agents, because failure to recognize this may lead to inadequate treatment.

The nerve agents are claimed to be both tasteless and odorless. Data are understandably scant.

The liquid nerve agents are all spontaneously volatile; that is, they evaporate spontaneously at room temperature. In the Tokyo subway attack, liquid sarin was deliberately spilled out on the floor of subway cars. None of

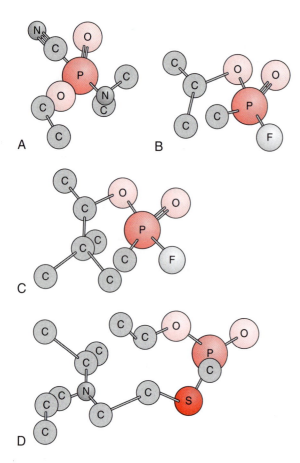

Figure 56-1. Molecular models of tabun (GA; *A*), sarin (GB; *B*), soman (GD; *C*), and VX *(D)*. (Courtesy of Offie E. Clark, U.S. Army Medical Research Institute of Chemical Defense, Aberdeen Proving Ground, Maryland.)

the affected patients actually came into physical contact with the liquid. They were affected by an evaporating nerve agent in the vapor phase.

G agents have the density of water and evaporate at about the same rate as water, freezing around 0°C and boiling around 150°C. A puddle of G agent outdoors probably evaporates in 24 hours, making these agents tactically "nonpersistent." VX, by contrast, is oily, with a consistency similar to that of motor oil, and evaporates slowly. Thus, although it poses less vapor hazard than the G agents, VX is tactically "persistent" and can contaminate an area far longer.

With the exception of certain polypeptide biological toxins, most notably botulinum, the nerve agents as a group are the most toxic substances known in biology. Toxicity data for poisons in the liquid or solid state are given by median lethal doses (LD$_{50}$s), the amount of the poison that would kill 50% of an exposed population. Toxicity data for vapors or aerosols are given by LCt_{50}s, the amount of the poison, measured as a product of

concentration × time, that would kill 50% of an exposed population. Data are given for the five classical nerve agents in Table 1. Mg × min/m^3 units are not familiar to most physicians. It may be more graphic to point out that an LD$_{50}$ of liquid VX would form a droplet just large enough to cover two columns on the Lincoln Memorial on the back of a U.S. penny.

PATHOPHYSIOLOGY

Like organophosphate insecticides, nerve agents act primarily as cholinesterase inhibitors. Antidotal blockade of cholinesterase inhibition by nerve agents saves exposed animals or patients, proving that this is the major pathophysiology of these agents, although they may have additional effects upon the nervous system. A recent mathematical analysis of data from multiple animal experiments supports this long-held view.[11] In summary, then, *nerve agents cause a life-threatening cholinergic crisis.*

It sometimes comes as a surprise to civilian physicians that all service members in NATO, most with no medical training, are nevertheless trained to recognize and to treat acute cholinergic crisis in themselves or in buddies. This is because the cholinergic crisis caused by nerve agents must be treated quickly and cannot wait until the patient reaches the care of a physician.[12,13]

The cholinergic system is the only neurotransmitter system in the nervous system that uses an enzymatic turn-off switch. To understand the pathophysiology of nerve agent poisoning, the clinician must recall that the cholinergic synapses, those using acetylcholine (ACh) as their neurotransmitter, carry the enzyme, acetylcholinesterase (AChE), on their postsynaptic membranes. AChE functions at cholinergic synapses as the turn-off switch for cholinergic transmission. It can be thought of as the governor that prevents cholinergic transmission from getting out of control. AChE blockade produces precisely this effect: uncontrolled cholinergic transmission.

Blockade of AChE, an enzyme with only one active site, by any of the organophosphates or nerve agents is essentially irreversible unless an oxime, a specific reactivator, is administered. AChE molecules inhibited by a nerve agent must be replaced by normal cell synthesis of AChE, which can take several months.

The cholinergic system classically divides into muscarinic and nicotinic synapses, named for the false neurotransmitters originally found to trigger them. Nerve agent poisoning turns all of these on, since AChE is the same in both major classes of synapses. Since antidotes work differentially, it is helpful to remember that certain cholinergic synapses, notably those in bronchial smooth muscle, exocrine neuroglandular synapses, and the vagus

Table 1: Chemical, Physical, Environmental, and Biological Properties of Nerve Agents

Properties	Tabun (GA)	Sarin (GB)	Soman (GD)	VX
CHEMICAL AND PHYSICAL				
Boiling point	230°C	158°C	198°C	298°C
Vapor pressure	0.037 mm Hg at 20°C	2.1 mm Hg at 20°C	0.40 mm Hg at 25°C	0.0007 mm Hg at 20°C
Density				
Vapor (compared to air)	5.6	4.86	6.3	9.2
Liquid	1.08 g/mL at 25°C	1.10 g/mL at 20°C	1.02 g/mL at 25°C	1.008 g/mL at 20°C
Volatility	610 mg/m^3 at 25°C	22,000 mg/m^3 at 25°C	3900 mg/m^3 at 25°C	10.5 mg/m^3 at 25°C
Appearance	Colorless to brown liquid	Colorless liquid	Colorless liquid	Colorless to straw-colored liquid
Odor	Fairly fruity	No odor	Fruity; oil of camphor	Odorless
Solubility				
In water	9.8 g/100 g at 25°C	Miscible	2.1 g/100 g at 20°C	Miscible < 9.4°C
In other solvents	Soluble in most organic solvents	Soluble in all solvents	Soluble in some solvents	Soluble in all solvents
ENVIRONMENTAL AND BIOLOGICAL				
Detectability				
Vapor	M8A1, M256A1, CAM, ICAD	M8A1, M256A1, CAM, ICAD	M8A1, M256A1, CAM, ICAD	M8A1, M256A1, CAM, ICAD
Liquid	M8, M9 papers	M8, M9 papers	M8, M9 papers	M8, M9 papers
Persistency				
In soil	Half-life: 1–1.5 days	2–24 hours at 5°C–25°C	Relatively persistent	2–6 days
On material	Unknown	Unknown	Unknown	Persistent
Decontamination of skin	M258A1, diluted hypochlorite, soap and water, M291 kit, RSDL	M258A1, diluted hypochlorite, soap and water, M291 kit, RSDL	M258A1, diluted hypochlorite, soap and water, M291 kit, RSDL	M258A1, diluted hypochlorite, soap and water, M291 kit, RSDL

Table 1: Chemical, Physical, Environmental, and Biological Properties of Nerve Agents—cont'd

Properties	Tabun (GA)	Sarin (GB)	Soman (GD)	VX
Biologically Effective Amount				
Vapor	LCt_{50}: 400 mg × min/m³	LCt_{50}: 100 mg × min/m³	LCt_{50}: 50 mg × min/m³	LCt_{50}: 10 mg × min/m³
Liquid	LD_{50} (skin): 1.0 g for a 70-kg man	LD_{50} (skin): 1.7 g for a 70-kg man	LD_{50} (skin): 350 mg for a 70-kg man	LD_{50} (skin): 10 mg for a 70-kg man

CAM, chemical agent monitor; ICAD, individual chemical agent detector; LCt_{50}, vapor or aerosol exposure necessary to cause death in 50% of the population exposed, LD_{50}, dose necessary to cause death in 50% of the population with skin exposure; M8 and M9, chemical detection papers; M8A1, chemical alarm system; M256A1, detection card; M258A1, self-decontamination kit; M291, decontamination kit; RSDL, reactive skin decontamination lotion.

nerve, are muscarinic whereas others, particularly sympathetic cholinergic synapses and skeletal neuromuscular junctions, are nicotinic. The brain has a roughly 9:1 mixture of cholinergic muscarinic and nicotinic synapses. The cholinergic system is the most widely distributed in human brain.

To understand how nerve agent poisoning works, it is helpful to consider two routes of exposure: exposure to vapor and exposure to liquid on the skin. The clinical syndromes differ in speed and order of symptoms; consequently, the treatment is somewhat different as well.

Exposure to nerve agent vapor is overwhelmingly more likely than exposure to liquid on the skin in both terrorist and battlefield scenarios. In this situation, the most vulnerable cholinergic synapses on the outside of the patient's body are those in the pupillary muscles, part of the parasympathetic nervous system. Small vapor molecules of a nerve agent pass unaltered through the cornea and interact directly with the pupillary muscle, causing miosis. It is hard to get significant vapor exposure without miosis. Patients complain of dim or blurred vision; about 10% may have nausea. In the Japanese subway attack, patients described looking at a cloudless sky and wondering why everything seemed dark.[10]

The next most accessible cholinergic synapses are those exocrine glands in the nose and mouth responsible for rhinorrhoea and salivation. These are the next symptoms to develop.

Once the patient inhales nerve agent vapor, exocrine glands in the respiratory passages pour excess secretions into those passages (bronchorrhea). Simultaneously, cholinergically innervated smooth muscle in respiratory passages constrict (bronchoconstriction). This causes respiratory distress strongly resembling that caused by an acute asthmatic attack.

Unhappily for the patient, however, the nerve agent easily crosses the alveolar–capillary barrier unchanged and enters the circulating blood from the lung. Blood passively carries the nerve agent everywhere in the body. For unclear reasons, the first symptoms tend to be gastrointestinal. Cholinesterase inhibition in the gastrointestinal tract causes parasympathetic hyperstimulation, leading to abdominal cramping, abdominal pain, nausea, vomiting, diarrhea, and increased bowel movements.

A bloodborne nerve agent more or less simultaneously causes cholinergic overstimulation in the heart and nervous system. Cardiac effects are unpredictable, because individuals possess their own balance of vagal and sympathetic inputs to the heart and muscarinic vagal inputs may cancel out nicotinic sympathetic inputs. In many patients there is an initial tachycardia, but this may not occur; in fact, either tachycardia or bradycardia, and either hypotension or hypertension, may occur.

In peripheral muscles, nerve agent poisoning causes cholinergic overload at neuromuscular junctions, which clinically manifests first as fasciculations and then as frank twitching, which moves joints. Untrained or even trained observers may mistake this clinical sign for grand mal seizures, and only an electroencephalogram can definitively distinguish them. Eventually, if twitching persists, adenosine triphosphate is depleted and the patient may develop flaccid paralysis. Crucially, in contrast to botulinum toxin, which causes flaccid paralysis early because of the failure of the presynaptic neuron to secrete ACh, nerve agents cause flaccid paralysis not initially but only after a period of overstimulation. The peripheral neuromuscular effect of a nerve agent can also worsen respiratory distress as the diaphragm becomes involved.

Nerve agent poisoning in the brain activates all cholinergic synapses essentially simultaneously. Since the cholinergic system is so widespread within the human brain, a large nerve agent challenge causes almost immediate loss of consciousness, effectively multicentric seizure activity, and then central apnea.

Death from nerve agent poisoning is almost always respiratory because of a combination of bronchorrhea and bronchospasm from direct muscarinic effects, central apnea from muscarinic and nicotinic effects in the brain, and paralysis of the muscles of respiration, notably the diaphragm, from direct nicotinic effects upon neuromuscular junction.

In a vapor challenge of sufficient magnitude, perhaps 0.5 LCt_{50} or higher, the sequence of symptoms can be so fast as to seem clinically simultaneous. Many patients have been described who, after a large vapor challenge, lost consciousness, seized, and developed all of the other symptoms essentially within seconds of exposure. In this situation, buddy aid becomes crucial, either on the battlefield or in a terrorist scenario where aid comes from the first responder.

Vapor nerve casualties, if removed from the source of contamination, or masked, and treated aggressively, either die or improve rapidly. Humans metabolize a circulating nerve agent quickly if it does not kill them. No depot effect is observed with vapor casualties.

The situation is quite different with the patient who gets a drop of liquid nerve agent on the skin. Some of the agent itself evaporates spontaneously. Nerve agents do not irritate skin, an important point in that patients do not, unless they suspect its presence, necessarily perform the most important decontaminating action, physical removal. That proportion that does not evaporate, varying according to temperature, humidity, and degree of skin moisture, retains its chemical integrity and begins its passage through the skin. It encounters and interacts with cholinergic synapses in a different order and tempo than nerve agent vapor. First, it encounters sweat glands in the skin, causing localized sweating, which may escape the patient's notice. Next, it travels through a subcutaneous layer, which varies from location to location in the body. For example, transit through this layer is much faster directly behind the ear than on the soles of the feet. In women the layer is thicker, and hence the transit time is elongated. In small children, the stratum corneum is much thinner, and transit time is reduced.[14] Beneath the skin, the agent encounters neuromuscular junctions in the underlying muscles, producing localized fasciculations that, again, may escape notice. Because muscle is well vascularized, the agent enters the bloodstream and goes systemic from the muscle, causing first gastrointestinal symptoms and then brain, smooth and skeletal muscle, heart, and respiratory symptoms. Only after all this does the nerve agent diffuse through the aqueous humors of the eye and involve the pupillary muscle, causing miosis to appear last.

The development of the full-blown cholinergic crisis after liquid-on-skin nerve agent challenge takes much longer than with vapor challenge. Even a lethal drop may require 30 minutes, rather than seconds, to manifest clinically, and a small, nonlethal drop may develop symptoms over 18 hours. As a result, if this route of exposure is suspected, the physician must treat longer and more aggressively than in uncomplicated vapor exposure, since the subcutaneous tissue forms a "depot" from which the agent is absorbed into the bloodstream and can cause symptoms for hours after exposure. Decontamination of the skin, if delayed more than a few minutes, does not catch all of the agent, and clinical symptoms must then be anticipated for hours after exposure.

Special mention must be made of a delayed neurobehavioral syndrome that has been seen non–dose dependently in a small proportion of nerve agent survivors. Some patients who have otherwise clinically recovered report new headache syndromes, difficulty sleeping, difficulty concentrating, mood disorders, and even changed personalities, lasting 3 to 6 weeks in most industrial cases but for several months in a few of the Tokyo survivors. This neurobehavioral syndrome overlaps with posttraumatic stress disorder and in some patients may be posttraumatic stress disorder.[15] The pathophysiology of this syndrome is not understood and may involve mild hypoxia or some other unspecified neurotoxicity of nerve agents.[16,17] Individual case reports have emphasized the treatment of symptoms with the expectation of full recovery.[18]

Before the Tokyo subway attack, it was assumed that few patients who had not been pretreated with a cholinesterase inhibitor, such as pyridostigmine bromide, which was given to troops in the 1991 Gulf War, would go into status epilepticus after nerve agent poisoning. This assumption proved to be false in Tokyo, where a small number of patients without a previous history of epilepsy went into prolonged seizures upon nerve agent vapor challenge.

LABORATORY DIAGNOSIS

In acute nerve agent poisoning, there is no time to await laboratory verification of the diagnosis. Laboratory diagnosis is most useful either in population screening, such as in workers at storage sites or research laboratories, or for forensic purposes to document past exposure to a cholinesterase inhibitor.

Since the actual site of action of a nerve agent is at tissue synapses, the gold standard would be to check the level of inhibition of synaptic cholinesterase. This is impractical, but good surrogates exist in circulating cholinesterases, of which the two most useful are plasma butyrylcholinesterase and red blood cell AChE. The latter is believed to be the best marker of past exposure to a cholinesterase inhibitor and forms the basis of commercially available kits used in agricultural workers exposed to pesticides. Unfortunately, patients vary enormously from day to day in their cholinesterase activity level, and interpretation of a single value without a baseline is problematic. In the U.S. Army, two baseline values drawn 14 days apart are required, and the standard for exposure to inhibitor is 10% reduction from the mean of the two baseline values.[19] The serum half-life of nerve agents is so short that no routinely available test for circulating nerve agents is available.

Blood for cholinesterase activity may be sent to the U.S. Army Medical Research Institute of Chemical Defense as a reference laboratory. See the ccc.apgea. army.mil Web site for a standard operating procedure for blood samples and the procedure for establishing chain of custody. The Centers for Disease Control and Prevention in Atlanta also has a reference laboratory.

DIFFERENTIAL DIAGNOSIS

Only two classes of chemical warfare or terrorist agents have the potential to cause a person not injured directly by the weapon suddenly to fall, lose consciousness, and seize. These are the nerve agents and the cyanides. Miosis is not usually seen in cyanide poisoning. While both can cause seizures, cyanide classically does not cause the huge increase in secretions seen in nerve agent poisoning. The cholinergic crisis seen in nerve agent poisoning is identical practically to that caused by insecticides or any other cholinesterase inhibitor; luckily, the treatment is identical, at least initially.

THERAPY

The five basic principles of nerve agent casualty treatment are (1) decontamination; (2) supportive care, particularly respiratory; two antidotal strategies, (3) anticholinergic and (4) oxime therapy; and (5) anticonvulsant therapy.[4,13]

Decontamination

Since decontamination is primarily the purview of the nonhospital responder, this vital subject is not discussed here at length. An important principle to emerge from animal studies[20] is that physical removal trumps all known decontamination solutions. In the civilian context, where water is not a limiting factor, copious amounts of water applied as quickly as possible are the preferred decontamination method, as long as it is accompanied by physical scrubbing.

In the Tokyo subway attack, all affected patients were exposed to vapor only. Patients were not disrobed before entering the hospital, and 10% of the emergency room staffs in some hospitals became miotic.[21] This was almost certainly due not to actual liquid contamination but to vapor that had become trapped in the patients' clothing, since the patients were not exposed to liquid sarin. Removing the patients' clothing would have avoided most of these symptoms in caregivers.

Supportive Care

Nerve agent casualties are most likely to die of respiratory distress. Intubation and oxygen may be required. The period of support is likely to be longer for liquid casualties than for vapor casualties. Mouth-to-mouth resuscitation should not be employed. The U.S. military fields a resuscitation device, individual, chemical, basically an Ambu bag fitted with a filter for a chemical agent, which is available for purchase by first responders.

It is important to point out that even in liquid casualties, for whom support is required longer than with vapor casualties, the period of support is far shorter than for the far *less* toxic organophosphate insecticides. This may seem counterintuitive, since insecticides are far less toxic by weight. The explanation lies in the much greater lipid solubility of insecticides, such as malathion and parathion. Patients poisoned with these agents off-gas insecticide for days and often require days of intensive care unit care with respiratory support. Because the military nerve agents are generally water soluble rather than lipid soluble, the period of support required is usually hours rather than days.

Isolated reports of patients from the Tokyo subway attack who failed to recover normal mental functioning highlight the real possibility of hypoxic encephalopathy complicating nerve agent poisoning. This reinforces the importance of respiratory support during the acute phase.[18]

Antidotal Therapy

The two antidotal strategies employed in nerve agent casualty care are synergistic and are used simultaneously.

Atropine

Atropine is an anticholinergic drug, similar to many in use, including scopolamine and trihexyphenidyl hydrochloride. It competes with ACh for the postsynaptic muscarinic receptor. A high-enough dose of atropine, even in the face of the huge excess of ACh produced by cholinergic crisis, prevents excess ACh from having deleterious effects by binding to the postsynaptic muscarinic receptor; it is as if even though there is too much ACh around it does not have its life-threatening effects.

Atropine does not work at nicotinic sites but can be life-saving because life-threatening effects, particularly respiratory, are mostly mediated by muscarinic synapses. Of all the anticholinergics in medicine, atropine has been universally adopted for this purpose because of its extremely good uptake via the IM route and its effectiveness over a huge temperature range. Field treatment is given via an IM autoinjector. In the United States, the IM autoinjector in the commonly fielded MARK 1 kit (used both by the military and by civilian agencies and fully U.S. Food and Drug Administration [FDA] approved; Figure 56-2) gives a dose of 2 mg of atropine. In 2003, pediatric doses of 0.5 and 1 mg were also approved; in 2004, a dose of 0.25 mg was approved.

The field doctrine in a severely nerve agent–poisoned adult is to use three autoinjectors or 6 mg of atropine to start and then to re-treat every 5 to 10 minutes. Re-treatment may be given either IM or IV. Figure 56-4 demonstrates the approved method of self-treatment using an autoinjector. No upper bound exists for atropine use. The endpoint for atropine administration should be the patient's ability to breathe comfortably on her or his own, without the complication of increased secretions. Do not use endpoints such as termination of miosis or cardiac status, which may mislead the treater.

Monotherapy with atropine has saved many patients. In the Iran–Iraq war, the Iranians had only limited amounts of oximes available at aid stations and no far-forward oxime therapy. They reported using much higher doses of atropine, sometimes as many as 50 to 100 mg at once in a severe casualty.[22] With good availability of oximes, U.S. doctrine states that probably only 15 to 20 mg of atropine will be necessary for a severe casualty, either IM or IV.

In a patient severely poisoned with a nerve agent who still has a beating heart, giving an IM atropine autoinjector before taking the time to intubate the patient is probably the best advice. Ventilation of a patient in with severe nerve agent poisoning probably is quite ineffective because of bronchospasm and bronchorrhea. Atropine, by contrast, works extremely quickly, within 1 minute in nonhuman primates, via the IM route.

Dosage recommendations for children are not universally accepted, but several have been proposed.[14,23]

To reduce by half the time needed to treat a casualty, the U.S. military has developed a dual-chamber autoinjector containing both atropine and the oxime 2-pralidoxime chloride (2-PAM Cl; Figure 56-3). Once this product, which the FDA has approved, is fielded, it will replace the MARK 1 autoinjector set. It contains an atropine dose of 2.1 mg.

Oximes

Oximes are a class of drugs that react with the AChE–nerve agent adduct. The result of this reaction is to cleave the nerve agent into two harmless and rapidly metabolized fragments, as well as to restore catalytic AChE activity. Since oximes, unlike atropine, react directly with AChE and not with the postsynaptic receptor, they work equally well, in theory, at both nicotinic and muscarinic sites.

Unlike the universal use of atropine, oximes vary by country. Most of Europe uses obidoxime (Toxogonin), manufactured in Germany by Merck. Iran used obidoxime in small quantities in caring for Iraq War casualties in 1984 to 1987. Obidoxime is not licensed in the United States,

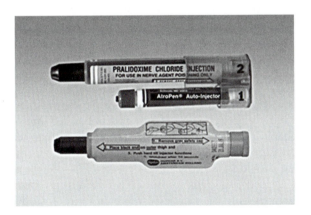

Figure 56-2. MARK 1 set as presently fielded, containing two autoinjectors. Autoinjector 1 contains 2 mg of atropine sulfate. Autoinjector 2 contains 600 mg of 2-pralidoxime chloride. Convulsive antidote for nerve agent autoinjector contains 10 mg of diazepam. Note its distinctive contour, which can be easily differentiated from the MARK 1 autoinjectors in low light conditions. (Courtesy of the Chemical Casualty Care Division, U.S. Army Medical Research Institute of Chemical Defense, Aberdeen Proving Ground, Edgewood Area, Maryland.)

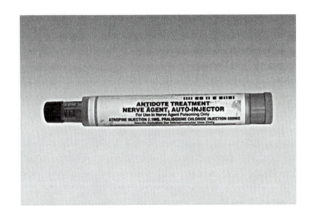

Figure 56-3. Autoinjector treatment nerve agent antidote containing 2.1 mg of atropine sulfate and 600 mg of 2-pralidoxime chloride. (Courtesy of the Chemical Casualty Care Division, U.S. Army Medical Research Institute of Chemical Defense, Aberdeen Proving Ground, Edgewood Area, Maryland.)

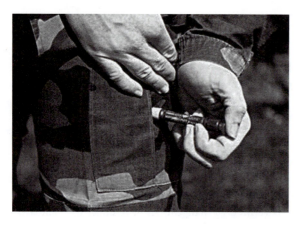

Figure 56-4. Autoinjector in use. (Courtesy of the Chemical Casualty Care Division, U.S. Army Medical Research Institute of Chemical Defense, Aberdeen Proving Ground, Edgewood Area, Maryland.)

partially because its synthesis involves a carcinogenic intermediate. In the United States, the licensed oxime is 2-PAM Cl. Israel uses TMB-4, another oxime developed in the United States but not licensed here. Canada presently uses 2-PAM Cl, but the Canadian Forces have petitioned to replace it with the Hagedorn oxime, HI-6. Japan uses 2-PAM iodide, rather than 2-PAM Cl, largely for cultural reasons; in Japan, the high baseline rate of thyroid disease predisposes physicians to treat with iodides where possible. 2-PAM iodide was used in Tokyo.

In the United States, 2-PAM Cl is usually found only at poison control centers. The 2-PAM Cl injector in the MARK 1 kit contains 600 mg of 2-PAM Cl. No pediatric injector has been fielded. The loading dose can be up to three MARK 1 kits, or 1800 mg of 2-PAM Cl. At doses of 2000 mg or greater (IM or IV), there is a substantial chance of triggering dangerous hypertension, so the rule in U.S. doctrine is not to give more than 1800 mg via autoinjector or 2000 mg IV per hour.[24] If treatment must be continued during that time, atropine alone is used. Pediatric use of 2-PAM Cl is IV in children too small to be treated with the autoinjector.[14] The 2-PAM Cl dose in the dual-chambered autoinjector is unchanged at 600 mg.

All oximes have the same limitation, a side reaction misleadingly titled "aging," that greatly constrains their use. After the nerve agent has bound to AChE, unless it is reactivated by oxime, and after a characteristic period has elapsed, the nerve agent moiety loses a side chain. The result is to charge the remaining complex negatively. Oximes cannot reactivate negatively charged complexes. The effect of the aging side reaction is to render oximes unable to reactivate AChE.

In the case of some nerve agents, the aging side reaction is so slow that it can be ignored clinically. For instance, VX, while the most toxic of the group, ages with a $t\frac{1}{2}$ of at least 22 days. Since the patient will probably die within minutes, this is only of academic interest. Sarin's aging $t\frac{1}{2}$ is 3 to 4 hours, tabun's is 13 to 14 hours, and soman's, the shortest, only 2 minutes.[25] Thus, if a rapidly aging agent such as soman were used, the patient would, in theory, gain nothing from oxime therapy unless the patient was treated within minutes. The United States and other countries have ongoing efforts to replace 2-PAM with more effective AChE reactivators, but none was close to FDA approval at the time of writing.[26–28]

Anticonvulsant Therapy

Nerve agent–induced status epilepticus does not respond to the usual anticonvulsants used for status. Animal experiments have clearly shown that these seizures do not stop without industrial-strength doses of phenytoin, phenobarbital, lamotrigine, carbamazepine, or valproic acid.[29,30] The reason for this may lie in the wide anatomical distribution of the cholinergic system within human brain. Effectively, status in nerve agent poisoning is extremely multicentric, and thus drugs that work, at least partly, by dampening the spread of seizure discharges are ineffective. Although anticholinergic medications are actually anticonvulsants in animal models of nerve agent–induced seizures, they only retain this activity temporarily, for about 20 minutes in guinea pigs, presumably because other neurotransmitter systems are recruited.[31–33]

The only class of anticonvulsant drugs effective in nerve agent–induced seizures is benzodiazepines. Since the U.S. military must only use FDA-approved drugs on-label (for the approved indications), it can only use a benzodiazepine for nerve agent–induced seizures that carries the indication for seizures, and the only benzodiazepine so labeled is diazepam. For this reason, the U.S. military fields 10-mg autoinjectors of diazepam (labeled as CANA, convulsive antidote for nerve agent), to all of its service members. Animal studies have shown that for full-blown nerve agent status epilepticus 10 mg will probably not suffice. Extrapolation to the human leads us to expect that the actual anticonvulsant dose of diazepam should be 30 to 40 mg.

Licensed physicians are not constrained to use benzodiazepines only for their on-label indication. A study of the entire benzodiazepine class has shown that the member of this class that stops the seizures fastest and at the lowest blood level administered IM, against all of the nerve agents, is midazolam.[32,34] Midazolam may even work via the nasal route.[35] The U.S. military has asked the FDA to consider on-label indication for midazolam against seizures, and an FDA-ordered Phase I clinical trail for safety is ongoing at the time of writing. For a civilian physician, it is best to remember that all benzodiazepines are effective and that midazolam is probably the best based upon animal data, although not specifically approved for this use.

In any event, it has been shown in animal models that stopping seizures in nerve agent poisoning are crucial for preventing neuronal loss, which can proceed either through apoptotic or through frankly necrotic pathways.[36] It may well be necessary to check the electroencephalogram of the patient emergently to make sure that seizures are not continuing, masked by flaccid paralysis. Once the patient is in the hospital and proper respiratory control has been established, it is probably safer to overmedicate with anticonvulsant than to undermedicate, although clinical experience with this condition is fragmentary.

In certain animal models, evidence shows that adding an anticholinergic drug to benzodiazepines may be synergistic.[37] This has not so far been adopted into acute human treatment protocols.

A recent study has shown that having atropine on board can lower the required dose of anticonvulsant, indicating that anticonvulsant is a synergistic antidote in nerve agent poisoning.[38]

CHRONIC NEUROLOGICAL SEQUELAE

Attention has classically focused upon the acute treatment of nerve agent poisoning, for the good reason that immediate treatment is the only thing that will save the patient's life. The UN team invited to Iran to document chemical weapons use by Iraq probably underestimated the impact of the nerve agents precisely because, by the time the UN team arrived, the nerve agent casualties were largely either dead or well.[3]

A review of the follow-up studies done on victims of the Tokyo sarin attack, including data up to 10 years after exposure, showed minor or no performance decrements in survivors. The one consistent finding was posttraumatic stress disorder.[39] In another retrospective review, the incidence of posttraumatic stress disorder was estimated as 8%.[40] Yet a third review of Japanese survivors found significant psychomotor and memory function deficits 7 years after exposure.[41] Perhaps the best summary at this point is that there is good evidence of neuropsychological dysfunction up to years after exposure, but how much of this is organic and how much is functional is still unclear.

Another recent review of neuroimaging studies of Tokyo sarin attack survivors suggested significant atrophy in the area of the insular cortex can result from exposure; the authors conjectured that this might lead to "greater subjective awareness of internal bodily status."[42]

There is no indication that survivors of nerve agent poisoning who have seized are at any greater risk for epilepsy than the general population, although data are fragmentary.[43]

There is likewise no indication that survivors of nerve agent poisoning are at increased risk of neuromuscular problems. One patient who survived the Tokyo attack has had documented neuropathy,[44] but causality is not proven.

As mentioned earlier, a portion of nerve agent survivors complain of nonspecific neurobehavioral changes, in some cases allegedly lasting for months. In some studies, this actually affected most patients. Most of the data come from the 1950s, when offensive munitions were still being tested. In one series of accidental exposures,[45] 51% of patients accidentally exposed to small doses of sarin or tabun (49 patients, 53 exposures) reported CNS effects ranging from sleep disturbances to mood changes and easy fatigueability. In another series of 72 workers exposed accidentally to sarin, 16 reported difficulty in concentration, mental confusion, giddiness, or insomnia.[46] Series like these could not be replicated today with modern imaging techniques. This appears to be idiosyncratic, not dose related, and may overlap with posttraumatic stress disorder. Recent animal studies, however, suggest that exposure to low doses of nerve agents can cause delayed behavioral change if stress is a factor at the time of exposure,[47] which may partly explain the link between psychological and physiological components.

The most significant long-term neurological effect of nerve agent exposure is hypoxic encephalopathy, which complicates nerve agent exposure because of the respiratory depression seen in nerve agent poisoning. Dissecting how much of the neuropathological picture seen in nerve agent exposure is due to hypoxic encephalopathy is extremely difficult.

It was previously thought that nerve agent intoxication in humans would produce only short-lived convulsions.[48,49] In the Tokyo subway attack, however, a few patients were found to seize clinically for prolonged periods after exposure.[50] The possibility of lasting status epilepticus added to hypoxic encephalopathy makes it even more difficult to distinguish between nerve agent direct toxicity to the brain, hypoxic encephalopathy, and status as causative in neurological dysfunction.

A patient who has survived a nerve agent attack is presumably at greater risk for severe problems in a subsequent exposure to a cholinesterase inhibitor because of the time that it takes for synapses to replace AChE. In one Tokyo survivor, the circulating red blood cell AChE level did not return to normal for 6 months.[17] This is particularly relevant for military members and for civilian first responders who might be at increased risk for reexposure.

PYRIDOSTIGMINE BROMIDE

During the late 1980s, the U.S. military increasingly worried about rapidly aging nerve agents such as soman. It was known that Iraq was then interested in obtaining the starting materials for the synthesis of soman, although Iraq had not used soman during the 1984 to 1987 war with Iran. Animal studies showed that, in the case of soman, the MARK 1 autoinjector kit containing atropine and 2-PAM Cl would not confer sufficient protection for a soldier exposed to soman because of the rapid aging of this toxin. Within 10 minutes after exposure, or five half-lives, one of the two legs of this standard treatment, oxime, would be rendered useless by aging.

To solve this problem, the military turned to the carbamate pyridostigmine, a reversible cholinesterase inhibitor. It had a long safety record, having been approved by the FDA for myasthenia gravis as far back as 1951. Because humans have a large excess of AChE, the reasoning went, if there were a strong likelihood of exposure to a rapid-aging nerve agent, pretreatment with enough pyridostigmine reversibly to inhibit a fraction of the AChE would allow a soldier to survive what would have been a lethal challenge of the agent. That AChE fraction would be unavailable for the agent to inhibit permanently and would come available if the patient were supported through the clinical crisis by the standard antidotes. Animal data were submitted to the FDA in 1991 showing that the protective ratio against soman was increased from 1.6 to 40 using pyridostigmine pretreatment. On the basis of this data, the FDA waived informed consent. Consequently, the military was able to order 100,000 coalition forces to take pyridostigmine bromide in the 1991 Gulf War. The data underlying this choice and the resultant side effect profile reported by unit physician assistants are summarized.[24] The waiver was withdrawn in 1992. In 2003, with a new war with Iraq looming, the FDA approved pyridostigmine for the specific purpose of pretreatment against soman. In the 2003 war with Iraq, pyridostigmine was present in theater but was not used. In the event of a war with an adversary equipped with a rapidly aging nerve agent, it is U.S. and NATO doctrine to issue pyridostigmine.

The dose of pyridostigmine usually taken in myasthenia is 60 mg every 8 hours and may go much higher. The nerve agent pretreatment dose is 30 mg every 8 hours. Once the patient has been exposed to the nerve agent, pyridostigmine is contraindicated. Pyridostigmine does not obviate the need for the standard antidotes; it merely converts what would have been a dead patient into a living but sick patient.

In general, pyridostigmine is a countermeasure strictly for battlefield use. Only a few civilian first-responder agencies have looked into making it available to their members, and none has mandated it.

NEUROPROTECTION

The microscopic damage caused to brain tissue by nerve agents resembles ischemic penumbra; the clinician sees both necrotic and apoptotic neurons. This superficial similarity stimulated interest in adapting neuroprotectants for a patient who has survived nerve agent exposure, to optimize the eventual neurological recovery. None of the neuroprotectants so far investigated is yet established for this indication.

Preliminary work has shown proof of concept using the experimental drug HU-211 or dexanabinol, a nonpsychotropic analogue of tetrahydrocannabinol.[51] In a rat model, dexanabinol reduced the size of the lesion produced in highly cholinergic cortex by 90% after exposure to a high dose of soman and subsequent status epilepticus. Unfortunately, dexanabinol could not exert this effect in thalamus. Dexanabinol is now under development as a neuroprotectant for head trauma. Dantrolene, a ryanodine agonist commonly used against malignant hyperthermia, synergized with diazepam in the same rat model.[52]

More recently, ketamine, a commonly used anesthetic agent that has proven to be protective in models of cardiac ischemia, has been shown to reduce the cross-sectional area of damage in soman exposures when combined with diazepam.[53]

BIOSCAVENGERS

A substantial research effort is under way in the medical chemical defense community to develop a circulating bioscavenger. Such a compound, either a human cholinesterase molecule or an altered human cholinesterase with one or two amino acids substituted so as to alter the active site, would detoxify the nerve agent entering a patient's circulation so that it would not be able to reach the tissue AChE and produce clinical symptoms. Several putative bioscavengers have been shown effective against multiple LD_{50}s of many nerve agents in animal models, including both rodents and nonhuman primates.[54]

No less than three bioscavenger efforts are under way. An investigational new drug application has already been submitted to the FDA on a plasma-derived butyrylcholinesterase.[55] Closely behind that product, which will be extremely expensive to produce, a recombinant butyrylcholinesterase raised in transgenic goats is also in development.[56] These two products detoxify the nerve agent on a stoichiometric basis; one enzyme molecule kills one nerve agent molecule. A more effective product would be a catalytic bioscavenger, killing multiple nerve agent molecules per enzyme molecule. Such a bioscavenger will most likely be a modified human enzyme with site-directed mutagenesis altering its active site. Several candidates have been shown to detoxify multiple LD_{50}s in multiple animal species.

USE OF A FIELD SEIZURE MONITOR

The clinical situation of a nerve agent survivor who has been saved from death by poisoning by the timely and judicious administration of antidotes as already described concerns military and civilian planners. Specifically, a patient who is no longer in respiratory distress, breathing comfortably on his or her own without increased secretions, may have still greatly abnormal mental status. Potential causes of diminished mental status may include hypoxia or postictal state, for which further administration of anticonvulsants would be relatively contraindicated. But the reason might also be that the patient remains in electrical status epilepticus, certainly a possibility if the level of adenosine triphosphate in the patient's muscles has diminished to the point that visible twitching is no longer seen. In this situation, timely administration of more anticonvulsant, which first responders have available, may be helpful. To distinguish these clinical situations, two programs are under way, one as a Small Business Innovative Research program under the U.S. Army and a second one sponsored by the National Institute of Neurological Disorders and Stroke, which are collectively funding four American companies to develop field seizure detectors. If successful, these items will be regulated as medical devices by the FDA. Once they are marketed, they may be useful not only to first responders dealing with nerve agent casualties but also to out-of-hospital seizure patients and possibly to head trauma patients.

CONCLUSION

Since nerve agents primarily target the nervous system, nonneurologists turn to their neurologist colleagues for expertise when the time comes to plan for a response to an attack using these agents. Battlefield experience clearly demonstrates that understanding the basic principles of treatment and assuring that enough antidotes are rapidly available in the event of a release can save many lives.

WHERE TO GO FOR INFORMATION

Most standard references, including treatment protocols, and a procedure for processing biological samples for the nation's reference laboratory, are available at the Chemical Casualty Care Division Web site, ccc.apgea.army.mil. References 4, 12, 13, and 25 are all available in their entirety. Non-U.S. government clinicians and agencies are welcome to use this Web site but must register to gain access to the reference materials. If you will have an acute need to access this material, you are strongly encouraged to register in advance. Clinical advice may be obtained from the U.S. Army Medical Research Institute of Chemical Defense 24 hours a day at (410) 436-3276.

DISCLAIMER

The opinions herein expressed are solely those of the author and not necessarily those of the U.S. Department of Defense, the U.S. Department of the Army, or the Joint Program Executive Office for Chemical/Biological Defense.

This paper is an update of previously published material (Newmark J. Nerve agents. *Neurol Clin.* 2005; 23:623–641). This material appears courtesy of the permission of the editor, Michael Dobbs.

REFERENCES

Note: The standard reference textbook, *Textbook of Military Medicine: Chemical and Biological Warfare,* from which references 4 and 25 are drawn, will be replaced in 2009 with a new and revised edition. It is in press at the Government Printing Office. When it is available, it will also be available on the Chemical Casualty Care Division Web site given earlier.

1. Gunderson CH, Lehmann CR, Sidell FR, Jabbari B. Nerve agents: a review. *Neurology.* 1992;42:946–950.
2. Yokoyama K, Yamada A, Nobuhide M. Clinical profiles of patients with sarin poisoning after the Tokyo subway attack. *Am J Med.* 1996;100:586.
3. Foroutan SA. Medical notes on chemical warfare, part I–XI. *Kowsar Med J.* 1996–1999;1(1)–4(1). (Original in Farsi.)
4. Sidell FR. Nerve agents. In: Sidell FR, Takafuji ET, Franz DR. *Medical Aspects of Chemical and Biological Warfare.* In: Zajtchuk R, Bellamy RF, eds. *Textbook of Military Medicine.* Washington, DC: U.S. Department of the Army Office of the Surgeon General and the Borden Institute; 1997.
5. Pelletiere SC, Johnson DV. *Lessons Learned: The Iran–Iraq War.* Carlisle Barracks, Pa: Strategic Studies Institute, U.S. Army War College; 1991.

6. Cordesman AH, Wagner AP. *The Lessons of Modern War.* vol 2: The Iran–Iraq War. Boulder, Colo: Westview Press; 1990.

7. Dingeman A, Jupa R. Chemical warfare in the Iran–Iraq conflict. *Strategy Tactics Mag.* 1987;113:51–52.

8. Barnaby F. Iran–Iraq War: the use of chemical weapons against the Kurds. *Ambio.* 1988;17:407–408.

9. Okumura T, Takasu N, Ishimatsu S, et al. Report on 640 victims of the Tokyo subway sarin attack. *Ann Emerg Med.* 1996;28:129–135.

10. Murakami H. *Underground.* P. Gabriel, trans. New York: Vintage Books; 2001.

11. Maxwell DM, Brecht KM, Koplovitz I, Sweeney RE. Acetylcholinesterase inhibition: does it explain the toxicity of organophosphorus compounds? *Arch Toxicol.* 2006;80(11):756–760.

12. Departments of the Army, Navy, and Air Force, and Commandant, Marine Corps. Field Manual: Treatment of Chemical Agent Casualties and Conventional Military Chemical Injuries. Serial Nos. Army FM 8-285, Navy NAVMED P-5041, Air Force AFJMAN 44-149, and Marine Corps FMFM 11-11. Washington, DC; December 1995. [A new version is in preparation but has not yet been promulgated.]

13. Chemical Casualty Care Division, U.S. Army Medical Research Institute of Chemical Defense. *Medical Management of Chemical Casualties Handbook,* 3rd ed. Aberdeen Proving Ground, Md; July 2000.

14. Rotenberg JS, Newmark J. Nerve agent attacks on children: diagnosis and management. *Pediatrics.* 2003;112:648–658; 22(4):239–244.

15. Kawana N, Ishimatsu S, Kanda K. Psychophysiological effects of the terrorist sarin attack on the Tokyo subway system. *Mil Med.* 2001;166(Suppl 2):23–26.

16. Murata K, Araki S, Yokoyama K, et al. Asymptomatic sequelae to acute sarin poisoning in the central and autonomic nervous system six months after the Tokyo subway attack. *J Neurol.* 1997;244:601–606.

17. McDonough JH. Performance effects of nerve agents and their pharmacological countermeasures. *Mil Psychol.* 2002;14:93–119.

18. Hatta K et al. Amnesia from sarin poisoning. *Lancet.* 1996;347:1343.

19. Evans ES, Olds KL, Weyandt TB. Pesticides. In: Deeter DP, Gaydos JC, eds. *Occupational Health: The Soldier and the Industrial Base.* In: Zajtchuk R, Bellamy RF, eds. *Textbook of Military Medicine.* Washington, DC: U.S. Department of the Army Office of the Surgeon General and Borden Institute; 1993:532–536.

20. Van Hooidonk C, Ceulen BI, Bock J, van Generen J. Chemical warfare agents and the skin: penetration and decontamination. Proceedings of the International Symposium on Protection against Chemical Warfare Agents, June 6–9, 1983, Stockholm, Sweden, pp 153–160.

21. Rodgers JC. Chemical incident planning: a review of the literature. *Accid Emerg Nurs.* 1998; 6:155–159.

22. Newmark J. The birth of nerve agent warfare: lessons from Syed Abbas Foroutan. *Neurology.* 2003;60(Suppl 1):A87–A88.

23. Foltin G, Tunik M, Curran J, et al. Pediatric nerve agent poisoning: medical and operational considerations for emergency medical services in a large American city. *Pedatr Emerg Care.* 2006;22(4):239–244.

24. Sidell FR. Clinical considerations in nerve agent intoxication. In: Somani SM, ed. *Chemical Warfare Agents.* New York: Academic Press; 1992:181.

25. Dunn MA, Hackley BE, Sidell FR. Pretreatment for nerve agent exposure. In: Sidell FR, Takafuji ET, Franz DR. *Medical Aspects of Chemical and Biological Warfare.* In: Zajtchuk R and Bellamy RF, eds. *Textbook of Military Medicine.* Washington, DC: U.S. Department of the Army Office of the Surgeon General and Borden Institute; 1997:181–196.

26. Kuca K, Cabal J, Kassa J, Jun D, Hrabinova M. A comparison of the potency of the oxime HLo-7 and currently used oximes (HI-6, pralidoxime, obidoxime) to reactivate nerve agent–inhibited rat brain acetylcholinesterase by in vitro methods. *Acta Medica (Hradec Kralove).* 2005;48:81–86.

27. Kuca K, Juna D, Musilek K. Structural requirements of cholinesterase reactivators. *Mini Rev Med Chem.* 2006;6:269–277.

28. Worek F, Szinicz L, Thiermann H. Estimation of oxime efficacy in nerve agent poisoning: a kinetic approach. *Chem Biol Interact.* 2005;157–158:349–352.

29. Shih T, McDonough JH, Koplovitz I. Anticonvulsants for soman-induced seizure activity. *J Biomed Sci.* 1999;6:86–96.

30. McDonough JH, Benjamin A, McMonagle JD, Rowland T, Shih TM. Effects of fosphenytoin on nerve agent–induced status epilepticus. *Drug Chem Toxicol.* 2004;27(1):27–39.

31. Shih TM, McDonough JH. Neurochemical mechanisms in soman-induced seizures. *J Appl Toxicol.* 1997;17:255–264.

32. McDonough J, McMonagle J, Copeland T, Zoeffel D, Shih T-M. Comparative evaluation of benzodiaepines for control of soman-induced seizures. *Arch Toxicol.* 1999;73:473–478.

33. McDonough JH Jr, Zoeffel LD, McMonagle J, Copeland TL, Smith CD, Shih TM. Anticonvulsant treatment of nerve agent seizures: anticholinergics versus diazepam in soman-intoxicated guinea pigs. *Epilepsy Res.* 2000;38(1):1–14.

34. Capacio BR, Byers CE, Merk KA, Smith JR, McDonough JH. Pharmacokinetic studies of intramuscular midazolam in guinea pigs challenged with soman. *Drug Chem Toxicol.* 2004;27(2):95–110.

35. Gilat E, Kadar T, Levy A, et al. Anticonvulsant treatment of sarin-induced seizures with nasal midazolam: an electrographic, behavioral, and histological study in freely moving rats. *Toxicol Appl Pharmacol.* 2005;209(1):74–85.

36. Shih TM, Duniho SM, McDonough JH. Control of nerve agent–induced seizures is critical for neuroprotection and survival. *Toxicol Appl Pharmacol.* 2003;188:69–80.

37. Koplovitz I, Schulz S, Shutz M, et al. Combination anticonvulsant treatment of soman-induced seizures. *J Appl Toxicol.* 2001;21(Suppl 1):S53–S55.

38. Shih TM, Rowland TC, McDonough JH. Anticonvulsants for nerve agent–induced seizures: the influence of the therapeutic dose of atropine. *J Pharmacol Exp Ther.* 2007;320:154–161.

39. Hoffman A, Eisenkraft A, Finkelstein A, Schein O, Rotman E, Duschnitsky T. A decade after the Tokyo sarin attack: a review of neurological follow-up of the victims. *Mil Med.* 2007;172:607–610.

40. Yanagisawa N, Morita H, Nakajima T. Sarin experiences in Japan: acute toxicity and long-term effects. *J Neurol Sci.* 2006;249:76–85.

41. Miyaki K, Nishiwaki Y, Maekawa K, et al. Effects of sarin on the nervous system of subway workers seven years after the Tokyo subway sarin attack. *J Occup Health.* 2005;47:299–304.

42. Yamasue H, Abe O, Kasai K, et al. Human brain structural change related to acute single exposure to sarin. *Ann Neurol.* 2007;61:37–46.

43. Duffy FH, Burchfiel JL, Bartels PH, Gaon M, Sim VM. Long-term effects of an organophosphate upon the human electroencephalogram. *Toxicol Appl Pharmacol.* 1979;47:161–176.

44. Himuro K, Murayama S, Nishiyama K, et al. Distal sensory axonopathy after sarin intoxication. *Neurology.* 1998;51(4):1195–1197.

45. Craig AB, Freeman G. Clinical Observations on Workers Accidentally Exposed to "G" Agents. Medical Laboratory Research Report 154. Edgewood Arsenal, Md: Medical Research Laboratory; 1953.

46. Brody BB, Gammill JF. Seventy-five Cases of Accidental Nerve Gas Poisoning at Dugway Proving Ground. Medical Investigational Branch Special Report 5. Dugway Proving Ground, Utah: Medical Investigational Branch; 1954.

47. Mach M, Grubbs RD, Price WA. Delayed behavioral and endocrine effects of sarin and stress exposure in mice. *J Appl Toxicol.* 2008;28(2):132–139.

48. Sidell FR. Soman and sarin: clinical manifestations and treatment of accidental poisoning by organophosphates. *Clin Toxicol.* 1974;7:1–17.

49. Grob D. The manifestations and treatment of poisoning due to nerve agents and other organic phosphate anticholinesterase compounds. *Arch Intern Med.* 1956;98:221–239.

50. Ohbu S, Yamashina A, Takasu N, et al. Sarin poisoning on Tokyo subway. *South Med J.* 1997;90:587–592.

51. Filbert MG, Forster JS, Smith CD, Ballough GP. Neuroprotective effects of HU-211 on brain damage resulting from soman-induced seizures. *Ann NY Acad Sci.* 1999:890:505–514.

52. Newmark J, Ballough GPH, Filbert MG. Dantrolene plus diazepam: a viable strategy for neuroprotection following soman-induced status epilepticus. *Neurology.* 2003;60(Suppl 1):A385.

53. Newmark J, Ballough GPH, Kan RK, Filbert MG. Pathology associated with nerve agent–induced seizures is greatly reduced by ketamine plus diazepam, a potential nerve agent neuroprotectant regimen. *Neurology.* 2007;68(Suppl 1):A379.

54. Cerasoli DM, Lenz DE. Nerve agent bioscavengers: protection with reduced behavioral effects. *Mil Psychol.* 2002;14:121–143.

55. Lenz DE, Maxwell DM, Koplovitz I, et al. Protection against soman or VX poisoning by human butyrylcholinesterase in guinea pigs and cynomolgus monkeys. *Chem Biol Interact.* 2005;157–158:205–210.

56. Cerasoli DM, Griffiths EM, Doctor BP, et al. In vitro and in vivo characterization of recombinant human butyrylcholinesterase (Protexia) as a potential nerve agent bioscavenger. *Chem Biol Interact.* 2005;157–158:363–365.

Human Incapacitants

Peter G. Blain

INTRODUCTION

An incapacitant reduces or abolishes the ability to perform an action or achieve a task. Until recently, the use of incapacitating agents was primarily in a military context but an expanding range of less-lethal technologies are being introduced for use by civil agencies in crowd control and dispersion or to render a single individual incapable of an aggressive response during a policing operation. Chemicals or drugs may be regarded as classical incapacitating agents, but partly because of the inherent delay with their onset of action, other more instant–acting technologies have been developed.[1] These include the discharge of an electrical charge into the body (e.g., the Taser) or the rapid transfer of kinetic energy to the body from the impact of a ballistic round (e.g., the plastic baton round or "rubber bullet"). The latter may also be used to deliver a personalized aerosol dose of a chemical or drug. Debate is ongoing about whether incapacitants contravene the Chemical Weapons Convention or are excluded as domestic law enforcement methods.[2]

The term *nonlethal* was initially applied to these devices but, as with any pharmacological agent, the level of effect required to incapacitate inevitably is lethal in some individuals. Consequently, reference to *less-lethal*

technologies is more realistic. The ideal incapacitant does not, and probably never will, exist.[3–5]

Rather than focus only on methods or chemicals that produce major incapacitation, such as loss of consciousness, behavioral change, or the capacity for voluntary action, techniques to disrupt specific abilities have also been developed. The human senses are obvious targets for disruption, and laser dazzling, auditory hyperstimulation, skin and mucous membrane irritation, and malodourants have all been trialed. Low-frequency noise or microwave heating has also been tested for crowd control.

In this chapter, chemical and drug incapacitants are primarily considered, although reference to other technologies is made.

PROPERTIES OF AN INCAPACITANT

An ideal incapacitant would have some of the following attributes:

- Rapidly produces total incapacitation, or disruption of a specific capability, in an individual or group
- Is reversible in time, or by specific treatment, without any residual adverse effects

- Produces predictable effects with little variation in extent or nature
- Does not compromise the survival or safety of an unattended incapacitated individual
- Is capable of deployment and targeted delivery

In many civilian situations, incapacitants (or less-lethal technologies) are now regarded as the preferred alternative to lethal force, occupying a position in the escalation of response between physical restraint and shooting. Increased use of the technologies demands that they are safe; otherwise, they will not be a credible option.

TYPES OF INCAPACITANTS

Most incapacitants are designed to alter the voluntary functioning of the body, causing loss of purposeful movement, directed thought, or conscious awareness. Consequently, drugs or chemicals (such as 3-quinuclidinyl benzilate, described later) that affect the nervous system are seen as the ideal, and these are discussed here in detail. However, other nonpharmacological or toxicological approaches have also been developed.

PHYSICAL INCAPACITANTS

Light

Rapidly flashing lights are known to produce a feeling of mild disorientation and unsteadiness. Indeed, a specific frequency (around 14 Hz) may induce seizures in predisposed individuals. Very high–intensity oscillating light can affect visual feedback coordination, and a sudden high-intensity flash, especially if accompanied by a similarly high-intensity bang, momentarily incapacitates by disorientation. This effect underlies the use of stun grenades (also known as flash bangs). More recently the capability of some lasers to produce dazzle has been used in battlefield weapons, but the potential irreversibility of retinal damage should limit the development of this technology.[6,7]

Handheld lasers can also be used to produce spot burning on the skin.

Noise

Loud or continuous white noise has been used to disorientate or facilitate interrogation. Although noise is distracting, only at high or low frequency can it be specifically incapacitating. A commercial device, available to the public in the United Kingdom, emits a high-frequency noise at 75 dB, which is irritating to teenagers but not older (over 25 years of age) people (the opposite effect to that from teenage music). The device has been especially popular with shopkeepers wishing to prevent or disperse groups of young people gathering around shop entrances and causing a "nuisance."

Very low–frequency sound waves (infrasonic) are capable of producing unpleasant abdominal pain, in particular, if specifically focused on an individual.

Microwaves

Microwaves produce a heating effect when directed onto tissue. Targeted microwaves have been trialed for dispersing crowds by causing sudden sharp pain on skin, but the potential risks with microwaves are considerable. For example, the effect of microwave irradiation on the human lens may result in cataract formation, and the heating effect may damage sensitive cells in the nervous system, gastrointestinal tract, etc.

Obnoxious Odors

Humans find some smells instinctively repellent, and this response has been trialed as a repelling dissuader rather than an incapacitant. Mercaptan and indole derivatives have an obnoxious smell and do cause revulsion, and even nausea, in exposed individuals. Most people take avoidance action, so this is not regarded as a real incapacitant but rather a repellent.[8]

Taser

The Taser (Thomas A. Swift's electric rifle) is a handheld gun that fires two barb-tipped projectiles, each connected to the device by an electrically conductive wire and propelled by compressed nitrogen charges, as used in paintball guns. The barbs penetrate and attach to the skin or clothing of the target, completing a circuit, and a high voltage, low amperage electric current is passed down the wires. Each cartridge contains a set of two electrodes and propellant for a single shot and so has to be replaced after firing. The type of cartridge determines the range, the maximum being about 35 feet (10.6 meters), as the barbs diverge, as well as require sufficient propellant energy for the distance. The barbed electrodes penetrate clothing and are shaped to prevent removal once in place. Early Taser models depended on penetration of the skin for effect, but newer versions use a "shaped pulse" to increase conduction.

The characteristics of the electrical output and wave form vary among Taser models and their intended use. A typical output (X26 Taser, Figure 57-1) may have an initial "arcing" voltage of 50,000 V, falling rapidly to 1200 V with a current of 2.1 mA. The pulse duration is 100 µsec at a rate of 19 pulses per second over a 5-second

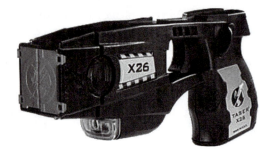

Figure 57-1. X26 Taser.

cycle. The two barbs are fired by compressed nitrogen at a speed of 55 meters per second for up to 9 meters, with the thin wires trailing behind connected to the gun. Each 9-mm barb at the tip of each wire weighs 1.6 grams and penetrates clothing and the outer layer of skin. Once a circuit through the device is made, a series of 100-μsec pulses at 19 per second is fired, each pulse carrying 100 μcoulombs of charge. The relationship between the effect of pulse length and current is described by a value called the chronaxie. Determined from the minimum current that triggers a nerve cell using a long pulse, the chronaxie is the minimum stimulus length to trigger a cell at twice the current required for the long pulse. The Taser pulses are designed to be just below the chronaxie of the nerves to skeletal muscle but much lower than that of heart muscle, which is about 3 msec (30 times that of skeletal muscle and the pulse length of 100 μsec of a Taser).

When an individual is "tasered," that person does not suddenly loose all muscle tone or control. Indeed, it is remarkable that most individuals are able to control their inevitable fall to the ground and usually do not suffer serious injury from striking the ground. Nevertheless, they are unable to get up again, or do anything constructive, until the application of current is stopped, when they can move purposely and stand up. Subjects are rarely incontinent. Most volunteers (usually police officers willing to experience the effects) describe being "tasered" as painful and frightening but with little residual effect. The barbs do need to be removed by a clinician using aseptic techniques; the wires are usually cut from the barbs when the subject is arrested. Several deaths have been reported in individuals who were detained after the use of a Taser. In many cases the subjects had been taking recreational drugs, such as phencyclidine, and this was subsequently determined to be the major factor in their death.[9] It still remains to be confirmed, however, whether in certain individuals, through disease or drug taking, the electric current may not precipitate a cardiac dysrhythmia.[10] The safe use of Tasers in children and the elderly is still unresolved.

CHEMICAL WARFARE AGENTS

Classical chemical warfare agents produce incapacitation but often of a lethal nature. Consequently, compounds not currently classified as chemical weapons in the Chemical Weapons Convention, but those with highly irritant properties (such as tear gases) or that produce severe nausea, vomiting, coughing, or sneezing have been considered as incapacitants. Similarly, psychoactive compounds or narcotic agents have also been classified as incapacitating and less-lethal agents.[11] These are considered here in more detail.

Irritant Incapacitants

Irritant incapacitants, also called riot control agents, lacrimators, and tear gases, are aerosol-dispersed chemicals that produce eye, nose, mouth, skin, and respiratory tract irritation. Tear gas is the common name for substances that, in low concentrations, cause pain in the eyes, flow of tears, and difficulty keeping affected eyes open. Some of these symptoms resolve within 30 minutes after exposure has ceased, but ocular and mucous membrane symptoms may persist for 24 hours. The lethal concentration is very high but the effective concentration is low, so there is a large safety ratio.

Among a long series of substances that are irritants, only three have been extensively used by civil agencies (Figure 57-2):

1. *1-Chloroacetophenone* (CN) is the most toxic lacrimator and may have accounted for at least five deaths that were probably the result of pulmonary injury, asphyxia, or both.[12,13] Readily apparent irritation occurs at 40 mg/m³. At higher concentrations, corneal epithelial damage and chemosis develop. The maximum safe dose for short-term inhalation is 500 mg/m³.[14] It is now little used, having been replaced by CS.
2. *2-Chlorobenzylidene malononitrile* (CS) is a lacrimator that is 10 times more potent than CN but is less toxic. It is now probably the most widely used in crowd control and by some police forces to disable individuals.
3. *Dibenz[b,f]-1,4-oxazepine* (CR) is the most potent lacrimator with the least systemic toxicity and is highly stable. CR is the parent compound of the antipsychotic drug loxapine. It is now most often used by military forces.

After World War I, when CN was used widely, military and law enforcement agencies used this compound until CS, a more potent and less toxic compound synthesized in 1928 by Corson and Stoughton (hence the acronym CS), replaced it in 1959. CN is still available in devices

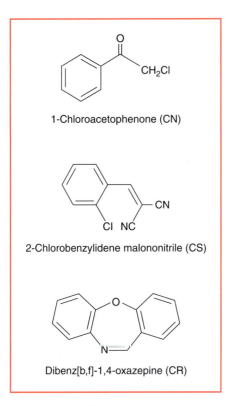

Figure 57-2. Structure of lacrimators.

for self-protection (Mace, United States), and military forces use CS in training as a confidence builder for demonstrating the effectiveness of the protective respirator used in personal protection against chemical warfare agents. The United States used CS extensively in Vietnam, primarily for tunnel denial. Worldwide, police forces (e.g., Ireland, France, Russia, the United Kingdom, and the United States) use CS for crowd control and to incapacitate individuals. CS devices are not available to the public in the United Kingdom.

The United States excludes these agents from international treaty provisions such as the Chemical Weapons Convention. They may be used in military situations only by presidential order. The United Nations has initiated action to include tear gas agents among chemical weapons banned under the Geneva Protocol.[14]

Physical and Chemical Properties

At room temperature, CS and CR are white solids, are stable when heated, and have a low vapor pressure. Consequently, they are generally dispersed as fine particles, or in solutions, as aerosols. Dispersion devices include small handheld spray cans, large spray tanks, grenades, and larger weapons.

All irritant incapacitants have low solubility in water but can be dissolved in organic solvents. Mace is a

1% solution of CN in a solvent propellant mixture of 4% kerosene, 5% 1,1,1-trichloroethane, and Freon 113. A 1-second spray releases 25 mg of CN, but evaporation of the organic solvent may concentrate the mixture in the eyes and intensify damage.[14] Other aerosol protectants available in some European countries may contain capsicum, an irritant compound that can be extracted from red peppers (Guardian; discussed later), or CS (Paralyzer). CS spray, used by U. K. police forces, is issued as a small cylinder containing 5% CS in a propellant, methyl isobutyl ketone, itself a potent irritant.[15,16]

High-temperature dispersion (greater than 700°C) of CS has been shown to produce several organic thermal degradation products through rearrangements and loss of cyano and chlorine substituents present on the parent CS compound. Hydrogen chloride and hydrochloric acid might also be air contaminants produced during high-temperature dispersion of CS.[17]

Hydrolysis of CN is very slow in water or if alkali is added. CS is rapidly hydrolyzed in water (half-life at pH 7 is about 15 minutes at room temperature) and extremely rapidly in an alkaline solution (half-life at pH 9 is about 1 minute). CR is hydrolyzed to a smaller extent in water. CN and CR are, therefore, difficult to decontaminate by decomposition under practical conditions, whereas CS may easily be inactivated by means of a water or alkaline solution. Hence, washing with soap and water inactivates CS, whereas CN and CR are only removed from the surface and runoff decontaminant may produce irritation if it enters the eyes or touches skin. Environmental contamination may be persistent and difficult to remove.

Mechanisms of Toxicity

The mechanism of biological activity is less well understood for riot control agents than for many other toxic chemicals. Fortunately, detailed knowledge of the mechanism of action is not required for appropriate immediate medical management.

The lacrimators are potent mucous membrane irritants and chemical activators of the lacrimal glands. Both CN and CS are SN2 alkylating agents (sulfur mustard, in contrast, is a SN1 alkylator) and react avidly with nucleophilic sites. Prime targets include sulfhydryl-containing enzymes, such as lactic dehydrogenase. In particular, CS reacts rapidly with the disulfhydryl form of lipoic acid, a coenzyme in the pyruvate decarboxylase system. Tissue injury and necrosis probably result from biochemical inhibition of important enzymes such as pyruvic decarboxylase.

CS has the ability to generate bradykinin both in vitro and in vivo.[18] Postmortem findings associated with CN include acute tracheobronchitis with necrosis of the respiratory mucosa and pseudomembrane formation, focal intraalveolar hemorrhage, early bronchopneumonia, pulmonary edema, cerebral edema, and fatty changes in the liver.[12,13]

Animals given lethal amounts of CS by intravenous or intraperitoneal administration developed increased blood thiocyanate concentrations hours later, indicating that the malononitrile portion of CS had been metabolized to cyanide. However, cyanide was not a factor in causing death (which was due to lung damage). A significant increase in blood concentration of thiocyanate has not been noted after aerosol administration of CS. Several databases mention this cyanogenic potential of CS and suggest incorrectly that treatment of a CS casualty might require therapy for cyanide poisoning (this recommendation is apparently based on the parenteral administration data). After receiving lethal amounts of CS by inhalation, animals died some 12 to 24 hours later from severe damage to airways; cyanide was not implicated in their deaths.

CN, occasionally in combination with the vomiting agent Adamsite, has caused deaths in people who stubbornly refused to leave a confined space. In every case, the agent was used in great excess. Death generally occurred hours after the initial exposure, and postmortem findings were of severe airway damage, similar to that seen in animals.

Toxicokinetics

CS reacts covalently with plasma macroproteins to form compounds that may have antigenic properties. On contact with water, CS hydrolyses into ochlorobenzaldehyde and malononitrile. The kidney excretes the ochlorobenzaldehyde as the metabolites o-chlorohippuric acid (major) and ochlorobenzoic acid (minor). The malononitrile is metabolized to thiocyanate. The cyano groups of CS are unlikely to cause systemic cyanide toxicity since a 1-minute exposure to an intolerable level (10 mg/m^3) produces less cyanide than two inhalations of a cigarette[19] and significant amounts of free cyanide do not appear in the plasma.[20]

The published data on the toxicokinetics of the other agents are limited.

Clinical Features

Acute Effects

The parameters *threshold concentration* (TC) and *incapacitating* or *intolerable concentration* (IC) are often used to express the efficiency of a tear gas. TC_{50} defines the concentration required to obtain no more than a perceptible effect on 50% of the population exposed to the gas for 1 minute. ICt_{50} is the concentration that incapacitates, or is intolerable to, 50% of the population exposed to the tear gas for a specified period. ICt_{50} is typically expressed as the product of the chemical concentration in air (mg/m^3) and the duration of exposure in minutes (i.e., in $\text{mg/m}^3 \times \text{min}$). TC_{50} and ICt_{50} values for CN, CS, and CR are listed in Table 1.

The irritating properties of tear gases depend on activation of sensory nerve endings in mucous membranes and skin. Sensitivity to tear gases varies considerably among individuals, and some groups, such as children, may be particularly susceptible. Factors influencing individual reactions are emotional state, motivation, physical activity, ambient temperature, and humidity. Generally, the sensations caused by exposure to tear gas are so disagreeable that the behavior of most victims is not predictable, although a brief period of rational behavior may occur. Some individuals are able to override this incapacitating effect.

The irritating effect remains as long as a sufficient concentration of tear gas is present but usually disappears quickly (15 to 30 minutes) after exposure has ceased.

The initial response to aerosolized CS is an increase in blood pressure and irregular respiration. Bypassing the pain receptors of the nose and upper airway by endotracheal administration of CS leads to a decrease in blood pressure and in respiration, as is seen after intravenous injection. This suggests that the initial pressor effect and irregular respiration are emotional responses to a noxious stimulus rather than the toxico- or pharmacological effects of CS. Pain can occur without tissue injury and may be bradykinin mediated. CS causes bradykinin release in vivo and in vitro, and elimination of bradykininogen in vivo abolishes the systemic response to CS.

Table 1: Threshold Concentration (TC_{50}) and Incapacitating Concentration (ICt_{50}) of CN, CS, and CR

	CN Concentration (mg/m³)	CS Concentration (mg/m³)	CR Concentration (mg/m³)
TC_{50} (eyes)	0.3	0.004	0.004
TC_{50} (airways)	0.4	0.023	0.002
ICt_{50}	20–50	3.6	0.7

CN = 1-chloroacetophenone; CR = dibenz[b,f]-1,4-oxazepine; CS = 2-chlorobenzylidene malononitrile.

A significant leukocytosis (more than 20×10^9 per liter) may occur after exposure to CN and can last several days.[20,21]

All tear gases cause almost instant pain in the eyes, excessive flow of tears, and contraction of the eyelids. The strongly irritating effect leads to incapacitation of exposed people as they focus on finding relief from the pain and discomfort. Apart from the effects on the eyes, most tear gases cause irritation in the nose, mouth, throat, and airways and sometimes to the skin, particularly in the moist and warm areas of the body. In situations of massive exposure, tear gas, which is swallowed, may cause vomiting. Serious systemic toxicity is rare and would only be likely to occur when these agents are used in very high concentrations within confined nonventilated spaces, such as in hostage release or storming a building.

Eyes The eye is the most sensitive organ to irritant agents, and contact with small amounts produces a sensation of conjunctival and corneal burning, leading to tearing, blepharospasm, and conjunctival injection. The severe blepharospasm causes the eyelids to close tightly and may produce transient "blindness." However, if the recipient opens the eyes, vision is nearly normal even if a significant concentration of the agent persists.

CS and CR both produce intense blepharospasm, pain, lacrimation, conjunctival erythema, periorbital edema, and a short-duration rise in intraocular pressure. Symptoms generally diminish within 30 minutes after exposure, but the persistence of symptoms depends on the concentration and duration of exposure. Recorded ocular injuries range from conjunctival irritation, ecchymosis, corneal edema, and loss of epithelium to necrotizing keratitis, coagulative necrosis, iridocyclitis, and deformities of the anterior chamber angle.[20]

Respiratory Tract CS and CR produce nasal irritation, rhinorrhoea and nasal congestion, bronchorrhea, sore throat, cough, sneezing, unpleasant taste, and burning of the mouth immediately after exposure. These effects rapidly resolve within minutes after cessation of exposure.

Prolonged heavy exposures (e.g., exposure in a closed space) can produce an acute laryngeotracheobronchitis.[21] An infant developed persistent wheezes, rales, cough, and bronchial secretions for 3 to 4 days after a 2- to 3-hour CS exposure in a house.[22] After 1 week of ampicillin and steroid therapy, the child developed a right upper lobe infiltrate that resolved over the next 10 days. In doses likely to occur during a riot (open space), pulmonary function tests in human volunteers indicate no adverse effects.[23]

Reactive airways dysfunction syndrome (RADS) may follow a high-level exposure to CS and other respiratory irritants such as CR.[24–26] Following the acute changes (eyes, face, throat, nasal passages), a paroxysmal cough, a feeling of tightness and burning in the chest, and an abnormal chest x-ray may be seen. The chronic changes last for several weeks (cough, shortness of breath) and may lead to RADS.[19] In most exposures to CS gas, only short-term health effects are observed. Any cough, shortness of breath, chest pain, sore throat, and fever generally resolve within 12 weeks.[27]

No evidence shows that CS causes permanent lung damage after one or several exposures to field concentrations. Following inhalation of lethal amounts, animals died from severe airway damage 12 to 24 hours after exposure, but survivors from large exposures had minimal or no pulmonary abnormalities. After multiple daily exposures (50 or more) to smaller amounts, animals developed laryngitis and tracheitis.

Nine U.S. Marines developed a transient pulmonary syndrome with symptoms of cough and shortness of breath.[28] Five of the nine presented with hemoptysis, and four presented with hypoxia. Symptoms were associated with strenuous physical exercise from 36 to 84 hours after heavy exposure of CS in a field training setting. Four of the nine Marines required intensive care observation as a result of profound hypoxia. All signs and symptoms resolved within 72 hours of hospital admission. One week after CS exposure, all nine Marines demonstrated normal lung function during spirometry before and after exercise challenge using cycle ergometry.

A 26-year-old female teacher, with no history of respiratory disease, developed asthma after repeated exposure to tear gas discharged in her classroom.[29] The clinical effects occurring during these repeated exposures were consistent with low-level RADS.

Gastrointestinal Tract Gastrointestinal effects usually do not occur with most riot control agents (the vomiting agent Adamsite is an exception), although there may be retching or vomiting if the agent concentration is high and the exposure is prolonged. Ingestion of CS leads to repeated episodes of abdominal cramping pain and diarrhea. Two such patients were treated with cathartics and antacids and recovered.[30]

Skin Burning and sometimes erythema occur after exposure to tear gases. Contact with the skin causes a tingling or burning sensation and may produce erythema, particularly if the skin is raw or freshly abraded (e.g., shortly after shaving). The erythema begins several minutes after exposure and generally subsides 45 to 60 minutes after termination of exposure.

Prolonged exposures, particularly associated with wet clothing or the use of petroleum jelly, can cause second-degree chemical burns.[21] The development of skin effects depends on the thickness of the stratum corneum at the site of contact, as well as the extent of exposure. Skin previously exposed to CR may become painful again on contact with water for up to 24 to 48 hours after exposure.[31] Cutaneous erythema usually resolves within 3 hours.

CN is a skin sensitizer and may produce an allergic contact dermatitis (pruritus, weeping, papulovesicular rash) within 72 hours of exposure.[21,32,33] Delayed cutaneous sensitivity can then develop to CN.[32]

A 30-year-old prisoner, who was sprayed with CS, was hospitalized 8 days later with erythroderma, wheezing, pneumonitis with hypoxemia, hepatitis with jaundice, and eosinophilia.[34] During the subsequent months, he continued to suffer from generalized dermatitis, recurrent cough and wheezing consistent with RADS, and eosinophilia. These abnormalities responded to brief courses of systemic corticosteroids but recurred when treatment was withdrawn. The dermatitis resolved gradually over 6 to 7 months, but the patient still had asthma-like symptoms a year following exposure. Patch testing confirmed sensitization to CS. The mechanism of the patient's prolonged reaction is unknown but may involve cell-mediated hypersensitivity, perhaps to adducts of CS (or a metabolite) and tissue proteins.

Three German police officers were exposed to CN after escape of the chemical from their personal tear gas canisters.[35] All of them showed localized dermatitis at the site of contact to CN, while widespread lesions appeared after 4 days in one case. Patch testing with the original involved tear gas dissolved in acetone (at 0.1-0.0001%) indicated an allergic reaction in two patients and an irritative reaction in the third.

Long-Term Health Effects of CR

Toxicological investigations have been unable to demonstrate effects of tear gases on genetic material or on fetal development in experimental animals or humans. The teratogenic potential of CR on fetal development in rats and rabbits has not been reported.

In animals exposed 5 days a week for 18 weeks and retained until 1 year after the start of exposure, CR, at high doses, affected survival, and a dose-related increase in the incidence of alveogenic carcinoma was noted in the mice when the high-dose group was excluded from the statistical analyses. This effect was not present when the incidence in all dosed groups was analyzed. Since bacterial and mammalian cell mutagenicity results did not suggest a carcinogenic potential, it was concluded that CR does not represent a carcinogenicity risk.

The long-term toxicity of CR has been studied by repeated skin application to mice. A solution of 0.02 mL of 5% CR in acetone was applied to the dorsal skin of mice after depilation for a total of 60 applications per mouse over a 12-week period. After an observation period of 80 weeks, the surviving animals were sacrificed for pathology. Some animals died before this point, but none of the deaths were attributed to CR. Several pathological changes were observed in the survivors, but these were randomly distributed between test and control animals. The conclusion was that CR does not cause long-term toxic effects after repeated skin application.[31]

Management of an Exposed Individual

The main effects of riot control agents are pain, burning, and irritation of exposed mucous membranes and skin. These effects do not differ appreciably from one agent to another except in the case of Adamsite, which may cause significant nausea and vomiting.

The effects of exposure under normal operational conditions (that is in the open air) generally are self-limiting and require no specific therapy. Most disappear in 15 to 30 minutes, although skin erythema may persist for an hour or longer.

Decontamination

Contaminated clothing should be removed and sealed in a plastic bag. Disposable rubber gloves should be used for personal protection when handling contaminated clothes. The eyes should be irrigated copiously with saline for 15 to 20 minutes. Contaminated skin should be washed thoroughly with copious amounts of water, alkaline soap and water, a mildly alkaline solution (sodium bicarbonate or sodium carbonate), or mild liquid soap and water. The use of sodium hypochlorite solution exacerbates the skin lesions and should not be employed. Only a saline irrigation should be used over vesiculated skin.

Decontamination of material and clothing after contamination with CS can be done with a sodium bicarbonate or carbonate 5% to 10% solution. If this method of decontamination cannot be accomplished (e.g., contaminated rooms and furniture), then the only other means is by intensive air exchange—preferably with hot air.

If clothing is to be washed, cold water should be used because hot water causes any residual CS to volatilize, leading to symptoms in attending staff.[36]

Exposure to High Concentrations

Exposure to high concentrations only occurs under exceptional circumstances such as prolonged exposure in a confined space or exposure in adverse weather (e.g., still, hot, humid air). In such circumstances, less than 1% of exposed people may have effects that are severe or prolonged enough to cause them to seek medical care. Those who do will most likely have eye, airway, or skin complaints. As no antidote to these agents exists, treatment mainly consists of symptomatic management.

Eyes   General care consists of use of a topical solution to relieve the irritation and topical antibiotics. The eyes should be examined for corneal abrasions. Treatment with oral analgesics, topical antibiotics, and mydriatics may be provided as needed.

Since these compounds are solids, it is possible for a particle or clumps of solid to become embedded in the cornea or conjunctiva and cause tissue damage. Medical care for eye pain after exposure should include thorough decontamination of the eyes and obsessive ophthalmological examination. The eye with ocular injuries should be carefully irrigated with isotonic saline, and the remaining powder should be removed with a cotton wool swab. Any remaining stromal particles should be removed with a needle tip under slit-lamp illumination.

Nose and Mouth   Contact with the mucous membranes of the nose produces a burning sensation, rhinorrhea, and sneezing; a similar burning sensation accompanied by increased salivation occurs after contact with the mouth. Treatment is symptomatic.

Respiratory Tract   The immediate priority is removal from exposure and establishment of a patent airway. The development of laryngeal edema, spasm, or both is a theoretical possibility. Patients with respiratory distress should be given humidified oxygen, undergo an evaluation of airway patency, and receive assisted ventilation if necessary. They may require an intravenous line, electrocardiogram monitoring, arterial blood gases, and serial chest x-rays. Bronchospasm may contribute to respiratory distress, and management includes oxygen administration (with ventilation, if necessary), bronchodilators such as inhaled $\beta2$ agonists (e.g., salbutamol), and antibiotics for specific infections.

Inhalation causes burning and irritation of the airways with bronchorrhea, coughing, and a perception of a "tight chest" or an inability to breathe. However, pulmonary function studies done immediately after exposure have shown minimal changes.

These agents may exacerbate chronic disease or unmask latent disease. Bronchospasm with wheezing and mild distress, continuing after exposure, may occur in a latent asthmatic, and more severe effects with respiratory distress may occur with chronic bronchitis or emphysema. Animal studies and limited human data indicate that maximal effects occur 12 hours after exposure.

These effects appear to be unlikely with CS or CN, even though these agents have been used widely in mixed populations. However, it should nevertheless be anticipated that airway problems may occur in individuals with lung disease, particularly if they are exposed to higher-than-average field use concentrations.

Skin   Early erythema requires reassurance, but no specific therapy exists unless exposure is severe and prolonged for more than 1 or 2 hours. Later-onset erythema, precipitated by a larger exposure in a hot and humid atmosphere, is usually more severe and less likely to resolve quickly; it may require the use of soothing compounds such as calamine, camphor, and mentholated creams. Small vesicles should be left intact, but larger ones ultimately break and should be drained. Irrigation of denuded areas several times a day should be followed by the application of a topical antibiotic. Large oozing areas have responded to compresses containing substances such as avena (colloidal oatmeal) and aluminum acetate (Burrow's solution).

Under conditions of high temperature, high humidity, and high concentration of agent, a severe dermatitis may start with erythema several hours after exposure and be followed by vesiculation. Generally, these are second degree burns not unlike, but more severe than, sunburn and are treated as a second-degree chemical burn. Firemen who entered contaminated buildings after summer riots developed these lesions from stirring up the contaminating particles. They later developed erythema and blisters on their exposed skin.

Hypersensitivity may develop. An individual developed generalized vesiculation and a high fever after an uneventful exposure to CS, but more than 20 years after his only and equally uneventful previous exposure.

Ingestion   Children occasionally ingest CS, and several adults have swallowed CS pellets. Aside from bouts of diarrhea and abdominal cramps, their recovery has been uneventful. In animals, the oral median lethal dose is about 200 mg/kg (which is about 14 grams for a 70-kg person), an amount unlikely to be ingested, even deliberately. A few animals fed lethal amounts (or greater) had gastric irritation or erosions, and several had signs of intestinal perforation. Recommended therapy after ingestion consists of cathartics, antacids, and observation.

Cardiovascular System   A transient increase in heart rate and blood pressure has occurred in people immediately before exposure to a riot control agent or immediately after onset of exposure. The heart rate and blood pressure returned to within the pretest range while exposure continued and may have been caused by the anxiety or the initial pain rather than a pharmacological effect of these agents. This "alarm" reaction may cause adverse effects in individuals with preexistent cardiovascular disease.

Analytical Detection

Analytical methods for identification of lacrimators include gas chromatography–mass spectrometry procedures, which provide a sensitivity level of 1 to 10 ng/mL.[37,38] Spectra data (ultraviolet, fluorescence, nuclear magnetic resonance, infrared, and mass) and a capillary gas–liquid chromatography–mass spectrometry method that differentiate and identify CN and CS are available.[37]

Conclusions

These agents incapacitate by causing severe, unpleasant irritation of sensory nerve endings in mucous membranes and, in rare situations, some tissue damage. The release of irritant incapacitants in a confined, unventilated space may expose an individual to very high concentrations of CN, CS, and CR. Some individuals may be more susceptible to high concentrations, possibly because of an existing medical condition such as asthma, and require intensive supportive medical treatment after exposure. There remains a real, but extremely small, risk that an individual may die during exposure to very high concentrations of these agents. Medical practitioners treating casualties should be aware of the methods for decontamination and of the medical management of individuals exhibiting continued severe eye, skin, or respiratory effects resulting from exposure to irritant incapacitants.

Adamsite

The effects of the vomiting agent Adamsite, also known as diphenylarenamine (DM), are similar to those of the other riot control agents except that DM has little irritancy to the skin. However, at higher concentrations DM causes nausea, vomiting, and a feeling of general malaise. The effects begin 3 to 4 minutes after the onset of exposure and can last for 1 or 2 hours.

Similar compounds include diphenylchlorarsine and diphenylcyanoarsine. All are sensory irritants and at high dose cause vomiting but after a latent period of several minutes. They were, therefore, considered a useful adjunct to more conventional chemical weapons, as vomiting would cause an individual to remove a respirator.

Pepper Spray

Pepper spray contains capsaicin (oleoresin capsicum) obtained from the peppers *Capsicum annum* and *Capsicum frutescence*. These contain a range of compounds, of which capsaicin is the most potent. Capsaicin acts directly by stimulating the release of substance P, a neuroactive endogenous peptide, which produces vasodilatation and inflammation but, more importantly, through its effect on type-C fibers, severe and long-lasting pain.

PSYCHOACTIVE INCAPACITANTS

3-Quinuclidinyl Benzilate

3-Quinuclidinyl benzilate (BZ) is a centrally acting drug with an anticholinergic action similar to atropine (Figure 57-3). It has a longer duration of action and is more potent than atropine but with less peripheral antimuscarinic activity compared to its central effects. BZ is absorbed by the respiratory route (ICt_{50} 100 mg $\times$ min/m^3).

The onset of an effect from BZ can take more than an hour and may not peak until after some 8 to 10 hours. However, the effects sometimes can persist for several days. BZ is absorbed through the lungs and rapidly crosses the blood–brain barrier. Individuals exposed to a high dose develop confusion and hallucinations and become delirious. While sufficiently lucid, they may report a dry mouth and blurred vision from loss of accommodation. With lower-dose exposure, the effects may be more subtle and initially only affect complex cognitive tasks or psychomotor skills. Features pathognomic of BZ poisoning have been described and include "woolgathering," where individuals pick at clothing, at their body, or in the air. Other sensory hallucinations have been reported.

The peripheral antimuscarinic effects of BZ are not as pronounced as the central effects but can include flushed, dry, warm skin and dilated pupils; sinus tachycardia and hyperthermia; urine retention; and diminished bowel activity. Essentially, the clinical signs are similar to those seen in atropine intoxication but with greater central than peripheral effect.

The treatment of BZ exposure follows the standard protocol for any patient exposed to an incapacitating agent: first protect yourself, then decontaminate the patient of any residual compound. BZ is disseminated as a small particle aerosol and so may be present on clothing,

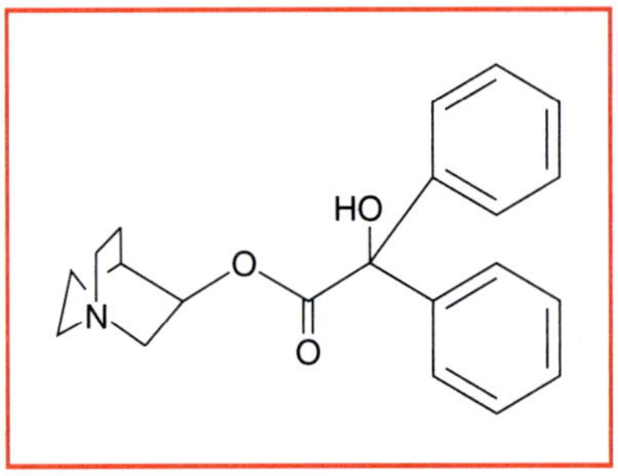

Figure 57-3. Structure of 3-quinuclidinyl benzilate.

which is removed and sealed in a plastic bag, or skin, which is washed with water. If severe delirium and agitation occur, then the patient may require sedation with a benzodiazepine. Successful management of BZ delirium with physostigmine has been reported. Physostigmine is a carbamate drug that reversibly inhibits acetylcholinesterase and so increases acetylcholine levels; acetylcholine then displaces the BZ from the muscarinic receptor. Of the three commonly used carbamates, physostigmine is the only one that easily crosses the blood–brain barrier and so acts directly on central BZ effects.

Hyperthermia occurs as a consequence of agitation, as well as from anticholinergic inhibition of sweating. Physical methods of cooling are preferable using water misting and fan-assisted evaporation from skin. Rhabdomyolysis (and renal failure) has been reported in cases with delirium, seizures, and hyperthermia.

Agent 15 is a compound reported in Iraq as similar to BZ, but it may be a structural analogue.

Other psychoactive agents have been assessed. Both the U.S. and U.K. military administered lysergic acid diethylamide (LSD) to volunteers in the 1950s as part of an appraisal of its potential as a chemical weapon or less-lethal incapacitant. LSD interacts with G protein–coupled receptors, including all dopamine and adrenoreceptor subtypes, and binds to many serotonin receptor subtypes. However, the functional (psychological) effects of these many interactions are so complex, and unpredictable, that LSD was judged too unreliable to be considered for military use as an incapacitant.

SEDATIVES AND ANESTHETIC AGENTS

Opioids

Opiates have long been recognized as powerful sedatives (or "calmative" agents), but with the major adverse effect of respiratory depression that would limit their safe use as incapacitants. However, more recently synthetic opioids, such as the fentanyls, have demonstrated greater potential. Fentanyl itself is widely used in clinical anesthetic practice, and some of its analogues are used in veterinary practice to sedate large animals. During the development of the fentanyls, several synthesized analogues were found to be so potent that their safe use in patients was questioned and many were shelved or found use only in animals. The best known of these include carfentanil, which is highly potent and has a high therapeutic index; sufentanil; remifentanil; and alfentanil (Figure 57-4).

The potential of fentanyls as mass incapacitants was powerfully demonstrated in October 2002 when a combination of compounds was used to end a siege in a Moscow theater. Chechen rebels had taken hostage the audience of several hundred people and placed explosives, and suicide bombers, around the auditorium. After several days of stand off, Russian Special Forces entered the theater after all the people in the auditorium had been rendered unconscious by the infiltration of a gas into the ventilation system. Those rebels not in the auditorium were shot. The unconscious hostages were removed and transported to hospital. Unfortunately, when some hostages had become unconscious, they had obstructed their airways and asphyxiated. Others died from gas-induced respiratory arrest. The few medical attendants in support of the operation were not briefed on the nature of the gas and had not deployed with an appropriate antidote. Out of some 800 people in the theater, about 120 were reported to have died as a direct result of the effects of the incapacitating gas.

Understandably, the Russian authorities were reluctant to identify the ingredients of the gas, but as the clinical features in the patients admitted to hospital were clearly of opiate poisoning, eventually they confirmed that a principle component was a fentanyl analogue. There has been much speculation as to the precise identity of this compound and whether any other chemical, such as a volatile anesthetic, was also used. The current consensus is that carfentanil, or a close analogue, was probably the main ingredient, but whether or not other incapacitants were present is not known. There has been speculation that 3-methylfentanyl dissolved in halothane (Kolokol-1 gas) was the active product used.[39]

This episode provided clear evidence of the potential usefulness of an incapacitant in a hostage situation. However, there was a high death rate in those incapacitated but, to a large degree, many of the fatalities resulted from a failure to get medical treatment quickly to the hostages while they were still in the auditorium. Sufficient quantities of the most appropriate antidote, naloxone, were not on site, and methods of supporting respiration were not available. Nevertheless, the gas had quickly induced narcosis in all those exposed without any of them apparently realizing what was happening to them and panicking. None of the suicide bombers had reacted.

Fentanyl was first synthesized by Janssen Pharmaceuticals and found to be more potent than morphine but safer (a higher therapeutic index). It is also more rapidly eliminated from the body, with an elimination half-life varying from 2 to 4 hours.

Substitution at the N4 position of the fentanyl molecule produces fentanyl analogues, many of which are even more potent (Table 2).

Most fentanyls are administered by either the intravenous or the intramuscular route. Some have been shown to be absorbable through the skin, but fentanyl itself is not well absorbed by inhalation as an aerosol, at least to achieve effective analgesia. Carfentanil is several

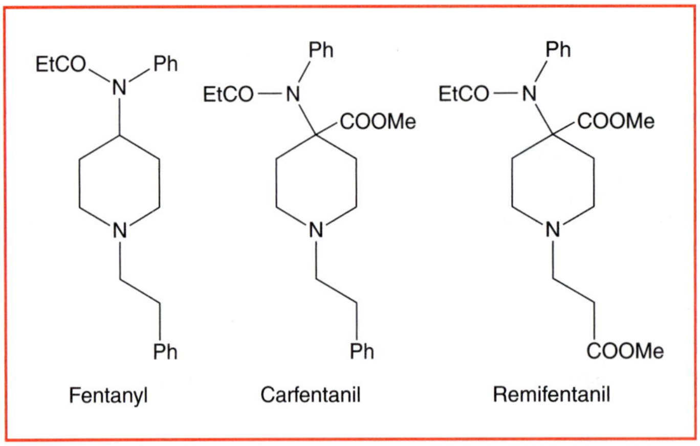

Figure 57-4. Structure of fentanyls.

thousand times more potent than fentanyl but still has a relatively high therapeutic ratio and so would be more effective as an incapacitant even with incomplete bioavailability. However, despite the high potency, it will always be difficult to produce safe incapacitation in every exposed individual, not least because of the variability in response within a population due to age, size, existing disease, and other more subtle (or unrecognized) factors. There is also a purely physical problem in distributing a gas in a large space quickly and evenly. Despite all these limitations, it still appears that fentanyl analogues come nearest to fulfilling the criteria for an effective incapacitating agent.[40]

Fentanyls and other opiates are widely used as analgesics in hospital anesthetic practice, but all have serious adverse effects, such as respiratory depression. It has been suggested that this occurs by direct inhibition of the respiratory rhythm–generating neurons in the pre-Boetzinger complex of the brainstem and that the 5-hydroxytryptamine-4a receptors (5-HT4a) on the respiratory pre-Boetzinger complex neurons are involved in generating the respiratory drive. Selective agonists stimulate respiratory activity. Rats

Table 2: Relative Potency of Opioid Drugs			
Drug	**Relative Potency**	**Lipid Solubility (Octanol-to-Water Ratio)**	**Therapeutic Index (LD$_{50}$ or Lowest ED$_{50}$)**
Meperidine	0.5	40	5
Morphine	1	1.4	70
Methadone	4	120	12
Alfentanil	75	150	1080
Remifentanil	220	18	33,000
Fentanyl	300	800	277
Sufentanil	4500	1800	25,211
Carfentanil	10,000	N/A	10,594

ED$_{50}$ = median effective dose; LD$_{50}$ = median lethal dose; N/A = data not available.
Adapted from Alavattam S. Sleep-Inducing Compounds. Final Report. Office of Counterproliferation, Biological and Chemical Warfare Assessments Division, Defense Intelligence Agency. Battelle Memorial Institute, Arlington, VA, 2005: p. 43.

treated with a 5-HT4a receptor–specific agonist overcame fentanyl-induced respiratory depression and maintained respiratory rhythm, without loss of any analgesic effect. Activation of these receptors raises intracellular adenosine 3′,5′-monophosphate, while fentanyls decrease levels. The use of a 5-HT4a agonist in preventing respiratory depression following opiate administration has not been demonstrated in man.[41]

Anesthetic Agents

Halothane is a highly volatile inhalational anesthetic agent. Although colorless, it has a sweet smell and would be noticeable in an atmosphere. Its effects are quick, peaking within 1 to 4 minutes and lasting for about 20 minutes, most of the dose being excreted unchanged via the lungs. It is more effective than other anesthetic gases, such as enflurane and nitrous oxide. Exposure produces drowsiness progressing to central nervous system depression with loss of respiratory drive. There may be hypotension and cardiac arrhythmias.

Ketamine is primarily a noncompetitive antagonist of N-methyl-d-aspartate (glutamate) receptors producing analgesia at low doses but also binds to opiate receptors at higher anesthetic doses. Ketamine produces a state described as dissociative anesthesia, a feeling of detachment from the body and the external world, often with intense hallucinations and memory loss. In anesthetic practice, it is administered either by the intravenous or the intramuscular route but is also effective orally, nasally, and by smoking. The principle adverse effects of hallucinogenesis and memory loss are also the main reasons ketamine has been assessed as an incapacitant, although the difficulty with standoff delivery is a more fundamental problem.

PERFORMANCE ENHANCEMENT

Understanding the mechanisms by which drugs and other agents can incapacitate an individual may also provide indications of how manipulation of such mechanisms might be used to enhance, rather than degrade, performance. Several drugs are marketed as cognitive enhancing, memory improving, or concentration intensifying, as well as some claiming to reduce impulsive behavior and risk taking. Other drugs maintain alertness and abolish sleepiness, even after a full 24 hours of exertion. While most of these medications are used to treat clinical conditions and improve the quality of life for patients with neuropsychiatric disorders or after brain injury, they do have the potential to extend or enhance the abilities of normal individuals.

Modafinil

Modafinil (2-benzhydrylsulphinylethanamide) is used in the treatment of narcolepsy to maintain wakefulness. The mechanism of action is not clear, although modafinil does inhibit the reuptake of dopamine and norepinephrine in the ventrolateral preoptic nucleus, an area of the hypothalamus involved in sleep induction. Another possible mechanism is via activation of orexinergic neurones in the hypothalamus (also called the hypocretin system), which increases dopamine and norepinephrine levels.

The ability of modafinil to promote wakefulness and alertness has led to its use in situations of sleep deprivation. The effects are not directly that of a stimulant, such as amphetamine, and there appear to be minimal adverse reactions or aftereffects. However, it is not the panacea for maintaining performance and negating the need for sleep. Subjects were able to maintain alertness and high-level performance (such as for flight control or covert operations) for more than 40 hours without sleep or rest but at the end of the exercise still required sufficient catch-up sleep.

γ-Hydroxybutyrate

γ-Hydroxybutyric acid (GHB) was originally developed as an anesthetic drug. It is a naturally occurring precursor of the structurally similar inhibitory neurotransmitter, γ-aminobutyric acid (GABA). GHB is an illegal drug that has gained notoriety for its use as an alternative to amphetamines (and by athletes mistakenly believing it significantly raises growth hormone levels and muscle bulk).

At low doses, GHB produces a state of euphoria and sensory awareness, but higher doses are associated with drowsiness, agitation, visual disturbances, respiratory depression, and amnesia. The latter effect has led to speculation about its use to incapacitate an individual following addition to a drink (or, in popular culture, as a "date rape" drug), since the subject loses self-control but has no later recollection. GHB concentrations peak after about 1 hour, although clinical effects appear rapidly, often within 10 minutes. The half-life of elimination is 20 to 30 minutes, but clinical effects may be present for more than 24 hours. The steep dose–response curve for GHB makes this addition to drink an extremely dangerous act, especially if alcohol is also consumed, as ethanol potentiates the effects of GHB. Ethanol and GHB compete for the same metabolic pathways. The clinical effects are potentiated by other central nervous system depressants, such as benzodiazepines and antipsychotic drugs.

Acute ingestion of a moderate dose of GHB causes nausea, drowsiness, confusion, euphoria, and amnesia, followed by urinary incontinence, tremors, and myoclonus and culminating in hypotonia and hypothermia. Agitation and aggression may occur. Ingestion of a high dose of GHB causes bradycardia, hypotension, and respiratory depression, progressing to respiratory failure, coma, and death.

GHB binds to $GABA_B$ receptors and inhibits norepinephrine release. The effects on dopamine are dose dependent; low doses inhibit release, but higher doses raise levels in the brain.

GHB is an endogenous compound, possibly a metabolite of GABA, and there appear to be GHB-specific binding sites in the cortex, substantia nigra, basal ganglia, and most densely, hippocampus. The latter may be related to the amnesia associated with GHB intake.

CONCLUSION

Intrinsic features of human physiology greatly limit the type of mechanism by which a human incapacitant might function. Pharmacological or chemical agents have to be absorbed into the body and then delivered, via the systemic circulation, to a target area, usually in the nervous system, to have an incapacitating action. This takes some time, at least equal to the blood circulation time but probably longer due to absorption delays and time for the toxic mechanism to result in functional incapacitation. In addition, such agents have to be safe when used in a range of scenarios so that they truly meet the criteria of an ideal nonlethal, reversible incapacitant. Pharmaceutical and bioactive compounds are unlikely to ever achieve this profile, and there will always be a tradeoff between effective dose and lethality.

The human nervous system relies on electrical conductance to achieve speed of motor response and maintain conscious activity. Interference with this electrical process is probably the most effective method of causing immediate, and hopefully reversible, incapacitation and underlies the development of the Taser as a less-lethal method of incapacitation. Inevitably, variations in the technology to deliver an electrical charge will be delivered that appear to have greater safety margins, but as with pharmacological agents, none of these will ever be risk free.

A genuine individual policing need, as well as in responding to civil disorder, exists for a method to incapacitate individuals that does not rely on lethal force and forms part of a gradual escalation from direct physical restraint, through levels of incapacitation, to—as the last resort—lethal force. No technology for law enforcement (or operational success in military conflict) can ever be absolutely safe, so a rigorous risk–benefit assessment must always precede deployment.[42]

REFERENCES

1. Davison N, Lewer N. Bradford Non-lethal Weapons Research Project. Research Report No. 8. Available at: http://www.brad.ac.uk/acad/nlw/research_reports/docs/BNLWRPResearchReportNo8 _Mar06.pdf. Accessed March 2008.
2. Wheelis M, Dando M. Neurobiology: a case study of the imminent militarization of biology. *Int Rev Red Cross.* 2005;87(859):553–568.
3. Pearson A. Incapacitating biochemical weapons. *Nonproliferation Rev.* 2006;13(2):151–188.
4. Klotz L, Furmanski M, Wheelis M. Beware the Siren's Song: Why "Non-Lethal" Incapacitating Chemical Agents Are Lethal. Available at: http://www.fas.org/bwc/papers/sirens_song.pdf. Accessed March 2008.
5. Wheelis M, Klotz L. Chemical Incapacitating Weapons Are Not Non-lethal. Federation of American Scientists Working Group on Biological Weapons. Available at: http://www.fas.org/bwc/papers/pp_chemical_incapacitants.pdf. Accessed March 2008.
6. North Atlantic Treaty Organization Research and Technology Organisation. The Human Effects of Non-Lethal Technologies: Final Report of NATO RTO HFM-073. Available at: http://www.rta.nato.int/Pubs/RDP.asp?RDP=RTO-TR-HFM-073. Accessed March 2008.
7. Marshall J. Blinding laser weapon. *BMJ.* 1997;315:1392.
8. Wright S. Future Sub-Lethal, Incapacitating and Paralysing Technologies: Their Coming Role in the Mass Production of Torture, Cruel, Inhumane and Degrading Treatment. Draft Paper presented to the Expert Seminar on Security Equipment & the Prevention of Torture. Available at: http://www.statewatch.org/news/2002/nov/torture.pdf. Accessed March 2008.
9. O'Brien AJ, McKenna BG, Simpson AIF. Health professionals and the monitoring of Taser use. *Psychiatr Bull.* 2007;31:391–392.
10. Cao M, Shinbane JS, Gillberg JM, Saxon LA. Taser-induced rapid ventricular myocardial capture demonstrated by pacemaker intracardiac electrograms. *J Cardiovasc Electrophysiol.* 2007;18(8):876–879.
11. Davison N. "Off the Rocker" and "On the Floor": The Continued Development of Biochemical Incapacitating Weapons. Bradford Science and Technology Report No. 8. Available at: http://www.brad.ac.uk/acad/nlw/research_reports/docs/BDRC_ST_Report_No_8.pdf. Accessed March 2008.
12. Stein AA, Kirwan WE. Chloroacetophenone (tear gas) poisoning: a clinicopathologic report. *J Forensic Sci.* 1964;9:374–382.
13. Chapman AJ, White C. Death resulting from lacrimatory agents. *J Forensic Sci.* 1978;23:527–530.
14. Beswick FW. Chemical agents used in riot control and warfare. *Hum Toxicol.* 1983;2:247–256.
15. Varma S, Holt PJ. Severe cutaneous reaction to CS gas. *Clin Exp Dermatol.* 2001;26:248–250.
16. Committees on Toxicity MaCoCiFCPatE, Department of Health. Statement on 2-Chlorobenzylidene Malononitrile (CS) and CS Spray. Available at: http://www.doh.gov.uk/pub/docs/doh/csgas.pdf. Accessed March 2008.
17. Kluchinsky TA Jr, Savage PB, Fitz R, et al. Liberation of hydrogen cyanide and hydrogen chloride during high-temperature dispersion of CS riot control agent. *Am Ind Hyg Assoc J.* 2002;63:493–496.
18. Cucinell SA, Swentzel KC, Biskup R, et al. Biochemical interactions and metabolic fate of riot control agents. *Fed Proc.* 1971;30:86–91.

19. Anonymous. Verdict on CS. *BMJ.* 1971;3:722.
20. Leopold IH, Lieberman TW. Chemical injuries of the cornea. *Fed Proc.* 1971;30:92–95.
21. Thorburn KM. Injuries after use of the lacrimatory agent chloroacetophenone in a confined space. *Arch Environ Health.* 1982;37:182–186.
22. Park S, Giammona ST. Toxic effects of tear gas on an infant following prolonged exposure. *Am J Dis Child.* 1972;123:245–246.
23. Beswick FW, Holland P, Kemp KH. Acute effects of exposure to orthochlorobenzylidene malononitrile (CS) and the development of tolerance. *Br J Ind Med.* 1972;29:298–306.
24. Brooks SM, Weiss MA, Bernstein IL. Reactive airways dysfunction syndrome (RADS): persistent asthma syndrome after high level irritant exposures. *Chest.* 1985;88:376–384.
25. Brooks SM, Weiss MA, Bernstein IL. Reactive airways dysfunction syndrome: case reports of persistent airways hyperreactivity following high-level irritant exposures. *J Occup Med.* 1985;27:473–476.
26. Hu H, Christiani D. Reactive airways dysfunction after exposure to teargas. *Lancet.* 1992;339:1535.
27. Wheeler H, Murray V. Treating CS gas injuries to the eye: poisons centre will monitor cases. *BMJ.* 1995;311:871.
28. Thomas RJ, Smith PA, Rascona DA, et al. Acute pulmonary effects from ochlorobenzylidenemalonitrile "tear gas": a unique exposure outcome unmasked by strenuous exercise after a military training event. *Mil Med.* 2002;167:136–139.
29. Bayeux-Dunglas M-C, Deparis P, Touati M-A, et al. Asthmé professionnel chez une enseignante après inhalation repetée de gaz lacrymogènes. *Rev Mal Respir.* 1999;16:558–559.
30. Sidell FR. Civil emergencies involving chemical warfare agents: medical considerations. In: Somani SM, ed. *Chemical Warfare Agents.* San Diego: Academic Press; 1992:341–356.
31. Holland P. The cutaneous reactions produced by dibenzoxazepine (CR). *Br J Dermatol.* 1974;90:657–659.
32. Frazier CA. Contact allergy to mace. *JAMA.* 1976;236:2526.
33. Penneys NS. Contact dermatitis to chloroacetophenone. *Fed Proc.* 1971;30:96–99.
34. Hill AR, Silverberg NB, Mayorga D, et al. Medical hazards of the tear gas CS: a case of persistent, multisystem, hypersensitivity reaction and review of the literature. *Medicine (Baltimore).* 2000;79:234–240.
35. Treudler R, Tebbe B, Blume-Peytavi U, et al. Occupational contact dermatitis due to 2-chloroacetophenone tear gas. *Br J Dermatol.* 1999;140:531–534.
36. Scott RAH. Treating CS gas injuries to the eye illegal: illegal "mace" contains more toxic CN particles. *BMJ.* 1995;311:871.
37. Wils ERJ, Hulst AG. Gas chromatographic–mass spectrometric identification of tear gases in dilute solutions using large injection volumes. *J Chromatogr.* 1985;330:379–382.
38. Ferslew KE, Orcutt RH, Hagardorn AN. Spectral differentiation and gas chromatographic–mass spectrometric analysis of the lacrimators 2-chloroacetophenone and o-chlorobenzylidene malononitrile. *J Forensic Sci.* 1986;31:658–665.
39. Alavattam S. Sleep-Inducing Compounds. Final Report. Office of Counterproliferation, Biological and Chemical Warfare Assessments Division, Defense Intelligence Agency. Battelle Memorial Institute, Arlington, VA, 2005: p. 43.
40. Lakoski JM, Murray WB, Kenny JM. The Advantages and Limitations of Calmatives for Use as a Non-Lethal Technique. Applied Research Laboratory. Pennsylvania State University; 2000.
41. Eilers H, Schumacher MA. Opioid-induced respiratory depression: are 5-HT4a receptor agonists the cure? *Mol Interv.* 2004;4(4):197–199.
42. British Medical Association Board of Science. The Use of Drugs as Weapons: The Concerns and Responsibilities of Healthcare Professionals. Available at: http://www.bma.org.uk/ap.nsf/AttachmentsByTitle/PDFdrugsasweapons/$FILE/Drugsasweapons.pdf. Accessed March 2008.

Page numbers followed by "f" denote figures; those followed by "t" denote tables